Clinical Decisions in Nephrology, Hypertension and Kidney Transplantation

Edgar V. Lerma • Mitchell Rosner
Editors

Clinical Decisions in Nephrology, Hypertension and Kidney Transplantation

Springer

Editors
Edgar V. Lerma, MD
Section of Nephrology
University of Illinois at Chicago College of Medicine
Chicago, IL USA

Mitchell Rosner, MD
Division of Nephrology
University of Virginia Health System
Charlottesville, Virginia USA

ISBN 978-1-4614-4453-4 ISBN 978-1-4614-4454-1 (eBook)
DOI 10.1007/978-1-4614-4454-1
Springer New York Heidelberg Dordrecht London

Library of Congress Control Number: 2012948592

Printed on acid-free paper

Springer is part of Springer Science+Business Media (www.springer.com)

To my mentors, colleagues, and friends at the University of Santo Tomas Faculty of Medicine and Surgery in Manila, Philippines, and Northwestern University Feinberg School of Medicine, who have guided me to where I am right now.

To all the medical students, interns, and residents at Advocate Christ Medical Center whom I have taught or learned from.

To my parents and my brothers, without whose unwavering love and support through thick and thin I would not have persevered and reached my goals in life.

Most especially, to my two lovely daughters Anastasia Zofia and Isabella Ann, whose smiles and laughter constantly provide me unparalleled joy and happiness; and my very loving and understanding wife Michelle, who has always been supportive of my endeavors and who sacrificed a lot of time and exhibited patience as I devoted a significant amount of time and effort to this project. Truly, they are my inspiration.

Edgar V. Lerma

To my wife Michelle who is my greatest inspiration and strength. Her support and smiles through the years has been my greatest asset.

To my children Max, Sam, and Anna who provide me with joy and inspiration. Perhaps, they will be the next generation of great teachers.

Finally, to my mentors in Nephrology, Mark Okusa and Kline Bolton. They have set a high benchmark for excellence, and their professionalism, high standards, and outstanding teaching serve as constant examples of the very best.

Mitchell Rosner

Preface

According to Merriam-Webster's Dictionary, "the Socratic approach" is a method of inquiry and instruction employed by Socrates especially as represented in the dialogues of Plato and consisting of a series of questionings, the object of which is to elicit a clear and consistent expression of something supposed to be implicitly known by all rational beings.

As a medical student trying to navigate the intricacies and complexities of internal medicine and various subspecialties, I was constantly intrigued and fascinated by the challenges of clinical problem solving. With the influence of my parents and my mentors, somehow this attitude was further cultivated in me.

As I went through my residency and fellowship years, I found two publications particularly appealing and stimulating. They were the following: Robert Schrier's "The Internal Medicine Casebook: Real Patients, Real Answers" and David Levine's "Caring for the Renal Patient." These were unique in the sense that unlike conventional textbooks, the chapters started off by presenting various clinical vignettes. A comprehensive discussion followed as the case continued to evolve. Salient features of diseases and conditions in question were highlighted. This method of instruction was truly appealing and kept me reading and wanting more.

A similar format was utilized by New England Journal of Medicine's Case Records of the Massachusetts General Hospital, which was originally developed and inspired by the works of Dr. Walter Cannon (ca. 1800) and Dr. Richard Cabot (ca. 1900).

As I became a teacher myself, I started employing these techniques of teaching to my junior medical students, interns, and residents.

In this book, I had the honor and privilege of collaborating with Dr. Mitchell Rosner who is well known in the realm of medical education. Prior to this collaboration, he has written numerous texts, including the "NMS Review for USMLE III," and is involved with medical education at the University of Virginia School of Medicine. We were fortunate that Richard Lansing of Springer provided encouragement and support for this collaboration.

The book is divided into several parts that highlight the typical content areas that are encountered in a typical clinical nephrology practice. Each chapter is started with a clinical case presentation centered on an important topic. The didactic discussion that follows draws on evidence-based literature—from diagnosis to the practicalities of management. The first part focuses on "Patient Assessment," which deals with nephrology-centered history and physical examination, as well as basic laboratory and ancillary diagnostic procedures. The next five parts focus on common problems/disease entities, namely glomerular diseases, fluid and electrolytes and acid–base disorders, acute kidney injury, and chronic kidney disease. Parts 7 and 8 deal with renal replacement therapies, namely dialysis (hemodialysis, peritoneal dialysis) and kidney transplantation. Parts 9–11 deal with hypertension and other systemic diseases involving the kidneys, namely diabetes, lupus nephritis, systemic viral illnesses, myeloma, and nephrolithiasis. There is also a chapter on kidney diseases with genetic predispositions.

We trust that this will be of great utility to all learners from all walks of life, especially those with an interest in the study of kidney disease, hypertension, and kidney transplantation—from medical students, interns, and residents to busy clinicians. For all allied health professionals, this would also be valuable as it is patient oriented, problem oriented, and it brings the reader to the latest updates in patient management.

Chicago, IL, USA — Edgar V. Lerma
Charlottesville, VA, USA — Mitchell Rosner

Acknowledgement

This book would not have been possible were it not for so many people. First, we would like to thank all of our contributing authors, who have spent countless hours in producing high-quality, up-to-the-last-minute information. We spent a significant amount of time communicating via telephone and e-mail as we reviewed the chapters and discussed recommendations, most of which were agreed upon, but, on occasion, disputed. We express our sincere gratitude for their openness to this very collegial collaboration, which has been a truly rewarding learning experience for us.

We appreciate the help and support of all the staff of Springer, most especially Joni Fraser, our Developmental Editor, and Richard Lansing, Editorial Director for Clinical Medicine, both of whom have been very patient with our procrastinations and stubbornness at times.

We thank all our teachers and mentors, who devoted their own time to educate and train us to become who we are. We thank all the medical students, residents, and fellows who in one way or another have given us inspiration to persevere in the teaching profession. Mostly, we thank all of our patients, who have been truly instrumental in our learning and devotion to medicine. On behalf of all the contributors to this book, we fervently hope that all our efforts will contribute to relieving your suffering and perhaps lead to your recovery.

Contents

Contributors

Maaz A. Abbasi Nephrology Private Practice, DeSoto, TX, USA

Maryam Afkarian Department of Medicine, Kidney Research Institute, Seattle, WA, USA

Hatem Amer Division of Nephrology and Hypertension, Department of Medicine, The William J. von Liebig Transplant Center, Mayo Clinic, Rochester, MN, USA

A. Eric Anderson Department of Medicine, University of Washington Medical Center, Seattle, WA, USA

Adriana Arcila Department of Pulmonary and Critical Care, University of Miami, Miami, FL, USA

James L. Bailey Medicine, Renal Division, Emory University, Atlanta, GA, USA

Scott D. Bieber Division of Nephrology, University of Washington, Seattle, WA, USA

Ian H. de Boer Department of Medicine/Nephrology, University of Washington, Seattle, WA, USA

William Burtnett Nephrology, University of Louisville, Louisville, KY, USA

Dawn J. Caster Division of Nephrology, Department of Internal Medicine, University of Louisville, Louisville, KY, USA

Harini A. Chakkera Nephrology and Hypertension, Mayo Clinic Arizona, Phoenix, AZ, USA

Kerry C. Cho Division of Nephrology, Department of Medicine, University of California San Francisco, San Francisco, CA, USA

Jorge Cerda Division of Nephrology, Department of Medicine, Albany Medical College, Capital District Renal Physicians, Albany, NY, USA

Jason Cobb Renal Division, Emory University School of Medicine, Atlanta, GA, USA

Shaun D. Conlon Nephrology, Emory University, Atlanta, GA, USA

Cynthia M. Cooper Inpatient Clinician Educator Unit, Department of Medicine, Massachusetts General Hospital, Boston, MA, USA

Fionnuala C. Cormack Division of Nephrology, Department of Medicine, University of Washington, Seattle, WA, USA

Lynn D. Cornell Department of Laboratory Medicine and Pathology, Mayo Clinic, Rochester, MN, USA

Miguel F. Palma Diaz Laboratory Medicine, Department of Pathology, David Geffen School of Medicine at UCLA, Los Angeles, CA, USA

Ziad M. El-Zoghby Division of Nephrology, Department of Internal Medicine, Mayo Clinic, Rochester, MN, USA

Jennifer A. Fillaus Internal Medicine, Nephrology, University of Nebraska Medical Center, Omaha, NE, USA

Marius C. Florescu Internal Medicine, Nephrology, University of Nebraska Medical Center, Omaha, NE, USA

Harold A. Franch Renal Division, Atlanta Veterans Affairs Medical Center and Emory University School of Medicine, Decatur, GA, USA

Hussain A. Gilani Nephrology, Emory University, Atlanta, GA, USA

Joni H. Hansson Section of Nephrology, Department of Medicine, Hospital of Saint Raphael, New Haven, CT, USA

Leah A. Haseley Department of Medicine, University of Washington Medical Center, Harborview Hospital, Seattle, WA, USA

German T. Hernandez Division of Nephrology and Hypertension, Department of Internal Medicine, Paul L. Foster School of Medicine, Texas Tech University Health Center at El Paso, El Paso, TX, USA

LaTonya J. Hickson Division of Nephrology and Hypertension, Department of Internal Medicine, Mayo Clinic, Rochester, Olmstead County, MN, USA

M. Rashid Ishaque Department of Nephrology, Harbin Clinic, Marietta, GA, USA

J. Ashley Jefferson Division of Nephrology, University of Washington, Seattle, WA, USA

Eric K. Judd Department of Nephrology, University of Alabama at Birmingham, Birmingham, AL, USA

Luis A. Juncos Division of Nephrology, Department of Medicine, University of Mississippi Medical Center, Jackson, MS, USA

Luis I. Juncos Department of Medicine, J. Robert Cade Foundation, Cordoba, Argentina

Claire M. Kennedy Department of Nephrology, Beaumont Hospital, Dublin, Ireland

Warren L. Kupin Division of Nephrology and hypertension, Department of Medicine, University of Miami, Miami, FL, USA

Sophia M. Rothberger Lannon Department of Obstetrics and Gynecology, University of Washington, Seattle, WA, USA

Janice P. Lea Division of Nephrology, Department of Medicine, Emory University of Medicine, Atlanta, GA, USA

Eleanor D. Lederer Medicine/Nephrology, University of Louisville, Louisville, KY, USA
Robley Rex VA Medical Centre, Louisville, KY, USA

Oliver Lenz Division of Nephrology and Hypertension, University of Miami, Miller School of Medicine, Miami, FL, USA

Edgar V. Lerma Section of Nephrology, Department of Medicine, University of Illinois at Chicago College of Medicine, Chicago, IL, USA

Kelly V. Liang Renal-Electrolyte Division, Department of Medicine, University of Pittsburgh, Pittsburgh, PA, USA

Kimberly P. Liang Rheumatology Division, Department of Medicine, University of Pittsburgh, Pittsburgh, PA, USA

Andrew Lin Nephrology, University of California San Francisco, San Francisco, CA, USA

Elizabeth C. Lorenz Department of Nephrology and Hypertension, Mayo Clinic, Rochester, MN, USA

Lowell J. Lo Department of Medicine, University of California-San Francisco, San Francisco, CA, USA

Lina Mackelaite Division of Nephrology, University of Louisville, Louisville, KY, USA

Colm C. Magee Consultant Nephrologist, Beaumont Hospital, Dublin 9, Ireland

Tahsin Masud Renal Division, Emory University School of Medicine, Atlanta, GA, USA

Shikha Mehta Department of Nephrology, University of Alabama at Birmingham, Birmingham, AL, USA

Clifford D. Miles Internal Medicine, Nephrology, University of Nebraska Medical Center, Omaha, NE, USA

Vibha S. Nayak Department of Medicine, Nephrology, University of Louisville, Louisville, KY, USA

Grace J. No Department of Nephrology, University of California, San Francisco, CA, USA

Suzanne M. Norby Division of Nephrology, Department of Medicine, College of Medicine, Mayo Clinic, Rochester, MN, USA

Luis M. Ortega Internal Medicine/Nephrology and Hypertension, Allegheny General Hospital, Temple University School of Medicine, WPAHS Campus, Pittsburgh, PA, USA

Mark G. Parker Division of Nephrology and Transplantation, Maine Medical Center, Portland, ME, USA

Raimund H. Pichler Division of Nephrology, Department of Medicine, University of Washington, Seattle, WA, USA

Troy J. Plumb Internal Medicine, Nephrology, University of Nebraska Medical Center, Omaha, NE, USA

Vishal N. Ratkalkar Department of Medicine (Nephrology), Medical College of Wisconsin, Milwaukee, WI, USA

Kevin R. Regner Department of Medicine (Nephrology), Medical College of Wisconsin, Milwaukee, WI, USA

Robert E. Richard Department of Hematology, VA–Puget Sound Health Care System, University of Washington School of Medicine, Seattle, WA, USA

Rudolph A. Rodriguez Department of Nephrology, Puget Sound Veterans Affairs Medical Center, Seattle, WA, USA

Mitchell H. Rosner Department of Medicine, University of Virginia, Charlottesville, VA, USA

Ankit Sakhuja Internal Medicine, Medical College of Wisconsin, Milwaukee, WI, USA

Scott L. Sanoff Department of Medicine, Division of Nephrology, University of Virginia, Charlottesville, VA, USA

Sejal P. Sarolia Humble, TX, USA

Lynn E. Schlanger Department of Nephrology, Veteran Affairs Medical Center at Atlanta, Decatur, GA, USA

Neha Sehgal Division of Nephrology, Medical College of Wisconsin, Milwaukee, WI, USA

Shirin Shafazand Division of Pulmonary, Critical Care and Sleep Medicine, University of Miami, Miller School of Medicine, Miami, FL, USA

Shamik Shah Department of Nephrology, Apollo Hospitals, Gujarat, India

Lena Sibulesky Department of Transplantation, Mayo Clinic Florida, Jacksonville, FL, USA

M. Salman Singapuri Division of Nephrology, Department of Medicine, Emory University of Medicine, Atlanta, GA, USA

C. John Sperati Division of Nephrology, Department of Medicine, Johns Hopkins University School of Medicine, Baltimore, MD, USA

Leslie F. Thomas Nephrology and Hypertension, Mayo Clinic Arizona, Phoenix, AZ, USA

Denyse Thornley-Brown Department of Internal Medicine (Nephrology), University of Alabama at Birmingham, Birmingham, AL, USA

Ashita J. Tolwani Department of Nephrology, University of Alabama at Birmingham, Birmingham, AL, USA

Rebecca L. Toonkel Department of Pulmonary and Critical Care, University of Miami, Jackson Memorial Hospital, Miami, FL, USA

J. Kevin Tucker Department of Medicine/Renal Division, Boston, MA, USA

Nina Vasavada Department of Medicine, University of Louisville, Louisville, KY, USA

Brahm Vasudev Medical College of Wisconsin, Milwaukee, WI, USA

Monica Vasudev Allergy and Clinical Immunology, Medical College of Wisconsin, Milwaukee, WI, USA

Hani M. Wadei Department of Transplantation, Mayo Clinic, Jacksonville, FL, USA

James C. Wasserman Department of Medicine, Main Medical Center, Portland, Cumberland County, ME, USA

Kambiz Zandi-Nejad Nephrology, Harvard Vanguard Medical Associates, Beth Israel Deaconess Medical Center, Harvard Medical School, Boston, MA, USA

Part I

Patient Assessment

Approach to the Patient with Renal Disease

1

Jennifer A. Fillaus and Troy J. Plumb

Case One

A 35-year-old man presents with a 1-week history of progressive shortness of breath and an episode of hemoptysis earlier today. For the past 2 days he has had decreased urine volume and dark colored urine. He has no past medical history and takes no medications. Blood pressure is 145/85 mmHg. Pulse is 110 beats per minute. Temperature is 36.8°C. Pulse oximetry is 87% on room air. He is anxious and slightly pale. Pulmonary exam reveals bibasilar crackles. The remainder of his exam is unremarkable. His laboratory data is notable for a hemoglobin level of 10.9 g/dL and serum creatinine of 2.7 mg/dL. His chest X-ray shows bilateral pulmonary infiltrates.

What is your approach to diagnosis and management in this patient?

Case Two

A 55-year-old woman is referred to your office because of a serum creatinine of 2.5 mg/dL noted on routine labs 3 weeks prior. She denies dysuria, gross hematuria, or change in urine output. She urinates at least two times per night. She is obese and has chronic back pain. She is not taking any prescription medications. Blood pressure is 135/78 mmHg. Pulse is 82 beats per minute. She has trace to 1+ edema to her mid-shin. Remainder of her physical exam is unremarkable. Repeat serum creatinine is 2.6 mg/dL. Urine sediment is a bland.

What is your approach to diagnosis and management of this patient?

Patients with kidney disease can have a myriad of presentations. Patients may be completely asymptomatic and have only elevated blood pressure or lab abnormalities such as an increase in serum creatinine, decreased glomerular filtration rate (GFR), or microscopic hematuria and proteinuria. Alternatively, patients may present with overt signs and symptoms related to uncontrolled blood pressure, nephrotic syndrome, volume overload, changes in urination, or as part of a systemic disease.

When patients present with abrupt onset signs or symptoms of systemic disease along with kidney involvement it is often relatively simple to determine when the kidney disease began and thus what may have been the etiology for the injury. Likewise, when an otherwise healthy patient (especially younger patient) presents with decreased GFR and active urine sediment, it is clear that they have active kidney disease and a tissue biopsy will likely be required. However, oftentimes patients present having not seen a physician in many years, without historical laboratory studies and with an unclear duration of

J.A. Fillaus, D.O. • T.J. Plumb, M.D. (✉)
Internal Medicine, Nephrology, University of Nebraska Medical Center, 983040 Nebraska Medical Center, Omaha, NE 68918-3040, USA
e-mail: tplumb@unmc.edu

E.V. Lerma and M. Rosner (eds.), *Clinical Decisions in Nephrology, Hypertension and Renal Transplantation*,
DOI 10.1007/978-1-4614-4454-1_1, © Springer Science+Business Media New York 2013

edema, diabetes, or hypertension. Such patients require a methodical approach in determining the etiology and treatment plan. This approach must be sensitive to cost, and the sensitivity and specificity of the various testing modalities. This chapter focuses on the approach to the patient who presents with kidney dysfunction with a focus on the key features of the history, physical exam, laboratory, and imaging that can be helpful in narrowing the differential diagnosis and determining the acuity and activity of kidney disease. This information can be extremely helpful in determining the etiology of disease, guiding the diagnostic workup, and determining a treatment plan. In many cases a kidney biopsy will still be required to make the diagnosis. The information gathered using a systematic approach will provide important clinical correlation to the pathologic findings in these cases.

History

The first step in approaching all patients with abnormal renal function tests is a detailed history. Patient history needs to include a detailed review of systems with a focus on the urinary system as well as on obtaining pertinent history of symptoms of systemic diseases with known renal involvement.

Urologic History

Has the patient had any previous urinary tract infections, previous episodes of pyelonephritis, history of vesicoureteral reflux, episodes of nephrolithiasis, or known renal cystic diseases? Each patient also needs a voiding history. Ask the patient about changes in the color of the urine. Gross hematuria may present as tea- or cola-colored urine as is often seen in glomerular disease and nephrolithiasis. Patients with nephrotic syndrome may have foamy urine. Patients with bladder outlet obstruction (e.g., secondary to BPH) may complain of smaller urine volumes, incomplete sensation of bladder emptying, weaker urine stream, or even dribbling at completion of voiding. The first sign of renal disease may also be a decrease in the ability to concentrate urine, the earliest symptom of which may be new onset or increasing nocturia, sometimes noted in patients with tubulointerstitial disease and polycystic kidney disease.

Volume Status

Has the patient noticed weight gain with associated lower extremity edema, orthopnea, or periorbital edema? Conversely, is there a history of poor oral intake, emesis, diarrhea, or high output from ostomy or drains? Are there symptoms of orthostasis or syncope?

Systemic Diseases

The clinician should carefully assess the patient for symptoms of systemic disease processes with associated kidney involvement. Ask the patient about any fevers, night sweats, oral ulcers, rashes, and arthralgias as these symptoms correlate with autoimmune disease and vasculitis. The presence of dyspnea, hemoptysis, or upper respiratory symptoms should prompt evaluation for pulmonary-renal syndromes. New onset of easy bruising or petechiae may indicate thrombocytopenia from a thrombotic microangiopathy (TMA). Any history of, or risk factors for, chronic infections such as hepatitis B and C as well as HIV should be obtained.

When the renal dysfunction appears to be chronic, obtain history for chronic diseases including diabetes, hypertension, peripheral vascular disease, tobacco abuse, and known malignancy. If the patient has diabetes, include in your history the duration, degree of control, and whether he or she has retinopathy and neuropathy. Detailed history of hypertension should include duration, baseline blood pressures, and medications. If the patient has cardiovascular disease, note if any recent angiographic procedures have occurred that would place the patient at risk for contrast-induced nephropathy or atheroembolic disease. Ask about exercise tolerance and symptoms of claudication which may be helpful in determining vascular causes of renal disease.

Family History

In cases of chronic renal dysfunction, family history can also be very helpful if hereditary kidney diseases such as Alport syndrome, polycystic kidney disease, or inherited interstitial kidney diseases are suspected. In all such cases, a detailed pedigree should be obtained as well as past medical records of affected individuals.

Medications

Particular attention needs to be given to medications including prescription, over-the-counter, and herbal medications. Medications commonly associated with acute and chronic kidney injury are diuretics (especially consider in the context of history of volume losses), nonsteroidal anti-inflammatory drugs, angiotensin converting enzyme inhibitors, angiotensin receptor blockers, highly active antiretroviral therapies, chemotherapeutic agents, calcineurin inhibitors, and lithium [1, 2]. Be sure to review records from any recent hospitalizations for exposure to nephrotoxic medications, especially aminoglycosides, vancomycin, acyclovir, and amphotericin [1–3]. Certain medications are associated with the development of interstitial nephritis such as penicillins and cephalosporins, or proton pump inhibitors [3–5]. Review the intake of over-the-counter medications, herbal medications, and supplements. Patients often do not perceive these substances as being potentially harmful and thus may not report them.

Physical Exam

Head

Careful exam of the eyes can give clues to systemic disease processes. Ocular findings may include arteriovenous nicking in long-standing hypertension and cotton wool spots and retinal hemorrhages in association with systemic lupus erythematosus (SLE). Scleritis or uveitis is seen in collagen vascular diseases, vasculitis, and tubulointerstitial nephritis and uveitis syndromes. Proptosis and orbital pseudotumor should prompt suspicion for an underlying diagnosis of granulomatosis with polyangiitis or cyroglobulinemia. Lens rupture can be seen in Alport syndrome [6].

Oral exam findings may provide helpful clues to the presence of systemic diseases with renal involvement. Enlarged and friable "strawberry gums" are a characteristic finding in patients with granulomatosis with polyangiitis. Oral ulcerations may be found in SLE and Henoch–Schonlein purpura (HSP). Periodontal disease is often associated with bacteremia and subsequent risk of endocarditis. Examine the tongue for the presence of macroglossia in patients with suspected amyloidosis [7].

Volume Status/Cardiovascular

Assessment of volume status is of critical importance. Vital signs should be taken in the supine, seated, and standing position to evaluate for the presence of orthostasis. Orthostasis, tachycardia, dry mucus membranes, and flat neck veins all lend support to a diagnosis of hypovolemia. Hypervolemia will manifest as edema (periorbital, peripheral, or anasarca), pulmonary crackles, elevated jugular venous pressure, and cardiac gallops.

The presence of a friction rub is an indicator of uremic pericarditis or of cardiac tamponade and requires emergent attention. In the proper setting, a new murmur may be suggestive of endocarditis.

In addition to assessment of volume status, careful vascular exam should include auscultation over bilateral carotid arteries and aorta, renal, and femoral arteries for evidence of bruits. Palpate peripheral pulses and examine extremities for evidence of hypoperfusion.

Pulmonary

In a patient with renal disease and dyspnea, upper respiratory symptoms, or hemoptysis, prompt evaluation for pulmonary-renal syndromes should be initiated. The most common pulmonary renal syndromes are anti-glomerular basement membrane (GBM) antibody mediated, anti-neutrophil cytoplasmic antibody (ANCA) positive (granulomatosis with polyangiitis, microscopic polyangiitis, Churg–Strauss syndrome), and autoimmune associated (SLE) [8]. However, even severe volume overload due to kidney failure can manifest as hemoptysis and dyspnea. The physical exam will be notable for the presence of pulmonary crackles, rhales, or rhonchi.

Abdomen/Genitourinary

The presence of hepatomegaly will alert the clinician to potential liver disease and the possibility of associated secondary glomerular diseases including membranous nephropathy (MN) associated with hepatitis B, membranoproliferative glomerulonephritis (MPGN), and cryoglobulinemia in association with hepatitis C [9]. Palpation of enlarged kidneys is noted in patients with polycystic kidney disease. Pertinent genitourinary findings include a distended bladder and prostatic hypertrophy.

Skin/Joints

Examine the skin and joints to evaluate for systemic diseases with renal involvement. Look for the characteristic rashes of SLE, palpable purpura as can be seen in cryoglobulinemia and HSP, petechiae as seen in TMAs, and embolic phenomenon seen in endocarditis and atheroembolic disease. The presence of inflammatory arthritis will also give clues to the diagnosis of underlying collagen vascular diseases.

Laboratory Findings

When evaluating a patient with abnormal kidney function, one of the most important initial goals is to determine if they have an acute or a chronic process and if the renal function is rapidly deteriorating or is relatively stable. The rate of decline in kidney function, as measured by serum creatinine or GFR, will be an important determinant of the urgency of the workup. A patient with rapidly progressive renal disease will likely need immediate biopsy and possibly even hospitalization to expedite evaluation, whereas a patient with a chronic course can have an evaluation carried out over many days. The only way to determine whether the renal failure is acute or chronic is to do a review of prior lab testing. Many times patients will be unaware of previous laboratory values or even of the significance of abnormalities. Every effort should be made to review previous laboratory data, including serum creatinine values and urinalysis. In cases where no previous data is available, a kidney ultrasound may be helpful in sorting out an acute versus chronic process as is discussed below.

Serum creatinine is the most widely used laboratory test for determining kidney function and estimating GFR. When considered alone, creatinine is an imperfect marker for estimating renal function [10]; this will be discussed in detail in Chap. 2. Despite limitations of this test, changes in serum creatinine (and estimated GFR) are used both in the diagnosis and management of patients with renal dysfunction. If a patient presents with an unknown baseline or with rapidly changing renal function, a repeat creatinine level should be obtained followed by serial measurement.

A fresh urine specimen should be obtained for dipstick testing and microscopic exam of the sediment. Pertinent findings on urinalysis include the presence of hematuria or proteinuria. If proteinuria is present it should be quantified via a spot urine protein-to-creatinine ratio [11]. While patients with tubulointerstitial disease often have proteinuria less than 1 g per 24 h and patients with glomerular disease frequently present with proteinuria greater than 2 g per 24 h, there is often significant overlap in these presentations.

Microscopic exam of the urine sediment must be performed on all patients with kidney disease. Active urinary sediment is characterized by the presence of dysmorphic red blood cells (RBCs) and cellular casts (granular, white blood cell (WBC), and RBC). Active urinary sediment

Table 1.1 Laboratory evaluation for secondary causes of kidney disease

Complete blood count	
Schistocytes	TMA
Peripheral eosinophils	AIN, atheroembolic disease
Liver function tests	Underlying liver disease
Serum complements	
Low C3 and C4	Lupus nephritis, MPGN type I, cryoglobulinemia
Low C3 and normal C4	PIGN, endocarditis-associated glomerulonephritis, shunt nephritis, hepatitis B, HUS, MPGN type II (dense deposit disease), atheroembolic renal disease
Antinuclear antibody, anti-double-stranded DNA	Lupus nephritis
Anti-neutrophil cytoplasmic antibody	Pauci immune glomerulonephritis, granulomatosis with polyangiitis, MPA, Churg–Strauss syndrome
Anti-glomerular basement membrane antibody	Anti-GBM nephritis, Goodpasture's disease
Hepatitis B surface antigen	MN, MPGN, cryoglobulinemia
Hepatitis C virus antibody	MPGN, MN, cryoglobulinemia
Human immunodeficiency virus	HIV-associated nephropathy/collapsing FSGS
Serum protein electrophoresis with immunofixation	Multiple myeloma-cast nephropathy, AL amyloidosis, LCDD
Urine protein electrophoresis with immunofixation	Multiple myeloma-cast nephropathy, AL amyloidosis, LCDD
Quantitative serum free light chains	Multiple myeloma-cast nephropathy, AL amyloidosis, LCDD
Hemoglobin A1c	DN
Blood cultures	Endocarditis-associated glomerulonephritis
Urine eosinophils	AIN Atheroembolic disease

Abbreviations: *TMA* thrombotic microangiopathy, *AIN* allergic interstitial nephritis, *MPGN* membranoproliferative glomerulonephritis, *PIGN* post-infectious glomerulonephritis, *HUS* hemolytic-uremic syndrome, *MPA* microscopic polyangiitis, *MN* membranous nephropathy, *LCDD* light chain deposition disease, *DN* diabetic nephropathy

is indicative of acute tubulointerstitial or glomerular disorders and should prompt immediate evaluation. In patients with evidence of active kidney disease, further laboratory testing (see Table 1.1) may be useful in determining the etiology, but renal biopsy will often be required to confirm the diagnosis and potential response to treatment.

Findings of chronic, slowly progressive renal dysfunction and the presence of inactive urinary sediment are consistent with chronic kidney disease (CKD). If a modifiable primary disease process is not identifiable, then therapy is aimed at slowing progression and managing sequelae of CKD. Goals of therapy in slowing progression of kidney disease include blood pressure control, proteinuria reduction, dietary sodium and protein restriction, control of the components of metabolic syndrome, and tobacco cessation. Once patients have reached CKD stage 3 and higher, screening for sequelae of CKD should be performed. This is discussed in a later chapter.

Renal Ultrasound

Renal ultrasonography when combined with clinical and laboratory findings is an extremely useful tool in the diagnosis of patients with kidney disease. Any person presenting with abnormal renal function tests should have a kidney ultrasound. The ultrasound may actually make the diagnosis (as in polycystic kidney disease or acute obstruction) or give valuable data in regard to potential etiologies or aid in identifying the chronicity of kidney disease.

Kidney length correlates with body height and is not gender specific [12]. In the adult, normal kidney length averages 10–12 cm. The presence of normal sized kidneys does not exclude the possibility of chronic disease. Normal sized kidneys can be present in patients with any type of kidney disease. Small, atrophic kidneys correlate with duration and severity of chronic disease. Smooth bilateral renal enlargement may be present in diabetes, HIV, lymphoma, amyloidosis, and renal edema (such as seen in acute glomerulonephritis or pyelonephritis [12]).

Renal echogenicity is a sensitive but nonspecific marker for parenchymal renal disease [13]. The normal cortex is hypoechoic when compared with liver or spleen. An increase in cortical echogenicity is considered to be indicative of renal disease (a proxy for fibrous tissue deposition). Medullary echogenicity may be seen in chronic interstitial nephritis (particularly analgesic nephropathy), uric acid deposition, and nephrocalcinosis [12].

Urinary obstruction typically results in hydronephrosis, a dilation of the collecting system. Ultrasound can help indicate the duration and cause of obstruction. In cases of acute obstruction, the cortex is intact, whereas chronic obstruction can lead to cortical thinning. It is important to examine the entire urinary tract when hydronephrosis is present as the location of obstruction may be suggested. Failure to visualize the proximal ureter suggests obstruction at the ureteropelvic junction whereas a dilated ureter indicates downstream obstruction. A large post-void bladder indicates urinary retention, whereas an empty bladder with dilation of the distal ureters suggests obstruction at the bladder inlet [12]. Obstruction without ureteral dilation may also occur in retroperitoneal fibrosis, cancers involving the retroperitoneum, and transplanted kidneys.

Care must be taken in interpretation of the ultrasound findings as calyceal dilation in the absence of obstruction may be seen in reflux nephropathy, papillary necrosis, brisk diuresis, and pregnancy. Renal venous engorgement may be mistaken as hydronephrosis and doppler flow can be helpful in distinguishing these entities [12].

Cases Revisited

Case 1

Case 1 represents a rapidly progressive glomerulonephritis and highlights the importance of prompt diagnosis and treatment in a potentially life-threatening situation. Using the approach outlined above, the patient's history of hemoptysis and gross hematuria alerted the clinician to the presence of a pulmonary renal syndrome. Review of previous labs from this patient's primary care office showed him to have a baseline serum creatinine of 0.9 mg/dL. Urine sediment was active with the presence of RBC casts. Protein-to-creatinine ratio was 2. Renal ultrasound showed normal-appearing kidneys bilaterally.

Due to his acute kidney injury, active sediment, and concern for alveolar hemorrhage, the patient was directly admitted for further evaluation and treatment. Further laboratory data was obtained which included serum for ANCA, anti-GBM antibody level, complement C3 and C4, and ANA. A renal biopsy was performed which revealed a diffuse proliferative glomerulonephritis with linear deposition of IgG along the glomerular basement membrane. Serum for anti-GBM antibody was positive, confirming the diagnosis of Goodpasture's disease.

Case 2

Case 2 illustrates just how important meticulous history taking is. Further history was obtained which revealed that she had been taking 800 mg of ibuprofen three times daily for the past several years due to her chronic back pain. She reported taking no other over-the-counter or herbal substances. There were no constitutional symptoms or family history of renal diseases. Her exam was unremarkable. Previous laboratory data was not available. The urine sediment was bland. Protein excretion was 1 g via spot ratio. Renal ultrasound showed small (9 cm) bilateral kidneys with increase in cortical echogenicity. No masses, cysts, or hydronephrosis were noted. A presumptive diagnosis of chronic tubulointerstitial disease was made and the patient was advised to discontinue her ibuprofen. Her creatinine and proteinuria were routinely monitored and treatment focused on slowing CKD progression and management.

Conclusion

The patient with kidney disease may be completely asymptomatic or may present with symptoms related to kidney disease or a systemic syndrome. Regardless of the presentation it is important to have a systematic approach to each patient which includes a detailed history, physical exam, and pertinent laboratory and renal imaging studies. Determination of the acuity, activity, or progressive nature of the kidney disease will help guide the need for prompt or emergent evaluation and therapy.

Key Points

Pertinent history for all patients being evaluated for kidney disease should include:

- History of urinary system symptoms including gross hematuria (cola-colored urine), flank pain, urinary frequency, and nocturia
- Medication history including prescribed, over-the-counter, and herbal medications
- Detailed family history of kidney diseases
- History of symptoms of systemic disease associated with renal involvement (e.g., SLE)
- Symptoms of volume overload or depletion

Important physical exam findings in patients being evaluated for renal dysfunction

- Head
  - Ocular findings: AV nicking, cotton wool spots, scleritis, uveitis, lens rupture
  - Oral findings: Gingival hyperplasia, oral ulcers, periodontal disease, macroglossia
- Cardiovascular
  - Hypovolemia
  - Hypervolemia
  - Vascular exam
- Pulmonary
  - Tachypnea, crackles, rales, rhonchi
  - Abdominal/GU
  - Bruits over aorta or renal arteries suggest vascular disease
  - Organomegaly
    - Hepatomegaly
    - Enlarged palpable kidneys
  - Distended urinary bladder
  - Prostatic enlargement
- Skin and Joints
  - Rashes
  - Purpura
  - Petechiae
  - Inflammatory arthritis

Findings associated with active kidney disease:

- New onset or worsening hypertension
- New onset or worsening edema
- Abrupt change in GFR
- Proteinuria
- Active urine sediment: Dysmorphic red blood cells, cellular casts (RBC, WBC, granular)

References

1. John R, Herzenberg AM. Renal toxicity of therapeutic drugs. J Clin Pathol. 2009;62(6):505–15.
2. Perazella MA. Drug-induced renal failure: update on new medications and unique mechanisms of nephrotoxicity. Am J Med Sci. 2003;325(6):349–62.
3. Vandecasteele SJ, De Vriese AS. Recent changes in vancomycin use in renal failure. Kidney Int. 2010; 77(9):760–4.
4. Praga M, Gonzalez E. Acute interstitial nephritis. Kidney Int. 2010;77(11):956–61.
5. Geevasinga N, Coleman PL, Webster AC, Roger SD. Proton pump inhibitors and acute interstitial nephritis. Clin Gastroenterol Hepatol. 2006;4(5):597–604.
6. Izzedine H, Bodaghi B, Launay-Vacher V, Deray G. Oculorenal manifestations in systemic autoimmune diseases. Am J Kidney Dis. 2004;43(2):209–22.
7. Summers SA, Tilakaratne WM, Fortune F, Ashman N. Renal disease and the mouth. Am J Med. 2007; 120(7):568–73.
8. Papiris SA, Manali ED, Kalomenidis I, Kapotsis GE, Karakatsani A, Roussos C. Bench-to-bedside review: pulmonary-renal syndromes—an update for the intensivist. Crit Care. 2007;11(3):213.
9. Lai AS, Lai KN. Viral nephropathy. Nat Clin Pract Nephrol. 2006;2(5):254–62.

10. Stevens LA, Coresh J, Greene T, Levey AS. Assessing kidney function—measured and estimated glomerular filtration rate. N Engl J Med. 2006;354(23):2473–83.
11. Levey AS. Clinical practice. Nondiabetic kidney disease. N Engl J Med. 2002;347(19):1505–11.
12. O'Neill WC. Sonographic evaluation of renal failure. Am J Kidney Dis. 2000;35(6):1021–38.
13. Moghazi S, Jones E, Schroepple J, et al. Correlation of renal histopathology with sonographic findings. Kidney Int. 2005;67(4):1515–20.

2 Assessment of Renal Function

Clifford D. Miles

Case 1

Mrs. P is a 62-year-old African-American female with type II diabetes mellitus. She weighs 78 kg, and has previously had an above-knee amputation of the right leg. She is being seen in clinic for an annual examination, and inquires about her kidney function.

Introduction

The assessment of renal function is an important aspect of medical care. While the kidneys perform many essential roles for the body, the excretion of waste by-products of metabolism is the most fundamental. The glomerulus is a specialized tuft of capillaries that serves as a filter. Its size- and charge-selectivity allow for the free passage of water and small, nonpolar molecules while retaining the cellular elements and large proteins (e.g., albumin) in the serum (see Fig. 2.1). The glomerular filtration rate (GFR) is the parameter by which renal function is expressed. As this is difficult to measure directly, many methods of approximating the GFR have been developed. Serial determination of GFR is the best method of following patients with kidney disease as it serves as the basic parameter for staging severity of kidney disease.

Glomerular Filtration Rate

A human kidney has approximately one million nephrons. Each nephron produces filtrate at a rate dictated by the plasma flow, pressure gradient, surface area, and intrinsic permeability of the glomerular filtration barrier. The GFR of the body is the sum of all the individual nephrons' filtering capacity. GFR can be assessed in terms of clearance, defined as the volume of plasma from which a given substance is completely filtered into the urine per unit time. Mathematically,

$$C_x = U_x V / P_x,$$

where C_x is the clearance of substance x, U_x is the concentration of x in the urine, V is the urinary flow rate, and P_x is the plasma concentration of x. By convention, GFR is typically reported in mL/min.

Ideal substances to calculate GFR are freely filtered through the glomerulus, and neither absorbed, metabolized, nor secreted along the course of the nephron. Inulin is the classic exogenous marker used for this purpose, though it is expensive, difficult to assay, and needs to be administered by continuous IV infusion to

C.D. Miles, M.D., M.S. (✉)
Internal Medicine, Nephrology, University of Nebraska Medical Center, 983040 Nebraska Medical Center, Omaha, NE 68198-3040, USA
e-mail: cdmiles@unmc.edu

E.V. Lerma and M. Rosner (eds.), *Clinical Decisions in Nephrology, Hypertension and Renal Transplantation*,
DOI 10.1007/978-1-4614-4454-1_2, © Springer Science+Business Media New York 2013

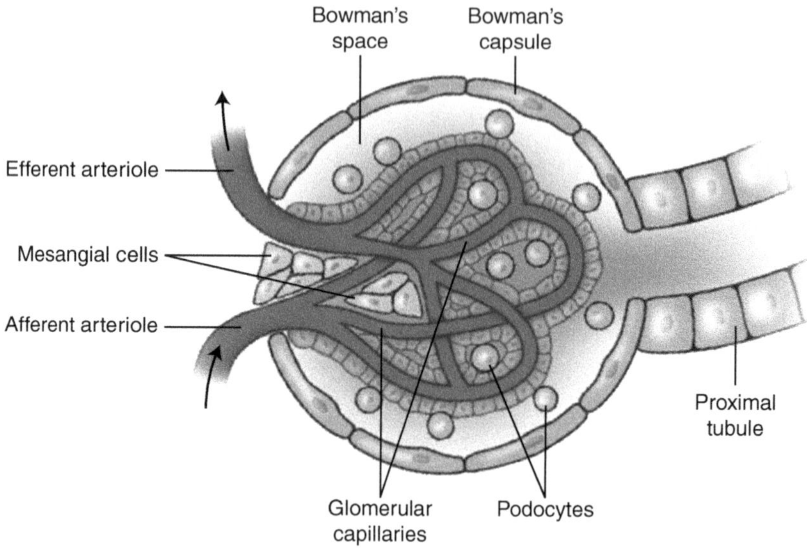

Fig. 2.1 The Glomerulus. The glomerulus is a specialized tuft of capillaries that serves as a filter. Blood flows to the glomerulus via the afferent arteriole and then distributes through the network of capillaries. The capillary endothelium, glomerular basement membrane, and podocyte-derived epithelium make up the filtration barrier. Its size- and charge-selectivity allow for the free passage of water and small, nonpolar molecules while retaining the cellular elements and large proteins in the serum. The filtrate (urine) collects in Bowman's space, and then exits into the proximal tubule of nephron

perform clearance studies. Various radionuclides can be utilized to measure GFR, including ^{125}I-iothalamate, ^{99m}Tc-diethylenetriaminepentaacetic acid (Tc-DTPA), and ^{51}Cr-ethylenediaminetetraacetic acid (Cr-EDTA). In addition, nonradioactive forms of radiocontrast dyes, like iothalamate, can be used to perform clearance measurements. Methods include standard urinary clearance analysis, but also plasma disappearance protocols, which avoid the cumbersome duty of timed urine sample collection [1]. One published protocol involves the bolus infusion of iothalamate, followed by serial plasma concentration measurements, which are then used to calculate the GFR (as iothalamate is cleared exclusively by the kidneys). The authors of this protocol stress that more blood samples and longer duration are important to attain accurate and precise GFR measurements, ultimately recommending eight samples over 6 h to ensure reliable results [2]. Thus, as with inulin, these plasma disappearance assays tend to be tedious and expensive and their use remains largely restricted to the research setting.

Creatinine

Creatinine is an organic waste compound generated in the body by the metabolism of phosphocreatine, primarily in skeletal muscle. The day-to-day production of creatinine is relatively constant, and it is freely filtered by the glomerulus, and not absorbed along the nephron. Thus, the plasma concentration of creatinine is inversely related to GFR—i.e., higher creatinine levels correlate with reduced renal function (see Fig. 2.2). Note that the relationship between creatinine concentration and GFR is not linear, such that small changes in plasma concentration at low levels (e.g., from 0.8 to 1.2 mg/dL) can signify major changes in GFR. Meanwhile seemingly large changes in plasma creatinine at the right end of the creatinine to

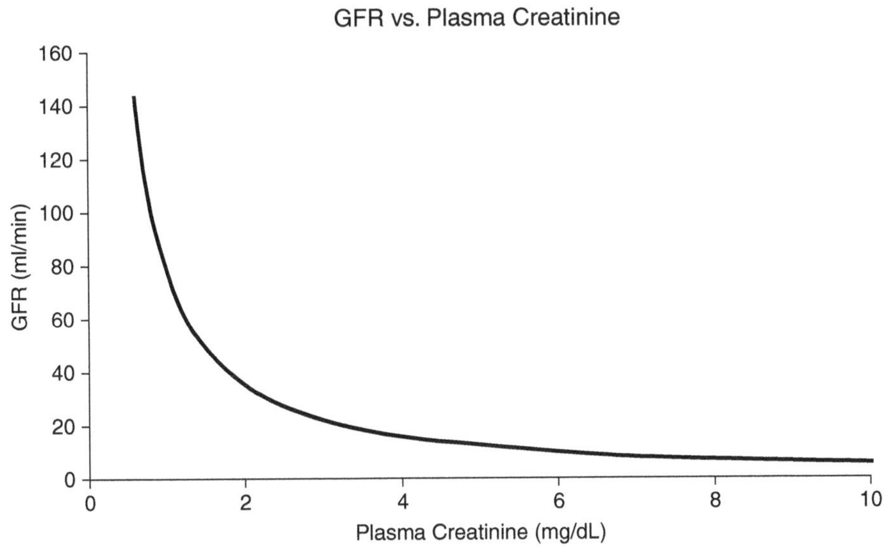

Fig. 2.2 Relationship between plasma creatinine concentration and glomerular filtration rate. With impaired glomerular filtration, clearance of creatinine from the plasma is reduced. Thus, plasma concentration of creatinine is inversely related to GFR—i.e., higher creatinine levels correlate with reduced renal function. The relationship between creatinine concentration and GFR is not linear. Note at the *left end* of the curve that small changes in plasma creatinine concentration at low levels (e.g., from 1.0 to 2.0 mg/dL) can signify major changes in GFR. Meanwhile seemingly large changes in plasma creatinine at the *right end* (e.g., 4–8 mg/dL) correspond to clinically insignificant changes in GFR

Table 2.1 Factors associated with changes in plasma creatinine concentration

Factor	Direction of change	Mechanism
Decline in renal function	↓	Reduced clearance
Male gender	↑	Higher relative muscle mass
African-American race	↑	Higher relative muscle mass
Diet high in meat products	↑	Absorption from intestine
Malnutrition	↓	Reduced generation
Amputation	↓	Reduced generation
Cimetidine, trimethoprim	↑	Blockade of tubular secretion

GFR curve (e.g., 4–7 mg/dL) correspond to clinically insignificant changes in GFR. In addition, creatinine generation tends to be higher in men and African Americans, and declines with age, all related to differences in relative muscle mass [3]. Other factors influencing plasma creatinine concentration are listed in Table 2.1. One should appreciate that a plasma creatinine concentration of 1.4 mg/dL may be normal in a young, muscular African-American male, but signify considerable renal insufficiency in a patient who is older, poorly nourished, or has had an amputation. This indicates that assessment of kidney function must not rely on single creatinine measurements.

Between 10 and 40% of the creatinine in the final urine is derived from tubular secretion (typically, as kidney function worsens the percentage of total creatinine found in the urine due to tubular secretion increases). Thus, it is not an ideal substance to calculate GFR. However, because it is endogenously produced, and is cheap and easy to measure, it is the most widely used laboratory measurement to estimate kidney function.

Creatinine Clearance

The creatinine clearance (CrCl) can be calculated from easily obtainable data, by substituting into the above formula:

$$C_{\text{creat}} = U_{\text{creat}} V / P_{\text{creat}}.$$

Standard practice is to have the patient collect a 24-h urine specimen, and have the plasma creatinine checked on the same day.

Case 1 Continued

The clinic nurse knew that Mrs. P was worried about her kidneys, and so had asked her to submit a 24-h urine collection. She turned in a jug with 1,400 mL of urine, which had a creatinine concentration of 85 mg/dL. Plasma creatinine that day was 1.4 mg/dL.

Using the data supplied from the case, it can be shown that this patient's CrCl is

$$C_{\text{creat}} = (85\,\text{mg/dL}) \times (1{,}400\,\text{mL}/24\,\text{h}) / (1.4\,\text{mg/dL}) = 85{,}000\,\text{mL}/24\,\text{h}$$

To convert to conventional mL/min, one must divide by 1,440, the number of minutes in a day. Thus, the patient in the example has a calculated CrCl of 59 mL/min.

The most common error using this method is an incomplete urine collection. Adequacy of the collection can be verified by assessing the total creatinine in the sample. Men excrete on average 20–25 mg/kg body mass of creatinine daily; women excrete 15–20 mg/kg. The patient's urine collection in the example had:

$$\text{Total creatinine} = (85\,\text{mg/dL}) \times (1{,}400\,\text{mL}) \times (1\,\text{dL}/100\,\text{mL}) = 1{,}190\,\text{mg}.$$

As she weighed 78 kg, this represents 15.3 mg/kg, so it was likely an adequate collection.

To avoid the cumbersome collection of a 24-h urine sample, and the likelihood of it being done improperly, estimation (regression) formulae for the CrCl have been developed. The most commonly used formula to estimate the CrCl is the Cockcroft–Gault equation [4]. It is based on the plasma creatinine concentration, and takes into account the age, weight, and gender:

$$\text{CrCl} = (140 - \text{age}) \times (\text{weight}) / (72 \times P_{\text{creat}}),$$

with age expressed in years, weight in kg, and P_{creat} in mg/dL. The result is multiplied by 0.85 if the patient is female. Returning again to our example, one can calculate Mrs. P's CrCl using the Cockcroft–Gault equation:

$$\text{CrCl} = \{[(140 - 62) \times 78\,\text{kg}] / (72 \times 1.4\,\text{mg/dL})\} \times 0.85 = 51.3\,\text{mL/min}.$$

At relative extremes of body habitus, it is recommended that this result be normalized for body surface area (BSA). This is done by dividing the "standard" BSA of 1.73 m^2 by the patient's BSA, and multiplying the CrCl by the result. If Mrs. P's BSA is 1.5 m^2, then

$$(1.73/1.5) \times 51.3\,\text{mL/min} = 59.2\,\text{mL/min}/1.73\,\text{m}^2.$$

As mentioned above, creatinine is secreted along the course of the nephron. The proportion of creatinine in the final urine due to secretion varies from 10% to as high as 40%. In general, individuals with lower GFR have higher relative secretion rates. Thus, CrCl overestimates true GFR, and the degree of overestimation tends to be greater as renal function worsens. In recent years, several formulae have been developed to try to more accurately calculate GFR.

Creatinine-Based Estimation Formulae for GFR

The Modification of Diet in Renal Disease (MDRD) study was a prospective study of the effects of protein restriction and blood pressure control on progression of renal disease. Data from 1,628 subjects enrolled in the trial included a directly measured baseline GFR (using ^{125}I-iothalamate), and other demographic and serum variables. Using stepwise linear regression analysis, a formula was developed that more accurately predicted GFR than the

Cockcroft–Gault equation [5]. A simplified version of the formula, the four variable MDRD equation (or abbreviated, aMDRD), was subsequently published, and has become one of the most commonly employed tools for estimating renal function [6]:

$$\mathrm{GFR} = 175 \times P_{\mathrm{Creat}}^{-1.154} \times \mathrm{Age}^{-0.203} \times (0.742 \text{ if female}) \times (1.21 \text{ if Black}).$$

The result is again in mL/min, normalized to BSA in square meters. While the MDRD formula was originally derived from a predominantly white population with nondiabetic kidney disease, it has since been validated in African Americans, diabetics, and renal transplant recipients. However, it has been noted that the MDRD formula does not perform as well in subjects with normal or near-normal renal function, where it tends to underestimate measured GFR [7].

The Chronic Kidney Disease Epidemiology Collaboration (CKD-EPI) sought to develop a more accurate GFR estimation formula, again based on plasma creatinine. Data from ten studies (8,254 participants) was pooled to derive the new equation, which was subsequently validated using data from an additional 16 studies (3,896 participants) [8]. The mean GFR of the group used for development of the formula was 68 mL/min, compared to 40 mL/min for the MDRD equation. The CKD-EPI formula was shown to be both more accurate and more precise than the MDRD formula among individuals with GFR >60 mL/min. Online calculators for the MDRD and CKD-EPI equations can be found at http://www.kidney.org/professionals/kdoqi/gfr_calculator.cfm

Note that inputs for both of these equations to predict GFR include serum creatinine concentration, age, race, and gender.

Case 1 Revisited

By employing either the aMDRD or the CKD-EPI formula, it can be shown that Mrs. P's estimated GFR is 46 mL/min/1.73 m^2. Note that this result is less than the CrCl, either calculated from the urine collection or estimated with the Cockcroft–Gault equation. Furthermore, as an amputee, one should suspect that her creatinine-based GFR/CrCl calculations may *over*estimate her renal function due to reduced expected creatinine generation.

Case 2

Mrs. P's son is 24 years old. He became concerned about his own kidney function after talking with his mother, especially since he knew from his Army physical that his plasma creatinine was also 1.4 mg/dL. However, using the CKD-EPI calculator, one can quickly show that his estimated GFR is 81 mL/min/1.73 m^2. He further discloses that he weighs 100 kg and exercises vigorously 5 days per week. Thus, one should suspect that his creatinine generation is relatively high, and his GFR estimate may be spuriously low.

At the current time, the aMDRD formula is the most widely used equation for estimation of renal function. It tends to be more accurate *and* more precise compared to the Cockcroft–Gault equation, directly estimates GFR rather than creatinine clearance, and does not require the measurement of body mass, such that laboratories can more easily report automated eGFR values to help aid in the detection and monitoring of chronic kidney disease.

Cystatin C

The above equations all rely on serum creatinine concentration. Other potential markers have been evaluated, with the most attention recently given to cystatin C. Cystatin C is a small protein produced at a constant rate by all nucleated cells. As it is freely filtered by the glomerulus and not reabsorbed, its serum concentration, like creatinine, is inversely related to renal function. Other factors that appear to be associated with increased cystatin C concentration include male gender, increasing weight and height, and smoking [9]. As with creatinine, equations have been developed to estimate GFR based on serum concentration of cystatin C, incorporating variables such as gender and age, and perhaps an equation that includes both creatinine and cystatin C will eventually come into use for estimating GFR [10]. At the current time, assays for cystatin C remain available in only a limited number of laboratories, and hence it is not a commonly used marker for assessing renal function.

Key Points

1. Plasma creatinine concentration is the most widely used test to estimate kidney function, but it has distinct limitations and should be interpreted with caution. Age, gender, race, and relative muscularity all have an effect on creatinine generation.
2. Many formulae have been developed to more accurately estimate kidney function, most based on plasma creatinine, and including variables such as age, gender, and race. The aMDRD formula for estimating GFR is the most widely used, and online calculators are readily available.
3. All equations assume a steady state—i.e., the plasma creatinine concentration is not rapidly rising or falling.

References

1. Rolin HA, Hall PM. Evaluation of glomerular filtration rate and renal plasma flow. In: Jacobsen HR, Striker GE, Klahr S, editors. The principles and practice of nephrology. 2nd ed. St. Louis, MO: Mosby-Year Book; 1995. p. 8–13.
2. Agarwal R, Bills JE, Yigazu PM, Abraham T, Gizaw AB, Light RP, Bekele DM, Tegegne GG. Assessment of iothalamate plasma clearance: duration of study affects quality of GFR. Clin J Am Soc Nephrol. 2009;4:77–85.
3. Stevens LA, Levey AS. Measurement of kidney function. Med Clin North Am. 2005;89:457–73.
4. Cockcroft DW, Gault MH. Prediction of creatinine clearance from serum creatinine. Nephron. 1976;16:31–41.
5. Levey AS, Bosch JP, Lewis JB, Greene T, Rogers N, Roth D. A more accurate method to estimate glomerular filtration rate from serum creatinine: a new prediction equation. Modification of Diet in Renal Disease Study Group. Ann Intern Med. 1999;130:461–70.
6. Levey AS, Coresh J, Greene T, Stevens LA, Zhang Y, Hendriksen S, Kusek JW, Van Lente F, Chronic Kidney Disease Epidemiology Collaboration. Using standardized serum creatinine values in the modification of diet in renal disease study equation for estimating glomerular filtration rate. Ann Intern Med. 2006;145:247–54.
7. Poggio ED, Wang X, Greene T, Van Lente F, Hall PM. Performance of the modification of diet in renal disease and Cockcroft-Gault equations in the estimation of GFR in health and in chronic kidney disease. J Am Soc Nephrol. 2005;16:459–66.
8. Levey AS, Stevens LA, Schmid CH, Zhang Y, Castro AF, Feldman HI, Kusek JW, Eggers P, Van Lente F, Greene T, Coresh J, Chronic Kidney Disease Epidemiology Collaboration. A new equation to estimate glomerular filtration rate. Ann Intern Med. 2009;150:604–12.
9. Knight EL, Verhave JC, Spiegelman D, Hillege HL, De Zeeuw D, Curhan GC, DeJong PE. Factors influencing serum cystatin C levels other than renal function and the impact on renal function measurement. Kidney Int. 2004;65:1416–21.
10. Stevens LA, Coresh J, Schmid CH, Feldman HI, Froissart M, Kusek J, Rossert J, Van Lente F, Bruce RD, Zhang Y, Greene T, Levey AS. Estimating GFR using serum cystatin C alone and in combination with serum creatinine: a pooled analysis of 3418 individuals with CKD. Am J Kidney Dis. 2008;51:395–406.

Approach to Renal Diagnostic Testing

3

Marius C. Florescu

Case 1

A 65-year-old man with hypertension and coronary artery disease but no previous kidney disease is seen by the renal consult service for decreased urine output and increased serum creatinine 1 day after undergoing a right hemicolectomy for colon cancer. The patient is in the intensive care unit and his blood pressure is 120/80 mmHg. His urine output for the last 24 h was 250 mL despite receiving 4 L of intravenous fluids. He is alert and oriented. Examination of the chest reveals faint crackles at both lung bases; the abdomen is slightly distended with decreased but present bowel sounds. He has trace lower extremity and sacral edema. His urine output did not increase following 200 mg of intravenous furosemide.

What is the differential diagnosis?

What tests you want to order to determine the etiology of acute kidney injury (AKI)?

What do you expect to see on urine microscopic examination?

Case 2

A 40-year-old man is seen in the renal clinic for proteinuria noted by his physician on urinalysis during his annual physical examination. He has no past medical history and takes no medications. There is no family history of renal disease. Physical examination is normal. Blood pressure is 155/90. Urinalysis shows microscopic hematuria and proteinuria. Serum creatinine is 0.9 mg/dL; his spot urine protein-to-creatinine ratio is 2.

What do you expect to see on microscopic examination of the urine?

What is the significance of dysmorphic red blood cells?

What is the differential diagnosis of his renal disease?

What further tests do you want to order to determine the etiology of his renal disease?

Case 3

A 55-year-old woman is admitted to the hospital for abdominal pain. Three months ago she had a total hysterectomy and chemotherapy for uterine carcinoma. Her serum creatinine is 3 mg/dL (it was 0.8 mg/dL 1 month ago). She has no prior kidney disease. She has no gross hematuria. Her vitals are within normal limits and she appears to be moderately fluid overloaded. She has diffuse abdominal pain to moderate palpation. Her urine output is 1,000 mL/24 h.

What is the differential diagnosis of her AKI?

What tests do you want to order to determine the etiology of her AKI?

Her renal ultrasound shows no evidence of hydronephrosis. Do you think this finding

M.C. Florescu, M.D. (✉)
Internal Medicine, Nephrology, University of Nebraska Medical Center, 983040 Nebraska Medical Center, Omaha, NE, 68918-3040, USA
e-mail: mflorescu@unmc.edu

E.V. Lerma and M. Rosner (eds.), *Clinical Decisions in Nephrology, Hypertension and Kidney Transplantation*, DOI 10.1007/978-1-4614-4454-1_3, © Springer Science+Business Media New York 2013

excludes urinary obstruction? What test can diagnose urinary obstruction missed by the renal ultrasound?

Case 4

A 60-year-old man is seen in the renal clinic for evaluation of difficult-to-control hypertension despite being compliant with his prescribed medications. He has hypertension for 5 years, hypercholesterolemia, and coronary artery disease. He voices no complaints and his physical examination is within normal limits. His serum creatinine increased from 1 mg/dL 1 year ago to 2 mg/dL last week. The patient had a renal ultrasound with Doppler showing bilateral normal kidney size, increased resistive indexes bilaterally, blunting of the Doppler waveform on the right kidney, and increased velocity of blood flow in the midsegment of the right renal artery.

What is the significance of the ultrasound findings?

Does he have renal artery stenosis?

Does he need any further tests?

There is a large diversity of renal diseases and the approach to diagnose them should be tailored for each particular condition. Physicians caring for patients with renal disease should understand the role of each test to maximize the diagnostic yield and to avoid unnecessary risk and expenditure. Urinalysis, including urine microscopy and dipstick, should be performed for all patients evaluated for renal disease. Spot urine or 24-h urine collection for protein, albumin, creatinine, urea nitrogen, and electrolytes can offer further valuable diagnostic data. There are numerous renal imaging methods, each presenting different primary indications, advantages, and disadvantages.

Urinalysis

The trained nephrologist should perform a complete urinalysis (including microscopic urinary examination) in all patients with renal disease. In order to maximize the clinical correlation, microscopic examination of the urine sediment should be performed by the treating nephrologist and not by a laboratory technician [1].

The urine should be examined within 1 h of voiding. Before collection the external genitalia need to be washed and wiped dry. The urine should be collected after discarding the first portion (midstream) and then centrifuged at 3,000 rpm for 5 min [2]. The sediment is used for the microscopic examination and the supernatant for dipstick. Strenuous exercise should be avoided for 72 h prior to urine collection to avoid exercise-induced proteinuria or hematuria. In women, urinalysis should not be done during menstruation to avoid blood contamination.

1. *Color*. Normal urine is clear and yellow. The color of the urine can range from light to dark depending on how dilute or concentrated the urine may be. Red urine can be observed in several conditions [3]. Initial testing of red urine is centrifugation to determine whether the color is from the supernatant or the sediment. If the sediment is red and the supernatant is clear then the diagnosis is hematuria. If the supernatant is red, then the supernatant should be tested for heme pigments with a urine dipstick. If the test is positive then the diagnosis is either hemoglobinuria or myoglobinuria. If the supernatant is heme negative then the diagnosis can be beeturia, porphyria, and use of phenazopyridine. Table 3.1 shows different urine colors and their diagnostic significance.
2. *Turbidity*. Normal urine is transparent. Turbid urine can be caused by an increased concen-

Table 3.1 Urine color and diagnostic significance [3]

Urine color	Condition
Red sediment	Hematuria
Red supernatant Heme negative	Beeturia, phenazopyridine, porphyria
Red supernatant Heme positive	Myoglobinuria—clear plasma Hemoglobinuria—red plasma
Black upon standing	Alkaptonuria—homogentisic aciduria
Black	Hemoglobinuria
Green	Methylene blue, propofol, amitriptiline, triamterene
White	Pyuria, chyluria, propofol

Table 3.2 Urine odor and rare metabolic disorders

Urine odor	Condition
Mousy	Phenylketonuria
Sweet, fruity	Ketones
Sweaty feet	Isovaleric acidemia
Maple syrup	Maple syrup urine disease
Pungent	Urinary tract infection due to ammonia production
Fishy	Hypermethioninemia

tration of any urine particle. The most common causes of turbid urine are urinary tract infections, hematuria, and contaminated urine. A non-turbid urine does not equate with the absence of renal disease.

3. *Odor*. There are some rare metabolic conditions that are associated with characteristic urine odors as presented in Table 3.2.
4. *Relative density*.
   (a) Specific gravity: Depends on the number and weight of the particles dissolved in the urine. It is influenced by the presence of proteins, glucose, and contrast. In normal urine, under physiologic conditions, specific gravity will vary from 1.000 to 1.030 depending on volume and hydration status.

   A specific gravity of 1.000–1.003 is associated with very dilute urine as seen in diabetes insipidus or water intoxication. A specific gravity of 1.010 is called isosthenuric because it has the same specific gravity as plasma. It is found in conditions with impaired ability to concentrate or dilute the urine like acute tubular necrosis and chronic kidney disease. Isosthenuria can also be found in subjects with normal kidney function. When the specific gravity is above 1.032, glycosuria should be suspected and above 1.040 the presence of an extrinsic substance like contrast should be suspected.

   (b) Osmolality: Depends only on the number of particles dissolved in the urine. The specific gravity generally varies with osmolality. However, large molecules such as proteins, glucose, or contrast, which cause large changes in specific gravity, cause relatively minor changes in osmolality due to their large molecular weight.

   The urine osmolality is more reliable in assessing the solute concentration of the urine than the specific gravity. The urine osmolality varies with volume status and interpreting the urine osmolality should be done only considering the clinical state. Urine osmolality is clinically relevant in patients with hypo- or hypernatremia and polyuria.
5. *pH*. It is measured by dipstick. The pH indicator covers the pH range between 5.0 and 9.0. The dipstick pH measurement is significantly less accurate for pH values less than 5.5 and above 7.5. Urine pH ranges between 4.5 and 8.0. The urine pH is important clinically in patients with metabolic acidosis and to determine if renal acidification mechanisms are intact.

   Urine pH can be influenced by urinary infections with any urease-producing pathogen (such as *Proteus mirabilis*). Urease production can increase the urine pH above 7.0.
6. *Hemoglobin*. It is detected by dipstick through the pseudoperoxidase activity of the heme moiety of the hemoglobin. This method can detect hemoglobinuria equivalent to 1–2 red blood cells per high-powered field. The test is also positive in hemoglobinuria following intravascular hemolysis, rhabdomyolyis with myoglobinuria, or high concentration of bacteria with pseudoperoxidase activity such us staphylococci and streptococci. False negative reactions can be caused by ascorbic acid.
7. *Glucose*. The test is sensitive to urine glucose concentrations of 0.5–20 g/L. False negative reactions can occur in the presence of ascorbic acid.

   Glucosuria can be caused by the inability of the kidney to reabsorb the filtered glucose despite normal plasma levels (renal glucosuria) or urinary spillage caused by elevated plasma glucose as seen in diabetes mellitus. Glucosuria occurs in normal kidneys when the plasma glucose is above 180 mg/dL (above the renal threshold for tubular reabsorption). Renal glucosuria is usually seen as part of the Fanconi syndrome (proximal tubular dysfunction), which includes hypophosphatemia, hypouricemia, renal tubular acidosis, aminoaciduria, and glucosuria with normal serum glucose.

8. *Protein*. Physiologic proteinuria does not exceed 150 mg of proteins/24 h.
   (a) The urine dipstick detects mainly albumin. Urine proteins such as light chains can be missed even when they are in significant quantity. The test becomes positive when proteinuria exceeds 15–30 mg/dL (approximately 300–500 mg/day depending on urine volume). It is important to understand that the dipstick measures the urinary protein concentration and not the urinary protein excretion. The semiquantitative results of the dipstick are expressed on a scale from + (15–30 mg/dL) to ++++ (300–600 mg/dL), and should be used as a rough guide because protein concentration in the urine changes with urine volume; a concentrated urine will increase apparent albumin excretion and a diluted urine will decrease apparent albumin excretion.

   The regular dipstick is insensitive to detect microalbuminuria, which is the earliest manifestation of diabetic nephropathy. When testing for microalbuminuria, special sensitive dipsticks should be used. Microalbumin dipsticks can detect urine albumin concentrations as low as 2 mg/dL. False positive results for proteinuria by urine dipstick can occur for up to 24 h after iodinated contrast administration [4].

   (b) Sulfosalicylic acid test detects all urinary proteins. Three percent sulfosalicylic acid is added to an equal volume of urine. The acidification causes precipitation of protein in the sample (seen as increasing turbidity), which is subjectively graded as trace, 1+, 2+, 3+, or 4+. A positive sulfosalicylic test associated with a negative dipstick for proteins suggests non-albumin proteins in the urine, usually immunoglobulin light chains (Bence Jones proteins). Radiocontrast agents can cause a false positive reaction with sulfosalicylic acid [3]. The sulfosalicylic test has been replaced with quantitative measurement of proteinuria.

   (c) Quantitative measurement of proteinuria.

   Collection of urine for a 24-h period allows for an accurate measurement of protein and/or albumin excretion. However, this method is cumbersome, especially in the ambulatory setting, and very often the urine is not correctly collected leading to inaccurate results.

   A single voided urine specimen can be used as alternative to the 24-h urine collection. Standard expression of protein-to-creatinine ratio is in grams/24 h. Hence, when urine protein and creatinine are expressed in the same units (e.g., mg/dL) the ratio is the estimated 24-h urine protein excretion. For example, a patient with a urinary protein concentration of 250 mg/dL and a urinary creatinine concentration of 100 mg/dL has a protein-to-creatinine ratio of 2.5 and an estimated 24-h urine protein excretion of 2.5 g. The same ratio can be applied to urine albumin excretion. However, urinary albumin ratios are often reported in micrograms of albumin to mg of creatinine. For example, a patient with a urinary albumin concentration of 20 mg/dL and a urinary creatinine concentration of 100 mg/dL has an albumin-to-creatinine ratio of 0.2, and an estimated 0.2 g of albumin in 24 h. However, in many labs, the albumin-to-creatinine ratio is reported in μg/mg. Hence, using the above example, urinary albumin is 20,000 μg/dL and urinary creatinine is 100 mg/dL. Hence, the ratio becomes 200 μg albumin/mg creatinine, which is equivalent to a 24-h albumin excretion of 200 mg.

The spot urine protein-to-creatinine ratio is reliable for quantifying proteinuria even in pregnant proteinuric patients, in pediatric population, and in kidney transplant population [5–8].

(d) Qualitative analysis of proteinuria can be done using electrophoresis or immunofixation. Immunofixation is more sensitive in detecting monoclonal proteins than electrophoresis and is preferred for evaluating urinary Bence Jones proteinuria [9, 10]. When evaluating a patient for suspected monoclonal gammopathy, it is important to order urine protein electrophoresis with immunofixation.

(e) Some urinary proteins may predict the severity and the prognosis of different glomerular diseases. Urinary excretion of Beta-2 microglobulin predicted that the prognosis of idiopathic membranous nephropathy and urinary excretion of IgG and alpha-1 microglobulin were markers of renal outcome and response to therapy. Fractional excretion of IgG predicted the progression and the response to therapy in crescentic IgA nephropathy. Those are novel urinary markers of glomerular damage but they are not yet available in clinical practice [11–13].

9. *Leukocyte esterase*. Evaluates the presence of leukocytes by detecting the indoxyl esterase activity released from the lysed neutrophil granulocytes and macrophages. This is why very commonly there is a negative microscopy for white blood cells but a positive dipstick for leukocyte esterase. A positive reaction suggests the presence of urinary tract infection.
10. *Nitrites*. The dipstick detects the presence of bacteria that possess nitrate reductase activity which reduces nitrates to nitrites. The nitrate reductase activity is present in most Gram-negative uropathogenic bacteria but absent in Pseudomonas, Staphylococcus, and Streptococcus.
11. *Bile pigments*. The detection of urinary urobilinogen and bilirubin has lost the clinical value being replaced by measuring plasma liver enzymes.
12. *Ketones*. The dipstick detects acetoacetate and acetone but not beta-hydroxybutyrate. The test is positive in diabetes ketoacidosis, fasting, and recent vomiting.

Key Points

- Urinalysis and urine microscopy should be done in all patients with renal disease.
- Urine microscopy should be performed by the treating nephrologist.
- Urine dipstick for proteins can miss monoclonal proteinuria.
- When evaluating a patient for suspected monoclonal gammopathy, order urine protein electrophoresis with immunofixation.
- Urine dipstick for proteins is insensitive to detect microalbuminuria—the earliest manifestation of diabetes nephropathy.
- Dysmorphic red blood cells and red blood cell casts are hallmarks of glomerular disease.

Urine Microscopy

Microscopic examination of the urine sediment is an essential part of renal disease evaluation. It allows the detection of elements that cannot be found on urine dipstick such as red and white blood cell casts and crystals. Approximately 10 mL of freshly voided urine should be centrifuged at 3,000 rpm for 5 min. Most of the supernatant should be gently discarded. The pellet should be resuspended in the remaining supernatant and a drop added to the glass microscope slide.

It is very important to remember that in normal urine one high power field can contain 0–2 red blood cells, 0–4 white blood cells, and occasional casts [14]. The urine sediment should be evaluated by a trained clinician to maximize the diagnostic yield [1]. The elements seen during the urine microscopic evaluation are cells, casts, crystals, and bacteria.

1. *Bacteria*. In most cases bacteriuria is caused by urine contamination. Urinary infection is suspected when numerous urine leukocytes are present along with bacteria [15].
2. *Cells*.
   (a) Erythrocytes: The presence of RBCs is called hematuria. Hematuria can be benign or it can reflect a serious disease. Hematuria can be continuous or intermittent. It can be classified as microscopic or may be grossly visible. Microscopic hematuria is defined as more than two red blood cells per high power field.

   Causes of hematuria include glomerular diseases, malignancies, and kidney stones. It is very important to differentiate if the hematuria originates in the glomerulus (glomerular diseases) versus the urinary tract (infection, stone, malignancy). Dysmorphic red blood cells and red blood cell cast are pathognomonic for hematuria of glomerular origin. The combination of red blood cell casts, dysmorphic red blood cells, and proteinuria strongly suggests a glomerular disease.

   (b) Leukocytes: Neutrophils are the leukocytes most frequently seen in the urine. They are larger than red blood cells, have a granular cytoplasm, and have multilobated nuclei. The presence of leukocytes in the urine is called pyuria. Neutrophils are markers of urinary tract infection.

   Eosinophils and lymphocytes can be identified in the urine using the Wright's stain. While eosinophils may be present in patients with acute interstitial nephritis, they are also present in other disorders such as glomerulonephritis, prostatitis, and atheroembolic diseases [16].

   (c) Renal tubular cells derive from the tubular epithelium. They are 1.5–3 times larger than white cells and have a round, large nucleus. Tubular cells are difficult to differentiate from lower urinary tract cells.

   Tubular cells are markers of tubular damage and they are found in acute tubular necrosis, acute interstitial nephritis, and acute cellular rejection [17]. Many times they are associated with tubular cell casts.

   (d) Uroepithelial cells line the urinary tract from the renal calyces to the bladder. This epithelium is multilayered with small cells (diameter 13–20 μm) in the deep layers and large cells (diameter 20–40 μm) in the superficial layers.

   Large amounts of deep-layer cells are found in urologic neoplasms. Superficial layer cells are found in urinary tract infections.

   (e) Squamous cells derive from the urethra. In large amounts they indicate urine contamination from genital secretions.
   (f) Podocytes: In normal urine, podocytes are absent or present in very small amounts [18]. Urinary podocyte excretion increases in active renal disease and decreases with successful treatment [19, 20]. Recent data suggests that podocyturia may be a better marker of ongoing glomerular damage than proteinuria [21]. Recently, podocyturia was shown to be a highly sensitive and specific marker for preeclampsia [22]. Currently, there is no commercially available test to detect and quantify the urine podocytes.
3. *Casts*.

   Casts are urine entities with cylindrical shape and regular margins. They form inside the distal renal tubules or collecting ducts. Their matrix is formed of Tamm–Horstfall glycoprotein secreted by the cells of the thick ascending limb of the loop of Henle. Different materials can be trapped inside a cast; hence many types of casts exist. Some of them can be seen in normal urine and others are diagnostic of significant renal diseases.

   (a) Hyaline casts are colorless and do not indicate renal disease.
   (b) Red cell casts clearly indicate that the hematuria is of glomerular origin and suggests glomerulonephritis or vasculitis. The cast can contain a few or very abundant erythrocytes.
   (c) White cell casts are associated with pyuria in tubulointerstitial diseases or acute

pyelonephritis but can be found in many glomerular diseases [23].

(d) Epithelial cell casts contain variable amounts of tubular cells recognized by their large nucleus. They are seen in acute tubular necrosis and acute glomerulonephritis [23].

(e) Fatty casts are seen in patients with significant proteinuria. The epithelial cells forming these casts are degenerated and loaded with lipid droplets giving the characteristic Maltese cross appearance under polarized light.

(f) Granular casts are formed of degenerated cells and are found in a large variety of renal diseases.

(g) Waxy casts are considered to be the last stage of degeneration of granular casts and are seen in advanced renal diseases.

(h) Broad casts are wider that the other casts suggesting that they formed in severely damaged and dilated tubules and are seen in advanced renal failure.

An overview of the clinical significance of urinary casts is shown in Table 3.3.

4. *Crystals*.

Examination of the urine for crystals is indicated in renal stone disease, rare metabolic diseases, or drug toxicity. In asymptomatic patients finding a few uric acid, calcium oxalate, or calcium phosphate crystals is not considered pathologic. The significance of crystals should be interpreted in the appropriate clinical setting.

Table 3.3 Clinical significance of urinary casts

Cast type	Clinical significance
Hyaline	Normal subject
Red cell	Glomerular bleeding—proliferative or necrotizing glomerulonephritis
White cell	Acute interstitial nephritis, acute pyelonephritis, proliferative GN
Epithelial cell	ATN, acute interstitial nephritis
Granular	ATN
Fatty	Severe proteinuria, nephrotic syndrome
Waxy	CKD
Broad	CKD

ATN acute tubular necrosis, *CKD* chronic kidney disease

(a) Uric acid crystals form in acidic urine and can have a wide spectrum of appearances ranging from rhomboids to barrels. They have a polychromatic appearance under polarized light.

(b) Calcium oxalate crystals: There are two types: monohydrate—dumbbell shaped which polarizes light and bihydrate—bipiramidal which does not polarize light.

(c) Calcium phosphate crystals can have different shapes ranging from prisms, needles, and star shaped.

(d) Triple Phosphate crystals contain magnesium ammonium phosphate and have the shape of "Coffin lids." They are found in alkaline urine and strongly polarize light.

(e) Cholesterol crystals look like transparent thin plates with sharp edges. They are markers of severe proteinuria.

(f) Cystine crystals look like hexagonal plates with irregular sides and are found only in acid urine. Their presence is always pathologic and is a hallmark of cystinuria.

(g) Crystals due to drugs: In the setting of drug overdose, volume depletion, hypoalbuminemia, and favorable pH conditions some drugs can crystallize in the urine. Drugs more commonly known to cause urine crystals are sulfadiazine, amoxicillin, ciprofloxacin, acyclovir, indinavir, and vitamin C.

Patterns of Urinary Findings in Renal Disease

Many renal diseases are associated with distinct patterns of urinary findings. These patterns are very important in diagnosing renal diseases and are presented in Table 3.4.

Case 1 Revisited

The differential diagnosis includes prerenal disease caused by third spacing and possible inadequate fluid resuscitation, acute tubular necrosis, and urinary tract obstruction as a complication of his surgery. Bladder outlet obstruction and

Table 3.4 Urine microscopy patterns and their clinical significance

Renal disease	Urinary pattern
Nephrotic syndrome	Fatty casts, few tubular cells
Nephritic syndrome	Erythrocyte casts, dysmorphic red blood cells, tubular cells, rare epithelial casts
Acute tubular necrosis	Epithelial cell casts, muddy brown granular casts, numerous tubular cells
Urinary tract infection	Leukocytes, bacteria
Prerenal disease, urinary tract obstruction, chronic renal failure	Few cells with little or no casts, no proteinuria

abdominal compartment syndrome are also in the differential.

What tests should we order to evaluate his AKI? Microscopic examination of the urine sediment can show evidence of ATN such us muddy brown granular casts and numerous epithelial cells or may reveal normal urine sediment consistent with obstruction or prerenal disease.

Urinalysis may show new-onset proteinuria suggesting ATN. A renal ultrasound can exclude obstruction and give important information about the renal blood perfusion. In this case, careful review of the operative flow sheet revealed that the patient had a period of 20 min where his systolic blood pressure was less than 90 mmHg. His urine sediment revealed numerous muddy brown granular casts, and a diagnosis of ischemic ATN was made.

Case 2 Revisited

This patient has new-onset subnephrotic proteinuria and microscopic hematuria. This is highly suggestive for glomerular disease. The absence of edema makes the nephrotic syndrome unlikely. On urine microscopic examination we would expect to see dysmorphic red blood cells, red blood cell casts, and possibly a few epithelial cell casts. Dysmorphic red blood cells are suggestive of glomerular bleeding, hence the diagnosis of nephritis or vasculitis. The presence of red blood cell casts confirms the glomerular source of bleeding. The absence of dysmorphic red blood cells or red blood cell casts does not exclude nephritis or vasculitis.

The renal diseases that can cause the urinary findings discussed above include IgA nephropathy, membranoproliferative glomerulonephritis (GN) with or without cryoglobulinemia, postinfectious GN, lupus nephritis, pauciimmune rapidly progressive GN, and Goodpasture disease/syndrome.

Further tests include renal ultrasound, antinuclear antibody (ANA), anti-neutrophil cytoplasmic antibody (ANCA) panel, human immunodeficiency virus (HIV), hepatitis B and C serology, cryoglobulins, anti-glomerular basement membrane (GBM) antibody. Renal biopsy will establish the final diagnosis and will provide valuable prognostic data.

In this case, further laboratory testing was negative, the renal ultrasound was normal, and a kidney biopsy was consistent with IgA nephropathy.

Table 3.5 Renal diseases and the appropriate imaging techniques

Acute renal failure	Ultrasound
Renal stone	Noncontrast CT
Renal mass	Contrast CT or MRI
Hematuria	CT
Retroperitoneal fibrosis	Contrast CT
Renal artery stenosis	CT angiography or MRA
Papillary necrosis	Contrast CT

Renal Imaging

A large number of renal imaging techniques are available and a proper understanding of these techniques is mandatory for an accurate and effective diagnosis of renal diseases (see Table 3.5).

Regardless of the technique used to image the kidney, some simple notions of renal anatomy should be emphasized. The kidneys are located in the superior retroperitoneum with the upper poles directed medially and the lower poles laterally. A normal kidney should be about 3–4 vertebral bodies in length. The renal outline is smooth and well demarcated. Renal enhancement should begin 30 s after intravenous contrast administration and should be symmetric. Asymmetry in renal enhancement can suggest renal artery stenosis. The ureters should enhance after 5 min.

Renal Ultrasonography

Renal ultrasound provides a relatively inexpensive and noninvasive method to assess renal location, size, and vasculature. It is the test of choice to evaluate patients with AKI, to exclude urinary obstruction [24].

(a) Kidney size: The renal size varies in adults and normally is between 9 and 12 cm in length. Kidney size can be easily measured with the renal ultrasound.

(b) Renal echotexture: Echotexture describes the quantity of echoes generated within an organ. Structures that produce no echoes (like fluids) appear black on ultrasound. Structures which produce more echoes appear light gray or white on ultrasound. In regard to the kidney, an increase in echoes or echogenicity is associated with increased collagen deposition, and hence chronic kidney disease. The normal renal cortex appears hypoechoic or dark by ultrasound.

When compared to the echogenicity of the liver, the renal cortex should be isoechoic or hypoechoic [25]. An increase in echogenicity of the renal cortex is often found in diseases affecting the renal parenchyma. Because it contains fat, the renal sinus is more echogenic than the renal cortex. The renal pelvis and the proximal ureter are anechoic.

(c) Urinary obstruction is inferred by the presence of a dilated collecting system and proximal ureter and is called hydronephrosis. Very rarely will the renal ultrasound identify the cause or location of the obstruction. In order to produce the hallmark image of obstruction, the collecting system must be able to dilate. In conditions like retroperitoneal fibrosis and retroperitoneal cancers, the collecting system often cannot dilate and the ultrasound can miss the diagnosis of urinary obstruction. If the clinical suspicion of urinary obstruction persists a nuclear renal scan can aid in the diagnosis.

(d) Renal calculi appear as echogenic structures with an acoustic shadow. The renal ultrasound is not the test of choice for renal calculi detection.

(e) Renal cysts: Renal ultrasound identifies renal masses as cystic or solid. Cystic masses can be simple or complex. Simple cysts are anechoic (no internal structures), fluid filled (black), and have a very thin wall. They are common and are typically benign.

Complex cysts can contain septations, calcifications, and nodules and present internal echoes. Complex cysts can be benign or malignant. A CT or an MRI evaluation is necessary for further diagnosis.

(f) Solid renal mass: The renal ultrasound is less sensitive than CT or MRI in diagnosing renal masses. A renal ultrasonography depicting an exophytic renal mass is presented in Fig. 3.1.

(g) Renal vasculature: Doppler investigation is used to evaluate the renal vasculature. This test is mainly used to investigate a possible renal artery stenosis. Ultrasound evaluation can detect a blood flow velocity change caused by the presence of stenosis as well as a change in the normal arterial waveform downstream from the lesion. A normal renal artery waveform presents a rapid systolic upstroke and an early systolic peak.

An increase in the systolic velocity and the presence of a tardus (slow systolic acceleration) and parvus (rounded systolic peak) waveform distal to the stenosis are suggestive of the presence of renal artery stenosis. These findings require a skilled operator and a long examination time. Renal artery stenosis suggested by the above findings needs to be confirmed by a CT angiogram, magnetic resonance angiography (MRA), or renal angiogram.

Doppler examination of the renal arteries is used to calculate the resistive indexes.

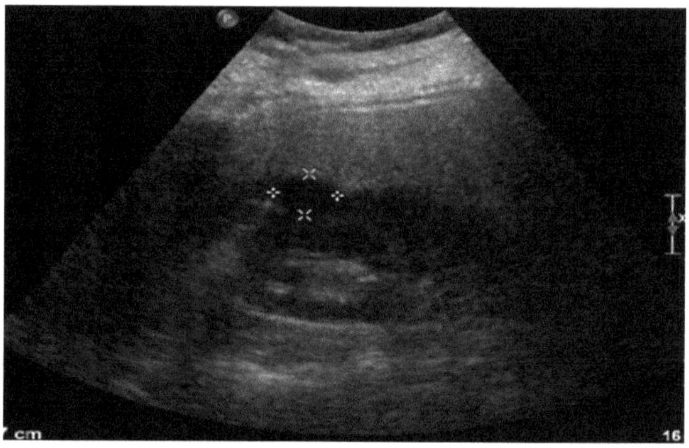

Fig. 3.1 Renal ultrasound showing the contour of the kidney with an exophytic mass (*stars*)

The resistive index is calculated using the following formula:

(Peak systolic velocity – End diastolic velocity)/Peak systolic velocity.

The normal value is <0.7. It is elevated in numerous conditions such as ATN, transplant rejection, urinary obstruction, and chronic kidney disease. An elevated resistive index associated with decreased kidney size may signal advanced intrarenal vascular disease and predicts a decreased response to treatment [26, 27]. A new renal ultrasound technique, contrast-enhanced sonography, might be useful to evaluate renal graft status because of its capability to evaluate cortical capillary blood flow [28].

(h) Bladder: The urine-filled bladder can be easily evaluated with the ultrasound. Doppler evaluation can identify the presence of urine flowing from the ureters into the bladder, the so-called ureteral jets.

Plain Radiography

It is nowadays rarely performed. It used to be the initial study for suspected renal stones but it is poor at detecting radiolucent uric acid stones, small stones, or stones overlying bony structures and now has been replaced with spiral CT.

Intravenous contrast urography (abdominal X-ray after intravenous contrast injection) has been replaced by CT or MRI and now it is very rarely used.

Table 3.6 Indications for renal CT

Renal masses: Cystic or noncystic
Noncontrast helical CT is the diagnostic of choice for renal stones
Evaluate and stage renal cell carcinoma
Diagnose renal vein thrombosis
Early diagnosis of polycystic kidney disease
Evaluate retroperitoneal masses

Retrograde Pyelography

It is performed by placing a catheter into the ureter through direct cystoscopic guidance. The catheter is advanced into the renal pelvis and contrast is injected as the catheter is retracted. This technique is used when the ureters are poorly visualized through other techniques or samples of urine are needed for cytology evaluation.

Computed Tomography

The indications for renal computed tomography (CT) are presented in Table 3.6.

The renal CT can be performed with or without intravenous contrast.

(a) Noncontrast CT is the test of choice for nephrolithiasis. Suspected renal hemorrhage is evaluated by noncontrast CT because the contrast might obscure the blood.

(b) Contrast CT: The kidneys should be similar in size and show similar enhancement and excretion of contrast. Delayed excretion can be a sign of urinary obstruction or a renal dis-

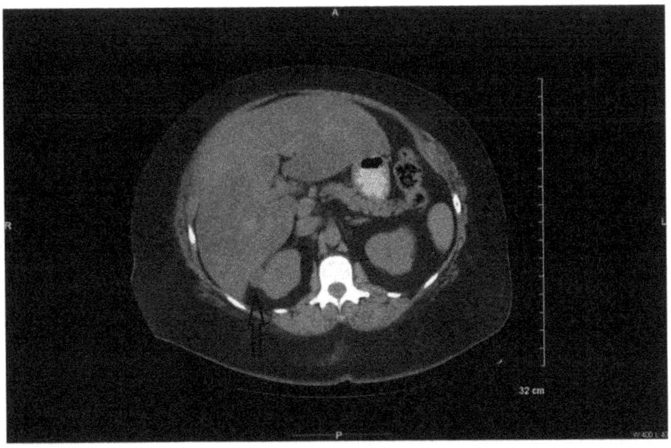

Fig. 3.2 Same lesion as in Fig. 3.1 seen on noncontrast renal CT (*arrow*)

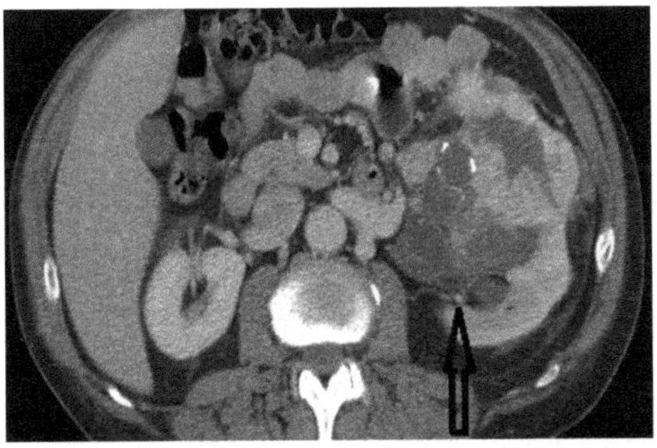

Fig. 3.3 Left renal cell carcinoma (*arrow*). Intravenous contrast renal CT (courtesy of Dr. Michael Feloney)

ease such as acute tubular necrosis. Figure 3.2 shows the CT image of the same renal mass depicted by renal ultrasonography and Fig. 3.3 shows a large renal cell carcinoma.

CT urography has largely replaced the intravenous pyelogram. It is used for evaluation of renal masses, collecting system, and ureteral abnormalities. A diuretic can be administered after the intravenous contrast to increase the urine output to better distend the collecting system and the ureters and offer a better image.

CT angiography can produce images similar to angiography but it is less invasive. Contrast is administered intravenously and the CT is timed for maximal enhancement of the aorta. The image is reconstructed showing the aorta and its branches. CT angiography is used to evaluate renal arteries in potential renal donors and to assess renal artery stenosis [29].

Magnetic Resonance Imaging

MRI is very rarely used as the first test for renal imaging, most of the time being used as an adjunct to a previous renal imaging technique. Magnetic resonance urography and MRA can also be performed.

CT and MRI offer comparable results and the choice is more of a local preference. MRI might be preferred over CT in patients with contrast allergy or to decrease the radiation exposure in children. A new approach has been to use Blood Oxygenation Level Dependence (BOLD) imaging to demonstrate renal medullary hypoxia in the evaluation of renal artery stenosis [30] and renal transplant rejection [31]. This is a promising but still experimental MRI technique.

Measurement of Glomerular Filtration Rate with CT and MRI

CT or MRI can be used to measure GFR. These techniques are new but reliable and yield comparable results but have not gained widespread acceptance [32, 33].

Renal Arteriography

Renal angiography has largely been replaced by CTA and MRA. It is still used for therapeutic interventions such as renal artery angioplasty and stenting and renal artery embolization therapy. The technique is slightly superior to CT or MRI

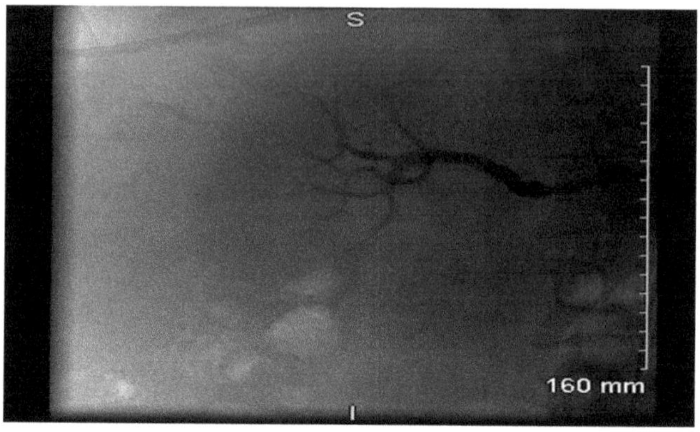

Fig. 3.4 Right renal arteriogram. Normal renal arteriogram

mainly in detecting small accessory renal arteries. The arteriography requires accessing the arterial system usually through the femoral artery. Figure 3.4 shows a normal renal arteriography.

Radionuclide Scintigraphy

A radiotracer is administered to the patient and a gamma ray camera captures the photons emitted by the radiotracer within the patient and generates an image.

Indications for the use of renal scintigraphy:

(a) Assessment of renal function: Renal scintigraphy is the investigation of choice before total nephrectomy or nephron-sparing surgery for renal malignancies to predict the postoperative renal function.

(b) Urinary obstruction: Scintigraphy is the test of choice when the ultrasound evidence for obstruction is questionable but the clinical suspicion of obstruction is high.

(c) Scintigraphy is superior to other imaging modalities in the evaluation of renal flow and function. The renal radiotracer uptake and excretion by the kidney evaluate the renal function. By comparing the uptake and excretion of each kidney a split function of each kidney can be calculated. If obstruction is suspected, a loop diuretic is injected intravenously while the radiotracer is still present in the renal pelvis. If the obstruction is present, the renal pelvis activity will persist. Without obstruction the radiotracer will rapidly wash out from the renal pelvis and the activity will drop.

(d) Vesicoureteral reflux can be diagnosed and evaluated by radioisotope cystography. The radiotracer is placed into the bladder and its reflux in the ureters is detected by the gamma camera.

Case 3 Revisited

The differential diagnosis includes urinary obstruction caused by the presence of malignancy, chemotherapy-related nephrotoxicity, and membranous nephropathy associated with malignancy. The diagnostic tests include urinalysis and microscopic examination of the urine, renal ultrasound, spot urine protein-to-creatinine ratio. When urinary obstruction is high in the differential diagnosis and there is the possibility that hydronephrosis might not develop, a renal scan is the test of choice to exclude obstruction.

In this case, urinalysis and microscopic examination of the urine were unremarkable. A renal ultrasound showed no evidence of obstruction but suggested the presence of retroperitoneal lymphadenopathy, which was confirmed by a noncontrast CT scan of the abdomen and pelvis. Renal scintigraphy with the administration of a loop diuretic showed persistent tracer in the renal pelvis suggesting urinary obstruction. Following bilateral percutaneous nephrostomy tube placement the serum creatinine returned to 0.9 mg/dL.

Case 4 Revisited

The blunting of the waveform and the increased velocity of the right renal artery are highly suggestive of renal artery stenosis, but its presence needs to be confirmed by CT angiography or MRA. The presence of the renal artery stenosis however does not mandate angioplasty and stenting of the renal artery in all patients.

Key Points

- Renal ultrasound is the test of choice for acute renal failure to exclude urinary obstruction.
- Complex cysts diagnosed with a renal ultrasound can be benign or malignant and a CT or an MRI evaluation is necessary for further diagnosis.
- Noncontrast CT is the test of choice for nephrolithiasis.
- CT and MRI offer comparable results and the choice is more of a local preference.
- When the renal ultrasound fails to show obstruction but urinary obstruction is high in the differential diagnosis and there is the possibility that hydronephrosis might not develop, a renal scan is the test of choice.

References

1. Tsai JJ, Yeun JY, Kumar VA, Don BR. Comparison and interpretation of urinalysis performed by a nephrologist versus a hospital-based clinical laboratory. Am J Kidney Dis. 2005;46(5):820–9.
2. European Confederation of Laboratory Medicine. European urinalysis guidelines. Scand J Clin Lab Invest Suppl. 2000;231:1–86.
3. Baran RB, Rowles B. Factors affecting coloration of urine and feces. J Am Pharm Assoc. 1973;13:139.
4. Morcos SK, el-Nahas AM, Brown P, Haylor J. Effect of iodinated water soluble contrast media on urinary protein assays. BMJ. 1992;305:29.
5. Schwab SJ, Lyle Christensen R, Dougherty K, Klahr S. Quantitation of proteinuria by the use of protein-to-creatinine ratios in single urine samples. Arch Intern Med. 1987;147(5):943–4.
6. Robert M, Sepandj F, Liston RM, Dooley KC. Random protein-creatinine ratio for the quantitation of proteinuria in pregnancy. Obstet Gynecol. 1997;90(6):893–5.
7. Kim HS, Cheon HW, Choe JH, Yoo KH, Hong YS, Lee JW, Kim SK. Quantification of proteinuria in children using the urinary protein-osmolality ratio. Pediatr Nephrol. 2001;16(1):73–6.
8. Steinhäuslin F, Wauters JP. Quantitation of proteinuria in kidney transplant patients: accuracy of the urinary protein/creatinine ratio. Clin Nephrol. 1995;43(2):110–5.
9. Graziani M, Merlini G, Petrini C. Guidelines for the analysis of Bence Jones protein. IFCC Committee on Plasma Proteins; SIBioC Study Group on Proteins. Clin Chem Lab Med. 2003;41(3):338–46.
10. Levinson SS. Urine protein electrophoresis and immunofixation electrophoresis supplement one another in characterizing proteinuria. Ann Clin Lab Sci. 2000;30(1):79–84.
11. Branten AJW, du Buf-Vereijken PW, Klasen IS, Bosch FH, Feith GW, Hollander DA, Wetzels JF. Urinary excretion of beta 2-microglobulin and IgG predict prognosis in idiopathic membranous nephropathy: a validation study. J Am Soc Nephrol. 2005;16:169–74.
12. D'Amico G, Bazzi C. Urinary protein and enzyme excretion as markers of tubular damage. Curr Opin Nephrol Hypertens. 2003;12(6):639–43.
13. Bazzi C, Rizza V, Raimondi S, Casellato D, Napodano P, D'Amico G. In crescentic IgA nephropathy, fractional excretion of IgG in combination with nephron loss is the best predictor of progression and responsiveness to immunosuppression. Clin J Am Soc Nephrol. 2009;4:929–35.
14. Wright WT. Cell counts in urine. AMA Arch Intern Med. 1959;103:76.
15. Vickers D, Ahmad T, Coulthard MG. Diagnosis of urinary tract infection in children: fresh urine microscopy or culture? Lancet. 1991;338(8770):767–70.
16. Nolan 3rd CR, Kelleher SP. Eosinophiluria. Clin Lab Med. 1988;8(3):555–65.
17. Fogazzi GB, Saglimbeni L, Banfi G, Cantú M, Moroni G, Garigali G, Cesana BM. Urinary sediment features in proliferative and non-proliferative glomerular diseases. J Nephrol. 2005;18(6):703–10.
18. Vogelmann SU, Nelson WJ, Myers BD, Lemley KV. Urinary excretion of viable podocytes in health and renal disease. Am J Physiol Renal Physiol. 2003;285(1):F40–8. Epub 2003 11.
19. Donghai Yu, Petermann A, Kunter U, Rong S, Shankland SJ, Floege J. Urinary podocyte loss is a more specific marker of ongoing glomerular damage than proteinuria. J Am Soc Nephrol. 2005;16(6):1733–41.
20. Nakamura T, Ushiyama C, Suzuki S, Hara M, Shimada N, Sekizuka K, Ebihara I, Koide H. Urinary podocytes for the assessment of disease activity in lupus nephritis. Am J Med Sci. 2000;320(2):112–6.
21. Sato Y, Wharram BL, Lee SK, Wickman L, Goyal M, Venkatareddy M, Chang JW, Wiggins JE, Lienczewski C, Kretzler M, Wiggins RC. Urine podocyte mRNAs mark progression of renal disease. J Am Soc Nephrol. 2009;20(5):1041–52.
22. Garovic VD, Wagner SJ, Turner ST, Rosenthal DW, Watson WJ, Brost BC, Rose CH, Gavrilova L, Craigo P,

Bailey KR, Achenbach J, Schiffer M, Grande JP. Urinary podocyte excretion as a marker for preeclampsia. Am J Obstet Gynecol. 2007;196(4): 320e.1–7.
23. Fogazzi GB, Saglimbeni L, Banfi G, Cantú M, Moroni G, Garigali G, Cesana BM. Urinary sediment features in proliferative and non-proliferative glomerular diseases. J Nephrol. 2005;18(6):703–10.
24. Webb JA. Ultrasonography in the diagnostic of renal obstruction. BMJ. 1990;301:944.
25. Katzberg RW. Urography into the 21st century: new contrast media, renal handling, imaging characteristics, and nephrotoxicity. Radiology. 1997;204(2):297–312.
26. Ikee R, Kobayashi S, Hemmi N, Imakiire T, Kikuchi Y, Moriya H, Suzuki S, Miura S. Correlation between the resistive index by Doppler ultrasound and kidney function and histology. Am J Kidney Dis. 2005; 46(4):603–9.
27. Moghazi S, Jones E, Schroepple J, Arya K, McClellan W, Hennigar RA, O'Neill WC. Correlation of renal histopathology with sonographic findings. Kidney Int. 2005;67:1515–20.
28. Jimenez C, Lopez MO, Gonzalez E, Selgas R. Ultrasonography in kidney transplantation: values and new developments. Transplant Rev (Orlando). 2009;23(4):209–13. Epub 2009 4.
29. Wittenberg G, Kenn W, Tschammler A, Sandstede J, Hahn D. Spiral CT angiography of renal arteries: comparison with angiography. Eur Radiol. 1999;9(3): 546–51.
30. Juillard L, Lerman LO, Kruger DG, Haas JA, Rucker BC, Polzin JA, Riederer SJ, Romero JC. Blood oxygen level-dependent measurement of acute intra-renal ischemia. Kidney Int. 2004;65(3):944–50.
31. Sadowski EA, Fain SB, Alford SK, Korosec FR, Fine J, Muehrer R, Djamali A, Hofmann RM, Becker BN, Grist TM. Assessment of acute renal transplant rejection with blood oxygen level-dependent MR imaging: initial experience. Radiology. 2005;236(3):911–9.
32. Krier JD, Ritman EL, Bajzer Z, Romero JC, Lerman A, Lerman LO. Noninvasive measurement of concurrent single-kidney perfusion, glomerular filtration, and tubular function. Am J Physiol Renal Physiol. 2001;281(4):F630–8.
33. Nilsson H, Wadström J, Andersson L-G, Raland H, Magnusson A. Measuring split renal function in renal donors: can computed tomography replace renography? Acta Radiol. 2004;45:474–80.

Part II

Glomerular Diseases

Approach to the Patient with Nephrotic Syndrome

4

Leslie F. Thomas and Harini A. Chakkera

Case 1

A 50-year-old woman with no significant past medical history acutely develops bilateral lower extremity pitting edema. A thorough evaluation of cardiac and hepatic functions is unremarkable; however, urinalysis reveals significant proteinuria. Further testing shows an elevated serum creatinine level of 1.8 mg/dL, low serum albumin level of 2.2 g/dL, and hyperlipidemia (total cholesterol 385 mg/dL, triglycerides 480 mg/dL, LDL 245 mg/dL, and HDL 44 mg/dL). Urinary protein measures 5.2 g in a 24-h collection. The clinical diagnosis of nephrotic syndrome is made.

Introduction

Nephrotic syndrome is characterized by proteinuria exceeding 3.5 g/1.73 m^2/day, hypoalbuminemia, edema, hyperlipidemia, and lipiduria [1, 2]. Diseases leading to nephrotic syndrome are diverse and include common conditions such as diabetes mellitus as well as less commonly encountered genetic disorders. Kidney-specific conditions and systemic disease states may each promote the development of the nephrotic syndrome. This chapter outlines basic themes surrounding the diagnosis and treatment of nephrotic syndrome. It is also important to distinguish nephrotic-range proteinuria from the nephrotic syndrome. In patients with nephrotic-range proteinuria, total urine protein exceeds 3.5 g/day but other manifestations such as hypoalbuminemia, edema, hyperlipidemia, and lipiduria may be absent.

Question: How Does Nephrotic-Range Proteinuria Occur?

Pathophysiology

The pathophysiological events of nephrotic syndrome are summarized in Fig. 4.1 [3]. Normally, small-molecular-weight proteins are filtered across the glomerular filtration barrier (GFB), enter the glomerular filtrate, and are subsequently removed from the filtrate via actions of the proximal tubular epithelium, thereby preventing the occurrence of proteinuria. Changes to one or more of the elements of the GFB may increase the rate of passage of humoral proteins into the filtrate. If the rate of passage across an abnormally functioning GFB is high enough, the reabsorptive capacity of the proximal tubule will be exceeded, and proteinuria will ensue. Diseases in which the GFB is abnormal demonstrate the shared histopathologic finding of effacement, or fusion, of the foot processes of the glomerular visceral epithelial cell, the podocyte, as depicted in Fig. 4.2 [4]. Additionally, in states of protein

L.F. Thomas, M.D. (✉) • H.A. Chakkera, M.D., M.P.H.
Nephrology and Hypertension, Mayo Clinic Arizona, 5777 E Mayo Blvd, Phoenix, AZ 85054, USA
e-mail: thomas.leslie@mayo.edu

E.V. Lerma and M. Rosner (eds.), *Clinical Decisions in Nephrology, Hypertension and Kidney Transplantation*, DOI 10.1007/978-1-4614-4454-1_4, © Springer Science+Business Media New York 2013

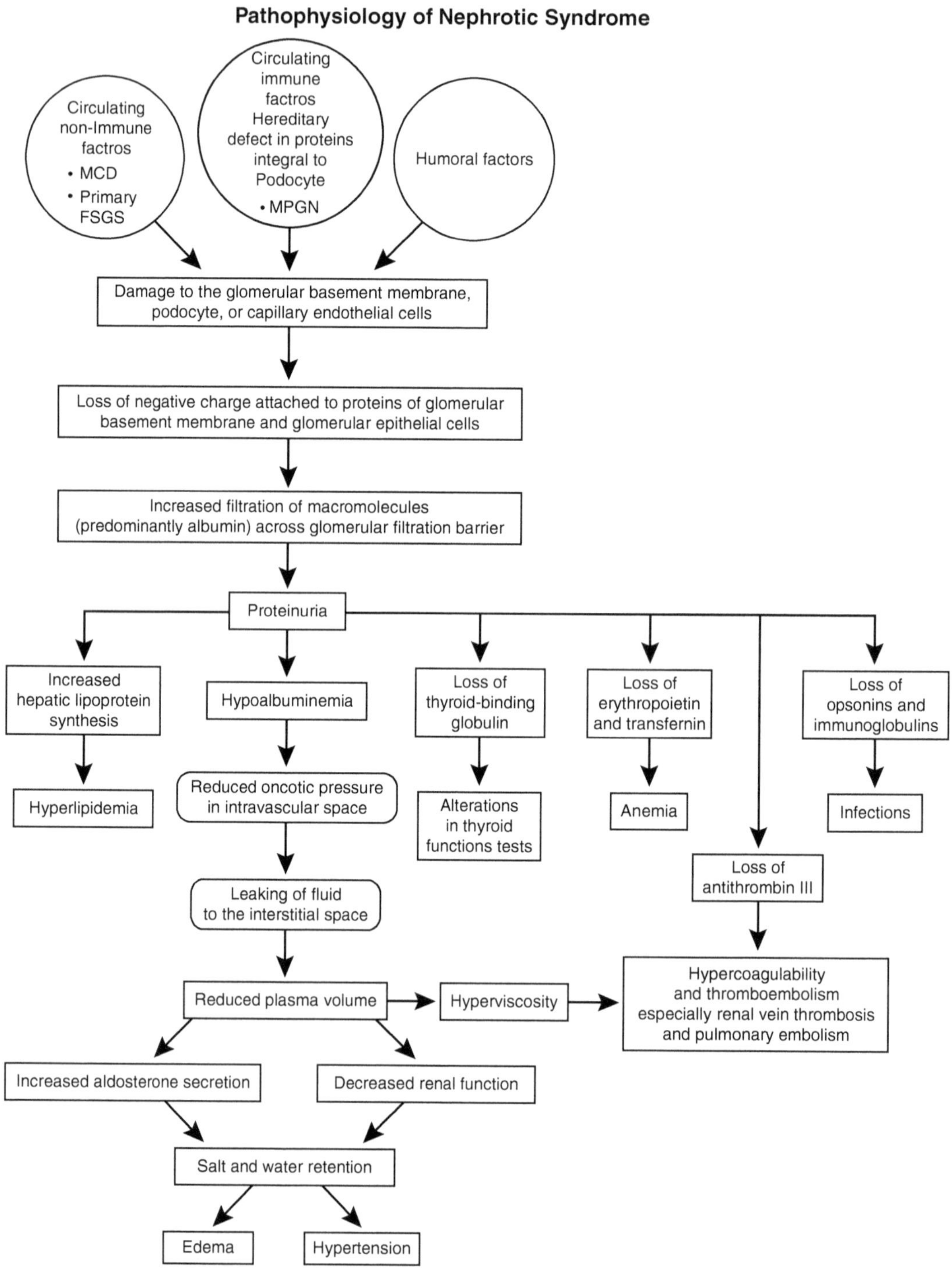

Fig. 4.1 Pathophysiology of nephrotic syndrome. Modified with permission from Macmillan Publishers Ltd [3], copyright 1988

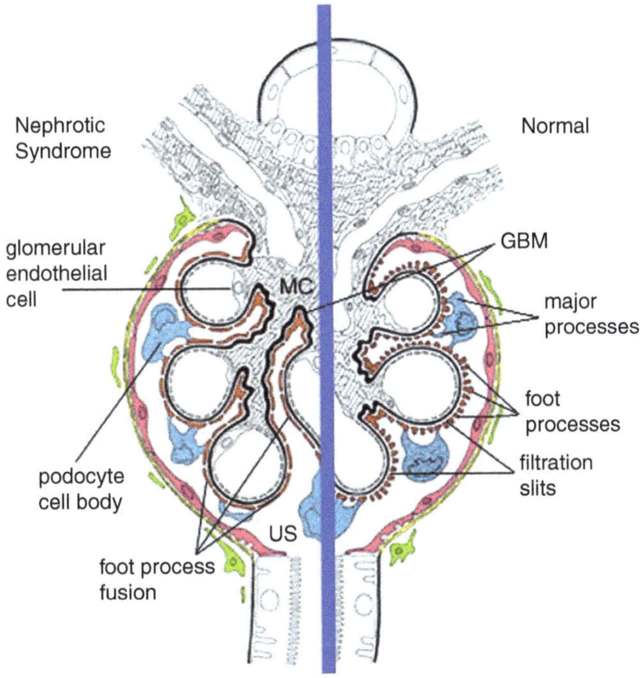

Fig. 4.2 Podocyte effacement and fusion in the nephrotic syndrome. The normal glomerular structure (*right*) includes loops of capillaries, composed of fenestrated endothelium, and surrounded by a basement membrane and podocytes and their foot processes. Glomerular changes seen in the nephrotic syndrome (*left*) include foot process effacement and fusion. *GBM* glomerular basement membrane, *MC* mesangial cells, *US* urine space. Reprinted by permission from Macmillan Publishers Ltd [4], copyright 2000

overproduction (e.g., multiple myeloma, amyloidosis, etc.) and in states associated with proximal tubular epithelial dysfunction (e.g., Fanconi syndrome), nephrotic-range proteinuria may occur without significant alteration to the GFB.

Question: What Is the Differential Diagnosis of Nephrotic Syndrome?

Nephrotic syndrome may result from both congenital and acquired conditions. In recent years, much progress has been made in the study of the components that comprise the GFB and of how specific alterations in the endothelial, basement membrane, and epithelial (podocyte) layers may contribute to the development of disease. Studying congenital diseases of the GFB has increased our understanding of these structural components. For example, congenital nephrotic syndrome (Finnish type) results from a defect in *NPHS1*, the gene coding for the protein nephrin, located at 19q13.1. Familial and sporadic steroid-resistant nephrotic syndrome occurs secondary to a defect in the *NPHS2* gene, located at 1q25-q31, which encodes the protein podocin. Neonatal nephrotic syndrome results from a mutation in the gene encoding CD2-associated protein. Common to the aforementioned congenital diseases resulting in nephrotic syndrome is an abnormality or absence of proteins that bridge the gap between foot processes, resulting in fusion of the foot processes. In addition to congenital disorders, which present soon after birth, genetic defects have also been found to associate with diseases that present later in life. Familial focal segmental glomerular sclerosis (FSGS) typically presents during or after the second decade of life with progressive proteinuria and may result from defects in genes encoding various proteins including α-actinin-4 and transient receptor potential cation 6 (TRPC6). Most recently, podocyte-secreted angiopoietin-like-4 was found to play a key role in steroid-sensitive minimal change disease (MCD).

In addition to inherited glomerular defects, nephrotic-range proteinuria can be seen with virtually any acquired glomerular disease. Early studies attempted to delineate the distribution of various disease states resulting in nephrotic syndrome [5, 6]. With the increase in prevalence of diabetes mellitus, the most common cause of nephrotic-range proteinuria worldwide is believed to be diabetic nephropathy although individuals presenting with slowly progressive proteinuria in the setting of a long-standing history of diabetes mellitus seldom undergo renal biopsy for confirmation. A multitude of systemic diseases other than diabetes mellitus may also promote the development of nephrotic syndrome, including systemic lupus erythematosus (SLE) and multiple myeloma. These conditions are discussed in detail in Section IX of this book. Among the primary renal diseases that may lead to nephrotic syndrome, MCD, primary FSGS, and membranous nephropathy (MN) are most commonly encountered. Other glomerular diseases that may also present with nephrotic syndrome include IgA nephropathy and membranoproliferative glomerulonephritis [7]. Table 4.1 describes the clinical and pathologic presentation of each of the more commonly encountered disorders.

MCD accounts for the vast majority of pediatric cases and a substantial minority of adult cases of nephrotic syndrome. Its name derives from the relatively normal appearance of the renal parenchyma by light microscopy, yet electron microscopy reveals diffuse podocyte effacement. As mentioned above, recent data implicates podocyte-secreted angiopoietin-like-4 in leading to loss of the GBM charge barrier as well as podocyte foot process effacement.

At present, FSGS is the most common cause of nephrotic syndrome and is also the most common primary glomerular disease leading to end-stage renal disease (ESRD) in the United States. The FSGS pattern of glomerular injury may develop from a variety of causes. Recently, the presence of high-risk alleles of myosin heavy chain 9 on chromosome 22 has been proposed to be a factor contributing to the higher propensity of African-American males to develop the disease [8]. Secondary FSGS occurs in the setting of glomerular hyperfiltration, as seen in obesity, hypertension, or previous glomerular injury related to another renal disorder. Interestingly, patients with the secondary form of FSGS may manifest nephrotic-range proteinuria in the absence of hypoalbuminemia or edema. Several distinct histological variants of FSGS have been described (classic, collapsing, tip, perihilar, and cellular) and may be associated with different clinical outcomes [9]. For example, individuals with tip variant lesions tend to have better renal function while those with the collapsing variant of FSGS are more resistant to therapy and have the worst renal prognosis [10].

MN differs from MCD and primary FSGS due to the presence of complement (C3) and IgG deposits within the glomerular basement membrane, demonstrated by immunofluorescence microscopy. MN can be either a primary disorder or secondary to a variety of other causes. A major step forward in the understanding of primary MN occurred with the recent discovery of an antigenic target, the phospholipase A2 receptor (PLA2R) [11]. Anti-PLA2R antibody is present in a substantial proportion of patients with primary MN and may represent a way to differentiate it from secondary MN. In addition, anti-PLA2R antibody titers decline as individuals with MN enter remission; thus, the anti-PLA2R antibody level may eventually be useful as a marker of disease activity.

Nephrotic syndrome may also develop in patients who have had a kidney transplant, as a result of recurrence of the primary renal disease, de novo glomerular disease, effects of immunosuppressive agents such as mTOR inhibitors (sirolimus, everolimus), and chronic allograft nephropathy [12–14]. Native kidney diseases more likely to recur within the allograft include diabetes mellitus, primary FSGS, MN, SLE, and amyloidosis. Recurrent primary FSGS is the most common clinically significant example of post-transplant nephrotic syndrome with an overall reported recurrence rate as high as 50% and may occur at any time after transplantation, from minutes to years [15]. Patients at the highest risk for recurrence include pediatric patients, those who presented with a rapid course initially, and those who have lost a prior allograft to recurrent FSGS. Unfortunately, the rate of graft loss within the first 5 years after recurrence of FSGS is high, ranging between 20 and 50% [16].

Table 4.1 Clinical features of disorders presenting with nephrotic syndrome

Congenital nephrosis	Nephrotic syndrome appears shortly after birth
	Abnormal nephrin in congenital nephrotic syndrome (Finnish type)
	Abnormal podocin in familial and sporadic steroid-resistant nephrotic syndrome
	Abnormal CD2-associated protein in neonatal nephrotic syndrome
Minimal change disease	Usually mild or benign case of nephrotic syndrome; onset may be rapid
	Spontaneous remission may occur; ESRD is uncommon
	Relapsing disease more common in adults than children
	Primary disease (majority of cases)
	Secondary disease can be associated with:
	Medications (lithium, NSAIDS)
	Hodgkin's disease and lymphoproliferative disorders
	HIV infection
	Heroin use
	Insect bites
Focal segmental glomerulosclerosis (FSGS)	*Primary disease*
	Sudden-onset nephrotic syndrome
	Prior history of kidney disease usually absent
	High incidence of recurrence post kidney transplant
	Pathology: Normal size glomeruli on LM, diffuse effacement of foot processes on EM
	Secondary disease
	Slowly progressive proteinuria with less severe edema
	Associated with obesity, reflux nephropathy, sickle cell disease, diabetes mellitus, pregnancy
	Pathology: Glomerular hypertrophy, foot processes not diffusely involved, and evidence of prior kidney injury often present
	Familial disease
	Progressive proteinuria during or after the second decade of life
	May result from defects in genes encoding various proteins including protein α actinin-4 and transient receptor potential cation 6 (TRPC6)
Membranous nephropathy	Presentation varies based on underlying disorder
	Primary disease
	Anti-PLA2R antibody may be present
	Secondary disease
	Rheumatologic disorders (systemic lupus erythematosus, Sjögren's syndrome, rheumatoid arthritis)
	Infections (hepatitis B and C, syphilis, parasitic infections)
	Solid organ malignancies
	Medications (gold, penicillamine, NSAIDS, hydralazine, hydrochlorothiazide, trimethadione)
	Pathology
	Thickened glomerular capillary basement membrane with "spike" pattern
	Diffuse granular capillary wall staining with antibodies to IgG and C3 on IF
	Subepithelial glomerular basement membrane deposits on EM

NSAIDS nonsteroidal anti-inflammatory drugs, *IF* immunofluorescence, *EM* electron microscopy

Question: What Are the Relationships Between Nephrotic-Range Proteinuria and the Other Cardinal Features of Nephrotic Syndrome?

Hypoalbuminemia

The hypoalbuminemia associated with nephrotic syndrome primarily occurs as a result of ongoing excessive urinary protein excretion. However, urinary losses of only a few grams of albumin per day do not completely explain the resultant decrease in serum albumin because hepatic albumin synthesis can easily surpass urinary losses in most situations [17]. Furthermore, the manifestation of nephrotic-range proteinuria does not universally associate with hypoalbuminemia, as can be seen with obesity-associated FSGS in which the serum albumin is usually normal [18, 19]. These findings highlight our incomplete understanding of the process by which hypoalbuminemia develops.

Edema

Factors influencing the development of edema in patients with nephrotic syndrome are also not fully elucidated. Classical teaching suggests that hypoalbuminemia results in decreased oncotic pressure with associated alterations in transcapillary pressure gradients, thus favoring the passage of water into the interstitial space. Decreased oncotic pressure would potentially also contribute to a decrease in the effective circulating volume with subsequent activation of the renin angiotensin aldosterone system (RAAS) and enhanced renal sodium avidity. However, while decreased oncotic pressure may be an important component of edema formation in nephrotic syndrome, independent renal sodium avidity also plays an important role.

Hyperlipidemia

Similarly, the causal link between nephrotic-range proteinuria and the advent of dyslipidemia is not completely understood. Part of our current understanding derives from the repeated observation that apoB100-containing lipoproteins (VLDL, IDL, and LDL) undergo increased production and decreased catabolism by the liver. In sum, the serum concentrations of plasma triglycerides, VLDL, IDL, LDL, and Lp(a), increase while the concentration of HDL may not change significantly [20].

Question: What Are the Specific Tests You Would Order to Help Establish a Diagnosis?

Investigations

The investigational approach to nephrotic syndrome includes establishing the diagnosis of nephrotic syndrome, determining the degree of renal insufficiency, obtaining a pathologic diagnosis, and ascertaining whether a secondary etiology exists. In the patient described above, the diagnosis of nephrotic syndrome is confirmed by the presence of edema on exam and by the demonstration of hypoalbuminemia, hyperlipidemia, and nephrotic-range proteinuria in a 24-h urine collection. Of note, a spot urine protein-to-creatinine ratio in an early morning sample can also be utilized to quantitate the degree of proteinuria. The degree of renal insufficiency is assessed by measuring or estimating the glomerular filtration rate (GFR). Multiple methods for determining or estimating GFR exist and include iothalamate clearance, 24-h urine creatinine clearance, and various estimating equations [21, 22]. An evaluation for secondary causes includes searching for underlying infections, metabolic disorders, and malignancy. Commonly ordered diagnostic tests are listed in Table 4.2.

Question: How Is Nephrotic Syndrome Treated?

Management

The approach to management of nephrotic syndrome is twofold: therapy aimed at managing the proteinuria, edema, dyslipidemia, and other com-

Table 4.2 Diagnostic evaluation of nephrotic syndrome

Patient history
• Medication or toxin exposure
• Pregnancy
• Risk factors for human immunodeficiency virus (HIV) or viral hepatitis
• History of diabetes, systemic lupus erythematosus, or other systemic illness
• Signs and symptoms suggestive of malignancy
Laboratory tests
Urine
• Urinalysis
• Urine spot protein/creatinine ratio, confirm with 24-h urine protein collection
• Urine protein electrophoresis and immunofixation
Serum
• Complete blood count, electrolytes, glucose, lipid profile, liver tests, albumin
• Cryoglobulins
• Hepatitis B and C viral serologies
• HIV serology
• Syphilis antibody
• Antinuclear antibody, rheumatoid factor, complement levels (C_3, C_4, CH_{50})
• Thyroid-stimulating hormone
• Serum immunofixation, serum free light chains
Renal Biopsy—confirmatory diagnostic test

plications of nephrotic syndrome and therapy tailored to an individual's underlying disease process.

Proteinuria. Control of hypertension is critical to reduce proteinuria, and antihypertensive agents from multiple classes are employed. In particular, angiotensin converting enzyme (ACE) inhibitors and angiotensin II receptor blockers (ARBs) are used to reduce urinary protein excretion via relatively increased efferent arteriole dilatation and decreased intraglomerular pressure. Addition of an aldosterone receptor antagonist may further reduce proteinuria [23]. These medications are generally started at low doses and titrated up as tolerated, with the goal of reducing proteinuria as much as possible. Although they are generally considered to be safe, well tolerated, and effective, increasing doses or combining drugs from more than one of the above categories raises the risk of complications from therapy [24]. Common adverse effects include hyperkalemia and decreased GFR, and serum creatinine and potassium levels should be checked within 1–2 weeks of initiating or titrating these medications. Typically, a decrease in GFR of up to 30% may be tolerated and should not necessarily lead to dose reduction or medication discontinuation.

Edema. Successful treatment of edema in nephrotic syndrome includes strict adherence to a low sodium diet (<2 g/day) along with diuretic therapy. Diuresis is generally best accomplished with loop diuretic therapy. Twice-daily dosing of short-acting loop diuretics (furosemide, bumetanide) is essential to facilitate a net negative sodium and volume balance over a 24-h period. Thiazide-type diuretics (metolazone), which act in the distal convoluted tubule, may also be employed for further sequential blockade of sodium reabsorption in the distal nephron. Aldosterone antagonists (spironolactone, eplerenone) can be added if diuresis is not adequate with blockade of more proximal nephron segments. Salt-poor albumin solutions may be infused intravenously, and some data suggest that the combination of albumin and furosemide may be more effective at promoting a diuresis than furosemide alone [25]. However, this process is both cumbersome and expensive and should not be employed in routine cases. A rapid reduction in volume balance is not recommended, as this may promote intravascular volume depletion, hypotension, and worsening renal function. Also, hypokalemia and hypomagnesemia can occur with diuretic use; frequent laboratory monitoring is warranted.

Hyperlipidemia. Multiple types of lipid alterations have been described in patients with nephrotic syndrome, and HMG-CoA reductase inhibition ameliorates the dyslipidemias associated with nephrotic syndrome [20, 26, 27]. Therefore, unless a contraindication exists, treatment with an HMG-CoA reductase inhibitor (statin) is recommended for all patients with nephrotic syndrome.

Disease-specific management varies and depends upon the underlying process. For primary glomerular diseases such as MCD, FSGS, and MN, induction and maintenance therapy with immunosuppressive agents is commonly employed. Corticosteroids, azathioprine, chlorambucil, cyclophosphamide, and cyclosporine have classically been used, and newer agents such as tacrolimus, mycophenolate mofetil, and rituximab have also shown promise [28]. Due to potential long-term side effects and toxicity of these medications, their use should be directed by experienced nephrologists and reserved for patients for whom close follow-up is possible.

Outcomes

The long-term prognosis for patients with nephrotic syndrome is disease specific and even may differ for patients with the same pathologic diagnosis. In general, adverse prognostic factors include male sex, uncontrolled hypertension, a more severe degree of proteinuria, and decrease in renal function at presentation.

MCD is the most treatable cause of idiopathic nephrotic syndrome, and spontaneous remission may occur. However, relapses are common, and a small percentage of individuals with MCD are resistant to treatment. In contrast, spontaneous remission is less common in patients with primary FSGS, in whom the risk of progression to ESRD is highest. Primary MN has a better prognosis than primary FSGS. In general, approximately one-third of patients will undergo spontaneous complete or partial remission, and one-third will progress to ESRD [29, 30]. A thorough search for secondary causes of these disorders, as outlined in Table 4.2, should be conducted since outcomes depend on appropriate treatment of a secondary cause, if present.

Key Points

Nephrotic syndrome is characterized by proteinuria exceeding 3.5 g/1.73 m^2/day, hypoalbuminemia, edema, hyperlipidemia, and lipiduria.

Proteinuria in nephrotic syndrome occurs primarily as a result of alterations to the glomerular filtration barrier. In addition, non-glomerular processes including systemic protein overproduction and proximal tubular dysfunction may also contribute to nephrotic-range proteinuria.

The differential diagnosis of nephrotic syndrome includes primary renal disorders such as MCD, primary FSGS, and MN, as well as renal disorders arising from systemic disease, the most common of which is diabetic nephropathy.

ACE inhibitors, ARBs, diuretics, and statins are the mainstays of nonspecific therapy aimed at the management of proteinuria, edema, and hyperlipidemia associated with nephrotic syndrome.

Disease-specific therapy varies based on the underlying process and may include the use of immunosuppressive agents to treat primary glomerular diseases.

References

1. Orth SR, Ritz E. The nephrotic syndrome. N Engl J Med. 1998;338(17):1202–11.
2. Hull RP, Goldsmith DJ. Nephrotic syndrome in adults. BMJ. 2008;336(7654):1185–9.
3. Bernard DB. Extrarenal complications of the nephrotic syndrome. Kidney Int. 1988;33(6):1184–202.
4. Somlo S, Mundel P. Getting a foothold in nephrotic syndrome. Nat Genet. 2000;24(4):333–5.
5. Korbet SM, Genchi RM, Borok RZ, Schwartz MM. The racial prevalence of glomerular lesions in nephrotic adults. Am J Kidney Dis. 1996;27(5):647–51.
6. Haas M, Meehan SM, Karrison TG, Spargo BH. Changing etiologies of unexplained adult nephrotic syndrome: a comparison of renal biopsy findings from 1976–1979 and 1995–1997. Am J Kidney Dis. 1997;30(5):621–31.
7. Swaminathan S, Leung N, Lager DJ, et al. Changing incidence of glomerular disease in Olmsted County, Minnesota: a 30-year renal biopsy study. Clin J Am Soc Nephrol. 2006;1(3):483–7.
8. Kopp JB, Smith MW, Nelson GW, et al. MYH9 is a major-effect risk gene for focal segmental glomerulosclerosis. Nat Genet. 2008;40(10):1175–84.
9. D'Agati V. Pathologic classification of focal segmental glomerulosclerosis. Semin Nephrol. 2003;23(2):117–34.
10. Thomas DB, Franceschini N, Hogan SL, et al. Clinical and pathologic characteristics of focal segmental glomerulosclerosis pathologic variants. Kidney Int. 2006;69(5):920–6.
11. Beck Jr LH, Bonegio RG, Lambeau G, et al. M-type phospholipase A2 receptor as target antigen in idiopathic membranous nephropathy. N Engl J Med. 2009;361(1):11–21.
12. Padiyar A, Bodziak KA, Hricik DE, Augustine JJ. Clinical predictors of proteinuria after conversion to sirolimus in kidney transplant recipients. Am J Transplant. 2010;10(2):310–4.
13. Sirolimus and proteinuria in renal transplant patients: evidence for a dose-dependent effect on slit

diaphragm-associated proteins. Stallone G, Infante B, Pontrelli P, Gigante M, Montemurno E, Loverre A, Rossini M, Schena FP, Grandaliano G, Gesualdo L. Transplantation. 2011 May 15;91(9):997–1004.
14. Loriga G, Ciccarese M, Pala PG, et al. De novo everolimus-based therapy in renal transplant recipients: effect on proteinuria and renal prognosis. Transplant Proc. 2010;42(4):1297–302.
15. Hariharan S, Adams MB, Brennan DC, et al. Recurrent and de novo glomerular disease after renal transplantation: a report from Renal Allograft Disease Registry (RADR). Transplantation. 1999;68(5):635–41.
16. Vinai M, Waber P, Seikaly MG. Recurrence of focal segmental glomerulosclerosis in renal allograft: an in-depth review. Pediatr Transplant. 2010;14(3): 314–25.
17. Ballmer PE, Weber BK, Roy-Chaudhury P, et al. Elevation of albumin synthesis rates in nephrotic patients measured with [1–13C]leucine. Kidney Int. 1992;41(1):132–8.
18. Praga M, Borstein B, Andres A, et al. Nephrotic proteinuria without hypoalbuminemia: clinical characteristics and response to angiotensin-converting enzyme inhibition. Am J Kidney Dis. 1991;17(3):330–8.
19. Praga M, Hernandez E, Morales E, et al. Clinical features and long-term outcome of obesity-associated focal segmental glomerulosclerosis. Nephrol Dial Transplant. 2001;16(9):1790–8.
20. Marsh JB. Lipoprotein metabolism in the nephrotic syndrome. Front Biosci. 2002;7:e326–38.
21. Stevens LA, Coresh J, Greene T, Levey AS. Assessing kidney function—measured and estimated glomerular filtration rate. N Engl J Med. 2006;354(23):2473–83.
22. Levey AS, Stevens LA, Schmid CH, et al. A new equation to estimate glomerular filtration rate. Ann Intern Med. 2009;150(9):604–12.
23. Bomback AS, Kshirsagar AV, Amamoo MA, Klemmer PJ. Change in proteinuria after adding aldosterone blockers to ACE inhibitors or angiotensin receptor blockers in CKD: a systematic review. Am J Kidney Dis. 2008;51(2):199–211.
24. Mann JF, Schmieder RE, McQueen M, et al. Renal outcomes with telmisartan, ramipril, or both, in people at high vascular risk (the ONTARGET study): a multicentre, randomised, double-blind, controlled trial. Lancet. 2008;372(9638):547–53.
25. Dharmaraj R, Hari P, Bagga A. Randomized cross-over trial comparing albumin and frusemide infusions in nephrotic syndrome. Pediatr Nephrol. 2009;24(4):775–82.
26. Vaziri ND, Liang K. Effects of HMG-CoA reductase inhibition on hepatic expression of key cholesterol-regulatory enzymes and receptors in nephrotic syndrome. Am J Nephrol. 2004;24(6):606–13.
27. Olbricht CJ, Wanner C, Thiery J, Basten A. Simvastatin in nephrotic syndrome. Simvastatin in Nephrotic Syndrome Study Group. Kidney Int Suppl. 1999;71:S113–6.
28. Appel GB, Waldman M, Radhakrishnan J. New approaches to the treatment of glomerular diseases. Kidney Int. 2006;70(S104):S45–50.
29. Polanco N, Gutierrez E, Covarsi A, et al. Spontaneous remission of nephrotic syndrome in idiopathic membranous nephropathy. J Am Soc Nephrol. 2010;21(4): 697–704.
30. Fervenza FC, Sethi S, Specks U. Idiopathic membranous nephropathy: diagnosis and treatment. Clin J Am Soc Nephrol. 2008;3(3):905–19.

Approach to the Patient with Hematuria

5

Vishal N. Ratkalkar and Kevin R. Regner

Case 1

An 83-year-old man presents with painless gross hematuria. The patient's history is notable for a 50 pack-year history of smoking. He is afebrile with a blood pressure of 128/64. Physical examination is notable for an enlarged prostate but shows no rash, edema, or abnormal abdominal findings. Serum creatinine is within normal limits. A dipstick urinalysis shows 3+ blood and trace proteinuria.

Case 2

A 38-year-old woman presents with new-onset lower extremity edema. One month ago, she was seen by her primary care physician with complaints of headache and fatigue. A dipstick urinalysis showed 2+ blood, and she was treated for a urinary tract infection. She subsequently developed new-onset lower extremity edema 1 week ago. On examination, she is afebrile with a blood pressure of 164/102. There is 2+ pretibial edema but no rash or abnormal abdominal findings. Her serum creatinine is 1.56 mg/dl. A dipstick urinalysis shows 3+ blood and 2+ protein.

V.N. Ratkalkar, M.D. • K.R. Regner, M.D. (✉)
Department of Medicine (Nephrology), Medical College of Wisconsin, 8701 Watertown Plank Road, Milwaukee, WI 53226, USA
e-mail: kregner@mcw.edu

Introduction

Hematuria is a common sign of genitourinary disease involving the kidneys, ureters, bladder, prostate, or urethra (Table 5.1). Patients can present with either "gross" hematuria that is visible to the naked eye or with hematuria detectable only under microscopic examination or by urinary dipstick analysis. Notably, 1 ml of blood/l of urine is sufficient to produce gross hematuria. In most cases, gross hematuria is an indication for a detailed diagnostic evaluation. Microscopic hematuria has been defined as ≥3 red blood cells (RBCs) per high power field (HPF) upon examination of the urinary sediment from 2 of 3 properly collected and centrifuged urine specimens [1]. In contrast to gross hematuria, the approach to asymptomatic microscopic hematuria remains controversial. However, the diagnostic approach to both types of hematuria requires consideration of both benign and malignant processes involving the kidneys and urinary tract.

The prevalence of hematuria is variable and depends upon the characteristics of the patients screened and whether hematuria is detected by dipstick or by urine microscopy. Therefore, estimates of the prevalence of hematuria in adults range from 0.19 to 16.1% [1, 2]. In patients selected for referral to a hematuria clinic, the underlying etiology for hematuria could not be established in up to 60% of patients [3]. Urinary tract infection (13%), bladder cancer (11.9%), urolithiasis (3.6%), renal cancer (0.6%), prostate

E.V. Lerma and M. Rosner (eds.), *Clinical Decisions in Nephrology, Hypertension and Kidney Transplantation*, DOI 10.1007/978-1-4614-4454-1_5,

Table 5.1 Causes of hematuria

Non-glomerular hematuria
Malignancy
Bladder cancer
Prostate cancer
Transitional cell carcinoma
Renal cell carcinoma
Urinary tract infection
Urolithiasis
Glomerular hematuria
Glomerulonephritis (GN)
IgA nephropathy
Post-infectious GN
Membranoproliferative GN
Lupus nephritis
Necrotizing crescentic GN
Hereditary glomerular disease
Thin basement membrane nephropathy
Alport's Syndrome

cancer (0.4%), and urothelial cancer (0.1%) were the underlying urologic causes of hematuria in the remainder of cases. Renal parenchymal disease was identified in approximately 10% of cases [3]. The incidence of bladder cancer was four times higher in the setting of gross hematuria in comparison to microscopic hematuria. The American Urological Association Best Practice Policy outlined the following factors as high risk for urological malignancy in patients with hematuria: age >40 years; history of smoking; occupational exposure to chemicals or dyes (aromatic amines, benzenes); gross hematuria; history of urological disease, irritative voiding symptoms, or urinary tract infection; analgesic abuse; and prior pelvic irradiation [4]. Obviously, those patients falling into high-risk subsets would require a more aggressive diagnostic approach to exclude malignancy as the cause.

Renal parenchymal causes of hematuria include glomerulonephritis (GN) and hereditary glomerular disease (Table 5.1). Glomerulonephritis can be primary (no clear associated etiology) or secondary to a number of systemic diseases. The most common causes of GN presenting with hematuria include IgA nephropathy, necrotizing crescentic GN, lupus nephritis, post-infectious GN, and membranoproliferative GN [5]. Hereditary glomerular diseases include Alport's syndrome and thin basement membrane nephropathy (TBMN). Alport's syndrome is most commonly due to an X-linked mutation in the *COL4A5* gene resulting in defective α5 chains of type IV collagen and subsequent alterations in the glomerular basement membrane [6]. Autosomal recessive and autosomal dominant Alport's syndrome occur less frequently. Both types of autosomal Alport's syndrome can be due to mutations in either the *COL4A3* or the *COL4A4* gene which produce defects in the α3 or α4 chains of type IV collagen. Hematuria and sensorineural hearing loss are common presenting signs of Alport's syndrome [6]. TBMN is typically transmitted in an autosomal dominant pattern and presents with isolated hematuria [7].

Case 1

In this case, the patient's age and history of cigarette smoking increase his risk for urologic malignancy. He has no signs or symptoms of a urinary tract infection or urolithiasis. There was no family history of hematuria or kidney disease. The absence of hypertension and renal dysfunction decreases the likelihood of an underlying renal parenchymal disease. Taken together, these findings should raise concern that malignancy is the most likely cause for hematuria. It is important to look at the urine under microscopy. The absence of dysmorphic red blood cells or red blood cell casts increases the likelihood that the hematuria is not secondary to GN. Furthermore, the absence of significant proteinuria also argues against a glomerular source for the proteinuria.

Case 2

The patient in this case is <40 years old and has no significant risk factors for urologic malignancy and no current symptoms to suggest urinary tract infection or urolithiasis. Renal parenchymal disease should be strongly considered, especially in the context of hypertension, proteinuria, and elevated serum creatinine. Once again, the presence of dysmorphic red blood cells or red blood cell casts would argue that the source is the glomerulus in this case. There was no family history of hematuria or renal failure to suggest a hereditary glomerular disease. Therefore, glomerulonephritis should be strongly suspected.

Diagnostic Approach

Initial Evaluation

The initial approach to hematuria involves a stepwise evaluation to confirm the presence of hematuria and to ascertain the most likely source of urinary tract bleeding (Fig. 5.1). First, a complete history and physical examination should be performed in all patients. Historical elements of particular importance include recent unintentional weight loss, fever, dysuria, flank or abdominal pain, hearing loss, or skin rash. The family history should be reviewed for documentation of Alport's syndrome, TBMN, nephrolithiasis, polycystic kidney disease, or hematuria of undetermined etiology. Medications should be reviewed with particular attention to recent use of anticoagulants, aspirin, or nonsteroidal anti-inflammatory drugs (NSAIDS). Notable physical findings include costovertebral angle tenderness radiating to the groin in patients with nephrolithiasis, sensorineural hearing loss in Alport's syndrome, flank masses in renal cancer, organomegaly in polycystic kidney disease, and palpable purpura in some types of glomerulonephritis.

Hematuria is often initially detected by dipstick urinalysis. Dipstick reagent strips detect the heme peroxidase activity of RBC hemoglobin, free hemoglobin, and myoglobin. The sensitivity and specificity of dipstick tests for the detection of ≥5 RBCs/HPF range from 86 to 100% and 64

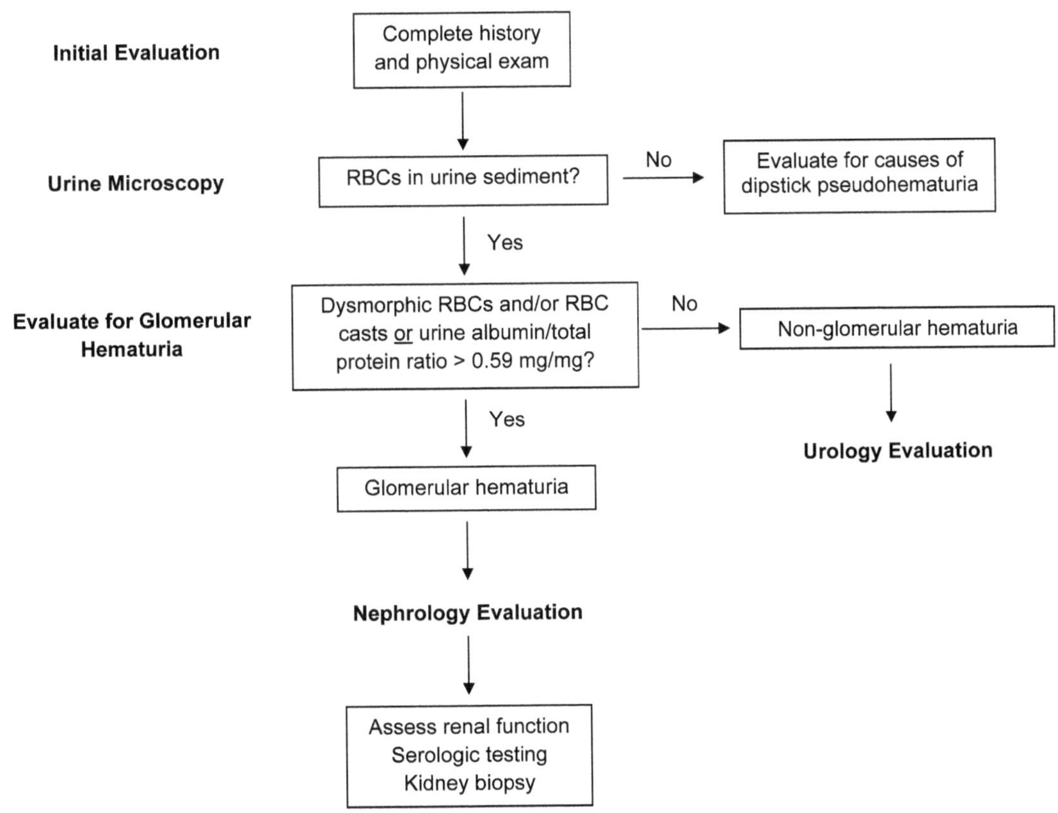

Fig. 5.1 Initial evaluation of hematuria

to 94%, respectively [8]. However, dipstick tests for hematuria should be interpreted with caution as a variety of factors can produce false positive and false negative results. Dipstick pseudohematuria is defined as a positive dipstick result for hematuria without the presence of RBCs on urine microscopy [10]. Myoglobin and free hemoglobin in the urine can both result in a pseudohematuria and require additional evaluation in the appropriate clinical contexts. Vigorous exercise and highly concentrated urine can also lead to pseudohematuria. In these cases, repeat testing after resting or hydration is indicated. Very dilute (specific gravity <1.007) urine can cause RBC lysis giving rise to false negative urine microscopy [1, 10]. Therefore, careful interpretation of the dipstick and microscopic urinalyses requires consideration of patient factors, urine specific gravity, and urine pH. In all cases, it is critical to view the urine sediment under the microscope.

Urine Microscopy

Microscopic examination of the urine is performed to confirm the presence of RBCs in the urine and to determine the anatomical origin of the RBCs [1, 10]. A clean-catch midstream urine sample is collected, and 10 ml of urine is spun in a conical centrifuge tube for 5 min at 2,000 rpm. After centrifugation, the tube is inverted and cleared of the supernatant fluid and the pellet is carefully resuspended without excessive agitation. A drop of this specimen is placed onto a microscope slide with a pipette and should be sufficient in size such that the coverslip floats on the specimen. The urine sediment should then be examined under low-power magnification prior to moving on to high-power examination of individual fields. The presence of ≥3 RBCs/HPF is considered pathological [1].

Evaluate for Glomerular Hematuria

Urine RBC morphology can help distinguish glomerular causes of hematuria from non-glomerular causes. Non-glomerular hematuria is characterized by normal-appearing RBCs on urine microscopy. In contrast, glomerular hematuria is defined by the presence of dysmorphic RBCs and/or RBC casts. Urine RBC casts are pathognomonic of glomerulonephritis. Dysmorphic RBCs are differentiated from normal RBCs by the presence of cellular blebs or spicules. Greater than 80% dysmorphic RBCs has been shown to have high specificity but low sensitivity for glomerular disease [8]. Therefore, this cutoff value is most useful for ruling in a glomerular source of hematuria.

Urine microscopy is operator dependent and not always readily available. Therefore, the urine albumin-to-total protein ratio has been proposed as a novel method of differentiating glomerular from non-glomerular hematuria. A urine albumin-to-total protein ratio of >0.59 mg albumin/mg total protein was shown to be highly sensitive and specific for glomerular bleeding compared with phase contrast microscopy of the urinary sediment [11]. Of note, this test is not useful in patients with a urine total protein concentration of <5 mg/dl. Other laboratory findings that are suggestive of a glomerular cause for hematuria include proteinuria (>300 mg/g creatinine) and/or elevated serum creatinine.

Nephrology Evaluation

Patients with glomerular hematuria, as determined by the presence of RBC casts or dysmorphic RBCs on microscopic urinalysis or elevated urine albumin-to-total protein ratio, should be referred to a nephrologist. Renal function should be assessed by measurement of serum creatinine and proteinuria quantified by 24-h urine collection or spot urine protein-to-creatinine ratio. Laboratory testing for lupus (antinuclear antibody, anti-double-stranded DNA antibodies, and serum complement C3 and C4), post-infectious GN (blood cultures, anti-streptolysin O titer, and serum C3 complement), small vessel vasculitis (anti-neutrophil cytoplasmic antibodies and antibodies to proteinase 3 and to myeloperoxidase), viral infections (serologic testing for hepatitis B and C viruses and human immunodeficiency virus), and Goodpasture's syndrome (anti-glomerular basement membrane antibody) may assist in the diagnosis of GN. Patients with acute kidney injury in the setting of suspected GN should be emergently evaluated for rapidly progressive glomerulonephritis (see Chap. 6). Ultimately, a kidney biopsy may be necessary to establish the diagnosis in cases of glomerular hematuria.

Kidney biopsies are typically performed by percutaneous approach under the guidance of real-time ultrasound [12]. The lower pole of the kidney is identified, and a 14–16-gauge biopsy needle is used to obtain 2–3 cores of tissue from the renal cortex and the tissue is examined with an operating microscope to confirm the presence of glomeruli. The specimens are then evaluated by a renal pathologist after staining and preparation for light, immunofluorescence, and electron microscopy. Common complications of kidney biopsy include perinephric hematoma formation (2.1%) and transient gross hematuria (3.1%). Major complications such as arteriovenous fistula formation and bleeding requiring invasive intervention occur in <1% of native kidney biopsies [12].

Urology Evaluation

Patients with gross hematuria or persistent non-glomerular microscopic hematuria should be referred for urological evaluation (Fig. 5.2) [1]. A urine culture should be performed on a clean-catch midstream urine sample. If the urine culture is positive the patient should be treated with the appropriate antibiotics. A repeat urinalysis should then be performed to confirm resolution of the hematuria. In high-risk patients or patients with persistent hematuria, further examination of the urinary tract is warranted. Low-risk patients should first undergo radiologic imaging of the upper urinary tract followed by urine cytology and cystoscopy depending on the patient's age and risk factors for malignancy [4]. The American Urological Association has recommended cystoscopy for evaluation of hematuria in all patients over the age of 40 and in patients <40 years old with risk factors for bladder cancer [4]. High-risk patients should be referred for complete evaluation of the urinary tract including upper tract radiologic imaging, urine cytology, and cystoscopy (Fig. 5.2) [4].

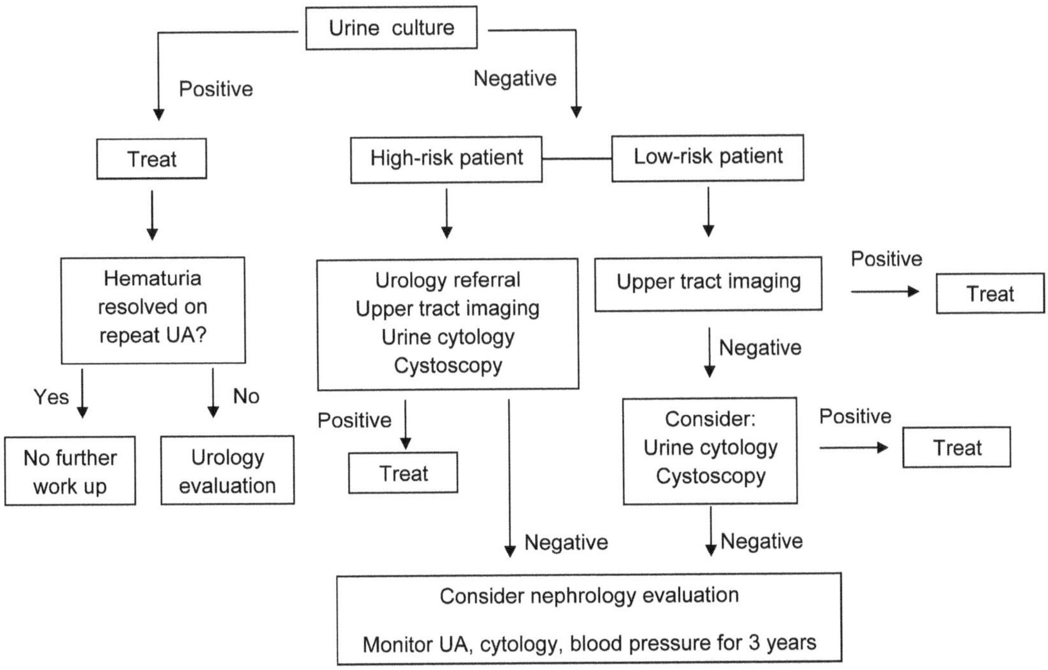

Fig. 5.2 Evaluation of gross hematuria or persistent non-glomerular microscopic hematuria

Radiologic imaging of the urinary tract is most useful for detecting urolithiasis, cysts, and tumors of the kidney and ureters. Cystoscopy is the preferred method for detection of bladder cancer [4]. Radiologic techniques for urinary tract imaging include intravenous urography (IVU), ultrasound (US), computed tomography (CT), and magnetic resonance imaging (MRI) [8]. Each of these modalities has unique advantages and disadvantages which need to be accounted for based on patient factors, local expertise, and clinical context. The major disadvantage of IVU is its inability to differentiate cystic lesions from solid masses; therefore, an indeterminate mass detected on IVU requires additional radiologic follow-up [4, 8]. US is less costly than IVU and is useful in the characterization of renal cysts but is less sensitive for solid lesions <3 cm [4, 8]. CT detects renal cysts and solid masses and is also useful for detection of urolithiasis and intra-abdominal pathology outside of the urinary tract [4, 8]. MRI can characterize small renal masses and differentiate solid from cystic masses and is advantageous when exposure to radiation and iodinated contrast is contraindicated [8, 9].

Case 1

Microscopic examination of the patient's urine showed >100 RBCs/HPF. No dysmorphic RBCs or RBC casts were found. He had no significant proteinuria. These findings were consistent with a nonglomerular cause for hematuria. The patient was referred to a urologist and underwent a CT scan of the abdomen and pelvis which revealed an irregular bladder mass. A cystoscopy was performed which showed a 3 cm lesion over the posterior bladder wall. Biopsy of this lesion confirmed the diagnosis of high-grade invasive urothelial carcinoma.

Case 2

In this case, the patient was found to have a urine protein excretion of 1.3 g/day. Microscopic examination of the patient's urine showed 26–50 RBCs/HPF with >80% dysmorphic RBCs and numerous RBC casts. These findings, in the setting of concurrent renal dysfunction, were strongly suggestive of a glomerular cause for hematuria. The patient was referred to a nephrologist for further evaluation. At that time, serologic testing was notable for an elevated anti-streptolysin O titer and markedly decreased serum C3 concentration. A renal biopsy was performed which demonstrated a proliferative glomerulonephritis with diffuse endocapillary proliferation on light microscopy and glomerular deposition of IgG and C3 on immunofluorescence microscopy consistent with a final diagnosis of post-streptococcal GN.

Prognosis

The prognosis of hematuria depends upon the underlying cause. However, a large proportion of patients with hematuria have no readily identifiable cause despite an extensive urologic and renal evaluation. Urologic malignancy develops rarely (<1%) in this situation [13]. However, the American Urological Association recommendations state that such patients be followed closely for 3 years with serial urinalysis, urine cytology, and screening for hypertension, proteinuria, and renal dysfunction [4]. Indications for reevaluation include positive urine cytology, gross hematuria, new-onset hypertension, proteinuria, or renal dysfunction.

Key Points

1. Hematuria is a sign of a number of benign and malignant disorders involving the kidneys or the urinary tract.
2. Patients with gross hematuria should undergo complete urologic evaluation. The approach to microscopic hematuria requires a stepwise evaluation of the kidneys and urinary tract.
3. Urine microscopy should be performed to confirm the presence of urine RBCs in patients with dipstick hematuria.
4. Patients with RBC casts or dysmorphic RBCs on urine microscopy should be evaluated for glomerular causes of hematuria. An elevated

urine albumin/total protein ratio in the setting of hematuria is also suggestive of glomerular hematuria.

5. Patients with non-glomerular hematuria should undergo a urologic evaluation which may include radiologic imaging of the upper urinary tract, urine cytology, and cystoscopy.

References

1. Grossfeld GD, Litwin MS, Wolf JS, Hricak H, Shuler CL, Agerter DC, Carroll PR. Evaluation of asymptomatic microscopic hematuria in adults: the American Urological Association best practice policy. Part I: Definition, detection, prevalence, and etiology. Urology. 2001;57:599–603.
2. Woolhandler S, Pels RJ, Bor DH, Himmelstein DU, Lawrence RS. Dipstick urinalysis screening of asymptomatic adults for urinary tract disorders: I. Hematuria and proteinuria. J Am Med Assoc. 1989;262:1214–9.
3. Khadra MH, Pickard RS, Charlton M, Powell PH, Neal DE. A prospective analysis of 1,930 patients with hematuria to evaluate current diagnostic practice. J Urol. 2000;163:524–7.
4. Grossfeld GD, Litwin MS, Wolf JS, Hricak H, Shuler CL, Agerter DC, Carroll PR. Evaluation of asymptomatic microscopic hematuria in adults: the American Urological Association best practice policy. Part II: Patient evaluation, cytology, voided markers, imaging, cystoscopy, nephrology evaluation, and follow-up. Urology. 2001;57:605–10.
5. Swaminathan S, Leung N, Lager DJ, Melton 3rd LJ, Bergstralh EJ, Rohlinger A, Fervenza FC. Changing incidence of glomerular disease in Olmsted County, Minnesota: a 30-year renal biopsy study. Clin J Am Soc Nephrol. 2006;1:483–74.
6. Heidet L, Gubler M. The renal lesions of Alport syndrome. J Am Soc Nephrol. 2009;20:1210–5.
7. Tryggvason K, Patrakka J. Thin basement membrane nephropathy. J Am Soc Nephrol. 2006;17:813–22.
8. Rodgers M, Nixon J, Hempel S, Aho T, Kelly J, Neal D, Duffy S, Kleijnen J, Westwood M. Diagnostic tests & algorithms used in the investigation of haematuria: systematic reviews & economic evaluation. Health Technol Assess. 2006;10:1–276.
9. O'Donoghue PM, McSweeney SE, Jhaveri K. Genitourinary imaging: current and emerging applications. J Postgrad Med. 2010;56:131–9.
10. Rao PK, Jones JS. How to evaluate 'dipstick hematuria': what to do before you refer. Cleve Clin J Med. 2008;75:227–33.
11. Ohisa N, Yoshida K, Matsuki R, Suzuki H, Miura H, Ohisa Y, Murayama N, Kaku M, Sato H. Comparison of urinary albumin—total protein ratio to phase-contrast microscopic examination of urine sediment for differentiating glomerular and nonglomerular bleeding. Am J Kidney Dis. 2008;52:235–41.
12. Whittier WL, Korbet SM. Timing of complications in percutaneous renal biopsy. J Am Soc Nephrol. 2004;15:142–7.
13. Madeb R, Golijanin D, Knopf J, Davis M, Feng C, Fender A, Stephenson L, Messing EM. Long-term outcome of patients with a negative work-up for asymptomatic microhematuria. Urology. 2010;75:20–5.

Suggested Reading

Grossfeld GD, Litwin MS, Wolf JS, Hricak H, Shuler CL, Agerter DC, Carroll PR. Evaluation of asymptomatic microscopic hematuria in adults: the American Urological Association best practice policy. Part II: Patient evaluation, cytology, voided markers, imaging, cystoscopy, nephrology evaluation, and follow-up. Urology. 2001;57:605–10.

Rodgers M, Nixon J, Hempel S, Aho T, Kelly J, Neal D, Duffy S, Kleijnen J, Westwood M. Diagnostic tests & algorithms used in the investigation of haematuria: systematic reviews & economic evaluation. Health Technol Assess. 2006;10:1–276.

Swaminathan S, Leung N, Lager DJ, Melton 3rd LJ, Bergstralh EJ, Rohlinger A, Fervenza FC. Changing incidence of glomerular disease in Olmsted County, Minnesota: a 30-year renal biopsy study. Clin J Am Soc Nephrol. 2006;1:483–7.

Ohisa N, Yoshida K, Matsuki R, Suzuki H, Miura H, Ohisa Y, Murayama N, Kaku M, Sato H. Comparison of urinary albumin–total protein ratio to phase-contrast microscopic examination of urine sediment for differentiating glomerular and nonglomerular bleeding. Am J Kidney Dis. 2008;52:235–41.

6 Approach to the Patient with Rapidly Progressive Glomerulonephritis

Ziad M. El-Zoghby

Case 1

Mr. A, a 68-year-old male with no history of renal disease, was evaluated for upper respiratory symptoms including cough and postnasal drip. A 10-day course of amoxicillin was prescribed for presumed sinusitis. After 2 weeks, his symptoms did not improve, and levofloxacin was started. One month after the initial presentation, he presented to the emergency department with progressive dyspnea, abdominal pain, and nausea. Serum creatinine level is 7.1 mg/dL (1 month ago, serum creatinine was 1.0 mg/dL), and he is admitted to the hospital for urgent evaluation. On exam, he is afebrile, and blood pressure is 162/90 mmHg. Scattered bilateral pulmonary crackles were noted on exam, and chest X-ray revealed bilateral nodular pulmonary infiltrates. Urinalysis showed 3+ protein with renal epithelial cells, granular casts, 50 red blood cells (RBCs) per high power field (HPF) with many dysmorphic RBCs, and RBC casts on microscopy.

What is the cause of Mr. A's acute kidney injury?

What investigations are needed to determine the diagnosis?

How should Mr. A be treated?

Case 2

Mrs. C is a 70-year-old previously healthy female who presents to the emergency department with a 1-week history of anorexia, nausea, and occasional vomiting. She also reports decreased urine output and darker urine over the past few days. Serum creatinine is elevated at 10.1 mg/dL (serum creatinine 2 months ago was 0.9 mg/dL), and she is admitted to the hospital. Urinalysis shows >100 RBCs per HPF with many dysmorphic RBCs. Anti-glomerular basement membrane (anti-GBM) antibody level is >8 units (normal <1), perinuclear anti-neutrophil cytoplasmic antibody (p-ANCA) and anti-myeloperoxidase (anti-MPO) antibody levels are positive. Antinuclear antibody (ANA) is weakly positive while anti-double-stranded DNA antibody (anti ds-DNA), rheumatoid factor, cytoplasmic central anti-neutrophil cytoplasmic antibody (c-ANCA), and anti-proteinase 3 antibody (PR3) are negative. C-reactive protein and sedimentation rate are both significantly elevated.

Based on the serologic testing, what is Mrs. C's most likely diagnosis?

Are further tests required to confirm the diagnosis?

How is her condition treated, and what is her prognosis?

Z.M. El-Zoghby, M.D. (✉)
Division of Nephrology, Department of Internal Medicine, Mayo Clinic, 200 First Street SW, Rochester, MN 55905, USA
e-mail: zoghby.ziad@mayo.edu

E.V. Lerma and M. Rosner (eds.), *Clinical Decisions in Nephrology, Hypertension and Kidney Transplantation*, DOI 10.1007/978-1-4614-4454-1_6, © Springer Science+Business Media New York 2013

Introduction

Rapidly progressive glomerulonephritis (RPGN) is a clinical syndrome characterized by (1) an acute and progressive loss of kidney function over days to weeks and (2) the presence of an active urinary sediment (dysmorphic RBC and RBC casts) reflecting an underlying glomerular inflammatory process. Histologically, RPGN is characterized by the presence of extra-capillary glomerular epithelial cell crescents. Thus, the terms crescentic glomerulonephritis and RPGN are sometimes used interchangeably. Generally, the number and extent of crescents seen on renal biopsy correlate with the severity of the kidney injury [1]. RPGN is relatively uncommon among kidney diseases and accounts for a small proportion of patients with end-stage renal disease (ESRD) [2]. However, RPGN must be recognized promptly because if left untreated, the disease has significant morbidity and usually progresses to ESRD and/or death [3].

Pathophysiology

RPGN itself is not a specific renal disease and occurs as a consequence of different etiologies which can lead to significant glomerular inflammation that induce crescent formation. The exact mechanisms of crescent formation are not completely understood but appear to result from a nonspecific inflammatory response to severe injury and disruption of the glomerular capillary wall. Anti-GBM antibodies, ANCA-associated vasculitis, and immune complex deposition are among the known initiating factors that commonly lead to glomerular basement membrane injury. Subsequent to this severe glomerular basement membrane injury, lymphocytes and macrophages from the blood inside the glomerular capillary loops, along with pro-inflammatory cytokines and fibrinogen, leak into the extra-capillary glomerular space (Bowman's space) causing a reaction leading to the formation of crescents by glomerular parietal epithelial cells [2]. In the initial acute phase, the crescents are "cellular," principally formed by proliferative parietal epithelial cells and macrophages. Composition of the crescents shifts over time to fibroblasts and fibrin, and the crescents become "fibro-cellular" and ultimately "fibrous." At this late stage, the process is irreversible, and aggressive therapy may no longer be indicated because it will expose patients to potentially serious side effects without substantial benefit.

Classification of RPGN

Crescentic glomerulonephritis can be divided into three main groups (Table 6.1).

- Type I, or anti-GBM, refers to the presence of IgG antibodies to type IV collagen present in the glomerular basement membrane. 40–60%

Table 6.1 Classification and causes of RPGN

Anti-GBM antibody (type I)	Immune complex (type II)	Pauci-immune (type III)
Renal-limited anti-GBM disease	Post-infectious	ANCA positive
With pulmonary hemorrhage (Goodpasture's syndrome)	Lupus nephritis	Microscopic polyangiitis (MPA)
	Henoch–Schönlein purpura	Wegener's granulomatosis (WG)
	IgA nephropathy	Churg–Strauss (CS)
	Type II cryoglobulinemia	ANCA-negative or idiopathic
	MPGN	
	Membranous nephropathy (rare)	
	Other	

MPGN membranoproliferative glomerulonephritis, *GBM* glomerular basement membrane

Table 6.2 Frequency of different types of crescentic glomerulonephritis in consecutive native renal biopsy

Age group (in years)	*N*	Anti-GBM (%)	Immune complex (%)	Pauci-immune (%)	Other (%)
All	632	15	24	60	1
1–20	73	12	45	42	0
21–60	303	15	35	48	3
61–100	256	15	6	79	0

Reprinted with permission from Macmillan Publishers Ltd [4]

of cases also have alveolar involvement causing pulmonary hemorrhage (Goodpasture's syndrome). The pathognomonic renal pathological finding is linear staining for IgG along the glomerular capillary walls on immunofluorescence. Anti-GBM disease is the most aggressive type of RPGN, with renal biopsy findings that include widespread (diffuse as well as global) crescent formation in the glomeruli in almost all patients [4]. Type I is the least common cause of RPGN, accounting for approximately 6–20% of cases.

- Type II, or immune complex crescentic glomerulonephritis, refers to the presence of immune deposits associated with a specific systemic or renal disease. The most common diseases in this category are lupus nephritis, post-infectious glomerulonephritis, Henoch–Schönlein purpura, cryoglobulinemia, and IgA nephropathy. Disease severity and outcomes are variable depending on the underlying disease. Type II RPGN is more common among children and young adults.
- Type III, or pauci-immune crescentic glomerulonephritis, is characterized by crescentic and necrotizing glomerulonephritis with the absence of immune deposits. Approximately 70–90% of patients with pauci-immune glomerulonephritis have systemic small vessel vasculitis associated with circulating autoantibodies to neutrophil cytoplasmic antigens (ANCA). When examined by indirect immunofluorescence microscopy, ANCA show a perinuclear (p-ANCA) or cytoplasmic (c-ANCA) staining pattern. The two major antigen specificities for ANCA are myeloperoxidase (MPO) and proteinase 3 (PR3). While there is some overlap, anti-MPO antibodies are found in most p-ANCA vasculitis while anti-PR3 antibodies are found in most c-ANCA vasculitis [5]. The remaining patients are ANCA negative (classified also as idiopathic pauci-immune glomerulonephritis) [6]. Type III is the most common type of RPGN in adults, especially older adults.

While the proportions of the three types of RPGN vary among studies of different populations, type I is consistently the most infrequent and Type III the most common. Thus, among 632 consecutive native renal biopsy specimens with crescentic glomerulonephritis in one series, the frequencies of type I, II, and III were 15, 24, and 60%, respectively [4]. As shown in Table 6.2, these frequencies vary based on the age group, with type II being more common among children. In a Japanese survey of 1,772 patients diagnosed with RPGN between 1989 and 2007, approximately 62% were associated with pauci-immune GN and 6.1% with anti-GBM [7]. Similarly, in a Chinese study of 106 consecutive patients with biopsy-proven crescentic glomerulonephritis, the proportions of type I, II, and III were 16, 40.6, and 43.4%, respectively [8].

Of note, approximately 5% of patients with ANCA and 21–43% of patients with anti-GBM are "double-antibody" positive, with evidence of both anti-GBM and ANCA antibodies [9, 10]. The prognostic significance of this entity is unclear but seems to be poor, similar to type I RPGN [11]. One study reported patient and renal survival rates of 52 and 26% at 1 year, respectively [10].

Clinical Presentation

The clinical presentation of RPGN depends on the type and severity of the underlying disease and can vary significantly. Some patients have an indolent course with nonspecific symptoms of

Table 6.3 Characteristics of the different types of RPGN

RPGN type	Mean age (range)	M:F	Creatinine (mg/dL)	Proteinuria (g/day; range)	% With any crescents	% With >50% crescents
Anti-GBM	52 (14–84)	1:1	9.7±7.2	1.7 (0.2–16.2)	97%	85%
Immune complex	33 (4–77)	1:1.6	4.9±3.8	4.4 (0.3–22)	<61%	<13%
Pauci-immune	56 (2–92)	1:0.9	6.5±4	1.9 (0.11–18)	90%	50%

M:F = male:female ratio
Adapted with permission from Macmillan Publishers Ltd [4]

malaise and fatigue while others presents with classic symptoms of acute glomerulonephritis (hypertension, decreased urine output, and edema). Initially, as in Case 1 described above, patients may develop upper respiratory symptoms that do not resolve after adequate treatment with antibiotics, followed by gradual onset of fatigue, nausea, and vomiting that triggers further evaluation leading to the diagnosis. At presentation, serum creatinine is often above 3 mg/dL and may exceed 20 mg/dL (Table 6.3). Patients with Goodpasture's syndrome, ANCA-associated vasculitis (AAV), or systemic lupus erythematosus (SLE) can have pulmonary involvement with respiratory symptoms including shortness of breath, cough, and hemoptysis [12]. Pulmonary hemorrhage can be severe enough to cause respiratory failure requiring intubation. These patients are initially seen by the nephrologist in the intensive care unit and usually require urgent treatment with plasmapheresis and high-dose intravenous corticosteroids. Patients with vasculitis or SLE can present with musculoskeletal symptoms, skin rashes, epistaxis, purpura, and mental status changes. Proteinuria is usually present to varying degrees but is rarely in the nephrotic range (Table 6.3). Urinalysis shows active sediment: hematuria with dysmorphic RBC and RBC casts.

Investigations

The suspicion of RPGN (acute rise in serum creatinine and active urinary sediment) should trigger an urgent nephrology consult, and serological tests should be ordered to identify the underlying cause. These tests include serum complement levels (C3 and C4); cryoglobulins; rheumatoid factor; ANA; anti-ds-DNA; p-ANCA, c-ANCA, anti-MPO, and anti-PR3 antibodies; anti-GBM antibody; hepatitis B and C serologies; and monoclonal protein studies. Renal biopsy is mandatory and should be done as soon as possible in the absence of contraindications. When present, coagulation abnormalities should be reversed prior to the biopsy. If a patient is anticoagulated, empiric treatment should be initiated, especially in severe cases, and the biopsy delayed until it can be safely performed. Histologic findings do not change rapidly after treatment initiation, and tissue diagnosis can still be obtained several days later. Besides identifying the cause of RPGN, the biopsy provides valuable information on the severity and degree of irreversible damage, thereby aiding the therapeutic medical decision by weighing the risks and benefits of treatment. A kidney ultrasound is not helpful to establish the diagnosis; however, it is usually done to exclude other conditions such as urinary tract obstruction and to assess the anatomy and size of the kidneys prior to the biopsy.

Differential Diagnosis

Patients with RPGN have a significant acute decline in kidney function thus the differential diagnosis is broad and includes all causes of acute kidney injury. Acute tubular necrosis and acute interstitial nephritis are the most common differential diagnoses to consider, but the clinical presentation and presence of active urinary sediment usually point toward a glomerular process. Of note, an acute thrombotic microangiopathic process can present similarly to RPGN with active urinary sediment although this process is not classified as RPGN due to the absence of crescents on histology. Appropriate serologic tests can narrow the diagnosis to a specific type of RPGN, but definite diagnosis is confirmed by kidney biopsy. A complete list of drugs ingested should be obtained from the patient since certain drugs (hydralazine, allopurinol, minocycline, and propylthiouracil) are known to induce MPO-ANCA-positive disease, and discontinuation of the causative drug usually reverses the process if done early in the course of the disease [13].

Management

The treatment of RPGN depends on the underlying diagnosis. For example, post-infectious glomerulonephritis does not require specific therapy and usually recovers spontaneously while anti-GBM disease requires immediate treatment with plasmapheresis in addition to aggressive immunosuppression. Crescentic IgA nephropathy may or may not be treated with immunosuppression based on the severity of the presentation and the number of crescents on biopsy. For aggressive disease, and in most patients admitted to the hospital, treatment generally consists of high-dose intravenous corticosteroid pulses (such as 1 g/day of methylprednisolone) followed by oral corticosteroid and a cytotoxic agent—typically oral or intravenous cyclophosphamide [14, 15]. Plasmapheresis (7–14 daily treatments) is indicated for anti-GBM disease to remove the autoantibodies as well as in patients with pulmonary hemorrhage (such as that seen in SLE or AAV) or severe renal failure [16]. Oral steroids are commonly tapered after 1 month and continued for 4–6 months based on clinical response. Cyclophosphamide can be given intravenously monthly or orally daily, with dose adjustment based on kidney function. Close monitoring of the WBC count is mandatory. Cyclophosphamide dose is reduced if WBC count drops below 3,000 cells/mm [3]. Because of potential serious side effects, cyclophosphamide is usually discontinued after 3–6 months (12 months at most) and replaced by another immunosuppressive agent such as azathioprine, methotrexate, or mycophenolate mofetil [17–19]. Rituximab, a B-cell-depleting anti-CD 20 monoclonal antibody, has been investigated in AAV and SLE as an induction agent and appears to be a promising alternative option to cyclophosphamide [14, 20–22].

Maintenance immunosuppression beyond 6 months is not needed in anti-GBM disease as recurrence is rare. On the other hand, patients with lupus nephritis and Wegener granulomatosis (WG) (more recently referred to as granulomatosis with polyangiitis [Wegener's] [23]) require longer courses of immunosuppression while those with microscopic polyangiitis will be treated for 12 months after remission in the absence of recurrence [24–27].

Patients treated with corticosteroids and immunosuppression receive prophylactic treatment to prevent complications. Calcium and vitamin D supplements are given to prevent osteoporosis, and a proton pump inhibitor or a histamine-2 receptor blocker is prescribed for gastric protection during the duration of corticosteroid exposure. In addition, low-dose sulfamethoxazole/trimethoprim (or dapsone in patients allergic to sulfa drugs) is given for *Pneumocystis jiroveci* prophylaxis. During the period of exposure to cyclophosphamide, some prescribe fluconazole or nystatin for Candida prophylaxis and acyclovir for herpes zoster prophylaxis.

In the absence of kidney function recovery, kidney transplantation remains the best renal replacement therapy option. Generally, it is suggested that the underlying disease be quiescent for 6–12 months before proceeding with transplantation. The risk of recurrent disease is small and does not preclude transplantation [28, 29].

Outcomes

Untreated, RPGN progresses to ESRD and death [30]. Outcomes have dramatically improved with current available therapies, but prognosis depends on the underlying disease, severity at presentation, and how quickly the treatment is initiated [15, 27]. For example, one study from Japan reported all cases of RPGN diagnosed between 1990 and 2007 in which patient survival was 79–86% and renal survival at 6 months was 73–82%, during the different time periods studied [7]. In a systematic review of AAV, remission rates ranged from 30 to 93% in WG, 75 to 89% in microscopic polyangiitis (MPA), and 81 to 91% in Churg–Strauss syndrome (CSS). The 5-year patient survival rates were 74–91%, 45–76%, and 60–97%, respectively [31]. Higher serum creatinine level and pulmonary hemorrhage at presentation are predictors of higher mortality in AAV [32]. For lupus nephritis, a recent study showed that patients with crescents have a worse renal outcome compared to those without crescents although patient survival was similar [33]. For anti-GBM disease, 1-year patient and renal survival is 75–100% and 82–84%, respectively, based on recent series although among those who require dialysis at presentation, patient and renal survival at 1 year is lower at 65 and 8%, respectively [34].

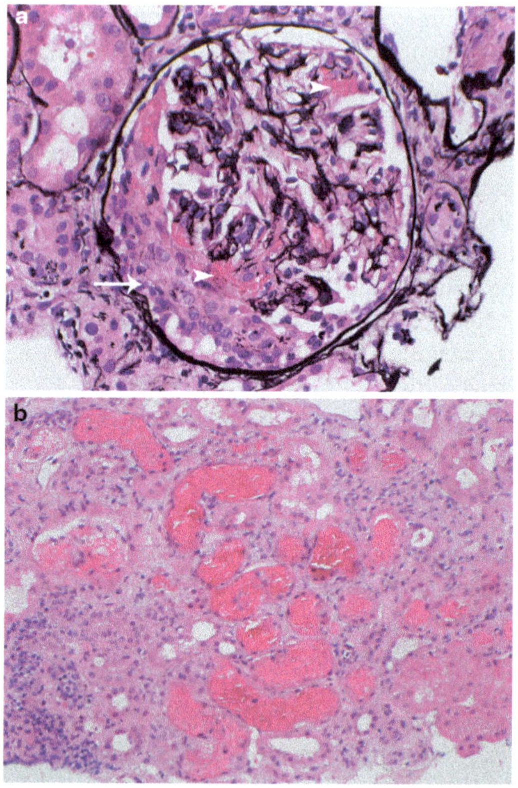

Fig. 6.1 (**a**) Cellular crescent (*arrow*) and fibrinoid necrosis (*arrowhead*) in patient 1 with ANCA vasculitis (Silver stain, original magnification 400×). (**b**) Red blood cell casts in the lumen of multiple tubules (H&E stain, original magnification 200×). Courtesy of Dr. Samih Nasr

Case 1 Follow-Up

The presence of hematuria with dysmorphic RBCs on urinalysis suggests a glomerular process. Serological tests showed normal complement C3 and C4 levels and negative ANA, cryoglobulin, anti-ds-DNA, and anti-GBM antibodies. C-reactive protein and sedimentation rate were both significantly elevated. c-ANCA titer was positive and anti-PR3 antibodies were elevated while p-ANCA and anti-MPO antibodies were negative. This was consistent with WG, and renal biopsy showed diffuse pauci-immune crescentic and necrotizing glomerulonephritis (Fig. 6.1). Mr. A began high-dose intravenous methylprednisolone for 3 days followed by oral prednisone and cyclophosphamide. Because the disease was aggressive with initial serum creatinine 7.1 mg/dL and crescents present in 9 out of 12 glomeruli on renal biopsy, he was treated more aggressively and also underwent plasmapheresis. He did not require dialysis, and kidney function gradually improved. Four months later, serum creatinine was 1.8 mg/dL; CRP, ESR, and urinalysis were normal; and c-ANCA and PR3 antibodies were negative. He completed 6 months of prednisone and cyclophosphamide and was then switched to azathioprine for long-term maintenance immunosuppression.

Case 2 Follow-Up

Based on the presentation, Mrs. C has RPGN due to anti-GBM disease. The serology was also positive for p-ANCA (double antibody positive) which can be present in approximately 30% of the cases as noted previously. Her kidney biopsy showed a necrotizing and crescentic glomerulonephritis with crescents present in 15 out of 20 glomeruli (Fig. 6.2a). Immunofluorescence staining showed linear IgG antibodies along the glomerular capillary walls (Fig. 6.2b). Serum creatinine peaked at 11.3 mg/dL, and she required two sessions

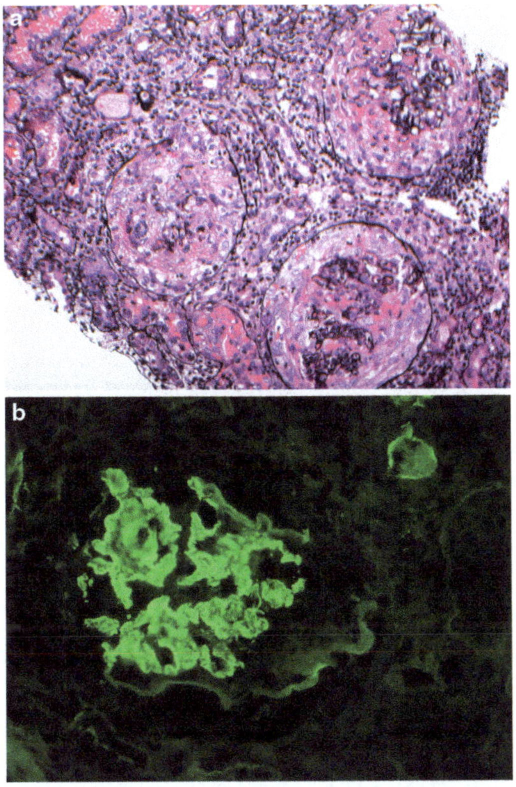

Fig. 6.2 (**a**) Three glomeruli with crescents in patient 2 with anti-GBM disease (Silver stain, original magnification 300×). (**b**) Immunofluorescence showing linear anti-IgG antibody deposition in the glomerular capillary walls. Courtesy of Dr. Sanjeev Sethi

of hemodialysis. She was treated with high-dose intravenous methylprednisolone for 3 days followed by oral prednisone and cyclophosphamide along with ten sessions of daily plasma exchange. Anti-GBM antibody became undetectable, and cyclophosphamide was stopped after 2 months due to leukopenia. Prednisone was gradually tapered over 6 months. At 1 year, anti-GBM antibody was undetectable, serum creatinine was 2.1 mg/dL, and urine sediment was normal with 24-h urine total protein of 450 mg.

Key Points

- RPGN is a clinical syndrome that should be suspected in the presence of a rapid increase in serum creatinine and active urinary sediment.
- RPGN should be promptly recognized and treated because it is associated with significant morbidity and ESRD if left untreated.
- RPGN is classified into three types: (1) anti-GBM disease; (2) immune complex glomerulonephritis; and (3) pauci-immune glomerulonephritis.
- Clinical manifestations are variable, depending on underlying cause, type of organ involved, and disease severity.
- Diagnostic evaluation includes serological testing and kidney biopsy.
- Treatment depends on the cause of RPGN but usually consists of corticosteroids and immunosuppressive agents.
- Plasmapheresis is indicated with type I RPGN or in the presence of pulmonary hemorrhage or severe kidney injury.

References

1. Berden AE, Ferrario F, Hagen EC, et al. Histopathologic classification of ANCA-associated glomerulonephritis. J Am Soc Nephrol. 2010;21(10):1628–36.
2. Couser W. Rapidly progressive glomerulonephritis: classification, pathogenetic mechanisms, and therapy. Am J Kidney Dis. 1988;11(6):449–64.
3. Jennette JC, Falk RJ. Small-vessel vasculitis. N Engl J Med. 1997;337(21):1512–23.
4. Jennette JC. Rapidly progressive crescentic glomerulonephritis. Kidney Int. 2003;63(3):1164–77.
5. Falk RJ, Jennette JC. ANCA small-vessel vasculitis. J Am Soc Nephrol. 1997;8(2):314–22.
6. Chen M, Kallenberg CGM, Zhao M-H. ANCA-negative pauci-immune crescentic glomerulonephritis. Nat Rev Nephrol. 2009;5(6):313–8.
7. Koyama A, Yamagata K, Makino H, et al. A nationwide survey of rapidly progressive glomerulonephritis in Japan: etiology, prognosis and treatment diversity. Clin Exp Nephrol. 2009;13(6):633–50.
8. Lin W, Chen M, Cui Z, Zhao MH. The immunopathological spectrum of crescentic glomerulonephritis: a survey of 106 patients in a single Chinese center. Nephron Clin Pract. 2010;116(1):c65–74.
9. Denton M, Magee C, Niles J. Rapidly progressive glomerulonephritis. Ann Intern Med. 2002;137(5 Part 1):W1.
10. Levy JB, Hammad T, Coulthart A, Dougan T, Pusey CD. Clinical features and outcome of patients with both ANCA and anti-GBM antibodies. Kidney Int. 2004;66(4):1535–40.
11. Rutgers A, Slot M, van Paassen P, van Breda VP, Heeringa P, Tervaert JWC. Coexistence of anti-glomerular basement membrane antibodies and myeloper-

oxidase-ANCAs in crescentic glomerulonephritis. Am J Kidney Dis. 2005;46(2):253–62.
12. Papiris S, Manali E, Kalomenidis I, Kapotsis G, Karakatsani A, Roussos C. Bench-to-bedside review: pulmonary-renal syndromes—an update for the intensivist. Crit Care. 2007;11(3):213.
13. Wiik A. Drug-induced vasculitis. Curr Opin Rheumatol. 2008;20(1):35–9.
14. Bomback AS, Appel GB. Updates on the treatment of lupus nephritis. J Am Soc Nephrol. 2010;21(12): 2028–35.
15. Falk RJ, Jennette JC. ANCA disease: where is this field heading? J Am Soc Nephrol. 2010;21(5): 745–52.
16. Jayne DRW, Gaskin G, Rasmussen N, et al. Randomized trial of plasma exchange or high-dosage methylprednisolone as adjunctive therapy for severe renal vasculitis. J Am Soc Nephrol. 2007;18(7): 2180–8.
17. Hiemstra TF, Walsh M, Mahr A, et al. Mycophenolate mofetil vs azathioprine for remission maintenance in antineutrophil cytoplasmic antibody–associated vasculitis. J Am Med Assoc. 2010;304(21):2381–8.
18. Jayne D, Rasmussen N, Andrassy K, et al. A randomized trial of maintenance therapy for vasculitis associated with antineutrophil cytoplasmic autoantibodies. N Engl J Med. 2003;349(1):36–44.
19. Pagnoux C, Mahr A, Hamidou MA, et al. Azathioprine or methotrexate maintenance for ANCA-associated vasculitis. N Engl J Med. 2008;359(26):2790–803.
20. Jones RB, Cohen Tervaert JW, Hauser T, et al. Rituximab versus cyclophosphamide in ANCA-associated renal vasculitis. N Engl J Med. 2010;363(3):211–20.
21. Melander C, Sallée M, Trolliet P, et al. Rituximab in severe lupus nephritis: early B-cell depletion affects long-term renal outcome. Clin J Am Soc Nephrol. 2009;4(3):579–87.
22. Stone JH, Merkel PA, Spiera R, et al. Rituximab versus cyclophosphamide for ANCA-associated vasculitis. N Engl J Med. 2010;363(3):221–32.
23. Falk RJ, Gross WL, Guillevin L, et al. Granulomatosis with polyangiitis (Wegener's): an alternative name for Wegener's granulomatosis. J Am Soc Nephrol. 2011;22(4):587–8.
24. Jayne D. Current management of lupus nephritis: popular misconceptions. Lupus. 2007;16(3):217–20.
25. Lionaki S, Jennette J, Falk R. Anti-neutrophil cytoplasmic (ANCA) and anti-glomerular basement membrane (GBM) autoantibodies in necrotizing and crescentic glomerulonephritis. Semin Immunopathol. 2007;29(4):459–74.
26. Ortega LM, Schultz DR, Lenz O, Pardo V, Contreras GN. Review: lupus nephritis: pathologic features, epidemiology and a guide to therapeutic decisions. Lupus. 2010;19(5):557–74.
27. Pallan L, Savage CO, Harper L. ANCA-associated vasculitis: from bench research to novel treatments. Nat Rev Nephrol. 2009;5(5):278–86.
28. Choy BY, Chan TM, Lai KN. Recurrent glomerulonephritis after kidney transplantation. Am J Transplant. 2006;6(11):2535–42.
29. Fairhead T, Knoll G. Recurrent glomerular disease after kidney transplantation. Curr Opin Nephrol Hypertens. 2010;19(6):578–85.
30. Hoffman GS. Therapeutic interventions for systemic vasculitis. J Am Med Assoc. 2010;304(21):2413–4.
31. Mukhtyar C, Flossmann O, Hellmich B, et al. Outcomes from studies of antineutrophil cytoplasm antibody associated vasculitis: a systematic review by the European League Against Rheumatism systemic vasculitis task force. Ann Rheum Dis. 2008;67(7):1004–10.
32. Hogan SL, Falk RJ, Chin H, et al. Predictors of relapse and treatment resistance in antineutrophil cytoplasmic antibody-associated small-vessel vasculitis. Ann Intern Med. 2005;143(9):621–31.
33. Yu F, Tan Y, Liu G, S-x W, W-z Z, M-h Z. Clinicopathological characteristics and outcomes of patients with crescentic lupus nephritis. Kidney Int. 2009;76(3):307–17.
34. Levy JB, Turner AN, Rees AJ, Pusey CD. Long-term outcome of anti-glomerular basement membrane antibody disease treated with plasma exchange and immunosuppression. Ann Intern Med. 2001;134(11): 1033–42.

7 Interpretation of the Renal Biopsy

LaTonya J. Hickson and Lynn D. Cornell

Case

An 84-year-old female with a history of hypertension presents to the emergency department complaining of shortness of breath. On exam, blood pressure is 180/90 mmHg. Cardiac exam is normal, breath sounds are diminished in both lung bases, and +2 pitting edema is present. Chest X-ray reveals bilateral pleural effusions, and she is hospitalized for suspected acute congestive heart failure. Serum creatinine is elevated to 1.8–1.9 mg/dL from 1.2 mg/dL measured 5 months previously. A urinalysis shows 9.9 g of total protein excretion per day, 31–40 red blood cells per high power field of which greater than 25% were dysmorphic, 11–20 white blood cells per high power field, lipiduria, and granular casts. Nephrology is consulted. Renal ultrasound demonstrates normal sized kidneys, patent renal veins, and no evidence of hydronephrosis. Initial serologic studies are negative including antinuclear antibody, erythrocyte sedimentation rate, C-reactive protein, antibodies to hepatitis B and C viruses, anti-neutrophil cytoplasmic antibodies (ANCA), and anti-glomerular basement membrane (GBM) antibody titers. C3 is normal, and C4 is mildly reduced at 11 mg/dL (normal 14–40 mg/dL). No monoclonal protein is detected by serum or urine protein electrophoresis studies. To determine the diagnosis, a renal biopsy is recommended.

What are the indications for renal biopsy in this case?

What are the risks associated with a renal biopsy?

What do you think the renal biopsy will demonstrate in this patient?

Purpose of and Indications for Renal Biopsy

An invaluable tool with multiple utilities, the renal biopsy aids in the diagnosis of renal parenchymal diseases, determines disease extent and activity for prognostic and treatment purposes, and, when repeated, documents disease progression over time. Oftentimes, the modality of treatment is determined by renal biopsy findings. For example, the management of a patient with acute renal failure due to acute tubular necrosis or acute or chronic renal failure from advanced nodular diabetic glomerulosclerosis may be predominantly supportive. In contrast, the presence of active necrotizing crescentic lesions such as in a pauci-immune glomerulonephritis combined with other clinical findings may prompt clinicians to initiate immunosuppressive therapies such as

L.J. Hickson, M.D.
Division of Nephrology and Hypertension, Department of Medicine, 200 First Street SW, Rochester, MN 55901

L.D. Cornell, M.D. (✉)
Division of Anatomic Pathology,
Department of Laboratory Medicine and Pathology,
Mayo Clinic, 200 First Street SW,
Rochester, MN 55905, USA
e-mail: cornell.lynn@mayo.edu

E.V. Lerma and M. Rosner (eds.), *Clinical Decisions in Nephrology, Hypertension and Kidney Transplantation*,
DOI 10.1007/978-1-4614-4454-1_7, © Springer Science+Business Media New York 2013

Table 7.1 Indications for renal biopsy

Elevated serum creatinine or blood urea nitrogen
May be acute, subacute, or chronic
Proteinuria
Often a sign of increased glomerular basement membrane permeability to plasma proteins
May be asymptomatic (lower levels) or symptomatic (higher levels)
Nephrotic syndrome
Proteinuria at >3.5 g/day
Hypoalbuminemia
Edema
Hyperlipidemia
Hematuria
Sign of glomerular inflammation or structural anomaly, tubulointerstitial disease, or urologic disease
May be gross or microscopic
Nephritic syndrome
Glomerular hematuria (red blood cell casts, dysmorphic red blood cells)
Proteinuria
Renal dysfunction
Hypertension
Edema

corticosteroids and cyclophosphamide with or without plasma exchange therapy. Moreover, the degree of disease activity may influence management choices: the presence of extensive tubulointerstitial fibrosis along with fibrocellular crescents on the renal biopsy of a patient with pauci-immune glomerulonephritis might suggest a less aggressive therapeutic approach.

Common indications for renal biopsy include reduced renal function (acute, subacute, or chronic), proteinuria, nephrotic syndrome, hematuria, and nephritic syndrome (Table 7.1). Proteinuria, especially at higher levels (>1 g/day), is usually a sign of increased glomerular basement membrane permeability to plasma proteins. Proteinuria may also be found with sub-optimally controlled hypertension, tubular proteinuria, and following vigorous exercise. Nephrotic syndrome is characterized by the presence of proteinuria greater than or equal to 3.5 g/24 h (nephrotic-range proteinuria), hypoalbuminemia, hyperlipidemia, and edema. Hematuria may be visible to the naked eye (gross hematuria) or seen only under the microscope. The term glomerular hematuria refers to the presence of dysmorphic red blood cells, which are damaged as they pass through the damaged glomerular basement membrane. When these cells become adherent to Tamm–Horsfall protein within tubules, red blood cell casts are formed. The presence of dysmorphic hematuria or red blood cell casts should alert the clinician to investigate intrinsic renal processes, for which a renal biopsy is usually necessary to obtain a diagnosis. The clinical picture of "nephritic syndrome" occurs when glomerular hematuria is accompanied by proteinuria, renal dysfunction, edema, and hypertension.

In general, the presence of progressive proteinuria, nephrotic-range proteinuria with or without nephrotic syndrome, hematuria, and nephritic syndrome should alert the clinician to an underlying renal disease process and need for appropriate laboratory testing and consideration of a renal biopsy. In the patient described in the case vignette, features of nephritic syndrome were found and prompted a renal biopsy.

Value of Renal Biopsy

The renal biopsy usually results in a definitive diagnosis. In a prospective study of 276 patients with a variety of clinical presentations of renal disease, renal biopsy altered patient management 43% of the time [1]. In patients with systemic diseases that cause renal disease, such as diabetes mellitus, a renal biopsy can confirm the clinical diagnosis and predict prognosis of the disease, it may reveal a different diagnosis, or both. For example, in a study of over 3,575 renal biopsies that showed diabetic glomerulosclerosis, 27% demonstrated other glomerular, tubulointerstitial, or vascular diseases not directly attributable to diabetes, including 8% of cases with glomerular disease other than and in addition to diabetic glomerulosclerosis [2]. These findings have been supported in other smaller case series as well [3, 4].

In some transplant centers, protocol allograft biopsies are performed at set intervals of time post kidney transplant. Protocol renal allograft biopsies allow clinicians to monitor for subclinical renal disease including subclinical rejection, polyoma (BK) virus nephropathy, calcineurin inhibitor toxicity, recurrence of primary renal disease, and early transplant glomerulopathy. In two reported series, the utilization of surveillance biopsies allowed early detection and treatment of recurrent primary renal diseases in transplant recipients with recurrent membranous nephropathy and membranoproliferative glomerulonephritis [5–7].

Safety of Renal Biopsy Procedure

A renal biopsy is generally performed on a fasting patient in the outpatient setting under ultrasound or computed tomography guidance, which allows for visualization of the target organ and its surroundings. The skin and subcutaneous tissue over the area of the biopsy is anesthetized. An automated biopsy device with a 16- to 18-gauge needle retrieves the tissue samples. Generally, 2–3 renal biopsy cores measuring 1–2 mm in diameter and 10–20 mm in length are obtained from the lower pole of the kidney. Depending upon provider preference, patients are instructed to lie flat from 3 to 24 h post procedure to minimize bleeding risks. Antiplatelet and anti-thrombotic agents are held anywhere from 3 to 7 days prior to procedure and several days to 2 weeks following the procedure, depending on the indications for these therapies. A normal International Normalized Ratio (INR) value is sought with values <1.5 accepted in some patients on chronic anticoagulation therapy. These precautions will minimize the risk of post-biopsy bleeding. Patients with acute renal failure, severe hypertension, anemia, and uremia are at the highest risk of bleeding [8]. Other studies revealed an association between female gender, younger age, higher baseline partial thromboplastin time, and systemic autoimmune diseases with an increased risk of native kidney bleeding [9, 10]. Relative contraindications to biopsy may include severe uncontrolled hypertension, anatomic abnormalities which may increase the risk of bleeding, significantly atrophic kidneys (<9 cm), and active bleeding disorders that are not correctable. Solitary kidney was at one time considered a relative contraindication, but biopsies have been performed safely in patients with only one kidney [11]. However, caution should be exercised in this patient group. Postrenal biopsy complication rates are variable, ranging from transient gross hematuria (0.4–16%) or hematoma formation (10–30%) to less common events such as significant bleeding requiring red blood cell transfusion (1–6%), arterial embolization, arteriovenous fistula formation, and nephrectomy (0.1–3.0%), and death (0–0.1%) [8–15]. Successful use of CT-guided renal biopsies revealed adequate tissue sampling and low complication rates [12]. Given the use of modern techniques involving automated needles and real-time ultrasound or CT, the renal biopsy procedure is generally accepted to be safe with low incidence of serious complications.

Tissue Processing

At the time of biopsy, the tissue specimen should be examined for the presence of renal cortex, indicated by the presence of glomeruli. A dissecting microscope or magnifying glass can assist in identification of glomeruli, which appear similar to small raspberries. If renal cortex is not obtained, then the sample will likely be inadequate for diagnosis, and the patient will require repeat biopsy.

Routine tissue handling of renal biopsies requires that tissue be sent for light microscopy (LM), immunofluorescence (IF), and electron microscopy (EM). Tissue samples for these studies require different fixation and transport procedures. The routine stains performed are hematoxylin and eosin, periodic acid-Schiff, Masson trichrome, and Jones-methenamine silver. Each stain highlights particular anatomic structures and disease processes (Table 7.2). Additional special stains (such as Congo red for amyloidosis), immunohistochemical stains, in situ hybridization, and other studies may also be performed on the LM sample depending on the features of the particular case.

Routine IF for native biopsies usually consists of stains for IgG, IgA, IgM, kappa and lambda light chains, complement components C3 and C1q,

Table 7.2 Common light microscopy special stains of the renal biopsy[a]

Stain	Main staining features on kidney biopsy
Hematoxylin and Eosin (H&E)	Highlights red blood cells, thrombi, glomerular capillary loop thickness
	Calcium oxalate deposits visible on H&E stain when examined under polarized light
Periodic Acid-Schiff (PAS)	Basement membrane stain; glomerular basement membrane thickening or duplication, tubular basement membrane thickening/tubular atrophy
	Hyalinosis, in arterioles or in glomeruli, stains positively
	Mesangial matrix/mesangial sclerosis positive
	Normal proteinaceous casts stain positively by PAS
	Immune complex deposits usually positive, amyloid negative by PAS
Jones-methenamine silver	Basement membrane stain; glomerular basement membrane thickening, duplication, "spikes," or other irregularities
	Glomerular necrosis or thrombi apparent on silver stain
Masson trichrome	Highlights fibrosis as blue
	Immune complex deposits visible and appear red on trichrome stain
Congo red	Amyloid stains positively (red) by Congo red and shows "apple-green" birefringence when examined under polarized light
Von Kossa	Phosphate stain; highlights calcium phosphate deposits in kidney
Ziehl–Neelsen (AFB)	Special stain for acid-fast bacilli
Grocott's Methenamine Silver (GMS)	Special stain for fungus

[a]In addition to these special stains, hundreds to thousands of immunoperoxidase and in situ hybridization tests are available clinically and on a research basis for specific molecules to evaluate for inflammatory infiltrates, activation markers on cells, specific infections, and other conditions

fibrin/fibrinogen, and albumin. Renal transplant biopsies require an additional immunofluorescence stain, C4d, to evaluate for antibody-mediated rejection.

The EM sample is fixed, processed, and embedded into blocks of an epoxy resin. Survey sections, cut at 1 μm and stained with toluidine blue, are used to evaluate the sample for the presence of glomeruli or other structures of interest, and those blocks are ultrathin-sectioned and stained with a heavy metal (lead/uranium) for examination under the electron microscope. The pathologist or the electron microscopist photographs representative areas of glomeruli, the tubules and interstitium, and vascular components of the EM sample.

Interpretation and Report of the Renal Biopsy

The pathologist examines the LM, IF, and EM samples, together with consideration of the clinical history and laboratory results, to arrive at a diagnosis. Clinical information and laboratory results are essential for an accurate and complete diagnosis and determination of the etiology of the disease pattern on biopsy. For example, calcium oxalate crystals seen on biopsy may be due to a number of inherited or acquired conditions, including primary hyperoxaluria, ingestion of ethylene glycol or heavy ingestion of oxalate-containing foods, or an effect of previous gastric bypass surgery. Helpful clinical information includes presenting features of the renal disease and indication for renal biopsy, personal medical history, family history, and medications the patient is taking currently and was taking in the past (including nonprescription medications like non-steroidal anti-inflammatory drugs). Radiographic features, renal ultrasound, CT, or MRI scan, are also helpful to the pathologist in some diseases. Depending on the clinical presentation, laboratory tests are usually indicated prior to or at the time of renal biopsy (Table 7.3).

On the tissue sample, the pathologist examines and describes each of the four anatomic compartments of the kidney—glomeruli, tubules,

Table 7.3 Basic clinical and laboratory information to obtain at the time of renal biopsy

Clinical History
Recent infection, joint pain (arthralgias), rash, gross hematuria, abdominal pain, malignancy, or connective tissue disease
Drug exposure (gold, penicillamine, NSAIDs, antibiotics, chemotherapeutic agents, etc.)
Travel history
Personal history of renal dysfunction or proteinuria (during prior work, health benefit, or sport physical examination)
Family history of renal disease
Renal function and proteinuria
Serum creatinine, blood urea nitrogen
Urinalysis with microscopy
24-h urine collection for total protein and/or spot urine protein:creatinine ratio
Other general tests
Complete blood count with differential, serum albumin, electrolyte panel, prothrombin time, partial thromboplastin time
Renal ultrasound
Serologic and other laboratory tests
Hepatitis B and C virus serologies
Human immunodeficiency virus serology
Anti-streptolysin antibodies
Antinuclear antibody and antibody to double-stranded DNA
Antineutrophil cytoplasmic antibodies (ANCA) with antibodies to myeloperoxidase and proteinase 3
Anti-glomerular basement membrane (anti-GBM) antibody
Complement levels (total, C3, and C4)
Rheumatoid factor
Cryoglobulin level
C-reactive protein
Serum protein electrophoresis and immunofixation
Urine protein electrophoresis and immunofixation
Serum free light chains

interstitium, and vessels—and determines which is the primary compartment affected by the disease process. The pathologist describes the specific pattern of injury in the kidney and forms a diagnosis or differential diagnosis based on available clinical and laboratory information and additional special studies on the tissue sample. The pathologist's role is not only to determine the pattern of injury but also to establish the cause of the injury seen on the biopsy sample. Many different diseases may give the same pattern of injury. For example, a pattern of nodular glomerulosclerosis seen on light microscopy may be due to diabetes mellitus, smoking and hypertension, or monoclonal immunoglobulin deposition disease. A pattern of interstitial nephritis may be caused by an allergic drug reaction, a systemic autoimmune disease, an infection, or other conditions.

In the past several years, there has been a movement towards establishing "critical values" or critical diagnoses in anatomic pathology, similar to critical values in laboratory medicine [16, 17]. Critical diagnoses are those with immediate clinical consequences or with significant discrepant findings compared to the outside pathologist on a consultation case. On renal biopsy, examples of critical diagnoses are diffuse crescentic glomerulonephritis (e.g., anti-GBM nephritis, diffuse active lupus nephritis, ANCA-associated glomerulonephritis) and acute rejection in a renal transplant patient. These findings should prompt immediate reporting to the nephrologist.

The renal biopsy report describes the pathological features of different compartments of the kidney and results of the special studies performed, as well as the clinical history, as the basis of the conclusions made by the pathologist. [18]. Additional laboratory studies may be recommended as well. If an accepted classification system exists, the most recent classification system should be used in the appropriate disease, for example the Oxford classification of IgA nephropathy or the International Society of Nephrology/Renal Pathology Society (ISN/RPS) 2003 classification for lupus nephritis [19, 20]. The report should include information about adequacy of the sample, with an adequate sample generally considered to contain at least ten glomeruli for light microscopy and additional glomeruli for immunofluorescence and electron microscopy, and, on renal allograft biopsies, the presence of arteries. Because sampling errors may occur, focal lesions are more likely to be detected and thus classified correctly on a larger tissue sample. For example, in cases of proliferative lupus nephritis in a "moderate" disease activity group (20–60% glomerular involvement), based on sampling error only, 55% of patients with just ten glomeruli on a kidney biopsy sample will be classified correctly [21].

Case Revisited

In our case patient, renal biopsy confirmed the presence of a membranoproliferative glomerulonephritis pattern, consistent with type I cryoglobulinemic glomerulonephritis given the presence of monoclonal IgM lambda deposition (see Fig. 7.1). Due to the association of type I cryoglobulinemia with underlying lymphoproliferative and plasma cell proliferative disorders, the patient was referred to hematology for extensive evaluation although no concomitant disease was identified. The patient was treated with steroids and rituximab, an anti-CD20 monoclonal antibody, with improvement in renal function and proteinuria. In this example, the diagnosis of cryoglobulinemic glomerulonephritis was solely reliant on renal biopsy, as cryoglobulins were never identified in the blood during initial assessment, illustrating the importance of a tissue diagnosis.

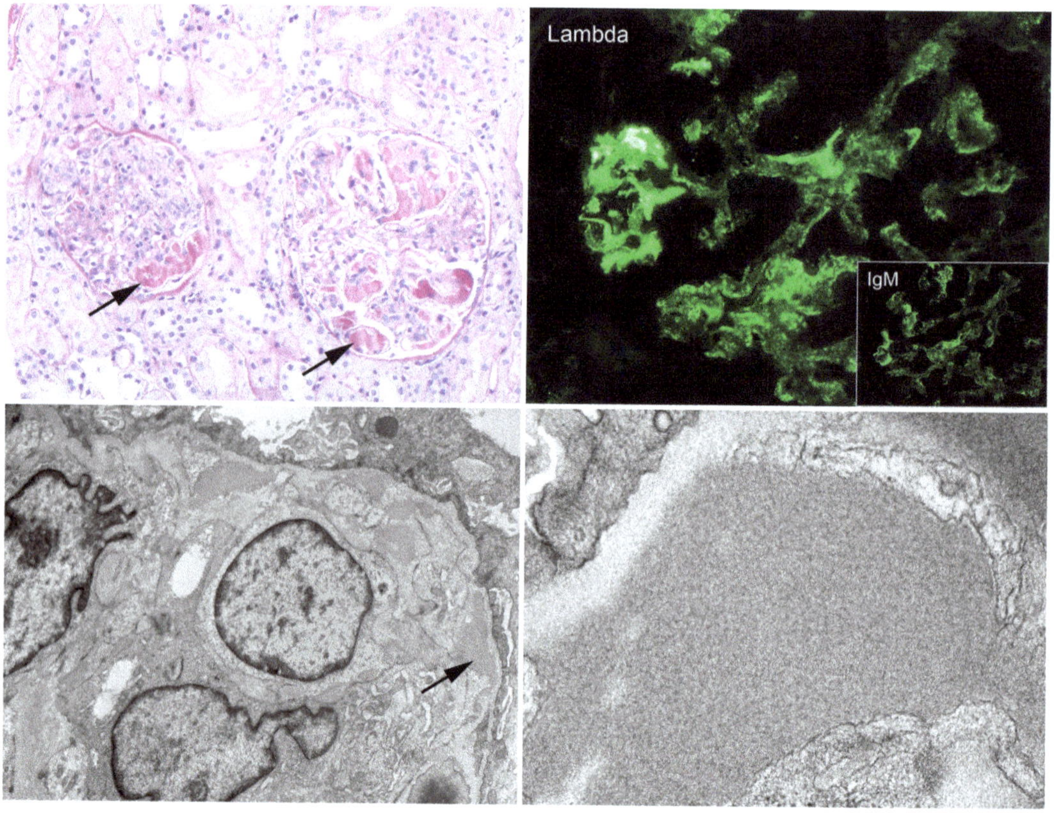

Fig. 7.1 Renal biopsy from case patient: By light microscopy (*upper left*), the glomeruli show numerous PAS-positive immunoglobulin "pseudothrombi" (*arrows*) within glomerular capillary lumens, compatible with cryoglobulinemia (periodic acid-Schiff stain). By immunofluorescence (*upper right*), there is granular mesangial and glomerular basement membrane staining for lambda light chain and IgM (*inset*), along with staining of the immunoglobulin "pseudothrombi." Staining for kappa light chains and other immunoreactants was negative. This immunofluorescence staining pattern is suggestive of type I cryoglobulinemia. By electron microscopy (*lower panels*), mesangial and subendothelial (*arrow*, *lower left*) immune complex deposits are seen; on higher magnification, the deposits show a vaguely curvilinear substructure in areas (*lower right*), suggestive of cryoglobulinemia

Key Points

1. Kidney biopsy is an invaluable tool in the diagnosis, prognostication, surveillance, and management of renal parenchymal diseases.
2. A variety of clinical features such as glomerular hematuria, renal dysfunction, persistent or progressive proteinuria, or nephrotic syndrome may prompt the clinician to perform a renal biopsy.
3. A focused history, physical examination, and serologic tests are important adjuncts to the renal biopsy in the diagnosis of glomerular disease processes.
4. Renal biopsy is generally a safe procedure when appropriate precautions are taken.
5. Adequate tissue sample and techniques for light microscopy, immunofluorescence, and electron microscopy preparation are required to provide an optimal, informative renal biopsy report.

References

1. Richards NT, Darby S, Howie AJ, Adu D, Michael J. Knowledge of renal histology alters patient management in over 40% of cases. Nephrol Dial Transplant. 1994;9(9):1255–9.
2. Hickson LJ, El-Zoghby Z, Pflueger A, et al. Non-diabetic renal disease in diabetic patients. In: American Society of Nephrology Annual Meeting, Denver, Colorado; 2010
3. Pham TT, Sim JJ, Kujubu DA, Liu IL, Kumar VA. Prevalence of nondiabetic renal disease in diabetic patients. Am J Nephrol. 2007;27(3):322–8.
4. Mak SK, Gwi E, Chan KW, et al. Clinical predictors of non-diabetic renal disease in patients with non-insulin dependent diabetes mellitus. Nephrol Dial Transplant. Dec 1997;12(12):2588–91.
5. El-Zoghby ZM, Grande JP, Fraile MG, Norby SM, Fervenza FC, Cosio FG. Recurrent idiopathic membranous nephropathy: early diagnosis by protocol biopsies and treatment with anti-CD20 monoclonal antibodies. Am J Transplant. 2009;9(12):2800–7.
6. Lorenz E, Sethi S, Leung N, Dispenzieri A, Ferevenza F, Cosio F. Recurrent membranoproliferative glomerulonephritis after kidney transplantation. Kidney Int. 2010;77(8):721–8.
7. Stegall M, Park W, Larson T, et al. The histology of solitary renal allografts at 1 and 5 years after transplantation. Am J Transplant. 2011;11(4):698–707.
8. Shidham GB, Siddiqi N, Beres JA, et al. Clinical risk factors associated with bleeding after native kidney biopsy. Nephrology. 2005;10(3):305–10.
9. Manno C, Strippoli GF, Arnesano L, et al. Predictors of bleeding complications in percutaneous ultrasound-guided renal biopsy. Kidney Int. 2004;66(4):1570–7.
10. Stratta P, Canavese C, Marengo M, et al. Risk management of renal biopsy: 1387 cases over 30 years in a single centre. Eur J Clin Invest. 2007;37(12):954–63.
11. Mendelssohn DC, Cole EH. Outcomes of percutaneous kidney biopsy, including those of solitary native kidneys. Am J Kidney Dis. 1995;26(4):580–5.
12. Margaryan A, Perazella MA, Mahnensmith RL, Abu-Alfa AK. Experience with outpatient computed tomographic-guided renal biopsy. Clin Nephrol. 2010; 74(6):440–5.
13. Maya ID, Allon M. Percutaneous renal biopsy: outpatient observation without hospitalization is safe. Semin Dial. 2009;22(4):458–61.
14. Soares SM, Fervenza FC, Lager DJ, Gertz MA, Cosio FG, Leung N. Bleeding complications after transcutaneous kidney biopsy in patients with systemic amyloidosis: single-center experience in 101 patients. Am J Kidney Dis. 2008;52(6):1079–83.
15. Waldo B, Korbet SM, Freimanis MG, Lewis EJ. The value of post-biopsy ultrasound in predicting complications after percutaneous renal biopsy of native kidneys. Nephrol Dial Transplant. 2009;24(8): 2433–9.
16. Association of Directors of Anatomic and Surgical Pathology. Critical diagnoses (critical values) in anatomic pathology. Am J Surg Pathol. 2006;30(7):897–9.
17. Huang EC, Kuo FC, Fletcher CD, Nose V. Critical diagnoses in surgical pathology: a retrospective single-institution study to monitor guidelines for communication of urgent results. Am J Surg Pathol. 2009;33(7):1098–102.
18. Chang A, Gibson IW, Cohen AH, Weening JJ, Jennette JC, Fogo AB. A Position Paper on Standardizing the Nonneoplastic Kidney Biopsy Report. Clin J Am Soc Nephrol. 2012 Jul 12. [Epub ahead of print] PubMed PMID: 22798541.
19. Roberts IS, Cook HT, Troyanov S, et al. The Oxford classification of IgA nephropathy: pathology definitions, correlations, and reproducibility. Kidney Int. 2009;76(5):546–56.
20. Weening JJ, D'Agati VD, Schwartz MM, et al. The classification of glomerulonephritis in systemic lupus erythematosus revisited. J Am Soc Nephrol. 2004;15(2):241–50.
21. Corwin HL, Schwartz MM, Lewis EJ. The importance of sample size in the interpretation of the renal biopsy. Am J Nephrol. 1988;8(2):85–9.

Interpretation of Serologic Testing in Glomerular Diseases

8

Kelly V. Liang and Kimberly P. Liang

Case

A 69-year-old Caucasian male was admitted to the hospital with progressive dyspnea, decreased urine output, and hemoptysis and was found to have anemia, acute kidney injury, and bilateral pulmonary infiltrates. Antibodies to cytoplasmic antinuclear cytoplasmic antibody (c-ANCA) and proteinase 3 (anti-PR3 Ab) were positive, and perinuclear antinuclear cytoplasmic antibody (p-ANCA) and antibodies to myeloperoxidase (anti-MPO Ab) were negative. A diagnosis of Wegener granulomatosis (WG) was made. His course was complicated by respiratory failure and renal failure requiring hemodialysis. Treatment consisted of cyclophosphamide (CYC), corticosteroids, plasmapheresis, and intravenous immunoglobulin (IVIG). Ultimately, dialysis was discontinued, and serum creatinine level (Cr) was stabilized at 1.6–1.8 g/dL 4 months after presentation. After 6 months, immunosuppression was changed from CYC to azathioprine, and prednisone was tapered and discontinued after 1 year.

Fifteen months after the initial presentation, the patient was seen in clinic for routine follow-up. At that time, Cr was 1.61 g/dL, and anti-PR3 Ab was still positive.

What is the sensitivity and specificity of these autoantibodies in the diagnosis of vasculitides?

What is the utility of monitoring serial c-ANCA, p-ANCA, anti-PR3, and anti-MPO antibodies?

Do elevations in these autoantibodies predict flares of vasculitis?

Overview of Serologic Tests for Glomerulonephritis

Serologic Testing for Nephrotic Syndrome

As discussed in a prior chapter, nephrotic syndrome may be caused by primary glomerular diseases (typically minimal change disease, idiopathic membranous nephropathy, and primary focal segmental glomerulosclerosis) or secondary systemic diseases. Various serologic tests are routinely ordered to help exclude secondary causes of nephrotic syndrome [1]. Common laboratory tests for nephrotic syndrome are summarized in Table 8.1, along with the disorders suggested by abnormal tests [1, 2]. Although serologic tests are useful in narrowing the differential diagnosis, a renal biopsy is necessary to determine a definitive diagnosis and offers additional prognostic information.

K.V. Liang, M.D. (✉)
Renal-Electrolyte Division, Department of Medicine, University of Pittsburgh, A915 Scalfe Hall, 3550 Terrace Street, Pittsburgh, PA 15261, USA
e-mail: liangk@upmc.edu

K.P. Liang, M.D.
Rheumatology Division, Department of Medicine, University of Pittsburgh, Pittsburgh, PA 15261, USA

E.V. Lerma and M. Rosner (eds.), *Clinical Decisions in Nephrology, Hypertension and Kidney Transplantation*, DOI 10.1007/978-1-4614-4454-1_8, © Springer Science+Business Media New York 2013

Table 8.1 Serologic evaluation of nephrotic syndrome in adults [1, 56]

Laboratory test	Suggestive disorder
Serum protein electrophoresis (with immunofluorescence) Urine protein electrophoresis (with immunofluorescence)	Monoclonal protein disorder, e.g., primary amyloidosis, light chain deposition disease, multiple myeloma
Anti-streptococcal antibodies (antistreptolysin O antibody, anti-DNAse B, antihyaluronidase)	Poststreptococcal glomerulonephritis (GN) or postinfectious GN
Cryoglobulin	Mixed cryoglobulinemia
Syphilis serology	Membranous nephropathy secondary to syphilis
Hepatitis B and C virus serology	Membranous nephropathy secondary to hepatitis B Membranoproliferative GN secondary to hepatitis C
Human immunodeficiency virus (HIV) serology	Focal segmental glomerulosclerosis (FSGS), usually collapsing variant (commonly presents with severe nephrotic syndrome and renal dysfunction and may rapidly progress to end-stage renal disease)
Fasting plasma glucose and hemoglobin A1c (HbA1c)	Diabetic nephropathy (nodular glomerulosclerosis) secondary to diabetes mellitus

Table 8.2 Kidney diseases featuring hypocomplementemia [56, 57]

Lupus nephritis
Acute poststreptococcal GN or postinfectious GN
GN associated with subacute bacterial endocarditis
"Shunt" nephritis
Cryoglobulinemia
Membranoproliferative GN
Atheroemboli
Hereditary or acquired complement deficiencies
Heavy chain deposition disease

GN glomerulonephritis

Serologic Testing for Nephritic Syndrome (Acute Glomerulonephritis)

Similar to nephrotic syndrome, acute glomerulonephritis (GN) may represent a primary renal disease or secondary systemic disease. In combination with the history and physical examination, serologic studies can be helpful in narrowing the differential diagnosis. In particular, serum complement levels can direct the initial approach to patients presenting with acute GN. Low complement levels suggest activation of complement pathway(s) (classical, alternative, or mannose-binding lectin complement pathways), leading to consumption of C3 and/or C4 in excess of production of complement components. However, normal serum complement levels do not necessarily exclude complement activation because production of complement components may match the consumption rate. Therefore, repeated measurements may be useful. With persistent hypocomplementemia, the differential diagnosis includes systemic diseases such as systemic lupus erythematosis (SLE), subacute bacterial endocarditis (SBE), cryoglobulinemia, shunt nephritis, or postinfectious glomerulonephritis or a primary glomerular disease such as membranoproliferative GN (MPGN). Table 8.2 outlines systemic and renal diseases classified according to low or normal serum complement levels [3].

A number of additional antibodies and serologies provide significant diagnostic information in patients presenting with acute GN. In particular, pulmonary–renal syndromes may be differentiated by the presence of autoantibodies that play a pathogenetic role in diseases such as Goodpasture's syndrome, Wegener granulomatosis (WG) (more recently referred to as granulomatosis with polyangiitis [Wegener's] [4]), microscopic polyangiitis (MPA), Churg–Strauss syndrome (CSS), and renal-limited vasculitis (RLV) [5, 6]. Table 8.3 outlines the types of GN suggested by various abnormal serologic tests [2, 3].

Table 8.3 Serologic evaluation of nephritic syndrome in adults [2, 3]

Laboratory test	Suggestive disorder
C3, C4, CH_{50}	Helpful in narrowing diagnostic possibilities (see Table 8.2)
Anti-glomerular basement membrane (GBM) antibodies	Goodpasture's syndrome or anti-GBM disease
Anti-double-strand DNA (dsDNA) antibodies	Systemic lupus erythematosus (SLE)
Cryoglobulins	Cryoglobulinemia
Hepatitis B and C serology	Mixed cryoglobulinemia
Blood cultures	Subacute bacterial endocarditis Acute poststreptococcal GN or postinfectious GN
Anti-streptozyme antibodies	Acute poststreptococcal GN or postinfectious GN
Antineutrophil cytoplasmic antibodies (ANCA)	Goodpasture's syndrome Wegener granulomatosis (WG) (or Granulomatosis with Polyangiitis [Wegener's]) Microscopic polyangiitis (MPA) Churg–Strauss syndrome (CSS) Renal-limited vasculitis (RLV)

Serologic Testing in Anti-glomerular Basement Membrane Disease (Goodpasture's Syndrome)

Anti-glomerular basement membrane (GBM) antibodies suggest Goodpasture's syndrome if pulmonary involvement is present (pulmonary–renal syndrome) or anti-GBM disease if only renal involvement is apparent. Anti-GBM antibodies target the non-collagenous (NC1) domain of the alpha-3 chain of type IV collagen (α3 ([V]) NC1) found in the aspect of the lamina densa of the GBM in the kidney and alveolar basement membrane in the lung [6]. The characteristic immunofluorescence finding on renal biopsy in anti-GBM disease is diffuse, intense linear staining for IgG, especially IgG1 and IgG4. Antibody–antigen interactions as well as autoreactive T-cell activation leads to an inflammatory response resulting in proliferative GN, breaks in the GBM, and extracapillary proliferation with crescent formation [7, 8]. In the lungs, this inflammatory response produces pulmonary hemorrhage and hemoptysis. Although approximately 90% of patients with anti-GBM disease or Goodpasture's syndrome have circulating anti-GBM antibodies [9], the antibody level does not necessarily correlate with pulmonary or renal disease activity and decreases over time in most patients [7, 8, 10]. In addition, up to 5–10% of patients who undergo kidney transplantation for Alport's syndrome develop anti-GBM disease in the allograft [11, 12].

While most other serologic studies are negative or normal in Goodpasture's syndrome, 10–38% of patients will exhibit positivity for both anti-GBM antibodies and ANCA, with most having positivity for anti-MPO antibody. Several studies suggest that the disease course in patients who are double positive for anti-GBM antibodies and ANCA is similar to those who have anti-GBM disease, with a much poorer prognosis in those with severe renal failure than those who are only ANCA-positive [5, 13]. However, other studies have reported that double positive dialysis-dependent patients are still more likely to recover renal function than those with only anti-GBM antibody positivity [14–17]. Treatment for double positive patients generally is the same as that for anti-GBM disease, including high-dose steroids, CYC, and plasmapheresis. Therefore, in patients presenting with rapidly progressive crescentic GN, it is important to test for both anti-GBM antibodies and ANCA because of the potential implications for both treatment and prognosis.

Serologic Testing in ANCA-Associated Vasculitis

Antineutrophil cytoplasmic antibodies are frequently positive in the small-vessel vasculitides including WG, MPA, CSS, and RLV, with the majority of patients testing positive for either c-ANCA or p-ANCA. WG and MPA often present with pulmonary–renal syndrome while CSS is typically associated with asthma. All of these disorders may be associated with leukocytoclastic vasculitis, a skin finding characterized by "palpable purpura," raised petechiae or purpura which do not blanch upon palpation. Most commonly, WG patients are positive for c-ANCA (typically anti-PR3 Ab), whereas MPA patients are positive for p-ANCA (anti-MPO Ab). However, these autoantibodies are not mutually exclusive, and approximately 15–20% of patients with ANCA-associated vasculitis (AAV) are negative for ANCA.

WG commonly presents with necrotizing pauci-immune GN, leading to renal failure. ANCA (usually c-ANCA and anti-PR3 Ab) is positive in 90–95% with WG, which is diagnosed based on the following American College of Rheumatology (ACR) 1990 Criteria [18]: (1) nasal or oral inflammation (painful or painless oral ulcers, purulent or bloody nasal discharge), (2) abnormal chest X-ray (nodules, fixed infiltrates, cavities, etc.), (3) abnormal urinary sediment (microscopic hematuria or RBC casts), and (4) biopsy showing granulomatous inflammation in the artery or perivascular area. The presence of at least two of these four criteria provides 88% sensitivity and 92% specificity for the diagnosis of WG.

Like WG, MPA is also a necrotizing small-vessel vasculitis that presents with pauci-immune GN, commonly progressing to renal failure. Unlike WG, MPA presents without upper airway respiratory involvement and instead is characterized by pulmonary capillaritis leading to pulmonary hemorrhage in patients with pulmonary involvement [19]. Granulomatous inflammation is absent on biopsy. In MPA, 70–80% of patients are ANCA-positive, which are usually p-ANCA and anti-MPO Ab rather than c-ANCA and anti-PR3 Ab.

In contrast to MPA, patients with polyarteritis nodosa (PAN), which is a vasculitis of medium-sized arteries, are generally ANCA-negative. Since PAN spares small vessels, it does not present clinically with a necrotizing pauci-immune crescentic GN as seen in the other small-vessel AAVs. Rather, PAN presents with renal infarcts, renal artery vasculitis, and visceral microaneurysms [19].

While CSS also may present with necrotizing pauci-immune GN, the diagnosis is based on the following ACR criteria [20]: (1) asthma (history of wheezing), (2) eosinophilia (>10%), (3) mononeuropathy (multiplex) or polyneuropathy, (4) migratory or transient pulmonary opacities, (5) paranasal sinus abnormality, and (6) biopsy showing eosinophils in extravascular areas and granulomatous inflammation. The presence of at least four of these six criteria provides 85% sensitivity and 99.7% specificity for the diagnosis of CSS. The proportion of patients with ANCA positivity ranges from 20 to 80% in various studies. Approximately 75% of ANCA-positive patients with CSS demonstrate positive p-ANCA (anti-MPO Ab) though some cases are positive for c-ANCA [21–23]. Studies have shown conflicting results for a correlation between ANCA titers and clinical disease activity, and ANCA titers may remain positive despite clinical remission [23, 24]. In addition to ANCA titers, other helpful laboratory markers include the presence of eosinophilia (as high as 50% of the total peripheral leukocyte count), elevated erythrocyte sedimentation rate (ESR), both of which may correlate with disease activity [9]. Elevated serum IgE levels and IgE-containing circulating immune complexes (CIC) are often found, whereas serum complement, hepatitis markers, ANA, and cryoglobulins are usually negative [25–28].

RLV presents as a crescentic necrotizing pauci-immune GN commonly leading to renal failure. Because inflammation is limited to the kidneys, the pulmonary and other systemic disease manifestations present in WG, MPA, and CSS are absent. In RLV, ANCA is positive in 80–100% and is usually p-ANCA (anti-MPO Ab) [1, 19].

ANCA Assays

ANCA serology may be tested using two different assays: (1) indirect immunofluorescence (IIF) and (2) enzyme-linked immunosorbent assay (ELISA) [29]. IIF uses alcohol fixed buffy coat leukocytes and distinguishes between c-ANCA vs. p-ANCA. C-ANCA staining by IIF shows heavy staining in the cytoplasm while the multilobulated nuclei are nonreactive. p-ANCA staining by IIF shows staining limited to the perinuclear region while the cytoplasm remains nonreactive. This test is considered more sensitive but less specific for the AAVs. In contrast, the ELISA is more specific for AAVs and uses purified specific antigens to distinguish between anti-PR3 vs. anti-MPO antibodies. Using a combination of IIF and ELISA testing for ANCA increases the sensitivity of AAV diagnosis; hence, it is most useful to obtain serologic tests for ANCA assays using both IIF (c-ANCA/p-ANCA) and ELISA (anti-PR3/anti-MPO) [30]. For this reason, some laboratories currently will run the more sensitive IIF assay first (c-ANCA/p-ANCA), and then if positive, the corresponding ELISA tests (anti-PR3/anti-MPO) will be tested automatically. Moreover, the predictive value of ANCA testing varies based on the clinical presentation and is most useful for excluding pauci-immune crescentic GN (PI-CGN) in patients who present with milder degrees of renal dysfunction, while positive ANCA serologies are most useful in confirming PI-CGN in those with more severe renal failure and rapidly progressive GN [29, 31].

In addition to the AAVs, ANCA are associated with a number of other diseases besides anti-GBM disease as discussed previously. Drug-induced ANCA-associated vasculitis can occur with propylthiouracil, hydralazine, and minocycline, among others. Table 8.4 shows other ANCA and disease associations in addition to the vasculitides [29].

Table 8.4 ANCA disease associations [29]

Disease (% positivity)	Typical ANCA pattern
Wegener's granulomatosis (WG) (90–95%)	c-ANCA (PR3)
Microscopic polyangiitis (MPA) (70–80%)	p-ANCA (MPO)
Churg–Strauss syndrome (CSS) (20–70%)	p-ANCA (MPO)
Renal-limited vasculitis (RLV) (80–100%)	p-ANCA (MPO)
Anti-GBM disease (10–40%)	p-ANCA (MPO)
Drug-induced AAV Drugs for hyperthyroidism Propylthiouracil (PTU) Methimazole Carbimazole Hydralazine Antibiotics Minocycline Rifampicin Cefotaxime Isoniazid Penicillamine Allopurinol Procainamide Thiamazole Clozapine Phenytoin Indomethacin Tumor necrosis factor (TNF) inhibitors (e.g., infliximab, adalimumab, etanercept) [58]	p-ANCA (MPO, elastase, lactoferrin), rarely c-ANCA (PR3)
Nonvasculitic rheumatic disorders Rheumatoid arthritis Systemic lupus erythematosus Inflammatory myopathies Juvenile chronic arthritis Reactive arthritis Relapsing polychondritis Scleroderma Antiphospholipid syndrome	p-ANCA or atypical patterns[a]
Autoimmune gastrointestinal disorders (60–80%) Inflammatory bowel disease Primary sclerosing cholangitis Autoimmune hepatitis	p-ANCA
Cystic fibrosis	ANCA against bactericidal/permeability-increasing protein (BPI)

[a]Atypical ANCA patterns may be due to antibodies directed against lactoferrin, elastase, cathepsin G, bactericidal/permeability-increasing protein (BPI), among others [30]

ANCA Testing and Disease Flares

Whether rises in ANCA titers predict disease flares in AAV has been a longstanding controversy.

One of the largest and most rigorous studies evaluating this question was a prospective, observational cohort study of 156 patients with WG enrolled in a clinical treatment trial during periods of active disease [32]. Serum samples were drawn and ANCA assays performed at 3-month intervals. Overall, ANCA levels were only weakly associated with disease activity across patients, with changes in ANCA levels explaining less than 10% of the variation in disease activity. Decreases in ANCA levels were not significantly associated with shorter time to remission, and increases in ANCA levels were not associated with relapse. The proportion of patients who experienced relapses within 1 year of an elevation in ANCA titer was only about 40%. However, other studies have suggested that persistently high or rising titers of ANCA are associated with increased risk for disease relapse [33, 34]. Even in these studies, however, the relationship between the onset of rising ANCA titer and disease flare was not strong. In a prospective study of 100 ANCA-positive patients followed for 2 years, relapse did not occur in 43% of those with a rise in ANCA titers and in 29% of those with anti-PR3 antibodies, [33]. Generally, if a patient was ANCA-positive during disease activity, ANCA-negativity is consistent with disease remission. However, persistent ANCA-negativity does not definitely indicate disease remission in all cases, as shown by a study which reported that 13 of 37 patients with AAV having flares were ANCA-negative at the time of relapse [33]. Therefore, monitoring of ANCA titers may be useful in following patients, but decisions to alter immunosuppressive therapy should take into consideration whether clear clinical signs of active disease are present [29].

Serologic Testing in Lupus Nephritis

Lupus nephritis (LN) is characterized by changes in several serologic markers, including high titers of anti-dsDNA antibodies (Ab), antinuclear Ab (ANA), low serum complement levels, and high levels of anti-C1q antibodies. These parameters are useful adjuncts to other clinical signs of LN such as elevated creatinine and the presence of hematuria, particularly dysmorphic red blood cells and red blood cell casts, on urinalysis. Approximately 70–80% of patients with active SLE have high-avidity IgG anti-dsDNA Ab [35]. There is a well-recognized association of high titers of IgG anti-dsDNA antibodies and nephritic activity, lending support for its utility in monitoring for LN disease activity [36–41]. In addition, anti-dsDNA Ab have been found in glomerular deposits of immune complexes in renal biopsies of subjects with active LN, which underscores a pathogenic role for these antibodies in LN [38, 42]. However, some studies have reported exceptions to this correlation, suggesting that elevated anti-dsDNA Ab is not a pre-requisite for disease flare [42, 43]. This phenomenon may be attributable to current sensitive assays that may be more likely to detect low avidity antibodies, which previously would have been missed and may not be as highly associated with disease flares.

The methods currently used by clinical laboratories to quantitate anti-dsDNA Ab differ in the ability to detect high affinity and low affinity anti-dsDNA Ab [35, 44]. Anti-dsDNA Ab are found to be elevated in more patients with SLE when the assay used detects both high affinity and low affinity anti-dsDNA Ab [35]. The most specific assay for SLE and active LN (Farr assay) may miss milder forms of the disease in which patients have only low avidity anti-dsDNA [44, 45]. Despite this caveat, studies suggest that the Farr technique is superior to other techniques in correlating with measures of SLE global disease activity, as well as renal and vasculitis involvement [41, 45]. However, because the Farr method requires the use of a radioactive antigen, its routine use has been limited [35].

In addition to anti-dsDNA, anti-C1q antibodies have been shown to be associated with SLE and LN disease activity [46–50]. In a study of 38 patients with SLE undergoing renal biopsy for suspected LN, all but one patient with proliferative LN were positive for anti-C1q (97.2%) compared with 35% of control SLE patients with inactive LN and 25% of SLE patients without LN. Anti-C1q Ab strongly decreased with successful treatment. These findings suggest a pathogenic role of anti-C1q in LN [47]. More recent studies underscore the clinical utility of anti-C1q Ab by demonstrating positive correlations between anti-C1q Ab and global SLE activity scores, anti-dsDNA Ab, and anticardiolipin Ab, and negative correlations between anti-C1q Ab and complement levels [46, 50]. Specifically, anti-C1q Ab has been shown to have strong associations with LN [48, 49], being present in 60% of patients with LN vs. only 14% of SLE patients without LN, and in 89% of patients with active LN vs. 0% of patients with inactive nephritis [49]. Furthermore, it has been suggested that monitoring anti-C1q titers in SLE patients could be important for predicting renal flares [48].

Antiphospholipid Antibodies

Antiphospholipid Ab syndrome (APLS) is characterized by the presence of antibodies directed against either phospholipids or plasma proteins bound to anionic phospholipids. There are three main types of antiphospholipid (APL) antibodies: anticardiolipin Ab, lupus anticoagulant (LAC), and beta-2 glycoprotein I Ab. APLS may be either primary or secondary to other rheumatic diseases, infections, and drugs. Primary clinical features of APLS include venous and arterial thromboses, recurrent fetal losses, and thrombocytopenia, in association with positivity for APL Ab on at least two occasions checked at least 12 weeks apart [51]. Renal involvement is characterized by noninflammatory occlusion of renal blood vessels of various sizes, from glomerular capillaries to the main renal arteries and veins, and the typical histopathology resembles that seen in thrombotic microangiopathies, such as hemolytic uremic syndrome, thrombotic thrombocytopenic purpura, and scleroderma. Treatment for APLS and acute renal failure is the same as that in APLS not involving the kidneys. Moderate intensity anticoagulation with warfarin (target international normalized ratio (INR) 2.0–3.0) is the standard of care [52]. In addition, in patients with acute renal failure or catastrophic APLS, plasmapheresis and corticosteroids may be effective, along with chronic anticoagulation [53].

Patients on maintenance hemodialysis have a high prevalence of APLS, placing them at greater risk for vascular access thrombosis, particularly of arteriovenous grafts [54]. There is no association between the development of APLS and age, gender, or dialysis duration [55]. In patients with renal transplants, circulating APL Ab can damage the allograft if not treated with anticoagulation [54].

Case Revisited

The patient's Cr remained relatively stable at 1.6–1.7 g/dL, and proteinuria declined to <500 mg/day. Repeat serologic tests 4 months later showed decreased but still equivocally positive anti-PR3 Ab of 0.8 U. Azathioprine alone was continued as maintenance immunosuppression, and renal function progressively improved. Twenty-one months after initial presentation, Cr was 1.28 g/dL, and anti-PR3 Ab remained stable at 0.7 U.

Key Points

- Serologic testing is a useful adjunct to the clinical history and physical examination in the evaluation and management of glomerular disorders, including both nephrotic and nephritic syndromes, and should be obtained as part of the initial work-up of patients presenting with acute renal failure and/or nephrotic-range proteinuria.
- In a patient suspected to have Goodpasture's syndrome, both anti-GBM and ANCA serologies should be obtained.
- ANCA serologies are particularly useful to differentiate among the pulmonary–renal syndromes and small-vessel vasculitides. IIF (p-ANCA/c-ANCA) is more sensitive but less specific than ELISA (anti-MPO/anti-PR3); thus, a positive IIF result should be confirmed by obtaining ELISA as well.
- Although useful in the diagnosis and monitoring of disease activity in the small-vessel

vasculitides, fluctuations in ANCA titers should not be used to alter immunosuppressive therapy unless there are clear changes in clinical signs of active disease.
- Serologic markers characteristic of lupus nephritis are anti-dsDNA Ab, anti-C1q Ab, and low serum complement levels.

References

1. Rose B. Serologic tests in the evaluation of nephrotic syndrome. UpToDate [Webpage]. 2011; 18.3. Accessed January 28, 2011.
2. Jennette J, Falk R. Glomerular clinicopathologic syndromes. In: Greenberg A, editor. Primer on kidney diseases. 4th ed. Philadelphia, PA: Elsevier Saunders; National Kidney Foundation; 2005. p. 150–64.
3. Madaio MP, Harrington JT. The diagnosis of glomerular diseases: acute glomerulonephritis and the nephrotic syndrome. Arch Intern Med. 2001;161(1):25–34.
4. Falk RJ, Gross WL, Guillevin L, et al. Granulomatosis with Polyangiitis (Wegener's): an alternative name for Wegener's Granulomatosis. Arthritis Rheum. 2011;63(4):863–4.
5. Saxena R, Bygren P, Arvastson B, Wieslander J. Circulating autoantibodies as serological markers in the differential diagnosis of pulmonary renal syndrome. J Intern Med. 1995;238(2):143–52.
6. Jara LJ, Vera-Lastra O, Calleja MC. Pulmonary-renal vasculitic disorders: differential diagnosis and management. Curr Rheumatol Rep. 2003;5(2):107–15.
7. Pusey CD. Anti-glomerular basement membrane disease. Kidney Int. 2003;64(4):1535–50.
8. Kluth DC, Rees AJ. Anti-glomerular basement membrane disease. J Am Soc Nephrol. 1999;10(11):2446–53.
9. Brenner B. Brenner and Rector's the kidney. 8th ed. Philadelphia, PA: Elsevier; 2011.
10. Hudson BG. The molecular basis of Goodpasture and Alport syndromes: beacons for the discovery of the collagen IV family. J Am Soc Nephrol. 2004;15(10):2514–27.
11. Pettersson E, Tornroth T, Miettinen A. Simultaneous anti-glomerular basement membrane and membranous glomerulonephritis: case report and literature review. Clin Immunol Immunopathol. 1984;31(2):171–80.
12. Kalluri R, Weber M, Netzer KO, Sun MJ, Neilson EG, Hudson BG. COL4A5 gene deletion and production of post-transplant anti-alpha 3(IV) collagen alloantibodies in Alport syndrome. Kidney Int. 1994;45(3):721–6.
13. Levy JB, Hammad T, Coulthart A, Dougan T, Pusey CD. Clinical features and outcome of patients with both ANCA and anti-GBM antibodies. Kidney Int. 2004;66(4):1535–40.
14. Jayne DR, Marshall PD, Jones SJ, Lockwood CM. Autoantibodies to GBM and neutrophil cytoplasm in rapidly progressive glomerulonephritis. Kidney Int. 1990;37(3):965–70.
15. O'Donoghue DJ, Short CD, Brenchley PE, Lawler W, Ballardie FW. Sequential development of systemic vasculitis with anti-neutrophil cytoplasmic antibodies complicating anti-glomerular basement membrane disease. Clin Nephrol. 1989;32(6):251–5.
16. Weber MF, Andrassy K, Pullig O, Koderisch J, Netzer K. Antineutrophil-cytoplasmic antibodies and antiglomerular basement membrane antibodies in Goodpasture's syndrome and in Wegener's granulomatosis. J Am Soc Nephrol. 1992;2(7):1227–34.
17. Kalluri R, Meyers K, Mogyorosi A, Madaio MP, Neilson EG. Goodpasture syndrome involving overlap with Wegener's granulomatosis and anti-glomerular basement membrane disease. J Am Soc Nephrol. 1997;8(11):1795–800.
18. Leavitt RY, Fauci AS, Bloch DA, et al. The American College of Rheumatology 1990 criteria for the classification of Wegener's granulomatosis. Arthritis Rheum. 1990;33(8):1101–7.
19. Jennette JC, Falk RJ, Andrassy K, et al. Nomenclature of systemic vasculitides. Proposal of an international consensus conference. Arthritis Rheum. 1994;37(2):187–92.
20. Masi AT, Hunder GG, Lie JT, et al. The American College of Rheumatology 1990 criteria for the classification of Churg-Strauss syndrome (allergic granulomatosis and angiitis). Arthritis Rheum. 1990;33(8):1094–100.
21. Choi YH, Im JG, Han BK, Kim JH, Lee KY, Myoung NH. Thoracic manifestation of Churg-Strauss syndrome: radiologic and clinical findings. Chest. 2000;117(1):117–24.
22. Solans R, Bosch JA, Perez-Bocanegra C, et al. Churg-Strauss syndrome: outcome and long-term follow-up of 32 patients. Rheumatology (Oxford). 2001;40(7):763–71.
23. Sinico RA, Di Toma L, Maggiore U, et al. Prevalence and clinical significance of antineutrophil cytoplasmic antibodies in Churg-Strauss syndrome. Arthritis Rheum. 2005;52(9):2926–35.
24. Hellmich B, Gross WL. Recent progress in the pharmacotherapy of Churg-Strauss syndrome. Expert Opin Pharmacother. 2004;5(1):25–35.
25. Hellmich B, Ehlers S, Csernok E, Gross WL. Update on the pathogenesis of Churg-Strauss syndrome. Clin Exp Rheumatol. 2003;21(6 Suppl 32):S69–77.
26. Abril A, Calamia KT, Cohen MD. The Churg Strauss syndrome (allergic granulomatous angiitis): review and update. Semin Arthritis Rheum. 2003;33(2):106–14.
27. Lhote F, Guillevin L. Polyarteritis nodosa, microscopic polyangiitis, and Churg-Strauss syndrome. Clinical aspects and treatment. Rheum Dis Clin North Am. 1995;21(4):911–47.
28. Guillevin L, Cohen P, Gayraud M, Lhote F, Jarrousse B, Casassus P. Churg-Strauss syndrome. Clinical study and long-term follow-up of 96 patients. Medicine (Baltimore). 1999;78(1):26–37.

29. Stone JH. Clinical spectrum of antineutrophil cytoplasmic antibodies. UpToDate [Webpage]. 2011; 18.3. Accessed March 29, 2011.
30. Hagen EC, Daha MR, Hermans J, et al. Diagnostic value of standardized assays for anti-neutrophil cytoplasmic antibodies in idiopathic systemic vasculitis. EC/BCR Project for ANCA Assay Standardization. Kidney Int. 1998;53(3):743–53.
31. Jennette JC, Wilkman AS, Falk RJ. Diagnostic predictive value of ANCA serology. Kidney Int. 1998;53(3):796–8.
32. Finkielman JD, Merkel PA, Schroeder D, et al. Antiproteinase 3 antineutrophil cytoplasmic antibodies and disease activity in Wegener granulomatosis. Ann Intern Med. 2007;147(9):611–9.
33. Boomsma MM, Stegeman CA, van der Leij MJ, et al. Prediction of relapses in Wegener's granulomatosis by measurement of antineutrophil cytoplasmic antibody levels: a prospective study. Arthritis Rheum. 2000;43(9):2025–33.
34. Han WK, Choi HK, Roth RM, McCluskey RT, Niles JL. Serial ANCA titers: useful tool for prevention of relapses in ANCA-associated vasculitis. Kidney Int. 2003;63(3):1079–85.
35. Reichlin M. Antibodies to DNA, Sm, and RNP. UpToDate 2011; 19.1. Accessed April 17, 2011.
36. Hahn BH. Antibodies to DNA. N Engl J Med. 1998;338(19):1359–68.
37. ter Borg EJ, Horst G, Hummel EJ, Limburg PC, Kallenberg CG. Measurement of increases in anti-double-stranded DNA antibody levels as a predictor of disease exacerbation in systemic lupus erythematosus. A long-term, prospective study. Arthritis Rheum. 1990;33(5):634–43.
38. Schur PH, Sandson J. Immunologic factors and clinical activity in systemic lupus erythematosus. N Engl J Med. 1968;278(10):533–8.
39. Cervera R, Khamashta MA, Font J, et al. Systemic lupus erythematosus: clinical and immunologic patterns of disease expression in a cohort of 1,000 patients. The European Working Party on Systemic Lupus Erythematosus. Medicine (Baltimore). 1993;72(2):113–24.
40. Bootsma H, Spronk P, Derksen R, et al. Prevention of relapses in systemic lupus erythematosus. Lancet. 1995;345(8965):1595–9.
41. Nossent JC, Huysen V, Smeenk RJ, Swaak AJ. Low avidity antibodies to double stranded DNA in systemic lupus erythematosus: a longitudinal study of their clinical significance. Ann Rheum Dis. 1989;48(8):677–82.
42. Deshmukh US, Bagavant H, Fu SM. Role of anti-DNA antibodies in the pathogenesis of lupus nephritis. Autoimmun Rev. 2006;5(6):414–8.
43. Gladman DD, Urowitz MB, Keystone EC. Serologically active clinically quiescent systemic lupus erythematosus: a discordance between clinical and serologic features. Am J Med. 1979;66(2):210–5.
44. Smeenk RJ, van den Brink HG, Brinkman K, Termaat RM, Berden JH, Swaak AJ. Anti-dsDNA: choice of assay in relation to clinical value. Rheumatol Int. 1991;11(3):101–7.
45. Neogi T, Gladman DD, Ibanez D, Urowitz M. Anti-dsDNA antibody testing by Farr and ELISA techniques is not equivalent. J Rheumatol. 2006;33(9):1785–8.
46. Zhang CQ, Ren L, Gao F, Mu FY, You YQ, Liu YH. Anti-C1q antibodies are associated with systemic lupus erythematosus disease activity and lupus nephritis in northeast of China. Clin Rheumatol. 2011;30(7): 967–73.
47. Trendelenburg M, Lopez-Trascasa M, Potlukova E, et al. High prevalence of anti-C1q antibodies in biopsy-proven active lupus nephritis. Nephrol Dial Transplant. 2006;21(11):3115–21.
48. Marto N, Bertolaccini ML, Calabuig E, Hughes GR, Khamashta MA. Anti-C1q antibodies in nephritis: correlation between titres and renal disease activity and positive predictive value in systemic lupus erythematosus. Ann Rheum Dis. 2005;64(3):444–8.
49. Sinico RA, Radice A, Ikehata M, et al. Anti-C1q autoantibodies in lupus nephritis: prevalence and clinical significance. Ann N Y Acad Sci. 2005;1050:193–200.
50. Oelzner P, Deliyska B, Funfstuck R, Hein G, Herrmann D, Stein G. Anti-C1q antibodies and antiendothelial cell antibodies in systemic lupus erythematosus - relationship with disease activity and renal involvement. Clin Rheumatol. 2003;22(4–5):271–8.
51. Miyakis S, Lockshin MD, Atsumi T, et al. International consensus statement on an update of the classification criteria for definite antiphospholipid syndrome (APS). J Thromb Haemost. 2006;4(2):295–306.
52. Crowther MA, Ginsberg JS, Julian J, et al. A comparison of two intensities of warfarin for the prevention of recurrent thrombosis in patients with the antiphospholipid antibody syndrome. N Engl J Med. 2003;349(12):1133–8.
53. Kaplan AA. The use of apheresis in immune renal disorders. Ther Apher Dial. 2003;7(2):165–72.
54. Appel G. Antiphospholipid syndrome and the kidney. UpToDate [Webpage]. 2011. Accessed April 24, 2011.
55. Brunet P, Aillaud MF, San Marco M, et al. Antiphospholipids in hemodialysis patients: relationship between lupus anticoagulant and thrombosis. Kidney Int. 1995;48(3):794–800.
56. Madaio MP, Harrington JT. Current concepts. The diagnosis of acute glomerulonephritis. N Engl J Med. 1983;309(21):1299–302.
57. Nast C, Appel G. A Case of Lupus Nephritis. Clin J Am Soc Nephrol. 2008;3(1):296–306.
58. Saint Marcoux B, De Bandt M. Vasculitides induced by TNFalpha antagonists: a study in 39 patients in France. Joint Bone Spine. 2006;73(6):710–3.

Part III

Fluid and Electrolyte Disorders

Hyponatremia

9

Cynthia M. Cooper

Case

A 29-year-old woman with a history of depression, treated with fluoxetine, presents with a 1 month history of increasing lethargy and 1 week history of altered mental status with slurred speech and confusion. Her family reports that the woman is obsessed with her body image and that she has been trying to lose weight by vomiting each morning and drinking more than 2 gallons of water a day to curb her appetite. In the emergency room, she is found to be somnolent, waking only briefly to stimulation. Her vital signs are normal with a heart rate of 65 bpm and blood pressure of 117/56 mmHg. Pupils are equal and responsive. Face is symmetric. She withdraws all limbs symmetrically to noxious stimuli. Serum sodium is 121 mmol/L. Urine sodium is <10 mmol/L. Urine osmolality is 60 Osm/L.

Hyponatremia is defined as a serum sodium concentration of <135 mmol/L and is the most common electrolyte abnormality in hospitalized patients. Mild hyponatremia (<135 mmol/L) occurs in 15–22% of these patients. Moderate hyponatremia (<130 mmol/L) occurs in 1–7% of hospitalized patients and more severe degrees of hyponatremia (<125 mmol/L) in < 1% [1–4].

C.M. Cooper, M.D. (✉)
Inpatient Clinician Educator Unit, Department of Medicine, Massachusetts General Hospital, 55 Fruit Street, Boston, MA 02114, USA
e-mail: ccooper1@partners.org

Pathophysiology

Water shifts between intracellular and extracellular spaces to balance total body osmolality. The main extracellular osmoles are sodium salts, e.g., NaCl and $NaHCO_3$, with a smaller contribution of glucose and urea (serum osmolality (millimoles per kilogram of water) = 2 × sodium + glucose/18 + blood urea nitrogen/2.8) [5, 6]. The main intracellular osmoles are potassium salts. The serum sodium concentration, unlike intracellular potassium concentration, can be clinically measured and reflects the distribution of water between the intracellular and extracellular spaces to balance osmoles [7, 8]. Thus, hyponatremia may be due to excessive solute loss or to a gain of water.

Most commonly, hyponatremia is due to the intake and subsequent retention of water, resulting in dilution of total body osmoles, e.g., hypoosmolar hyponatremia. Hyponatremia may also occur due to water shifting between the intracellular and extracellular spaces in response to an effective extracellular osmole, e.g., hyperosmolar hyponatremia.

Hypoosmolar hyponatremia occurs with the addition of electrolyte-free water in excess of electrolyte-free water loss. A key point is that the development of hypoosmolar hyponatremia requires the addition of water through intake [7]. Impaired water clearance alone, e.g., through diminished renal water clearance, is not sufficient to produce hyponatremia. Patients with anuric end-stage renal disease, the extreme example of

E.V. Lerma and M. Rosner (eds.), *Clinical Decisions in Nephrology, Hypertension and Kidney Transplantation*, DOI 10.1007/978-1-4614-4454-1_9, © Springer Science+Business Media New York 2013

impaired renal water clearance, will not develop hyponatremia without water intake.

The body has a daily obligate water loss through sweat and transdermal evaporative losses. Under usual conditions, the volume of sweat is about 500–700 mL/day, with a highly variable sodium concentration of 20–60 mEq/L, in adults [9]. These losses are increased by fever, exercise, and dermatologic conditions, e.g., erythroderma or burns, which increase dermal water losses. Gastrointestinal losses of fluid with electrolyte concentrations less than serum, e.g. vomiting or osmotic diarrheas, also lead to increased water loss. In both health and disease, without water intake, the body will lose total body water and become hypernatremic. Thus the development of hyponatremia necessarily must include the addition of water to the body, either through a patient's own water intake or through the administration of electrolyte-free water through medications, intravenous fluids, or intracorporeal procedures (e.g., hysteroscopy, cystoscopy).

The body defends its tonicity through tight control of water loss through the kidney. Osmoregulator neurons in the posterior hypothalamus respond to minute increases in osmolality by secreting arginine vasopressin or antidiuretic hormone (ADH). In response to a water load, ADH secretion is suppressed, allowing the dilute urine entering the collecting ducts of the kidneys to remain dilute through the terminal portions of the nephron [10]. With increases in osmolality, ADH is secreted and acts on the cells of the collecting ducts (through the vasopressin type-2 receptor) to allow intracellular aquaporins to fuse with the apical surface. The cells, now permeable to water, allow for the resorption of water down the medullary concentration gradient as the urine flows past these cells. This resorption results in maximally concentrated urine and limits the loss of free water from the system.

Clinical Consequences

The clinical consequences of hyponatremia all include neurological symptoms and reflect the sensitivity of the central nervous system to changes in cellular volume that occur with changes in extracellular osmolality. Severe acute hyponatremia (serum sodium <125 mmol/L) results in cellular edema and has severe and potentially fatal neurologic consequences. Patients can present with marked confusion, seizures, coma, and respiratory arrest. Milder symptoms of hyponatremia include mild encephalopathy, impaired memory, muscle cramps, and weakness. Chronic mild hyponatremia may be asymptomatic though several studies report an increased risk of falls and fractures in patients with chronic hyponatremia compared to those with normal serum sodium levels [11]. Recent data also links chronic hyponatremia to an increased risk for osteoporosis.

Chronic hyponatremia is a marker for morbidity and mortality in other systemic diseases including congestive heart failure and cirrhosis [12–14]. This is likely due to the fact that hyponatremia is a marker of more severe underlying disease.

Investigations

Hyponatremia exists when the ratio of serum sodium content, the numerator, over serum water content, the denominator, results in a serum sodium concentration of <135 mmol/L. Note that this concentration does not give clinical information about the etiology, physiologic impact, nor the absolute values of total body sodium or water content for a specific patient. Furthermore, in the vast majority of cases, hyponatremia reflects an abnormality of water handling.

In health, the body is able to maintain tonicity over a wide range of daily water intakes. As noted above, the body has an obligate water loss through the skin. This daily water loss is often increased in illness such that a minimum daily water intake is necessary to prevent hypernatremia. Conversely, the body in health has a huge capacity for electrolyte-free water clearance such that large volumes of water either through oral or other forms of intake can be quickly cleared through the production of dilute urine [8].

The first assessment in hyponatremia is the absence or presence of ADH effect assessed through measurement of the urine osmolality. Hyponatremia with a maximally dilute urine

(UOsm 50-70 mOsm/L) points to an etiology of water intoxication either through the patient's own intake or through the administration of intravenous water to a hospitalized patient.

ADHeffectispresentwithaUOsm>100mOsm/L. Patients with evidence of ADH effect can subsequently be characterized by volume status to assess the etiology of ADH secretion [1].

Hypovolemic Hyponatremia

ADH secretion is a physiologic response to marked hypovolemia. As Fig. 9.1 demonstrates, at normal blood volume, ADH secretion is suppressed when serum osmolality falls below 280 mOsm/L [15]. This threshold for suppression shifts to the left with increasing hypovolemia as cerebral baroreceptors stimulate ADH secretion despite normo- or hypotonicity. Most pathologic fluid losses are hypotonic or isotonic. As an example, both increased sweating due to fever and gastrointestinal losses due to vomiting or inflammatory diarrhea will result in hypernatremia in the absence of water intake. Note, also, that without water intake, isotonic volume loss due to hemorrhage or osmotic diarrhea, where osmoles and water are proportionately lost, will also ultimately result in hypernatremia due to ongoing obligate hypotonic losses. Thus, the development of hyponatremia in the setting of hypovolemia still requires the addition of water to the system through either oral or intravenous intake.

Hypervolemic Hyponatremia

Cerebral baroreceptors perceive effective arterial volume and respond to decreased stretch in the carotid arteries by lowering the osmotic threshold for ADH suppression (see above). In normal physiology, the perceived stretch in the carotid baroreceptors is an accurate surrogate for total body volume. This relationship, however, breaks down in the development of edematous states where carotid body stretch is diminished, not through true hypovolemia, but through derangements in the Starling forces which govern carotid artery stretch. Low effective arterial pressure of any etiology will result in non-osmotic ADH secretion and will limit the excretion of water. Congestive heart failure and cirrhosis both may result in low effective arterial pressure and, ultimately, hyponatremia due to retention of added water [16, 17].

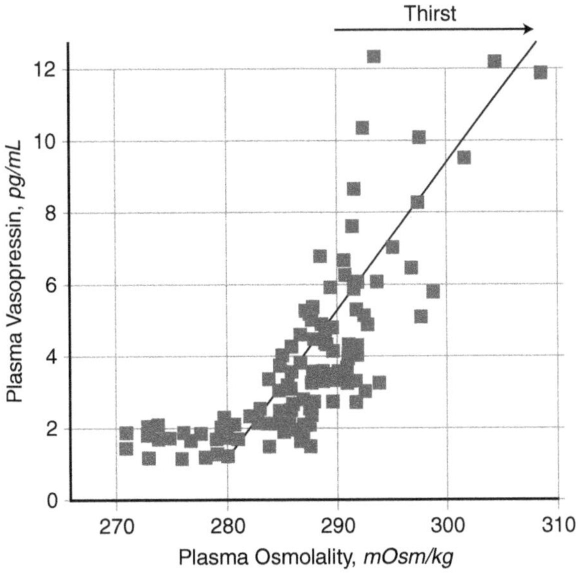

Fig. 9.1 The relationship of plasma vasopressin (adh) and thirst as a function of plasma osmolality. Reprinted from Am J Med, 72(2), robertson gl, aycinena p, zerbe rl., neurogenic disorders of osmoregulation, 339–53, copyright 1982, with permission from Elsevier

Normovolemic Hyponatremia

Water intoxication occurs when the intake of water outstrips the body's ability to excrete the water load. Normally, the kidneys are able to dilute the urine to an osmolality of ~60 mOsm/L and excrete 10–15 L of water a day given normal solute intake of ~600–900 mOsm/day. Rarely, a patient with psychosis may exceed this intake and, despite suppression of ADH and production of dilute urine, may become water intoxicated [18]. More commonly, patients with excessive water intake due to psychiatric disease also have abnormal ADH suppression with a higher urine osmolality for a given serum osmolality as compared to normal subjects [19, 20].

Malnourished patients or patients with poor dietary solute intake may develop hyponatremia with ingestion of smaller volumes of water. The kidney is unable to excrete pure water and, even at maximally dilute urine osmolality, requires that each liter of water have a "chaperone" of solute, primarily sodium, potassium, and urea. Patients with a diet that is primarily carbohydrate based, e.g., beer drinkers or tea-and-toast dieters, will have limited solute available to chaperone their water intake and will have impaired water excretion leading to hyponatremia [21].

The syndrome of inappropriate antidiuresis (SIAD) is defined as hyponatremia occurring in a clinically euvolemic patient with evidence of impaired water excretion, e.g., UOsm >100 mOsm/L [22]. Formal criteria have been developed and are detailed in Table 9.1.

In clinical practice, however, the distinction between hyponatremia due to extracellular volume depletion and SIAD is often uncertain and a trial of infusion of 1 L normal saline and assessment for correction in serum sodium is often necessary. In the case of volume depletion, the infusion of saline will lead to suppression of ADH secretion and a rise in serum sodium through excretion of free water in the urine. However, in those patients with SIAD and a urine osmoles of the infused solution are excreted in concentrated urine and free water is returned to the circulation through the actions of ADH on the collecting tubule.

Table 9.1 Diagnostic criteria for SIAD [22]

Essential features
Decreased effective osmolality (<280 mOsm/kg of water)
Urinary osmolality >100 mOsm/kg of water during hypotonicity
Clinical euvolemia
No clinical signs of volume depletion of extracellular fluid
No clinical signs of excessive volume of extracellular fluid
Urinary sodium >40 mmol/L with normal dietary salt intake
Normal thyroid and adrenal function
No recent use of diuretic agents
Supplemental features
Plasma uric acid <4 mg/dl
Blood urea nitrogen <10 mg/dl
Fractional sodium excretion >1%; fractional urea excretion >55%
Failure to correct hyponatremia after normal saline infusion
Correction of hyponatremia through fluid restriction
Abnormal result on test of water load
Elevated plasma AVP levels, despite the presence of hypotonicity and clinical euvolemia

Multiple drugs have been associated with the development of SIAD. A partial list is provided in Table 9.2.

In the absence of one of these drugs, a malignancy evaluation and a search for causes of CNS or pulmonary inflammation will demonstrate the etiology in most cases [23].

Management

Osmotic demyelination syndrome (ODS), previously called central pontine myelinolysis, is the feared complication of hyponatremia treatment [24]. Symptoms include lethargy and altered consciousness, mutism or dysarthria, spastic quadriparesis, and pseudobulbar palsy [25]. Retrospective reports of ODS point to rapid correction of hyponatremia (usually > 12 mmol/L in less than 24 h) as the common exposure predating its development [26]. The severity and duration of hyponatremia prior to correction are additional important risk factors.

Table 9.2 Drugs implicated in SIAD [22]

Nicotine
Chlorpropamide
Tolbutamide
Clofibrate
Cyclophosphamide
Ifosfamide
Vincristine
Narcotics
Barbiturates
Carbamazepine
Antipsychotics
Antidepressants
Acetaminophen
NSAIDs
MDMA ("ectasy")

Other factors which appear to increase the risk of ODS include malnutrition, alcoholism, cirrhosis, and hypokalemia.

Rate of Correction

The rate of correction of hyponatremia is based on two clinical decisions: symptoms and chronicity of the hyponatremia [27]. Patients with severe neurologic symptoms of hyponatremia, e.g., seizure or coma, should have their serum sodium rapidly raised by 1–2 mmol/L by infusing 3% saline. These recommended rates stem from data from case series given an absence of data from randomized trials. Most authorities concur that serum sodium should be raised until neurologic symptoms cease and that an increase in serum sodium of 4-5 mmol/L is sufficient to stop seizures and lower intracranial pressure.) is usually sufficient. The rate of correction should then be slowed to no faster than 0.5 mmol/L/h with a goal of no more than 8–10 mmol/L per 24 h [28].

In patient with chronic hyponatremia or hyponatremia of uncertain duration with minimal symptoms, the rate of correction should be much slower and can usually be achieved through limitation of water intake. As noted above, ongoing obligate hypotonic losses, e.g., through sweat, will raise the serum sodium concentration if water intake is less than this obligate loss. In patients with SIAD, the urinary osmolality provides the "ceiling" which dictates how much water the patient may take in without becoming hypotonic. For example, a urinary osmolality fixed at 300 mOsm/L, due to inappropriate ADH secretion, requires each liter of water to have a "chaperone" of 300 mOsm in order to be excreted. Patients who can increase their osmolal intake, typically through ingestion of salt and protein, will have sufficient osmolal "chaperones" to excrete their water intake and maintain a normal osmolality [8]. Arbitrarily choosing a fluid restriction rate of 1,000–1,500 mL/day is apt to fail as, in general, daily free water excretion will be less than this, especially if the urine is very concentrated. Providing fluids in excess of the daily free water loss will simply lower the serum sodium. Thus, an assessment of daily urine free water losses and assuming a value for non-renal free water loss is needed. Urine free water loss can be estimated by the following equation, which uses urine sodium, urine potassium, and plasma sodium to calculate the effective water clearance (utilizing urine electrolytes rather than urine osmolality reflects the effective water clearance as many of the osmotic particles found in the urine are not "effective" in the sense that they partition in all body compartments and do not determine the movement of fluid between body compartments (such as urea)):

$$\text{Urine free water loss} = \text{Urine volume}$$
$$(1 - (\text{Urine sodium} + \text{potassium}) / \text{plasma sodium})$$

For instance, if daily urine free water loss is 500 mL and non-renal water loss is 300 mL/day, then a fluid restriction less than 800 mL/day is required. Alternatively, a reasonable starting point is to restrict the water intake to 500 mL less than the daily urine output. Of note, if the urine sodium and potassium concentration is greater than the plasma sodium level, it is unlikely that fluid restriction will be successful. Compliance with such water restriction is difficult due the fact that thirst is stimulated and this leads to frequent failure of this therapy as the sole modality of sodium correction. Furthermore, even when effective, serum sodium values rise slowly and this therapy cannot be utilized for any patient with symptomatic hyponatremia (except as an adjunct).

Vaptan (Vasopressin Receptor Antagonists) Use

The vaptan drug class was developed to antagonize the effect of ADH in the kidney by blocking the vasopressin type 2 receptor [29]. Conivaptan was the first drug approved by the FDA for the treatment of euvolemic hyponatremia and hypervolemic hyponatremia in hospitalized patients. It is an intravenous drug which blocks both V1A (located on the vasculature and responsible for the vasopressor actions of ADH) and V2 receptors to lower urinary osmolality and increase urine volume [30]. Tolvaptan is an oral vaptan which selectively blocks V2 receptors [31]. They have both been shown in clinical trials to correct hyponatremia in SIADH and edematous states [32]. Tests of mental functioning improved after correction of hyponatremia in a tolvaptan trial. Neither drug has been shown to have a long-term effect on mortality [28].

Due to concern of its use leading to overly rapid correction of hyponatremia, conivaptan is only approved for use in hospitalized patients. Similarly, tolvaptan treatment should only be initiated or reinitiated in hospitalized patients. This restriction, along with the prohibitive cost of tolvaptan, ~$300/tablet, limit the utility of these drugs in clinical practice [33].

Case Revisited

The patient was admitted with hyponatremia in the setting of disordered eating and excessive water intake. Her urinary osmolality of 60 mmol/L is consistent with maximally dilute urine and, thus, no evidence of ADH activity. Clinically, she was euvolemic and her renal function was normal. She was diagnosed with euvolemic hyponatremia due to a combination of poor solute intake and excessive water ingestion. She was placed on a free water restriction and increased her dietary intake of sodium and protein through a supervised diet with special attention for signs of refeeding syndrome. Over the course of 72 h, her serum sodium increased to 135 mmol/L. She was transferred to an inpatient psychiatric bed for further treatment of her eating disorder.

References

1. Adrogue HJ, Madias NE. Hyponatremia. N Engl J Med. 2000;342(21):1581–9.
2. Anderson RJ, Chung HM, Kluge R, Schrier RW. Hyponatremia: a prospective analysis of its epidemiology and the pathogenetic role of vasopressin. Ann Intern Med. 1985;102(2):164–8.
3. Hawkins RC. Age and gender as risk factors for hyponatremia and hypernatremia. Clin Chim Acta. 2003;337(1–2):169–72.
4. Upadhyay A, Jaber BL, Madias NE. Incidence and prevalence of hyponatremia. Am J Med. 2006;119(7 Suppl 1):S30–5.
5. Milionis HJ, Liamis GL, Elisaf MS. The hyponatremic patient: a systematic approach to laboratory diagnosis. CMAJ. 2002;166(8):1056–62.
6. Gennari FJ. Current concepts. Serum osmolality. Uses and limitations. N Engl J Med. 1984;310(2): 102–5.
7. Rose BD. New approach to disturbances in the plasma sodium concentration. Am J Med. 1986;81(6): 1033–40.
8. Rose BD, Post TW. Clinical physiology of acid-base and electrolyte disorders. 5th ed. New York: McGraw-Hill, Medical Pub. Division; 2001.
9. McSwiney BA. The composition of human perspiration (Samuel Hyde Memorial Lecture): (Section of Physical Medicine). Proc R Soc Med. 1934;27(7): 839–48.
10. Schrier RW, Berl T, Anderson RJ. Osmotic and nonosmotic control of vasopressin release. Am J Physiol. 1979;236(4):F321–32.
11. Renneboog B, Musch W, Vandemergel X, Manto MU, Decaux G. Mild chronic hyponatremia is associated with falls, unsteadiness, and attention deficits. Am J Med. 2006;119(1):71. e1–8.
12. Bettari L, Fiuzat M, Felker GM, O'Connor CM. Significance of hyponatremia in heart failure. Heart Fail Rev. 2012 Jan; 17(1):17–26.
13. Chawla A, Sterns RH, Nigwekar SU, Cappuccio JD. Mortality and serum sodium: do patients die from or with hyponatremia? Clin J Am Soc Nephrol. 2011;6(5):960–5.
14. Kim WR, Biggins SW, Kremers WK, et al. Hyponatremia and mortality among patients on the liver-transplant waiting list. N Engl J Med. 2008;359(10):1018–26.
15. Robertson GL, Aycinena P, Zerbe RL. Neurogenic disorders of osmoregulation. Am J Med. 1982;72(2): 339–53.

16. Schrier RW. Water and sodium retention in edematous disorders: role of vasopressin and aldosterone. Am J Med. 2006;119(7 Suppl 1):S47–53.
17. Martin PY, Schrier RW. Pathogenesis of water and sodium retention in cirrhosis. Kidney Int Suppl. 1997;59:S43–9.
18. Illowsky BP, Kirch DG. Polydipsia and hyponatremia in psychiatric patients. Am J Psychiatry. 1988;145(6): 675–83.
19. Gillum DM, Linas SL. Water intoxication in a psychotic patient with normal renal water excretion. Am J Med. 1984;77(4):773–4.
20. Goldman MB, Luchins DJ, Robertson GL. Mechanisms of altered water metabolism in psychotic patients with polydipsia and hyponatremia. N Engl J Med. 1988;318(7):397–403.
21. Sanghvi SR, Kellerman PS, Nanovic L. Beer potomania: an unusual cause of hyponatremia at high risk of complications from rapid correction. Am J Kidney Dis. 2007;50(4):673–80.
22. Ellison DH, Berl T. Clinical practice. The syndrome of inappropriate antidiuresis. N Engl J Med. 2007;356(20):2064–72.
23. Schrier RW, Bansal S. Diagnosis and management of hyponatremia in acute illness. Curr Opin Crit Care. 2008;14(6):627–34.
24. Laureno R, Karp BI. Myelinolysis after correction of hyponatremia. Ann Intern Med. 1997;126(1):57–62.
25. Sterns RH, Cappuccio JD, Silver SM, Cohen EP. Neurologic sequelae after treatment of severe hyponatremia: a multicenter perspective. J Am Soc Nephrol. 1994;4(8):1522–30.
26. Sterns RH, Hix JK. Overcorrection of hyponatremia is a medical emergency. Kidney Int. 2009;76(6): 587–9.
27. Adrogue HJ. Consequences of inadequate management of hyponatremia. Am J Nephrol. 2005;25(3): 240–9.
28. Sterns RH, Nigwekar SU, Hix JK. The treatment of hyponatremia. Semin Nephrol. 2009;29(3):282–99.
29. Verbalis JG. AVP receptor antagonists as aquaretics: review and assessment of clinical data. Cleve Clin J Med. 2006;73 Suppl 3:S24–33.
30. Yeates KE, Morton AR. Vasopressin antagonists: role in the management of hyponatremia. Am J Nephrol. 2006;26(4):348–55.
31. Schrier RW, Gross P, Gheorghiade M, et al. Tolvaptan, a selective oral vasopressin V2-receptor antagonist, for hyponatremia. N Engl J Med. 2006;355(20): 2099–112.
32. Schrier RW. The sea within us: disorders of body water homeostasis. Curr Opin Investig Drugs. 2007;8(4):304–11.
33. Sterns R, Hix J. Hyponatremia: vasopressin antagonists in hyponatremia: more data needed. Nat Rev Nephrol. 2011;7(3):132–3.

Potassium Disorders

10

Kambiz Zandi-Nejad

Case 1 (Hypokalemia)

A 25-year-old otherwise healthy female with history of chronic constipation is found to have chronic hypokalemia. She denies any other gastrointestinal symptoms including nausea, vomiting, or diarrhea. She denies taking any medications. Family history is unremarkable as is her physical examination. Her BMI is 29. Lab results show:

Serum: Na 134, K 2.9, Cl 96, Total CO_2 33, Mg 1.3, Osmolality 278

Urine: Na 55, K 45, Cl 70, Cr 105, Ca 4, Osmolality 340

What is the most likely cause of her hypokalemia?

What is the best way to treat her hypokalemia?

Case 2 (Hyperkalemia)

A 54-year-old male with type 2 diabetes, hypertension, and chronic kidney disease (CKD) is found to be hyperkalemic during a routine follow-up visit. He has no complaints except for some muscle and body aches for the past few weeks after he started exercising in a gym. He has started naproxen for these aches. His prescription medications have remained the same for the past 2 years and include lisinopril (20 mg daily), metoprolol succinate (50 mg daily), and atorvastatin (10 mg daily). He states that his diet has remained the same. His blood pressure (BP) has been controlled and his HbA1C has been in the 6.8–7.2 range in the past 2 years. His potassium levels have been in the 4.8–5.2 range for the past 2 years. His exam shows BP of 130/80 and a pulse of 68. He appears to be euvolemic and his physical exam is unremarkable.

Serum: Na 137, K 5.9, Cl 100, Total CO_2 26, BUN 28, Creatinine 1.8, eGFR 42, Osmolality 282, HbA1C 6.9%. Normal CK and liver function tests.

Urine: Na 70, K 25, Osmolality 480.

What are the contributing factors to his hyperkalemia?

What is the most likely cause of recent rise in potassium level?

Introduction and Epidemiology

Hypokalemia

Hypokalemia is defined as serum potassium level of less than 3.5 mmol/L. It is a common finding in both inpatient (up to 20%) and outpatient (up to 30%) settings; mild hypokalemia (potassium level of 3.0–3.5 mmol/L) constitutes about three quarters of the cases [1, 2]. Consequences of hypokalemia are primarily manifested in the cardiovascular system, muscles, and kidneys.

K. Zandi-Nejad, M.D., F.A.S.N. (✉)
Nephrology, Harvard Vanguard Medical Associates, Beth Israel Deaconess Medical Center, Harvard Medical School, 133 Brookline Avenue, Boston, MA 02215, USA
e-mail: kzandi@bidmc.harvard.edu

E.V. Lerma and M. Rosner (eds.), *Clinical Decisions in Nephrology, Hypertension and Kidney Transplantation*, DOI 10.1007/978-1-4614-4454-1_10, © Springer Science+Business Media New York 2013

Hypokalemia is associated with significant morbidity and mortality and may increase mortality by up to tenfold in inpatient settings (primarily due to cardiovascular consequences, specifically arrhythmias) [1].

Hyperkalemia

Hyperkalemia is defined as serum potassium level of > 5.5 mmol/L. Approximately 10% of patients with hyperkalemia have significant hyperkalemia defined as potassium level ≥ 6.0 mmol/L [3–5]. Hyperkalemia is seen in 1–10% of all patients, with a higher prevalence in patients with CKD and end stage renal disease (ESRD) in whom the risk is tripled by treatment with angiotensin-converting enzyme inhibitors (ACE-I) or angiotensin receptor blockers (ARB). Consequences of hyperkalemia are primarily manifested in muscles and cardiovascular system. Although hyperkalemia has been associated with a mortality rate of 14–43%, the risk of death from hyperkalemia is reduced as CKD progresses and has been attributed to yet to be determined cardiac adaptation to the persistently high levels of potassium [3, 4].

Physiology/Pathophysiology

The total body potassium content is estimated at ~3,500 mmol, of which about 98% is intracellular (~75% in skeletal muscle) and results in intracellular and extracellular fluid potassium concentrations of about 150 and 4 mmol/L, respectively.

Normal potassium balance is critical for the normal function of excitable tissues. The serum potassium level is thus tightly kept in the 3.5–5 mmol/L range by *internal* and *external* potassium balance despite wide variation in daily potassium intake (30–150 mmol per day) [3, 4, 6].

Internal potassium balance refers to the distribution of potassium between intracellular and extracellular fluids across cell membrane. It occurs in minutes and plays a crucial role in maintaining normal serum potassium levels particularly when large amounts of potassium enter the circulation and extracellular fluid over a short period.

The intracellular accumulation of potassium against its electrochemical gradient is mediated by Na/K-ATPase through an energy consuming process. Of particular importance is the skeletal muscle Na/K-ATPase, the abundance and activity of which are among the major determinants of internal potassium balance capacity. Thus, whereas hypokalemia causes a significant decrease in Na/K-ATPase activity and skeletal muscle potassium content, hyperkalemia increases Na/K-ATPase activity, and muscle potassium content. Potassium exits the cells primarily through potassium channels down the electrochemical gradient [3, 4].

Major factors affecting internal potassium balance are as follows.

Insulin: Stimulates potassium uptake by skeletal muscle, cardiac muscle, liver, and fat through Na/K-ATPase activation. Potassium lowering effects of insulin are important both postparandially and at baseline; lack of basal insulin increases serum potassium level by about 0.5 mmol/L in normal subjects [7].

Sympathetic nervous system: Stimulation of beta-2 adrenergic receptors increases potassium uptake by cells (liver and muscle cells), whereas alpha adrenergic stimulation blunts the ability to buffer increases in potassium level [3, 4].

Acid–base abnormalities: For any given change in pH, acidemia has a stronger effect than alkalemia; it is primarily limited to inorganic acidoses such NH_4Cl infusion. The effect of respiratory acidosis is less than that of inorganic acidoses. The effect of respiratory and metabolic alkaloses on internal potassium balance is modest and comparable [6].

Osmolality: Hyperosmolarity (hypertonicity of extracellular fluid) enhances potassium efflux. This is primarily due to movement of water out of the cells which not only carries potassium along (solvent drag) but also increases intracellular potassium concentration and potassium movement out of the cells down its electrochemical gradient [3, 4, 8, 9].

Exercise: Intracellular depletion of ATP stores results in the opening of potassium channels (normally inhibited by ATP) and potassium efflux; the magnitude of this effect depends on the degree of exercise but is usually small. Of note, this increase in extracellular potassium acts as an arteriolar vasodilator and increases local blood flow to the exercising muscle [8].

External potassium balance maintains potassium excretion equal to potassium intake and requires several hours to complete. This is the major mechanism responsible for long-term potassium homeostasis. In a healthy person in steady state about 90–95% of the daily potassium intake is eliminated through kidneys and the rest in the stool (~5–10%); potassium excretion in the stool significantly increases in CKD and in diarrheal conditions.

Potassium excretion by the kidney is mainly regulated at the distal part of the nephron, namely the cortical collecting duct (CCD) and the connecting segment (CNT), primarily by principal cells. Urine flow rate, distal sodium delivery, intraluminal charge, aldosterone, vasopressin, chronic acid–base disorders, and serum potassium concentration affect potassium excretion by kidney primarily through their effects on principal cells of CCD and CNT (Fig. 10.1) [6].

Clinical Presentation and Consequences

Hypokalemia

The signs and symptoms associated with hypokalemia depend on the degree of hypokalemia, the rapidity with which it has developed, and the potentiating factors. In general symptoms become manifest when the potassium level is < 3.0 mmol/L [9] and include

- Vasoconstriction related to reduced tissue metabolism and oxygen consumption associated with hypokalemia.
- Elevation in blood pressure likely due to a combination of vasoconstriction and sodium retention.
- Electrocardiogram (ECG) abnormalities and cardiac dysrhythmias include flattened T wave, prominent U wave (U waves with amplitude more than T waves), PR interval prolongation, increase in QRS duration, and supraventricular and ventricular ectopic rhythm. Of note, several causes of hypokalemia can cause concomitant hypomagnesemia (e.g., diuretics or diarrhea) which in turn increases the

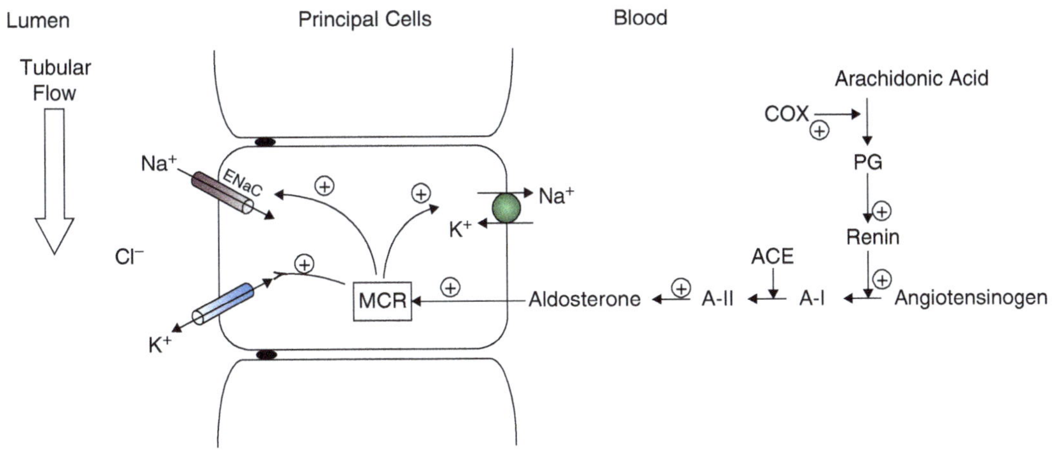

Fig. 10.1 Physiology of potassium handling by principal cells of distal nephron. *ENaC* epithelial sodium channel, *MCR* mineralocorticoid receptor, *A-I* angiotensin-I, *A-II* angiotensin-II, *ACE* angiotensin converting enzyme, *PG* prostaglandin, *COX* cyclooxygenase (Adapted with permission from Zandi-Nejad K, Tang CC. Disorders of potassium. In: McKean S, Bennett A, and Halasyamani L, editors. Hospital Medicine: Just the facts. New York: The McGraw-Hill; 2008. p. 484–494)

risk of dysrhythmias associated with hypokalemia.

Smooth muscle weakness manifesting as ileus, constipation, and urinary retention.

Skeletal muscle weakness which usually begins in the lower extremities (quadriceps muscle in particular) and advances upward to trunk, upper extremities, and respiratory muscles [9]. Of note, severe hypokalemia can result in rhabdomyolysis which in turn can increase potassium level and mask the underlying and initiating hypokalemia.

Kidneys may exhibit several functional and structural changes including increased ammoniogenesis (which occurs in proximal tubule cells and may be a contributing factor for hepatic encephalopathy in patients with advance liver disease), sodium retention, ESRD (aka hypokalemic nephropathy), and nephrogenic diabetes insipidus (NDI) [3, 4].

Reduction in insulin secretion which may play a role in thiazide-associated diabetes mellitus [10].

Hyperkalemia

The signs and symptoms associated with hyperkalemia depend on the degree of hyperkalemia, the rapidity with which it happens, and potentiating factors.

Skeletal muscle weakness tends to be flaccid, begins in lower extremities and progresses upward to involve trunk and upper extremity muscles including respiratory muscles . It should be remembered that muscle weakness may be due to a combination of hyperkalemia and underlying disease in familial hyperkalemic periodic paralysis.[4, 11]

ECG changes are usually seen with potassium level of more than 6.0 mmol/L and include tall, peaked, narrow-based T waves, prolonged PR interval, flattening of P waves, widening of the QRS complex, and finally sine waves due to eventual blending of QRS complex with T wave. Although these changes may be progressive, it is important to note that they may happen precipitously [6].

Impaired kidney acidifying ability due to interference with urinary excretion of ammonium (NH_4^+). Notably urinary (NH_4^+) excretion is increased in patients with type 4 RTA in response to the correction of hyperkalemia with an exchange resin [12, 13].

Approach and Investigation

Laboratory Tests

Initial laboratory tests should include complete blood count (CBC), electrolyte profile including calcium and magnesium, kidney function tests (BUN and creatinine), serum osmolality, and urine creatinine, osmolality, and electrolytes (Na^+, K^+, Cl^-).

Further laboratory investigation may be needed to diagnose the cause, which includes arterial blood gas, urinary pH, plasma renin activity, plasma aldosterone concentration, diuretic screen, and digoxin level (if applicable).

Transtubular Potassium Gradient

Transtubular potassium gradient (TTKG) is used to estimate potassium concentration and its gradient (urine to plasma) across the principal cells (at the end of CCD) and hence to assess the appropriateness of response of distal tubular potassium handling particularly by principal cells. It is calculated by using the following equation:

$$\text{TTKG} = [\text{urine potassium} / \text{plasma potassium}] / [\text{urine osmolality} / \text{plasma osmolality}]$$

It is valid only if the urine osmolality exceeds that of the plasma and if the urine sodium concentration is at least 25 mmol/L. Normal (or expected) values for TTKG vary and depend on the serum potassium level.

In patients with hypokalemia TTKG value of less than 2–3 is considered normal.

In patients with hyperkalemia TTKG value of more than 6–7 is considered normal.

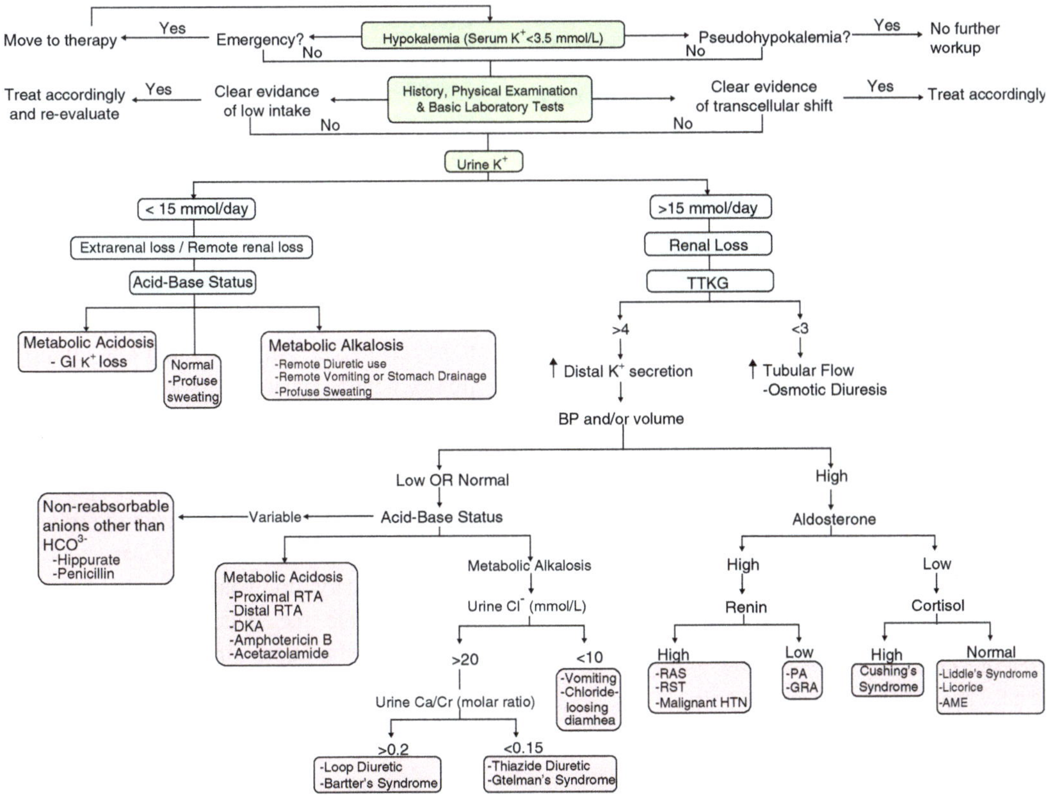

Fig. 10.2 Diagnostic approach to hypokalemia. *GI* gastrointestinal, *TTKG* transtubular potassium gradient, *BP* blood pressure, *RTA* renal tubular acidosis, *DKA* diabetic ketoacidosis, *RAS* renal artery stenosis, *RST* renin secreting tumor, *HTN* hypertension, *PA* primary aldosteronism, *GRA* glucocorticoid remediable aldosteronism, *AME* apparent mineralocorticoid excess (Adapted with permission from: Mount, DB, Zandi-Nejad, K. Disorders of potassium balance. In: Brenner BM, editor. Brenner and Rector's the kidney, 8th edition, Philadelphia, PA: W.B. Saunders; 2008)

Hypokalemia

The diagnosis of hypokalemia based on serum potassium level of ≤ 3.5 mmol/L is neither complete nor acceptable without the identification of the etiology. Although the cause of hypokalemia is usually obvious from the history, physical examination and basic laboratory tests, a systematic approach is preferred and will ascertain the etiology in most cases (Fig. 10.2) [3, 4].

1. The first step is to look for signs and symptoms suggestive of an emergency requiring immediate treatment such as progressive muscle weakness, ECG changes, dysrhythmias, and/or hepatic encephalopathy.
2. History should be directed at medications (diuretics, laxatives, antibiotics, chemotherapeutic agents, and beta-2 agonists), diet (e.g., low potassium intake, low calorie diet), dietary supplement (e.g., licorice), associated symptoms (e.g., vomiting, diarrhea), family history, and concomitant medical conditions (e.g., head injury, Cushing's syndrome). Timing and evolution of hypokalemia is of significant importance particularly in the inpatient setting; whereas it takes only minutes to hours to develop hypokalemia due to cellular shift, hypokalemia due to potassium loss usually requires days to develop.

   Physical examination should focus on blood pressure (including orthostatic blood

Table 10.1 Major causes of potassium shift into cells (Adapted with permission from Zandi-Nejad K, Tang CC. Disorders of potassium. In: McKean S, Bennett A, and Halasyamani L, editors. Hospital Medicine: Just the facts. New York: The McGraw-Hill; 2008. p. 484–494)

Insulin excess
Exogenous beta-2 adrenergic excess
Decongestants
Bronchodilators
Tocolytic agents
Endogenous beta-2 adrenergic excess
Head injury
Acute myocardial infarction
Alcohol withdrawal
Hypothermia
Hyperthyroidism
Theophylline
Caffeine
Barium intoxication
Cesium intoxication
Chloroquine intoxication
Verapamil intoxication
Familial hypokalemic periodic paralysis
Rapid and significant production of blood cells

pressure), volume status, and signs of associated disorders (e.g., Cushing's syndrome).

3. Rule out spurious hypokalemia. Spurious or pseudohypokalemia is a rare phenomenon usually seen in leukemic patients with high WBC count; it is due to potassium uptake by these cells at room temperature. Immediate separation of plasma/serum or immediate refrigeration of the sample will resolve the issue.
4. Transcellular redistribution with normal total body potassium content is next to consider (Table 10.1). The majority of these are due to increased cellular potassium uptake. However, inhibition of potassium efflux from cells may also cause hypokalemia (e.g., barium intoxication). Of note, excessive endogenous catecholamine release seen with stressful conditions such as head injury, acute myocardial infarction, and alcohol withdrawal should not be overlooked.
5. Hypokalemia associated with total potassium deficit may be due potassium loss through renal or non-renal routes. Urinary potassium excretion is important in differentiating the renal from non-renal potassium loss. In the presence of hypokalemia, daily urinary potassium excretion of more than 15 mmol is highly suggestive of renal potassium loss (Fig 10.2).
6. Extrarenal potassium loss is mainly due to gastrointestinal (GI) potassium loss or excessive sweating.

   The relatively high potassium content of lower GI tract explains hypokalemia seen with lower GI losses (both infectious and noninfectious), which is usually associated with metabolic acidosis (due to bicarbonate loss).

   The potassium content of gastric fluid is rather low and about 6-8 mmol/L. Thus hypokalemia associated with nasogastric suctioning or vomiting is mainly due to increased urinary potassium loss secondary to volume contraction and hypochloremic metabolic alkalosis associated with these conditions (in part driven by high aldosterone levels).

   Normal sweat contains only about 5–10 mmol/L of potassium (average of ~9 mmol/L). However, it may cause hypokalemia in conditions associated with excessive sweating. One such condition is intense physical exertion in hot climate in which sweat secretion may exceed 12 L/day.
7. Renal potassium loss: Although potassium loss by kidneys involves several mechanisms, it is mainly due to excessive potassium secretion by principal cells in the connecting segment and cortical collecting tubule of the distal nephron (Fig 10.3) [4, 6].

Hyperkalemia

The diagnosis of hyperkalemia based on serum potassium level of ≥ 5.5 mmol/L is neither complete nor acceptable without the identification of the etiology. Although the cause of hyperkalemia is usually multifactorial and obvious from the history, physical examination, and basic laboratory tests, a systematic approach is preferred and will help to ascertain the etiology in most cases (Fig 10.4) [3, 4].

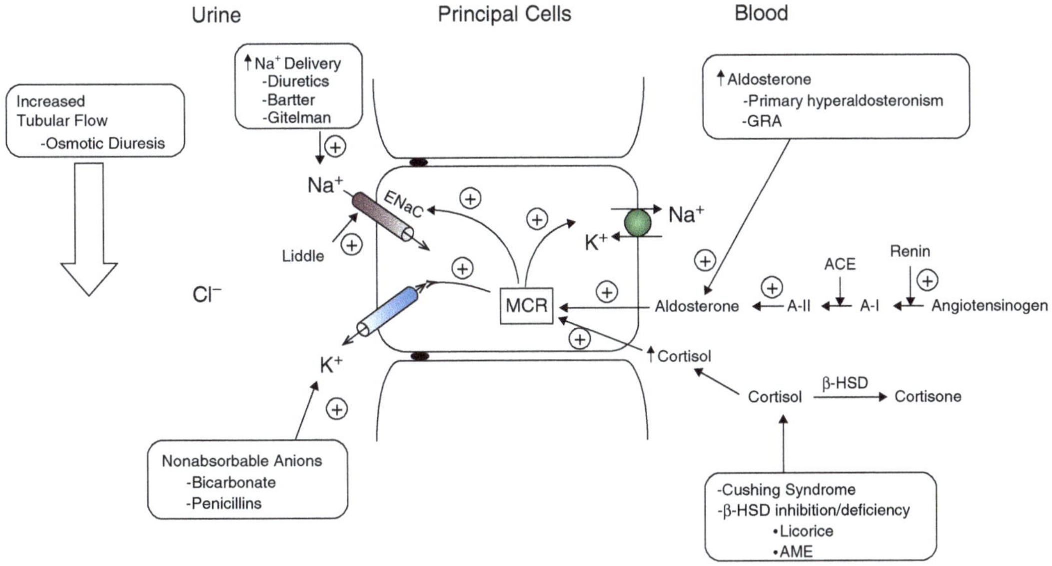

Fig. 10.3 Pathophysiology of hypokalemia due to renal potassium loss. *ENaC* epithelial sodium channel, *MCR* mineralocorticoid receptor, *A-I* angiotensin-I, *A-II* angiotensin-II, *ACE* angiotensin converting enzyme, *GRA* glucocorticoid remediable aldosteronism, *AME* apparent mineralocorticoid excess, *β-HSD* β-hydroxysteroid dehydrogenase (Adapted with permission from Zandi-Nejad K, Tang CC. Disorders of potassium. In: McKean S, Bennett A, and Halasyamani L, editors. Hospital Medicine: Just the facts. The McGraw-Hill: New York; 2008. p. 484–494)

1. First assess the need for emergency treatment (presence of ECG changes or potassium level ≥6.0–6.5 mmol/L).
2. Rule out spurious hyperkalemia (pseudohyperkalemia): Pseudohyperkalemia is a factitious rise in potassium level due to release of potassium during or after the sample is drawn. The most common causes are fist clenching, tourniquet use, hemolysis, severe thrombocytosis (potassium concentration increases by about 0.15 mmol/L for every 100,000 per mm^3 increase in platelet count), severe leukocytosis, erythrocytosis, and hereditary conditions affecting potassium efflux from red blood cells [3, 4].
3. History and physical examination should focus on risk factors for impaired kidney function, urine output, medications, sources of increased potassium load including diet and dietary supplements, blood pressure, and volume status.

   Several medications are frequent contributors: potassium-sparing diuretics, nonsteroidal anti-inflammatory medications (NSAIDs including COX-2 inhibitors), angiotensin-converting enzyme inhibitors (ACE-I), angiotensin-II receptor blockers (ARB), heparin and low molecular weight heparin (LMWH), and beta-blockers.
4. Increased potassium load may be endogenous or exogenous [6].

   Increased potassium load is an uncommon cause of hyperkalemia in the absence of impaired renal potassium excretion.

   The common sources for exogenous potassium are food and food supplements rich in potassium (e.g., salt substitute which has about 10–13 mmol of potassium chloride per gram), red blood cell transfusion (usually large amounts), and administration of potassium salts of medications (e.g., penicillin K or potassium phosphate).

   The major sources of endogenous potassium are GI bleeding, hematomas, tissue necrosis (e.g., rhabdomyolysis), and tumor lysis syndrome.

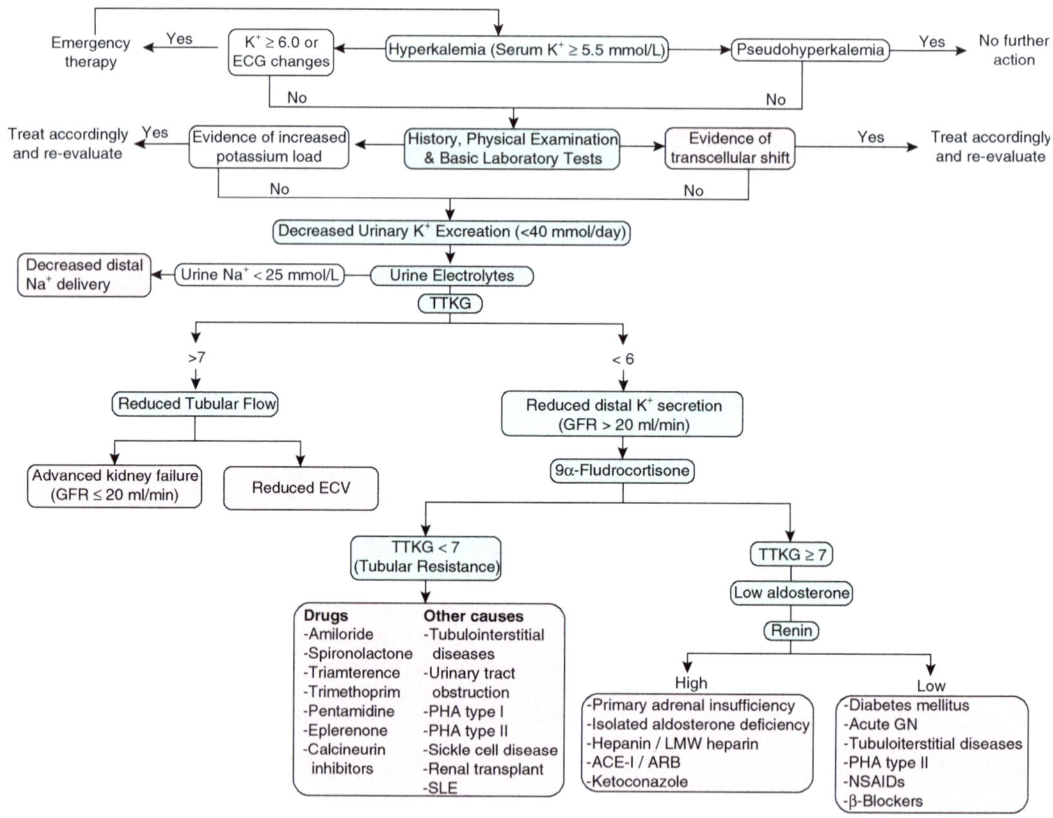

Fig. 10.4 Diagnostic approach to hyperkalemia. *TTKG* transtubular potassium gradient, *GFR* glomerular filtration rate, *ECV* effective circulatory volume, *acute GN* acute glomerulonephritis, *HIV* human immunodeficiency virus, *NSAIDs* nonsteroidal anti-inflammatory drugs, *LMW heparin* low molecular weight heparin, *ACE-I* angiotensin-converting enzyme inhibitor, *ARB* angiotensin II receptor blocker, *PHA* pseudohypoaldosteronism, *SLE* systemic lupus erythematosus (Adapted with permission from: Mount, D.B., Zandi-Nejad, K. Disorders of potassium balance. In: Brenner BM, editor. Brenner and Rector's the kidney, 8th edition, Philadelphia, PA: W.B. Saunders; 2008)

5. Transcellular redistribution with normal total body potassium content is next to consider (Table 10.2).
6. Reduced urinary potassium excretion (Figs. 10.4 and 10.5): In the absence of advanced kidney failure and low urine flow, a TTKG of less than 6 is suggestive of decreased potassium secretion by principal cells which primarily is due to either aldosterone deficiency or resistance. An increase in TTKG value to more than 7 in response to 9-alpha-fludrocortisone (a mineralcorticoid) is suggestive of aldosterone deficiency, whereas a lesser or no response indicates aldosterone resistance [3, 4, 6].

Table 10.2 Major causes of potassium shift out of cells (Adapted with permission from Zandi-Nejad K, Tang CC. Disorders of potassium. In: McKean S, Bennett A, and Halasyamani L, editors. Hospital Medicine: Just the facts. New York: The McGraw-Hill; 2008. p. 484–494)

Hypertonicity
Hyperglycemia
Mannitol
Beta-blockers (nonselective)
Insulin deficiency
Metabolic acidosis (nonorganic)
Digitalis toxicity
Exercise
Succinylcholine
Hyperkalemic periodic paralysis
Arginine hydrochloride infusion
ε-Aminocaproic acid

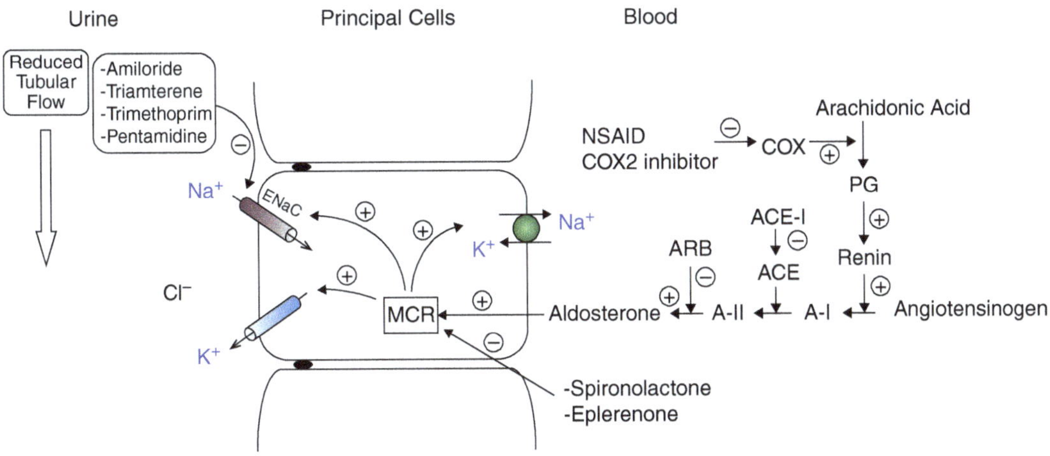

Fig. 10.5 Pathophysiology of hyperkalemia due to reduced renal potassium excretion. *ENaC* epithelial sodium channel, *MCR* mineralocorticoid receptor, *A-I* angiotensin-I, *A-II* angiotensin-II, *ACE* angiotensin converting enzyme, *ACE-I* angiotensin-converting enzyme inhibitor, *ARB* angiotensin II receptor blocker, *PG* prostaglandin, *COX* cyclooxygenase (Adapted with permission from Zandi-Nejad K, Tang CC. Disorders of potassium. In: McKean S, Bennett A, and Halasyamani L, editors. Hospital Medicine: Just the facts. The McGraw-Hill: New York; 2008. p. 484–494)

Hyporeninemic hypoaldosteronism is the most common form of aldosterone deficiency in adults. The usual presentation is in a patient with mild impairment of kidney function and hyperkalemia which is disproportionate to the level of kidney function impairment. It is commonly associated with mild non-anion gap metabolic acidosis [6].

Management

Hypokalemia

The goals of management are (1) to diagnose and prevent life-threatening consequences (e.g., cardiac dysrhythmias), (2) to replace any potassium deficit, and (3) to diagnose and manage/treat the underlying cause.

Potassium replacement is the mainstay of management and should be considered both in patients with true deficit and in those with hypokalemia due to transcellular shift. Potassium replacement should be done effectively but cautiously and with frequent monitoring of potassium level in order to avoid overcorrection and rebound hyperkalemia particularly in those with hypokalemia due to transcellular shift (e.g., hypokalemic thyrotoxic periodic paralysis) and in those with kidney function impairment.

Accurate estimation of potassium deficit and ongoing loss are thus important in guiding the management, in addition to the severity of hypokalemia, the rate of decline in potassium level, and the presence of associated conditions (e.g., hepatic encephalopathy). In the *absence* of abnormal transcellular redistribution, the potassium level drops by about 0.27 mmol/L for every 100 mmol reduction in total body potassium. In other words, loss of 400–800 mmol of total body potassium drops the plasma potassium level by approximately 2 mmol/L [14]. Again it has to be remembered that these are only estimates and frequent monitoring of potassium level is necessary to guide the treatment and the necessary adjustments.

Potassium replacement is necessary for patients' demonstrating symptoms and signs of hypokalemia (e.g., muscle weakness, ECG changes, cardiac dysrythmias) and in the following asymptomatic patients.

1. Patients' with moderate to severe hypokalemia (potassium level of less than 3.0 mmol/L);

2. High risk patients with potassium level of < 4.0 mmol/L. These are elderly patients (age > 65), patients' with organic heart disease, patients' on digitalis or antiarrhythmic medications, and patients with advance liver failure [15–17];
3. Patients' with moderate to severe hypertension and potassium level of < 4.0 mmol/L.

In cases of severe or symptomatic hypokalemia, the potassium level should be raised to a safe level rapidly (e.g., intravenous administration) followed by replacing the remaining deficit over days to weeks. Potassium replacement may be done through oral/enteral or intravenous routes. Whenever possible and appropriate, repletion through oral/enteral route is preferred. Intravenous potassium should be limited to patients with severe hypokalemia, symptomatic hypokalemia, high-risk patients, and patients unable to use oral/enteral route; it should be given as an adjunct to oral/enteral replacement with the exception of patients unable to use oral/enteral route. It is important to remember that rapid correction of hypokalemia through oral/enteral route is not only possible but may be even faster than intravenous replacement (mainly due to limitations in the rapidity with which intravenous potassium can be administered). In fact, it has been shown that an oral dose of 75 mmol of potassium chloride can increase potassium level by 1.0–1.4 mmol/L over 60–90 min [18].

The major potassium salts available are potassium chloride, potassium phosphate, and potassium bicarbonate or its precursors (potassium citrate, potassium acetate). The choice of potassium salt depends on the clinical situation. The following rules, however, are applicable in most circumstances.

Dietary potassium is primarily in the form of potassium citrate or potassium phosphate. It may be used as the first line of therapy in mild cases. However, it may not be effective in patients with concomitant chloride deficiency (e.g., diuretic use) given that both potassium phosphate and potassium citrate may actually increase renal potassium excretion by accentuating metabolic alkalosis associated with chloride deficiency and volume contraction.

Potassium phosphate should be reserved for patients with both potassium and phosphate deficiencies (e.g., patients with diabetic ketoacidosis or type 2 renal tubular acidosis). If given intravenously the dose should be limited to 50 mmol over 8 h to prevent hypocalcemia and metastatic calcification. In cases of moderate-to-severe hypokalemia it should be given along with another potassium salt.

Potassium bicarbonate or its precursors are primarily indicated for patients with concomitant hypokalemia and metabolic acidosis (e.g., patients with diarrhea, renal tubular acidosis).

Potassium chloride is the default salt of choice because it helps with the correction of chloride-responsive metabolic alkalosis *(please see above)* and may raise serum potassium level faster given that chloride is primarily an extracellular anion and therefore keeps more of the administered potassium in the extracellular fluid compartment [19].

Oral/enteral replacement. Potassium chloride is available in both liquid and tablet form. Liquid forms have immediate effect and are inexpensive but have poor taste and adherence. Effervescent potassium chloride (tablets for solution) has immediate effect but is more expensive than the elixir. Slow-release forms are less irritating to stomach and are better tolerated and therefore have higher risk of overdose and hyperkalemia. However, they have been associated with gastrointestinal erosions which is lower with microencapsulated forms [1, 9, 15, 20]. A dose of 40–100 mmol per day divided in 2–3 doses is effective in maintaining potassium level in desirable range in more than 90% patients with hypokalemia on diuretic therapy [1]. Larger doses or addition of a potassium sparing diuretic may be necessary in some patients; potassium chloride in doses of ≥ 2 mmol/kg may be toxic [20].

Intravenous replacement. Intravenous potassium chloride may be given through peripheral or central veins. A large central vein is preferred given that pain and phlebitis may be associated with potassium administration through a peripheral vein particularly when the rate of infusion is more than 10 mmol per hour. Femoral vein is superior to internal jugular or subclavian veins in most cases given that infusion through the upper body central veins may be associated with acute local rise in potassium and cardiac adverse effects [9, 21]. Potassium should be given in a dextrose-free solution in order to avoid endogenous insulin secretion and intracellular potassium relocation, which may transiently reduce potassium level by 0.2–1.4 mmol/L [22]. The usual concentration of potassium chloride is 20–40 mmol of potassium in 1 L of dextrose-free vehicle solution. Higher concentrations of up to 400 mmol/L may be used with extreme caution and only in the ICU setting; we recommend limiting the amount of potassium chloride per intravenous bag (e.g., 20 mmol per 100 mL) in order to avoid inadvertent administration of large doses [4, 9, 21].

The usual rate of administration is 10–20 mmol per hour. Higher infusion rates of up to 80 mmol per hour have been used in life-threatening conditions and may be associated with transient hyperkalemia [23]. ECG monitoring is recommended for infusion rates of more than 10 mmol per hour [24].

In addition to potassium supplementation, strategies to reduce potassium loss through the use of potassium-sparing diuretics (e.g., spironolactone, amiloride, triamterene) or other medications (e.g., ACE-I, ARB) should be considered. In patients with hypokalemia in the setting of metabolic alkalosis due to chloride-rich upper gastrointestinal loss (e.g., continuous nasogastric suction), proton pump inhibitors may be useful [25].

Magnesium deficiency enhances renal potassium excretion, it accompanies hypokalemia in many circumstances (e.g., diuretic use, diarrhea, Gitelman's syndrome) and is one of the common causes of refractory hypokalemia. Magnesium level should be measured in all patients with hypokalemia and corrected accordingly [6].

In patients with hypokalemia and chloride-responsive metabolic alkalosis, volume replacement may increase renal potassium loss by increasing bicarbonate excretion. Thus, in these patients, volume replacement should be done with extreme caution, along with potassium administration and with frequent monitoring of potassium level [6].

Hyperkalemia

The criteria for admission in hyperkalemia are not well defined. This is in part due to lack of universally accepted definition for mild, moderate, or severe hyperkalemia and in part because clinical consequences of hyperkalemia depend on other variables such as calcium level, acid–base status, and chronicity. As a rule the higher the potassium level and the faster the rise, the more urgent the treatment needs to be. In general any patient with hyperkalemia and associated symptoms and signs (e.g., ECG changes including tall, peaked T waves) needs to be treated urgently. In addition, patients with severe hyperkalemia (potassium level > 6–6.5 mmol/L) in the absence of symptoms and ECG findings require urgent management as well, given the limitations of ECG changes as an indicator of cardiac toxicity. Adequate management and serial monitoring of potassium level usually warrants admission. Serum potassium level should be repeated 1–3 h after initiation of the treatment and frequently thereafter as needed [3, 4].

Emergency treatment of hyperkalemia involves: antagonizing the effects of hyperkalemia on membrane potential, rapid reduction of potassium level through intracellular shift, and ultimately removing excess potassium from the body. Of note, low-risk patients with potassium level of < 5.8–6.0 mmol/L and no ECG changes may be treated with potassium removal strategies and frequent monitoring of the potassium level.

Antagonizing the Effects of Hyperkalemia on Membrane Potential

This is achieved by calcium administration and is effective even in patients with normal calcium levels. Calcium gluconate and calcium chloride are equally effective when used at equivalent millimolar doses of elemental calcium. Each mL of 10% calcium gluconate and calcium chloride has 8.9 mg (0.22 mmol) and 27.2 mg (0.68 mmol) of elemental calcium, respectively [26]. Whereas calcium gluconate may be given through a peripheral vein, calcium chloride should be administered through a central vein in order to avoid tissue necrosis associated with its extravasation.

The recommended dose is 10 mL of 10% calcium gluconate or 3–4 mL of 10% calcium chloride infused intravenously over 2–3 min under continuous ECG monitoring. The effect starts in 1–3 min and lasts for 30–60 min. The dose may be repeated every 5 min if ECG changes persist or recurs [27, 28].

In patients treated with digitalis, 10 mL of 10% calcium gluconate should be added to 100 mL of D5W (dextrose 5% in water) and infused intravenously over 20–30 min under continuous ECG monitoring. Avoid giving calcium in solutions containing bicarbonate, which may result in calcium carbonate precipitation [3, 4, 6].

Intracellular Potassium Shift

Insulin and Glucose

The potassium lowering effect is due to the effect of insulin on Na-K-ATPase and glucose is given only to prevent hypoglycemia (please see below). This is the most consistent and reliable method to redistribute potassium and is effective in almost all patients including patients with CKD and ESRD. Its potassium lowering effect starts in 10–20 min, peaks at 20–30 min, and lasts for 4–6 h. At its peak, it can drop the potassium level by 0.5–1.2 mmol/L. The dose can be repeated as necessary.

The recommended dose is 10 units of regular insulin given as an intravenous bolus and followed immediately by 50 mL of 50% dextrose. In order to avoid hypoglycemia, seen in up to 75% of patients about 1 h later [29], infusion of 10% glucose in water (D10W) at 50–75 mL/h is recommended; blood glucose level should be monitored hourly [30, 31].

Insulin without glucose maybe given to diabetic patients with blood glucose level equal to or more than 200–250 mg/dL with frequent monitoring of glucose level to ensure hypoglycemia does not develop. Administration of glucose without insulin is strongly discouraged given that endogenous insulin response could be quite variable and that hyperosmolar glucose administration may in fact increase potassium level.

Beta-2 Adrenergic Agonists

They should not be used as a single agent, particularly in patients with CKD and ESRD in whom up to 40% may be resistant to its potassium lowering effect, although some more recent studies have not confirmed this notion [4].

Albuterol (Salbutamol), a selective beta-2 agonist is the main agent used and studied. Intravenous and inhaled forms are effective in lowering potassium level. In its intravenous form, not available in the USA, 0.5 mg of albuterol is added to 100 mL of D5W and infused over 10–15 min. In its inhaled form 10–20 mg of albuterol is added to 4 mL of normal saline and nebulized over 10–20 min. With this method, its potassium lowering effect begins in 30 min, peaks at 90 min, and last for 2–6 h. At its peak it can lower potassium level by 0.5–1.0 mmol/L.

Although use of the inhaled albuterol was associated with small increase in heart rate (about 10 bpm) and no significant change in systolic or diastolic blood pressure, it should be used with extreme caution in high risk patients such as those with ischemic heart disease. Intravenous albuterol increases the heart rate by about 20 bpm [32, 33].

The effects of beta-2 adrenergic agonists and insulin are synergistic and the combination may drop the potassium level by 1.2–1.5 mmol/L. Use of epinephrine is not recommended and should be avoided.

Sodium Bicarbonate

The role of sodium bicarbonate in the *acute* treatment of hyperkalemia has been questioned. It has been shown that sodium bicarbonate infusion for up to 60 min (hypertonic or isotonic) had no effect on potassium level in a group of ESRD patients on hemodialysis (Fig 10.6) [34]. This finding has been confirmed by other studies [35, 36]. Of note, rapid increase in pH following administration of sodium bicarbonate may reduce the level of ionized calcium and attenuate/nullify the beneficial effects of calcium administration. However, sodium bicarbonate may be used in patients with concomitant hyperkalemia and severe acidosis where it is primarily indicated for acidosis treatment.

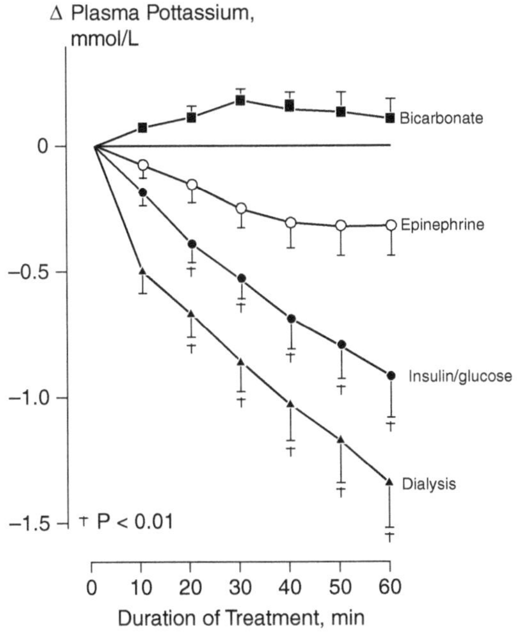

Fig. 10.6 Changes in serum potassium level during intravenous infusion of bicarbonate, epinephrine, or insulin and glucose and during hemodialysis (Adapted with permission from Blumberg A, Weidmann P, Shaw S, et al.: Effect of various therapeutic approaches on plasma potassium and major regulating factors in terminal renal failure, Am J Med 85:507–512, 1988)

Removal of Potassium from Body

Removal of body potassium is the mainstay of treatment in patients with excessive body potassium. Dialysis, particularly hemodialysis, and cation-exchange resins (Kayexalate®) are efficacious and are widely used for the treatment of hyperkalemia. However for the acute treatment of hyperkalemia, it is prudent that these measures only be used with other treatment options aimed at acutely lowering potassium level (mentioned above) given the usual logistic delay in the initiation of hemodialysis and the slow effect of Kayexalate® on potassium level.

Diuretics

Although their role in the acute treatment of hyperkalemia is quite limited, chronic administration of diuretics may be effective in patients with mild to moderate hyperkalemia.

Mineralocorticoids

Fludrocortisone in the dose of 0.1–0.3 mg per day may be used for the treatment of chronic hyperkalemia in patients with hypoaldosteronism [3, 4].

Cation-Exchange Resins

Sodium polystyrene sulfonate (Kayexalate®) is a cross-linked polymer that exchanges Na for K in the gastrointestinal tract (mainly colon). It has a slow onset of action and its full potassium-lowering effect may take up to 24 h or even longer to develop. Each gram of sodium polystyrene sulfonate binds 0.5–1.0 mmol of potassium in exchange for 2–3 mmol of sodium (the difference is due to the binding of other metals such as calcium and magnesium).

Traditionally sodium polystyrene sulfonate was given with 70% sorbitol in order to avoid concretion and colon impaction. However more recent data have linked sorbitol particularly 70% sorbitol to intestinal necrosis, an uncommon but frequently fatal complication primarily affecting colon and ileum. Although there are indications that sodium polystyrene sulfonate in 33% sorbitol (commercially available in the United States) is associated with lower risk, cases of intestinal necrosis with this preparation has been reported. As a result in 2009 Food and Drug Administration (FDA) recommended sodium polystyrene sulfonate NOT to be administered with sorbitol. Notably a case of intestinal necrosis following oral administration of sodium polystyrene sulfonate alone has been reported. Therefore, we strongly discourage the use of sodium polystyrene sulfonate (with or without sorbitol) in high risk patients including kidney transplant recipients, patients in postoperative period, patients with slow bowel transit, patients with ischemic bowel disease, and those with a history of bowel obstruction.

The efficacy of single-dose sodium polystyrene sulfonate to treat acute hyperkalemia has been challenged and is NOT recommended although it is commonly practiced. If indicated, sodium polystyrene sulfonate should be administered in repeated doses. The recommended dose is 15–30 g of sodium polystyrene sulfonate every 4–6 h. We recommend sodium polystyrene sulfonate (in powder form) to be administered with a laxative other than sorbitol (e.g., lactulose) [3, 4].

Renal Replacement Therapy [3, 4]

Hemodialysis is the preferred method, although all modes of renal replacement therapy (continuous hemodiafiltration, peritoneal dialysis, and hemodialysis) are effective in removing potassium from body.

An average hemodialysis session of 3–5 h removes 40–120 mmol of potassium of which about 15% is due ultrafiltration and the remaining from dialysis. Of the total potassium removed ~40% comes from extracellular space and ~60% from intracellular space. In the majority of the patients the greatest drop in potassium level (1.2–1.5 mmol/L) and the largest amount of potassium removal occur during the first hour of dialysis with potassium level reaching its nadir at about 3 h. However, potassium removal continues to the end of the dialysis session.

There exists a large variability in the amount of potassium removed which depends on the relative distribution of potassium between intracellular and extracellular spaces, the duration of dialysis, the type and characteristics of the dialyzer, blood and dialysate flow rates, and the plasma/dialysate potassium gradient. Factors affecting the relative distribution of potassium in favor of an intracellular shift (such as food consumption early in the dialysis session, and treatment with insulin/glucose and/or beta-2 agonists) can negatively impact the total amount of potassium removed by as much as 40%.

Plasma/dialysate gradient determined by the difference between plasma and dialysate potassium concentrations is a major determinant of the total potassium removed; the higher the gradient (the lower the dialysate potassium concentration), the more potassium is removed. Many nephrologists commonly use very low potassium dialysates (e.g., 0 or 1 mmol/L). The rapid drop in plasma potassium level associated with the use of these very low potassium dialysates however may have deleterious consequences.

Rebound hypertension: Is a significant increase in blood pressure 1 h after dialysis and is attributed to peripheral vasoconstriction.

Cardiac dysrhythmias: Some studies suggest a relation between dialysate potassium concentration, rate of plasma potassium decline, and cardiac dysrhythmias although the issue remains controversial.

We recommend the following when considering dialysate potassium concentration in patients treated for significant hyperkalemia.

Initiate dialysis with a 3 or 4 mmol/L potassium dialysate and reduce the concentration of dialysate bath in a stepwise fashion (e.g., drop the potassium concentration of dialysate by 1 mmol/L every hour).

Restrict the upfront use of dialysates with very low potassium concentration (0 or 1 mmol/L) to patients with life-threatening cardiac dysrhythmias.

When indicated, dialysates with very low potassium concentration should be used with caution particularly in high risk patients (elderly, patients with history of cardiac dysrhythmia, coronary/ischemic heart disease, left ventricular hypertrophy, systolic hypertension, and those treated with digitalis); continuous cardiac monitoring is strongly recommended for all patients.

Case 1 Follow-Up

What is the most likely cause of her hypokalemia?

Following the path provided in Fig 10.2, it is noted that

1. No clear evidence of transcellular redistribution or low potassium intake is present.
2. Urine K of > 15 mmol per day suggests renal loss.
3. TTKG of 12.7 confirms renal loss due to increased distal tubule potassium secretion.
4. Her high total CO_2 points toward metabolic alkalosis.
5. Urine chloride of > 20 mmol/L along with Ca/Cr ratio (both in mg) of less than 0.07 (0.04) suggests either Gitleman's syndrome or thiazide diuretic use.

6. A diuretic screen was positive for thiazide diuretics suggestive of diuretic abuse.

What is the best way to treat her hypokalemia?

Her treatment should include stopping the diuretic, and replacing the magnesium and potassium. Given the presence of alkalosis and chloride deficit, potassium chloride will be the potassium salt of choice and should be given orally.

Case 2 Follow-Up

What are the contributing factors for his hyperkalemia?

The cause of hyperkalemia is usually multifactorial. In this case CKD, ACE-I (lisinopril), and beta-blocker (metoprolol) are contributory (Figs. 10.4 and 10.5). Some degree of dietary indiscretion is likely to be contributing as well.

What is the most likely cause of recent rise in potassium level?

Although the above-mentioned factors are likely to play a role, they do not explain the sudden and recent rise in his potassium. In this case the factor that has tipped the balance in favor of hyperkalemia is NSAID (naproxen) use.

References

1. Gennari FJ. Hypokalemia. N Engl J Med. 1998;339(7):451–8.
2. Paltiel O, et al. Management of severe hypokalemia in hospitalized patients: a study of quality of care based on computerized databases. Arch Intern Med. 2001;161(8):1089–95.
3. Mount DB, Zandi-Nejad K. Disorders of potassium balance. In: Brenner BM, editor. Brenner & Rector's the kidney. Philadelphia: W.B. Saunders; 2008. p. 547–669.
4. Mount D, Zandi-Nejad K. Disorders of potassium balance. In: Taal MW et al., editors. Brenner & Rector's the kidney. Philadelphia: Elsevier Saunders; 2012. p. 640–688.
5. Stevens MS, Dunlay RW. Hyperkalemia in hospitalized patients. Int Urol Nephrol. 2000;32(2):177–80.
6. Zandi-Nejad K, Tang C. Disorders of potassium. In: McKean S, Bennett A, Halasyamani L, editors. Hospital medicine: Just the facts. New York: The McGraw-Hill; 2008. p. 484–94.
7. DeFronzo RA, et al. Influence of basal insulin and glucagon secretion on potassium and sodium metabolism. Studies with somatostatin in normal dogs and in normal and diabetic human beings. J Clin Invest. 1978;61(2):472–9.
8. Costanzo LS. Physiology. 4th ed. Philadelphia: Saunders Elsevier; 2010.
9. Rose B, Post T. Clinical physiology of acid–base and electrolyte disorders. 5th ed. New York: McGrraw-Hill; 2001. p. 794–930.
10. Shafi T, et al. Changes in serum potassium mediate thiazide-induced diabetes. Hypertension. 2008;52(6):1022–9.
11. Freeman SJ, Fale AD. Muscular paralysis and ventilatory failure caused by hyperkalaemia. Br J Anaesth. 1993;70(2):226–7.
12. Matsuda O, et al. Primary role of hyperkalemia in the acidosis of hyporeninemic hypoaldosteronism. Nephron. 1988;49(3):203–9.
13. Szylman P, et al. Role of hyperkalemia in the metabolic acidosis of isolated hypoaldosteronism. N Engl J Med. 1976;294(7):361–5.
14. Sterns RH, et al. Internal potassium balance and the control of the plasma potassium concentration. Medicine (Baltimore). 1981;60(5):339–54.
15. Cohn JN, et al. New guidelines for potassium replacement in clinical practice: a contemporary review by the National Council on Potassium in Clinical Practice. Arch Intern Med. 2000;160(16):2429–36.
16. Gabduzda GJ, Hall 3rd PW. Relation of potassium depletion to renal ammonium metabolism and hepatic coma. Medicine (Baltimore). 1966;45(6):481–90.
17. Jaeger P, Karlmark B, Giebisch G. Ammonium transport in rat cortical tubule: relationship to potassium metabolism. Am J Physiol. 1983;245(5 Pt 1):F593–600.
18. Nicolis GL, et al. Glucose-induced hyperkalemia in diabetic subjects. Arch Intern Med. 1981;141(1):49–53.
19. Villamil MF, et al. Anion effects on cation movements during correction of potassium depletion. Am J Physiol. 1975;229(1):161–6.
20. Su M, et al. Sustained-release potassium chloride overdose. J Toxicol Clin Toxicol. 2001;39(6):641–8.
21. Kruse JA, Carlson RW. Rapid correction of hypokalemia using concentrated intravenous potassium chloride infusions. Arch Intern Med. 1990;150(3):613–7.
22. Kunin AS, Surawicz B, Sims EA. Decrease in serum potassium concentrations and appearance of cardiac arrhythmias during infusion of potassium with glucose in potassium-depleted patients. N Engl J Med. 1962;266:228–33.
23. Seftel HC, Kew MC. Early and intensive potassium replacement in diabetic acidosis. Diabetes. 1966;15(9):694–6.
24. Kim GH, Han JS. Therapeutic approach to hypokalemia. Nephron. 2002;92 Suppl 1:28–32.
25. Eiro M, Katoh T, Watanabe T. Use of a proton-pump inhibitor for metabolic disturbances associated with anorexia nervosa. N Engl J Med. 2002;346(2):140.
26. Davey M, Caldicott D. Calcium salts in management of hyperkalaemia. Emerg Med J. 2002;19(1):92–3.

27. Ahmed J, Weisberg LS. Hyperkalemia in dialysis patients. Semin Dial. 2001;14(5):348–56.
28. Evans KJ, Greenberg A. Hyperkalemia: a review. J Intensive Care Med. 2005;20(5):272–90.
29. Allon M, Copkney C. Albuterol and insulin for treatment of hyperkalemia in hemodialysis patients. Kidney Int. 1990;38(5):869–72.
30. Allon M. Treatment and prevention of hyperkalemia in end-stage renal disease. Kidney Int. 1993; 43(6):1197–209.
31. Perazella MA. Approach to hyperkalemic end-stage renal disease patients in the emergency department. Conn Med. 1999;63(3):131–6.
32. Allon M. Hyperkalemia in end-stage renal disease: mechanisms and management. J Am Soc Nephrol. 1995;6(4):1134–42.
33. Liou HH, et al. Hypokalemic effects of intravenous infusion or nebulization of salbutamol in patients with chronic renal failure: comparative study. Am J Kidney Dis. 1994;23(2):266–71.
34. Blumberg A, et al. Effect of various therapeutic approaches on plasma potassium and major regulating factors in terminal renal failure. Am J Med. 1988;85(4):507–12.
35. Blumberg A, Weidmann P, Ferrari P. Effect of prolonged bicarbonate administration on plasma potassium in terminal renal failure. Kidney Int. 1992;41(2): 369–74.
36. Allon M, Shanklin N. Effect of bicarbonate administration on plasma potassium in dialysis patients: interactions with insulin and albuterol. Am J Kidney Dis. 1996;28(4):508–14.

Disorders of Calcium, Phosphorus, and Magnesium

11

J. Kevin Tucker and Denyse Thornley-Brown

Case 1

A 62-year-old man with chronic kidney disease (CKD) stage 3 undergoes an abdominal CT for workup of presumed diverticulitis. He is noted incidentally to have bilateral renal cysts and a solid mass in his right kidney. Biopsy of the mass confirms the diagnosis of renal cell carcinoma, and he is scheduled for elective nephrectomy. Prior to his scheduled nephrectomy, the patient is noted to have a serum calcium of 11.4 mg/dL with a serum albumin of 3.6 g/dL. How should this patient's hypercalcemia be approached? What management strategies should be employed?

Case 2

A 64-year-old man with a history of renal cell carcinoma, left nephrectomy, and partial right nephrectomy, spinal cord infarction with paraplegia, and chronic obstipation presents with abdominal pain and distention. In the emergency department, he is noted to be lethargic, bradycardic, and hypotensive. He requires intubation and mechanical ventilation for hypoxemic and hypercapnic respiratory failure. Electrolytes are sodium 133 mEq/L, potassium 4.2 mEq/L, chloride 100 mEq/L, and CO_2 22 mEq/L. The BUN is 46 mg/dL and the creatinine is 1.6 mg/dL. His electrocardiogram shows right bundle branch block and left fasicular block, and the QTc interval is 564 ms. The serum magnesium level is 8.9 mg/dL. How might this patient's hypermagnesemia have developed? What is the best management strategy for this patient?

Case 3

A 50-year-old Cambodian woman presents to her primary care physician with complaints of profound weakness, to the point that she is bedbound. Her past medical history is notable for chronic hepatitis B infection, for which she is treated with tenofovir. Laboratory studies are notable for sodium of 137 mEq/L, potassium of 2.5 mEq/L, chloride of 109 mEq/L, and CO_2 of 18 mEq/L. The BUN is 8 mg/dL, and the creatinine is 0.92 mg/dL. Calcium and phosphorus are 7.8 mg/dL and 0.5 mg/dL, respectively. The urinalysis shows 2+ glucose and a pH of 7.0. What is the explanation for this patient's hypophosphatemia and how should it be treated?

J.K. Tucker, M.D. (✉)
Department of Medicine/Renal Division,
75 Francis Street, Boston, MA 02115, USA
e-mail: jktucker@partners.org

D. Thornley-Brown, M.D.
Department of Internal Medicine (Nephrology),
University of Alabama at Birmingham,
Birmingham, AL 35294-0007, USA

E.V. Lerma and M. Rosner (eds.), *Clinical Decisions in Nephrology, Hypertension and Kidney Transplantation*,
DOI 10.1007/978-1-4614-4454-1_11, © Springer Science+Business Media New York 2013

Disorders of Calcium

Overview

Calcium balance is maintained through dynamic interactions among the intestinal tract, bone, and kidneys which are mediated through the hormonal influences of parathyroid hormone (PTH) and vitamin D. Disorders of calcium balance, therefore, may arise from perturbations in metabolism in any of these organs. The precise control of the extracellular calcium concentration is important for many cellular functions such as neuromuscular excitation and transmission of nerve impulses.

Calcium exists in the plasma in several different forms. Most of the circulating calcium, about 40–45%, is bound to protein, namely albumin, while the remainder is either free or in circulating complexes [1]. The free (ionized) form of calcium is the physiologically active form. In states of metabolic alkalosis, the ionized calcium may be low even when the total serum calcium is normal as more calcium is albumin bound. Similarly, in states of hypoalbuminemia the measured total calcium level may be low but the ionized calcium may be normal. The total calcium may be estimated in states of hypoalbuminemia by the equation

$$\text{Corrected calcium} = \text{Measured calcium}\left(\text{mg / dL}\right) - \text{serum albumin}\left(\text{g / dL}\right) + 4$$

Epidemiology

Asymptomatic hypercalcemia, defined as a total calcium concentration greater than or equal to 11.0 mg/dL, may be present in up to 3.9% of the general population [2]. Asymptomatic hypercalcemia occurs most commonly in the setting of primary hyperparathyroidism or malignancy, which together account for about 90% of all cases of hypercalcemia. The prevalence of primary hyperparathyroidism appears to have risen since the 1970s, but this increased prevalence is likely explained by the advent of routine serum calcium measurement [3]. Primary hyperparathyroidism occurs about three times more commonly in women than in men.

Table 11.1 Causes of hypercalcemia

Causes of hypercalcemia
Primary hyperparathyroidism
Humoral hypercalcemia of malignancy
Multiple myeloma
Sarcoidosis and other granulomatous diseases
Milk-alkali syndrome
Vitamin D intoxication
Familial hypocalciuric hypercalcemia
Thiazide diuretics
Immobilization
Paget's disease
Addison's disease
Thyrotoxicosis

Hypocalcemia, while rare in the general population, occurs frequently in critically ill patients. As many as 88% of ICU patients may have hypocalcemia as defined by an ionized calcium level of less than 1.16 mmol/L [4].

Etiology/Pathophysiology

Hypercalcemia may arise from a number of pathophysiologic mechanisms (see Table 11.1) which may be summarized as (1) increased mobilization of calcium from bone, (2) decreased urinary excretion of calcium, or (3) increased absorption of calcium from the gastrointestinal tract. Rarely, excessive calcium intake may contribute to the development of hypercalcemia. The two most common causes of asymptomatic hypercalcemia are primary hyperparathyroidism and malignancy.

Primary hyperparathyroidism accounts for about 50% of cases of asymptomatic hypercalcemia and is related to excess secretion of parathyroid hormone (PTH), either from a discrete adenoma or to diffuse four-gland hyperplasia. PTH stimulates calcium reabsorption from the kidney and the release of calcium from bone stores. The humoral hypercalcemia of malignancy is also caused by increased mobilization of calcium from bone, but in this case the endocrine mediator is not PTH but rather parathyroid hormone-related protein (PTHrP). A number of solid tumors including renal cell carcinomas, squamous cell lung cancers, breast cancers, and ovarian cancers are known to elaborate PTHrP leading to hypercalcemia (paraneoplastic syndrome). Multiple myeloma, a common malignancy-related cause of hypercalcemia, does not cause hypercalcemia through PTHrP but through the direct lytic destruction of bone by plasma cells, causing release of calcium from bone stores. Specific cytokines such as interleukin-6 are important in promoting bone resorption in this condition.

Decreased urinary excretion of calcium is an uncommon cause of hypercalcemia, but may occur with a commonly used medication: thiazide diuretics. The hypercalcemia associated with thiazides is typically mild and asymptomatic. However, thiazide use may unmask latent primary hyperparathyroidism. Lithium may also be associated with hypercalcemia and hypocalciuria. Familial hypocalciuric hypercalcemia (FHH) is a rare genetic disorder with autosomal dominant inheritance caused by inactivating defects in the extracellular calcium sensing receptor [5]. Affected individuals typically have mild degrees of hypercalcemia and are asymptomatic. In contrast to other causes of hypercalcemia, the urinary calcium excretion is not elevated in FHH [6]. Distinguishing between hyperparathyroidism and FHH is important since the hypercalcemia of FHH generally does not respond to parathyroidectomy.

Vitamin D intoxication, the milk-alkali syndrome and granulomatous diseases cause hypercalcemia through increased absorption of calcium from the gastrointestinal tract. The use of calcium and vitamin D for prevention of osteoporosis, for example, may lead to the development of hypercalcemia if the doses are excessive or in the presence of impaired renal function which limits renal calcium excretion. The milk-alkali syndrome is characterized by hypercalcemia and metabolic alkalosis, and it occurs most commonly in patients with concurrent CKD who are often taking a combination of some form of alkali (such as sodium bicarbonate) and high doses of calcium. The use of calcium carbonate as a calcium supplement and as a phosphate binder has led to an increased incidence of milk-alkali syndrome such that it now may account for up to 9% of cases of hypercalcemia [7]. Granulomatous diseases such as sarcoidosis may be associated with hypercalcemia through the elaboration of 1,25 (OH)-vitamin D by macrophages. The non-renal production of 1,25 (OH)-vitamin D leads to increased intestinal absorption of calcium causing hypercalcemia. Hypercalcemia may occur in as many as 10% of sarcoidosis patients [8].

In the non-acute care setting hypocalcemia is uncommon, but when it does occur it is most commonly caused by hypoparathyroidism, hypomagnesemia, vitamin D deficiency, or CKD.

Hypoparathyroidism may occur as a postsurgical complication in patients who have undergone parathyroidectomy for primary hyperparathyroidism or for secondary or tertiary hyperparathyroidism in the setting of CKD. Hypoparathyroidism may occur inadvertently as a surgical complication in patients undergoing thyroid surgery. The parathyroid gland may also be subject to hypofunction as the result of radiation to the neck. Hypomagnesemia causes hypocalemia through the effects of magnesium depletion on parathyroid gland function (inhibiting the release of PTH).

Severe deficiencies of vitamin D cause hypocalcemia as well as rickets and osteomalacia. While childhood vitamin D deficiency has become uncommon in North America with vitamin D fortification of milk products, hypovitaminosis D is still seen frequently in the frail elderly and in individuals who are not exposed to the sun for prolonged periods of time. Vitamin D deficiency occurs commonly in patients following gastrectomy or intestinal resection and in patients with other gastrointestinal disorders such as Crohn's disease and celiac sprue. It is also common following certain types of obesity surgery.

CKD may lead to hypocalcemia over months to years; thus patients who develop hypocalcemia in the setting of long-standing CKD are often asymptomatic despite their degree of hypocalcemia. Hypocalcemia may develop in CKD through several mechanisms. First, 25-OH vitamin D deficiency is common in patients with CKD. Second, decreased 1α hydroxylation of 25-OH vitamin D in the kidney leads to deficiency of

Table 11.2 Causes of hypocalcemia

Hypoparathyroidism
Vitamin D deficiency
Hypomagnesemia
Chronic kidney disease
Citrate toxicity
Alkalosis
Medications
Phenytoin
Phenobarbital
Laxatives
Phosphate enemas
Cinacalcet
Pancreatitis

1,25 (OH)-vitamin D, causing a reduction in intestinal absorption of calcium. Third, decreased renal clearance of phosphorus leads to hyperphosphatemia, with calcium levels falling as it precipitates with phosphorus. CKD patients with the nephrotic syndrome are also at risk of hypocalcemia because of the loss of vitamin D binding proteins in the urine. However, the diagnosis of hypocalcemia should be confirmed with measurement of the ionized calcium since these patients usually will have profound hypoalbuminemia which complicates the interpretation of the total calcium level.

Other less common causes of hypocalcemia are noted in Table 11.2. These include citrate toxicity as when administered with blood products (citrate is used as an anticoagulant in blood products) or as an anticoagulant for continuous renal replacement therapies; medications; alkalosis, metabolic, or respiratory; pancreatitis; and rare genetic disorders.

Clinical Features

The clinical presentation of the hypercalcemic patient is variable and relates to the underlying pathologic process and the rate of development of hypercalcemia. For example, the chronically hypercalcemic patient with primary hyperparathyroidism may be asymptomatic for years, and the diagnosis is made on routine laboratory evaluation. In contrast, the patient with a malignancy who becomes acutely hypercalcemic is much more likely to be symptomatic. The presenting features of patients with hypercalcemia include nausea, vomiting, abdominal pain, fatigue, polyuria, polydipsia, altered mental status, obtundation, and coma. On physical examination there may be signs of volume depletion such as orthostatic hypotension, dry mucous membranes, and decreased skin turgor.

In addition to confirming the diagnosis of hypercalcemia, the laboratory assessment of the hypercalcemic patient may show signs of acute kidney injury, resulting from the renal sodium wasting (calcium acts at the level of the loop of Henle to impair the function of the Na–K–2Cl transporter, similar to the actions of a loop diuretic) and impaired urinary concentration associated with hypercalcemia. The urine specific gravity may reflect a relatively dilute urine despite volume depletion because of the concentrating defect. Hypercalcemia can also cause renal vasoconstriction further impairing renal perfusion.

When patients with primary hyperparathyroidism become symptomatic, it is often due to the development of kidney stones, which are most commonly calcium oxalate stones. Ultrasound imaging or computed tomography imaging will easily diagnose these stones, which are often small and non-obstructing. Diffuse soft tissue calcification of the kidneys or *nephrocalcinosis* may also develop in patients with more prolonged hypercalcemia.

The hypocalcemic patient presents with signs and symptoms of neuromuscular irritability: Chvostek's sign, circumoral numbness, paresthesias, cramping, and seizures. Electrocardiographic findings include a prolonged QT interval and nonspecific ST-T wave abnormalities.

Diagnosis

The diagnosis of hypercalcemia and hypocalcemia should be confirmed by measuring the ionized calcium level. The importance of measuring the ionized calcium level has been confirmed by recent findings that have shown that the measured

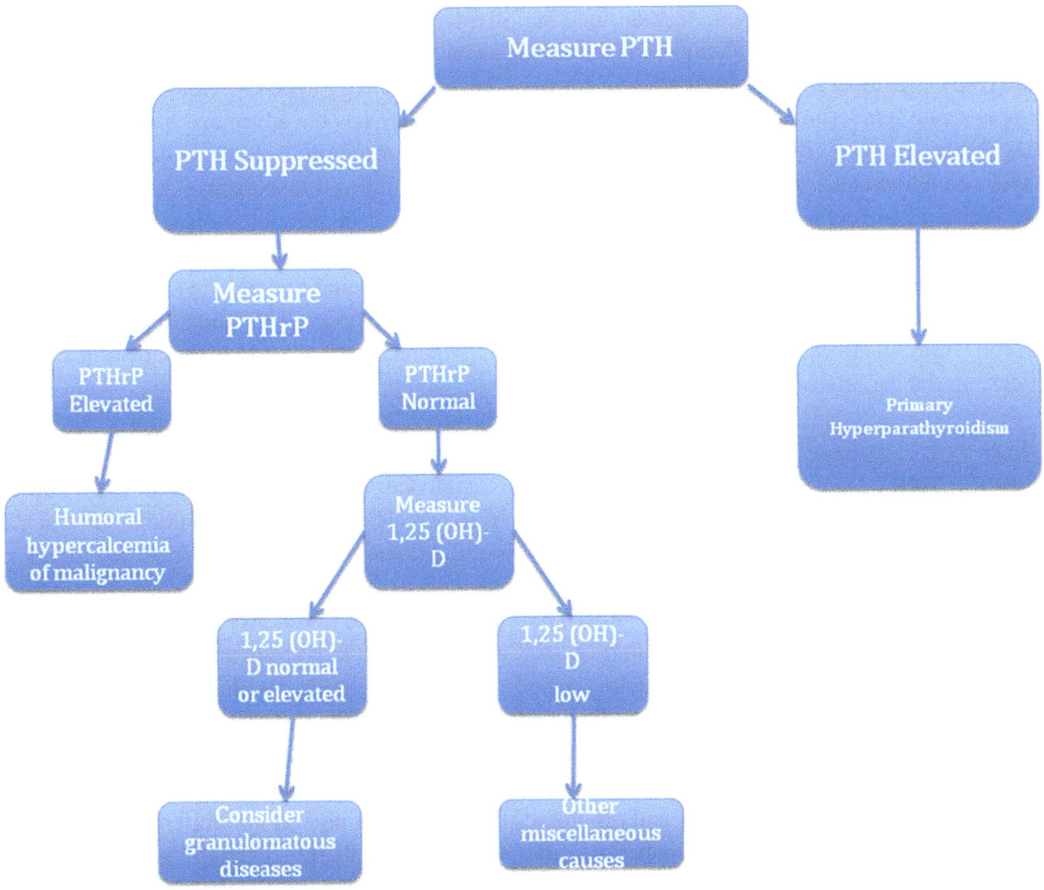

Fig. 11.1 Work-up of hypercalcemia

calcium level corrected for serum albumin is poorly predictive of ionized calcium levels, especially in patients with CKD. Furthermore, the serum albumin concentration is measured using differing methodologies: the Bromcresol green and the Bromcresol purple assays. There is enough variability in the albumin measurement depending upon the assay used that the patient may be classified as hypocalcemic or hypercalcemic with one assay but not with the other [9].

Once an abnormality of calcium is confirmed, the history may provide clues as to the etiology. Particular attention should be paid to diet and the use of medications and calcium supplements. Measurement of the PTH and 1,25 (OH)-vitamin D levels are important laboratory studies for understanding the underlying pathogenesis. Measurement of PTHrP in the correct clinical setting may be diagnostic of paraneoplastic hypercalcemia.

Differential Diagnosis

Other than the history, the PTH provides the most important clue as to the etiology of a calcium abnormality (See Fig. 11.1). In cases other than primary hyperparathyroidism, the PTH should be suppressed, although in some cases of FHH, PTH levels may be high normal or elevated (due to defects in the feedback loop of calcium at the mutated calcium sensing receptor). A low 24-h urine calcium or low ratio of calcium clearance to creatinine clearance may help to distinguish between the two disorders. If the PTH is suppressed and the calcium is elevated, then one of the other mechanisms of hypercalcemia must be causing the elevated serum calcium. The PTHrP, 1,25 (OH) vitamin D level, serum protein electrophoresis, and free serum light chains are useful in diagnosing humoral hypercalcemia of malignancy, granulomatous diseases, and plasma cell dyscrasias in patients with unexplained hypercalcemia. In addition to measuring the PTH, the serum magnesium level should be measured in patients with hypocalcemia since hypomagnesemia may itself cause hypocalcemia via its effects on the parathyroid gland.

Management

The management of the hypercalcemic patient should focus on restoring normal volume if the patient shows signs of volume depletion (which is present in these patients). The administration of isotonic saline will restore volume, correcting prerenal azotemia and restoring the GFR. *Saline Diuresis*: Once euvolemia has been achieved, a loop diuretic such as furosemide, may be given as adjunctive therapy to induce diuresis and promote urinary calcium excretion in those patients with volume overload. Routine use of loop diuretics should be avoided and may exacerbate hypercalcemia if volume is not adequately restored before their use. Electrolytes and volume status must be monitored closely when saline diuresis is attempted to control hypercalcemia, and it is usually only the first step towards more definitive management.

Calcitonin increases urinary calcium excretion and decreases resorption of calcium from bone. It is an effective adjunct therapy to saline diuresis, but the effect may be short-lived because of the development of tachyphylaxis. The usual starting dose of salmon calcitonin is 4 IU/kg subcutaneously or intramuscularly every 12 h [10].

The *bisphosphonates* are a group of medications that inhibit osteoclast-mediated bone resorption. The bisphosphonates that are currently available in the USA include pamidronate, etidronate, zoledronate, ibandronate, and alendronate. Pamidronate and zoledronate have been used most extensively for the treatment of humoral hypercalcemia of malignancy. Pamidronate is given in doses of 30, 60, or 90 mg, depending upon the degree of hypercalcemia, over 4–24 h. Zoledronate has the advantage of having a longer effect and requiring a shorter infusion time (4 mg over 15 min). All bisphosphonates must be used with caution in patients with CKD because the ideal dosing is not well understood, and there is the potential for renal toxicity [11]. Bisphosphonates should be considered the most definitive therapy for hypercalcemia outside of therapy of the underlying condition. The addition of calcitonin to bisphosphonates will lead to more rapid control of the hypercalcemia.

Glucocorticoids are effective in the treatment of hypercalcemia due to granulomatous diseases such as sarcoidosis. Prednisone in doses of 20–40 mg per day is usually effective in suppressing the production by macrophages of 1,25 (OH)-vitamin D that leads to hypercalcemia [12].

In states of hypocalcemia, the treatment depends upon the severity of the hypocalcemia, symptoms, and signs. In cases of mild chronic hypocalcemia associated with vitamin D deficiency, treatment with oral cholecalciferol or ergocalciferol along with oral calcium supplementation, will generally correct the hypocalcemia. Calcium carbonate is an inexpensive oral calcium supplement, and it is 40% elemental calcium by weight. For more refractory cases of hypocalcemia, as in patients who have undergone parathyroidectomy, calcitriol in doses of 0.25–1.0 μg daily may be used to increase oral calcium absorption from the gastrointestinal tract.

Symptomatic hypocalcemia with neuromuscular irritability or electrocardiographic manifestations requires replacement with intravenous calcium. Calcium gluconate is preferred as a calcium salt over calcium chloride because the latter is quite caustic in cases of extravasation. Calcium gluconate should be given intravenously in a dose of 1–2 g initially, followed by a slow infusion of calcium. Oral calcium supplements and oral calcitriol should also be given as soon as the patient is able to tolerate oral medications, thus allowing the maintenance of serum calcium levels and the gradual withdrawal of the intravenous infusion.

Prognosis

The prognosis for hypercalcemia and hypocalcemia depends primarily upon the underlying cause. Patients with hypercalcemia of malignancy have a poor prognosis: within 1 month, about 50% of these patients have died. The prognosis of hypocalcemia is generally good if the hypocalcemia is appropriately managed and if the patient is compliant with long-term oral calcium supplementation.

Complications

Patients with hyperparathyroidism are at risk of developing kidney stones, particularly calcium oxalate stones due, in part, to hypercalciuria. However, only about 7–20% of individuals with primary hyperparathyroidism will develop kidney stones. Strategies to reduce stone formation in patients with primary hyperparathyroidism, in addition to surgical treatment of the underlying process, include maintaining a urine flow rate of at least 2 L per day, reduction of dietary oxalate, and dietary sodium restriction since a high urinary sodium concentration increases urinary calcium excretion.

Case 1 Discussion

A 62-year-old man with renal cell carcinoma develops hypercalcemia with a calcium of 11.4 mg/dL. His hypercalcemia was confirmed by measuring the ionized calcium, which was 6.3 mg/dL (REF 4.5–5.3). The serum protein electrophoresis was normal. The PTH was appropriately suppressed at 11.1 pg/mL, and the PTHrP was elevated at 101 pg/mL. The patient was treated with 30 mg of intravenous pamidronate with resolution of his hypercalcemia prior to undergoing right nephrectomy. In this case, the paraneoplastic production of PTHrP by the renal cell carcinoma was cured by nephrectomy.

Disorders of Magnesium

Magnesium serves important cellular functions, including acting as an enzymatic cofactor in more than 300 enzymatic reactions that involve energy metabolism and nucleic acid synthesis [13]. In addition, magnesium is involved in regulating neuromuscular function, hormone receptor binding, gating of calcium channels, cardiac excitation, and neurotransmitter release, among other functions. Magnesium is stored in several body compartments: 60% in bone, 20% in muscle, and the rest in soft tissues [14]. Serum magnesium levels are tightly regulated even though less than 1% of total body magnesium is stored in serum and red blood cells. In the serum, magnesium exists in three states: ionized, protein bound, mainly to albumin, and complexed to anions such as citrate and phosphate [15].

Epidemiology

Hypermagnesemia occurs rarely in the USA. One study of routine magnesium measurements found magnesium abnormalities in 53% of specimens analyzed. Of the 1,033 specimens, hypomagnesemia occurred in 487 (47%), while hypermagnesemia was present in 59 (5.7%) [16]. Magnesium deficiency is common in hospitalized patients with a prevalence of 7–11%. Hypomagnesemia may occur concurrently in up to 40% of patients with other electrolytes abnormalities, particularly hypokalemia and hypophosphatemia [17].

Etiology/Pathophysiology

Hypermagnesemia may be seen in the setting of administration of magnesium containing antacids or cathartics to patients with CKD where the impaired GFR limits magnesium excretion. Obstetric patients can receive large doses of intravenous magnesium as treatment for preeclampsia or eclampsia and thus developed iatrogenic hypermagnesemia.

Table 11.3 Causes of hypomagnesemia

Malnutrition
Alcoholism
Diarrhea
Malabsorption
Proton pump inhibitors
Cisplatin
Amphotericin B
Cetuximab
Osmotic diuresis
Hypercalcemia
Gitelman syndrome

Hypomagnesemia may be related to one of three mechanisms (see Table 11.3): (1) dietary magnesium deficiency, (2) gastrointestinal losses, or (3) renal losses. Dietary magnesium deficiency is particularly common among alcoholic patients and patients with generalized protein-calorie malnutrition. Gastrointestinal magnesium losses may be caused by diarrhea or malabsorptive disorders such as inflammatory bowel disease. Diarrheal fluid is high in magnesium content, so that any cause of diarrhea may be associated with hypomagnesemia. Proton-pump inhibitors are an important but not well-known drug-induced cause of hypomagnesemia [18]. Although the mechanism by which proton pump inhibitors cause hypomagnesmia is not well understood, it is thought to be due to decreased absorption of magnesium from the gastrointestinal tract rather than to renal wasting.

Renal magnesium wasting is most commonly seen as a result of tubular toxicity caused by medications such as cisplatin and amphotericin B. More recently, drugs that target the EGF receptor, such as cetuximab, have been associated with renal magnesium wasting [19]. The renal tubular injury associated with leptospirosis may cause renal magnesium wasting [20]. Other causes of renal magnesium wasting include osmotic diuresis, hypercalcemia, and genetic tubular disorders such as Gitelman syndrome.

Clinical Features

The clinical manifestations of hypermagnesemia involve the neuromuscular system and the cardiovascular system. Mild hypermagesnemia with levels of 4–6 mg/dL may cause nausea, vomiting, flushing, urinary retention, ileus, and hyporeflexia. As the serum magnesium level approaches 7–9 mg/dL, respiratory depression occurs, the PR and QT intervals elongate, and the QRS complex widens. In the most severe cases of hypermagnesemia, there may be hypotension, complete heart block, and asystole. Because high levels of magnesium may inhibit acetylcholine release from the neuromuscular end plate, flaccid paralysis may develop in cases of severe hypermagnesemia. Paralysis of the respiratory muscles may lead to respiratory failure. Smooth muscle paralysis also may occur, causing urinary retention and ileus.

Clinically, hypomagnesemia is often asymptomatic. It is often suspected in association with other electrolyte abnormalities, specifically hypokalemia and hypocalcemia. Patients with hypomagnesemia who are symptomatic may have nonspecific symptoms such as anorexia, vomiting, tremors, ataxia, vertigo, or confusion. Hypomagnesemia is often suspected clinically in patients with a prolonged QT interval on electrocardiography. Severe hypomagnesemia may predispose to the development of ventricular arrhythmias, including *torsades de pointes*.

Differential Diagnosis

The distinction between hypomagnesemia caused by gastrointestinal losses or renal wasting is made by measuring urinary magnesium excretion through a 24-h urine or by calculating the fractional excretion of magnesium (FE_{Mg}). In states of hypomagnesemia the kidney should conserve magnesium to low levels. Thus, an $FE_{Mg} > 2\%$ or 24-h urinary magnesium excretion that exceeds about 30 mg indicates urinary magnesium wasting [21]. The FE_{Mg} is calculated using the following equation

$$FE_{Mg} = \left(U_{Mg} \times P_{Cr}\right) / \left[\left(P_{Mg} \times 0.7\right) \times U_{Cr}\right] \times 100.$$

U_{Mg} is the urinary magnesium concentration in mg/dL, P_{Cr} is the plasma creatinine concentration in mg/dL, P_{Mg} is the plasma magnesium concentration in mg/dL, and U_{Cr} is the urine creatinine concentration in mg/dL. The plasma magnesium concentration is corrected by a factor of 0.7 since about 30% of the measured total magnesium is bound to albumin and therefore not free to be filtered across the glomerular filtration barrier [21].

Management

Hypermagnesemia in patients with normal renal function may be treated with saline diuresis, just as in cases of hypercalcemia. However, saline diuresis will also increase the renal excretion of calcium, thereby potentially exacerbating the effects of hypermagnesemia through the development of hypocalcemia. The effects of hypermagnesemia may be blunted by the administration of intravenous calcium [22]. In cases of severe hypermagnesemia and renal failure, hemodialysis or continuous renal replacement with a magnesium-free dialysate or magnesium-free replacement fluid are very effective in lowering the serum magnesium concentration [23].

The hypomagnesemic patient usually requires magnesium repletion, either orally or intravenously. Patients with signs of ventricular arrhythmias associated with hypomagnesemia should be given 50 mEq of intravenous magnesium over 8–24 h. (One gram of magnesium sulfate contains 8.12 mEq of magnesium.) Hypomagnesemia is a major stimulus to reabsorption of magnesium in the thick ascending limb of the loop of Henle. Hence, the administration of intravenous magnesium removes the driving force for magnesium reclamation so that as much as 50% of an administered intravenous magnesium dose may be excreted in the urine. The repletion of intracellular magnesium stores may take several days, so repeated doses of intravenous magnesium as well as the concurrent administration of oral magnesium may be required in cases of severe magnesium deficiency.

Oral magnesium repletion is preferred for the asymptomatic patient. Magnesium oxide tablets provide 20.6 mEq of magnesium per 416 mg tablet. Sustained release preparations of magnesium chloride and magnesium lactate are also available, providing 5–7 mEq of magnesium per tablet. The major side effect of oral magnesium preparations that limits their utility is diarrhea. Amiloride, a potassium sparing diuretic that acts on the epithelial sodium channel in the cortical collecting segment of the distal nephron, may be used an adjunct to treat refractory hypomagnesemia induced by thiazide or loop diuretics since it enhances magnesium reabsorption in the cortical collecting tubule [24].

Complications

Complications of hypermagnesemia include confusion, diminished deep tendon reflexes, hypotension, respiratory failure, complete heart block, and asystole.

The complications associated with hypomagnesemia include electrolyte abnormalities, namely hypokalemia, and neuromuscular symptoms such as vertigo, ataxia, confusion, tremors, and seizures. Electrocardiographic findings include prolongation of the QT interval, and in severe cases, ventricular arrhythmias such as *torsades de pointes*.

Case 2 Discussion

A 64 year-old man with a history of renal cell carcinoma, left nephrectomy, and partial right nephrectomy, spinal cord infarction with paraplegia, and chronic obstipation presents with abdominal pain and distention. In the Emergency Department, he is noted to be lethargic, bradycardic, and hypotensive. He requires intubation for hypoxemic and hypercapnic respiratory failure. Electrolytes are sodium 133 mEq/L, potassium 4.2 mEq/L, chloride 100 mEq/L, and CO_2 22 mEq/L. The BUN is 46 mg/dL and the creatinine is 1.6 mg/dL. His electrocardiogram shows right bundle branch block and left fasicular block, and the QTc interval is 564 ms. The serum magnesium level was 8.9 mg/dL.

This patient developed hypermagnesemia in the setting of the use of oral magnesium salts for treatment of chronic obstipation. With worsening CKD, he developed hypermagnesemia complicated by lethargy, bradycardia, respiratory failure, and hypotension. He was intubated, placed on mechanical ventilation and admitted to an intensive care unit. He was given intravenous calcium and started on hemodialysis with vasopressor support, followed by continuous venovenous hemofiltration with a magnesium-free replacement fluid. Within 24 h, the patient's magnesium level had come down to normal range.

Disorders of Phosphorus

Overview

Phosphorus is critical to a number of cellular metabolic functions related to energy and metabolism including ammoniagenesis, glycolysis, and gluconeogenesis. The vast majority of phosphate stores are intracellular as creatinine phosphate and adenosine triphosphates, which serve as energy sources for a variety of biologic functions. Phosphorus is also a constituent of cell membranes in the form of phospholipids.

About 80% of phosphorus is stored in bone in the form of hyroxyapatite and only about 0.1% is found in extracellular fluid [25]. Within the serum, about 85% of inorganic phosphorus occurs as free inorganic phosphate ions ($H_2PO_4^-$ and HPO_4^{2}), while about 10% is protein bound and 5% is complexed to calcium, magnesium, or sodium [1, 25]. Phosphorus is absorbed from the gastrointestinal tract under the influence of vitamin D, while its renal excretion is controlled by PTH and the phosphaturic hormone fibroblast growth factor-23 (FGF-23).

Epidemiology

Hypophosphatemia that is not associated with other disorders that affect phosphate absorption or urinary excretion such as hyperparathyroidism occurs most often in the setting of alcoholism, malnutrition, and diabetic ketoacidosis. One study reported that 0.91% of hospitalized alcoholics were found to be severely hypophosphatemic (phosphorus less than or equal to 0.3 mmol/L [0.93 mg/dL]) on routine laboratory measurements, while 2.42% of septic patients, 10.4% of malnourished patients, and 14.6% of patients with diabetic ketoacidosis had severe hypophosphatemia [26]. Clinically significant hypophosphatemia occurs rarely in patients with primary hyperparathyroidism. Hypophosphatemia may also occur in the setting of the refeeding syndrome.

Hyperphosphatemia is a common finding in patients with CKD, including patients on dialysis. Hyperphosphatemia becomes most apparent at about stage 4 of CKD with a prevalence of about 40% among patients with a GFR of less than 20 mL/min [27].

Etiology/Pathophysiology

There are three mechanisms by which hypophosphatemia may occur: (1) decreased intestinal absorption, (2) increased urinary excretion, and (3) redistribution. Causes of hypophosphatemia are outlined in Table 11.4.

Decreased intestinal absorption occurs most commonly in the setting of severe malnutrition and alcoholism. Diarrhea, malabsorption, and the use of phosphate binding antacids may also lead to the development of hypophosphatemia. Because vitamin D and 1,25 (OH) vitamin D play a major role in controlling phosphorus homeostasis, deficiency of vitamin D may lead to hypophosphatemia.

Increased urinary excretion of phosphorus occurs in the setting of primary hyperparathyroidism and in the patients with end-stage renal

Table 11.4 Causes of hypophosphatemia

Diarrhea
Malabsorption
Vitamin D deficiency
Primary hyperparathyroidism
Post renal transplantation
Fanconi's syndrome
Imitinab
Post-obstructive diuresis
Glucosuria
Refeeding syndrome
Diabetic ketoacidosis
Hungry bones syndrome

disease and tertiary hyperparathyroidism who undergo renal transplantation. A more common cause of hypophosphatemia, however, is generalized proximal tubular dysfunction, also known as Fanconi's syndrome, in which urinary phosphate wasting occurs along with glucosuria, aminoacodiuria, and metabolic acidosis. In adults the most common cause of Fanconi's syndrome is multiple myeloma. However, a number of medications such as the cancer chemotherapeutic agent ifosfamide and the antiretroviral tenofovir [28] also cause Fanconi's syndrome [1]. Imitinab has been reported to cause hypophosphatemia by inducing Fanconi's syndrome as well as by causing bone turnover and phosphate release [29–31]. Post-obstructive diuresis and glucosuria are also associated with increased urinary losses of phosphorus.

The redistribution of phosphate from the extracellular to the intracellular compartment is the most common cause of hypophosphatemia. In diabetics with hyperglycemia, an osmotic diuresis causes increased urinary losses of phosphorus while at the same time, the hyperglycemia along with insulin therapy causes a further shift of phosphorus into cells. Similarly the refeeding of a severely malnourished patient, for example, a chronic alcoholic, will drive phosphorus from the extracellular into the intracellular compartment [32]. Respiratory alkalosis caused by hyperventilation may also lead to hypophosphatemia because of a shift of phosphorus into the intracellular compartment [25]. Finally the hungry bone syndrome, which often occurs in patients with end-stage renal disease undergoing parathyroidectomy for tertiary hyperparathyroidism, may lead to hypocalcemia and hypophosphatemia because the bones act as a massive reservoir for these ions, and they deposit in large quantities following parathyroidectomy.

Hyperphosphatemia occurs due to either impaired renal excretion of phosphorus, the rapid release of phosphorus from intracellular stores into the extracellular compartment, or increased intestinal absorption of phosphorus [1]. Table 11.5 lists causes of hyperphosphatemia. Impaired renal excretion of phosphorus occurs commonly in CKD but generally not until stage 4 [27].

Table 11.5 Causes of hyperphosphatemia

Chronic kidney disease
Hypoparathyroidism
Acromegaly
Hyperthyroidism
Volume depletion
Familial tumoral calcinosis
Tumor lysis syndrome
Rhabdomyolysis
Hemolysis
Hyperthermia
Vitamin D intoxication
Phosphate containing medications

Increased active reabsorption of phosphate in the kidney occurs in hypoparathyroidism, acromegaly, hyperthyroidism, volume depletion, and in familial tumoral calcinosis, a rare autosomal recessive disorder characterized by hyperphosphatemia and calcified soft-tissue masses. The rapid release of tissue stores of phosphorus occurs in tumor lysis syndrome, rhabdomyolysis, hemolysis, and hyperthermia. Finally, intestinal absorption of phosphorus leading to hyperphosphatemia occurs with the intake of large quantities of phosphate-containing enemas or laxatives or with vitamin D overdose [1].

Clinical Features

Phosphate depletion may cause any of a number of symptoms, and the symptoms generally occur at a phosphate level of <0.3 mmol/L (0.93 mg/dL). Patients with prolonged hyperventilation and patients who are recovering from diabetic ketoacidosis are often asymptomatic because there is often not a real phosphate depletion, just redistribution [33].

Clinical manifestations of phosphate depletion include proximal myopathy, weakness, bone pain, rhabdomyolysis, myocardial dysfunction, respiratory failure, failure to wean, tremors, neuropathy, and hemolysis.

Hyperphosphatemia may often be asymptomatic; however, patients with end-stage renal disease and chronic hyperphosphatemia often develop musculoskeletal symptoms such as bone pain and muscle weakness related to secondary or tertiary hyperparathyroidism. Pruritus is commonly noted in dialysis patients with hyperphosphatemia. Chronic hyperphosphatemia and elevation of the calcium × phosphorus product (>65–70) may also predispose dialysis patients to vascular calcification and the development of calcific uremic arteriolopathy.

Differential Diagnosis

Hypophosphatemia is caused by one of three mechanisms: (1) decreased intestinal absorption, (2) increased urinary excretion, and (3) redistribution. The diagnosis can usually be made by history with careful attention to diet, medications, and risk factors for redistribution of phosphorus. If the history is not revealing, the fractional excretion of phosphorus can be calculated to assess for urinary losses. In states of hypophosphatemia, the kidney should retain phosphorus such that the fractional excretion of phosphorus is < 5%.

Management

Mild chronic hypophosphatemia may typically be managed with oral phosphate repleation. Cow's milk is a good source of phosphorus as it contains about 1 mg (0.032 mmol) elemental phosphorus per mL [25]. Alternatively, phosphorus is commercially available as sodium or potassium phosphate. A typical dosing regimen would provide 15 mg/kg of oral phosphate in three to four divided doses to minimize diarrhea [34, 35].

Patients with severe or symptomatic hypophosphatemia will require intravenous repletion. A number of intravenous repletion protocols have been recommended. In one commonly used protocol 4.5 mmol/h is given for 3 h, with up to 90 mmol over a 24 h period [36]. More aggressive phosphate repletion protocols have been utilized in recent years, particularly in intensive care settings. A dose of 15 mmol of sodium phosphate administered over 2 h and repeated up to three times over 24 h has been shown to be effective in surgical intensive care unit patients with moderate hypophosphatemia [34, 37]. Weight-based and graded dosing regimens based upon the serum phosphate level have also been shown to be safe and effective [38, 39].

Severe hyperphosphatemia associated with the rapid release of phosphorus from intracellular stores and acute or chronic kidney dysfunction, as in tumor lysis syndrome, may require hemodialysis or continuous renal replacement therapy to lower the serum phosphorus. The time on dialysis is critical to phosphate removal; hence patients with severe hyperphosphatemia may require longer periods of dialysis or more frequent dialysis to control the serum phosphorus. Continuous renal replacement therapies are very effective at removing phosphorus such that most patients on these therapies require phosphorus repletion.

The management of chronic hyperphosphatemia associated with CKD centers around dietary phosphorus restriction and the use of phosphate binders. Phosphate binders are medications which are given with meals to bind dietary phosphorus within the gastrointestinal tract. Commonly used phosphate binders may be divided into calcium based and non-calcium based. Calcium carbonate and calcium acetate are the commonly used calcium-based binders. There has been increasing use in recent years of non-calcium-based binders because of concerns that the calcium-based binders may predispose to the development of soft tissue and vascular calcification; however, no mortality benefit has been shown with the use of non-calcium-based binders over calcium-based binders. The commonly used non-calcium-based binders in the USA are sevelamer hydrochloride, sevelamer carbonate, and lanthanum carbonate. Sevelamer carbonate has the advantage over the hydrochloride form of not causing the metabolic acidosis associated with the hydrochloride moiety [40]. Aluminum hydroxide is a very potent phosphate binder, but it is not recommended for long-term use because of the toxicities associated with aluminum tissue deposition.

Complications

The major complications of severe hypophosphatemia are muscular dysfunction, including myocardial dysfunction and respiratory failure, and hemolysis. The major complication of hyperphosphatemia is phosphate deposition in tissues due to its precipitation with calcium. A recently recognized cause of acute kidney injury, particularly in patients with preexisting CKD, is acute phosphate nephropathy due to the use of phosphate-containing bowel preparations for endoscopies [41].

Case 3 Discussion

A 50-year-old Cambodian woman presents to her primary care physician with complaints of profound weakness, to the point that she is bedbound. Her past medical history is notable for chronic hepatitis B infection, for which she is treated with tenofovir. Laboratory studies are notable for a sodium of 137 mEq/L, potassium of 2.5 mEq/L, chloride of 109 mEq/L, and CO_2 of 18 mEq/L. The BUN is 8 mg/dL and the creatinine is 0.92 mg/dL. Calcium and phosphorus are 7.8 mg/dL and 0.5 mg/dL, respectively. The urinalysis shows 2+ glucose and a pH of 7.0. What is the explanation for this patient's hypophosphatemia and how should it be treated?

This patient has profound hypophosphatemia associated with glucosuria and metabolic acidosis. Her presentation is consistent with Fanconi's syndrome, which is most likely caused by tenofovir. She was treated with intravenous phosphorus and oral vitamin D and tenofovir was discontinued. Her weakness gradually improved over several weeks.

References

1. Moe SM. Disorders involving calcium, phosphorus, and magnesium. Prim Care. 2008;35(2):215–37. v–vi.
2. PalmÉR M, Jakobsson S. ÅKerstrÖM G, Ljunghall S. Prevalence of hypercalcaemia in a health survey: a 14-year follow-up study of serum calcium values. Eur J Clin Invest. 1988;18(1):39–46.
3. Wermers RA, Khosla S, Atkinson EJ, Hodgson SF, O'Fallon WM, Melton 3rd LJ. The rise and fall of primary hyperparathyroidism: a population-based study in Rochester, Minnesota, 1965–1992. Ann Intern Med. 1997;126(6):433–40.
4. Zivin JR, Gooley T, Zager RA, Ryan MJ. Hypocalcemia: a pervasive metabolic abnormality in the critically ill. Am J Kidney Dis. 2001;37(4):689–98.
5. Pollak MR, Brown EM, Chou Y-HW, et al. Mutations in the human Ca2+-sensing receptor gene cause familial hypocalciuric hypercalcemia and neonatal severe hyperparathyroidism. Cell. 1993;75(7):1297–303.
6. Marx SJ. Familial hypocalciuric hypercalcemia. N Engl J Med. 1980;303(14):810–1.
7. Picolos MK, Lavis VR, Orlander PR. Milk-alkali syndrome is a major cause of hypercalcaemia among non-end-stage renal disease (non-ESRD) inpatients. Clin Endocrinol (Oxf). 2005;63(5):566–76.
8. Conron M, Young C, Beynon HL. Calcium metabolism in sarcoidosis and its clinical implications. Rheumatology (Oxford). 2000;39(7):707–13.
9. Labriola L, Wallemacq P, Gulbis B, Jadoul M. The impact of the assay for measuring albumin on corrected ('adjusted') calcium concentrations. Nephrol Dial Transplant. 2009;24(6):1834–8.
10. Wisneski LA. Salmon calcitonin in the acute management of hypercalcemia. Calcif Tissue Int. 1990; 46(Suppl):S26–30.
11. Stewart AF. Hypercalcemia associated with cancer. N Engl J Med. 2005;352(4):373–9.
12. Sharma OP. Hypercalcemia in granulomatous disorders: a clinical review. Curr Opin Pulm Med. 2000; 6(5):442–7.
13. Fawcett WJ, Haxby EJ, Male DA. Magnesium: physiology and pharmacology. Br J Anaesth. 1999;83(2): 302–20.
14. Elin RJ. Magnesium: the fifth but forgotten electrolyte. Am J Clin Pathol. 1994;102(5):616–22.
15. Elin RJ. Assessment of magnesium status. Clin Chem. 1987;33(11):1965–70.
16. Whang R, Ryder KW. Frequency of hypomagnesemia and hypermagnesemia. Requested vs routine. JAMA. 1990;263(22):3063–4.
17. Whang R, Oei TO, Aikawa JK, et al. Predictors of clinical hypomagnesemia. Hypokalemia, hypophosphatemia, hyponatremia, and hypocalcemia. Arch Intern Med. 1984;144(9):1794–6.
18. Regolisti G, Cabassi A, Parenti E, Maggiore U, Fiaccadori E. Severe hypomagnesemia during long-term treatment with a proton pump inhibitor. Am J Kidney Dis. 2010;56(1):168–74.
19. Izzedine H, Bahleda R, Khayat D, et al. Electrolyte disorders related to EGFR-targeting drugs. Crit Rev Oncol Hematol. 2010;73(3):213–9.
20. Khositseth S, Sudjaritjan N, Tananchai P, Ong-ajyuth S, Sitprija V, Thongboonkerd V. Renal magnesium wasting and tubular dysfunction in leptospirosis. Nephrol Dial Transplant. 2008;23(3):952–8.

21. Agus ZS. Hypomagnesemia. J Am Soc Nephrol. 1999;10(7):1616–22.
22. Mordes JP, Wacker WE. Excess magnesium. Pharmacol Rev. 1977;29(4):273–300.
23. Kelber J, Slatopolsky E, Delmez JA. Acute effects of different concentrations of dialysate magnesium during high-efficiency dialysis. Am J Kidney Dis. 1994;24(3):453–60.
24. Bundy JT, Connito D, Mahoney MD, Pontier PJ. Treatment of idiopathic renal magnesium wasting with amiloride. Am J Nephrol. 1995;15(1):75–7.
25. Gaasbeek A, Meinders AE. Hypophosphatemia: an update on its etiology and treatment. Am J Med. 2005;118(10):1094–101.
26. Camp MA, Allon M. Severe hypophosphatemia in hospitalized patients. Miner Electrolyte Metab. 1990;16(6):365–8.
27. Levin A, Bakris GL, Molitch M, et al. Prevalence of abnormal serum vitamin D, PTH, calcium, and phosphorus in patients with chronic kidney disease: results of the study to evaluate early kidney disease. Kidney Int. 2007;71(1):31–8.
28. Hall AM, Hendry BM, Nitsch D, Connolly JO. Tenofovir-associated kidney toxicity in HIV-infected patients: a review of the evidence. Am J Kidney Dis. 2011;57(5):773–80.
29. Francois H, Coppo P, Hayman JP, Fouqueray B, Mougenot B, Ronco P. Partial fanconi syndrome induced by imatinib therapy: a novel cause of urinary phosphate loss. Am J Kidney Dis. 2008;51(2): 298–301.
30. Berman E, Nicolaides M, Maki RG, et al. Altered bone and mineral metabolism in patients receiving imatinib mesylate. N Engl J Med. 2006;354(19): 2006–13.
31. Osorio S, Noblejas AG, Duran A, Steegmann JL. Imatinib mesylate induces hypophosphatemia in patients with chronic myeloid leukemia in late chronic phase, and this effect is associated with response. Am J Hematol. 2007;82(5):394–5.
32. Crook MA, Hally V, Panteli JV. The importance of the refeeding syndrome. Nutrition. 2001;17(7–8):632–7.
33. Kebler R, McDonald FD, Cadnapaphornchai P. Dynamic changes in serum phosphorus levels in diabetic ketoacidosis. Am J Med. 1985;79(5):571–6.
34. Brunelli SM, Goldfarb S. Hypophosphatemia: clinical consequences and management. J Am Soc Nephrol. 2007;18(7):1999–2003.
35. Shiber JR, Mattu A. Serum phosphate abnormalities in the emergency department. J Emerg Med. 2002;23(4):395–400.
36. Miller DW, Slovis CM. Hypophosphatemia in the emergency department therapeutics. Am J Emerg Med. 2000;18(4):457–61.
37. Rosen GH, Boullata JI, O'Rangers EA, Enow NB, Shin B. Intravenous phosphate repletion regimen for critically ill patients with moderate hypophosphatemia. Crit Care Med. 1995;23(7):1204–10.
38. Clark CL, Sacks GS, Dickerson RN, Kudsk KA, Brown RO. Treatment of hypophosphatemia in patients receiving specialized nutrition support using a graduated dosing scheme: results from a prospective clinical trial. Crit Care Med. 1995;23(9):1504–11.
39. Taylor BE, Huey WY, Buchman TG, Boyle WA, Coopersmith CM. Treatment of hypophosphatemia using a protocol based on patient weight and serum phosphorus level in a surgical intensive care unit. J Am Coll Surg. 2004;198(2):198–204.
40. Tonelli M, Pannu N, Manns B. Oral phosphate binders in patients with kidney failure. N Engl J Med. 2010;362(14):1312–24.
41. Markowitz GS, Stokes MB, Radhakrishnan J, D'Agati VD. Acute phosphate nephropathy following oral sodium phosphate bowel purgative: an underrecognized cause of chronic renal failure. J Am Soc Nephrol. 2005;16(11):3389–96.

Part IV

Acid–Base Disorders

Metabolic Acidosis

12

Warren L. Kupin

Case 1

A 24-year-old man with Type I Diabetes was found unconscious in his home. He had been depressed recently and was known to have become increasingly non-compliant with his insulin therapy and diet. Lying next to him was a glass bottle without a label on it with only a few drops of liquid in it. When he was brought to the ER he appeared to have labored breathing and a comprehensive blood panel, arterial blood gases, urinalysis, and a chest X-ray were performed. His test results are summarized in Table 12.1.

Case 2

A 30-year-old woman was seen by her primary care physician for an evaluation of a recent episode of nephrolithiasis. The stone passed spontaneously 2 weeks previously and she was now feeling well. Her X-rays showed no further signs of stone disease. Her past medical history is significant for long standing migraine headaches that have been quite severe. She has been taking Topiramate for the past 2 years which has successfully decreased her recurrent migraine episodes. A full biochemical profile was obtained and subsequently a blood gas was also ordered once the results were noted. Her test results are summarized in Table 12.1.

Introduction

The appropriate clinical diagnosis and management of acid–base disorders is an essential component of daily patient care and requires an organized systematic approach. This section will focus on the classification, differential diagnosis, and workup of patients with a primary metabolic acidosis and will be presented in a question and answer format with a detailed discussion of the clinical cases described above.

Are There Different Approaches Used to Describe and Define a Metabolic Acidosis?

There are three different methodologies currently employed in deciphering acid–base abnormalities: the Physiologic Concept by Van Slyke, the Base Excess Concept by Astrup, and the Strong Ion concept by Stewart [1]. The Physiologic Concept focuses primarily on the bicarbonate buffer system and is based on changes in the pH, pCO_2, and HCO_3^- concentrations as measured on the blood gas. It is assumed that changes in HCO_3^- directly reflect the H^+ balance in the body

W.L. Kupin, M.D. (✉)
Division of Nephrology and hypertension, Department of Medicine, University of Miami, Clinical Research Building, 1120 NW 14th Ave, Suite 360, Miami, FL 33136, USA
e-mail: WKupin@med.miami.edu

E.V. Lerma and M. Rosner (eds.), *Clinical Decisions in Nephrology, Hypertension and Kidney Transplantation*,
DOI 10.1007/978-1-4614-4454-1_12,

Table 12.1 Summary of laboratory results for Case 1 and Case 2

	Case 1	Case 2
Na (meq/L)	130	140
K (meq/L)	5.2	3.0
CL (meq/L)	96	110
HCO_3 (meq/L)	10	18
BUN (mg/dL)	30	10
Creatinine (mg/dL)	1.6	0.6
Glucose (mg/dL)	450	90
Anion gap	24	12
Measured serum osmolality (mosm/L)	310	288
Albumin (g/dL)	3.0	4.0
Arterial blood gas		
pO_2 (mmHg)	100	100
pCO_2 (mmHg)	24	35
HCO_3(mmHg)	10	18
pH	7.25	7.33
Base excess	−15	−7
Urine chemistry		
Na (meq/L)	40	35
K (meq/L)	20	20
Cl (meq/L)	70	90

and the directional change in HCO_3^- and pCO_2 is used to categorize the different subgroups of acid–base disorders [2]. In this approach the anion gap is used to identify the metabolic source of the acidosis. The Physiologic Concept requires only collection of a blood gas and an electrolyte profile. This approach is the most common one used clinically and will be the foundation of the concepts discussed in this section.

The Base Excess Concept is often used as a supplement to the Physiologic Concept and also focuses on determining the H^+ balance of the body. However the key role of the HCO_3^- concentration in the Physiologic Concept is replaced by a new term called the standard base excess (SBE) [3]. Almost all laboratories that report the results of a blood gas also automatically calculate and report an SBE value. This result provides an estimate of the amount of alkali that must be added or removed to each liter of blood to normalize the pH assuming that the pCO_2 is normal at 40 mmHg. How the Base Excess Concept can be used in the setting of a metabolic acidosis will be addressed later in this chapter.

The Strong Ion Concept is the newest of the three methods used to describe acid–base disorders and focuses on a completely distinct definition of H^+ balance compared to the Physiologic and Base Excess Concepts [4]. In this method, the theory holds that the pH is not determined solely by the HCO_3^- concentration but rather by the equilibrium balance between the major cations (Na^+, K^+, Ca^{2+}, and Mg^{2+}) and the major anions (Cl^-, SO_4^{2-}, lactic acid, and albumin) [5]. At the present time the Strong Ion Concept is not widely utilized due to the complexity of the calculations and the lack of clinical data showing superiority of this approach as compared with the Physiologic Concept in predicting morbidity and mortality [6].

What Is the Difference Between the Terms Acidosis and Acidemia?

The pH of the extracellular fluid (ECF) is tightly controlled by renal and respiratory mechanisms and remains within the range of 7.35–7.45. If there is an absolute plasma accumulation of protons (H^+) or a loss of plasma bicarbonate (HCO_3^-), then the pH of the blood will fall below 7.35 indicating the presence of Acidemia. However, there may be circumstances when these same two processes occur but there is another over-riding acid–base disorder in the form of an alkalosis elevating the blood pH > 7.45. In this circumstance, the presence of the alkalosis will mask the presence of an underlying acidemic state. This condition is defined as an Acidosis and not an Acidemia because the blood pH is not below 7.35 but yet there is an excessive accumulation of H^+. Although the two terms are often used interchangeably, physiologically they differ by the clinical presentation. All patients with a pH below 7.35 have an acidemia and an acidosis. Selected patients with a pH > 7.45 may have an acidosis superimposed on their alkalosis (alkalemia) but do not have an acidemia. In essence, acidoses represent processes where by academia represents the final state of the blood pH due to the various processes.

How Do You Diagnose a Metabolic Acidosis?

By definition, a metabolic acidosis is characterized by an excess of H^+ which may result from either the accumulation of nonvolatile acids and/or the loss of bicarbonate (HCO_3^-). The nonvolatile acids may be of endogenous (i.e., lactic acid, ketoacids) or exogenous (toxins) origin while the loss of HCO_3^- may be of gastrointestinal (diarrhea, ostomy output) or renal (renal tubular acidosis) etiologies. Regardless of the cause, all types of metabolic acidosis are associated with a decrease in the HCO_3^- concentration [7].

The systematic evaluation of a metabolic acidosis can be outlined into five key steps (Fig. 12.1). The first step in the diagnosis of any acid–base disorder is to establish the primary disorder that is present [8]. There can be only one primary acid–base disorder among the four options: metabolic acidosis, metabolic alkalosis, respiratory acidosis, or respiratory alkalosis. The initial clinical suspicion of a metabolic acidosis usually comes from the presence of a low serum bicarbonate concentration (<24 meq/L) on the electrolyte profile. One of the most frequent errors is to label a patient with an acidosis strictly on the basis of the low serum bicarbonate level. This can be completely misleading since a low bicarbonate may be a reflection of the renal response to a primary respiratory alkalosis. Therefore the differential diagnosis of a low bicarbonate level may be either a metabolic acidosis or a respiratory alkalosis making the blood gas the key determining factor as to which disorder is present.

A blood gas is the first and most essential test required to begin any discussion of an acid–base abnormality. The pH of the blood gas will correctly identify the primary acid–base abnormality in terms of acidemia or alkalemia. Whether or not it is a respiratory or metabolic disorder depends on the direction of change in the pCO_2 and the HCO_3^- that corresponds to any given pH (Table 12.2). There are two important rules of thumb in acid–base physiology: (1) no acid–base

Table 12.2 Diagnosis of a primary acid–base disorder based on the blood gas

	Respiratory alkalosis	Metabolic acidosis	Respiratory acidosis	Metabolic alkalosis
pH	<7.35	<7.35	>7.45	>7.45
HCO_3 (meq/L)	<24	>24	>24	<24
pCO_2 (mmHg)	<40	>40	>40	<40

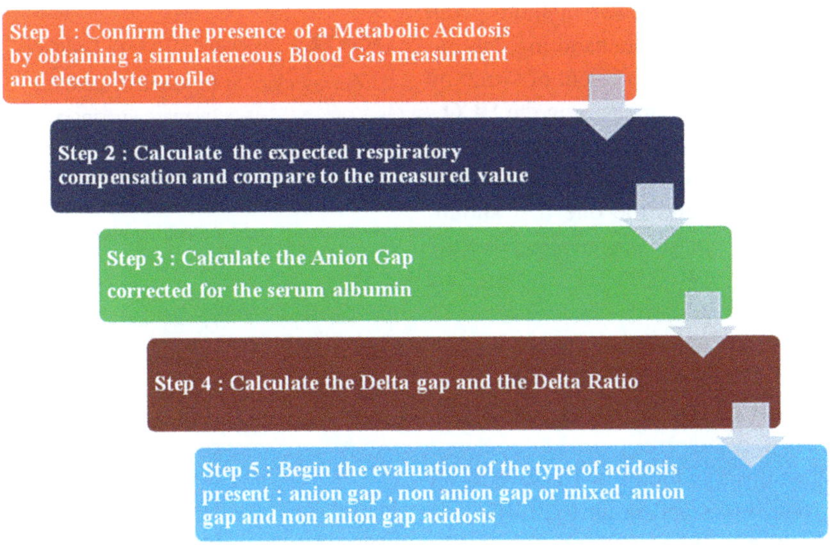

Fig. 12.1 Initial workup algorithm for a metabolic acidosis

disorder can ever overcorrect itself and (2) the compensatory mechanisms can never return the pH completely to normal. Whatever the pH is on the blood gas reflects the primary acid–base disorder. If the pH is in the normal range (7.35–7.45) in the setting of altered HCO_3^- and pCO_2 levels then there must be at least two distinct independent acid–base abnormalities present. Finally, the pO_2 concentration on the blood gas is not part of the evaluation of an acid–base abnormality and is not used to categorize the patients into any of the four primary disorders. However, a low pO_2 concentration may be hint that a lactic acidosis may be present.

Is There a Difference Between the HCO_3 Measured in Plasma or the HCO_3 Reported on the Blood Gas?

There can be occasional laboratory errors in the measurement of HCO_3 on routine serum samples which can lead to an erroneous diagnosis of a metabolic acidosis. The HCO_3^- measured in venous blood either from plasma or serum is a direct analytical measurement of HCO_3^- concentration, whereas the HCO_3^- reported on a blood gas is a mathematically derived value using the Henderson–Hasselbach equation with the measured pH and pCO_2 [9]. Periodically, a discrepancy may exist between these two methods given the variability of blood sample handling, laboratory preparation, and the coefficient of variation of the analyzer used when measuring the HCO_3^- in blood. Therefore the HCO_3^- value on the blood gas is a more accurate reflection of the true HCO_3^- concentration and the one that should be used for all calculations of the anion gap and the base deficit.

How Frequently Does a Metabolic Acidosis Occur in the Clinical Setting?

A metabolic acidosis is found in 10–15% of all emergency room visits and in up to 30–40% of hospitalized patients. When looking specifically at patients in the intensive care unit, 64% had an underlying metabolic acidosis [10]. The incidence of a metabolic acidosis in the community setting is likely a result of a chronic metabolic process leading to acidemia. In the National Health and Examination Survey (NHANES) III a cross section of 15,000 adults in the outpatient setting were studied and 1.9% were found to have a HCO_3^- of <22 meq/L suggestive of a metabolic acidosis [11]. Although a blood gas was not performed the data suggest that even outside of the hospital setting metabolic acidosis can be found in the general population.

What Are the Clinical Consequences of Having a Metabolic Acidosis?

The presence of an acute or chronic metabolic acidosis causes significant systemic complications (Table 12.3) [12]. In hospitalized patients, especially those in the intensive care unit, the impact of a metabolic acidosis will adversely affect morbidity and mortality. The blood pH is a separate and distinct integral component for the calculation of the APACHE score but in addition its peripheral effects will also indirectly influence other key elements influencing this score: the glascow coma scale, heart rate, potassium level, and respiratory rate [13].

Table 12.3 Systemic effects of metabolic acidosis

Cardiovascular	Impaired contractility
	Increased peripheral arterial vasodilation
	Increased sympathetic activity
	Decreased response to catecholamines
	Increased venous tone
	Pulmonary artery vasoconstriction
	Decreased threshold for arrhythmias
Neurologic	Obtundation/coma
Respiratory	Increased rate
	Shift of the oxygen/hemoglobin dissociation curve to the right
	Decreased 2,3 DPG production
Musculoskeletal	Increased bone resorption
Endocrine	Insulin resistance
	Increase protein catabolism

The most important systemic impact of a metabolic acidosis is on the cardiovascular system. As a result of impaired glycolysis and reduced ATP generation, a decrease in cardiac contractility occurs exacerbated by hypotension from increased arteriolar vasodilation. Although the sympathetic nervous system is activated in a metabolic acidosis there is increased resistance to the effects of catecholamines especially as the pH approaches 7.2. Central venous return is increased due to venoconstriction leading to an increased risk of pulmonary edema particularly in conjunction with the lower ejection fraction seen with an acidosis.

From a physiologic standpoint, the oxygen–hemoglobin dissociation curve is shifted to the right in metabolic acidosis which decreases the affinity of oxygen for hemoglobin allowing a greater release of oxygen to the tissues. This process is known as the Bohr Effect and is eventually offset by a gradual reduction in 2,3 DPG concentration in order to reestablish the normal dissociation curve (shift back to the left) [14]. Patients with persistent acidemia have markedly reduced 2,3 DPG levels.

Finally, long-term untreated metabolic acidosis leads to marked bone resorption and an increased risk of fractures. In children, impaired growth is a major consequence of acidosis which is reversible if treated early in its course. The loss of bone mass with chronic acidemia is a result of the constant leaching of carbonate from the bone in order to buffer the excess H^+ [15]. Overall, chronic metabolic acidosis leads to a hypercatabolic state.

What Compensatory Mechanisms Occur to Counteract the Development of a Metabolic Acidosis?

The abnormal buildup of H^+ in the ECF must be dealt with immediately to prevent dramatic and life threatening changes in the blood pH. A system of buffers exist both in the ECF and in the intracellular fluid (ICF) to sequester the H^+ and stabilize the pH until elimination of the acid can occur. After the buffering phase, both respiratory and renal mechanisms come into play to remove excess H^+ [16].

As the blood pH decreases and H^+ accumulates in the ECF, the presence of HCO_3^- provides the first line of defense with the formation of H_2CO_3 (carbonic acid). In the ICF, the presence of hemoglobin, proteins, and organophosphate complexes provides similar immediate buffering capacity. After the ECF and ICF buffers have initiated the first response, the pulmonary clearance of the volatile acid CO_2 takes over priority as the elimination of excess H^+ begins. In the lungs, the enzyme carbonic anhydrase catalyzes the removal of water (anhydrase) from H_2CO_3 which yields H_2O and CO_2. This CO_2 is expelled through increased respiration [17].

What Is Kussmaul Breathing?

The respiratory response to a metabolic acidosis is initiated directly through central chemoreceptors and indirectly through stimulation of peripheral chemoreceptors [18]. Central chemoreceptors are present in the respiratory center located on the ventrolateral surface of the medulla oblongata and detect changes in cerebrospinal fluid pH. Since H^+ cannot diffuse into the CSF, the change in CSF pH is a result of diffusion of pCO_2 into the CSF with local production of H^+ which then alters the pH and stimulates the chemoreceptor.

The peripheral chemoreceptors are located in the aortic body found along the aortic arch and in the carotid body located at the carotid bifurcation. The aortic chemoreceptors sense changes in pCO_2 only while the carotid chemoreceptors are stimulated by changes in H^+ as well as changes in pCO_2. Efferent signals from the peripheral chemoreceptors activate an increase in the respiratory rate and the depth of respiration. These signals stimulate the thoracic nerves (T1–T11) to increase the intercostal muscle activity to enhance the rate of respiration and the phrenic nerve (C3–C5) to increase diaphragmatic contractions in order to maximize the depth of respiration [19].

Kussmaul Breathing refers to the combination of rapid deep breathing that accompanies the pulmonary compensatory response to a metabolic acidosis [20]. It can be confused with tachypnea from respiratory distress such as from hypoxia, pulmonary edema or pneumonia, pain, CHF, or pulmonary embolism. In each of these circumstances the respiratory rate is rapid but shallow in an effort to improve oxygenation but not specifically to blow off CO_2 which is achieved more effectively by the depth of respiration rather than the rate. The absence of hypoxia, normal pulmonary findings on physical examination, and normal radiographic studies in addition to the unusual depth of each respiration should lead to the diagnosis of Kussmaul Breathing from an underlying metabolic acidosis.

Can the Pulmonary Response Be Predicted for Any Given Degree of Metabolic Acidosis?

Determining the clinically appropriate respiratory compensation to a metabolic acidosis is the second step in the investigation of a metabolic acidosis after obtaining the blood gas. The pulmonary response which follows the ECF and ICF buffering in a metabolic acidosis begins within minutes but takes approximately 12–24 h to reach its maximal effort. The predicted pCO_2 response for any level of acidemia can be mathematically determined and is the same for all individuals (Table 12.4) [21]. Of the four different formulas available the most commonly used one due to its accuracy is—expected pCO_2 (mmHg) $= (1.5 \times HCO_3) + 8 \pm 2$ (also known as Winter's Formula). There is a clearly defined physiologic limit to the amount of hyperventilation that can occur in the presence of a metabolic acidosis and in a healthy individual this is a pCO_2 of 8–12 mmHg [22]. In a patient with significant lung disease the maximal amount of hyperventilation will be limited.

After calculating the predicted pCO_2 and comparing it to the actual measured response it is now possible to determine if the patient is adequately compensating or if a mixed acid–base disorder is present. Hypothetically, if the pH is 7.32 and the HCO_3 is 15 meq/L then according to the formula—the expected pCO_2 should be $(1.5 \times 15) + 8 \pm 2 = 31 \pm 2$ mmHg. If the pCO_2 on the blood gas is in fact 31 mmHg then this patient is labeled as having an appropriate respiratory compensation. If the pCO_2 is 35 mmHg, a value higher than predicted and above the confidence limits of 29–33 mmHg, there is a presence of superimposed respiratory acidosis. Alternatively, if the pCO_2 was 26 mmHg, a level lower than predicted, then this patient has a superimposed respiratory alkalosis.

Table 12.4 Important formulas used in the diagnosis and evaluation of a metabolic acidosis

Respiratory compensation
1. pCO_2 (mmHg) $= (1.5 \times HCO_3) + 8 \pm 2$
2. $pCO_2 =$ last two digits of the pH
3. pCO_2 decreases by 1.25 for every 1 meq/L decrease in HCO_3
4. $pCO_2 = HCO_3 + 15$
Anion gap
$Na - (HCO_3 + Cl) = 12 \pm 4$ meq/L
Albumin correction for the anion gap
Decrease in anion gap (12) by 2.5 meq/L for every 1 g/dL decrease in albumin <4.5 g/dL
Delta anion gap
Calculated anion gap − anion gap corrected for albumin
Delta HCO_3
HCO_3 value (blood gas) − 24 meq/L (normal HCO_3 level)
Delta ratio
Delta anion gap − delta $HCO_3 = 0 \pm 6$ meq/L
Delta ratio
Delta anion gap/delta $HCO_3 = 1.0 \pm 0.2$
Calculated serum osmolality
$(2 \times Na) + glucose/18 + BUN/2.8$
Osmolar gap
Measured serum osmolality − calculated serum osmolality (normal <10 mosm/L)
Urine anion gap (used only in the presence of a non-anion gap metabolic acidosis)
(Urine Na + Urine K) − Urine Cl > −20 meq/L (adequate NH_4Cl generation)
Standard base excess
$0.9287 \times (HCO_3 - 24.4 + 14.83 \times [pH - 7.4]) = HCO_3^-$
Bicarbonate space
$[0.4 + (2.6/[HCO_3])] \times$ body weight (in kg)
Bicarbonate deficit
Standard base excess × (bicarbonate space × body weight)

As an example of how these combined disorders could occur clinically, maintenance of the respiratory compensation in metabolic acidosis requires a continued supply of energy (ATP) for the ongoing diaphragmatic hyperactivity. Over time many patients may tire and be unable to maintain the same level of respiratory rate leading to an elevation of the pCO_2 at a value higher than expected resulting in a superimposed respiratory acidosis. In the second example, a coexisting pneumonia or sepsis would cause additional hyperventilation (respiratory alkalosis) beyond the level that would be expected from the primary metabolic acidosis and result in a pCO_2 lower than predicted. Understanding how and when to use the compensatory formula for a metabolic acidosis is essential to being able to pick up hidden mixed disorders. Understanding these hidden mixed acid–base disorders is critical in identifying patients with subtle regulatory deficits that may subsequently develop a decompensation.

What Does the Anion Gap Indicate?

The third step in the evaluation of a metabolic acidosis is calculation of the anion gap (Table 12.4) [23]. Conceptually the term "anion gap" is a misnomer because there can never be an imbalance between the number of cations and the number of anions in the body based on the law of electrical neutrality. The anion gap is an artificial deficit because the equation does not take into consideration all the actual circulating cations and anions. The measured electrolytes used in the calculation: anion gap $= Na - (Cl + HCO_3)$, yield an average value of 12 ± 4 indicating a deficit of 12 meq/L of the sum between the unmeasured cations and the unmeasured anions. In reality this deficit is made up of those unmeasured anions and cations not used in the equation: K^+, Ca^{2+}, Mg^{2+}, PO_4^{3-}, and most importantly albumin [24].

The serum albumin plays a major role in determining the normal range of the anion gap especially for hospitalized patients. It is estimated that albumin typically accounts for 65% of the negative unmeasured anion charges in the normal person. Albumin is a polyvalent anion that contributes 2.5 meq/L of charge to the anion gap for every 1 g/dL of albumin concentration [25]. When the normal range for the anion gap is listed as 12 ± 4 meq/L it is assumed that the serum albumin is 4.5 g/dL. As the serum albumin falls from protein catabolism, cytokine release, malnutrition, nephrotic syndrome, cirrhosis, and other causes, the anion gap must decrease accordingly because of the loss of the negative charges contributed by albumin and the replacement of these charges by higher Cl^- and HCO_3^- levels. For example, if the anion gap is 12 meq/L for a patient with an albumin of 4.5 g/dL then when the albumin falls to 3.5 g/dL the expected anion gap for that patient is now $12 - 2.5 = 9.5$ meq/L. With an albumin of 2.0 g/dL, a level frequently seen in acute and chronically ill patients, the "normal" anion gap for that patient is now $12 - 5.0 = 7$ meq/L (two increments of 1 g/dL each decrease in albumin at a charge loss of 2.5 meq/L for each 1 g/dL).

A metabolic acidosis is defined as either the accumulation of nonvolatile acid (H^+) or the loss of HCO_3 leading to a relative excess of blood H^+ [26]. The anion gap is used to detect the presence of either endogenously or exogenously produced anionic organic or inorganic acids. In the presence of a circulating acid, HCO_3^- levels will be reduced as a consequence of their buffering capacity. The anion gap will increase because the other electrolytes (Na^+ and Cl^-) remain unchanged in their concentration. Even though HCO_3^- has been consumed the law of electrical neutrality is preserved because Na^+ is now free to bind to the anionic acid (such as lactate) in a molar equivalent to the amount of H^+ released by the acid molecule. All acids regardless of their origin will result in an increase of the anion gap. An anion gap >16 is usually considered to be clinically important and a gap >30 is highly associated with acidosis from an exogenous intoxication. A variety of mnemonics have been used in order to remember all the potential causes of an anion gap acidosis and these are listed in Table 12.5 [27].

Alternatively, the HCO_3^- may be low in the presence of a normal anion gap indicating loss of HCO_3^- from either a renal or GI source or the accumulation of H^+ due to a failure of renal excretion. The causes of a normal anion gap metabolic acidosis are listed in Table 12.6.

Table 12.5 Etiologies of an anion gap metabolic acidosis: CUTE DIMPLES

		Source	Acid
C	Cyanide	Occupational exposure Amygdalin (Apricot. peach kernels) Nitroprusside therapy	Lactic acid
U	Uremia	Kidney	Sulfuric acid Phosphoric acid Lactic acid
T	Toluene	Glue sniffing Industrial solvent Paints/dyes/varnishes	Hippuric acid
	Tylenol	Acetaminophen analgesics	Pyroglutamic acid
E	Ethylene glycol[a]	Antifreeze/coolant	Glycolic acid Glyoxalic acid Lactic acid
D	Diabetes	Diabetic ketoacidosis	β Hydroxybutyric acid Acetoacetic acid
	D-Lactate	Short bowel syndrome	D-Lactic acid
I	Isoniazid	Anti-tuberculosis therapy	Lactic acid
	Iron	Vitamin supplements	Lactic acid
M	Methanol[a]	Windshield wiper fluid Industrial solvent	Formic acid
	Metformin	Hypoglycemic therapy	Lactic acid
P	Propylene Glycol[a]	Medication solvent (Diazepam. Lorazepam)	Lactic acid
	Phenformin	Hypoglycemic agent	Lactic acid
L	L-Lactate	Mitochondria	Lactic acid
E	Ethanol	Alcoholic ketoacidosis	β Hydroxybutyric acid Acetoacetic acid
S	Salicylates	Aspirin Oil of wintergreen Bismuth subsalicylate	Salicylic acid

[a]Osmolar gap may be present

What Is the Renal Response to a Metabolic Acidosis?

The renal adaptation to control a metabolic acidosis is the third and last systemic mechanism that is present often requiring 3–5 days to reach maximal activity. The kidney's role in a metabolic acidosis is to achieve two main objectives—(1) enhance bicarbonate reabsorption and (2) increase net H^+ secretion. These processes are distinct and separate from each other with the proximal tubule being almost exclusively responsible for HCO_3 reclamation and the distal tubule having the sole capacity for net H^+ secretion [28].

In the proximal tubule the enzyme carbonic anhydrase is present both on the luminal surface and also inside the cells in order to catalyze the conversion of filtered HCO_3^- to CO_2. This allows the CO_2 to be absorbed into the cells and re-converted back to HCO_3^- which is added to the systemic circulation. Even though no new HCO_3^- is generated, this process is essential to reclaim and maintain the serum HCO_3^- concentration until the source of the acidosis is removed [29].

The intercalated cells of the distal tubule have ultimate responsibility for the secretion of H^+ into the urinary space. In order to add H^+ into the urine, buffers must be present to avoid lowering the urine pH to levels that would cause tissue injury. In addition, if the secreted H^+ were to remain in a free ionic form, no additional H^+ could be secreted against a high concentration gradient. The urine pH must be maintained >5.0 and the presence of a combination of a titratable acid (phosphoric acid—$H_2PO_4^-$ and HPO_4^{2-}) and a buffer system (NH_3/NH_4^+) prevents an extreme fall in the urine pH. Therefore, the urine pH is not a reliable indicator of the absolute amount of H^+ being secreted since the urine may contain a large quantity of buffered H^+ and the pH can be 5.5 [30].

The source of the $H_2PO_4^-$ and HPO_4^{2-} is through glomerular filtration and is a relatively fixed amount regardless of the acid–base status of the patient. The source of urinary NH_3 is from deamination of glutamine in the proximal tubule, a process that is pH sensitive and is the key regulator of renal acid excretion. Any cause of renal parenchymal injury especially tubulointerstitial diseases will inhibit renal ammoniagenesis and prevent the normal H^+ secretory function of the distal tubule due to lack of the NH_3 buffer in the urine. The most common cause of acidosis in Chronic Kidney Disease Stages 3–5 is a failure of ammoniagenesis from parenchymal injury [31].

What Is the Benefit of Measuring a Urinary Anion Gap?

A urine anion gap (UAG) is used only in the evaluation of a patient with a non-anion gap metabolic acidosis. A UAG has no application in the presence of a high anion gap acidosis. Once the diagnosis of a non-anion acidosis is made, clues to the etiology of this disorder can be obtained from the UAG [32]. The UAG is calculated from the electrolyte values on a random urine sample and is expressed as meq/L: $UAG = (Na + K) - Cl$.

This formula differs from the calculation of the serum anion gap by the elimination of the HCO_3^- concentration in the anion part of the equation since there is no appreciable HCO_3^- that reaches the final urine that is excreted in a healthy state. The UAG is a direct reflection of NH_4^+ production in the setting of a metabolic acidosis. Once formed in the distal tubule NH_4^+ is excreted as the chloride salt—NH_4Cl in the final urine [33].

In a steady state with a systemic pH of 7.40, minimal amounts of NH_4Cl will be produced and virtually all the Cl^- in the urine will be bound for electrical neutrality by a urinary Na^+ or K^+. The UAG will be −20–0 meq/L or even a slightly positive number. However, in the setting of a metabolic acidosis, a significant amount of Cl^- will be excreted as NH_4Cl. In the calculation of the UAG, there will be an excess concentration of Cl^- not accounted for by Na^+ or K^+ and the value will be a highly negative number often <−50 meq/L indicating large amounts of NH_4Cl and a well functioning distal tubule. Any UAG value <−20 is considered to be a result supporting adequate distal tubular function (Table 12.6) [34].

Patients with either a gastrointestinal cause of a non-anion gap metabolic acidosis or a Type II (proximal) renal tubular acidosis (RTA) will have a normal functioning distal tubule and the UAG will be a highly negative number (<−50 meq/L). In the presence of a Type I or Type IV distal RTA the UAG will be close to 0 or a positive number in spite of the presence of systemic acidemia indicating an ineffective distal tubule and the absence of NH_4^+ production.

What Is Meant by the Terms Delta Gap, Delta/Delta, and Delta Ratio?

The fourth step in the evaluation of a metabolic acidosis is to determine if there is another acid–base abnormality present in addition to a primary metabolic acidosis. The delta gap represents the difference between the change in the anion gap and the change in the HCO_3 concentration. This is why it is sometimes abbreviated and called the delta/delta as it is the delta change in the anion gap compared to the delta change in HCO_3^- [35].

Ideally, for every additional anion added to the blood making the anion gap increase, the H^+ from that anion was released and buffered by HCO_3 thereby lowering the HCO_3^- concentration. The delta or change in the anion gap should equal the delta or change in the HCO_3 levels and the difference would be equal to 0 for a patient with a high

Table 12.6 Differential diagnosis of a non-anion gap metabolic acidosis

		Urine anion gap (meq/L)
Gastrointestinal		<–20
Diarrhea		
Pancreatic fistula		
Ureteral diversions		
Renal tubular acidosis		
Proximal (Type II)		<–20
Storage diseases		
Myeloma/Fanconi's syndrome		
Heavy metals		
Drugs		
Carbonic anhydrase inhibitors		
Tenofovir		
Ifosphamide		
Amyloidosis		
Distal (Type I)		>–20 or any positive value
Drugs		
Amphotericin	Ifosphamide	
Lithium		
Autoimmune diseases		
SLE, Sjogren's, rheumatoid arthritis		
Obstructive uropathy		
Sickle cell anemia		
Hypergammaglobulinemia		
Distal (Type IV)		>–20 or any positive value
Diabetes mellitus		
Obstructive uropathy		
Drugs		
Trimethoprim	NSAIDs	
Amiloride	Pentamidine	
Spironolactone	Epleronone	
Triamterene	ACEI	
ARB	Cyclosporine/tacrolimus	
Heparin		

anion gap acidosis. It must be kept in mind that the anion gap must be corrected as usual for the albumin and the HCO_3 used should be the one from the blood gas. Given the variations on accuracy of measuring the anion gap the normal delta ratio has relatively a large confidence interval so the delta gap = delta (anion gap) − delta (HCO_3) = 0 ± 6. Therefore any delta gap value between −6 and +6 means there is no likely superimposed acid–base disorder on top of the metabolic acidosis [36].

For example, if the patient has an anion gap of 20 the delta anion gap is 20 − 12 (normal anion gap assuming an albumin of 4.5 g/dL) = 8 meq/L. Now the delta HCO_3^- is calculated. In this example the HCO_3^- is 17 meq/L. Therefore, the delta HCO_3 = 24 meq/L (normal HCO_3^- level) − 17 meq/L (measured HCO_3 level) = -7 meq/L. The delta gap can now be calculated as 8 (delta anion gap) − 8 (delta HCO_3) = -1! No second acid–base disorder is present and every acid H^+ and HCO_3 is accounted for. It is a simple high anion gap metabolic acidosis.

If the same patient had a HCO_3 of 10 meq/L with an anion gap of 20 and the delta anion gap of 8 then the delta HCO_3 would be

$24-10=14$ meq/L. The delta gap would be 8 (delta anion gap) − 14 (delta HCO_3) = −6! This means that the HCO_3 is much lower than can be accounted for by the accumulated H^+ demonstrating that there is a second cause for the metabolic acidosis other than a high anion gap acidosis and this would have to be an additional non-anion gap process.

Another calculation that has also been used to determine the presence of a secondary acid–base disorder is called the delta gap ratio [37]. In this case instead of subtracting the delta anion gap from the delta HCO_3, the values are placed in a ratio. In a patient with a simple high anion gap acidosis the delta anion gap is equal to the delta HCO_3 and the ratio will be equal to 1. In the first example in the preceding paragraph the delta anion gap was 8 meq/L and the delta HCO_3 was 8 meq/L so the delta ratio = 8/8 = 1. The confidence interval is 1 ± 0.2 so values of 0.8–1.2 are considered the same.

In the second example, the delta anion gap was 8 meq/L but the delta HCO_3 was 14 meq/L producing a delta ratio of 8/14 = 0.5. This indicates that something was lowering the HCO_3^- to a greater extent than could be accounted for by anion gap, namely, HCO_3 losses from GI or renal sources.

Performing a delta gap and delta ratio is a critical step in understanding acid–base disorders [38].

What Is an Osmolar Gap?

The osmolar gap is used in cases when an exogenous toxin may be present causing a high anion gap acidosis. There is no utility of calculating the osmolar gap in patients with a non-anion gap metabolic acidosis. The concept for calculating the osmolar gap is to find the difference between the measured serum osmolality and the osmolality calculated from the known determinants of the serum osmolality (Table 12.4) [39]. The serum osmolality is calculated by the following formula: $(2 \times Na) + (glucose/18) + (BUN/2.8)$. Some laboratories only reports the measured serum osmolality and the physician must personally determine the calculated osmolality from the variables listed above.

There are three important toxins that cause a high anion gap acidosis and result in the accumulation of active osmoles: ethylene glycol, methanol, and propylene glycol intoxication. None of these alcohols are acids directly but their metabolism leads to the accumulation of specific organic acids (Table 12.5). Ethanol and isopropyl alcohol both cause a high osmolar gap but do not cause a metabolic acidosis.

The osmolar gap can detect the presence of the parent alcohol compound before it is completely metabolized and generates excess H^+. If present, this would allow the opportunity to initiate specific therapeutic interventions that could prevent further enzymatic breakdown [40]. If the measured serum osmolality minus calculated osmolality is <10 mosm/L then there is no evidence for the presence of the parent compound of any of the three intoxicants. This does not exclude the likelihood that either of these agents could be causing the acidosis since all of the drug may have already been metabolized. If the osmolar gap is >10 mosm/L then there exists unmetabolized parent compound and a toxicology screen will likely determine which of the three alcohols is present. None of the organic acids that cause a high anion gap (lactic acid, ketoacids, salicylic acid, etc.) result in an osmolar gap.

The Blood Gas Report Always Lists Base Excess: What Does That Number Mean?

The base excess concept is defined as the amount of HCO_3^- required to achieve a normal pH with a pCO_2 of 40 mmHg for any given patient with a metabolic acidosis or alkalosis. The formula used is shown in Table 12.4 [41]. The answer is the amount of HCO_3^- in meq/L that needs to be supplemented in the case of an acidosis (a negative base excess value) or that exists in excess in the case of an alkalosis (a positive base excess value) [42]. Since the result is per liter the next question that needs to be answered is—what is the volume of distribution of HCO_3?

The volume of distribution of HCO_3^- varies with the HCO_3^- concentration due to recruitment of H^+ buffering by alternative systems (intracellular; bone carbonate). The estimated space for HCO_3^- can be determined by the formula: Bicarbonate space (% of total body weight) = [0.4 + (2.6/[HCO_3])] × body weight (in kg) [16]. For a 70 kg individual this means the HCO_3^- space can vary from 28% with a HCO_3 of 20 meq/L to 40% for a HCO_3 of 15 meq/L and 46% for a HCO_3 of 10 meq/L. This nonlinear relationship means that HCO_3 supplementation to correct the pH is significantly more than would be expected as the acidosis intensifies.

As an example, a 70 kg man with a pH of 7.30, a HCO_3 of 15 meq/L, and a pCO_2 of 31 mmHg has a base excess of 0.9287 × (HCO_3 − 24.4 + 14.8 3 × [pH − 7.4]) = −10 meq/L. The volume of distribution of HCO_3^- at a concentration of 15 meq/L is 40% of lean body weight as noted above. Therefore the total HCO_3 deficit is 10 meq/L × (0.4 × 70) = 280 meq which is the amount of HCO_3^- needed to return the serum HCO_3^- back to a level of 24 meq/L.

In a metabolic acidosis the Base Excess number should always be a negative value and helps to provide a clue to the magnitude of the underlying acid–base disorder.

When and How Is HCO_3^- Used to Treat a Metabolic Acidosis?

There are three methods to supplement HCO_3 in the setting of an acidosis: intravenous push, slow intravenous drip, and oral therapy. Current recommendations do not advise the use of rapid intravenous push HCO_3 unless there is a life threatening acidosis defined as a pH < 7.1 with the goal of treatment to raise the pH to approximately 7.2. This target is based on the physiologic consequences of an acidosis on the cardiovascular system being most significant at a pH < 7.2. Controversy however exists on the risks involved with excessive intravenous HCO_3 administration [43]. These concerns center on the following issues: volume overload from the excess sodium infusion, rapid decline in ionized calcium leading to impaired circulatory and cardiac function, and dissociation of the intracellular and extracellular pH resulting in increased intracellular lactic acid production [44]. For all other patients with pH > 7.2, the HCO_3 can be supplemented and the origin of the acidosis corrected at a much slower pace.

Oral HCO_3^- can be provided using a variety of agents all of which also provide either a Na^+ or a K^+ equimolar with the anion. The following list provides an overview of some of the options available for oral therapy:

Sodium bicarbonate tablets	650 mg tablets	7.7 meq HCO_3^- per tablet
Shohls' solution (sodium citrate)	1 mL	1 meq of HCO_3^-
Baking soda	1 mL	12 meq HCO_3^-
Polycitra (Na/K citrate)	1 mL	2 meq HCO_3^-

In addition to HCO_3^- supplementation, the majority of the organic acids that cause an anion gap acidosis represent potential sources of alkali. Consequently it is possible to overshoot into an alkalemia once the generation of the acidosis stops and the anions are metabolized to HCO_3 if the pH was already aggressively normalized by HCO_3 administration.

What Is the Effect of a Metabolic Acidosis on the Serum K^+ Concentration?

Experimentally, a predictable relationship exists between the change in the pH and the serum K^+ concentration. Metabolic acidosis has been associated with an increase in the K^+ level according to the formula: a decrease in pH of 1.0 = an increase of 0.6 meq/L in K^+ concentration. However this relationship was demonstrated in the setting of an inorganic acidosis (HCl infusion) and does not apply to the common clinical settings of organic acidosis (i.e., lactic acid, ketoacids, etc.) seen in the hospital or clinic setting [45].

The mechanism for this increase in K^+ was related to an exchange of H^+ across the cell membrane for intracellular K^+. This exchange is predicated on the inability of the accompanying anion associated with H^+ to enter the cell at the same time [46]. This would be true of HCl where the cell membrane is impermeable to Cl^-, trapping this ion in the extracellular space but allowing H^+ to enter the cell with an exchange for K^+. Most organic anions such as lactate and the ketoacids are freely permeable across the cell wall. There is no need for K^+ to efflux out of the cell since the inward movement of the acid molecule produced an electrically neutral event. Consequently, hyperkalemia is a non-predictable byproduct of a metabolic acidosis and may occur concomitantly due to other factors (cell lysis, tissue catabolism, hyperglycemia, insulin resistance, etc.) [47].

Summary Algorithm

The approach to a metabolic acidosis can now be outlined into a series of steps based on the above discussion (Figs. 12.1 and 12.2). The cases provided at the beginning of the chapter will now be approached using this sequence of steps.

Case 1 Discussion

Step 1: The blood gas confirms the presence of an acidemia with the pH of 7.25 and a decreased serum HCO_3 of 10 meq/L on the electrolyte profile. The HCO_3^- concentration on the blood gas and the HCO_3^- level on the electrolyte panel are identical confirming the validity of the plasma specimen which can now be used for Step 3.

Diagnosis After Step 1: Metabolic Acidosis

Step 2: The compensation formula for the predicted pCO_2 in the presence of a HCO_3^- of 10 meq/L is $(1.5 \times HCO_3) + 8 = (1.5 \times 10) + 8 = 15 + 8 = 23 \pm 2$ mmHg. The actual pCO_2 is 24 mmHg which is within the estimated range of 23–25 mmHg.

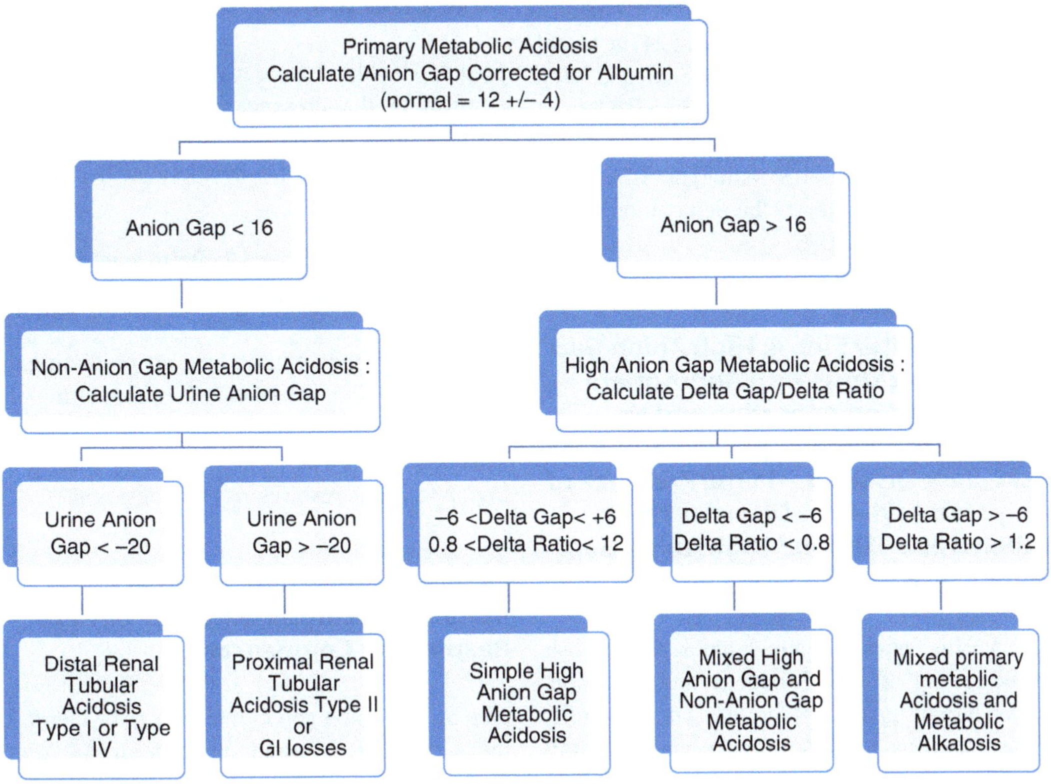

Fig. 12.2 Evaluation of metabolic acidosis: algorithm for steps 3 and 4

Diagnosis After Step 2: Metabolic Acidosis with Appropriate Respiratory Compensation

Step 3: Using the electrolyte panel, the anion gap is 24 meq/L; however, the serum albumin in this patient is abnormal and decreased to 3.0 g/dL. The anion gap must be corrected based on the low serum albumin. The albumin of 3.0 g/dL is 1.5 g/dL below the normal level of 4.5 g/dL and the anion gap must be corrected by $2.5 \times 1.5 = 3.7$. The expected normal anion gap for this patient is $12 - 3.7 = 9.3$ meq/L instead of 12 meq/L. The calculated anion gap of 24 is actually 27.7.

Diagnosis After Step 3: High Anion Gap Metabolic Acidosis with Appropriate Respiratory Compensation

Step 4: The delta anion gap is based on the correction of the expected normal anion gap for this patient with the serum albumin. The expected anion gap for an albumin of 3.0 g/dL is 9.3 meq/L. Since the anion gap was measured at 24 the actual delta anion gap is $24 - 9.3 = 14.7$ meq/L. The delta HCO_3^- is based on the serum HCO_3 of 10 meq/L compared to a normal level of 24 meq/L. The delta HCO_3 for this patient is 14 meq/L. Therefore the delta gap is the delta anion − delta $HCO_3 = 14.7 - 14 = +0.7$.

Diagnosis After Step 4: High Anion Gap Metabolic Acidosis with Appropriate Respiratory Compensation and No Evidence of a Superimposed Secondary Acid–Base Disorder—In the Presence of Only One Acid–Base Disorder This Is Labeled as a "Simple" High Anion Gap Metabolic Acidosis

Step 5: This patient has a high anion gap acidosis in the setting of Type I diabetes and an uncontrolled blood sugar of 450 mg/dL. The possibility of ketoacidosis is strongly suspected but it is essential to work through all the possibilities in the differential diagnosis (CUTE DIMPLES Table 12.5). Of particular concern in this case is the finding of an empty bottle nearby a comatose patient indicating the possibility of a toxic ingestion. Standard toxicology screening along with blood lactic acid , blood ketones, and urine ketone testing will cover the major etiologies of a high anion gap acidosis. While these results are pending, the osmolar gap can be checked to see if an unmetabolized intoxicant is present.

The calculated osmolality in this case is $(2 \times Na) + glucose/18 + BUN/2.8 = (2 \times 130) + (450/18) + (30/2.8) = 260 + 25 + 10 = 295$ mosm/L. The measured osmolality is 310 mosm/L so the osmolar gap is $310 - 295 = 15$ mosm/L. This is a positive finding (normal osmolar gap < 10 mosm/L) and confirms that this patient not only has uncontrolled diabetes and possible ketoacidosis but also has an unidentified ingestion such as ethylene glycol, methanol, or propylene glycol. Further intervention will be based on the toxicology findings appropriate to the compound detected.

Case 2 Discussion

Step 1: The blood gas demonstrates a pH of 7.33 confirming the presence of acidemia and the decreased HCO_3^- concentration of 18 meq/L supports the diagnosis of a metabolic acidosis.

Diagnosis After Step 1: Primary Metabolic Acidosis

Step 2: The compensation formula predicting the pCO_2 for a HCO_3^- of 18 meq/L in the setting of a metabolic acidosis is $(1.5 \times 18) + 8 = 35$ mmHg. This patient has a pCO_2 of 35 mmHg demonstrating appropriate respiratory compensation.

Diagnosis After Step 2: Primary Metabolic Acidosis with Appropriate Respiratory Compensation

Step 3: The anion gap in this case is 12 meq/L in the setting of a serum albumin of 4.0 g/dL. Consequently there is no evidence for the presence of an anion gap acidosis.

Diagnosis After Step 3: Primary Non-anion Gap Metabolic Acidosis with Appropriate Respiratory Compensation

Step 4: There is no delta gap or delta ration to calculate in the setting of a non-anion gap metabolic acidosis so this step is skipped.

Step 5: In the workup of a non-anion gap acidosis, the UAG should be used to try to identify whether the distal tubule of the kidney is functioning properly to produce $NH4^+$ and eliminate H^+. In this case the UAG can be calculated from the random urine Na^+, K^+, and Cl^- concentrations = (35 + 20) − 90 = −45 meq/L. This is a highly negative UAG > −20 which indicates the presence of adequate distal tubular function in the setting of a non-anion gap acidosis. The cause of the acidosis is now established as a loss of HCO_3— rather than impaired H^+ secretion.

The differential diagnosis for this HCO_3^- loss shifts to the gastrointestinal tract or the proximal tubule (Type II RTA). From the clinical history, the patient was recently started on Topiramate for migraine headaches. This drug has well-known inhibitory actions on carbonic anhydrase activity similar to acetazolamide which will inhibit the resorption of filtered HCO_3—in the proximal tubule. Patients on long-term Topiramate will have a chronic non-anion gap metabolic acidosis and run the risk of significant bone demineralization from ongoing buffering of H^+ by bone carbonate [48]. These patients will be at risk for calcium phosphate nephrolithiasis.

Conclusion

Metabolic acidosis is a common acid–base disorder seen encountered in clinical practice that significantly impacts patient morbidity and mortality. Utilizing a sequential approach (Figs. 12.1 and 12.2) in the recognition and classification of a patient with a metabolic acidosis is essential in order to correctly initiate a therapeutic plan and define any additional acid–base abnormalities that may be present.

References

1. Adrogué HJ, Gennari FJ, Galla JH, Madias NE. Assessing acid-base disorders. Kidney Int. 2009;76(12):1239–47.
2. Kraut JA, Madias NE. Metabolic acidosis: pathophysiology, diagnosis and management. Nat Rev Nephrol. 2010;6(5):274–85.
3. Schlichtig R. [Base excess] vs [strong ion difference]. Which is more helpful? Adv Exp Med Biol. 1997;411:91–5.
4. Rastegar A. Clinical utility of Stewart's method in diagnosis and management of acid-base disorders. Clin J Am Soc Nephrol. 2009;4(7):1267–74.
5. Story DA. Bench-to-bedside review: a brief history of clinical acid-base. Crit Care. 2004;8(4):253–8.
6. Dubin A, Menises MM, Masevicius FD, Moseinco MC, Kutscherauer DO, Ventrice E, Laffaire E, Estenssoro E. Comparison of three different methods of evaluation of metabolic acid-base disorders. Crit Care Med. 2007;35(5):1264–70.
7. Adrogué HE, Adrogué HJ. Acid-base physiology. Respir Care. 2001;46(4):328–41.
8. Preston R. Metabolic acidosis Acid base, fluids and electrolytes made ridiculously simple. Linwood, NY: Mcmaster, Inc.; 2002. p. 97–124.
9. Sood P, Paul G, Puri S. Interpretation of arterial blood gas. Indian J Crit Care Med. 2010;14(2):57–64.
10. Witte DI, Rodgers JL, Barrett DA. Anion gap: its use in quality control. Clin Chem. 1976;22:643–6.
11. Eustace JA, Astor B, Muntner PM, Ikizler TA, Coresh J. Prevalence of acidosis and inflammation and their association with low serum albumin in chronic kidney disease. Kidney Int. 2004;65:1031–40.
12. Handy JM, Soni N. Physiological effects of hyperchloraemia and acidosis. Br J Anaesth. 2008;101(2): 141–50.
13. Rosenberg AL. Recent innovations in intensive care unit risk-prediction models. Curr Opin Crit Care. 2002;8(4):321–30.
14. Bellingham AJ, Detter JC, Lenfant C. Regulatory mechanisms of hemoglobin oxygen affinity in acidosis and alkalosis. J Clin Invest. 1971;50(3):700–6.
15. Lemann J, Bushinsky DA, Hamm LL. Bone buffering of acid and base in humans. Am J Physiol. 2003;285:F811–32.
16. Fernandez PC, Cohen RM, Feldman GM. The concept of bicarbonate distribution space: the crucial role of body buffers. Kidney Int. 1989;36:747.
17. Pierce NF, Fedson DS, Brigham KL, et al. The ventilatory response to acute base deficit in humans. Time course during development and correction of metabolic acidosis. Ann Intern Med. 1970;72:633.
18. Corne S. Basic principles of control of breathing. Bshouty Z Respir Care Clin N Am. 2005;11(2): 147–72.
19. Burki NK, Lee LY. Mechanisms of dyspnea. Chest. 2010;138(5):1196–201.

20. Minagar A, Weiner WJ. Adolf Kussmaul and his respiratory sign. J Med Biogr. 2001;9(3):181–3.
21. Bushinsky DA, Coe FL, Katzenberg C, et al. Arterial PCO2 in chronic metabolic acidosis. Kidney Int. 1982;22:311.
22. Adrogué HJ, Madias NE. Secondary responses to altered acid-base status: the rules of engagement. J Am Soc Nephrol. 2010;21(6):920–3.
23. Gabow PA, Kaehny WD, Fennessey PV, Goodman SI, Gross PA, Schrier RW. Diagnostic importance of an increased serum anion gap. N Engl J Med. 1980; 303(15):854–8.
24. Kraut JA, Madias NE. Serum anion gap: its uses and limitations in clinical medicine. Clin J Am Soc Nephrol. 2007;2(1):162–74.
25. Carvounis CP, Feinfeld DA. A simple estimate of the effect of the serum albumin level on the anion gap. Am J Nephrol. 2000;20(5):369–72.
26. Ghosh AK. Diagnosing acid-base disorders. J Assoc Physicians India. 2006;54:720–4.
27. Gabow PA. Disorders associated with an altered anion gap. Kidney Int. 1985;27:472–83.
28. Morris CG, Low J. Metabolic acidosis in the critically ill: part 1. Classification and pathophysiology. Anaesthesia. 2008;63(3):294–301.
29. Reddy P. Clinical approach to renal tubular acidosis in adult patients. Int J Clin Pract. 2011;65(3):350–60.
30. Bagga A, Sinha A. Evaluation of renal tubular acidosis. Indian J Pediatr. 2007;74(7):679–86.
31. Laing CM, Unwin RJ. Renal tubular acidosis. J Nephrol. 2006;19 Suppl 9:S46–52.
32. Oh M, Carroll HJ. Value and determinants of urine anion gap. Nephron. 2002;90(3):252–5.
33. Kirschbaum B, Sica D, Anderson FP. Urine electrolytes and the urine anion and osmolar gaps. J Lab Clin Med. 1999;133(6):597–604.
34. Kim GH, Han JS, Kim YS, Joo KW, Kim S, Lee JS. Evaluation of urine acidification by urine anion gap and urine osmolal gap in chronic metabolic acidosis. Am J Kidney Dis. 1996;27(1):42–7.
35. Reddy P, Mooradian AD. Clinical utility of anion gap in deciphering acid-base disorders. Int J Clin Pract. 2009;63(10):1516–25.
36. Emmett M, Narins RG. Clinical use of the anion gap. Medicine. 1977;56:38–54.
37. Rastegar A. Use of the $\Delta AG/\Delta HCO_3^-$ ratio in the diagnosis of mixed acid-base disorders. J Am Soc Nephrol. 2007;18:2429–31.
38. Emmett M. Anion gap interpretation: the old and the new. Clin Pract Nephrol. 2006;2:4–6.
39. Poulose V. Factors influencing the serum osmolar gap. Chest. 2002;122(1):381.
40. Kraut JA, Kurtz I. Toxic alcohol ingestions: clinical features, diagnosis, and management. Clin J Am Soc Nephrol. 2008;3:208–25.
41. Kofstad J. Base excess: a historical review-has the calculation of base excess been more standardised the last 20 years? Clin Chim Acta. 2001;307(1–2):193–5.
42. Mizock BA. Utility of standard base excess in acid-base analysis. Crit Care Med. 1998;26(7):1146–7.
43. Kraut JA, Kurtz I. Controversies in the treatment of acute metabolic acidosis. NephSAP. 2006;5:1–9.
44. Sabatini S, Kurtzman NA. Bicarbonate therapy in severe metabolic acidosis. J Am Soc Nephrol. 2009;20:692–5.
45. Palmer BF. A physiologic-based approach to the evaluation of a patient with hyperkalemia. Am J Kidney Dis. 2010;56(2):387–93.
46. Wiederseiner JM, Muser J, Lutz T, et al. Acute metabolic acidosis: characterization and diagnosis of the disorder and the plasma potassium response. J Am Soc Nephrol. 2004;15:1589.
47. Magner PO, Robinson L, Halperin RM, Zettle R, Halperin ML. The plasma potassium concentration in metabolic acidosis: a re-evaluation. Am J Kidney Dis. 1988;11(3):220–4.
48. Mirza N, Marson AG, Pirmohamed M. Effect of topiramate on acid-base balance: extent, mechanism and effects. Br J Clin Pharmacol. 2009;68(5): 655–61.

13 Metabolic Alkalosis

Luis M. Ortega and Oliver Lenz

Case 1

A 32-year-old thin woman is complaining of weakness and light-headedness. She denies vomiting and intake of medications except vitamins. On physical examination she has a blood pressure of 100/60 mmHg with a heart rate of 95 beats/min and diminished skin turgor. The remainder of her exam is unremarkable. Laboratory data are shown in Table 13.1.

Case 2

A 68-year-old Caucasian male with a history of peripheral vascular disease and previous angina episodes presents with difficult to treat hypertension and an increase in his serum creatinine from 1.2 to 2.5 mg/dL after an angiotensin-converting enzyme inhibitor (ACEi) was started. He is currently taking four medications: a beta-blocker, a calcium channel antagonist, a diuretic, and the ACEi. On physical exam his blood pressure is 155/88 mmHg with a heart rate of 56 beats/min, he has pulmonary crackles bilaterally, and moderate bilateral lower extremity edema. Laboratory data are shown in Table 13.1.

Introduction

Metabolic alkalosis occurs when a primary pathophysiologic process leads to the net accumulation of base (bicarbonate) or the net loss of acid from the extracellular fluid (ECF). In the absence of other primary acid–base disorders, metabolic alkalosis is recognized by increases in both arterial blood pH, which is termed alkalemia, and serum bicarbonate concentration. The increase in arterial blood pH promptly depresses ventilation resulting in increased $PaCO_2$ and the buffering of alkalemia [1, 2].

Metabolic alkalosis is a common acid–base abnormality and is reported in up to 51% of hospitalized patients [3]. This is not surprising given that vomiting, diuretic use, and nasogastric suctioning are common events among hospitalized patients and are primary etiologies of metabolic alkalosis. The mortality associated with severe metabolic alkalosis has been reported to be up to 80% when the pH was greater than 7.65 [4].

Pathophysiology

Metabolic alkalosis is generated by the addition of HCO_3^- or the loss of H^+ from the ECF and maintained by an abnormal retention of bicarbonate.

L.M. Ortega, M.D. (✉)
Division of Nephrology and Hypertension, Allegheny General Hospital, Temple University School of Medicine, WPAHS Campus, 320 East North Avenue, Pittsburgh, PA 15212, USA
e-mail: lortega@wpahs.org

O. Lenz, M.D.
Division of Nephrology and Hypertension, Miller School of Medicine, University of Miami, Miami, FL 33136, USA
e-mail: OLenz@med.miami.edu

E.V. Lerma and M. Rosner (eds.), *Clinical Decisions in Nephrology, Hypertension and Kidney Transplantation*, DOI 10.1007/978-1-4614-4454-1_13, © Springer Science+Business Media New York 2013

Table 13.1 Laboratory data for case 1 and case 2

	Case 1	Case 2
Serum		
Na^+ (mEq/L)	133	142
K^+ (mEq/L)	3.1	2.9
Cl^- (mEq/L)	90	94
HCO_3^- (mmol/L)	33	34
BUN (mg/dL)	60	67
Creatinine (mg/dL)	1.4	2.5
Arterial blood gas		
pH	7.48	7.48
pCO_2 (mmHg)	46	47
pO_2 (mmHg)	98	99
HCO_3^- (mmol/L)	33	34
Urine		
pH	8.0	8.0
Na^+ (mEq/L)	52	15
K^+ (mEq/L)	50	50
Cl^- (mEq/L)	<15	52

A brief algorithm for the differential diagnosis of metabolic alkalosis is shown in Fig. 13.1, and common causes of metabolic alkalosis are listed in Table 13.2. In broad terms, metabolic alkalosis can be due to chloride depletion, disturbances of the renin–aldosterone axis, inherited or acquired tubular dysfunctions, metabolic alkalosis in combination with renal failure, and the administration of non-exchangeable anions. The normal kidney rapidly restores serum bicarbonate levels after alkali loading. If metabolic alkalosis is to persist then there must be interference with the expected urine loss of bicarbonate (maintenance). The three noteworthy mechanisms leading to the maintenance of metabolic alkalosis include chloride depletion, potassium depletion, and a reduced glomerular filtration rate (GFR).

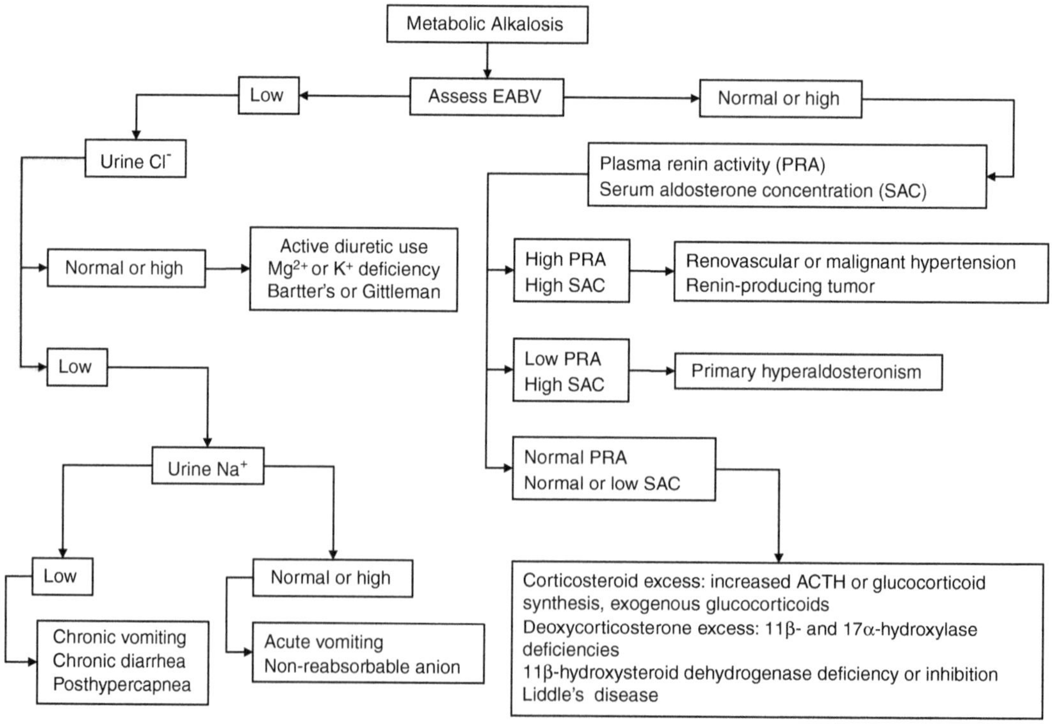

Fig. 13.1 Simplified algorithm for the differential diagnosis of metabolic alkalosis based on the patient's effective arterial blood volume (EABV). When measuring plasma renin activity and serum aldosterone concentration it may be difficult to interpret the result in the presence of a mineralocorticoid receptor antagonist, but it is not necessary to stop most other antihypertensive medications, and posture is not important. Although the cutoff is laboratory dependent, in patients with primary hyperaldosteronism plasma renin activity is usually very low, typically less than 1 ng/mL/h (0.28 ng/L/s), and serum aldosterone concentration is elevated, typically >15 ng/dL (416 pmoL/L), resulting in a ratio greater than 20

Table 13.2 Common causes of metabolic alkalosis

Chloride depletion (saline responsive)
Gastric losses: vomiting or nasogastric suctioning
Renal losses: diuretic therapy
Intestinal losses: chronic diarrhea, laxative abuse, villous adenoma
Posthypercapnea
Cystic fibrosis
Severe potassium depletion
Primary, secondary, or apparent mineralocorticoid excess
Primary hyperaldosteronism
Corticosteroid excess: increased ACTH or glucocorticoid synthesis, exogenous glucocorticoids
Deoxycorticosterone excess: 11β- and 17α-hydroxlase deficiencies
Renovasular disease or malignant hypertension
Congestive heart failure or liver cirrhosis with diuretic therapy
11β-hydroxysteroid dehydrogenase deficiency or inhibition (glycyrrhizic acid)
Tubular abnormalities
Gittleman and Bartter syndromes
Bartter-like syndromes (aminoglycosides, cystic fibrosis)
Liddle syndrome
Metabolic alkalosis maintained by renal failure
Hypercalcemia: milk-alkali syndrome or hypercalcemia of malignancy
Medications: carbenicillin, ampicillin, penicillin
Dietary: bicarbonate ingestion, recovery from starvation

Chloride Depletion

Common clinical scenarios leading to chloride depletion include vomiting, nasogastric suctioning, diuretic therapy, and chronic diarrhea [5]. Traditionally it was thought that volume depletion, which is common in these states of chloride depletion, is the driving factor, whereby an increased avidity to sodium results in an inability to eliminate sodium bicarbonate. However, more recent studies suggest that without chloride repletion the addition of sodium to the ECF will not normalize the alkalosis, even if volume depletion is corrected [6]. In animal studies the Cl^-–HCO_3^- exchange in the cortical collecting duct has been identified as a site that responds rapidly to changes in chloride delivery [7], and subsequent studies showed that pendrin, a member of the solute carrier 26 family, exhibits the function and distribution of such an anion exchanger [8].

Post-hypercapnic metabolic alkalosis also presents with a low urine chloride. These patients commonly developed an elevated serum bicarbonate in response to respiratory acidosis, but cannot excrete the accumulated bicarbonate after respiratory failure has resolved due to concomitant chloride depletion, for example, due to nasogastric suctioning in the intensive care unit [9].

Hypokalemia

Hypokalemia can occur as a consequence of the disease state that leads to metabolic alkalosis, such as in mineralocorticoid excess, and as a consequence of bicarbonaturia. In addition, hypokalemia per se can contribute to the maintenance of metabolic alkalosis. Two important mechanisms include the H^+–K^+ exchange in the distal convoluted tubule, which facilitates reclaiming potassium in hypokalemic states but also leads to a net loss of protons resulting in a net gain of bicarbonate, and the increased ammoniagenesis in response to hypokalemia-induced intracellular metabolic acidosis. The latter is caused by the shift of potassium from the intracellular to the extracellular compartment in response to hypokalemia and the accompanying H^+–K^+ exchange to maintain electroneutrality. The resulting increase in the synthesis of NH_3 leads to enhanced loss of protons as NH_4^+.

True or Apparent Mineralocorticoid Excess

In patients with metabolic alkalosis and volume expansion or hypertension, who commonly but not always also exhibit hypokalemia, the renin–aldosterone axis needs to be examined to identify cases of aldosterone excess. Stimulation of the mineralocorticoid receptor leads to metabolic alkalosis either as a consequence of hypokalemia, although hypokalemia may not be present in all cases, or the direct effect on proton excretion in the distal tubule. The tubular mechanisms involved include activation of the H^+/K^+ exchanger, activation of the H^+ pump, and the generation of an electrical gradient favoring H^+ excretion due to activation of the $3Na^+/2K^+$ ATPase.

Tubular Disorders

In Bartter's syndrome a variety of mutations have been identified in the thick ascending loop of Henle, leading to a primary inability to reabsorb sodium chloride. As a consequence these patients exhibit salt, potassium, and calcium wasting and a urinary concentration defect. Metabolic alkalosis follows both the chloride and potassium depletion via the mechanisms described above. In Gittleman's syndrome the defect is located in the distal convoluted tubule, affecting the thiazide-sensitive sodium chloride cotransporter. These patients, too, exhibit renal salt and potassium wasting, although usually milder than patients with Bartter's, but they retain calcium, and hence the urinary calcium may be a useful marker to distinguish between the two. The development of metabolic alkalosis follows the same mechanisms as in Barrter's syndrome. Bartter-like syndromes may be caused by medications, such as aminoglycosides, or severe electrolyte imbalances, such as hypokalemia or hypomagnesemia [10–14].

Reduced GFR

Although renal failure is a well-known cause for metabolic acidosis, a reduced GFR may contribute to the maintenance of metabolic alkalosis by reducing the filtered bicarbonate load. The pathophysiology of the milk-alkali syndrome, now also called calcium-alkali syndrome [15], is a good example. Hypercalcemia will contribute to renal failure via vasoconstriction and interstitial damage. Metabolic alkalosis ensues due to the alkali accompanying calcium supplements, which worsens hypercalcemia by interfering with tubular calcium elimination. Renal failure will impair both Ca^{2+} and HCO_3^- excretion, thus perpetuating the disorder.

Clinical Approach and Diagnosis

The diagnosis of metabolic alkalosis requires an elevated arterial pH (alkalemia), an elevated bicarbonate concentration (alkalosis), and an appropriate respiratory response resulting in a decreased pCO_2. It is important to obtain an arterial blood gas to exclude respiratory acidosis, which will also present with an increase in bicarbonate concentration, and to verify that no mixed disorder is present. The appropriateness of the respiratory response can be evaluated by calculating the expected pCO_2 as $40+0.7\times$(change in bicarbonate from a baseline of 24 mEq/L) [5]. For example, in a patient with metabolic alkalosis and a serum bicarbonate of 34 mEq/L the expected pCO_2 would be $40+0.7\times(34-24)=47$. If the actual pCO_2 is lower or higher than the expected value then a concomitant respiratory disorder is present.

Once the diagnosis of metabolic alkalosis has been confirmed, the underlying causes need to be elucidated (Fig. 13.1). The history and physical examination will reveal important clues, such as volume status, gastrointestinal losses, and medication use or abuse. In most cases, the volume status helps categorize the patients into two groups: hypervolemic patients with hypertension versus those with normal to low ECF and normal blood pressure.

In the hypervolemic, hypertensive group, examination of the renin–angiotensin system is the next step to establishing the diagnosis. Screening for the etiology is usually done by obtaining a morning blood sample for plasma renin activity and serum aldosterone levels. Plasma renin activity and serum aldosterone concentrations may be difficult to interpret in the presence of a mineralocorticoid receptor antagonist, so whenever possible these should be held, but it is not necessary to stop most other antihypertensive medications.

Although the cutoff is laboratory dependent, in patients with primary hyperaldosteronism plasma renin activity is usually very low, typically less than 1 ng/mL/h (0.28 ng/L/s), and serum aldosterone concentration is elevated, typically >15 ng/dL (416 pmol/L), resulting in a ratio greater than 20. The picture is similar in glucocorticoid-remediable aldosteronism (GRA), although the aldosterone-to-renin ratios commonly are slightly lower than what is seen in Conn's disease (primary hyperaldosteronism). In patients with a compelling history or family history, such as childhood hypertension or early hemorrhagic strokes, a dexamethasone suppression test can be performed (in patients with GRA, the aldosterone levels will be suppressed with dexamethasone and the blood pressure will improve), and genetic testing is available (International Registry for GRA) [16].

In cases with normal or low serum aldosterone concentrations and normal or low plasma renin activity one should consider exogenous sources of mineralocorticoids. Additional considerations are a deficiency in 11β-hydroxysteroid dehydrogenase (the enzyme that deactivates cortisol to cortisone that does not have mineralocorticoid activity), an excess of glucocorticoids that overwhelm the enzyme, as may be seen in Cushing's disease and syndrome, or the presence of inhibitors of this enzyme, such as glycyrrhizic acid [11]. Deficiencies in the 11β- or 17α-hydroxylase will produce a similar picture due to an excess of deoxycorticosterone [17]. Liddle's disease, which is characterized by constitutive expression of epithelial sodium channels, leading to excessive sodium reabsorption and consequently loss of potassium and protons, is an additional consideration [18].

In those with both elevated plasma renin activity and serum aldosterone concentrations renovascular hypertension should receive strong consideration. Renin-producing tumors are rare but remain part of the differential diagnosis. Patients with congestive heart failure or liver cirrhosis undergoing diuretic therapy may also appear volume expanded and have an increased plasma renin activity and serum aldosterone concentration, but these patients are usually hypotensive and have a low effective arterial blood volume, making the laboratory abnormalities a secondary phenomenon.

In normo- or hypovolemic cases determination of urinary electrolytes including sodium, chloride, and calcium offers additional clues. Those with an elevated urinary chloride will have a primary renal problem, such as diuretic use, Bartters' or Gittlemans syndromes, or Bartter-like diseases. As mentioned above, the urinary calcium may provide an important clue to the site of the lesion: it is usually high when the thick ascending limb of Henle is affected, while defects in the sodium chloride cotransporter lead to a low urinary calcium. Genetic testing is commonly required to demonstrate with certainty the underlying mutation. Diuretic abuse should always be considered in this scenario, and given that many patients do not admit to diuretic abuse a urine diuretic screen may be needed when the suspicion is high.

Patients with low urinary chloride concentrations most commonly have gastrointestinal losses, such as vomiting or diarrhea, and the urine sodium may help determine the duration of the disorder. Patients with cystic fibrosis may exhibit the same constellation due to excessive sodium chloride loss through the skin. Patients with intermittent diuretic abuse and intermittent vomiting may present similarly. Serial laboratory determinations showing fluctuations in the acid–base and volume status may be a clue to the diagnosis.

Treatment

Treatment is directed at two areas: Correction of existing deficits and prevention of continuing losses.

Conditions associated with a low ECF and low urine chloride concentrations are also referred to as saline or chloride responsive. Once any offending medications, such as loop or thiazide-like diuretics, have been removed, replacement of the chloride deficit is the primary intervention. This is commonly achieved with isotonic saline solutions. Potassium chloride should be added to replace any co-existing potassium deficits. The chloride deficit can be estimated as 0.2 × body-weight (kg) × desired chloride increase (mEq/L). Hence, in a man weighing 77 kg in whom one wants to increase the serum chloride by 10 mEq/L one would have to administer 154 mEq of chloride or 1 L of 0.9% saline. Note that this will correct the chloride deficit, but not necessarily the volume deficit, and additional fluids may be needed to control the latter. In patients with normal kidney function, bicarbonate and base equivalents will be excreted with sodium or potassium and metabolic alkalosis will be corrected due to the availability of chloride [5].

In the presence of pernicious vomiting or the need for nasogastric suctioning metabolic alkalosis will be maintained if losses are not corrected. Although proton pump inhibitors will blunt gastric acid production and decrease HCl losses, chloride losses still occur and require appropriate replacement. While congenital chloridorrhea can often be managed with adequate replacements and a proton pump inhibitor [19, 20], a surgical solution would be required in the presence of villous adenomas [19, 20].

The use of saline may not be possible despite a diminished effective arterial volume, such as in patients with severe congestive heart failure. Acetazolamide, a carbonic anhydrase inhibitor, may be used at doses of 250–500 mg daily in these cases and augment the elimination of sodium bicarbonate as long as the GFR is adequate.

In patients with chloride-resistant metabolic alkalosis one should aim at correcting the underlying problem, if possible. This is particularly true if medications or diet contribute to the disorder as in exogenous mineralocorticoid administration or licorice consumption. Metabolic alkalosis occurring as a consequence of potassium depletion can be corrected with oral KCl 40–60 mEq four or five times daily as needed. Any concomitant magnesium deficit will have to be corrected as well in order to make this strategy successful. In case of life-threatening cardiac arrhythmias or generalized profound muscle weakness intravenous KCl may be given at rates as high as 40 mEq/h; when concentrations greater than 20 mEq/L are used, a central venous catheter should be utilized. In the setting of true mineralocorticoid excess, aldosterone antagonists such as spironolactone or eplerenone should be part of the treatment plan, while in apparent mineralocorticoid excess and glucocorticoid-remediable hyperaldosteronism the addition of dexamethasone is required. Patients with Liddle's disease can be managed with blockers of the epithelial sodium channel, such as triamterene or amiloride.

The management of patients with Bartter's and Gittleman's syndromes can be challenging if salt and magnesium wasting are significant. Given that these are inherited disorders the tubular defect cannot be corrected, and treatment is aimed at managing symptoms and electrolyte deficiencies. Oral replacement of potassium and magnesium in combination with a potassium-sparing diuretic, such as amiloride, or a mineralocorticoid receptor antagonist, such as aldactone, is commonly employed; some patients require recurrent intravenous magnesium replacement to manage severe muscle cramps.

In cases of severe metabolic alkalosis, usually with a $pH > 7.55$, and in the presence of hepatic encephalopathy, arrhythmias, digitalis intoxication, or altered mental status, intravenous HCl can be used. The amount needed to correct alkalosis is calculated based on the following formula: $0.5 \times$ body weight (kg) $\times$ desired decrement in plasma bicarbonate (mEq/L). The infusion rate should not exceed 25 mEq/h, and a central venous catheter and intensive care monitoring are required. An alternative is the intravenous administration of ammonium chloride unless renal or hepatic insufficiencies are present. The advantage of NH_4Cl is that it can be infused into a peripheral vein. The infusion rate should not exceed 300 mEq in 24 h. In cases of advanced renal failure, dialysis is necessary. Exchange of bicarbonate for chloride by hemodialysis or peritoneal dialysis will correct metabolic alkalosis, and the dialysis solutions need to be modified accordingly.

Case Discussions

Case 1

What Acid–Base Disturbance Is Present?

The patient has an elevated pH (alkalemia) and an increased bicarbonate concentration (alkalosis); consequently, metabolic alkalosis is present. The expected pCO_2 is $40 + 0.7 \times$ delta bicarbonate $= 40 + 0.7 \times (33–24) = 46$. The expected and observed pCO_2 match, indicating that no additional respiratory disorder is present.

What Caused the Metabolic Alkalosis?

We have several clues. The patient has a diminished ECF based on the complaint of light-headedness combined with a low skin turgor, a low blood pressure with tachycardia, and a high BUN-to-creatinine ratio. Hence, chloride losses likely caused this condition. Given that the urine chloride is low, these likely are extra-renal losses. Since the patient does not appear to be receiving non-reabsorbable anions such as penicillin, vomiting is the likely explanation for the elevated urine sodium, which is discussed further below.

Why Is the Na^+ in the Urine Not Lower Despite the Diminished ECF?

For the urine Na^+ to be low filtered, Na^+ must be reabsorbed. Na^+ can be reabsorbed with Cl^-, and the urine Cl^- of less than 15 mEq/L suggests that this is in fact occurring. However, some Na^+ must be lost with another anion, and in the setting of alkalosis, when the serum bicarbonate exceeds the resorptive capacity of the proximal tubule, that anion likely is HCO_3^-. The high urine pH also suggests the presence of bicarbonate in this setting. One might expect the urine sodium to decrease if the vomiting were to continue for a longer time with more pronounced volume depletion.

Why Does the Patient Have Hypokalemia?

The presence of a significant amount of potassium in the patient's urine despite the presence of hypokalemia suggests renal potassium wasting. The latter is a consequence of the chloride deficiency and the activation of the renin angiotensin system.

What Maintains the Metabolic Alkalosis?

If there is continued metabolic alkalosis despite bicarbonaturia, there must be a continuous generation of HCO_3^-. If the source were exogenous there would be volume expansion, hence we must assume a non-renal endogenous generation of HCO_3^-. This happens with vomiting, when HCl in the stomach is regenerated. This involves the production of bicarbonate through carbonic anhydrase activity, and since the patient is vomiting no bicarbonate is utilized by the small bowel. Although some bicarbonate appears in the urine of this patient, the presence of a low ECF with chloride depletion further impairs the correction of the metabolic alkalosis.

Case 2

What Acid–Base Disorder Is Present?

The patient has an elevated pH (alkalemia) and an increased bicarbonate concentration (alkalosis); consequently, metabolic acidosis is present. The expected pCO_2 is $40+0.7\times$delta bicarbonate$=40+0.7\times(34-24)=47$. The expected and observed pCO_2 match, indicating that no additional respiratory disorder is present.

What Is the Cause of the Metabolic Alkalosis?

This patient has an increased ECF given that he has pulmonary crackles, edema, and hypertension. Both urine potassium and chloride are high, the urine pH is high, and urine sodium is low, suggesting that the patient is losing KCl and $NaHCO_3$ while retaining NaCl. Consequently, the possibility of mineralocorticoid excess must be examined. Given that the patient developed a significant worsening of his renal function after starting an ACEi, renovascular hypertension with bilateral renal artery stenosis leading to secondary hyperaldosteronism is the most likely scenario in this case.

What Additional Studies Are Needed in This Patient?

Imaging of the renal arteries will reveal the severity of the disease. Determinations of plasma renin activity and serum aldosterone may corroborate the suspected etiology: If primary hyperaldosteronism was present, then a low plasma renin activity and a high serum aldosterone concentration would be seen, while the plasma renin activity would be normal or high in a patient with renal artery stenosis.

References

1. Stone DJ. Respiration in man during metabolic alkalosis. J Appl Physiol. 1962;17:33–7.
2. Javaheri S, Kazemi H. Metabolic alkalosis and hypoventilation in humans. Am Rev Respir Dis. 1987;136:1011–6.
3. Hodgkin JE, Soeprono FF, Chan DM. Incidence of metabolic alkalemia in hospitalized patients. Crit Care Med. 1980;8:725–8.
4. Anderson LE, Henrich WL. Alkalemia-associated morbidity and mortality in medical and surgical patients. South Med J. 1987;80:729–33.
5. Galla JH. Metabolic alkalosis. J Am Soc Nephrol. 2000;11:369–75.
6. Rosen RA, Julian BA, Dubovsky EV, Galla JH, Luke RG. On the mechanism by which chloride corrects metabolic alkalosis in man. Am J Med. 1988;84:449–58.
7. Gifford JD, Ware MW, Luke RG, Galla JH. HCO3– transport in rat CCD: rapid adaptation by in vivo but not in vitro alkalosis. Am J Physiol. 1993;264:F435–40.
8. Wagner CA, Finberg KE, Stehberger PA, Lifton RP, Giebisch GH, Aronson PS, Geibel JP. Regulation of the expression of the Cl–/anion exchanger pendrin in mouse kidney by acid-base status. Kidney Int. 2002;62:2109–17.
9. Riccio JF, Irani FA. Posthypercapnic metabolic alkalosis: common and neglected cause. South Med J. 1979;72:886–7.
10. Simonetti GD, Mohaupt MG, Bianchetti MG. Monogenic forms of hypertension. Euro J pediatr 2011;14 March online first.
11. Sontia B, Mooney J, Gaudet L, Touyz RM. Pseudohyperaldosteronism, liquorice, and hypertension. J Clin Hypertens (Greenwich). 2008;10:153–7.
12. Kaufman AM, Kahn T. Potassium-depletion alkalosis in the rat. Am J Physiol. 1988;255:F763–70.
13. Chen YS, Fang HC, Chou KJ, Lee PT, Hsu CY, Huang WC, Chung HM, Chen CL. Gentamicin-induced Bartter-like syndrome. Am J Kidney Dis. 2009;54:1158–61.
14. Chadha V, Alon US. Hereditary renal tubular disorders. Semin Nephrol. 2009;29:399–411.
15. Patel AM, Goldfarb S. Got calcium? Welcome to the calcium-alkali syndrome. J Am Soc Nephrol. 2010;21:1440–3.
16. Litchfield WR, New MI, Coolidge C, Lifton RP, Dluhy RG. Evaluation of the dexamethasone suppression test for the diagnosis of glucocorticoid-remediable aldosteronism. J Clin Endocrinol Metab. 1997;82:3570–3.
17. Fraser R. Disorders of the adrenal cortex: their effects on electrolyte metabolism. Clin Endocrinol Metab. 1984;13:413–30.
18. Shimkets RA, Warnock DG, Bositis CM, Nelson-Williams C, Hansson JH, Schambelan M, Gill Jr JR, Ulick S, Milora RV, Findling JW, et al. Liddle's syndrome: heritable human hypertension caused by mutations in the beta subunit of the epithelial sodium channel. Cell. 1994;79:407–14.
19. Eiro M, Katoh T, Watanabe T. Use of a proton-pump inhibitor for metabolic disturbances associated with anorexia nervosa. N Engl J Med. 2002;346:140.
20. Aichbichler BW, Zerr CH, Santa Ana CA, Porter JL, Porter JL, Fordtran JS. Proton-pump inhibition of gastric chloride secretion in congenital chloridorrhea. N Engl J Med. 1997;336:106–9.

Respiratory Acidosis

14

Adriana Arcila and Shirin Shafazand

Case 1

C. S. is a 51-year-old, morbidly obese black male, with a history of tobacco smoking, crack cocaine abuse, chronic obstructive pulmonary disease (COPD) and an elevated left diaphragm following a left cervical blunt trauma. He was admitted for gradual exacerbation of his baseline shortness of breath. He reported increased cough and greenish sputum production. He had clinical symptoms and signs suggestive of obstructive sleep apnea. His physical examination was remarkable for morbid obesity, weighing 324 lbs (147.3 kg), increased respiratory rate of 30 breaths per minute, supraclavicular fullness, use of accessory respiratory muscles, and decreased breath sounds bilaterally at lung bases. His arterial blood gases (ABG) show pH 7.21, $PaCO_2$ 88 mmHg, $PaCO_2$ 45 mmHg, and HCO_3 32 mEq/L. His oxygen saturation while breathing room air was 76%.

Case 2

A. B. is a 45-year-old male who was found unarousable at home. It appeared that he had attempted to commit suicide, and a bottle of almost empty oxycodone pills was found by his bed. Nasogastric lavage did not recover any pills. The patient was admitted to the intensive care unit unresponsive with a respiratory rate of 8 breaths per minute. ABG showed pH 7.10, $PaCO_2$ 80 mmHg, PaO_2 45 mmHg, and HCO_3 27 mEq/L.

Introduction

Alveolar hypoventilation leads to an increase in the partial pressure of alveolar carbon dioxide ($PACO_2$). This translates to an increase in the arterial carbon dioxide ($PaCO_2$) with a subsequent decrease in the ratio of HCO_3 to $PaCO_2$ and therefore, decreased plasma pH [1]. "Acidemia" refers to a decrease in pH below 7.35. This is different from the term "acidosis," which refers to the underlying physiologic process (for respiratory acidosis an increase in $PaCO_2$ leading to an excess plasma H^+ and in the absence of other physiological processes, a decrease in plasma pH). Alveolar hypoventilation with subsequent hypercapnia (increased $PaCO_2$) and acidosis (increased H^+) occurs when there is a strong suppression of the respiratory drive, interfering with the lungs ability to expel carbon dioxide.

A. Arcila, M.D., B.A.
Division of Pulmonary, Critical Care and Sleep Medicine, University of Miami, Miami, FL 33136, USA

S. Shafazand, M.D., M.S. (✉)
Division of Pulmonary, Critical Care and Sleep Medicine, Miller School of Medicine, University of Miami, PO Box 016960 (D60), Miami, FL 33101, USA
e-mail: sshafazand@med.miami.edu

E.V. Lerma and M. Rosner (eds.), *Clinical Decisions in Nephrology, Hypertension and Kidney Transplantation*, DOI 10.1007/978-1-4614-4454-1_14, © Springer Science+Business Media New York 2013

Respiratory acidosis may be acute or chronic and may occur as a primary disorder or as a secondary disorder in response to a primary metabolic alkalosis. In this section, we will discuss the pathophysiology, etiology, and physiological response to respiratory acidosis.

Pathophysiology and Etiology

Carbon dioxide (CO_2) is the major source of acid in the body, with a large amount produced as a byproduct of metabolism of carbohydrates and fats [2]. CO_2 diffuses readily into the erythrocytes to combine with water and produce carbonic acid (H_2CO_3), the production of which is catalyzed by carbonic anhydrase. Carbonic acid dissociates slowly to H^+ and bicarbonate in the following chemical reaction

$$CO_2 + H_2O \leftrightarrow H_2CO_3 \leftrightarrow HCO_3^- + H^+.$$

Under normal physiologic conditions, the lungs are in charge of excreting the acid through ventilation, and under Le Chatelier's principle the equation is normally driven to the left due to efficient CO_2 production and excretion by the lungs. The lungs eliminate 12,500 mEq of H^+ daily, in comparison to 20–70 mEq of hydrogen ions excreted by the kidneys daily [2, 3].

CO_2 is excreted by the lungs during ventilation, at a rate that balances CO_2 production in the tissues. The normal range for $PaCO_2$ is 35–45 mmHg [2]. When there is an increase in $PaCO_2$, driving the equation to the right, there is a decrease in the bicarbonate (HCO_3) to $PaCO_2$ ratio, causing a decrease in the pH [4]. Acidemia occurs with pH decreases below 7.35 and severe academia is defined as a pH of less than 7.20. The hypercapnia and decrease in pH due to alveolar hypoventilation is the mechanistic cause of respiratory acidosis.

In acute respiratory acidosis, the initial response is cellular buffering, in which deoxygenated hemoglobin, as the principle buffering system, receives H^+ into its histidine residues, and bicarbonate is pumped actively out of the cell. Chloride shifts inside the cells, maintaining electroneutrality and the continued production of bicarbonate. This occurs over minutes to hours and results in plasma bicarbonate elevation of on average 1 mEq/L for each rise in $PaCO_2$ of 10 mmHg, acutely. Saturation of hemoglobin as a buffering system, leads to a rapid acidemia. The long-term compensatory response seen in chronic respiratory acidosis relies on the kidneys, with increased excretion of carbonic acid, reabsorption of bicarbonate, and elimination of acid and chloride in urine. The overall metabolic compensation by the kidneys increases plasma bicarbonate over a period of 3–5 days [5, 6]. In this chronic setting, plasma bicarbonate increases 3.5–4 mEq/L for every 10 mmHg increase in $PaCO_2$. Table 14.1 exemplifies the expected compensatory changes, starting with a patient with a normal acid base status, followed by acute and chronic phases of respiratory acidosis.

The central respiratory centers, located in the pons and the medulla, control alveolar ventilation. Ventilation is influenced and regulated by chemoreceptors for $PaCO_2$, PaO_2, and pH located in the brainstem, as well as by neural impulses from pulmonary-stretch receptors and impulses from the cerebral cortex.

Acute respiratory acidosis occurs with the rapid onset of ventilatory failure. Clinical situations which may precipitate acute ventilatory failure (Table 14.2) include depression of the central nervous system by disease or medications, neuromuscular impairment (e.g., Guillain-Barre syndrome, muscular dystrophy), upper or lower airway obstruction as in status asmathicus, COPD, alveolar processes such as pneumonia or pulmonary edema, abdominal hypertension, and ventilatory restrictions (e.g., rib fractures with flail chest) [2, 5–7].

The sum of the pressures of alveolar gas CO_2 ($PaCO_2$) and O_2 (PAO_2) is constant in patients

Table 14.1 Relation between pH, PaCO2, and HCO3 in respiratory acidosis

	pH	$PaCO_2$ (mmHg)	HCO_3 (mmol/L)
Normal acid base	7.40	40	24
Acute respiratory acidosis	7.21	70	27 (24+3)
Chronic respiratory acidosis	7.34	56	29 (24+5)

Table 14.2 Etiology of respiratory acidosis

CNS depressant	Opiates, sedatives, anesthetics Obesity-hypoventilation syndrome CNS disorders (cervical cord trauma/lesions at or above C4) Oxygen therapy in COPD
Neuromuscular disorders	Spinal cord and nerves: multiple sclerosis, poliomyelitis, phrenic nerve injuries, high cord lesions at or above C4, Guillain-Barre syndrome, botulism, tetanus End plate abnormalities: myasthenia gravis, muscle relaxants, succinylcholine chloride, toxins (curare, aminoglycosides, organophosphorus) Muscle: hypokalemia, hypophosphatemia, muscular dystrophy
Restrictive disorders	Pleural effusions, empyema, pneumothorax Kyphoscoliosis, scleroderma, ankylosing spondylitis, morbid obesity, pulmonary fibrosis, pulmonary edema, pneumonia
Defects in CO_2 transport	Congestive heart failure, cardiac arrest with CPR, extensive pulmonary embolism, severe anemia, carbonic anhydrase inhibitor (acetazolamide), high-dose loop diuretics, NSAIDs, salicylates

breathing room air and an increase in the CO_2 component is necessarily accompanied by a decrease in O_2 [4, 7]. The alveolar gas equation (shown below) mandates this decrease in partial pressure of alveolar oxygen (PAO_2) with elevation of partial pressure of arterial carbon dioxide ($PaCO_2$), up to a limit of 80–90 mmHg. When $PaCO_2$ increases two times, the alveolar O_2 (PAO_2) will halve. The resultant tissue hypoxemia is the life-threatening component of respiratory acidosis, more so than any rise in $PaCO_2$ [4].

$$P_AO_2 = \left(F_iO_2 \times \left(P_{atmos} - P_{H_2O}\right)\right) - \left(\frac{P_aCO_2}{RQ}\right).$$

F_iO_2 = fraction of inspired oxygen (usually as a fraction, but entered here as a percentage for ease of use); PaO_2 = partial pressure of oxygen in alveolar gas; F_iO_2 = fraction of inspired oxygen entered as a percentage (on room air this would be 21%); P_{atmos} = ambient atmospheric pressure, which is 760 mmHg at sea level; P_{H_2O} = water vapor pressure at 37 °C and is equal to 47 mmHg; RQ = respiratory quotient = ratio of CO_2 eliminated divided by the O_2 consumed, and its value is typically 0.8 but can range from 0.7 to 1.0.

Chronic respiratory acidosis is characterized by an increase in $PaCO_2$ above the upper limit of normal, with a near normal pH (but less than 7.35) and a concomitant increase in serum bicarbonate. A decrease in plasma chloride, as a result of chronic renal compensation is also noted. Chronic states of hypercapnia result from COPD, chronic upper airway obstruction, central nervous system depression, neuromuscular impairment (e.g., amyotrophic lateral sclerosis), abnormal chest wall mechanics, obesity-hypoventilation syndrome, severe restrictive ventilatory defects (e.g., interstitial pulmonary fibrosis), and thoracic cage anomalies.

Hypoventilation in COPD is attributed to a decreased response to hypoxia and hypercapnia, increased ventilation–perfusion mismatch causing increased dead space ventilation, and diaphragmatic muscle impairment due to fatigue and hyperinflation [2, 7]. Decompensation of this chronic hypercapnic state usually results from infection, narcotic use, and uncontrolled oxygen use and may lead to a life-threatening acidosis of respiratory origin. In extreme cases, a comatose state, known as hypercapnic encephalopathy, may ensue.

Diagnosis

Clinical manifestations of acute respiratory acidosis depend on the symptoms and signs of the underlying illness, the rate of development of hypercapnia, and severity of the acidemia. A patient with mild to moderate hypercapnia that has developed gradually will have symptoms such as gradual onset dyspnea, anxiety, and daytime hypersomnolence. A severe acute hypercapnia may cause delirium, sleepiness, and even an obtunded state, known as carbon dioxide narcosis. Cyanosis may be seen with accompanying hypoxemia. The patient may have asterixis, myoclonus, and seizures with increasing levels of $PaCO_2$. For the most part, the symptoms and signs of mild to moderate respiratory acidosis are subtle and diagnosis requires a clinical suspicion in the appropriate setting. Measurement of an arterial blood gas specimen is required for confirming any clinical suspicion and a low-threshold for ordering this test should be maintained. As discussed in other sections in this book, an algorithmic approach to the diagnosis of acid base disorders is the best approach. In acute respiratory acidosis, the pH will be decreased to less than 7.35 with an increase in $PaCO_2$ of greater than 45 mmHg, pointing towards a respiratory cause for the acidemia. In chronic respiratory acidosis, there will be an increase in serum bicarbonate along with an increase in $PaCO_2$.

A stepwise approach to the interpretation of simple acid base and respiratory acidosis in particular is suggested.

General Rule: Look at the direction of change in pH and $PaCO_2$. A primary metabolic acid base disorder is present if the pH is abnormal and pH and $PaCO_2$ change in the *same* direction. A primary respiratory acid base disorder is present if the $PaCO_2$ is abnormal and the $PaCO_2$ and pH change in the *opposite* direction.

Step 1: Look at pH.
- pH <7.35: acidemia
- pH 7.35–7.45: normal pH range or mixed acid base disorder
- pH >7.45: alkalemia

Step 2: Look at respiratory component, $PaCO_2$.
- $PaCO_2$ <35 mmHg: respiratory alkalosis or compensation for metabolic acidosis.
- $PaCO_2$ 35–45 mmHg: normal range.
- $PaCO_2$ >45 mmHg: respiratory acidosis or compensation for metabolic alkalosis.

Step 3: Determine whether there is adequate compensation, given the clinical history and probable chronicity of the underlying disease processes.

The following equations may be used to calculate expected changes in serum bicarbonate concentration and pH in respiratory acidosis.

- *Acute Respiratory Acidosis*:
  HCO_3^- increases 1 mEq for each 10 mmHg rise in $PaCO_2$.
  Expected change in $pH = 0.008 \times (PaCO_2 - 40)$.
- *Chronic Respiratory Acidosis*:
  HCO_3^- increases 3.5 mEq for each 10 mmHg rise in $PaCO_2$.
  Expected change in $pH = 0.003 \times (PaCO_2 - 40)$.

Acute respiratory acidosis will have both a low pH and an elevated $PaCO_2$ >45 mmHg. Electrolytes are minimally affected by respiratory acidosis. There may be a mild increase in serum ionized calcium due to decreased binding of calcium to albumin seen in acidemia. Acidemia may also cause potassium to shift outside the cell, but significant hyperkalemia rarely occurs in respiratory acidosis.

Once respiratory acidosis is confirmed by arterial blood gas evaluation, other diagnostic tests may be necessary to determine the underlying etiology and to guide therapy. Acute presentations of respiratory acidosis without a readily identifiable etiology, merits a toxicology evaluation, since central nervous system depression by opiates, barbiturates and benzodiazepines maybe responsible agents.

Patients with chronic hypoventilation and respiratory acidosis may also have hypoxemia with secondary polycythemia noted on peripheral blood count. Obese patients may have upper airway obstruction during sleep (obstructive sleep apnea) and chronic hypoventilation leading to daytime hypercapnia. A sleep history and formal sleep study may be warranted. Radiological imaging studies of the chest can show hyperinflation and diaphragm flattening in cases of severe obstructive airway disease, lung opacification in pneumonia, or elevation of the diaphragm with diaphragmatic dysfunction or atelectasis. Brain imaging will be helpful in identifying an acute stroke, trauma, or tumor that may be playing a role in depression of the respiratory drive. Respiratory muscle weakness may lead to chronic hypoventilation and respiratory acidosis. Specialized pulmonary function testing including the measurement of transdiaphragmatic pressures using an esophageal catheter (with an esophageal and a gastric balloon) may document respiratory muscle weakness.

Treatment

Treatment of respiratory acidosis is directed at management of the underlying etiology.

In acute respiratory acidosis, hypercapnia alone is usually not life threatening, but the resultant hypoxemia has serious consequences. Ensuring a patent airway and adequate oxygen administration is critical. Mechanical ventilation may be necessary with the provision of a minute ventilation that will permit a gradual decline of the $PaCO_2$ to the patient's baseline; allowing an adequate renal excretion of bicarbonate. A rapid decline in $PaCO_2$ may cause post-hypercapnic alkalosis with alkalinization of the cerebrospinal fluid, and, may in turn, cause seizures. In cases of severe bronchoconstriction (as seen in severe asthma or COPD exacerbation), bronchodilators, such as beta agonists, anticholinergic agents, and steroids, may be helpful. Heliox and oxygen mixture inhalation has also been used with some success in severe bronchoconstriction, unresponsive to standard therapy [8]. Sodium bicarbonate does not have a role in respiratory acidosis, except in the case of post-cardiac arrest, where pH is <7.1.

Central nervous system depressants, such as narcotics, may be reversed with the use of naloxone, a pure opioid antagonist that works by possibly displacing opioids from its receptors. It is used in increments of 0.1–0.2 mg every 2–3 min and a response should be obtained after 10 mg. Its half life is short between 30 and 80 min, with a faster onset of action with intravenous (IV) administration, of about 2 min and a shorter duration of action for IV route of 30–120 min. Flumazenil antagonizes the GABA/benzodiazepine receptor complex and may be useful in patients with benzodiazepine overdose. Patients will respond within 5 min of administering a cumulative dose of 5 mg; however, it should be used cautiously in patients with a history of chronic benzodiazepine use and those with a seizure history. Additionally, when using either medication, patients should be monitored closely for a sustained improvement in mental status and ventilation parameters [7].

The management of acute, superimposed on chronic, hypercapnic states relies on treating the underlying insult causing the decompensation. Patients with a COPD exacerbation exhibit an increased respiratory effort due to hyperinflation with a decrease in diaphragmatic excursion and increased intrinsic positive end expiratory pressure (PEEP). In some cases, reversal of these mechanisms may be achieved conservatively using noninvasive positive pressure ventilation (NIPV) [e.g., bi-level positive airway pressure (BPAP) ventilation or nasal continuous positive airway pressure ventilation (CPAP)] [9]. NIPV is also useful in improving PaO_2 and decreasing $PaCO_2$ in patients with obesity-hypoventilation syndrome and neuromuscular disorders [10–14]. Absolute contraindications to NIPV use include conditions requiring immediate intubation and mechanical ventilation including coma, cardiac arrest, respiratory arrest, intractable gastrointestinal bleeding, inability to protect the airway, status epilepticus, and potential for upper airway obstruction. The goals of NIPV therapy are to achieve adequate tidal volume between 5 and 7 mL/kg, reduce the respiratory rate to less than 25 breaths per minute and to maintain an oxygen saturation of greater than 90%. Response to therapy is monitored with serial ABG. Oxygen therapy may be needed in patients with hypercapnia, since they may also have hypoxemia. However, it must be used with caution, since it may worsen the ventilation–perfusion mismatch and cause worsened hypercapnia. For patients with chronic hypercapnia and hypoxemia, the threshold for oxygen saturation by pulse oximetry should be 88–90% with a PaO_2 target of 60–65 mmHg.

Case Discussion

Case 1

This patient is hypoxemic with acute decompensation of chronic respiratory acidosis. The patient received oxygen via nasal cannula at 4 L/min and he developed changes in mental status. He was subsequently managed with BPAP. He responded to BPAP with oxygen supplementation at 1 L/min.

Follow-up ABG showed: pH 7.39, $PaCO_2$ 50 mmHg, PaO_2 67 mmHg, and HCO_3 30 mEq/L. Pulmonary function tests showed severe restrictive ventilatory defect with reductions in lung capacity reflective of increased body mass and diaphragmatic dysfunction. Maximum inspiratory pressure (MIP) was 47% predicted and maximum expiratory pressure (MEP) was 33% predicted, consistent with a neuromuscular defect (diaphragm paralysis) contributing to the restrictive component. An urgent polysomnography prior to discharge showed severe obstructive sleep disordered breathing with apnea hypopnea index (AHI, a measure of severity of sleep apnea) of 159/h. In addition to compliance with oxygen and bi-level PAP therapy, he was enrolled in an aggressive weight management program and 1 year later was significantly improved without further hospital admissions.

Patient's initial arterial blood gas showed an acidemia, with a decreased pH of 7.21 and an elevated $PaCO_2$ of 88 mmHg, pointing towards a respiratory acidosis. The elevated HCO_3 of 32 mEq/L indicates the presence of a chronic respiratory acidosis, since the kidneys need approximately 3–5 days to elevate HCO_3 as part of the metabolic compensation. According to the acid base rules mentioned previously, in a simple acute respiratory acidosis, the expected HCO_3 should have been approximately 29 mEq/L (an approximate 1 unit increase of HCO_3 for every 10 mmHg increase in PCO_2, leading to an acute increase of 5 units in HCO_3: 24 + 5 = 29). HCO_3 of 32 mEq/L is not expected in an acute respiratory acidosis. This patient's history is suggestive of an acute on chronic respiratory acidosis. Obesity hypoventilation and COPD predispose to hypercapnia and chronic respiratory acidosis, and the recent COPD exacerbation led to an acute decompensation and worsening of pH and $PaCO_2$.

Once the patient was stabilized, his baseline $PaCO_2$ was 50 mmHg. According to the compensation formulas, his HCO_3 should increase chronically 3.5–4 mEq for every increase of 10 mmHg of $PaCO_2$. Thus his HCO_3 level at baseline is approximately 28 mEq/L (24 + 4 mEq/L). The acute COPD exacerbation, which increased his $PaCO_2$ from a baseline of 50–88 mmHg (38 units), increased his HCO_3 acutely by about 4 mEq/L, from his already elevated baseline of 28–32 mEq/L (acutely, there is an increase of 1 mEq HCO_3/every 10 mmHg increase of $PaCO_2$: 28 + 4 = 32).

Case 2

This is a case of a young patient with ingestion of opioid with subsequent severe central nervous suppression of respiratory drive leading to an acute respiratory acidosis. The increase in HCO_3 of 24–27 (27–24 = 3) is expected in an acute respiratory acidosis with the increase of $PaCO_2$ 40 mmHg above normal (80–40 = 40). pH has also decreased by 0.32 units below normal (7.40) to approximately 7.10, in accordance with the expected change $0.008 \times (PaCO_2 - 40)$. Due to the severe depression of his respiratory drive and his inability to clear secretions and protect his airway, he was intubated and placed on volume controlled ventilation, achieving adequate tidal volumes and saturations above 94%. He received a continuous intravenous infusion of naloxone and with improvement of consciousness and resumption of adequate spontaneous breathing switched to pressure support ventilation. The patient was following commands and successfully extubated 12 h later. His follow-up ABG was normal.

Summary

Respiratory acidosis is caused by alveolar hypoventilation, leading to increased CO_2 in the arterial blood. This acid–base disorder requires immediate diagnosis as it may be accompanied by life-threatening acidemia and hypoxemia. Respiratory acidosis occurs in clinical scenarios where there is a strong suppression of the respiratory drive, causing a delay in the lungs' ability to expel carbon dioxide effectively. Respiratory acidosis may be acute or chronic and is managed depending on the underlying clinical condition. The management includes the use of noninvasive and invasive mechanical support with intensive care monitoring. Prompt attention to correcting the acute acidemia and hypoxemia while addressing the underlying etiology will usually lead to favorable outcomes.

References

1. Adrogue HJ, Madias N. Secondary responses to altered acid-base status: the rules of engagement. J Am Soc Nephrol. 2010;21(6):920–3.
2. Miller's Anesthesia, 7th ed. Chapter 49-Perioperative acid-base balance. http://www.mdconsult.com/books. Accessed 11 Jan 2011.
3. West JB, Wagner PD. Pulmonary gas exchange. Am J Respir Crit Care Med. 1998;157:S82–S7.
4. Cruickshank S, Hirschauer N. The alveolar gas equation. Contin Educ Anaesth Crit Care Pain. 2004;4(1):24–7.
5. Adrogue HJ, Madias N. Management of life-threatening acid-base disorders: first of two parts. N Engl J Med. 1998;338(1):26–34.
6. Mason: Murray and Nadel's textbook of respiratory medicine, 5th ed. http://www.mdconsult.com/books. Accessed 28 Jan 2011.
7. Adrogue HJ. Diagnosis and management of severe respiratory acidosis: a 65-year-old man with a double-lung transplant and shortness of breath. Am J Kidney Dis. 2010;56(5):994–1000.
8. McGarvey JM, Pollack CV. Heliox in airway management. Emerg Med Clin North Am. 2008;26(4):905–20. viii. Review.
9. Ram FS, Picot J, Lightowler J, Wedzicha JA. Non-invasive positive pressure ventilation for treatment of respiratory failure due to exacerbations of chronic obstructive pulmonary disease. Cochrane Database Syst Rev. 2004;(1):CD004104. Review.
10. Naloxone: Drug information. http://www.uptodate.com. Accessed 11 Jan 2011.
11. Littleton SW, Mokhlesi B. The pickwickian syndrome-obesity hypoventilation syndrome. Clin Chest Med. 2009;30(3):467–78. vii-viii.
12. Adrogue HJ, Gennari FJ, Galla JH, Madias N. Assessing acid-base disorders. Kidney Int. 2009;76(12): 1239–47.
13. Piper AJ, Wang D, Yee BJ, Barnes DJ, Grunstein RR. Randomised trial of CPAP vs bilevel support in the treatment of obesity hypoventilation syndrome without severe nocturnal desaturation. Thorax. 2008;63(5):395–401.
14. Dabal LA, BaHammam AS. Obesity hypoventilation syndrome. Ann Thorac Med. 2009;4(2):41–9.

15 Respiratory Alkalosis

Rebecca L. Toonkel and Shirin Shafazand

Case 1

A. A. is a 27-year-old woman with asthma who presents to the emergency room with cough and dyspnea. The cough began approximately 2 weeks ago after the onset of "cold" symptoms. Her symptoms (sore throat, runny nose, and congestion) have resolved, but the cough has persisted. Since last night, she has felt increasing shortness of breath and "tightness" in her chest. She is breathing at a rate of 28 breaths per min and her oxygen saturation is 97% while breathing room air. Auscultation of the chest reveals diffuse expiratory wheezing. Electrolytes and complete blood cell counts are within normal limits, and the chest X-ray shows no pulmonary opacities. Analysis of the arterial blood gas reveals: pH 7.5, pCO_2 25 mmHg, and HCO_3^- 20 mEq/L.

R.L. Toonkel, M.D.
Division of Pulmonary, Critical Care and Sleep Medicine, Jackson Memorial Hospital, University of Miami, Miami, FL 33136, USA

S. Shafazand, M.D., M.S. (✉)
Division of Pulmonary, Critical Care and Sleep Medicine, Miller School of Medicine, University of Miami, PO Box 016960 (D60), Miami, FL 33101, USA
e-mail: sshafazand@med.miami.edu

Case 2

C. A. is a 76-year-old man with alcoholic liver cirrhosis who was found to be confused by family members and brought to the emergency department. The patient is arousable and follows simple commands. The family suspects that he has been drinking alcohol. He is breathing at a rate of 28 breaths per min but appears quite comfortable. The physical examination is essentially unremarkable except for the stigmata of chronic liver disease. His laboratory results are as follows: Na 133 mEq/L, K 3.3 mEq/L, Cl 115 mEq/L, pH 7.44, pCO_2 20 mmHg, and HCO_3^- 13 mEq/L.

Background and Definitions

Respiratory alkalosis occurs in 29–45% of hospitalized patients and is estimated to be present in approximately 26% of patients at the time of admission [1–3]. The prevalence of the disorder varies depending upon the underlying etiology and the type and timing of hospital admission. Among hospitalized patients, common etiologies include pain, fever, and hyperventilation while on a ventilator.

Sustained alveolar hyperventilation, iatrogenic or otherwise, is the cause of respiratory alkalosis. For the purposes of discussion, a number of important terms require definition. The term "*alkalosis*" refers to an underlying metabolic disorder resulting in an excess of plasma HCO_3^-.

E.V. Lerma and M. Rosner (eds.), *Clinical Decisions in Nephrology, Hypertension and Kidney Transplantation*, DOI 10.1007/978-1-4614-4454-1_15, © Springer Science+Business Media New York 2013

On the other hand, "*alkalemia*" refers to an elevation in the plasma pH. Therefore, in mixed disorders alkalosis and acidosis may occur concomitantly, but the primary disorder will determine whether the pH is elevated (alkalemia) or depressed (acidemia).

Similarly, the term "hyperventilation" is not synonymous with tachypnea (increased respiratory rate) or hyperpnea (increased minute ventilation). Hyperventilation, which can occur in the absence of either tachypnea or hyperpnea, is the clearance of CO_2 by the lungs at a rate faster than its production rate. Conversely, in the setting of increased CO_2 production, tachypnea and hyperpnea will occur without hyperventilation or subsequent hypocapnea.

Alveolar hyperventilation leads to a decrease in the partial pressure of alveolar carbon dioxide ($pACO_2$). This translates to a decrease in the arterial carbon dioxide ($paCO_2$) with a subsequent increase in the ratio of HCO_3^- to $paCO_2$ and therefore increased plasma pH. Alveolar hyperventilation with subsequent hypocapnea (decreased $paCO_2$) and alkalosis (excess HCO_3^-) occurs when a strong respiratory stimulus causes the lungs to expel more carbon dioxide than is produced metabolically in the tissues. Respiratory alkalosis may be acute or chronic and may occur as a primary disorder or as a compensatory disorder in response to a primary metabolic acidosis. In this section, we discuss the pathophysiology, etiology, and physiological response to respiratory alkalosis.

Pathophysiology

CO_2 is stored in the body primarily as HCO_3^- ion with an equilibrium maintained according to Le Chatelier's principle

$$CO_2 + H_2O \Leftrightarrow H_2CO_3 \Leftrightarrow HCO_3^- + H^+$$

CO_2 produced at the tissue level is combined with H_2O to form H_2CO_3 via the enzyme catalyst carbonic anhydrase. H_2CO_3 subsequently dissociates to form free H^+ and HCO_3^-. At the level of the lungs, the reaction is driven in the opposite direction as CO_2 is expelled. Respiratory alkalosis occurs when the lungs remove more CO_2 than is produced. Because CO_2 is highly diffusible, the partial pressure of CO_2 in the alveoli ($pACO_2$) and arterial blood ($paCO_2$) is equivalent under normal conditions at rest. Increased ventilation leads to a decrease in $pACO_2$ and subsequently also $paCO_2$, which in turn increases in the ratio of HCO_3^- to pCO_2 and therefore pH [4].

In order to maintain the integrity of protein structure and ultimately function, the pH of human tissue is tightly regulated. Peripheral chemoreceptors in the carotid bodies and central chemoreceptors in the brain sense pH and affect ventilation accordingly. In the setting of hyper- or hypoventilation, metabolic compensation occurs at the level of the kidneys with alterations in H^+ secretion and HCO_3^- reabsorbtion. Of note, this compensation is dependent on both renal function and volume status [5]. Because metabolic compensation by the kidney occurs over hours to days, expected changes in the HCO_3^- vary depending on the chronicity of the disorder. In the setting of an acute respiratory alkalosis, immediate but insufficient buffering occurs at the protein and cellular level with small decreases in HCO_3^- concentration. Over time, in the setting of chronic respiratory alkalosis, the kidneys retain H^+ and secrete HCO_3^- to more fully compensate. Examination of the peripheral arterial blood gas in conjunction with the clinical history allows the clinician to diagnose respiratory alkalosis and to determine its chronicity. An algorithmic approach is discussed below.

The onset and resolution of acute respiratory alkalosis is rapid. Experiments have shown that arterial pH begins to rise within 5–10 s of the initiation of forced hyperventilation, reaches a maximum by 5–10 min, and returns to normal within 5 min after cessation [6, 7]. On the other hand, augmented renal acid secretion begins almost immediately after the normalization of a chronically reduced $paCO_2$ but continues over many hours, leading to a brief period of metabolic acidosis [8].

Etiology

While clinicians often attribute hyperventilation to psychological causes, multiple organic etiologies of respiratory alkalosis are recognized [10]. These can be grouped broadly into categories including: pulmonary, central, hypoxia-related, drug-induced, endocrine, and miscellaneous (Table 15.1).

Mild acute respiratory alkalosis may occur frequently in clinical practice as a result of anxiety or pain. For example, atypical chest pain syndromes have also been implicated as initiators of a feedback cycle of anxiety, pain, and hyperventilation resulting in clinically evident respiratory alkalosis [11]. In the intensive care unit, respiratory alkalosis may occur as a result of over-ventilation or insufficient sedation and/or analgesia. Other causes, such as hyperthyroidism may lead to respiratory alkalosis by direct stimulation of chemoreceptors [12]. In addition, undiagnosed asthma (often mild and atypical) has been recognized as a common cause of previously labeled "idiopathic" hyperventilation [13]. In fact, as many as 80% of patients diagnosed with "pure hyperventilation" in the emergency room may have evidence of underlying asthma [14]. Finally, high levels of circulating progesterone during pregnancy and the second half of the menstrual cycle act both centrally and peripherally to induce a physiologically normal state of hyperventilation [15, 16].

When no underlying cause of chronic hyperventilation is determined, patients may be said to suffer from idiopathic hyperventilation. This entity was first described in 1938 and is thought to be a psychogenic syndrome related to stress and anxiety [17]. Patients are found to have daytime hyperventilation and respiratory alkalosis with normalization during sleep. Hyperventilation syndrome is a diagnosis of exclusion and therefore should only be made after an exhaustive search has revealed no other underlying cause [11].

Table 15.1 Etiologies of respiratory alkalosis

Pulmonary
Pneumonia
Pulmonary edema
Asthma
Chronic obstructive pulmonary disorder (COPD)
Pulmonary embolism
Interstitial lung disease
Central
Pain
Anxiety
Stroke
Trauma
Subarachnoid hemorrhage
Meningitis
Encephalitis
Hypoxia-related
High altitude
Anemia
Right to left shunt
Drug-induced
Salicylates
Nicotine
Catecholamines
Progesterone
Methylxanthines
Endocrine
Pregnancy
Hyperthyroidism
Miscellaneous
Fever
Mechanical ventilation
Gram-negative septicemia (early)
Hepatic failure

Clinical Signs and Symptoms

In 1908, Haldane and Poulton published the first description of clinical symptoms associated with hyperventilation [18]. Paresthesias, diaphoresis, circumoral numbness, and even tetany have been described. Symptoms are often attributed to serum electrolyte abnormalities as acute hypocapnea leads to decreased serum levels of potassium and phosphate due to intracellular shifts and decreased ionized calcium levels due to enhanced protein binding. Other symptoms, such as vertigo, syncope, and seizures have been attributed to cerebral vasoconstriction with decreased cerebral blood flow [19] or decreased cardiac index and increased systemic vascular resistance in the setting of acute hypocapnea [20].

While many symptoms are described in association with hyperventilation, most are nonspecific and not easily reproducible [21]. Normal values for $paCO_2$ are generally accepted to be between 37 and 43 mmHg and symptoms are thought to occur in the range of 14–29 mmHg with no clearly defined threshold. That said, the end tidal CO_2 in many normal individuals has been shown to fall within this range during the course of daily living, suggesting a broad spectrum of normal values [22].

Respiratory Alkalosis

Acute

HCO_3^- 2 meq/L for each 10 mmHg ↓ $paCO_2$

$HCO_3^- = 0.2(\Delta\ paCO_2)$

Expected Δ pH = 0.008 x (40 – $paCO_2$)

Chronic

HCO_3^- ↓ 5 meq/L for each 10 mmHg ↓ $paCO_2$

$\Delta\ HCO_3^- = 0.5(\Delta\ paCO_2)$

Expected Δ pH = 0.003 x (40 – $paCO_2$)

Fig. 15.1 Expected compensatory changes in respiratory alkalosis

Diagnosis and Treatment

Alkalemia is typically recognized at an arterial pH greater than 7.44 and is attributed to a primary respiratory disorder when the partial pressure of CO_2 in the arterial blood ($paCO_2$) is less than 36 mmHg [23]. With normal lungs function, the partial pressure of CO_2 measured at end expiration (end tidal CO_2 or $p_{ET}CO_2$) is roughly equivalent to $pACO_2$ and therefore also $paCO_2$. While this suggests that $p_{ET}CO_2$ can be used as a noninvasive surrogate for $paCO_2$, with exercise or with ventilation–perfusion mismatch (especially in the case of large amounts of dead space) this relationship does not hold and $p_{ET}CO_2$ may significantly underestimate $paCO_2$ [24]. Transcutaneous CO_2 measurement via skin electrodes is also possible and may be useful for following trends, but is not felt to be accurate enough for precise measurement [11]. For these reasons, and because of the relative ease of measuring $paCO_2$, direct examination of peripheral arterial blood gas remains the gold standard.

The diagnosis of respiratory alkalosis, like all acid–base disorders, requires a systematic approach to the interpretation of the arterial blood gas (Fig. 15.1). First, one must determine if the primary disorder is an alkalemia (pH >7.44) or acidemia (pH <7.35). If alkalemia is present, the next step is to determine if the primary etiology of the alkalemia is respiratory (pCO_2 <36 mmHg) or metabolic (HCO_3^- >26 mEq/L). Once the diagnosis of primary respiratory alkalosis has been made, one can determine if the disorder is acute or chronic by calculating the expected compensatory change in plasma HCO_3^-. In the acute setting, the plasma HCO_3^- concentration will fall approximately 2 mEq/L for each 10 mmHg decrease in the $paCO_2$. On the other hand, if the alkalosis is chronic, the HCO_3^- concentration will decrease approximately 5 mEq/L for each 10 mmHg decrease in the $paCO_2$ [9]. Finally, one must determine if the primary respiratory alkalosis (acute or chronic) is the only disorder present or if there is a concomitant metabolic acidosis or alkalosis also present. Due to the mechanical requirement of alveolar hyper- or hypoventilation for the development of respiratory driven acid–base disorders, respiratory alkalosis, and acidosis cannot occur simultaneously. To determine if a metabolic disorder is also present, it is important to remember that a compensatory metabolic acidosis drives the HCO_3^- down (in the same direction as the $paCO_2$), if the HCO_3^- is elevated or not decreased as much as predicted, a concomitant metabolic alkalosis is present. On the other hand, if the HCO_3^- is lower than predicted, a concomitant metabolic acidosis may be present. Of note, a HCO_3^- less than 12 mEq/L is unusual in pure respiratory alkalosis with metabolic compensation and should prompt investigation for sources of concomitant metabolic acidosis [4].

Treatment for respiratory alkalosis per se is rarely necessary unless arterial pH is severely elevated and is usually directed at addressing the underlying cause. Recognizing and treating the potentially serious underlying medical conditions that may cause respiratory alkalosis is of considerable importance. When hyperventilation is triggered by anxiety, rebreathing of exhaled CO_2 may be of benefit both physiologically and psychologically. In hospitalized patients, controlling pain or fever is often sufficient. In the case of patients undergoing mechanical ventilation, respiratory alkalosis may be corrected by decreasing the tidal volume delivered or, if the patient is not breathing spontaneously, the respiratory rate. For patients breathing spontaneously with low (lung protective) tidal volumes, increased sedation and/or analgesia may be required. In rare cases of severe respiratory alkalemia, carbonic anhydrase inhibitors such as acetazolamide may be used to decrease plasma pH by partially blocking renal resorption of HCO_3^-. If the PCO_2 is corrected rapidly in patients with chronic respiratory alkalosis, acidemia may develop due to the persistent renal compensatory drop in serum bicarbonate.

Case Discussions

Case 1

A. A. is experiencing an asthma exacerbation and her arterial blood gas is consistent with acute respiratory alkalosis (pH 7.5, pCO_2 25 mmHg, and HCO_3^- 20 mEq/L), which may be diagnosed using the algorithm discussed above. The pH of 7.50 (>7.44) is consistent with alkalemia as the primary disorder. The pCO_2 of 25 (<36) is consistent with a respiratory disorder as the etiology. The HCO_3^- 20 mEq/L suggests that this an acute respiratory alkalosis because we would expect a change in HCO_3^- of approximately 2 mEq/L for every 10 mmHg change in pCO_2 (expected 24—observed 21 = 3) based on the pCO_2 change of 15 (expected 40—observed 25 = 15). Treatment should be directed towards managing the underlying asthma exacerbation, using a combination of inhaled bronchodilators and a course of corticosteroids.

Case 2

C. A. has chronic liver disease and hyperventilation. At first glance, the HCO_3^- is low and lactic acidosis is certainly in the differential diagnosis of someone with decompensated end stage liver disease. However, the patient is not acidemic and, contrary to what one might expect in metabolic acidosis secondary to lactic acidosis, the anion gap of 5 [133–(115 + 13)] is not elevated, even when considering and correcting for the patient's likely hypoalbuminemic state. The pH of 7.44 is in the normal range and one is immediately alerted to the possibility of a mixed acid–base disorder. However, in chronic respiratory alkalosis, the pH can return to near normal in the presence of functioning kidneys that have had adequate time for compensatory mechanisms. The clinical scenario of a liver patient with increased respiratory rate, but no apparent distress is in keeping with chronic respiratory alkalosis, as patients with liver cirrhosis have various stimuli that promote increased respiration (e.g., ascites, chronic pain/anxiety, increased levels of progesterone, ammonia, vasoactive intestinal peptide, and glutamine can stimulate respiration) and the chronicity of their underlying disease allows for adequate compensatory responses. The arterial blood gas results are in keeping with the expected decrease in HCO_3^- of 5 mEq/L for every 10 mmHg decrease in pCO_2: change in HCO_3^- of 11 (24−13 = 11) versus change in pCO_2 of 20 (40–20 = 20).

Conclusion

Sustained alveolar hyperventilation is the cause of respiratory alkalosis. A broad differential diagnosis serves as the underlying etiology of hyperventilation. The most important factor in managing respiratory alkalosis is recognizing the many potentially life-threatening disorders that cause this acid–base abnormality and to treat the underlying disease.

References

1. Mazzara JT, Ayres SM, Grace WJ. Extreme hypocapnia in the critically ill patient. Am J Med. 1974;56(4):450–6.
2. Hodgkin JE, Soeprono FF, Chan DM. Incidence of metabolic alkalemia in hospitalized patients. Crit Care Med. 1980;8(12):725–8.
3. Palange P, Carlone S, Galassetti P, Felli A, Serra P. Incidence of acid-base and electrolyte disturbances in a general hospital: a study of 110 consecutive admissions. Recenti Prog Med. 1990;81(12):788–91.
4. Nadel JA, Murray JF, Mason RJ. Murray and Nadel's textbook of respiratory medicine. 4th ed. Philadelphia: Elsevier Saunders; 2005.
5. Harrison TR, Braunwald E. Harrison's principles of internal medicine. 15th ed. New York: McGraw-Hill; 2001.
6. Lepper EH, Martland M. Variations in the p(H) and bicarbonate of the plasma and of the alveolar CO(2) during forced breathing. Biochem J. 1927;21(4): 823–30.
7. Brown Jr EB. Physiological effects of hyperventilation. Physiol Rev. 1953;33(4):445–71.
8. Gennari FJ, Goldstein MB, Schwartz WB. The nature of the renal adaptation to chronic hypocapnia. J Clin Invest. 1972;51(7):1722–30.
9. Krapf R, Beeler I, Hertner D, Hulter HN. Chronic respiratory alkalosis. The effect of sustained hyperventilation on renal regulation of acid-base equilibrium. N Engl J Med. 1991;324(20):1394–401.
10. Gardner WN. Hyperventilation. Am J Respir Crit Care Med. 2004;170(2):105–6.
11. Gardner WN. The pathophysiology of hyperventilation disorders. Chest. 1996;109(2):516–34.
12. Engel LA, Ritchie B. Ventilatory response to inhaled carbon dioxide in hyperthyroidism. J Appl Physiol. 1971;30(2):173–7.
13. Osborne CA, O'Connor BJ, Lewis A, Kanabar V, Gardner WN. Hyperventilation and asymptomatic chronic asthma. Thorax. 2000;55(12):1016–22.
14. Saisch SG, Wessely S, Gardner WN. Patients with acute hyperventilation presenting to an inner-city emergency department. Chest. 1996;110(4):952–7.
15. Damas-Mora J, Davies L, Taylor W, Jenner FA. Menstrual respiratory changes and symptoms. Br J Psychiatry. 1980;136:492–7.
16. Hannhart B, Pickett CK, Moore LG. Effects of estrogen and progesterone on carotid body neural output responsiveness to hypoxia. J Appl Physiol. 1990;68(5):1909–16.
17. Kerr WJ, Gliebe PA, Dalton JW. Physical phenomena associated with anxiety states: the hyperventilation syndrome. Cal West Med. 1938;48(1):12–6.
18. Haldane JS, Poulton EP. The effects of want of oxygen on respiration. J Physiol. 1908;37(5–6):390–407.
19. Raichle ME, Plum F. Hyperventilation and cerebral blood flow. Stroke. 1972;3(5):566–75.
20. Kazmaier S, Weyland A, Buhre W, Stephan H, Rieke H, Filoda K, et al. Effects of respiratory alkalosis and acidosis on myocardial blood flow and metabolism in patients with coronary artery disease. Anesthesiology. 1998;89(4):831–7.
21. Saltzman HA, Heyman A, Sieker HO. Correlation of clinical and physiologic manifestations of sustained hyperventilation. N Engl J Med. 1963;268:1431–6.
22. Rafferty GF, Saisch SG, Gardner WN. Relation of hypocapnic symptoms to rate of fall of end-tidal PCO2 in normal subjects. Respir Med. 1992;86(4): 335–40.
23. Arbus GS, Herbert LA, Levesque PR, Etsten BE, Schwartz WB. Characterization and clinical application of the "significance band" for acute respiratory alkalosis. N Engl J Med. 1969;280(3):117–23.
24. Jones NL, Robertson DG, Kane JW. Difference between end-tidal and arterial PCO2 in exercise. J Appl Physiol. 1979;47(5):954–60.

Mixed Acid–Base Disorders

16

Oliver Lenz

Case 1

A 55-year-old man presents with a 3-day history of severe nausea and vomiting following an alcohol binge. He says that he has not been able to take anything by mouth for the past 3 days, and he complains about diffuse abdominal pain. On admission his blood pressure is 129/77 mmHg with a heart rate of 77 bpm supine and 105/62 mmHg with a heart rate of 92 bpm standing up. He is a febrile. He looks emaciated, has poor skin turgor, and dry mucous membranes. His bowel sounds appear diminished, and an abdominal X-ray shows small bowel ileus. On admission to the emergency room the laboratory data shown in Table 16.1 are obtained. What, if any, acid–base disturbance is present?

Case 2

A 27-year-old woman with a history of type 1 diabetes since age 14 is brought to the emergency room after she collapsed on the dance floor of a local club at 4 AM. On arrival, she has a blood pressure of 110/66 mmHg with a heart rate of 100 bpm. She is unable to stand up. Her temperature is 38.3°C (101 F), and she has dry mucous membranes. She is awake and moaning but does not give coherent answers. A friend who accompanies her says that she was dancing in the club for the past 8 h, consumed several alcoholic beverages, and possibly some ecstasy. Initial laboratory data are shown in Table 16.1.

Introduction

Mixed acid–base disorders are common, particularly in the critically ill patient. For the clinician it is important to recognize whether more than one acid–base abnormality is present, given that each disorder represents an underlying pathophysiologic entity that may warrant a different therapeutic approach. Consider a patient with respiratory acidosis and metabolic alkalosis. If the clinician failed to recognize the respiratory component he might treat only the metabolic alkalosis and be surprised by the sudden drop in pH or the worsening respiratory status after large-volume fluid resuscitation.

Several approaches exist to analyze acid–base disorders, the most popular ones being the method based on the Henderson-Hasselbalch equation utilizing pCO_2, bicarbonate, and the anion gap, the method using standardized base excess, and the strong ion theory proposed by Stewart. Although most acid–base disorders can be accurately identified with any of the three methods, each approach has advantages and disadvantages [1–3]. The bicarbonate-based methodology was

O. Lenz, M.D. (✉)
Division of Nephrology and Hypertension, Miller School of Medicine, University of Miami, 1120 NW 14th Street, Room 809A (R126), Miami, FL 33136, USA
e-mail: olenz@med.miami.edu

E.V. Lerma and M. Rosner (eds.), *Clinical Decisions in Nephrology, Hypertension and Kidney Transplantation*, DOI 10.1007/978-1-4614-4454-1_16, © Springer Science+Business Media New York 2013

Table 16.1 Laboratory data for case 1 and case 2

	Case 1	Case 2
Serum		
Glucose (mg/dl)	67	233
Na^+ (mEq/l)	136	145
K^+ (mEq/l)	3.1	5.3
Cl^- (mEq/l)	88	82
HCO_3^- (mmol/l)	24	31
BUN (mg/dl)	57	67
Creatinine (mg/dl)	1.3	1.7
Albumin (g/dl)	2.5	4.7
Ketones	+++	+
Arterial blood gas		
pH	7.40	7.32
pCO_2 (mmHg)	40	62
pO_2 (mmHg)	95	82
HCO_3^- (mmol/l)	24	31
Urine		
pH	6.5	6.5
Na^+ (mEq/l)	<15	20
K^+ (mEq/l)	33	37
Cl^- (mEq/l)	<15	<15
Ketones	+++	+

+ weakly positive
+++ strongly positive

Table 16.2 Stepwise approach to complex acid–base disorders

Step 1: identify a primary disorder
(a) Check the pH
Low: academia
High: alkalemia
(b) Analyze the change in pCO_2 and HCO_3^- in connection with the pH
pH ↑, pCO_2 ↑, and HCO_3^- ↑: metabolic alkalosis
pH ↑, pCO_2 ↓, and HCO_3^- ↓: respiratory alkalosis
pH ↓, pCO_2 ↓, and HCO_3^- ↓: metabolic acidosis
pH ↓, pCO_2 ↑, and HCO_3^- ↑: respiratory acidosis
Step 2: assess if there is an appropriate compensation for the primary disorder[a]
Step 3: calculate the anion gap[a]
Step 4: calculate the $\Delta AG / \Delta HCO_3^-$ ratio[a]

[a]See Table 16.3 for relevant equations

chosen for the following discussion because its conceptual framework can be readily fitted to the pathophysiology of the underlying acid–base disturbances.

In the preceding chapters the predicted responses to primary acid–base disorders were discussed, namely the expected change in pCO_2 when a primary metabolic disorder is present, and the expected change in HCO_3^- when a primary respiratory disorder is present. In the current chapter we use the previously discussed approaches in the analysis of complex acid–base disorders and highlight the utility of the anion gap and the delta anion gap to delta bicarbonate ratio.

Clinical Approach and Diagnosis

Whenever one is faced with complex acid–base disorders it is important to utilize all available clinical data. The history and physical examination are key elements in the analysis, because they reveal clues as to what might be expected on the arterial blood gas. Consider a patient with severe vomiting for several days presenting with signs and symptoms of volume depletion: one might reasonably expect to find a metabolic alkalosis. Let us further assume the arterial blood gas analysis shows a pH of 7.4 with a normal HCO_3^- and normal pCO_2. One could either conclude that the initial assumption was wrong and there is no metabolic alkalosis or that an equally significant metabolic acidosis caused the laboratory data to appear normal. In other words, laboratory data and mathematical equations do not substitute for clinical judgment. Another important prerequisite to the successful analysis of complex acid–base disorders is the realization that more than one metabolic disorder can exist in the same patient, but the patient can only present with a single respiratory disorder.

A stepwise approach to mixed acid–base disorders is shown in Table 16.2. In the first step, a primary disorder is identified based on the change in pH, pCO_2, and HCO_3^-. In a patient with more than one disorder the analysis with yield the same result no matter which one is picked first. Note that pCO_2 and HCO_3^- change in the same direction as the pH in metabolic disorders, while in the setting of alkalosis they change in opposite direction of the pH.

In the second step we analyze whether the expected physiologic compensation for the identified primary disorder is present. The relevant equations are shown in Table 16.3: For metabolic

Table 16.3 Commonly used formulas to examine mixed acid–base disorders

1. Expected pH from pCO_2 and HCO_3^-:
$pH = 6.1 + \log\frac{[HCO_3^-]}{0.03 \times pCO_2}$ or $pH = 7.62 - \log\frac{pCO_2}{[HCO_3^-]}$
2. Expected pCO_2 from HCO_3^- in metabolic disorders:
(a) Metabolic acidosis
$pCO_2 = 1.5 \times [HCO_3^-] + 8 \pm 2$
(b) Metabolic alkalosis
$pCO_2 = 40 + 0.7 \times \Delta[HCO_3^-] \pm 2$
3. Expected HCO_3^- from pCO_2 in respiratory disorders
(a) Respiratory acidosis
acute: $[HCO_3^-] = 24 + 0.1 \times \Delta pCO_2$ chronic: $[HCO_3^-] = 24 + 0.35 \times \Delta pCO_2$
(b) Respiratory alkalosis
acute: $[HCO_3^-] = 24 - 0.2 \times \Delta pCO_2$ chronic: $[HCO_3^-] = 24 - 0.5 \times \Delta pCO_2$
4. Serum anion gap
$AG = [Na^+] - [Cl^-] - [HCO_3^-] + 2.5 \times \Delta[\text{Albumin}]$
5. Delta–delta ratio

For the formulas shown the following units are used: pCO_2 (mmHg), Na^+ (mEq/l), Cl^- (mEq/l), HCO_3^- (mmol/l or mEq/l), Albumin (g/dl). The delta pCO_2 is the absolute difference between the current and the reference pCO_2, i.e., the value is always positive. pCO_2 of 40 mmHg is usually used as the reference value if the patient's pre-morbid baseline is not known. Delta albumin is calculated by subtracting the current value from the reference value, i.e., the value will be negative if the current albumin concentration exceeds the reference value. An albumin concentration of 4.5 g/dl is usually used as the reference value if the patient's pre-morbid baseline is not known. The delta–delta ratio is calculated from the absolute changes in anion gap and HCO_3^-, i.e., the value is always positive. An anion gap of 12 mEq/l and a HCO_3^- of 24 mmol/l are usually used as the reference values if the patient's pre-morbid baseline data are not known.

disorders we expect a respiratory compensation and thus a change in pCO_2, while for respiratory disorders we expect a metabolic compensation resulting in a change in HCO_3^-. This may be best illustrated with a few examples (Table 16.4). In case 3 the pH is above 7.4, i.e., there is alkalemia. The bicarbonate is increased, indicating a metabolic alkalosis. The appropriate compensation is hypoventilation leading to a rise in pCO_2, and the expected pCO_2 can be calculated as

$$pCO_2 = 40 + 0.7 \times \Delta[HCO_3^-] = 40 + 0.7 \times (31 - 24) = 45.$$

If the pCO_2 were higher than expected, then we would diagnose a concomitant respiratory acidosis. If the pCO_2 were lower, then an additional respiratory alkalosis would be present. The same arguments hold true for case 4 after the expected pCO_2 is computed according to equation 2(a) in Table 16.3. In case 5, alkalemia is present, and the pCO_2 is decreased, suggesting respiratory

Table 16.4 Laboratory data illustrating primary acid–base disorders with appropriate compensation

	Case 3	Case 4	Case 5	Case 6
	Metabolic alkalosis	Metabolic acidosis	Respiratory alkalosis (chronic)	Respiratory acidosis (chronic)
Arterial blood gas				
pH	7.46	7.32	7.43	7.33
pCO_2 (mmHg)	45	32	26	61
HCO_3^- (mmol/l)	31	16	17	31

alkalosis. The appropriate compensation is renal retention of bicarbonate, and the expected serum bicarbonate can be calculated as

$$[HCO_3^-] = 24 - 0.5 \times \Delta pCO_2 = 24 - 0.5 \times (40 - 26) = 17.$$

If the observed serum bicarbonate were higher, then we would diagnose a concomitant metabolic alkalosis, and if it were lower, a metabolic acidosis. The same arguments hold true for case 6 after the expected bicarbonate concentration has been calculated using equation 3(a) in Table 16.3. Note that a margin of error of ±2 is acceptable with these calculations.

Table 16.5 Causes of an elevated serum anion gap

Metabolic acidosis
Laboratory error
Severe volume depletion
Hyperalbuminemia
Metabolic alkalosis
Respiratory alkalosis
Severe hyperphosphatemia
Anionic paraproteins

The increase in serum anion gap in severe volume depletion can in most cases be explained by the increase in serum albumin concentration. The increase in anion gap by hyperventilation is usually very small

The third step requires calculation of the serum anion gap. To maintain electroneutrality, the sum of negative and positive charges must be equal, i.e., the sum of charges provided by circulating anions—chloride, bicarbonate, anionic proteins, inorganic phosphate, sulfate, and organic anions—and cations—sodium, potassium, calcium, magnesium, and cationic proteins—must be the same. In routine laboratory testing only sodium, potassium, chloride, and bicarbonate are measured, and the remaining ions are lumped together as unmeasured anions (UA) and unmeasured cations (UC). In addition, potassium is commonly omitted to facilitate the calculation and because potassium's low serum concentration contributes little to the overall amount of cations. The anion gap, AG = UC–UA, can be calculated by rearranging the equation to the formula $AG = [Na^+] - [Cl^-] - [HCO_3^-]$. This formula assumes that albumin, an important anionic protein, has a normal serum concentration. Given that this may not be the case, particularly in critically ill patients, and given that albumin's contribution to the anion gap is about 2.5 mEq/l for each 1 g/dl albumin [4], the formula can be expanded to the one shown in Table 16.3. If an anion gap greater than 20 mEq/l is detected, then an additional anion gap metabolic acidosis can be diagnosed. For a list of common causes of an anion gap metabolic acidosis, see the chapter on metabolic acidosis. Anion gaps between 12 and 20 may be due to metabolic acidosis, but other causes need to be considered and additional laboratory testing may be required (Table 16.5). If a normal anion gap is found then the next step is omitted.

The fourth step requires calculating the $\Delta \text{anion gap} / \Delta[HCO_3^-]$ ratio, also known as the delta–delta ratio. One might assume that for every unit increase in the concentration of an organic acid one unit of bicarbonate is consumed. However, the ratio is more variable and depends on the nature of the organic acidosis and the time in the course of the disease, and recent data suggest that one should use the ratio as one of several pieces of evidence to make a final diagnosis [5]. In patients with diabetic ketoacidosis the mean ratio found is close to 1, but it may be close to 1.6 in patients with lactic acidosis [6, 7], and the standard deviation in most case series was high. A prudent approach may be to look for an additional acid–base disorder if the delta–delta ratio is <0.8 or >1.2 in patients with ketoacidosis, or <1.2 or >2.0 in patients with lactic acidosis, while keeping the clinical scenario in mind. If the delta–delta ratio is larger than expected, then the serum bicarbonate did not drop as much as expected, and a concomitant metabolic alkalosis may be present. Conversely, if the delta–delta ratio is smaller than expected, then the serum bicarbonate decreased more than expected, and a concomitant non-anion gap metabolic acidosis may be present.

Case Discussion

Case 1

Based on the clinical scenario there is a high likelihood that the patient has a metabolic alkalosis: He had several days of vomiting with little to no oral intake, providing both a risen for the generation of a metabolic alkalosis, i.e., proton loss in the gastric fluid, and the maintenance of metabolic alkalosis, i.e., chloride depletion, as can be seen by the low urine chloride and the signs and symptoms of volume depletion. Having not eaten for 3 days it can be expected that he will also have ketoacidosis, and this again is supported by the presence of ketones in both the serum and the urine. Without having done any calculations, yet, the clinical picture has alerted us that a mixed acid–base disorder may be present. Using the stepwise approach, steps 1 does not yield any evidence for an acid–base abnormality, i.e., pH, pCO_2, and HCO_3^- are all within the normal range, and step 2 becomes obsolete. However, based on the clinical presentation it is still safe to assume that a mixed acid–base disorder is present, rather than concluding that the patient does not have any acid–base disorder. Step 3 sheds additional light on the situation: the anion gap is

$$AG = [Na^+] - [Cl^-] - [HCO_3^-] + 2.5 \times \Delta[\text{Albumin}].$$
$$= 136 - 88 - 24 + 5 = 29$$

This is clearly suggestive of an anion gap metabolic acidosis. Although ketones are positive, it may be prudent at this point to look for other unmeasured anions (it is always critical to exclude toxic ingestions). The abdominal pain may indicate another reason for having an anion gap metabolic acidosis, e.g., lactic acidosis due to bowel obstruction or necrotizing pancreatitis, and given that the patient is alcohol-dependent, methanol or ethylene glycol intoxications should be considered. Finally, in step 4 we calculate the delta–delta ratio. We do not know any baseline data, so let us assume the change in anion gap is 29–12 = 17 and the change in bicarbonate is 24–24 = 0. Although we cannot calculate the delta–delta ratio because a division by zero does not yield a mathematically useful result, it is evident that the change in bicarbonate is much smaller than expected, suggesting the presence of a metabolic alkalosis. These findings support our initial hypotheses and guide the management of the patient: The nature of the anion gap needs further investigation, and if the patient has significant liver impairment he may not be able to convert the ketone bodies into bicarbonate and the metabolic acidosis may become very apparent when volume expansion with isotonic saline is administered.

Case 2

In the analysis of case 2 let us start right away with the stepwise approach. The pH is decreased, and both pCO_2 and HCO_3^- are increased, so step 1 suggests that the patient has a respiratory acidosis. In step 2 we calculate the appropriate response and evaluate the rise in serum bicarbonate. The question is: Is this an acute or a chronic respiratory acidosis? This again illustrates that we must take the clinical presentation into account. The patient is a young woman, we have no knowledge of an underlying respiratory disorder, and she appears to have tolerated strenuous exercise, i.e., dancing for several hours, just fine. Consequently, this is likely an acute event, and we expect $[HCO_3^-] = 24 + 0.1 \times \Delta pCO_2 = 26\,\text{mmol/l}$. The actual bicarbonate, however, is 39 mEq/l, so an additional metabolic alkalosis is likely. The clinical picture fits to this: She has an elevated temperature, appears volume depleted, and her urine chloride is low, suggesting extra-renal chloride losses, such as from sweating. In the third step we calculate the anion gap, which is 145–88–31 = 26, suggesting the presence of an anion gap metabolic acidosis. While ketoacidosis is a possibility given the history of type 1 diabetes, elevated blood sugar, and positive ketones in serum and urine, other anions need to be considered given her altered mentation and possible substance abuse. In the last step we evaluate the delta–delta ratio. The change in anion gap is 26–12 = 14, and we expect a drop in bicarbonate by 14 to 10 mmol/l. This is not what we see: The bicarbonate actually is increased, suggesting that the previously diagnosed metabolic alkalosis is quite severe.

Key Points

Following the stepwise approach provides an important framework for the analysis of mixed acid–base disorders. After identifying a primary disorder, analysis of the compensatory mechanism, the anion gap, and the delta anion gap to delta bicarbonate ratio will provide clues as to whether additional acid–base disorders are present. However, it is paramount to take into consideration the patient's history, physical examination, and all other ancillary data, because at each step of the analysis there are potential pitfalls: The arterial blood gas analysis may look normal although a complex acid–base disorder is present, the anion gap may be influenced by factors other than an anion gap metabolic acidosis, and the expected values for the delta–delta ratio can vary significantly between individuals.

References

1. Kurtz I, Kraut J, Ornekian V, Nguyen MK. Acid-base analysis: a critique of the Stewart and bicarbonate-centered approaches. Am J Physiol Renal Physiol. 2008;294:F1009–F31.
2. Rastegar A. Clinical utility of Stewart's method in diagnosis and management of acid-base disorders. Clin J Am Soc Nephrol. 2009;4:1267–74.
3. Boniatti MM, Cardoso PR, Castilho RK, Vieira SR. Acid-base disorders evaluation in critically ill patients: we can improve our diagnostic ability. Intensive Care Med. 2009;35:1377–82.
4. Figge J, Jabor A, Kazda A, Fencl V. Anion gap and hypoalbuminemia. Crit Care Med. 1998;26:1807–10.
5. Rastegar A. Use of the DeltaAG/DeltaHCO3- ratio in the diagnosis of mixed acid-base disorders. J Am Soc Nephrol. 2007;18:2429–31.
6. Oh MS, Carroll HJ, Goldstein DA, Fein IA. Hyperchloremic acidosis during the recovery phase of diabetic ketosis. Ann Intern Med. 1978;89:925–7.
7. Paulson WD. Anion gap-bicarbonate relation in diabetic ketoacidosis. Am J Med. 1986;81:995–1000.

Part V

Acute Kidney Injury

17 Acute Kidney Injury: Definitions and General Approach

Ashita J. Tolwani

Case 1

A 75-year-old male presents to the Emergency Department with orthostatic hypotension, tachycardia, fever and 3-day history of vomiting, dyspnea, and green sputum production. Past medical history is significant for diabetes mellitus type II and chronic kidney disease (CKD) with baseline creatinine 1.5 mg/dL. His home medications include enalapril, glyburide, and hydrochlorothiazide. He is resuscitated with crystalloids and started on broad-spectrum antibiotics. He remains hypotensive and is admitted to the medical intensive care unit (MICU) on a norepinephrine infusion of 5 mcg/min with the diagnosis of sepsis from pneumonia. His admission creatinine is 1.8 mg/dL. Within 24 h, he develops worsening hypoxia and requires intubation and mechanical ventilation. Forty-eight hours after admission, his serum creatinine increases to 2.2 mg/dL, and his urine output declines to 0.4 mL/kg/h for the past 24 h. He has generalized edema and signs of fluid overload on his chest radiograph. Urinalysis shows 1+ proteinuria, no glucose, and is leukocyte esterase negative. Urine microscopy shows 1–5 coarse granular casts and 1–5 renal tubular epithelial cells per high power field.

What are his risk factors for developing acute kidney injury (AKI)? Does this patient have AKI?

Introduction

Acute renal failure (ARF) is defined as a decrease in kidney function, occurring over a period of hours to days, resulting in the accumulation of creatinine, urea, and other metabolic waste products (azotemia). It can occur in the setting of previously normal renal function or in patients with preexisting renal disease (acute-on-chronic renal failure). ARF is often accompanied by reductions in urine volume with associated salt and water retention and metabolic disturbances, such as metabolic acidosis and hyperkalemia. Anuria is defined as urine output less than 50 mL/day; oliguria is urine output less than 400 mL/day.

Characterizing the epidemiology of ARF has been problematic due to variations in the definition of ARF, differences in the causes and settings of ARF, and dissimilarities among patients developing ARF. Over recent years, there has been increasing recognition that relatively small rises in serum creatinine are associated with morbidity and mortality [1, 2]. For this reason the term "acute kidney injury" (AKI) has been coined to recognize the importance of the disease as a spectrum of injury extending from less severe forms to more advanced injury, such as that requiring renal replacement therapy (RRT).

A.J. Tolwani, M.D., M.Sc. (✉)
Department of Nephrology, University of Alabama at Birmingham, THT 643, 1530 3rd Ave. S, Birmingham, AL 35294-0006, USA
e-mail: atolwani@uab.edu

E.V. Lerma and M. Rosner (eds.), *Clinical Decisions in Nephrology, Hypertension and Kidney Transplantation*,
DOI 10.1007/978-1-4614-4454-1_17, © Springer Science+Business Media New York 2013

Epidemiology

The incidence of AKI varies widely and is dependent on the population studied and definition used. It accounts for 1% of hospital admissions in the USA [3]. The incidence of hospital-acquired AKI is 5–7%, exceeding that of community-acquired AKI by five to tenfold, and has nearly doubled over the last two decades [4]. Acute tubular necrosis (ATN) remains the most common cause of hospital-acquired AKI and is often multifactorial (sepsis, postsurgical, contrast agents, medications). In the intensive care unit (ICU), 5–20% of patients develop AKI, of which approximately 6% require some form of RRT during their ICU stay [5]. The incidence of ICU-related AKI has also increased over the last few decades. This is probably related to the rising incidence of sepsis-related hospital admissions; increased prevalence of risk factors for AKI, including older age, CKD, diabetes mellitus, and congestive heart failure; and expanded use of intravenous radiocontrast agents.

Definition and Staging

The major obstacle to research in AKI has been the lack of a uniform definition, which has led to conflicting reports in the literature. Because of this lack of standardization, in 2002, the Acute Dialysis Quality Initiative (ADQI) workgroup devised the RIFLE definition and staging system for AKI, categorizing AKI into three grades of increasing severity: "Risk" (defined as oliguria more than 6 h or a serum creatinine increase of at least 50%), "Injury," and "Failure" (both defined by a greater increase in serum creatinine, or duration and severity of oliguria, compared to the "Risk" group) (Table 17.1). These categories—R, I, and F—were associated with two clinical outcomes: renal "loss" and "end stage renal disease" (ESRD) [6]. Loss and ESRD were defined by the need for RRT for greater than 4 weeks and greater than 3 months, respectively. After emerging data demonstrated that even small alterations in renal function lead to adverse outcomes, the Acute Kidney Injury Network (AKIN) modified the RIFLE staging system and used the term AKI instead of ARF to encompass the entire spectrum of acute kidney dysfunction (Table 17.1) [7]. The AKIN workgroup defined AKI as a reduction in kidney function occurring over no more than 48 h manifest by an absolute increase in serum creatinine level ≥0.3 mg/dL or a relative increase in serum creatinine level ≥50%; or documented oliguria <0.5 mL/kg/h for more than 6 h despite adequate fluid resuscitation [7]. In addition, they categorized all patients requiring RRT for AKI in stage III. Multiple studies have validated the utility of these criteria to various populations, showing a correlation between more severe RIFLE stages and worse clinical outcomes [8, 9].

Table 17.1 RIFLE and AKIN criteria for AKI

RIFLE		AKIN		Both
Stage	sCr/GFR	Stage	sCr/GFR	Urine output
R	Increase in sCr of 1.5–2-fold from baseline or GFR decrease >25%	I	Increase in sCr of 1.5–2-fold from baseline or increase in sCr of ≥0.3 mg/dL	<0.5 mL/kg/h for 6 h
I	Increase in sCr of two to threefold from baseline or GFR decrease >50%	II	Increase in sCr of two to threefold from baseline	<0.5 mL/kg/h for 12 h
F	Increase in sCr > threefold from baseline or GFR decrease >75% or sCr ≥4 mg/dL with an acute rise of ≥0.5 mg/dL	III[a]	Increase in sCr >threefold from baseline or sCr ≥4 mg/dL with an acute rise of ≥0.5 mg/dL	<0.3 mL/kg/h for 24 h or anuria for 12 h
L	Persistent renal failure for >4 weeks			
E	Persistent renal failure for >3 months			

AKI acute kidney injury, *AKIN* acute kidney injury network, *GFR* glomerular filtration rate, *RIFLE* risk(R), injury (I), failure (F), loss (L), End-stage kidney disease (E), *Scr* serum creatinine

[a]Individuals who receive renal replacement therapy (RRT) are considered to have met the criteria for stage III irrespective of the stage they are in at the time of RRT

Case 1 Revisited

What Are His Risk Factors for Developing AKI?

The patient has multiple risk factors for developing AKI, placing him at high risk. These include older age, diabetes, CKD, and hypovolemia. Furthermore, enalapril and hydrochlorothiazide can be potentially nephrotoxic in the setting of volume depletion. However, the major risk is the development of sepsis. Early and appropriate resuscitation are key to lowering the risk for the development of AKI.

Does This Patient Have AKI?

He meets the definition of AKI since he has a sustained increase in his creatinine of greater than 0.3 mg/dL over a 48-h period. Given his drop in urine output to 0.4 mL/kg/h in 24 h, he currently classifies as having RIFLE class "I" or AKIN stage II AKI.

What is the most likely cause of his AKI? What further tests will help confirm the diagnosis?

Pathophysiology and Differential Diagnosis

Causes of AKI can be broadly divided into three categories: prerenal, intrinsic, and postrenal (Table 17.2).

Prerenal AKI

Prerenal AKI (also known as "prerenal azotemia") results from decreased renal perfusion, leading to a reduction in glomerular filtration rate (GFR) with no structural renal injury. Any condition that decreases effective circulating volume can result in prerenal AKI, including hypovolemia, cirrhosis, early sepsis, inadequate perfusion pressure due to heart failure, and medications such as

Table 17.2 Causes of acute kidney injury

Prerenal
Volume depletion (renal losses, GI losses, hemorrhage)
Decreased cardiac output (heart failure, pulmonary embolus)
Systemic vasodilation (sepsis, anaphylaxis, anesthetics)
Afferent arteriolar vasoconstriction
Hypercalcemia
Drugs (NSAIDs, amphotericin B, calcineurin inhibitors, radiocontrast agents)
Hepatorenal syndrome
Efferent arteriolar vasodilation (ACEIs, ARBs)
Renal artery occlusion
Post-renal
Intrinsic (stone, blood clots)
Extrinsic (retroperitoneal or pelvic malignancy)
Intrinsic
Acute tubular necrosis
Ischemic
Nephrotoxic
Drugs (aminoglycosides, lithium, amphotericin B, pentamidine, cisplatin, ifosfamide, radiocontrast agents)
Pigment (rhabdomyolysis, intravascular hemolysis)
Acute interstitial nephritis
Drug-induced (penicillins, cephalosporins, NSAIDs, proton-pump inhibitors, allopurinol, rifampin, sulfonamides)
Infection-related causes (pyelonephritis, viral nephritides)
Autoimmune diseases (Sjögren's syndrome, sarcoidosis, SLE)
Malignancy (lymphoma, leukemia)
Acute glomerulonephritis (postinfectious, cryoglobulinemia, RPGN)
Vascular
Macrovascular (bilateral renal artery, bilateral renal vein thrombosis)
Microvascular (atheroembolic disease, HUS, TTP, scleroderma, malignant hypertension)
Intratubular obstruction
Paraprotein (myeloma)
Crystals (tumor lysis syndrome, ethylene glycol, acyclovir, indinavir, methotrexate)

ACEIs angiotensin-converting enzyme inhibitors, *ARBs* angiotensin II receptor blockers, *NSAIDs* nonsteroidal anti-inflammatory drugs, *SLE* systemic lupus erythematosus, *RPGN* rapidly progressive glomerulonephritis, *HUS* hemolytic uremic syndrome, *TTP* thrombotic thrombocytopenic purpura nonsteroidal anti-inflammatory drugs (NSAIDS). Prerenal AKI is associated with a bland urinalysis, low urinary sodium, low fractional excretion of sodium and urea, and high urine osmolality (Table 17.3). These urinary indices are indicative of the renal response to decreased perfusion. If not treated, sustained renal hypoperfusion can progress to ischemic ATN.

Postrenal AKI

Oliguria/anuria may be caused by obstruction occurring anywhere from the renal pelvis to the external urethral meatus. Obstruction may be intraluminal, associated with lesions within the wall of the urinary tract (such as tumors) or extrinsic to the urinary tract. Obstruction may occur at the level of the bladder or urethra (lower tract obstruction) or at the level of the ureters or renal pelvis (upper tract obstruction). To cause AKI, upper tract obstruction must be bilateral or affect a solitary functioning kidney. If postrenal AKI is not treated promptly, the elevated tubular pressure can cause CKD due to irreversible injury.

Intrinsic AKI

Intrinsic processes that result in AKI are categorized according to the structural component of the kidney that is the primary site of histologic injury (Table 17.2). Intrinsic AKI includes tubular injury, interstitial injury, glomerular injury, vascular disease, and intratubular obstruction. The important distinction between intrinsic AKI and pre- and postrenal AKI is the presence of structural injury to the kidney in intrinsic AKI.

Tubular Injury

The most common cause of hospital-acquired AKI is ATN. This condition is usually induced by ischemia or toxins. Prerenal azotemia and ischemic ATN represent a continuum. Patients at risk for moving from prerenal azotemia to ATN include those with prolonged systemic hypotension and those with decreased effective renal perfusion for prolonged periods. Unlike prerenal AKI, the GFR does not improve with the restoration of renal blood flow (such as with restoration of intravascular volume with intravenous fluids). Ischemic ATN is frequently reversible, but if the ischemia is severe enough to cause cortical necrosis, irreversible renal failure can occur. Additionally, multiple medications and toxins may induce tubular damage (Table 17.2). The urine sediment in ATN commonly demonstrates many tubular epithelial cells and coarse granular casts, often described as "muddy brown" casts. ATN is characterized by failure to maximally dilute or concentrate urine (isosthenuria) due to tubular injury. In prerenal azotemia, urine osmolality is usually greater than 500 mOsm/kg, whereas in intrinsic renal disease, urine osmolality is less than 300 mOsm/kg. However, exceptions exist as seen in Table 17.3.

Interstitial Injury

Acute interstitial nephritis (AIN) results from lymphocytic infiltration of the interstitium. AIN is usually the result of an allergic reaction to a drug, but it may also be caused by autoimmune disease, infection, or infiltrative disease (Table 17.2). The classic triad of fever, rash, and eosinophilia is seen in only 10–30% of patients who have AIN [10]. The urine findings in AIN include sterile pyuria, white blood cell casts, non-nephrotic-range proteinuria, hematuria, and eosinophiluria. These urinary findings may or may not be accompanied by signs and symptoms of a more systemic allergic response.

Glomerular Injury

Acute glomerulonephritis refers to a specific set of renal diseases in which an immunologic mechanism triggers inflammation and proliferation of glomerular tissue that can result in damage to the basement membrane, mesangium, or capillary endothelium. Often, constitutional signs and symptoms are noted. Acute glomerulonephritis frequently accompanies systemic disorders such as systemic lupus erythematosus, hepatitis, vasculitis, and pulmonary renal syndromes. Serologic assays and kidney biopsy will identify most causes. Urinary findings range from moderate to severe proteinuria (nephrotic category), dysmor-

Table 17.3 Diagnostic findings in AKI

Condition	BUN/creatinine ratio	Urine sodium (mEq/L)	FENa (FEUrea)	Urine osmolality (mOsm/kg H_2O)	Urinalysis
Prerenal	>20:1	<20	<1% (<35%)	>500	Specific gravity >1.020; Normal or hyaline casts
ATN	10:1	>40	>1%[a] (>35%)	<300	Specific gravity ~1.010; muddy brown casts and tubular epithelial cells
AIN	Variable	>20	>1% (>35%)	<300	Hematuria, white blood cells, white blood cell casts, eosinophiluria
Acute GN	Variable	<20	<1% (<35%)	>500	Dysmorphic red blood cells and red blood cell casts
Intratubular obstruction	Variable	Variable	Variable	Variable	Crystalluria[b] or Bence-Jones proteinuria
Acute vascular syndromes	Variable	>20	Variable	Variable	Hematuria
Postrenal	>20:1	>20	Variable	Variable	Variable

AKI acute kidney injury, *ATN* acute tubular necrosis, *Acute GN* acute glomerulonephritis, *AIN* acute interstitial injury, *FENa* fractional excretion of sodium, *FEUrea* fractional excretion of urea, *BUN* blood urea nitrogen
[a]FENa can be low in radiocontrast nephropathy and pigment nephropathy
[b]Calcium oxalate crystals with ethylene glycol; uric acid crystals in tumor lysis syndrome

phic erythrocytes, and erythrocyte casts (nephritic category). Early recognition of this syndrome is extremely important because it can be fatal and result in irreversible kidney damage without prompt and aggressive treatment.

Vascular Injury

Microvascular or macrovascular disease (major renal artery occlusion or severe abdominal aortic disease) can cause AKI. The classic microvascular diseases often present with microangiopathic hemolysis and AKI occurring from glomerular capillary thrombosis, often with accompanying thrombocytopenia. Typical examples of these diseases are thrombotic thrombocytopenic purpura (TTP), hemolytic uremic syndrome (HUS) and hemolysis, elevated liver enzymes, and low platelets syndrome (HELLP). Atheroembolic disease is another important cause of irreversible AKI. Patients with atherosclerotic disease who undergo an invasive vascular procedure are at increased risk for AKI induced by atheroemboli.

Intratubular Obstruction

Intratubular obstruction from precipitation of either protein or crystals within the tubular lumen also can cause AKI. Examples include tubular obstruction from precipitated monoclonal light chains in multiple myeloma, uric acid from tumor lysis syndrome, calcium oxalate deposition from ethylene glycol, and drugs (Table 17.2).

Diagnosis

The basic diagnostic approach to patients with AKI is to assess whether the patient has prerenal, postrenal, or intrinsic AKI. This involves obtaining a detailed history and examination, as well as analysis of laboratory and radiology findings.

Medical Chart Review and Physical Examination

A thorough review of the patient's history often reveals possible contributing factors of AKI, such as nephrotoxin exposure, hypotension, predisposing conditions for AKI (CKD and diabetes), and obstructive symptoms. Distinguishing between acute and chronic kidney injury is extremely important since the approach, evaluation, and management differ. The most useful determination of chronicity of kidney failure is the knowledge of previous creatinine measurements. The physical examination is directed toward the assessment of volume status, identification of findings of systemic disease, and evidence of obstruction, such as a palpable bladder or flank pain.

Laboratory Testing

The diagnosis of AKI is primarily determined by increasing levels of blood urea nitrogen (BUN) and creatinine, often along with a decreased urine output. It is important to understand that the rise in serum creatinine is often seen several days after the renal insult making this a relatively late marker of AKI. For this reason, a search for both blood and urine biomarkers that can accurately detect the earliest stages of AKI is ongoing. Two promising markers are kidney injury molecule-1 (KIM-1) and neutrophil gelatinase-associated lipocalin (NGAL).

Microscopic evaluation of the urine sediment from a freshly voided urine sample is essential to the evaluation of AKI. Prerenal azotemia is characterized by abnormal sediment or by occasional hyaline casts. Dysmorphic red blood cells and red blood cell casts suggest glomerulonephritis and should lead to serological testing for autoimmune disorders or vasculitis. Sterile pyuria or white blood cell casts should raise the possibility of interstitial nephritis. "Muddy brown" casts (heavily pigmented casts resulting from tubular cell debris) and/or tubular epithelial cell casts are typically seen in patients with ATN. Eosinophiluria, which is often used to screen for interstitial nephritis, has limited specificity and positive predictive value, since it can be seen in other conditions associated with AKI such as acute glomerulonephritis and atheroembolic renal disease, as well as other common diseases in acutely ill patients, such as pyelonephritis and prostatitis [10].

Both the urinary sediment and the urinary indices in combination with serum values can often be extremely helpful in determining the cause of AKI. The fractional excretion of sodium (FENa) is used to determine whether tubular function is intact. Calculating the FENa is useful in AKI only in the presence of oliguria (i.e., in determining if the cause of decreased urine output is due to volume depletion or tubular injury). Values of less than 1% are seen in prerenal AKI, whereas values greater than 1% are seen in ATN. Exceptions to this rule are ATN caused by radiocontrast nephropathy, severe burns, acute glomerulonephritis, and rhabdomyolysis, which can initially present with FENa <1% but where tubular injury is prevalent. A frequent problem in the interpretation of the FENa is the concomitant use of diuretics, which may result in a high FENa despite a low effective circulating volume. In patients who are receiving diuretics, a fractional excretion of urea (FEUrea) can be obtained, since urea transport is not affected by diuretics [11, 12]. The formula for calculating the FEUrea is as follows: $FEUrea = (U_{urea}/P_{urea})/(U_{Cr}/P_{Cr}) \times 100$. FEUrea of less than 35% is suggestive of a prerenal state. The various serum and urinary findings used in diagnosing the major causes of AKI are shown in Table 17.3. Renal biopsy should be considered when no apparent cause of AKI is found or to achieve tissue diagnosis of a suspected glomerulonephritis associated with AKI.

Biomarkers for AKI

Serum creatinine is widely used in the diagnosis of AKI and is considered to be specific but generally an insensitive biomarker of renal dysfunction. With the recognition of the importance of small changes in serum creatinine of >0.3 mg/dL, the sensitivity of serum creatinine to detect early renal injury has improved. However, significant renal tubular injury can occur before such small increments in creatinine have occurred. Serum creatinine concentration is greatly influenced by changes in muscle mass and tubular secretion, body weight, race, age, sex, total body volume, drugs, muscle metabolism, and protein intake. For these reasons it is generally considered a poor marker of early AKI and an even poorer reflection of kidney function because patients with AKI are not in steady state and serum creatinine lags far behind renal injury. Novel biomarkers for the early detection of AKI have recently been developed.

The most promising of these include NGAL, interleukin (IL)-18, KIM-1, Cystatin C, and L-fatty acid binding protein (FABP) [13, 14].

Radiologic Evaluation

Renal ultrasonography is most often performed to rule out obstructive uropathy as the cause of AKI. Unfortunately, renal ultrasonography is neither highly sensitive nor specific for obstructive uropathy, but accuracy increases with serial examinations. Useful information about renal size, echotexture (parenchymal density), and renal vascular status (with Doppler evaluation) can be obtained. Reduced kidney size and cortical thickness are characteristic of CKD. However, kidney size can be preserved in patients with longstanding diabetes or other infiltrative disorders such as HIV nephropathy and multiple myeloma. A renal ultrasound should be performed on all patients with AKI.

Case 1 Revisited

What Is the Cause of His AKI?

The patient most likely has multifactorial AKI. On initial presentation he had evidence of prerenal AKI with volume depletion from vomiting, fever, and diuretic use. His physical exam findings of orthostatic hypotension and tachycardia support this. However, despite volume repletion his renal function worsened and urine sediment demonstrates coarse granular casts consistent with ATN. Thus, he no longer has a prerenal state and most likely has progressed to ATN from sepsis and hypotension in the setting of volume depletion and diuretic and enalapril use.

What Further Tests Will Help Confirm the Diagnosis?

A renal ultrasound should be performed to rule out an obstructive cause. Besides examination of the urine sediment, further urine indices such as urine osmolality and FENa may be helpful. However, given his diuretic use, the FEUrea is preferred.

How should he be managed?

Management

Treatment for intrinsic AKI is largely supportive, including adjusting medication dosages, providing appropriate nutritional support, and correcting volume status, hyperkalemia, and acidosis. Any potentially nephrotoxic drugs should be stopped. The leading indications for dialysis are volume overload, hyperkalemia, uremia, metabolic acidosis, and removal of certain harmful toxins and drugs.

Prognosis

The mortality rate estimates for AKI vary from 10 to 90%, dependent upon the patient population studied [15–17]. ICU patients presenting with AKI and multiorgan failure have been reported to have mortality rates of over 50% [5, 18]. If RRT is required the mortality rate has been reported as high as 80% [17–19].

Complications

Increasing severity of AKI can result in uremia, metabolic acidosis, hyperkalemia, volume overload, and other electrolyte disorders, causing increased risk of prolonged hospitalization and much higher mortality. Supportive management must focus on avoiding and treating these complications.

Preventive Measures

Because few measures exist to actively treat AKI, clinicians should try to prevent it. Issues to consider are correcting volume status, avoiding exposure to nephrotoxins, and preparing for high-risk procedures such as those using contrast agents with prophylactic strategies. Early AKI can be potentially reversible through simple interventions such as fluid volume replacement, discontinuing and/or avoiding potentially nephrotoxic agents, relief of urinary tract obstruction and earlier recognition of conditions causing rapid progression of AKI.

Case 1 Revisited

How Should He Be Managed?

Correcting his hemodynamic derangements, treating sepsis, and avoiding any further nephrotoxic medications are essential. Since he has developed fluid overload on chest radiograph, he no longer has volume depletion and has progressed to ATN. Continuing crystalloids will only worsen his volume overload and decrease his ability to be weaned to extubation. Besides supportive care, he may require RRT to treat the complications of his ATN.

Key Points

- AKI is a common clinical problem that is associated with increased morbidity and mortality.
- Small increments in serum creatinine are an independent risk factor for mortality.
- The most common cause of in-hospital AKI is ATN resulting from multiple insults such as sepsis, hypotension, and use of nephrotoxic agents.
- Risk factors for AKI include increased age, diabetes, CKD, and left ventricular dysfunction.
- Given the high mortality of AKI and the lack of specific pharmacological therapies, every effort should be made to prevent AKI through prompt recognition of the risk factors of AKI, accurate assessment of volume status, and avoidance of nephrotoxin insults.
- Obstruction is an immediately curable cause of AKI and should be excluded in each patient with AKI.

References

1. Lassnigg A, Schmidlin D, Mouhieddine M, et al. Minimal changes of serum creatinine predict prognosis in patients after cardiothoracic surgery: a prospective cohort study. J Am Soc Nephrol. 2004;15(6):1597–605.
2. Chertow GM, Burdick E, Honour M, Bonventre JV, Bates DW. Acute kidney injury, mortality, length of stay, and costs in hospitalized patients. J Am Soc Nephrol. 2005;16(11):3365–70.
3. Kaufman J, Dhakal M, Patel B, Hamburger R. Community-acquired acute renal failure. Am J Kidney Dis. 1991;17(2):191–8.
4. Lameire N, Van Biesen W, Vanholder R. The changing epidemiology of acute renal failure. Nat Clin Pract Nephrol. 2006;2(7):364–77.
5. Uchino S, Kellum JA, Bellomo R, et al. Acute renal failure in critically ill patients: a multinational, multicenter study. JAMA. 2005;294(7):813–8.
6. Bellomo R. Defining, quantifying, and classifying acute renal failure. Crit Care Clin. 2005;21(2):223–37.
7. Mehta RL, Kellum JA, Shah SV, et al. Acute Kidney Injury Network: report of an initiative to improve outcomes in acute kidney injury. Crit Care. 2007;11(2): R31.
8. Ricci Z, Cruz D, Ronco C. The RIFLE criteria and mortality in acute kidney injury: a systematic review. Kidney Int. 2008;73(5):538–46.
9. Bagshaw SM, George C, Dinu I, Bellomo R. A multicentre evaluation of the RIFLE criteria for early acute kidney injury in critically ill patients. Nephrol Dial Transplant. 2008;23(4):1203–10.
10. Rossert J. Drug-induced acute interstitial nephritis. Kidney Int. 2001;60(2):804–17.
11. Carvounis CP, Nisar S, Guro-Razuman S. Significance of the fractional excretion of urea in the differential diagnosis of acute renal failure. Kidney Int. 2002; 62(6):2223–9.
12. Diskin CJ, Stokes TJ, Dansby LM, Radcliff L, Carter TB. The comparative benefits of the fractional excretion of urea and sodium in various azotemic oliguric states. Nephron Clin Pract. 2010;114(2):c145–c50.
13. Parikh CR, Devarajan P. New biomarkers of acute kidney injury. Crit Care Med. 2008;36(4 Suppl): S159–S65.
14. Coca SG, Parikh CR. Urinary biomarkers for acute kidney injury: perspectives on translation. Clin J Am Soc Nephrol. 2008;3(2):481–90.
15. Liano F, Junco E, Pascual J, Madero R, Verde E. The spectrum of acute renal failure in the intensive care unit compared with that seen in other settings. The Madrid Acute Renal Failure Study Group. Kidney Int Suppl. 1998;66:S16–24.
16. Liano F, Pascual J. Epidemiology of acute renal failure: a prospective, multicenter, community-based study. Madrid Acute Renal Failure Study Group. Kidney Int. 1996;50(3):811–8.

17. Metcalfe W, Simpson M, Khan IH, et al. Acute renal failure requiring renal replacement therapy: incidence and outcome. QJM. 2002;95(9):579–83.
18. Brivet FG, Kleinknecht DJ, Loirat P, Landais PJ. Acute renal failure in intensive care units–causes, outcome, and prognostic factors of hospital mortality; a prospective, multicenter study. French Study Group on Acute Renal Failure. Crit Care Med. 1996;24(2):192–8.
19. Mehta RL, Pascual MT, Soroko S, et al. Spectrum of acute renal failure in the intensive care unit: the PICARD experience. Kidney Int. 2004;66(4):1613–21.

Prerenal Azotemia

18

Luis I. Juncos and Luis A. Juncos

Case 1

A 71-year-old man with a history of colon cancer status post right hemicolectomy with colostomy 6 months earlier, presented with a 3-day history of orthostatic dizziness. He reports that the content of the colostomy bag over the last 5 days has been watery, foul smelling, and has to be emptied every 2–3 h. He has diabetes mellitus, hypertension, and chronic kidney disease and is treated with metformin and enalapril. His blood pressure and pulse while lying down were 96/75 mmHg and 96 beats per minute (bpm), respectively. Standing up his blood pressure was 80/65 mmHg and his pulse was 112 bpm. His oral mucosa and axillae were dry, neck veins were not distended, lungs were clear, and he had no ventricular gallops. At admission his serum creatinine was 4.1 mg/dL (up from his baseline of 1.8), urine Na was 35 mEq/L, and fractional excretion of sodium (FENa) was 1.76.

What mechanisms are contributing to the decline in his renal function?

L.I. Juncos, M.D., Ph.D., M.S.
Department of Medicine, J. Robert Cade Foundation, Cordoba, Argentina 5003

L.A. Juncos, M.D. (✉)
Division of Nephrology, Department of Medicine, University of Mississippi Medical Center, 2500 North State St., Jackson, MS 39216, USA
e-mail: ljuncos@umc.edu

What diagnostic and/or therapeutic measures should be undertaken?

Case 2

A 62-year-old woman with a past history of bicuspid aortic stenosis was seen with progressive dyspnea on exertion (now limiting her day-to-day activities) and orthopnea. She reports no chest pain, dizziness, or syncope. Previous imaging studies have shown cardiomegaly with a thickened and calcified bicuspid aortic valve having an orifice area of 0.72 cm^2. She was offered but refused surgery. Physical examination revealed a blood pressure of 110/70, pulse of 116 bpm, and a respiratory rate of 28/min. She had engorged neck veins and pulsus parvus et tardus. Auscultation of the chest revealed agrade I/VI holosystolic murmur at the apex and a grade IV/VI systolic ejection murmur at the base, along with bilateral crepitant rales in the lower lung fields. The patient also had tender hepatomegaly and 2+ pedal edema. Chest X-ray and an EKG showed cardiomegaly and evidence of left ventricular hypertrophy, respectively. Initial laboratory findings were plasma creatinine 3.1 mg/dL, BUN 112 mg/dL, sodium 124 mEq/L, bicarbonate 22 mEq/dL, chloride 94 mEq/L, potassium 4.1 mEq/L, normal urinalysis, and urine Na 8 mEq/L.

What are the likely mechanisms for her renal failure?

What are the major complications that may occur as a result of treating her symptoms?

E.V. Lerma and M. Rosner (eds.), *Clinical Decisions in Nephrology, Hypertension and Kidney Transplantation*, DOI 10.1007/978-1-4614-4454-1_18, © Springer Science+Business Media New York 2013

Introduction

Prerenal azotemia refers to a decline in renal function/glomerular filtration rate (GFR) that occurs when effective renal perfusion or glomerular filtration pressure is reduced, and there is no structural damage to the kidney. This can result from any process associated with hypovolemia, peripheral vasodilation, decreased cardiac output, or abnormal intrarenal hemodynamics. Thus, it is a common form of acute kidney injury (AKI); it is present in 2–48% of hospitalized patients (depending on the diagnostic criteria used and the characteristics of the population studied) and accounts for up to 75% of all cases of AKI [1–5]. Recognizing its presence and identifying its cause is of critical importance because it is usually reversible if rapidly and appropriately treated. However, if this prerenal state is severe or prolonged, as occurs with delayed or unsuccessful therapy, it may lead to ischemic acute tubular necrosis (ATN) because prerenal azotemia and ATN lie along a continuum of renal hypoperfusion [5, 6].

Etiology/Pathophysiology

In order for the kidneys to maintain water and electrolyte homeostasis, and eliminate metabolic waste, they need to filter large volumes of blood; thus they receive approximately 20% of the cardiac output. Moreover, the body has several complementary mechanisms that help maintain this high level of renal blood flow (RBF) and GFR [5–8] when systemic perfusion is compromised. A reduction in absolute or effective systemic perfusion is sensed by pressure receptors in the thorax, which in turn increase the activity of the sympathetic nervous system and the renin angiotensin system, and cause release of vasopressin [6]. The increased activity of these systems results in systemic vasoconstriction and in renal salt and water retention, which together tend to correct the low perfusion pressure thus improving renal perfusion.

Locally, the kidney also contributes to the preservation of its blood flow and GFR via its inherent autoregulatory ability. That is, it maintains near constant RBF and GFR throughout a wide range of blood pressures [6–8]. Renal autoregulation is mediated through intrinsic mechanisms, namely, myogenic responses of the afferent and efferent arteriole and tubuloglomerular feedback (TGF).These mechanisms respond in tandem to changes in perfusion pressure; they adjust the vascular tone of the glomerular arterioles to keep RBF and GFR stable (Fig. 18.1) [6–8]. For instance, if renal perfusion pressure falls, the afferent arteriole dilates via myogenic-induced vasodilation and inhibition of TGF. This decrease in preglomerular resistance allows for more of the perfusion pressure to reach the glomerulus and in this way maintains RBF, glomerular capillary pressure, and consequently GFR. As renal perfusion pressure becomes more compromised, maintenance of RBF becomes increasingly dependent on the activity of renal vasodilators (e.g., prostaglandins and nitric oxide) [6–9]. In addition, the increased angiotensin II causes preferential constriction of the efferent arteriole, thus maintaining glomerular capillary pressure even during mild to moderate falls in RBF. Thus, prerenal azotemia develops if (a) the degree of renal hypoperfusion overrides the maximal capacity of the compensatory mechanisms or (b) the compensatory mechanisms are altered by either disease or drug.

The causes of prerenal azotemia can be categorized into those in which there is (a) reduced renal perfusion, (b) abnormal intrarenal hemodynamics causing glomerular capillary pressure to fall, or (c) a combination of both (Table 18.1). *Reduced renal perfusion* may arise from absolute or relative intravascular volume depletion, impaired cardiac function, or vascular obstruction (e.g., renal artery stenosis). *The intrarenal hemodynamic* patterns that reduce GFR are intense afferent arteriolar vasoconstriction and excessive efferent arteriolar vasodilation. Intense vasoconstriction of afferent arterioles may be the result of disease processes (e.g., hepatorenal syndrome or increased renal venous pressure) or medications (e.g., calcineurin inhibitors, NSAIDS, radiocontrast), whereas excessive vasodilation of efferent arterioles is seen with angiotensin-converting

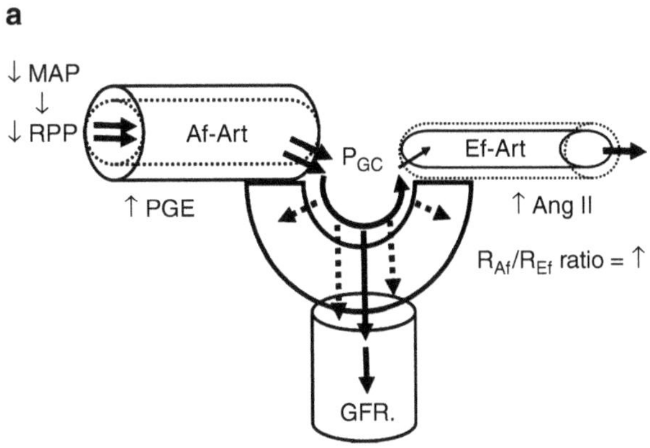

Fig. 18.1 The two main mechanisms by which renal perfusion is maintained in the setting of reduced renal perfusion pressure are (1) afferent arteriole vasodilation due to autoregulatory and renal vasodilators (e.g., prostaglandins) and (2) angiotensin II-induced vasoconstriction of the efferent arteriole

Table 18.1 Causes of prerenal azotemia

Decreased renal perfusion
Hypotension
Intravascular volume depletion
Gastrointestinal losses—vomiting, diarrhea, bleeding
Renal losses—diuretics, osmotic diuresis
Skin losses—diaphoresis, burns
Fluid sequestration (third Spacing)—crush injury, intestinal obstruction, peritonitis/pancreatitis, obstruction of major veins
Decreased effective renal blood flow
Decreased cardiac function—heart failure, acute myocardial infarction, pulmonary embolism, pericardial tamponade
Nephrotic syndrome
Peripheral vasodilation—sepsis, cirrhosis, vasodilators, anaphylaxis, arteriovenous fistulas
Selective renal/regional ischemia
Aortic dissection
Arterial thrombosis/embolism
Renal artery stenosis
Abnormalities in intrarenal hemodynamics
Preglomerular vasoconstriction
NSAIDS
Intravenous radiographic contrast
Calcineurin inhibitors
Hepatorenal syndrome
Increased renal vein pressure—abdominal compartment syndrome, renal vein thrombosis, CHF, portal hypertension
Postglomerular vasodilation
ACE inhibitors
Angiotensin receptor blockers
Sepsis

enzyme inhibitors (ACEI), angiotensin receptor blockers (ARB), and sepsis [5, 10]. Note that these medications are usually well-tolerated under normal conditions. However, when administered in conditions in which RBF/GFR are being maintained by compensatory afferent arteriolar vasodilation or efferent arteriolar vasoconstriction (such as volume depletion), they can significantly impair renal function (Figs. 18.2 and 18.3). Finally, several diseases affect renal perfusion via a combination of the above mechanisms. For instance, hepatorenal syndrome causes peripheral vasodilation and preglomerular vasoconstriction, thus leading to profound renal hypoperfusion [10]. Renal hypoperfusion in congestive heart failure (CHF) is the result of decreased cardiac output, combined with preglomerular vasoconstriction and venous congestion [11]. Sepsis causes peripheral vasodilation and postglomerular vasodilation, thus decreasing glomerular filtration pressure and consequently GFR.

Clinical Presentation and Diagnosis

Prerenal azotemia presents as an increase in serum creatinine and BUN, and most often with oliguria due to avid tubular reabsorption of sodium. The initial assessment of patients with suspected prerenal azotemia starts with a thorough history, review of recent medical history, and physical exam. The diagnostic goals in such

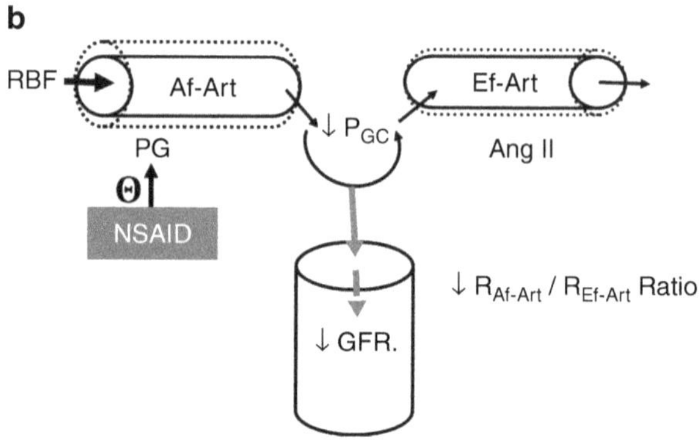

Fig. 18.2 The loss of vasodilatory prostaglandins prevents hypotension-induced vasodilation of afferent arterioles causing RBF and GFR to fall

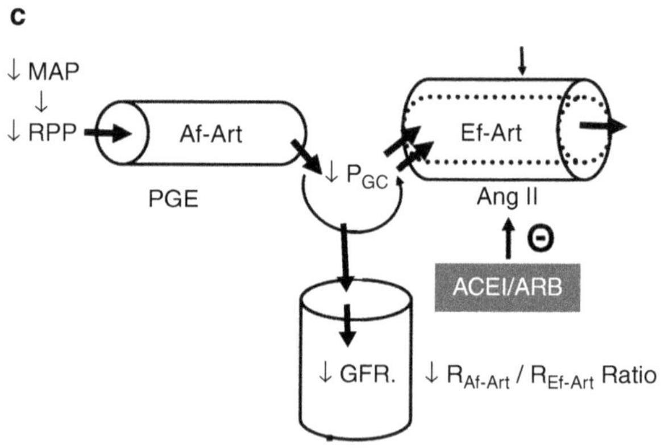

Fig. 18.3 Blockade of the renin–angiotensin system prevents angiotensin II-induced efferent arteriole constriction, thus reducing glomerular capillary pressure. While this effect is beneficial in various forms of chronic renal disease, it can hamper renal preservation of GFR in states in which renal perfusion is compromised

patients are (a) to assess the volume status, (b) to establish the presence of a condition associated with renal hypoperfusion, and (c) to determine the causative etiology so that therapy can be initiated promptly.

Azotemia in the presence of orthostatic dizziness, thirst, orthostatic changes in blood pressure, tachycardia, longitudinal tongue furrows, dry axillae, and mucous membranes, suggest volume depletion [12]. The causative etiology of the volume depletion is suggested by a history of hemorrhage, vomiting, diarrhea, or diuretic use. The history may also uncover factors that render some clinical findings less reliable; for instance, diuretic use may prevent oliguria, and the presence of autonomic neuropathies or use of vasodilators can cause orthostatic hypotension that is unrelated to hypovolemia.

Prerenal azotemia in the presence of adequate or excessive volume indicates decreased effective circulatory volume, as seen in CHF, liver disease, etc. (Table 18.1) [10, 11, 13]. Dyspnea, orthopnea, paroxysmal nocturnal dyspnea, nocturia, and edema suggest decompensated CHF. A history of hepatitis, use of alcohol or illicit drugs, transfusions, jaundice, easy bruising, ascitis, collateral abdominal circulation, and edema suggest liver cirrhosis. It is important to remember that not only do these conditions cause prerenal azotemia but also do their treatment. For instance, excessive or too rapid diuresis in the setting of CHF can cause intravascular volume depletion precipitating prerenal azotemia [12]. Differentiating these types of prerenal states is usually straightforward; but at times it may be helpful to determine filling pressures (by echocardiogram or central venous catheterization).

No history is complete without a careful search for overt or covert ingestion of drugs that may precipitate prerenal azotemia. Diuretics and laxatives can lead to excessive fluid loss and thus volume depletion, whereas other drugs can directly affect glomerular hemodynamics leading to prerenal azotemia. For instance, NSAIDs, cyclosporine, and intravenous contrast can cause excessive vasoconstriction of afferent arterioles, while ACE inhibitors and ARB vasodilates efferent arterioles; both actions cause a decrease in glomerular capillary pressure and thus GFR.

Laboratory Studies

Serial monitoring of serum electrolytes not only allows for monitoring of AKI-induced electrolyte imbalances but may also point to its etiology. For instance, BUN and creatinine levels that fluctuate in response to hemodynamic changes suggest prerenal azotemia, whereas a continuous rise suggests intrinsic AKI. ABUN/creatinine ratio of >20 is also considered to indicate prerenal azotemia. However, this ratio also increases as a result of increased urea production (e.g., gastrointestinal bleeding and hypercatabolic states), decreased protein anabolism (e.g., corticosteroids, tetracyclines), or decreased creatinine production. Conversely, the ratio may not rise, despite the presence of a prerenal state, if BUN production is low (e.g., liver disease, low protein intake). Hence, it is not a reliable marker for prerenal azotemia.

Urine Studies

Careful analysis of the urine and determination of the urinary indices can be quite useful in differentiating prerenal azotemia from intrinsic AKI. The urinalysis provides us with clues of whether there is parenchymal injury [14]. The urinary diagnostic indices determine whether the renal tubules are avidly reabsorbing salt, as would be expected in most cases of prerenal azotemia but not in intrinsic renal failure because of the tubular injury [15–20]. In prerenal azotemia, proteinuria is scant or absent and the sediment is usually normal, although occasionally it shows hyaline or fine granular casts [14]. In contrast, intrinsic renal disease is characterized by proteinuria (up to <1 g/day) and cellular or large brown granular casts in the sediment.

The FENa is the most sensitive urinary index; it corresponds to sodium excretion adjusted for creatinine clearance. The renal failure index (Table 18.2) offers similar results. The remaining

Table 18.2 Laboratory values and indices in prerenal and acute kidney injury

Diagnostic index	Prerenal	Intrinsic renal
BUN/serum creatinine ratio	>20	<10
Urine creatinine/plasma creatinine	>40	<20
Urinalysis	Normal or hyaline casts	Muddy brown granular casts
Proteinuria	Absent or scant	Present <1 g/day
Urine specific gravity	>1.020	~1.010
Urine osmolality (mosmol/kg H_2O)	>500	<350
U_{Na} (mEq/L)	<20	>20
$\text{FENa}\dfrac{\text{UNa}}{\text{PNa}}\div\dfrac{\text{UCr}}{\text{PCr}}\times 100$	<1	>2
$\text{Renal failure index}\dfrac{\text{UNa}}{\text{UCr}\div\text{PCr}}$	<1	>1
FE urea	<35%	>50
FE uric acid	<7	>15
FE lithium	<7	>20
Low molecular weight protein	Low	High
Brush-border enzymes	Low	High
Novel biomarkers	None	Kim1, cystatin C, NGAL, IL-18,others

indices (e.g., urine sodium concentration, specific gravity, and osmolality) are less sensitive and specific. Despite their usefulness, urinary indices have important limitations. For instance, the FENa may be >1% in patients with prerenal azotemia who are receiving diuretics, or those that have bicarbonaturia or chronic kidney disease [2, 21]. In the first two circumstances, the fractional excretion of urea may be more sensitive and specific. Conversely, an FENa <1% may be seen in patients with a variety of intrinsic renal diseases including contrast nephropathy, glomerulonephritis, and obstruction.

Therapeutic Trial

Because all of the diagnostic criteria have limitations and may render conflicting results, a therapeutic trial of fluid repletion in patients with evidence of volume depletion may be of great value [22, 23]. For instance, 500—1,000 mL of 0.9% normal saline may be infused over a period of about 30 min. This may be repeated if the clinical picture continues to suggest a volume deficit. A positive response, indicated by improvements in hemodynamics, urine output, and BUN and/or serum creatinine, validate the diagnosis of prerenal azotemia. This type of trial would of course be contraindicated in CHF and should be used cautiously in any edematous state.

Management/Outcomes

Despite the fact that prerenal azotemia is usually readily reversible, its presence is associated with a greater than twofold higher risk of hospital mortality, compared to non-AKI patients. If it progresses to ATN with intrinsic renal structural damage, the risk of death increases to greater than sixfold in hospital mortality. Thus, it is imperative that the underlying cause and the pathophysiologic status of the patient be promptly identified, so that appropriate treatment can be initiated. The goals of therapy in prerenal azotemia are to (a) normalize renal perfusion, (b) correct or remove the causative factors, (c) prevent/treat any complications, and (d) avoid further insults (e.g., hypotension, nephrotoxins). Table 18.3 summarizes the overall strategy in managing these patients.

Table 18.3 General management of prerenal azotemia

Treat or reverse underlying causes—volume depletion, CHF, cirrhosis
Normalize hemodynamics and maintain euvolemia—avoid hypotension/hypovolemia
Avoid nephrotoxins—NSAIDS, aminoglycosides, radiocontrast, ACEI/ARBs when indicated
Adjust medication dosages if necessary
Provide adjuvant therapy—antibiotics, nutrition, supportive care

In patients with true volume depletion, treatment is aimed at replenishing the intravascular volume deficit, correcting any water and electrolyte abnormalities, and replacing ongoing losses. The composition of the fluids should be based upon the clinical picture; blood products for hemorrhage, crystalloids for urinary or gastrointestinal losses, while colloids may be beneficial in hepatic cirrhosis. Patients with decompensated cardiac failure, liver cirrhosis, and sepsis will need meticulous management of their volume status and may require more intense hemodynamic monitoring and support. CHF patients may require preload and after load reducing agents, inotropic support, and occasionally mechanical support (e.g., intraaortic balloon pumps, ventricular assist devices). If volume overload is refractory to diuretic therapy, ultrafiltration can be used to reduce venous congestion, and this may result in improved cardiac hemodynamics and renal function. Septic patients may need volume resuscitation and vasopressors, in addition to general supportive measures. Cirrhotic patients can present particularly challenging problems. Prerenal azotemia in these patients may be due intravascular volume depletion (overzealous use of diuretics), tense ascitis, infection (e.g., spontaneous bacterial peritonitis), or full blown hepatorenal syndrome. Treatment should be directed to the underlying pathophysiologic state; gentle volume replenishment in patients with intravascular depletion, large volume paracentesis with intravenous albumin administration if tense ascitis is present.

Case 1 Revisited

This patient has several risk factors for acute renal failure; he has chronic kidney disease, diabetes mellitus, and is prone to dehydration due to his hemicolectomy. In addition, he is on an ACEI which impairs a key renal compensatory mechanism-efferent arteriole vasoconstriction. While this is an appropriate medication for him (which he was tolerating when he was not ill), it can precipitate a fall in GFR when his renal perfusion pressure is compromised. The patient's current clinical presentation suggests volume depletion, both by history and physical findings. While his urinary indexes were not consistent with volume depletion, they were likely influenced by his CKD rendering them less accurate. Thus, the factors that are most likely causing his prerenal azotemia are volume depletion (the etiology of which was his diarrhea) in a patient with chronic kidney disease on an ACEI. He has no evidence of fluid overload, so prompt volume repletion is indicated; he was hydrated with 0.9% normal saline (5 L in the first 24 h). In addition, he received ciprofloxacin (for his diarrhea) and his ACEI and metformin were held. He rapidly responded to volume replenishment; his blood pressure and creatinine quickly improved, and his diarrhea resolved within 3 days.

Case 2 Revisited

This patient suffers from severe symptomatic aortic stenosis, thus her prognosis is poor in the absence of valve replacement surgery. Her exam was consistent with volume overload, but she also had an elevated BUN and plasma creatinine, which were due to either a severe fall in renal perfusion or the presence of chronic kidney disease. The very low urine sodium, benign urine sediment, and lack of proteinuria suggest that the kidney is normal and responding to a fall in perfusion. Thus, her clinical presentation of volume overload with prerenal azotemia suggests low effective renal perfusion due to decreased cardiac output and intrarenal vasoconstriction. The first goal is to reduce venous congestion in an attempt to improve her cardiac and renal function. She was managed with a sodium restricted diet, a loop diuretic, digoxin, and an ACEI. Luckily her vascular congestion, and subsequently her renal function, improved on this regimen; her BUN and plasma creatinine fell to 89 and 1.7 mg/dL, respectively. Although she responded to this therapy, it can potentially decrease intravascular volume and/or blood pressure enough to further impair renal perfusion and thus GFR. If the patient would have been resistant to the diuretics, a trial of inotropic agents or ultrafiltration could have been considered. She subsequently accepted aortic valve replacement.

Key Points

- Prerenal failure is a frequent condition caused by renal hypoperfusion or abnormal hemodynamics causing decreased GFR.
- It occurs when the normal physiologic responses to decreases in renal perfusion are either overwhelmed or abnormal.
- Common causes include volume depletion, arterial hypotension, CHF, liver cirrhosis, and medications that interfere with renal responses to hypovolemia.
- A careful history, physical examination, laboratory studies (including urinary indexes), and a fluid challenge (if appropriate) are all important in establish the diagnosis.
- Urinalysis is usually bland, while urinary indices are usually consistent with the presence of profound sodium retention.
- The FENa is the most sensitive and specific of the urinary indices, but loses its usefulness when the renal concentrating ability is lost (diuretics, chronic kidney disease) or bicarbonaturia. FE urea may be more helpful in these settings.
- Prompt, appropriate therapy that restores renal perfusion is important in order to prevent progression to ATN. Addressing the causative etiology, avoiding secondary insults, and providing appropriate adjuvant care are important in the general management of prerenal azotemia.

References

1. Waikar SS, Curhan GC, Wald R, et al. Declining mortality in patients with acute renal failure, 1988 to 2002. J Am Soc Nephrol. 2006;17:1143.
2. Xue JL, Daniels F, Star RA, et al. Incidence and mortality of acute renal failure in Medicare beneficiaries, 1992 to 2001. J Am Soc Nephrol. 2006;17:1135.
3. Uchino S, Kellum JA, Bellomo R, et al. Acute renal failure in critically ill patients: a multinational, multicenter study. JAMA. 2005;294:813.
4. Liangos O, Wald R, O'Bell JW, et al. Epidemiology and outcomes of acute renal failure in hospitalized patients: a national survey. Clin J Am Soc Nephrol. 2006;1:43.
5. Lameire N, Van Biesen W, Vanholder R. Acute renal failure. Lancet. 2005;365:417.
6. Rose BD. Pathophysiology of renal disease. 2nd ed. New York: McGraw Hill; 1987.
7. Steinhausen M, Endlich K, Wiegman DL. Glomerular blood flow. Kidney Int. 1990;38:769.
8. Schnermann J, Briggs JP, Weber PC. Tubuloglomerular feedback, prostaglandins, and angiotensin in the autoregulation of glomerular filtration rate. Kidney Int. 1984;25(1):53–64.
9. Schrier RW. An odyssey into the milieu intérieur: pondering the enigmas. J Am Soc Nephrol. 1992;2:1549.
10. Henriksen JH, Bendtsen F, Gerbes AL, Christensen NJ, Ring-Larsen H, Sørensen TI. Estimated central blood volume in cirrhosis: relationship to sympathetic nervous activity, beta-adrenergic blockade and atrial natriuretic factor. Hepatology. 1992;16(5):1163–70.
11. Heywood JT, Fonarow GC, Costanzo MR, Mathur VS, Wigneswaran JR, Wynne J, ADHERE Scientific Advisory Committee and Investigators. High prevalence of renal dysfunction and its impact on outcome in 118,465 patients hospitalized with acute decompensated heart failure: a report from the ADHERE database. J Card Fail. 2007;13(6):422–30.
12. Kaufmann H. Consensus statement on the definition of orthostatic hypotension, pure autonomic failure and multiple system atrophy. Clin Auton Res. 1996;6:125.
13. Damman K, Navis G, Voors AA, Asselbergs FW, Smilde TD, Cleland JG, van Veldhuisen DJ, Hillege HL. Worsening renal function and prognosis in heart failure: systematic review and meta-analysis. J Card Fail. 2007;13(8):599–608.
14. Perazella MA, Coca SG, Kanbay M, et al. Diagnostic value of urine microscopy for differential diagnosis of acute kidney injury in hospitalized patients. Clin J Am Soc Nephrol. 2008;3:1615.
15. Miller TR, Anderson RJ, Linas SL, et al. Urinary diagnostic indices in acute renal failure: a prospective study. Ann Intern Med. 1978;89:47.
16. Espinel CH, Gregory AW. Differential diagnosis of acute renal failure. Clin Nephrol. 1980;13:73.
17. Esson ML, Schrier RW. Diagnosis and treatment of acute tubular necrosis. Ann Intern Med. 2002;137:744.
18. Dixon BS, Anderson RJ. Nonoliguric acute renal failure. Am J Kidney Dis. 1985;6:71.
19. Steiner RW. Interpreting the fractional excretion of sodium. Am J Med. 1984;77:699.
20. Chalasani N, Clark WS, Wilcox CM. Blood urea nitrogen to creatinine concentration in gastrointestinal bleeding: a reappraisal. Am J Gastroenterol. 1997; 92:1796.
21. Dossetor JB. Creatininemia versus uremia. The relative significance of blood urea nitrogen and serum creatinine concentrations in azotemia. Ann Intern Med. 1966;65:1287.
22. Schierhout G, Roberts I. Fluid resuscitation with colloid or crystalloid solutions in critically ill patients: a systematic review of randomised trials. BMJ. 1998;316(7136):961–4.
23. Wilkes MM, Navickis RJ. Patient survival after human albumin administration. A meta-analysis of randomized, controlled trials. Ann Intern Med. 2001;135(3): 149–64.

Post-renal Failure

19

Luis I. Juncos and Luis A. Juncos

Case 1

A 63-year-old male was seen for worsening hypertension and mild ankle edema. He was asymptomatic except for irregular urine output over the last few weeks. His blood pressure was 160/95 mmHg (no orthostatic changes), heart, lungs, and abdomen were normal, his prostate was modestly enlarged; and he had 1+ ankle edema. His serum potassium was 6.6 mEq/L, bicarbonate 15 mEq/L, and creatinine 5.8 mg/dL. His creatinine was 0.8 mg/dL 2 years earlier and 1.2 mg/dL 6 months earlier. He had 1+ proteinuria, microscopic hematuria, and his fractional excretion of sodium (FENa) was 1.5%. Ultrasound showed an empty bladder, bilateral hydronephrosis and hydroureters, and moderate cortical thinning of the right kidney.

What are the next diagnostic and therapeutic steps?

What complications may arise upon treating the obstruction?

L.I. Juncos, M.D., Ph.D. M.S.
Department of Medicine, J. Robert Cade Foundation, Cordoba, Argentina 5003

L.A. Juncos, M.D. (✉)
Division of Nephrology, Department of Medicine, University of Mississippi Medical Center, 2500 North State St, Jackson, MS 39216, USA
e-mail: ljuncos@umc.edu

Case 2

A 58-year-old female presented with 1 day of asymptomatic gross hematuria. Her aortic valve was replaced 7 years earlier, and she had a kidney transplant 2 years earlier. Her blood pressure was 130/85 mmHg and pulse 95 (no orthostatic changes). Her heart and lungs were normal. Her allograft was palpable, but not tender, in the right lower quadrant. Her serum creatinine was 3.2 mg/dL (up from her baseline of 1.0) and her INR was 7.0 (she is on warfarin). Her urine was grossly bloody. Ultrasound of the allograft showed moderate hydronephrosis of "similar magnitude to her previous ultrasound" obtained 2 years earlier, with a mildly dilated proximal ureter; the distal segment was not visible.

How would you proceed in evaluating this patient?

Introduction

Urinary tract obstruction (UTO) refers to structural or functional impediment to urine flow along the urinary tract. It leads to increased pressure within the urinary tract which, if left uncorrected, causes renal injury. UTO may be acute or chronic, partial or complete, and unilateral or bilateral. In acute UTO, the renal impairment is usually reversible if the obstruction is relieved early. However, if the obstruction is left untreated, it may cause progressive and irreversible loss of

E.V. Lerma and M. Rosner (eds.), *Clinical Decisions in Nephrology, Hypertension and Kidney Transplantation*, DOI 10.1007/978-1-4614-4454-1_19, © Springer Science+Business Media New York 2013

renal function. In fact, UTO remains an important cause of chronic kidney disease (CKD). Because recovery of renal function is inversely related to the duration and degree of obstruction, early diagnosis and treatment are crucial. The term "obstructive uropathy" refers to the structural or functional changes that hinder urine flow, while "obstructive nephropathy" refers to the functional or structural changes in the kidney that result from obstructive uropathy.

Epidemiology

UTO is fairly common and can affect persons of any age. It is the most common cause of CKD in children, and accounts for ~1.5% of end-stage renal disease in the USA and 3–5% in Europe. Moreover, hydronephrosis (a dilated urinary tract) is present in ~3% of the population at autopsy; but its true prevalence is likely higher because transient or treated hydronephrosis may not be detected at autopsy. Men and women are equally affected, but the incidences by age are different between genders. In women it presents a bimodal curve which peaks at 20–40 years of age (mainly pregnancy-related UTO) and again at 50–70 years (due to pelvic tumors). In men, the prevalence increases with age, largely due to prostatic enlargement; about 80% of men over 60 have symptoms of UTO [1–7].

Etiology

Obstruction of the urinary tract can be due to acquired or congenital causes and may affect either the upper or lower urinary tract. In addition, the acquired causes may be the result of intrinsic or extrinsic factors (Table 19.1) [1–7].

Acquired Urinary Tract Obstruction

Intrinsic Causes

Intraluminal and intramural processes may lead to intrinsic obstruction. Intraluminal obstruction may result from intrarenal or extrarenal causes.

Table 19.1 Causes of urinary tract obstruction

Acquired causes
Upper tract lesions
Intrinsic
Intraluminal
Intrarenal
Uric acid crystals
Sulfonamides
Acyclovir
Indinivir
Methotrexate
Multiple myeloma
Extrarenal
Blood clots
Pyogenic debris
Ureteral stones
Edema
Papillary necrosis
Intramural
Structural: transitional cell cancer
Functional: adynamic ureter
Extrinsic
Reproductive system: pregnancy, prolapse, tumors
Vascular lesions: aneurysms, aberrant vessels
Gastrointestinal tract: crohn's disease, diverticulitis, tumors, abscesses
Diseases of the retroperitoneum: hematomas, retroperitoneal fibrosis, tuberculosis, lymphoceles
Lower tract lesions
Bladder neck obstructions
BPH
Bladder carcinoma
Urethral stricture
TCC of the bladder
Stones: bladder
Bladder infection
Malpositioned Foley catheter
Blood clots
Functional
Neuropathy: neurogenic bladder
Ganglionic blocking agents
Anticholinergic agents
Congenital causes
Upper tract lesions
Ureteropelvic junction narrowing/obstruction
Ureterovesical junction narrowing/obstruction and reflux
Ureterocele
Retrocaval ureter
Lower tract lesions

(continued)

Table 19.1 (continued)

Bladder neck obstruction
Ureterocele
Anterior/posterior urethral valves
Urethral stricture
Meatal stenosis
Phimosis

Intrarenal causes often relate to deposition of crystals (uric acid, sulfonamides, acyclovir, indinivir, methotrexate) or casts (multiple myeloma) within the tubules that block urine flow. Renal calculi are the most common cause of extrarenal intraluminal obstruction. Other caused include blood clots (e.g., from renal trauma, and tumors) or sloughed papilla from papillary necrosis. In transplanted kidneys, the ureter can develop strictures due to ischemia, rejection, inflammation, or various infections.

Intramural obstruction can result from structural or functional causes. Structural causes include tumors of the urinary tract (e.g., transitional cell cancer), and ureteral or urethral strictures (infections, previous procedures, etc.). Functional obstruction may result from an adynamic ureter, vesicourethral reflux, or neurologic abnormalities from medications (e.g., anticholinergic agents, levodopa) or disease (e.g., diabetes mellitus, multiple sclerosis, Parkinson's disease, spinal cord injury, or stroke).

Extrinsic Causes

The most common cause of extrinsic UTO in women is pregnancy, where the gravid uterus may compress the ureter at the pelvic brim. In fact, two-thirds of pregnant women have evidence of ureteral dilatation in their third trimester (though hormonal effects on smooth muscle tone may also contribute). This is usually inconsequential and resolves shortly after delivery, but occasionally may cause acute kidney injury (AKI). Other causes include pelvic tumors (e.g., carcinoma of the cervix), abscesses, endometriosis, pelvic inflammatory disease, and uterine prolapse. In men, benign prostatic hypertrophy and carcinoma of the prostate are leading causes of UTO. Other processes that may lead to obstruction include various tumors (via extension or metastasis), lymphomas, abscesses, inflammatory diseases (e.g., Crohn's disease and diverticulitis), or retroperitoneal fibrosis.

Congenital Causes of UTO

Congenital causes of UTO can occur anywhere along the urinary tract. Its clinical course depends on severity and time of onset. If it occurs early during development, the kidney will not develop. If it is bilateral and severe, then renal failure and a high likelihood of death follows. However, if it appears later during gestation and is partial or unilateral, enough renal function may be present to allow for survival [8, 9]. Some cases of UTO may not present until adulthood [10]. Common causes of congenital obstruction are listed in Table 19.1.

Pathophysiology

Obstructing the urinary tract initiates pathways that alter glomerular hemodynamics and tubular function. The initial rise in tubular pressure is transmitted up to the proximal tubule reducing net glomerular filtration pressure and, consequently, GFR. The rise in tubular pressure is accompanied by afferent arteriolar vasodilation (via prostaglandins), which raises renal blood flow (RBF) and glomerular capillary pressure, but not enough to offset the rise in tubular pressure; thus GFR remains low. This early "hyperemic phase" lasts 2–5 h and is followed by a vasoconstrictive phase brought on by increases in renal angiotensin II, thromboxane A2, vasopressin, and 20-HETE and decreases in nitric oxide and bradykinins. This imbalance between vasoconstrictors and vasodilators constricts the afferent arterioles and decreases the ultrafiltration coefficient, thereby reducing RBF and GFR. In addition, tubular expression of chemoattractant factors increase, promoting leukocyte infiltration, and result in altered tubular function (impairment in urine concentration) and ultimately in interstitial fibrosis [1, 6, 8].

Tubular abnormalities are also common with UTO [1, 5, 6]. Initially, the urinary indices have a prerenal pattern (due to enhanced sodium reabsorption). However, this is soon replaced by a marked inability to concentrate the urine; maximum osmolarity reaching ~350 mOsm/kg. This concentrating defect is common and may be persistent, even after relieving the obstruction. It results from reduced medullary tonicity, decreased expression of sodium transporters and water channels (aquaporins) and decreased GFR in juxtamedullary nephrons [11]. There may also be defective acidification and abnormalities in potassium excretion. The abnormal acidification may range from persistent hyperchloremic metabolic acidosis to defects that are only apparent during acid loading. The mechanisms causing the abnormal acidification may include (a) impaired distal acidification (due to a fall in H^+-ATPase activity, and in the secretion and tubular response to aldosterone) and (b) increased bicarbonate excretion (although bicarbonaturia is not a consistent finding in humans). The decrease in potassium excretion is attributed to the decreased aldosterone levels or activity. After relief of bilateral renal obstruction, there is a marked increase in net and fractional excretion of potassium mainly due to increased delivery of sodium to the distal nephron. Recovery of tubular function is often reversible, but may be slow, and at times quite delayed [1].

Clinical Presentation and Diagnosis

The clinical presentation of UTO varies greatly depending on the duration, site, and degree of obstruction. For instance, patients with acute high-grade UTO may present with pain, anuria, and AKI, whereas those with chronic partial obstruction may be asymptomatic or have only subtle urinary symptoms. Because of its variable presentation and potential reversibility of renal impairment, UTO should be considered in any patient with unexplained renal failure.

The diagnostic approach to a patient who may have UTO starts with the history and physical, which may not only suggest the presence of UTO but also point toward the etiology, thus streamlining the diagnostic evaluation. The information obtained should include type and duration of symptoms, changes in previous symptoms, history of renal calculi, previous surgeries, and medication use. Some of the more common clinical presentations and their relationship to the type of obstruction are listed in Table 19.2 [1–5].

Pain is a common complaint and results from stretching of the collecting system or renal capsule. The severity depends on the rate, thus patients with acute obstruction can present with typical renal colic, whereas those with chronic obstruction may be asymptomatic. As shown in Table 19.2, the location and characteristics can help determine the site and type of obstruction. The other more frequent complaints are urinary tract symptoms. Urine output may oscillate between polyuria and oliguria, or even present as anuria. Hesitancy, decreased urine stream, and dribbling are associated with bladder outlet obstruction. Recurrent urinary tract infection may be the only complaint.

As with other forms of AKI, the physical exam should begin by assessing volume status. Obstructive nephropathy may be associated with

Table 19.2 Relationship between clinical presentation and type of UTO

Presentation	Cause
Pain	
Flank pain and tenderness	Acute upper ureteral or pelvic obstruction
Pain that radiates to the groin	Acute lower ureteral obstruction
Flank pain during micturition	Vesicoureteral reflux
Pain induced by fluid loading	Pelviureteral junction obstruction
Bladder symptoms	
Decreased caliber of stream, hesitancy, dribbling, nocturia	Lower urinary tract obstruction
Recurrent urinary tract infections	More common with lower UTO
Polyuria, sodium wasting, renal tubular acidosis	Chronic partial obstruction Postobstructive diuresis
Acute kidney injury	High-grade bilateral obstruction
Chronic kidney injury	Partial bilateral obstruction

new onset or worsening hypertension, due to increased volume (bilateral obstruction) or increased angiotensin II (unilateral obstruction). However, it may also be associated with hypotension when partial obstruction has caused polyuria. Abdominal exam may find a flank or suprapubic mass (hydronephrosis and distended bladder, respectively). A pelvic exam in women and rectal exam in all patients are essential to assess for masses or an enlarged prostate in men. Evidence of uremia may also be present. Bladder catheterization may reveal a large amount of residual urine. Depending on the cause of the obstruction, the urinalysis may show hematuria, low-grade proteinuria, pyuria, bacteriuria, or crystalluria. As mentioned before, the urine indices initially resemble prerenal indices, but convert to that of intrinsic failure when the concentrating defects became clinically significant.

Radiologic Evaluation

The radiographic finding most characteristic of UTO is hydronephrosis, which is readily seen with several tests. However, no single imaging study can establish or exclude UTO with certainty; there are conditions in which hydronephrosis is present in the absence of UTO, or conversely, UTO may be present but hydronephrosis has not developed yet. Thus, the use of complementary techniques, as shown in Table 19.3, may be needed [12–16].

Ultrasound is an inexpensive and safe test, with a high sensitivity and specificity for hydronephrosis (~ 90%), and is thus the preferred initial study to assess for UTO. It reveals renal size and cortical thickness. Its false-positive rate (nonobstructive hydronephrosis) is between 10 and 20%. False negatives (nondilated obstructive nephropathy)

Table 19.3 Radiographic assessment of UTO

Test	Useful for	Disadvantages
Renal ultrasound	Dilation of urinary tract	Does not localize UTO
	Size of kidney	Does not discern obstructive versus nonobstructive hyronephrosis
	Condition of cortex	
Intravenous urography	Defines the anatomy	Risk of contrast nephropathy
	Ureter well visualized	Delayed/decreased excretion during renal dysfunction
	Locates the obstruction	
Computed tomography	Dilation of urinary tract	More costly and cumbersome
	Presence of stones	
	Condition of cortex	
	Defines the anatomy	
	Locates the obstruction	
	Provides etiology information	
Magnetic resonance urography	Same as CT	Costly and cumbersome
Isotopic renography	Differential function	Poor anatomical definition
Diuresis renography	Discerns nonobstructive versus obstructive hydronephrosis	Poor renal function limits its use
		Cumbersome
Antegrade pyelography (nephrostograms)	Defines the anatomy	Invasive
	Locates the obstruction	Usual complications of percutaneous techniques
Retrograde pyelography	Defines the anatomy	Invasive
	Locates the obstruction	Cumbersome
Others	Pressure flow studies	
	Cystoscopy	
	Urodynamic studies	
	Excretory urograms	

are less common. Despite its usefulness in detecting hydronephrosis, it oftentimes does not reveal the etiology. A plain film of the kidneys, ureters, and bladder (KUB) is sometimes obtained in conjunction to look for urolithiasis [13]. However, noncalcium containing stones, such as uric acid, may not be shown on plain films.

Intravenous urography (IVU) defines the anatomy (especially of the ureter) and the location of the obstruction. However, it may cause contrast nephropathy and the delayed or decreased excretion of contrast makes it less useful in patients with renal failure. The use of this diagnostic test has decreased because of the development of better imaging techniques such as helical computed tomography.

Helical computed tomography (CT) has a high sensitivity for hydronephrosis and stones and is useful at determining the site and nature of the obstruction. It is particularly good at discovering extrinsic causes of UTO. Adding intravenous contrast enhances its diagnostic value, but should be avoided in patients with renal impairment.

Magnetic resonance urography is similar or superior to CT at identifying dilated urinary tracts, urolithiasis, and in providing information about the degree and site of the obstruction. It is less user-dependent and provides semiquantitative estimates of renal function. Thus its use is likely to increase [14].

Diuresis renography tests whether furosemide, given 20–30 min after injecting a radioisotope,"washes out" the isotope; washout is limited in UTO thus differentiating UTO from nonobstructive hydronephrosis. The test is less useful when renal function is diminished because of delayed isotope excretion and diuretic resistance.

Antegrade and retrograde pyelography can be both diagnostic and therapeutic in relieving the UTO. Antegrade or "nephrostograms" are usually performed after a percutaneous nephrostomy (PCN) tube has been placed into the renal pelvis. In retrograde pyelography, the ureter is catheterized via cystoscopy. These studies are useful to further establish the site and characteristics of the obstruction. Retrograde pyelography is especially useful in nondilated UTO [15–19].

Management

Several issues need to be considered when treating UTO; location of the lesion, underlying cause, degree of renal impairment, and the likelihood of renal recovery. The treatment starts with general measures, early relief of the obstruction and supportive care (volume and electrolyte management), later followed by specific therapy [18, 19].

Conservative management (pain control, hydration, etc.) is appropriate in cases in which the UTO is self-limited (e.g., small renal stones). However, complete bilateral UTO with AKI is an emergency that requires prompt intervention to maximize the chances of renal recovery. The site of obstruction dictates the intervention. Obstructions above the bladder usually require PCN, given its high technical success rate and low complication rate (abscess, infection, hemorrhage). Retrograde placement of ureteral stent via cystoscopy is an appropriate alternative approach in certain cases. For UTO at the bladder or below, placing a urethral catheter into the bladder will alleviate the obstruction, until definitive therapy is carried out. Specific therapy varies greatly depending on the etiology. It is aimed directly at correcting the underlying causative lesion, when possible. For instance, urethral obstruction by an enlarged prostate may require use of α-adrenergic blockers, 5α-reductase inhibitors, or urologic intervention. Urologic intervention may be needed for intraluminal obstruction (e.g., calculi) if severely impaired renal function or persistent infection are present. Thus, specific therapies often require consultation with other specialists (e.g., Urologist and Oncologist).

After relief of bilateral obstruction (and sometimes unilateral obstruction), there is often a period of marked natriuresis and diuresis. This *postobstructive diuresis* usually results from appropriate physiologic response to volume expansion and accumulation of electrolytes, urea and natriuretic factors that occur while the obstruction is present. However, it can also be due the tubular dysfunction which, if not managed correctly, may lead to severe, life-threatening depletion of volume and electrolytes. Thus frequent, careful clinical assessments of the patient's volume status and serum electrolytes are needed to guide intravenous fluid therapy with the goal of preventing volume depletion and electrolyte imbalances, while not perpetuating the diuresis (due to excessive administration of intravenous fluids). Intravenous fluid replenishment is needed once the patient's volume status is approaching euvolemia. Because the urine sodium concentration is ~80 mEq/L, 0.45% normal saline, given at a rate slightly slower than the urine output is an appropriate starting fluid. It may be necessary to add K^+, Mg^{2+}, Ca^{2+}, PO_4^{3-}, and HCO^{3-} to replace deficits.

Prognosis

Outcome data for UTO are scarce and will depend on the cause, duration, and severity of the UTO. Recovery of renal function after relief of UTO is more likely when it is resolved within 1–2 weeks. Patients with more chronic obstruction (12 weeks) are likely to have more severe and irreversible disease. Nevertheless, some patients with prolonged UTO (>69 days) may still recover. Because recovery of renal function cannot be predicted with certainty at the time of diagnosis, a trial of decompression followed by monitoring of renal function is warranted in most patients.

Case 1 Revisited

This patient has obstruction of both distal ureters (hydroureter with an empty bladder), which is chronic; he is asymptomatic, has cortical thinning of the right kidney, and his creatinine was already increased 6 months earlier. However, there appeared to be salvageable parenchyma, the cortex of the left kidney was preserved, and the right was thinned but not atrophic. The first step is to decompress the kidneys by placing either (PCN) tubes, or retrograde ureteral catheters, followed by further evaluation to identify the etiology. In this case, bilateral PCNs were placed, which resulted in very brisk nephrostomy output bilaterally. The creatinine fell to 1.4 mg/dL over several days. His urine output remained brisk for ~3 days, most of which was appropriate diuresis, though he required bicarbonate and potassium replenishment. Cystoscopy was performed and biopsies obtained, which revealed transitional cell cancer.

Case 2 Revisited

This kidney transplant patient presented with gross hematuria in the presence of a high INR and AKI. Her ultrasound showed hydronephrosis reportedly similar to that seen to a previous ultrasound (pyelectasis vs. obstruction). Because of her poor renal function, contrast studies should be avoided and diuresis renography would be of limited value. Moreover, retrograde studies are difficult in transplanted kidneys because the ureteric buds are difficult to visualize. However, the presence of a dilated ureter makes obstruction highly likely, thus she was given vitamin K and fresh frozen plasma and a PCN was placed the next morning when her INR was in a safe range. Her creatinine improved to near baseline. Her distal portion of the ureter was subsequently found to have significant stenosis which was managed with ureteral stents.

Key Points

- UTO is a common cause of AKI and CKD.
- It is caused by a very wide variety of conditions which can obstruct or compress the ureter.
- It should be looked for in all cases of unexplained renal failure because if detected and treated in time, UTO is usually reversible.
- The presence of UTO and AKI is a medical urgency; because renal recovery correlates with duration of obstruction.
- Therapy is divided into general measures which may include pain control and rapid decompression of the kidney via the placement of PCN tubes.
- Following relief of obstruction, patients may develop a postobstruction diuresis, resulting in prerenal AKI and electrolyte abnormalities if not managed carefully.

References

1. Khlar S. Obstructive nephropathy. Intern Med. 2000;39(5):355–61.
2. Rule AD, Lieber MM, Jacobsen SJ. Is benign prostatic hyperplasia a risk factor for chronic renal failure. J Urol. 2005;173:691–969.
3. Tseng TY, Stoller ML. Obstructive uropathy. Clin Ger Med. 2009;25(3):437–43.
4. Truong LD, Gaber L, Eknoyan G. Obstructive uropathy. Contrib Nephrol. 2011;169:311–26.
5. Siddiqui MM, McDougal WS. Urologic assessment of decreasing renal function. Med Clin North Am. 2011;95(1):161–8.
6. Klahr S, Morrissey J. Obstructive nephropathy and renal fibrosis. Am J Physiol Renal Physiol. 2002;283: F861–F75.
7. Ravanon R, Tomson CRV. Natural history of postobstructive nephropathy: a single-center retrospective study. Nephron Clin Pract. 2007;105:c165–c70.
8. Chevalier RL, Thornhill BA, Forbes MS, Kiley SC. Mechanisms of renal injury and progression of renal disease in congenital obstructive nephropathy. Pediatr Nephrol. 2010;25(4):687–97.
9. Ingraham SE, McHugh KM. Current perspectives on congenital obstructive nephropathy. Pediatr Nephrol. 2011;26(9):1453–61.
10. Halachmi S, Pillar G. Congenital urological anomalies diagnosed in adulthood-management considerations. J Pediatr Urol. 2008;4:2–7.
11. Nielson S, Kwon TH, Frokiaer J, Agre P. Regulation and dysregulation of aquaporins in water balance disorders. J Intern Med. 2007;261:53–64.
12. Reddy S. State of the art trends in imaging renal of colic. Emerg Radiol. 2008;15:217–25.
13. Webb JAW. Ultrasonography and Doppler studies in the diagnosis of renal obstruction. BJU Int. 2000;86 Suppl 1:25–32.
14. Theony HC, Binser T, Roth B, Kessler TM, Vermathen P. Noninvasive assessment of acute ureteral obstruction with diffusion-weighted MR imaging: a prospective study. Radiology. 2009;252(3):721–8.
15. Uppot RN, Gervais DA, Mueller PR. Interventional uroradiology. Radiol Clin North Am. 2008;46:45–64.
16. Uppot RN. Emergent nephrostomy tube placement for acute urinary obstruction. Tech Vasc Interv Radiol. 2009;12:154–61.
17. Adamo R, Saad WEA, Brown DB. Management of nephrostomy drains and ureteral stents. Tech Vasc Interv Radiol. 2009;12:193–204.
18. Abdel-Kadar K, Palevsky P. Acute kidney injury in the elderly. Clin Geriatr Med. 2009;25(3):331–58.
19. Tseng TY, Stoller ML. Medical and medical/urologic approaches in acute and chronic urologic stone disease. Med Clin North Am. 2011;95(1):169–77.

Acute Tubular Necrosis

20

Shamik Shah and Jorge Cerdá

Case

A 55-year-old Indian woman known to have diabetes mellitus for 10 years was transferred to a tertiary care hospital from a community hospital with a history of high grade fever for 1 week, decreased urine output for 3 days, and a 1-day history of altered sensorium. She had been treated at the community hospital for the past 2 days with intravenous crystalloids and antibiotics with no improvement in her symptoms.

On current examination at the tertiary hospital, she is drowsy and only arousable to painful stimuli. The respiratory rate is 42 breaths/min; heart rate, 115 beats/min; blood pressure, 80/54 mmHg; and she is afebrile. She weighs 45 kg and is 5 ft tall. The physical examination is remarkable for anicteric sclera; equal reacting pupils; no lymphadenopathy; normal heart sounds with no murmur or rub; clear lung fields with occasional basilar rales; and a soft, non-tender abdomen.

S. Shah, M.B.B.S., M.D., D.N.B. (Nephrology)
Department of Nephrology, Apollo Hospitals,
1-A GIDC Estate, Bhat, Gandhinagar 380054,
Gujarat, India
e-mail: Shamik.shah@gmail.com

J. Cerdá, M.D., F.A.C.P., F.A.S.N. (✉)
Division of Nephrology, Department of Medicine,
Capital District Renal Physicians, Albany Medical College,
62 Hackett Blvd., Albany, NY 12209, USA
e-mail: cerda@nycap.rr.com

Laboratory studies on admission to the outside hospital were as follows:

Blood urea nitrogen (BUN), 38 mg/dL; serum creatinine, 1.9 mg/dL (was 0.7 mg/dL 6 weeks ago); serum sodium, 139 mEq/L; random blood sugar of 522 mg/dL, normal serum acetone; urinalysis showed 2+ protein, specific gravity 1.022, 30–40 RBCs/hpf, and plenty of WBCs/hpf.

Current laboratory studies are as follows:

BUN, 58 mg/dL; serum creatinine, 3.7 mg/dL albumin, 3 g/dL; aspartate aminotransferase (AST), 35 U/L; alanine aminotransferase (ALT), 19 U/L; lactate dehydrogenase (LDH), 352 IU/L; alkaline phosphatase, 77 U/L; and bilirubin, 0.2 mg/dL. The white blood cell count is 33.8×10^3 mL; hemoglobin, 6.6 mg/dL; hematocrit, 21.4%; platelet count, 264×10^3μL; and INR 1.6. Urinalysis demonstrates 1+ protein, specific gravity 1.010; several scattered muddy-brown granular casts; urine sodium (spot sample), 47 mEq/L; and urine osmolality, 290 mOsm/kg. The arterial blood gas shows pH 7.36; pCO_2, 45 mmHg; bicarbonate, 24 mEq/L; and pO_2, 117 mmHg with FiO_2 of 0.54 on a high-flow face mask.

Blood and urine cultures obtained at the community hospital grew more than 10^5/mL colony counts of *Escherichia coli*. A bedside renal ultrasound shows mildly enlarged kidneys with grade II–III increase in parenchymal echogenicity, minimal left hydroureteronephrosis, and mild hepatomegaly.

What is the most likely etiology of the acute kidney injury?

How should this be treated?

E.V. Lerma and M. Rosner (eds.), *Clinical Decisions in Nephrology, Hypertension and Kidney Transplantation*,
DOI 10.1007/978-1-4614-4454-1_20, © Springer Science+Business Media New York 2013

Introduction

The syndrome of acute kidney injury (AKI) is quite common in hospitalized patients [1, 2]; its frequency may range from 1% on hospital admission to 2–5% during hospitalization and be as high as 15% after cardio-pulmonary bypass. The two most common causes of AKI are (1) Prerenal azotemia in two presentations: volume-responsive (such as in volume-contracted patients due to gastroenteritis) or volume non-responsive (such as in patients with congestive heart failure or decompensated cirrhosis); and (2) What has historically been known as acute tubular necrosis (ATN), a clinicopathologic syndrome of intrinsic AKI secondary to ischemic or toxic insults. This chapter will focus on ATN.

Etiology

The causes of ATN are broadly classified into the following categories:

1. Renal hypoperfusion
   (a) Hypovolemia
   - Gastrointestinal losses (vomiting or diarrhea)
   - Skin losses (excessive sweating, burn injury)
   - Hemorrhage

   (b) Hypotensive shock
   - Hypovolemic (hemorrhage, major trauma)
   - Distributive (hyperdynamic shock in sepsis)
   - Fluid translocation (for example, into muscle in crush syndrome, or intrabdominal in acute pancreatitis)

   (c) Edematous states
   - Congestive heart failure (cardiorenal syndrome)
   - Severe liver failure (fulminant liver failure or decompensated liver cirrhosis)
   - Nephrotic syndrome
   - Abdominal compartment syndrome, such as in tense ascites, toxic megacolon, or large retroperitoneal bleed, may cause AKI by direct renal compression and loss of intrarenal perfusion gradient. A similar mechanism may occur in pericardial tamponade.
2. Direct intrarenal ischemia (renal artery occlusion, atheroembolism)
3. Exogenous toxins and nephrotoxic drugs
   (a) Antibiotics (Aminoglycosides, pentamidine), antivirals (foscarnet, cidofovir)
   (b) Macromolecules causing osmotic injury (high molecular weight starches, IV immunoglobulin preparations, mannitol)
   (c) Radiocontrast iodinated dyes
   (d) Chemotherapeutic agents (Cisplatin)
   (e) Poisons (ethylene glycol)
   (f) Drugs affecting intrarenal hemodynamics (non-steroidal anti-inflammatory drugs, converting enzyme inhibitors, and angiotensin II receptor blockers)
4. Endogenous toxins
   (a) Endotoxemia and inflammatory injury (sepsis)
   (b) Myoglobin (rhabdomyolysis)
   (c) Hemoglobin (incompatible blood transfusion)
   (d) Uric acid (acute uric acid nephropathy) caused by tumor lysis syndrome is primarily due to intratubular precipitation of urate crystals and tissue deposition of calcium phosphate; it may lead to ATN

Pathophysiology

The pathogenesis of ATN [3] is believed to involve multiple pathways:

1. Vascular abnormalities: In comparison to cortical tubules, the S3 segment of the proximal convoluted tubule and the thick ascending loop of Henle (mTAL) are exposed to relatively low tissue oxygen tension but have the high-energy requirement related to sodium transport. Postischemic congestion worsens the relative hypoxia leading to prolonged cellular injury and cell death.
   (a) Effects on renal hemodynamics: There is a local imbalance of vasoactive substances, with enhanced release of vasoconstrictors

such as endothelin and decreased abundance of vasodilators such as endothelium-derived nitric oxide (NO). As a result, there is marked congestion and hypoperfusion of the outer medulla that persists even when cortical blood flow improves during reperfusion after an ischemic insult.

(b) Effects on the microvasculature: Disruption of the actin cytoskeleton and junctional complexes has been documented in experimental AKI, resulting in endothelial cell swelling, blebbing, death, and detachment of viable cells. Affected vascular territories are prone to prolonged vasoconstriction. Furthermore, ischemic injury leads to a marked upregulation of angiostatin, a widely known antiangiogenic factor that induces apoptosis of endothelial cells. There is also an increased endothelial expression of a variety of adhesion molecules that promote endothelial–leukocyte interactions.

2. Tubular changes
   (a) Alterations in tubule dynamics
   - Obstruction: The conversion of Tamm Horsfall protein into an obstructing gel-like polymer is enhanced by the increased luminal sodium concentration typically encountered in the distal tubule in AKI. This provides an ideal environment for cast formation along with desquamated tubule cells and brush border membranes.
   - Backleak: Movement of the glomerular filtrate across damaged tubules into the interstitium and back into the circulation has been shown to occur. However, it may account for a very minor component of the decrease in glomerular filtration rate (GFR) in humans.
   - Tubuloglomerular feedback: The increased delivery of sodium chloride to the macula densa as a result of cellular abnormalities in the ischemic proximal tubule induces afferent arteriolar constriction via A1 adenosine receptor (A1AR) activation and thereby decreases GFR.
   - Changes in tubule cell metabolism: A profound reduction in ATP content invariably occurs after an ischemic insult. This results in a drop in intracellular calcium, causing an increase in proteases, phosphatases, and cytoskeletal degradation. The reduction in ATP also causes the generation of reactive oxygen species. Collectively, reactive oxygen species cause renal tubule cell injury by oxidation of proteins, peroxidation of lipids, damage to DNA, and induction of apoptosis.

   (b) Changes in tubular structure: The initiation phase leads to sublethal injury, with loss of brush borders and disruption of cell polarity and the cytoskeleton. The extension phase is characterized by cell death, desquamation, luminal obstruction, and an inflammatory response.
3. Inflammation: Inflammatory cascades that are initiated by endothelial dysfunction are augmented by a “maladaptive response” of the ischemic proximal tubular cells. These include proinflammatory cytokines (e.g., TNF-α, IL-6, IL-1β, TGF-β) and chemotactic cytokines [e.g., monocyte chemoattractant protein-1 (MCP-1), IL-8, RANTES].

Diagnosis

Except for a renal biopsy, there is no clinical “gold-standard” test able to provide a diagnosis of ATN. The diagnosis is suggested by identifying risk factors in the context of a detailed history and physical examination and supported by laboratory and radiographic data. Risk factors for ATN are outlined in Table 20.1.

History and Physical Examination

The patient’s history is very important in the diagnosis of ATN. It frequently reveals recent hypotension, sepsis, or volume depletion, as well as exposure to nephrotoxic agents. The history is also important in establishing risk factors for the development of

Table 20.1 Risk factors for the development of acute tubular necrosis

1. Advanced age
2. Diabetes mellitus
3. Existing renal dysfunction
4. Use of non-steroidal anti-inflammatory drugs
5. Reduced effective arterial blood volume
(a) Volume depletion
(b) Congestive heart failure
(c) Liver disease
(d) Nephrotic syndrome

ATN. Physical examination is often nonspecific: patients may have signs of volume overload, or rarely, of uremia. Otherwise, the physical examination findings are more likely to reflect the underlying disease process. For example, in a patient with rhabdomyolysis, physical examination may disclose tender "doughy" muscles, with significant edema of the involved extremities.

Urinalysis

Urinalysis in a patient with ATN usually shows muddy-brown granular casts, renal tubular epithelial casts, and renal tubular epithelial cells. Also, in these patients urinary indices usually show an isotonic and isosmotic urine (urinary specific gravity and osmolality similar to plasma), urine sodium above 40 mEq/L, high fractional excretion of sodium and urea, and a low urine-to-plasma creatinine ratio. Such indices have low specificity and can be affected by concurrent medications such as diuretics.

In patients with sepsis, urinary markers may actually suggest a "prerenal" picture when in reality the patient has undergone severe parenchymal injury. Based on urinary markers alone, their low urinary sensitivity and specificity in patients with sepsis makes discrimination between "prerenal" and "renal" AKI impossible.

Serum Markers

BUN and Serum Creatinine

The problems with the use of BUN and serum creatinine as AKI biomarkers have been well described. BUN, serum creatinine, and urine output do not provide insight into the cause of AKI and cannot distinguish between prerenal AKI and ATN. As GFR declines, tubular secretion of creatinine increases and delays the increase in serum concentration. Also, administration of intravenous fluids blunts the rise in serum creatinine [4, 5]. Sepsis has been shown to decrease creatinine production. Medications may alter serum creatinine levels. BUN is not a reliable biomarker because in addition to the excretory function of the kidneys, it is directly related to the volume status of the patient, protein intake, degree of liver dysfunction, and hypercatabolism.

A considerable body of research led to the development of new biomarkers through genomic and proteomic analysis of urine and serum [6]. In recent years, a variety of biomarkers have been identified in various patient cohorts. These include L1 cell adhesion molecule, Kidney Injury Molecule 1 (KIM 1), Urinary NHE3, Urinary IL-18, NGAL, and sulfated HNK-1 epitope. Most, if not all, have a unique rate of rise, peak, and decrease in relation to the injury. These biomarkers offer promise for of earlier diagnosis, thus making early intervention possible and eventually the achievement of better outcomes.

Ultrasound

Ultrasound is the imaging modality of choice in patients with ATN. The advantages are that it is non-interventional and can be done at the bedside. However, its diagnostic utility is somewhat limited—other than ruling out the presence of obstruction—and is observer dependent.

Renal Biopsy

In most patients, a renal biopsy is not performed, and hence diagnosis is made on purely clinical basis. Multiple animal experimental studies have described the typical characteristics of ischemia–reperfusion injury including ATN [7]. Conversely, human renal biopsy reports or post-mortem assessments are scarce and in these studies, the presence of tubular necrosis is relatively uncommon. Most frequently, human specimens show heterogeneous histopathological findings. Characteristically, lesions of ATN are patchy, affect predominantly the S3 segment of the proximal convoluted tubule and the thick ascending loop of Henle, and coexist with significant areas of tubular cell apoptosis and inflammation [7]. In sepsis-induced AKI, the nature of the "typical lesion" is unclear [8, 9]. Therefore, although ATN is commonly mentioned as the common denominator of most cases of AKI, more information is needed on the human histopathology of AKI. Not uncommonly, renal biopsies show unexpected findings such as acute interstitial nephritis, glomerulonephritis or, perhaps in our case, acute pyelonephritis, or a mixed picture. Given these facts and the well-known unreliability of urinalysis findings, new initiatives to perform renal biopsies more frequently in patients with AKI are warranted.

Differential Diagnosis

Often, the terms "acute renal failure" and "acute tubular necrosis" are used interchangeably. It is important to note that ATN is a form of AKI caused by ischemic or toxic insult to the tubular epithelial cells, but that other forms of renal injury are also possible.

Important points in the differential diagnosis of ATN are outlined in Table 20.2.

Management

Supportive Measures

- Maintenance of stable hemodynamics and adequate renal perfusion
- Correction of electrolyte derangements and acidosis
- Avoidance of further nephrotoxic insults like NSAIDS, aminoglycosides, and radiocontrast

Pharmacological Approaches

Although a variety of pharmacological agents have been tried, none have been effective in the management of human ATN. The lack of efficacy may be related to either lack of effectiveness or lateness of administration, when renal parenchymal lesions are extensive.

A list of pharmacological agents that have been tried in ATN [10] and have been unsuccessful is presented in Table 20.3.

Prognosis

Historically, ATN was considered to be a condition from which full recovery was expected and was thus taken as a marker of disease severity. However, multiple recent studies have shown that AKI is an important independent predictor of mortality, which not uncommonly leads to the

Table 20.2 Differential diagnosis of acute tubular necrosis

Test	Prerenal azotemia	Acute tubular necrosis
Response to fluid repletion	Return of renal function to baseline in 24–72 h	No response
BUN/creatinine ratio	>20	<10
Rate of rise of serum creatinine	<0.3–0.5 mg/dL/day	>0.3–0.5 mg/dL/day
Urine sodium	<20 mEq/L	>40 mEq/L
Fractional excretion of sodium	<1%	>2%
Fractional excretion of urea	<35%	>35%
Urine osmolality	>500 mOsm/L	<450 mOsm/L
UCr/PCr	>40	<20
Urinary sediment	Normal; occasional hyaline or granular casts	Renal tubular epithelial cells: muddy-brown granular casts

Table 20.3 Pharmacotherapy of acute tubular necrosis proven to be ineffective

1. Renal vasodilators
(a) Dopamine
(b) Fenoldopam
(c) Natriuretic peptides
(d) Theophylline
(e) Endothelin receptor blockers
(f) Calcium channel blockers
2. Loop diuretics
3. *N*-Acetylcysteine
4. Mannitol
5. Statins
6. Ascorbic acid
7. Erythropoietin

development of chronic kidney disease (CKD). In patients with isolated ATN without other comorbid conditions, mortality ranges from 5 to 25%. Mortality rates increase steeply in patients with comorbid conditions like advanced age, male gender, oliguria, sepsis, multi-organ dysfunction, mechanical ventilation, and increased severity of illness scores.

In patients with AKI, the loss of the normal autoregulation of renal blood flow and glomerular pressures has important consequences. As renal blood flow becomes linearly dependent on perfusion pressure, multiple hypotensive insults worsen tissue damage and may eventually determine CKD or end-stage renal dysfunction. Therefore, renal functional recovery is critically dependent on the avoidance of subsequent hypotension episodes (i.e., intradialytic hypotensive damage).

Early Prediction/Prevention

1. Clinical risk scores: Numerous predictive scores for specific population subsets have been developed. These scores are reasonably accurate in predicting the development of AKI. However, these scores are generated in single-center studies and remain unvalidated for application to the general population.
2. Serum/urinary biomarkers: New research and novel scientific methods have produced several new serum and urinary biomarkers [6], which will help in AKI diagnosis. Some of these are: L1 cell adhesion molecule, KIM 1, Urinary NHE3, Urinary IL-18, NGAL, and sulfated HNK-1 epitope.

Key Points

- ATN is common in hospitalized patients.
- It is an independent risk factor for death and the development of CKD.
- No effective prevention strategy or therapeutic modality is available at present.

Case Revisited

A clinical diagnosis of oliguric AKI due to urosepsis was made on the basis of a history of fever with leukocytosis and urine sediment consistent with acute pyelonephritis (pyuria, absence of abundant brown granular casts). Initially the urinalysis suggested a prerenal cause for her AKI given the high specific gravity. After appropriate cultures were obtained, she was started on intravenous crystalloids, short acting insulin infusion, and broad-spectrum antibiotics. But despite treatment, she did not improve and was transferred to a tertiary hospital with worsening status.

The renal ultrasound ruled-out obstruction. The increased echogenicity suggested an element of underlying chronicity, but the increased echogenicity might have also been attributable to severe pyelonephritis. Laboratory studies demonstrated worsening AKI with urinalysis and urine indices more suggestive of ATN, including dipstick-positive proteinuria, muddy-brown granular casts on urinalysis, and an elevated urine sodium concentration (>20 mEq/L). The urine-specific gravity and osmolality are also consistent with the concentrating deficit that occurs in patients with ATN. One possible explanation for the evolution from a prerenal state to ATN may include persistent sepsis and hemodynamic instability.

Norepinephrine was added when blood pressure failed to stabilize with intravenous fluids. Over the course of the next few hours, the patient's respiratory status deteriorated and she was intubated and mechanically ventilated. She developed fluid overload (*cardiogenic* pulmonary edema) and *non-cardiogenic* edema due to sepsis-induced acute inflammatory lung injury (ALI). The estimated pO_2/FiO_2 ratio of 216 (estimating an FiO_2 of 0.54 with a high-flow face mask) and the tachypnea with relative hypercarbia without metabolic acidosis indicate that a component of ALI was present [11]. When ALI develops, excessive administration of fluids not uncommonly worsens cardiogenic pulmonary edema and precipitates acute respiratory distress requiring mechanically assisted ventilation[4], as in this case. During the next 24 h, she remained oliguric with a positive fluid balance of 3 L. Blood gas analysis showed metabolic acidosis and hyperkalemia of 5.6 mEq/L. She was started on continuous renal replacement therapy (CRRT), which she tolerated well. Her metabolic acidosis was corrected, electrolyte levels normalized, and blood pressure stabilized. She remained on CRRT for 2 days and switched to intermittent hemodialysis (IHD) as soon as she became hemodynamically stable. Subsequently, leukocyte counts normalized, inotropes were stopped, and she was successfully weaned off the ventilator after 6 days. She was transferred to a step-down unit and then to the general medical ward as her condition improved. However, she remained oliguric for 12 days before her urine output improved. During this period, she was treated with IHD on alternate days. On the 13th day after hospitalization, she started passing more than a liter of urine, which increased to 3 L per day in the next few days. During this period, her recovery was supported with intravenous fluids and potassium supplementation. She was discharged home with normal kidney function 3 weeks after her initial hospital admission.

References

1. Chertow GM, Burdick E, Honour M, Bonventre JV, Bates DW. Acute kidney injury, mortality, length of stay, and costs in hospitalized patients. J Am Soc Nephrol. 2005;16(11):3365–70.
2. Cerda J, Lameire N, Eggers P, Pannu N, Uchino S, Wang H, et al. Epidemiology of acute kidney injury. Clin J Am Soc Nephrol. 2008;3(3):881–6.
3. Devarajan P. Update on mechanisms of ischemic acute kidney injury. J Am Soc Nephrol. 2006;17(6): 1503–20.
4. Cerda J, Sheinfeld G, Ronco C. Fluid overload in critically ill patients with acute kidney injury [review]. Blood Purif. 2010;29:331–8.
5. Macedo E, Bouchard J, Soroko SH, Chertow GM, Himmelfarb J, Ikizler TA, et al. Fluid accumulation, recognition and staging of acute kidney injury in critically-ill patients. Crit Care. 2010;14(3):R82.
6. Parikh CR, Devarajan P. New biomarkers of acute kidney injury. Crit Care Med. 2008;36(4 Suppl): S159–65.
7. Sharfuddin AA, Molitoris BA. Pathophysiology of ischemic acute kidney injury. Nat Rev Nephrol. 2011;7(4):189–200.
8. Langenberg C, Bagshaw SM, May CN, Bellomo R. The histopathology of septic acute kidney injury: a systematic review. Crit Care. 2008;12(2):R38.
9. Bellomo R, Wan L, Langenberg C, May C. Septic acute kidney injury: new concepts. Nephron Exp Nephrol. 2008;109(4):e95–100.
10. Jo SK, Rosner MH, Okusa MD. Pharmacologic treatment of acute kidney injury: why drugs haven't worked and what is on the horizon. Clin J Am Soc Nephrol. 2007;2(2):356–65.
11. Liu KD, Matthay MA. Advances in critical care for the nephrologist: acute lung injury/ARDS. Clin J Am Soc Nephrol. 2008;3(2):578–86.

21 Specific Etiologies

Eric K. Judd, Shikha Mehta, and Ashita J. Tolwani

Introduction

In many cases of acute kidney injury (AKI), it is possible to identify a specific cause. While the previous chapters reviewed the general approach to AKI and its broad causes, this chapter focuses on specific etiologies of AKI. Five cases are presented and each meant to highlight a unique etiology of AKI. The case of contrast induced nephropathy is particularly useful when evaluating AKI in a hospitalized patient given the prevalence of contrast exposure in the hospital. Although hepatorenal syndrome and tumor lysis syndrome are less common causes of AKI, they frequently appear in the differential diagnosis and reviewing the presented cases should assist the reader in diagnosing or excluding these syndromes. In addition to presenting diagnostic criteria, each case discussion includes a brief review of the epidemiology, pathophysiology, prevention/management, and prognosis of the specific AKI etiology.

E.K. Judd, MD(✉)
Department of Nephrology, University of Alabama at Birmingham, ZRB 624, 1530 3rd Ave. S, Birmingham, AL 35294, USA
e-mail: ejudd@uab.edu

S. Mehta, M.D. • A.J. Tolwani, M.D., M.Sc.
Department of Nephrology, University of Alabama at Birmingham, Birmingham, AL 35294-0006, USA

Drugs/Nephrotoxins

Case 1

Mr. K is a 47-year-old Caucasian male with past medical history of hypertension, hyperlipidemia, and chronic kidney disease (baseline serum creatinine 1.5 mg/dL), who was admitted to the hospital with new onset left-sided chest pain. EKG at the time of admission showed ST elevation in the lateral leads, consistent with a myocardial infarction. He emergently underwent an angiogram via right femoral artery and had a percutaneous intervention performed. He received intravenous sodium bicarbonate during and after the procedure. Post intervention his chest pain resolved. On day 3 after admission, he started complaining of right thigh pain, which worsened over the next few hours. On physical exam his right thigh was swollen. He had preserved lower extremity pulses. His creatinine at that time was 1.5 mg/dL and he was making 30 ml/h of urine. He was prescribed narcotics for his pain. On day 4, his urine output declined to 5–10 ml/h and creatinine increased to 2.4 mg/dL. He was also noted to have a significant drop in hemoglobin to 7 g/dL and was transfused with blood products and started on intravenous 0.9% saline. Overnight he became anuric, and a nephrologist was consulted. At the time of consultation, his right thigh was extremely swollen and he had a diminished right femoral pulse. Laboratory investigations demonstrated serum creatinine of 3.5 mg/dL and

E.V. Lerma and M. Rosner (eds.), *Clinical Decisions in Nephrology, Hypertension and Kidney Transplantation*,
DOI 10.1007/978-1-4614-4454-1_21, © Springer Science+Business Media New York 2013

urinalysis with specific gravity 1.010, pH 5.3, 0–5 WBCs, 0–2 RBCs, 3+ blood, few granular casts, no bacteria. A Foley catheter was placed with no urine output.

For the case above, what is the etiology of AKI?

What diagnostic and/or therapeutic measures should be undertaken?

Epidemiology

Drug and toxin induced nephrotoxicity is an important cause of AKI in the community and hospital. In a large prospective multicenter observational study in the United States known as the Program to Improve Care in Acute Renal Dysfunction (PICARD) study, the incidence of nephrotoxic AKI was as high as 25% [1]. Among older adults the incidence of nephrotoxic AKI may be as high as 66%. The etiology of nephrotoxic AKI has changed over the last few decades. Compared to 30 years ago, patients are now older, are on multiple medications, have a higher incidence of diabetes, and are exposed to more diagnostic and therapeutic procedures. Currently, the common causes for nephrotoxic AKI are radiocontrast agents, aminoglycosides and other antibiotics, rhabdomyolysis, calcineurin inhibitors, nonsteroidal anti-inflammatory drugs (NSAIDs), and other over-the-counter medications. Some of the more common agents are shown in Table 21.1.

Pathogenesis of Nephrotoxic Kidney Injury

Nephrotoxicity of a drug/toxin or its metabolites can be a result of hemodynamic changes, direct injury to cells and tissue, inflammatory-mediated tissue injury or intratubular obstruction. Some of the mechanisms of AKI are outlined below and in Table 21.2 [2–29].

Table 21.1 Drug/toxins induced nephrotoxicity

Prerenal	ACE-inhibitors, Angiotensin Receptor Blockers (ARBs), Nonsteroidal Anti-inflammatory Drugs (NSAIDS), Cox-2 Inhibitors, Calcineurin Inhibitors (Tacrolimus, Cyclosporine), Diuretics, Interleukin-2, Interferon	Thrombotic microangiopathy	Clopidogrel, Cyclosporine, Mitomycin, Bleomycin, Tacrolimus, Sirolimus, Ticlopidine, Quinine, Lithium, Indinavir, Gemcitabine, Valacyclovir, Bevacizumab
Acute tubular necrosis	Aminoglycosides, amphotericin, Foscarnet, Cisplatin, Sucrose, Immunoglobulin, Mannitol, Hexastarch, Dextran, Lithium, Pentamidine, Streptozocin, NSAIDS, Acetaminophen, Myoglobin[a], Heme[a], Bilirubin[a], Paraprotein	Obstructive -crystal induced nephropathy	Acyclovir, Indinavir, Atazanavir, Foscarnet, Triamterene, Ascorbic Acid, Methotrexate, Sulfonamides, Sodium Phosphate
Acute interstitial nephritis	NSAIDS, Penicillin, Penicillamine, Rifampin, Sulfonamides, Ciprofloxacin, Allopurinol, Cephalosporins, Phenytoin, Proton-Pump Inhibitor, Ethylene Glycol, Paraprotein, Acyclovir, Lithium, Gold, Diuretics, Indinavir, Mesalamine, Triamterene, Valproic Acid	Tubular dysfunction	Aminoglycosides, Amphotericin B, Cisplatin, Foscarnet, Isofosfamide, Pentamidine, Streptozocin, Aristocholic Acid
		Nephrotic syndrome	NSAIDS, Penicillamine, Lithium, Interleukin 2, Gold, Interferon alpha and beta, Pamidronate, Sirolimus
Vascular injury (cholesterol emboli)	Heparin, Warfarin, Streptokinase	Rhabdomyolysis/ hemolysis	Statins, Ethanol, Quinine, Quinidine, Sulfonamides, Mephenytoin. Hydralazine

[a]Endogenous pigment

Table 21.2 Mechanism, clinical features, and treatment of nephrotoxic AKI

Drug	Mechanism	Clinical features	Prevention/treatment
Aminoglycosides	• Accumulate in the lysosomes and mitochondria of PT cells • Interferes with protein synthesis and mitochondrial function • ATN • Dose dependent toxicity	• Non-oliguric AKI 5–10 days after dosing • Potassium, magnesium wasting • Urine with ATN casts • Renal biopsy-ATN with myeloid bodies	• Monitor drug levels • Single daily dosing • Replete electrolytes • Use the least toxic aminoglycoside • Avoid other nephrotoxins • Treatment is to stop the drug
Amphotericin	• Binds to cell membranes and forms aqueous pores, increasing permeability • Tubulotoxic effect may be mediated by the detergent deoxycholate used to solubilize amphotericin • Constriction of afferent arteriole • ATN • Dose dependent toxicity	• Loss of ability to concentrate urine • Hypokalemia, Hypomagnesemia • Distal renal tubular acidosis • Urine with ATN casts	• Maintain high urine flow rate with saline as pre-medication • Liposomal amphotericin-B is less nephrotoxic as compared to conventional amphotericin • AKI is usually reversible after stopping the drug but sometimes the distal tubular acidosis persists
NSAIDS	• Decreased renal perfusion • ATN • Papillary necrosis • AIN	• Urine with ATN casts	• Avoid NSAIDs in patients high risk for AKI
Acetaminophen Intoxication	• 5% metabolized to *N*- acetylimidoquinone which causes both renal and hepatic cell injury • ATN	• AKI usually occurs 3–4 days after ingestion • Urine with ATN casts • Hepatitis	• *N*- acetylcysteine can be protective for hepatic injury but not for AKI • Usually recovers in 1–4 weeks
Ethylene Glycol Intoxication	• Metabolized into glycoaldehyde and glyoxylate which are toxic to tubular cells • Metabolized to oxalate which causes intratubular obstruction	• Anion gap acidosis • Osmolar gap • Hypocalcemia • Urine microscopy with oxalate crystals and ATN	• Inhibition of alcohol dehydrogenase with intravenous ethanol or fomepizole • Hemodialysis for drug removal
Intravenous-Immunoglobulin	• Certain products of IVIG are sucrose-based • Sucrose is taken up by the tubular cell which leads to an increased osmotic load and ATN	• Hyponatremia • Urine with ATN casts	• Adequate hydration • Slow infusion • Split dose in patients with CKD • Avoid sucrose-based compounds • Spontaneous resolution 4–10 days after discontinuation

Table 21.2 (continued)

Cisplatin	• PT cell damage • Vasoconstriction • Pro-inflammatory state • ATN	• Anemia • Hypomagnesemia • Salt wasting • Fanconi's syndrome	• Intravenous hydration • Decrease the dose • Discontinue if AKI occurs
Pigment Induced	• Massive volume depletion • Free radical mediated injury to the tubular cells • Intratubular obstruction from precipitation of myoglobin or heme • ATN	• Elevated creatine kinase in rhabdomyolysis • Increased LDH and haptoglobin in hemolysis • Urine: ATN casts • Urinalysis: Blood, no RBCs	• Aggressive and early volume resuscitation • Maintain electrolyte balance
Oral sodium phosphate	• Intratubular obstruction with calcium phosphate deposition • Inflammation • ATN	• Hypocalcemia • Hyperphosphatemia	• Avoid oral phosphate bowel preparations in patients at high risk of AKI • Dialysis for hyperphosphatemia
Intravenous Acyclovir	• Direct tubular toxicity • Intratubular acyclovir crystals • AIN	• Urine microscopy with needle shaped birefringent crystals	• Dosing based on renal clearance • Usually reversible in few days after stopping the drug

AIN acute interstitial nephritis, *AKI* acute kidney injury, *ATN* acute tubular necrosis, *CKD* chronic kidney disease, *GFR* glomerular filtration rate, *LDH* lactate dehydrogenase, *NSAIDS* nonsteroidal anti-inflammatory drugs, *PT* proximal tubule

Change in Intra-glomerular Hemodynamics

The kidney has the unique ability to autoregulate the intraglomerular pressure by maintaining the afferent and efferent arteriole to preserve the glomerular filtration rate (GFR). Intraglomerular pressure is sustained either by prostaglandin-induced vasodilatation in the afferent arteriole, as in case of volume depletion, or angiotensin mediated vasoconstriction in the efferent arteriole, or both. Drugs with anti-prostaglandin activity such as NSAIDs or those with anti-angiotensin like activity (angiotensin-converting enzyme inhibitors (ACEi), angiotensin receptor blockers (ARB)) can interfere with the kidney's ability to autoregulate and can decrease the GFR in the setting of volume depletion or decreased effective arterial circulation. Prolonged exposure to these drugs may sometimes lead to ischemic tubular necrosis. Other drugs such as calcineurin inhibitors can also lead to dose-dependent vasoconstriction of the afferent arteriole, leading to decreased GFR.

Tubular Cell Toxicity

Proximal renal tubular cells are responsible for absorbing more than 90% of the glomerular filtrate and are exposed to a high concentration of circulating toxins, drugs and their metabolites, making them prone to their toxic effects. Tubular cells also have transport pathways which may engender site specific toxicity. Drugs and toxins that cause tubular toxicity do so by impairing mitochondrial function, causing oxidative stress, generating free radicals, or interfering with tubular transport (Table 21.2). Exposure to hyperosmolar substances such as intravenous immunoglobulin and mannitol can lead to vacuolization injury and tubular damage.

Inflammation

Drugs can cause inflammation in the interstitium, glomerulus, vasculature, and tubules, leading to fibrosis and permanent scarring. The most common cause of drug-induced inflammation-mediated AKI is acute interstitial nephritis (AIN), which is usually a result of an idiosyncratic, non-dose-dependent allergic reaction to a drug. Drugs that cause AIN are thought to bind to antigens on the kidney or act as a hapten after binding to the interstitial matrix or tubular basement membranes, inducing an immune reaction [30, 31].

Glomerulonephritis is an inflammatory condition caused primarily by an immune mediated mechanism and is often associated with nephrotic range proteinuria. For instance, NSAIDs are believed to cause immunological hypersensitivity and nephrotic syndrome with minimal change disease. However, in some cases, NSAIDs can lead to immune deposits and membranous nephropathy, the pathogenesis of which is unclear [32–34]. The mechanism by which lithium causes minimal change disease is also not clear [35–37].

Endothelial Cell Injury

Drugs causing thrombotic microangiopathy do so by different mechanisms but result in a final common pathway of endothelial cell injury. Sirolimus (mammalian target of rapamycin inhibitor) and vascular endothelial cell growth factor (VEGF) antibody inhibit VEGF action which is essential for endothelial cell survival. Calcineurin inhibitors and antineoplastic agents cause direct endothelial cell toxicity. Quinine exposure results in immune mediated endothelial cell injury. The underlying mechanism for thrombotic microangiopathy due to ticlopidine and clopidogrel is still evolving [38–43]. Most recently bevacizumab (an anti-VEGF chemotherapeutic agent) has been associated with thrombotic thrombocytopenic purpura (TTP).

Crystal Induced Nephropathies

Many drugs have a propensity to precipitate within renal tubules to form crystals or stones leading to intratubular obstruction or nephrolithiasis. Examples of these medications include acyclovir, methotrexate, triamterene, and indinavir. The predisposing factors for precipitation of these substances are volume depletion, preexisting chronic kidney disease (CKD), other nephrotoxic drugs, and/or metabolic derangements (Table 21.2) [44–48]. Typically, crystallization occurs at high dosages of these medications.

Podocytopathies

Pamidronate and sirolimus are thought to cause podocyte damage by non-immunological mechanism and the toxicity usually presents itself as proteinuria [49–52].

Pigment Induced Kidney Injury

Rhabdomyolysis is a syndrome in which myocyte injury leads to the release of intracellular myoglobin and creatine kinase into the circulation. In cases of intravascular hemolysis, large amounts of hemoglobin are released in circulation. Both myoglobin and hemoglobin cause release of non-protein heme pigment which can cause renal injury secondary to direct toxicity, tubular obstruction, and alterations in GFR.

Clinical Presentation

Patients may present with oliguric or non-oliguric AKI, asymptomatic azotemia, proteinuria, AIN, Fanconi's syndrome, obstruction, nephrogenic diabetes insipidus, or electrolyte abnormalities. In the hospital setting, an elevation in serum creatinine or electrolyte abnormalities may be the first presentation. It is important to monitor serum creatinine frequently in patients exposed to potentially nephrotoxic medications.

Evaluation and Differential Diagnosis

A careful and thorough history, including drug or medication exposure and physical examination will help provide the initial clues as to the nephrotoxic agent. One should look for underlying risk factors such as age, history of CKD, volume depletion, or use of other nephrotoxic agents. The time line of drug exposure and the cumulative dose is crucial, especially with certain drugs such as aminoglycosides, which can cause cumulative toxicity. Certain serum and urine indices are helpful in teasing out the etiology of AKI (Table 21.3). A renal biopsy can be very helpful in patients with a complicated clinical picture. It is important to know that drugs like cimetidine, trimethoprim, probenicid, amiloride, spironolactone, and triamterene are competitively secreted by the tubules and can elevate serum creatinine in the absence of direct nephrotoxicity. Drugs such as ascorbic acid, flucytosine, levodopa, methyldopa, and certain cephalosporins interfere with laboratory determination of creatinine.

Prevention and Treatment

The key to treatment of drug/toxin induced AKI is prevention, early recognition and intervention. One should recognize patients at high risk, use appropriate dosing for renally excreted drugs, monitor renal function closely when introducing any drug with nephrotoxic potential, take precautions such as hydration prior to administering certain drugs such as amphotericin, and monitor drug levels. Most episodes of drug induced AKI are reversible with function returning to baseline after discontinuation of the drug (Table 21.2). In certain cases removing the drugs and its metabolites with dialysis may protect the kidney from further injury. Once a patient develops acute tubular necrosis (ATN), treatment is supportive and may include renal replacement therapy.

Pigment induced kidney injury can be prevented by early and aggressive fluid resuscitation.

In patients with drug induced AIN, discontinuation of the potential causative agent is mainstay of therapy, and renal function typically begins to recover in 5–7 days, depending on the half-life of the drug. Steroids may be employed in cases where there is no improvement in kidney function [53, 54].

The most important step in treating drug-induced thrombotic microangiopathy is to stop the offending agent. Role of plasma exchange therapy is controversial.

Crystal induced injury can be prevented and treated with intravenous volume repletion and stopping the offending agent. Urine alkalinization can help prevent crystalluria and AKI in patients receiving methotrexate, sulfonamides, or triamterene, since these drugs are more soluble in an alkaline pH.

Table 21.3 Clinical presentation and laboratory findings

Etiology/tests	Prerenal AKI	ATN	AIN	Intratubular obstruction	Thrombotic microangiopathy	Nephrotic syndrome	Pigment-induced injury
Time Course	Slow rise in serum Cr	Rapid rise in Cr	History of at least 3–5 day exposure or prior exposure	Rapid rise in Cr	Variable	Variable	Rapid rise in Cr
Urinalysis	SG >1.015, Normal or Hyaline Casts	SG 1.010, Muddy Brown Casts, Tubular Epithelial Cells	WBC casts, WBCs, Hematuria	Crystalluria, Benign Urinalysis, or ATN like picture	Hematuria	Proteinuria, Lipid Casts	SG 1.010, Heme Positive, Bilirubin, Myoglobinuria, Muddy Brown Casts, Tubular Epithelial Cells
BUN/Cr ratio	>20:1	10:1	Variable	Variable	Variable	Variable	Variable
FeNa (%)	<1	>2	>1	Variable	Variable	Variable	>2
Urine Sodium (mmol/L)	<20	>40	>20	Variable	>20	Variable	>40
Urine osmolality (mosm/kg)	>500	<450	Variable	Variable	Variable	Variable	Variable
Other Findings			Eosinophilia, Fever, Rash		Elevated LDH, Thrombocytopenia, Hemolytic Anemia	Hypoalbuminemia, hyperlipidemia, Edema	Elevated CK or Elevated Bilirubin, Hemolysis

AKI acute kidney injury, *ATN* acute tubular necrosis, *AIN* acute interstitial nephritis, *SG* specific gravity, *BUN* blood urea nitrogen, *FeNa* fractional excretion of sodium, *Cr* creatinine, *LDH* lactate dehydrogenase, *CK* creatine kinase, *WBC* white blood cell

Glomerulopathies are sometimes reversible after stopping the drug as in case of minimal change disease secondary to NSAIDs, whereas in other cases like focal segmental glomerulosclerosis caused by pamidronate, the damage is irreversible.

In conclusion, at the first sign of renal dysfunction, the patient medication list should be reviewed to identify offending agents and drug–drug interactions. The offending medication should be discontinued, further renal insults avoided, adequate blood pressure and hydration maintained, and all other potential nephrotoxins discontinued.

Case 1 Revisited

The differential diagnosis of AKI in this case includes contrast induced nephropathy (CIN), rhabdomyolysis and cholesterol emboli. Mr. K has underlying diabetes and CKD which increases his risk for AKI from the radiocontrast agent after his heart catheterization. However, the typical presentation of CIN is within 24–48 h and his serum creatinine was at baseline after 48 h. Also, in CIN the urinalysis is typically normal. Cholesterol emboli usually present 5–7 days after intervention with a gradual increase in serum creatinine. Physical exam findings of cholesterol emboli include livedo reticularis and evidence of embolic phenomena. Urinalysis shows eosinophiluria along with peripheral eosinophilia.

The key to the diagnosis in this patient is the swollen thigh and urinalysis with 3+ blood on dipstick and minimal red cells, suggesting the presence of pigment nephropathy. The diagnosis was confirmed by a creatine kinase level of 50,000 U/ml and positive urine myoglobin. These findings suggest that he developed rhabdomyolysis with compartment syndrome likely from bleeding in his thigh, leading to muscle breakdown and production of myoglobin. Treatment includes aggressive hydration, monitoring of electrolyte status, acid base status, and volume status. In extreme cases dialysis is required. The overall prognosis for patients with pigment induced AKI is favorable. Most patients recover sufficient kidney function to be dialysis-independent and may even recover near normal kidney function.

Key Points

- Many drugs/toxins can cause nephrotoxicity since the kidney is responsible for excretion of many drugs and their metabolites.
- Drugs/toxins induced kidney damage can manifest very differently.
- It is important to recognize the nephrotoxic potential of the drug/toxins and precautions should be taken to avoid kidney injury.
- Discontinuation of the drug is mainstay of therapy.

Contrast Induced Nephropathy

Case 2

Mr. K is a 45-year-old Caucasian man with past medical history of hypertension and diabetes who presented to the emergency department with chest pain. On exam, he was afebrile, with blood pressure 150/95 mmHg and pulse 96 beats/min. Physical exam was otherwise unremarkable. EKG showed ST segment elevation consistent with myocardial infarction. He underwent an emergent coronary angiography with percutaneous intervention. Admission laboratory tests were significant for an elevated WBC of 12,000 cells/μL, elevated serum creatinine of 1.8 mg/dL and random glucose of 368 mg/dL. Next morning his serum creatinine was 2.4 mg/dL, and nephrology was consulted. Further investigation into his past records revealed a baseline serum creatinine of 1.6 mg/dL with 3+ protein by urine dipstick. His home medications included enalapril 5 mg daily, amlodipine 10 mg daily, and over-the-counter naproxen for back pain. He received intravenous sodium bicarbonate before and after the procedure for contrast nephropathy prophylaxis. Current laboratory investigation shows 3+ proteinuria on urinalysis with fractional excretion of sodium of 0.09%.

What is the cause of patient's AKI?
What are his risk factors for this diagnosis?
What is the management?

Introduction

Contrast induced nephropathy (CIN) is the third most common cause of AKI in the hospital [55, 56]. Although CIN is reversible in most cases, it is associated with increased morbidity and mortality and can pose a significant clinical and economic burden.

Definition

CIN is defined as a rise in serum creatinine within the first 24 h after contrast exposure, peaking up to 5 days afterwards [57]. Until very recently CIN was defined as an increase in absolute serum creatinine of 0.5–1.0 mg/dL or as a proportional increase in serum creatinine of 25–50% from the baseline, leading to wide differences in the reported incidence and implications of CIN in various studies. Some studies have used a rise in serum cystatin C by 15–25% as a marker of AKI after contrast exposure. The development of RIFLE (Risk of renal dysfunction, Injury to the kidney, Failure of kidney function, Loss of kidney function, and End-stage renal disease) criteria and Acute Kidney Injury Network Criteria (AKIN) criteria for AKI should allow for a more uniform definition of CIN in the future [58–60].

Incidence of CIN

The incidence of CIN varies from 0% to over 50% depending on the definition used to define CIN, predisposing risk factors, radiocontrast agent, type of radiographic procedure, differences in clinical settings, prophylaxis protocols, and the study design.

The incidence of CIN is very low (2%) in the general population [61]. One study showed the incidence of CIN is <1% in patients with glomerular filtration rate (GFR) >45 ml/min/1.73 m^2 BSA who underwent non-emergent computed tomography [62]. The incidence of CIN varies from 4 to 38% in patients with CKD and diabetes [63–65], and can be as high as 50% in diabetic patients with advanced kidney disease undergoing coronary angiography [66].

Risk Factors for CIN

The most important and well-established patient risk factor for contrast induced AKI is CKD, particularly in combination with diabetes and advanced age. Other risk factors include advanced heart failure, decreased renal perfusion from hypovolemia, elevated fasting glucose independent of preexisting diabetes, anemia, use of nephrotoxic drugs, and multiple myeloma (Table 21.4). There are certain peri-procedural risk factors and procedures associated with a higher risk of CIN as compared to others. Patients undergoing percutaneous coronary intervention are at higher risk of developing CIN as compared to those undergoing non-emergent contrast enhanced procedures. Some studies have shown increased risk of CIN with increasing volume of contrast. Newer (iso-osmolar nonionic) contrast agents have a lower risk of CIN when compared to first generation contrast agents (hyperosmolar ionic agents), but not when compared to second generation low-osmolar agents [67–79].

Table 21.4 Risk factors for contrast induced nephropathy[a].

Patient risk factors	Procedural risk factors
• Chronic Kidney disease (GFR <60 ml/min/1.73 m^2 BSA) • Diabetes Mellitus (type 1 or type 2) • Volume depletion • Nephrotoxic drug use (Cyclosporine, NSAIDS, aminoglycosides, diuretics) • Other comorbidities: anemia, hypoalbuminemia, paraproteinemia • Heart Failure • Age	• Higher volume of contrast • First generation contrast agents • Emergent procedure • Length of procedure • Intra-arterial administration of contrast agent • Peri-procedural hemodynamic instability

[a]Adapted from McCullough et al. [11]

Identifying Patients at Risk for CIN

Various risk models have been used to predict the effects of baseline and peri-procedural characteristics for CIN in patients undergoing coronary interventions (Table 21.5). These models have been validated in a few studies to predict short term and long term outcomes [80, 81]; however, these risk models have not been studied in patients undergoing other contrast (non-coronary) enhanced procedures. Currently, the American College of Radiology recommends checking a serum creatinine prior to intra-arterial administration of contrast in patients with personal or family history of kidney disease, diabetes, para proteinemia, collagen vascular disease, prior renal surgery, or on certain drugs (metformin, NSAIDS, or nephrotoxic antibiotic); (guidelines can be found at *www.acr.*org). The European Society of Urogenital Radiology recommends measuring the serum creatinine level within 7 days prior to administration of contrast media in high risk patients (patients with estimated GFR <60 ml/min per 1.73 m^2 BSA or elevated serum creatinine), diabetic patients, patients receiving intra-arterial contrast media and those with a history suggesting a reduced GFR. In patients undergoing emergent procedures serum creatinine should always be measured if the delay in the examination will not harm the patient, or these patients should be assumed to be high risk and treated appropriately [82].

Table 21.5 Contrast-induced nephropathy (CIN) risk score[a]

Risk factors	Assigned score
Hypotension with systolic blood pressure <80 mm Hg for at least 1 h with inotropic support	5
Intra-aortic Balloon Pump	5
Congestive Heart Failure Class III/IV	5
Age >75 years	4
Anemia:	3
Hematocrit <39% for men	
Hematocrit <36% for women	
Diabetes	3
Contrast media volume	1 for each 100 ml of contrast
Serum creatinine >1.5 mg/dL or estimated glomerular filtration rate (eGFR) <60 ml/min/1.73 m^2	4 for serum creatinine criteria
	2 for eGFR 40–60
	4 for eGFR 20–40
	6 for eGFR <20

Total calculated score	% Risk of CIN	% Risk of dialysis
≤5	7.5	0.04
6–10	14.0	0.12
11–16	26.1	1.09
≥16	57.3	12.6

[a]Adapted from Mehran et al. [80]

Pathophysiology

There are three generations of iodinated contrast media which vary in their osmolality and ionic content and the risk for CIN (Table 21.6) [83]. Radiocontrast agents use di-iodinated or tri-iodinated rings which create a sufficient radio-opaque concentration in the blood stream. The cations used to carry iodide anions in early ionic hyperosmolar formulations are sodium, the sugar meglumine, or both, which easily disassociate into charged particles in the solution. This creates a solution which is very hypertonic relative to blood since both the anions (iodide) and cations (sodium or meglumine) are osmotically active. The newer nonionic contrast agents still use iodine as a radiocontrast agent, but they are attached to different side chains which do not disassociate readily in solution, decreasing the number of osmotically active particles and hence osmolality of the dye.

Table 21.6 Types and properties of radiocontrast agents

Iodinated radio contrast agents	Osmolality (mosm/kg)	Polarity
First generation agents	1,400–1,800	Ionic
Diatrizoate, Ioxathalmate		
Second generation agents	500–800	
Iohexol, Iopadimol, Ioversol, Iopromide		Nonionic
Ioxaglate		Ionic
Third generation agents	Approximately 290	Nonionic
Iodixanol		

Current understanding of the pathogenesis of CIN involves a complex interplay of various mechanisms. Mechanisms of CIN include the following:

1. Vasoconstriction and decrease in renal blood flow: Several studies have shown a decrease in renal blood flow [84–86], which can last for at least 4 h after the administration of contrast. Various animal studies have demonstrated an increase in release of vasoconstrictors—endothelin [85, 87–89] and adenosine [90, 91]—and decreased production of the vasodilator nitric oxide in response to contrast [92–94], especially with higher osmolality agents. Some investigators have also reported a role of calcium influx in contrast mediated vasoconstriction [95].
2. Medullary hypoxia: Studies have demonstrated a selective decrease in medullary blood flow after administration of contrast, leading to a further decrease in the already hypoxic outer medulla, making it more susceptible to injury [96, 97]. The reduction of medullary blood flow and reduced oxygen tissue can lead to necrotic changes in the tubular cells [98].
3. Oxidative stress: Hypoxia induced by contrast media may lead to the generation of reactive oxygen species which in turn can cause tubular membrane oxidative damage [99, 100].
4. Direct tubular cytotoxicity: Patients exposed to first generation high osmolality contrast agents can develop direct tubular injury from osmotic nephrosis. Osmotic nephrosis is a form of renal tubular injury characterized by vacuolization and swelling of proximal tubular cells in response to hyperosmolar substances [101].

Clinical Features

A rise in serum creatinine is noted within a period of 24–48 h after exposure to intravenous contrast media. The renal failure is non-oliguric in the vast majority of patients. Kidney damage may be limited to a transient rise in serum creatinine which returns to baseline in 3–5 days, or as persistent renal failure, especially in patient with preexisting renal disease combined with diabetes. Patients with CIN may have a benign urinalysis with a fractional excretion of sodium <1% in most cases [102]. The diagnosis of CIN is based on the time line in relation to contrast exposure and clinical course of the disease. Other causes of AKI should be taken into consideration based on the history and physical exam (Table 21.7).

Prevention

Multiple strategies have been tried to prevent CIN, given its associated clinical and economic burden. High risk patients should be proactively identified and alternative methods of imaging should be considered if possible. All potential nephrotoxic agents should be discontinued 24 h before administration of contrast media, such as nonsteroidal anti-inflammatory drugs. Despite numerous trials there has been little evidence to support the use of specific pharmaco-therapeutic agents to prevent CIN.

Contrast Agent and Volume

Studies have shown that the volume of contrast agent used for contrast-enhanced procedures is an independent risk factor for CIN; hence the lowest possible volume of contrast agent should

Table 21.7 Differential diagnosis for contrast induced nephropathy in the hospital

Etiology	Typical findings
Acute tubular necrosis	Clinical history, FeNa >1.0%, muddy brown casts
Acute interstitial nephritis	Exposure to nephrotoxic drug, time frame for rise in serum Cr is gradual after the exposure, eosinophilia, eosinophiluria, WBC casts, normal complements
Atheroembolic disease	Delayed onset of renal failure, long protracted course, presence of other embolic lesions, transient eosinophilia, eosinophiluria, hypocomplementemia
Others: prerenal causes, postrenal causes, nephrotoxic agents	Variable

FeNa fractional excretion of sodium, *Cr* creatinine, *WBC* white blood cell be used [66, 68, 77, 103, 104]. Repetitive studies requiring contrast should be spaced several days apart [71]. In patients with advanced CKD, a low volume of contrast (<10 ml) for fistulograms has been used safely [105]. Table 21.6 summarizes the characteristics of the commonly used radiocontrast media.

All generations of contrast agents seem to carry a similar risk of CIN in low risk patients. But in high risk patients, nonionic, lower osmolality agents (second-generation agents) have been associated with lower incidence of CIN when compared to ionic, high osmolality agents (first generation agents) [68, 72, 106]. Iodixonol (290 mosm/kg), a nonionic iso-osmolar agent has been associated with a lower incidence of CIN as compared to Iohexol (844 mosm/kg) in high risk patients [107], but no advantage was noted when it was compared to other nonionic low osmolar agents such as Iopamidol (795 mosm/kg) [108–110].

Hydration

There has been a general consensus in multiple studies that hydration is beneficial and reduces the incidence of CIN in high risk patients. The amount and rate at which fluid is given should be determined on an individual basis and the volume status of patient. A reasonable infusion rate is 1 ml/kg/h of 0.9% saline given 6 h before and continued for 6 h after contrast administration. There is conflicting evidence as to whether intravenous isotonic sodium bicarbonate is superior to intravenous normal saline hydration [111–121]. However, intravenous hydration, with normal saline or sodium bicarbonate, is clearly superior to oral hydration in high risk patients [122].

N-Acetylcysteine

Acetylcysteine, also known as mucomyst, is a thiol-based antioxidant which scavenges oxygen free radicals and behaves as a vasodilator by increasing the biologic effects of nitric oxide. The first beneficial effects of *N*-acetylcysteine were reported by Tepel et al., and since then numerous trials have been published about the benefits and its role in preventing CIN [123–126]. Other trials have not reported any significant risk reduction in the incidence of CIN [127–130]. In one of the largest meta-analyses, *N*-acetylcysteine reduced the risk of CIN when compared with saline alone by 38% [131]. The results of *N*-acetylcysteine for contrast induced nephropathy trial, which randomized 2,308 patients to receive *N*-acetylcysteine vs. placebo, showed no difference in the rate of CIN between the two groups; however the study population was at low risk for CIN [132]. Considering its high safety profile, many centers use *N*-acetylcysteine in conjunction with hydration to prevent CIN. The role of intravenous *N*-acetylcysteine therapy is controversial and currently not recommended.

Hemofiltration and Hemodialysis

Hemodialysis has been shown to remove contrast effectively from the blood circulation in small studies [133, 134]; however, it does not prevent the adverse effects of contrast such as vasoconstriction and AKI [135–137]. Therefore, prophylactic dialysis cannot be recommended.

Other Agents

Some agents with vasodilator properties may be associated with reduced incidence of CIN, while others have not shown any benefit, but these results need to be validated in larger studies before they are incorporated in practice. Theophylline, an adenosine antagonist has been shown to reduce the risk of CIN since adenosine is involved in the pathophysiology of CIN [131, 138]. Fenoldapam, a dopamine-1 agonist, did not reduce the incidence of CIN in a randomized controlled trial after angiography [139]. Iloprost, a prostacyclin analog, was recently shown to be associated with a lower incidence of CIN in patients with CKD undergoing angiography [140]. A randomized controlled trial testing a nonselective endothelin receptor antagonist showed detrimental effects on renal function after administration of contrast as compared to hydration alone [141].

Administration of the antioxidant ascorbic acid protected patients undergoing high risk coronary procedure from CIN in a randomized controlled trial [142]. Subsequent studies have failed to show an advantage of ascorbic acid over standard therapy in preventing CIN [143, 144]. Statins with their antioxidant and anti-inflammatory properties have been tested in multiple studies, and have shown a protective effect in preventing CIN but the data needs to be confirmed in larger studies [145]. Atrial natriuretic peptide has shown to decrease the incidence of CIN when compared to Ringer's solution in one recent prospective study [146].

Forced diuresis with furosemide or mannitol or administration of dopamine for prevention of CIN either was found to be harmful or conferred no benefit.

Prognosis

CIN has been associated with an increased in-hospital mortality and morbidity in many retrospective and observational studies [74, 147–150]. McCullough et al. reported in-hospital mortality rates of 1.1% for patients without CIN as compared to 7.1% for patients with CIN, and 35.7% for patients with CIN requiring dialysis in a group of 1,826 patients undergoing percutaneous coronary interventions [77]. Levy et al. reported a 5.5-fold increased risk of death in patients who developed CIN, after adjusting for comorbid diseases [148]. In a retrospective analysis of CIN and long term events, Solomon et al. reported a higher incidence rate of adverse events in patients who developed CIN after adjusting for co-morbidities, but the study was not powered to show the association with increased mortality, incidence of end stage renal disease (ESRD) requiring dialysis, stroke, or myocardial infarction [151]. CIN also has major economic implications, with average in-hospital cost reported to be approximately US $10,000 [152].

Treatment

There is no standard treatment for CIN. After establishing the correct diagnosis, treatment is primarily supportive while waiting for the recovery of kidney function.

Case 2 Revisited

Our patient Mr. K had a baseline serum creatinine of 1.6 mg/dL with an estimated GFR of 44 ml/min/1.73 m^2 BSA along with diabetes. He underwent an emergent percutaneous coronary intervention procedure. The volume of contrast agent used was 200 ml. According to the Mehran risk score (Table 21.5), his risk score was 7 and his risk for CIN was 14.0% with only 0.12% chance of needing dialysis. He likely did develop CIN, since the rise in serum creatinine was noted to be within 24 h of the administration of contrast agent. It is unlikely to be atheroembolic disease or acute interstitial nephritis (AIN) considering the rapidity of AKI and lack of physical exam and urinary findings. In addition, he did not have any risk factors for AIN. His urinalysis did not show any muddy-brown casts and fractional excretion of sodium was less than 1% which makes acute tubular necrosis from other causes less likely. CKD, diabetes, use of naproxen in conjunction with an angiotensin converting enzyme inhibitor, and emergent coronary procedure with percutaneous intervention are some of the underlying risk factors which predisposed Mr. K to develop CIN. His serum creatinine peaked at 3.6 mg/dL and then returned to baseline in 6 days. He did not require renal replacement therapy, but his hospital course was prolonged.

Key Points

- CIN is the third leading cause of AKI in the hospital.
- The incidence of CIN varies from <1 to 50% depending on the various risk factors with patients with diabetic kidney disease and CKD being at the highest risk.
- The elevation of creatinine in patients who develop CIN is seen within 24–48 h. Other causes of AKI should be considered.
- Appropriate preventive strategies should be applied to patients at high risk for CIN.
- Hydration with normal saline or sodium bicarbonate is the most widely accepted preventive intervention.

Hepatorenal Syndrome

Case 3

A 45 year-old man is brought to the hospital by his family for 2 days of "not acting like himself." Further history reveals heavy alcohol use for the past 30 years with prior hospitalizations for hepatic encephalopathy and cirrhosis. There is no record of prior kidney disease and his baseline creatinine is 0.7 mg/dL. The family denies fever, syncope, trauma, vomiting, diarrhea, or medication use other than his prescribed medications (furosemide 40 mg twice daily, lactulose 30 ml twice daily, and folate 1 mg daily). Physical exam reveals a jaundiced, chronically ill appearing man with the following vital signs: Temperature 97.5 F, heart rate 95 beats/min, blood pressure 100/55 mmHg, respiratory rate 14 breaths/min, and initial weight 75 kg. Shifting dullness is detected on abdominal exam and 1+ pitting edema noted on bilateral lower extremities. Initial laboratory values include:

- *Blood studies*: sodium 130 mEq/L, potassium 2.5 mEq/L, chloride 96 mEq/L, bicarbonate 28 mEq/L, blood urea nitrogen 34 mg/dL, creatinine 1.6 mg/dL, albumin 3.0 g/dL, leukocyte count 5,000 cells/μL, hemoglobin 7.5 g/dL, total bilirubin 8 mg/dL, alanine aminotransferase (ALT) 120 (normal 15–58 U/L), aspartate aminotransferase (AST) 200 (normal 15–40 U/L), and prothrombin time 23 s (INR 2.0).
- *Urine studies*: protein <6 mg/dL, sodium 10 mEq/L, potassium 60 mEq/L, creatinine 60 mg/dL, Urinalysis with specific gravity of 1.025, no blood or protein, and 0–2 red blood cells per high power field.

What causes of his renal injury must you consider?

What is the first step in management?

Do you need any additional diagnostic tests?

Introduction

AKI in cirrhosis is often an ominous sign. AKI can be due to the usual spectrum of causes seen in patient populations. However, hepatorenal syndrome is the most feared. Once hepatorenal syndrome (HRS) is diagnosed, 3 month survival can be as low as 10% (for Type 1 HRS) [153, 154]. Despite advances in identifying the causes of HRS, few medical therapies exist to alter its mortality. Liver transplant remains the only cure for HRS and medical therapy such as terlipressin, midodrine, transjugular intrahepatic portosystemic shunt (TIPS), paracentesis, albumin infusion, and renal replacement therapy, only serve as a bridge to liver transplant. Given the grim prognosis of HRS, it is important to consider a thorough differential of AKI in cirrhotic patients before diagnosing HRS. In fact, prerenal azotemia and acute tubular necrosis (ATN) may be much more common than HRS in the cirrhotic patient.

Incidence

Gines et al. [153] reported the 1-year probability of HRS in patients with cirrhosis at 18% and the 5-year probability at 39%. However, this study was published 3 years before the standardization of the diagnostic criteria for HRS by the International Ascites Club in 1996. A later multicenter, retrospective study in 2002 of 423 patients with cirrhosis and AKI found HRS (either Type 1 or 2) to be the cause of AKI in 20 cases (6.6%). In this study the majority of AKI was either ATN (35%) or prerenal failure (32%) [155].

Definition

Hepatorenal syndrome is a potentially reversible, functional renal impairment that occurs in patients with advanced liver cirrhosis or those with fulminant hepatic failure. It is characterized by marked reduction in glomerular filtration rate (GFR) and renal plasma flow (RPF) in the absence of other causes of renal failure. The hallmark of HRS is intense renal vasoconstriction with predominant peripheral arterial vasodilation. Notably, tubular function is preserved with the absence of proteinuria and lack of tubular histologic changes [156]. Two subtypes of HRS have been identified: [157]

- Type 1 HRS is a rapidly progressive renal failure that is defined by doubling of initial serum creatinine to a level >2.5 mg/dL or by 50% reduction in creatinine clearance to a level <20 ml/min in less than 2 weeks.
- Type 2 HRS is a moderate, steady renal failure with a serum creatinine of >1.5 mg/dL.

In type 1 HRS, a precipitating factor frequently is identified, whereas type 2 HRS arises spontaneously and is the main underlying mechanism of refractory ascites [156].

Pathophysiology

The pathophysiology of HRS is complex and while understanding of the details is still evolving, the principle mechanism has been known since 1970. Epstein et al. [158] demonstrated that splanchnic and systemic vasodilation together with intense renal vasoconstriction is the pathophysiologic hallmark of HRS.

Four interrelated pathways have been implicated in the pathophysiology of HRS: [156]

1. Peripheral arterial vasodilation with hyperdynamic circulation and subsequent renal vasoconstriction
2. Stimulation of the renal sympathetic nervous system (SNS)
3. Cardiac dysfunction contributing to the circulatory derangements and renal hypoperfusion
4. Action of different cytokines and vasoactive mediators on the renal circulation and other vascular beds.

Splanchnic Vasodilation and Renal Vasoconstriction

Portal hypertension in cirrhosis leads to decreased effective circulating volume, largely due to splanchnic blood pooling from increased draining pressures through a cirrhotic liver combined with increased vasodilator production. Decreased effective circulating volume triggers a compensatory cascade upregulating RAAS, the SNS, and vasopressin secretion. In summary, splanchnic (the primary driver) and peripheral vascular beds both dilate causing a hyperdynamic circulation, which leads to compensatory renal vasoconstriction mechanisms.

Renal Sympathetic Stimulation

Experimental data from both humans and dogs [159, 160] suggest the presence of a hepatorenal reflex where the renal SNS is stimulated by increases in hepatic sinusoidal pressure or reduction in sinusoidal blood flow. The degree that this mechanism contributes to HRS may vary by patient and is not known.

Cardiac Dysfunction

Cardiac output increases as early compensation for decreased effective circulating volume; therefore as the liver disease advances, less cardiac reserve is available to respond to stressors (infection, bleeding, hypovolemia, etc.) and a relative drop in cardiac output can precipitate HRS. It is important to note that the low afterload state seen in cirrhosis can mask cardiac dysfunction.

Cytokines and Vasoactive Mediators

Nitric oxide (NO) production is increased in cirrhosis as a result of upregulation of endothelial NO synthase (eNOS) activity from increased shear stress in the splanchnic and systemic circulation as well as endotoxin-mediated eNOS activation [161, 162]. Patients with cirrhosis and ascites have higher NO plasma concentrations than normal individuals or those with compensated cirrhosis [156]. Other implicated vasodilators (mainly in the splanchnic circulation) include carbon monoxide and endogenous cannabinoids [154, 163–166].

Precipitating Factors

In type 1 HRS a precipitating factor which worsens renal vasoconstriction can be identified in over 70–100% of patients (outlined in Fig. 21.1). Gines et al. [167] propose that subclinical bacterial infections can act as precipitating factors. Bacterial translocation, the passage of bacteria from the intestinal lumen to the mesenteric lymph nodes, may elicit an inflammatory response with increased cytokine production (mainly tumor necrosis factor α and interleukin-6) leading to splanchnic vasodilation without an overt infection [167]. Twenty to thirty percent of patients with spontaneous bacterial peritonitis (SBP) develop HRS despite appropriate treatment and resolution of infection [168, 169]. The extent to which intra-abdominal hypertension (IAH) or abdominal compartment syndrome contribute to

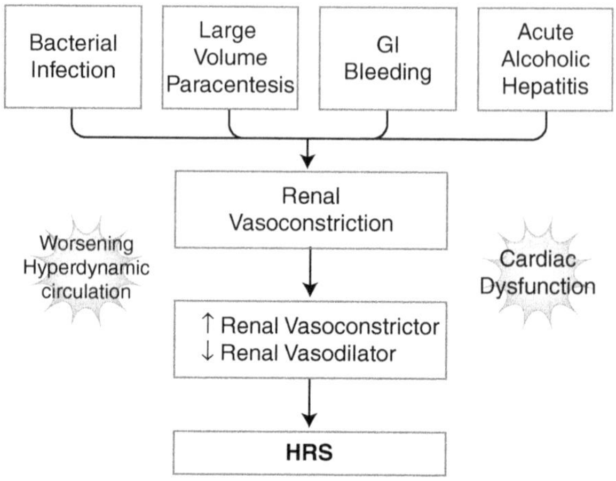

Fig. 21.1 Precipitating factors in HRS [156]

HRS as precipitating factors is not known, yet speculated to be under recognized in the critical care setting [170].

Clinical Features

Hepatorenal syndrome occurs in advanced cirrhosis or fulminant hepatic failure. Besides ascites, patients will display stigmata of chronic liver disease: hepatic encephalopathy (as in the clinical case above), palmar erythema, spider angiomas, jaundice, splenomegaly, edema, and bleeding tendencies. The increased peripheral vasodilation causes a low blood pressure with a widened pulse pressure. The urine output is drastically reduced in type 1 and poorly responsive to high dose diuretics in type 2 with daily urine output often less than 500 ml. Typically, patients are hyponatremic (serum sodium <130 meq/L).

Diagnosis

Both types of HRS require a rise in serum creatinine above 1.5 mg/dL. Please see the definition section above for the specific diagnostic distinctions of type 1 and 2 HRS. The International Ascites Club first defined the diagnostic criteria for HRS in 1996 [154]. It was revised in 2007 (displayed in Table 21.8) [157] with three notable distinctions:

- Volume expansion should be performed with albumin rather than saline.
- HRS can be diagnosed in the setting of an ongoing bacterial infection as long as septic shock is excluded.
- Minor criteria were removed.

Table 21.8 Revised diagnostic criteria of HRS [157]

• Cirrhosis with ascites
• Serum creatinine > 1.5 mg/dL
• No improvement in serum creatinine after 2 days of diuretic withdrawal and volume expansion with albumin (albumin 1 g/kg of body weight per day up to a maximum of 100 g/day)
• Absence of Shock
• No current or recent treatment with nephrotoxic drugs
• Absence of proteinuria >500 mg/day, microhematuria (>50 RBCs per HPF), and/or abnormal renal ultrasound

In general, other causes of AKI must be excluded in order to make the diagnosis of HRS. Diuretic withdrawal and volume expansion are used to exclude a prerenal cause. The absence of shock and nephrotoxic drugs decreases the likelihood of ATN or acute interstitial nephritis (AIN). Acute glomerular diseases seen in cirrhotic patients, such as cryoglobulinemia, membranoproliferative glomerulonephritis (MPGN), or Hepatitis C related membranous glomerulonephritis, can be excluded by the absence of significant proteinuria or hematuria.

The original diagnostic criteria contained minor criteria, which are not needed to make the diagnosis of HRS but may be helpful in supporting the diagnosis. These minor criteria included: serum sodium less than 130 mEq/L, urine osmolality >serum osmolality, urine sodium <10 mEq/L, and urine output <500 ml/day. Low urine sodium and relatively high urine osmolality are seen in renal hypoperfusion states with functioning tubules. These markers were originally used to distinguish between ATN and HRS, yet low sensitivity and specificity limited their diagnostic accuracy.

Differential Diagnosis

The differential diagnosis for AKI in patients with cirrhosis (Table 21.9) includes all the causes of AKI described in detail throughout this section. Intra-abdominal hypertension and abdominal compartment syndrome perhaps deserve more discussion as they pertain to patients with chronic ascites.

Intra-Abdominal Hypertension

Intra-abdominal pressure (IAP) is a steady-state pressure concealed within the abdominal cavity. Normal IAP is 5–7 mmHg, yet in morbid obesity normal values can be as high as 9–14 mm Hg [171]. IAP typically is expressed in mmHg; however, bladder pressure measurements are in cmH_2O, necessitating conversion (1 mmHg = 1.36 cmH_2O).

Intra-abdominal hypertension (IAH) is defined by a sustained or repeated pathologic increase in IAP ≥ 12 mmHg. An Intra-abdominal pressure >20 mmHg with associated new organ dysfunction/failure defines abdominal compartment syndrome (ACS). Because of its location deep within the posterior retroperitoneal space, the kidney is especially vulnerable to the deleterious effects of increased IAP resulting in AKI [170]. The pathophysiology of AKI in IAH/ACS is still not known but proposed mechanisms include increases in pressure transmitted directly to the kidney itself, or increased renal venous pressure transmitted to the peritubular capillaries decreasing solute reabsorption and glomerular filtration rate through tubular glomerular feedback.

Abdominal compartment syndrome is seen primarily in the critical care setting, often following an abdominal surgery. However, high intra-abdominal pressures may contribute to AKI in patients with cirrhosis and can act to precipitate HRS or independently cause AKI.

Management

Management for HRS differs between type 1 and type 2, and given the dismal prognosis of patients with type 1 HRS, aggressive therapy usually is indicated only for patients who are waiting for a

Table 21.9 Causes of acute kidney injury in patients with cirrhosis[a]

Prerenal causes	Intravascular volume depletion and hypotension
	Gastrointestinal fluid loss (NG suction) or pooling of fluid (pancreatitis, bowel disease)
	Trauma, surgery, or burns
Decreased effective intravascular volume	Congestive heart failure or other cause of decreased cardiac output
	Nephrotic syndrome
	Infection—sepsis (potential source SBP)
	Anaphylaxis, Anesthetic agents
HRS Types 1 and 2	
Intra-abdominal hypertension	Abdominal compartment syndrome
Atheroembolism	Renal artery or vein occlusion by thrombosis
Intrinsic causes	Tubular necrosis
	Ischemia (as a result of above mentioned prerenal cause)
	Toxic (as a result of drugs, organic solvents (CCl4, ethylene glycol), heavy metals (mercury, cisplatin), heme pigments (rhabdomyolysis), myeloma light chain, intravenous contrast
Interstitial nephritis	Related to drugs, infection, cancer, sarcoidosis
Postrenal causes	Upper urinary tract obstruction (ureteral obstruction from one or both kidneys)
	Lower urinary tract obstruction (bladder outlet obstruction)

[a]Adapted from Wadei et al. [156]

liver transplant or undergoing evaluation to determine candidacy for transplantation [156].

General management includes withholding diuretics, continuing a low sodium diet, initiating a less than 1 L/day free water restriction for hyponatremic patients, excluding other causes for AKI, and looking for precipitating factors (especially SBP). A therapeutic paracentesis is performed for patients with tense ascites in order to reduce abdominal pressures. Albumin is infused if >5 L of peritoneal fluid is removed to avoid precipitating volume contraction. Patients with type 2 HRS are typically less sick and can be managed as an outpatient. Patients with type 1 HRS, however, require inpatient care with frequent monitoring of fluid intake, chemistries, and urine output. Beyond general management there are four major therapeutic interventions: pharmacologic treatment with vasoconstrictors, TIPS, renal replacement therapy, and liver transplantation. Of these interventions, liver transplantation is the only one that positively affects long-term mortality.

Vasoconstrictor Therapy

Initial pharmacologic therapy was targeted at renal vasodilation, rather than vasoconstriction, in order to combat the renal vasoconstriction seen in HRS. However, studies involving renal vasodilators (dopamine, fenoldopam, and prostaglandins) and renal vasoconstrictor antagonists (saralasin, angiotensin-converting enzyme inhibitors, and endothelin antagonists) did not show any benefit, and pharmacologic attempts to target renal vasoconstriction in HRS have been largely abandoned [156].

Studies using vasoconstrictors designed to interrupt the splanchnic vasodilation have shown benefit and are now the most promising pharmacologic agents for managing HRS. Studied vasoconstrictors include vasopressin analogs (omipressin and terlipressin), somatostatin analog (octreotide), and the alpha adrenergic agonists (midodrine and norepinephrine). Terlipressin is the most studied vasoconstrictor and multiple small randomized trials [172] as well as a meta-analysis [173] showed improved renal function with reversal of HRS type 1 (serum creatinine <1.5 mg/dL for up to 15 days); though 3 month survival was unchanged [174]. Given these findings terlipressin with albumin infusion is considered first line therapy for HRS.

Terlipressin, however, is not available in all countries, including the United States. In these countries alternatives including vasopressin, midodrine, and octreotide have been used. Esrailian et al. [175] performed a retrospective study to support the efficacy of midodrine and octreotide. Of the 81 patients studied, 60 were treated with octreotide and midodrine and a significant difference in sustained creatinine reduction was reported as well as a 30 day reduction in mortality (43% vs. 71%) [175]. Without further data, midodrine and octreotide appear to be reasonable alternatives to terlipressin. Table 21.10 summarizes specific vasoconstrictor dosing.

Transjugular Intrahepatic Portosystemic Shunt

TIPS is a nonsurgical method of portal decompression previously used as an alternative therapy for cirrhotic patients bleeding from esophageal or gastric varices who do not respond to endoscopic and medical treatment. An interventional radiologist will place a side-to-side portacaval shunt that connects the portal and hepatic veins within the hepatic parenchyma. TIPS reduces portal pressure and returns some of the volume of blood

Table 21.10 Pharmacologic therapy for hepatorenal syndrome[a]

Therapy	Regimen and comments
Terlipressin	0.5–1 mg every 4–6 h intravenously, with an increase up to 2 mg every 4–6 h until serum creatinine decreases to 1–1.2 mg/dL; usual duration of therapy is 5–15 days
Midodrine	7.5 mg orally three times daily with an increase to 12.5 mg three times daily if needed; given in association with octreotide
Octreotide	100 μg subcutaneously three times daily with an increase to 200 μg three times daily if needed; given in association with midodrine
Albumin	Intravenous administration of albumin together with vasoconstrictor drugs (1 g of albumin/kg of body weight on day 1, followed by 20–40 g/day)

[a]Adapted from Gines and Schrier [167] with data from [173–180]

pooled in the splanchnic circulation to the systemic circulation [181].

Small prospective studies [182, 183] evaluating TIPS in HRS did show improved renal function as well as survival (Type 1 & 2 with 3 month survival of 81%) [183]. However, few patients with HRS are well enough to undergo the procedure. TIPS is contraindicated in advanced cirrhosis, which often accompanies HRS, since it can cause worsening liver failure and hepatic encephalopathy. It may benefit a select group of patients by prolonging survival long enough to receive a liver transplant or to avoid dialysis.

Renal Replacement Therapy

Initiation of dialysis is controversial in untreated patients who have HRS type 1 and are not candidates for liver transplantation because of the dismal chance of survival and the high morbidity and mortality rates associated with dialysis [156]. In a retrospective study by Keller et al. [184], 7 (44%) of 16 patients who had HRS and received renal replacement therapy survived compared with only 1 (10%) of 10 who did not receive dialysis. However, prolonged patient survival is incurred at the cost of increased morbidity and hospital stay, with 33% of the days gained spent in the hospital [185]. The decision to initiate dialysis in these patients should be individualized [156].

In patients awaiting a liver transplantation who have failed pharmacologic therapy or TIPS and have an indication for dialysis (intractable metabolic acidosis, volume overload, hyperkalemia), renal replacement therapy may be a reasonable option as a bridge to liver transplantation.

Liver Transplantation

Liver transplantation remains the best treatment for suitable candidates with HRS because it offers a cure to both the diseased liver and the renal dysfunction [156]. Following liver transplantation evidence of resolving HRS is present in the first month (but may be delayed up to 3 months) with return of renal sodium excretion and normalization of hemodynamic abnormalities [186, 187]. Long term renal function, however, may not normalize. In a study by Gonwa et al. [188], 7% of patients with HRS ultimately developed end stage renal disease compared with 2% in those without HRS.

Prognosis

The prognosis for patients with cirrhosis and renal failure is poor [155, 167]. The overall survival rate is approximately 50% at 1 month and 20% at 6 months, and HRS is associated with the worst prognosis [167]. Untreated type 1 HRS carries a grim prognosis: Mortality is as high as 80% in 2 weeks and only 10% of patients survive 3 months (see Fig. 21.2) [153, 154]. Patients with type 2 HRS have a much better median survival, approximately 6 months [189].

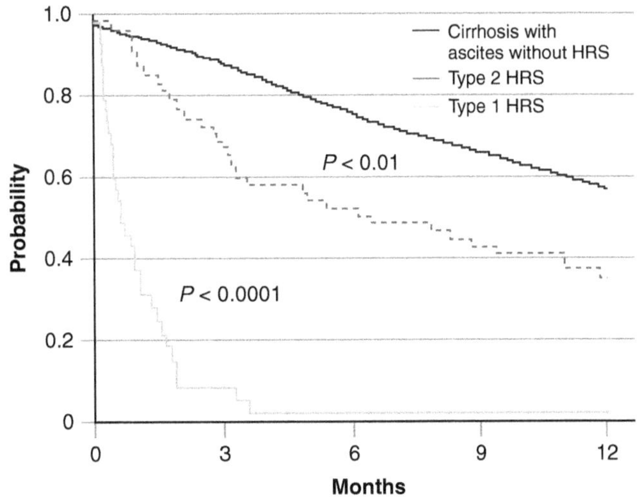

Fig. 21.2 Actuarial probability to survive in cirrhotic patients with different renal impairments: non-azotemic patients; patients with hepatic renal syndrome (HRS) type 2; and patients with HRS type 1. Adapted from Alessandria et al. [193]

Preventive Measures

Once HRS is diagnosed, little can be done to alter the 3–6 month mortality, aside from liver transplantation. Therefore, in patients at risk for developing HRS (advanced cirrhosis with refractory ascites), preventive measures should be considered. One strategy is to avoid potential precipitating factors of HRS type 1. Gines and Schrier [167] suggest that even the reduction of subclinical intestinal bacterial translocation reduces gut inflammation and ameliorates the hemodynamic abnormalities predisposing cirrhotic patients to develop HRS [190, 191]. Fernadez et al. showed that long-term administration of norfloxacin (400 mg per day) for primary SBP prophylaxis reduces the risk of HRS and improves survival [192]. Furthermore, once SBP is diagnosed, administration of albumin 1.5 g/kg on day 1 and 1 g/kg on day 3 reduces the risk of developing HRS [169]. Other preventive measures include judicious use of diuretics, rapidly correcting hypovolemia in gastrointestinal bleeding, and avoiding nonsteroidal anti-inflammatory drugs and aminoglycosides.

Revisiting Case 3

The patient's history, physical exam, and laboratory data fit with cirrhosis and hepatic encephalopathy. His creatinine on presentation is greater than two times his baseline and there is no history of volume loss or nephrotoxin use. The low blood pressure with a slightly widened pulse pressure and borderline tachycardia are consistent with the partially compensated low systemic vascular resistance physiology seen in advanced cirrhosis. He has both ascites and peripheral edema on exam, pointing away from profound volume contraction. There is no sign of overt infection with no fever, infectious symptoms, or elevated white blood cell count. His chemistry supports ongoing diuretic use with hypokalemia and mildly elevated bicarbonate, and the near hyponatremia is consistent with the relatively low renal perfusion state seen in cirrhosis causing chronic upregulation of vasopressin. His urine studies also support poor renal perfusion with functioning tubules given the high urine specific gravity and low urine sodium. Notably no blood or protein is detected on urinalysis, pointing away from intrinsic renal injury. At this point the patient has AKI (RIFLE injury by creatinine) that does not appear intrinsic but may be pre- or postrenal in cause. Though he is at risk for HRS, other causes of AKI must be excluded before making this diagnosis.

Case 3 Continued

The patient was admitted to the medical ward where his diuretic was held and potassium repleted. He underwent a paracentesis with removal of 3 L of clear yellow fluid. Albumin was started at 25 g every 8 h and a renal ultrasound was obtained showing normal sized kidneys without cysts, masses, or hydronephrosis. Over the next 2 days, he remained afebrile with stable blood pressures of 100s/50s mm Hg. His total intake and output was matched when including his paracentesis, yet his urine output dropped from 600 ml/day on day 1 to 400 ml/day on day 2. His serum blood urea nitrogen and creatinine trended up from admission (BUN/Cr of 38/1.8 on day 1–54/2.6 on day 2). His hemoglobin remained stable and after 2 days is 7.2 g/dL.

Now it is appropriate to diagnose his AKI as HRS. Despite 2 days of volume expansion with albumin, he is now oliguric with a worsened creatinine above 1.5 mg/dL, which effectively excludes prerenal AKI. There is no evidence of postrenal AKI with a normal renal ultrasound. There is no evidence of shock with stable blood pressures and hemoglobin.

The rapidity of his renal failure (less than 2 weeks) and rise in creatinine over 2.5 mg/dL is consistent with type 1 HRS and warrants initiation of a vasoconstrictor. It would also be reasonable to continue infusing albumin and to start norfloxacin at 400 mg daily in an attempt to reduce gut inflammation. If the patient develops tense ascites, a therapeutic paracentesis would be indicated to reduce intra-abdominal pressures.

Key Points

- Hepatorenal syndrome is a functional renal failure caused by intrarenal vasoconstriction which occurs in patients with end-stage liver disease and circulatory dysfunction. The circulatory dysfunction is characterized by splanchnic vasodilation with a relatively low and insufficient cardiac output [157].
- HRS may occur spontaneously with worsening liver function or secondary to a precipitating event such as a bacterial infection (most commonly SBP).
- Two types of HRS exist. Type 1 is a rapidly progressive renal failure with a median survival of 1 month, and type 2 is a moderate, steady renal failure with a median survival of 6 months.
- Current medical therapies for HRS including vasoconstrictors, albumin, TIPS, and RRT can prolong short-term survival but have not been shown to change long term survival (> 6 months).
- Preventive measures can improve short-term survival and include: albumin infusion in SBP, daily norfloxacin prophylaxis, nephrotoxin avoidance, and early reversal of hypovolemia from gastrointestinal bleeding.
- Liver transplant remains the only treatment of HRS that assures long-term survival.

Tumor Lysis Syndrome

Case 4

A 19-year-old man presents to the emergency room with 12 h of intense abdominal pain. He reports one week of nausea with non-bloody vomiting, lethargy, muscle cramps, and four pound weight loss in the past week despite abdominal swelling. He denies fever, chills, diarrhea, or the use of any medications. Physical exam reveals a thin, ill appearing young man with normal vital signs except for a heart rate of 112 beats per minute. His abdomen is firm and tense. Diffuse abdominal tenderness limits palpation, yet no rebound noted. His extremities have trace edema, yet his lungs are clear. No facial masses or peripheral adenopathy is discovered. Initial laboratory values include:

- *Renal function panel*: sodium 138 mEq/L, potassium 5.7 mEq/L, chloride 98 mEq/L, bicarbonate 22 mEq/L, blood urea nitrogen 44 mg/dL, creatinine 2.1 mg/dL, albumin 3.8 g/dL, calcium 7.6 mg/dL, phosphorus 6 mg/dL.
- *Complete blood count*: leukocyte count 18,000 cells/μL, hemoglobin 15.5 g/dL, platelet count 200,000 cells/μL.
- *Other laboratory data*: uric acid 9 mg/dL, lactate dehydrogenase 850 (normal 0–250 U/L), total bilirubin 0.9 mg/dL, alanine transaminase (ALT) 45 (normal 15–58 U/L).
- *Urinalysis*: specific gravity 1.020, no blood, 0–2 red blood cells per high power field, trace protein.

Electrocardiogram results are normal without T wave peaking or QRS prolongation. A computed tomography (CT) scan of the abdomen without contrast reveals multiple large abdominal masses in the ileum, stomach, and mesentery.

Introduction

Tumor lysis syndrome (TLS) is characterized by a constellation of metabolic derangements caused by massive and abrupt release of intracellular components into the blood following rapid lysis of malignant cells. It is typically seen after initiating cytotoxic therapy for hematologic malignancies with large tumor burden or cell counts as in acute lymphoblastic leukemia (ALL), Burkitt lymphoma, or acute myeloid leukemia (AML). The release of intracellular metabolites, including nucleic acids, proteins, phosphorus, and potassium, can overwhelm normal homeostatic mechanisms potentially leading to hyperuricemia, hyperkalemia, hyperphosphatemia, hypocalcemia, and uremia [194]. These metabolic derangements place patients at risk for AKI, cardiac arrhythmias, seizures, and even death.

Prevention and management consists primarily in identifying high risk patients, implementing appropriate prophylactic measures, and vigilant monitoring of electrolyte levels in patients undergoing chemotherapy. High risk patients may require more active therapies including rasburicase and dialysis.

Epidemiology

TLS occurs most frequently in patients with non-Hodgkin's Lymphoma (NHL), particularly Burkitt lymphoma. Other hematologic malignancies associated with TLS include acute myeloid leukemia (AML) and acute lymphoblastic leukemia (ALL). The syndrome is less frequently seen in chronic lymphocytic leukemia (CLL), indolent NHL, and promyelocytic leukemia. A multicenter retrospective study examined the incidence of hyperuricemia and TLS in 788 patients (433 adults, 322 children) with acute leukemia or NHL. Hyperuricemia was defined as >6.5 mg/dL in children and >7.5 mg/dL in adults. The overall incidence of hyperuricemia and TLS was 18.9% and 5.0% respectively. Rates were further reported for each hematologic malignancy: 14.7% and 3.4% in AML, 21.4% and 5.2% in ALL, 19.6% and 6.1% in NHL [195].

The incidence of renal complications in patients with TLS varies among reports reflecting differences in underlying malignancy, type and intensity of therapy, and patient characteristics [196]. In the above mentioned study by Annemans et al. [195], among the 5% of patients who developed TLS, 45% had AKI, 25% required dialysis, and 15% died as a result of TLS complications. In a study evaluating the efficacy and safety of rasburicase, 387 adults and 682 pediatric patients with malignancies presented either with or at risk for hyperuricemia and TLS. In this population AKI was noted in 7% of adults and 3% of pediatric patients on presentation, and the majority with AKI required dialysis (71% and 59%, respectively) [197]. Collectively, these data suggest that AKI is a common complication of TLS with incidence ranging from 7 to 45% in the adult population.

Pathophysiology

In malignancies with high proliferative rate, large tumor burden, and high sensitivity to chemotherapy, the initiation of cytotoxic chemotherapy, cytolytic antibody therapy, and/or radiation therapy can cause rapid lysis of tumor cells with a massive release of intracellular contents [194]. Tumor lysis can also occur in the absence of chemotherapy if the tumor burden is excessive and cell turnover is rapid. The release and subsequent catabolism of purine based nucleic acids can result in hyperuricemia. Both hyperuricemia and hyperphosphatemia have been implicated in causing AKI.

Hyperuricemia

Purines are catabolized to hypoxanthine; then xanthine oxidase facilitates further catabolism to uric acid (see Fig. 21.3). Uric acid is poorly soluble in water and solubility decreases with acidity; at a pH of 5 (the typical pH of urine), the solubility is 15 mg/dL [198]. Rapid tumor lysis and the resulting purine catabolism exceeds the renal clearance capacity of uric acid, which is normally 500 mg/day [199]. The precipitation of uric acid in renal tubules can lead to tubular obstruction and AKI. Crystal-independent causes of AKI from uric acid, even with mild increases (5.7±2 mg/dL), have been proposed and include renal vasoconstriction,

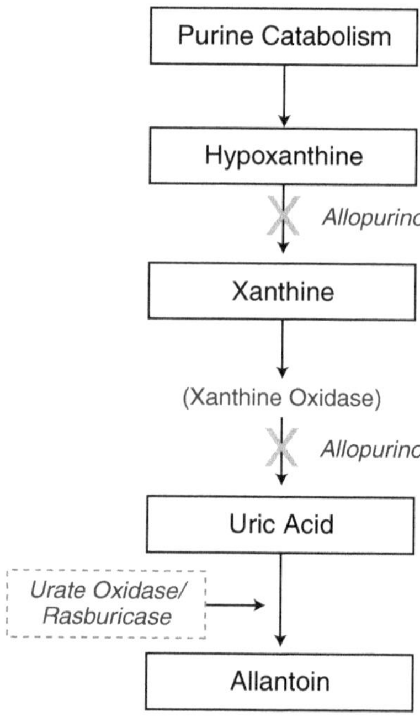

Fig. 21.3 Purine catabolism pathway. The enzyme urate oxidase exists in most other mammals. Rasburicase is a recombinant form of urate oxidase [194]

alterations in renal autoregulation through inhibition of nitric oxide synthase 1, decrease in endothelial cell nitric oxide, and stimulation of the renin–angiotensin system [200].

Hyperphosphatemia

The level of phosphorus in malignant cells can be up to four times the level found in normal cells and rapid release of these stores leads to hyperphosphatemia [194]. Renal injury from hyperphosphatemia is thought to be crystal related from calcium-phosphate precipitation in renal tubules. Risk of calcium-phosphate precipitation increases when the calcium phosphorus product exceeds 70 [201]. Hyperphosphatemia has also been implicated as the cause of AKI in acute phosphate nephropathy seen in patients receiving oral sodium phosphorus solution as a bowel preparation for colonoscopy [201].

Clinical Features

The clinical features of TLS result from the effects of each metabolic derangement. Adverse skeletal and cardiac muscle manifestations are seen in hyperkalemia including cardiac arrhythmias, weakness, and paresthesias [203]. Early symptoms of hyperphosphatemia include muscle cramps and lethargy; however, in severe cases nausea, vomiting, diarrhea, and seizures have been reported. Hypocalcemia, primarily caused by phosphorus binding, causes similar symptoms with muscle cramps, tetany, arrhythmias, and seizures. Increased serum uric acid is often asymptomatic, yet can precipitate gouty attacks.

Diagnosis

Diagnostic criteria for TLS were last modified by Cairo and Bishop in 2004 and are displayed in Table 21.11. The diagnosis of TLS can be made based on laboratory findings or clinical condition. Laboratory TLS is defined as having two or more of the serum values of uric acid, potassium, phosphorus, or calcium listed in Table 21.11 within a time frame extending from 3 days before to 7 days after the initiation of chemotherapy.

Table 21.11 Cairo-bishop definition of laboratory and clinical TLS [199]

Serum Values in Laboratory TLS	• Uric acid ≥8 mg/dL or 25% increase from baseline • Potassium ≥6 mEq/L or 25% increase from baseline • Phosphorus ≥6.5 mg/dL (children) or ≥4.5 mg/dL (adults) or 25% increase from baseline • Calcium ≤7 mg/dL or 25% decrease from baseline
Clinical TLS	• Serum creatinine ≥1.5 times the upper limit of normal for the age-adjusted normal range • Cardiac arrhythmia or sudden death • Seizure

Clinical TLS includes the presence of one or more clinical states from Table 21.11 that requires intervention. Although the Cairo and Bishop criteria are widely used, whether hypocalcemia should be included in the criteria is debated because it is a secondary abnormality to hyperphosphatemia [196].

Management and Preventive Measures

General principles for the management of patients at risk for or presenting with TLS are aggressive volume expansion, established treatments of hyperkalemia and secondary hypocalcemia, and preventive therapy for hyperuricemia.

Given the potential severity of TLS complications and the known causal relationship with oncologic therapies, preventive measures make up the core of management. Patients are stratified into low, intermediate, or high risk for developing TLS (outlined in Table 21.12). Guidelines from 2008 recommend that low risk patients undergo close monitoring with other preventive measures including volume expansion left up to clinical judgment; intermediate risk patients receive hydration with initial preventive hyperuricemic therapy using allopurinol (rasburicase can be used in pediatric patients); and high risk patients receive hydration and rasburicase [194].

Volume Expansion

Volume depletion can further increase uric acid or calcium-phosphate crystal precipitation in

Table 21.12 Patient risk stratification for developing TLS [194, 196]

High Risk	• *NHLs*: Burkitt lymphoma, Lymphoblastic lymphoma, B-ALL • *Acute Leukemias*: ALL with ≥100,000 WBC/μL, AML with ≥50,000 WBC/μL (monoblastic)
Intermediate Risk	• *NHL*: DLBCL • *Acute Leukemias*: ALL with 50,000–100,000 WBC/μL, AML with 10,000–50,000 WBC/μL • CLL with 10,000–100,000 WBC/μL (treated with fludarabine) • Other malignancies including CML, multiple myeloma, and solid tumors with rapid proliferation with expected rapid response to therapy
Low Risk	• *NHL*: Indolent NHL • *Acute Leukemias*: ALL with ≤50,000 WBC/μL, AML with ≤10,000 WBC/μL • CLL with ≤10,000 WBC/μL • Remainder of patients

NHL non-Hodgkin lymphoma, *B-ALL* B-cell acute lymphoblastic lymphoma, *ALL* acute lymphoblastic leukemia, *AML* acute myeloid leukemia, *DLBCL* diffuse large B-cell lymphoma, *CLL* chronic lymphocytic leukemia, *CML* chronic myeloid leukemia

renal tubules. Volume expansion remains one of the most important interventions in patients at risk of or with TLS because it maintains renal blood flow and urine flow promoting urinary excretion of potassium, uric acid, and phosphate [204]. Recommended intravenous fluid use is at least twice maintenance fluid requirements started 24–48 h before induction therapy to maintain urine output of 3–5 ml/kg/h in children or 80–100 ml/m²/h in adults [196]. Intravenous fluid rates may need to be decreased to avoid volume overload in patients with heart failure, particularly in elderly patients. Patients with oliguria require early evaluation by a nephrologist to assist with fluid management and to determine the need for renal replacement therapy.

Hypouricemic Agents

Hyperuricemia may be the main contributor to AKI in TLS. In a study conducted in 100 adults with aggressive non-Hodgkin lymphoma, AKI was avoided by preventing hyperuricemia [205]. Two main therapeutic interventions are used to prevent or reduce serum uric acid levels, xanthine oxidase inhibition and urate oxidase introduction. Urinary alkalinization has been recommended in the past to reduce precipitation of uric acid crystals in the renal tubules; however, the higher urine pH caused an increase in calcium-phosphate crystal deposition [196]. This side effect combined with lack of efficacy data have led to the removal of urine alkalinization from the guidelines.

Allopurinol

Allopurinol in its active form, oxypurinol, acts as a competitive inhibitor of xanthine oxidase, seen in Fig. 21.3. Early studies following the introduction of allopurinol in 1965 demonstrated efficacy in reducing the incidence of uric acid—obstructive uropathy in patients at risk for TLS [206]. Historically the standard of care for TLS prevention was oral allopurinol with hydration. Recently, intravenous (IV) formulations of allopurinol have also been well tolerated and effective. In a study of 460 patients (210 pediatric and 250 adult) who were unable to take oral allopurinol, IV allopurinol use in the prophylactic setting prevented the rise of serum uric acid in 93% of adults and 92% of pediatric patients [207]. Allopurinol dosing is summarized in Table 21.13.

Table 21.13 Hypouricemic agent dosing [199]

Allopurinol	• *Oral*: 100 mg/m²/dose every 8 h (10 mg/kg/d divided every 8 h); maximum of 800 mg/d • *Intravenous*: 200–400 mg/m²/d in 1–3 divided doses; maximum of 600 mg/d • *Dose adjustments*: dose reduction of 50% or more in renal failure, reduce 6-mercaptopurine and/or azathioprine doses by 65–75% with concomitant allopurinol
Rasburicase	• *Intravenous*: 0.20 mg/kg/day in high risk patients, 0.15 mg/kg/day in intermediate risk patients, and 0.05–0.10 mg/kg/day in low risk patients • *Length of Treatment*: Average duration of therapy is 2 days but can range from 1 to 7 days [194] • *Contraindications*: glucose-6-phosphate dehydrogenase deficient patients, patients with a known history or anaphylaxis or hypersensitivity reactions

There are, however, several limitations to allopurinol use. Allopurinol acts to decrease uric acid production, yet it cannot actively reduce pre-existing high levels of serum uric acid. Therefore, allopurinol use is limited to prevention. Also, the inhibition of xanthine oxidase blocks the catabolism of xanthine and hypoxanthine, increasing their levels. High xanthine levels could lead to xanthine crystal precipitation in renal tubules, also contributing to acute obstructive uropathy. Lastly, allopurinol interacts with purine-based chemotherapeutic agents. It reduces the clearance of 6-mercaptopurine and azathioprine, which are frequently used in leukemia treatment. Allergic reactions to allopurinol can be severe and life-threatening.

Rasburicase

Most mammals possess the enzyme urate oxidase, which converts uric acid to allantoin. The urine solubility of allantoin is 5–10 times higher than uric acid and allantoin crystal precipitation is largely nonexistent. Humans, however, lack this enzyme due to a nonsense mutation in the coding region. A recombinant version of the enzyme has been created, namely, rasburicase.

Rasburicase, unlike allopurinol, is effective in reducing high uric acid levels because it acts to directly catabolize uric acid further into allantoin. In a phase 2 study of 131 patients aged less than 21 years with newly diagnosed leukemia or lymphoma, plasma uric acid levels were rapidly reduced, median decrease from 9.7 to 1 mg/dL after 4 h [208]. The efficacy was compared with allopurinol in a study of 275 adults with hematologic malignancies at risk of TLS where patients were randomly assigned to one of 3 arms (rasburicase, allopurinol, or rasburicase plus allopurinol) [209]. Normalization of plasma uric acid levels was superior (87% vs. 66%) and time to control of uric acid levels was shorter (4 h vs. 27 h) in the rasburicase arm than the allopurinol arm [209]. The current FDA approved rasburicase dose is 0.20 mg/kg/d for up to 5 days, yet several studies suggest that a shorter schedule may be sufficient to treat most patients. A median of three doses was sufficient in Groupe d'Etude des Lymphomes de l'Adulte Trial on Rasburicase Activity in Adult Lymphoma (GRAAL1) study [205]. Dosing recommendations are summarized in Table 21.13. It is important to note when following plasma uric acid levels in patients receiving rasburicase, the enzyme remains active ex vivo and can falsely lower uric acid in blood samples not sent to the lab on ice.

The safety profile for rasburicase is good, though cases of hypersensitivity and methemoglobinemia have been reported with rasburicase [210, 211]. Rasburicase is also contraindicated in patients with glucose-6-phosphate dehydrogenase or catalase deficiencies [212]. Guidelines from 2008 recommend rasburicase use only in high risk patients or pediatric patients with intermediate risk of developing TLS. Yet following the results of the multicenter phase III study by Cortes et al. [209] in 2010 and the data linking even mild hyperuricemia with AKI, rasburicase use may expand and potentially replace allopurinol for the prevention and treatment of TLS.

Hemodialysis

Hemodialysis should be considered in every patient with TLS. In cases where metabolic derangements fail conservative therapy and renal function is worsening (rising creatinine and falling urine output) hemodialysis may be lifesaving. The efficacy of Rasburicase in rapidly lowering uric acid has reduced the need to dialyze for hyperuricemia; however, hyperphosphatemia, hyperkalemia, and symptomatic hypocalcemia remain as indications for dialysis. Furthermore, with ongoing cell lysis daily dialysis may be required until the metabolites stabilize.

Electrolyte Management

Electrolyte derangements seen in TLS include hyperkalemia, hyperphosphatemia, and hypocalcemia. In addition to the established measures for treating these disturbances, it is useful to restrict potassium and phosphorus intake and avoid medications that antagonize the renin–angiotensin–aldosterone system (RAAS). Administration of intravenous calcium should be restricted to symptomatic patients due to the risk of worsening calcium-phosphate precipitation and AKI.

Prognosis

Tumor lysis syndrome carries a poor overall prognosis. In the multicenter retrospective study by Annemans et al. [195] among the 5% of patients who developed TLS, 15% died as a result of TLS complications.

No data exist for the long-term consequences of AKI in patients with TLS [196]. It is known, however, that even mild AKI is associated with worsened outcomes. A review of hospitalized patients with 10–24% increase in serum creatinine had a relative risk of death of 1.8 compared to controls [213]. No studies to date have evaluated the renal recovery from urate nephropathy. In a study with acute phosphate nephropathy from oral sodium phosphate solution 19% developed end-stage renal disease and the remainder developed moderate chronic kidney disease [202].

Case 4 Discussion

The patient presented was found to have Burkitt lymphoma, a highly aggressive B-cell neoplasm. Rapid tumor growth is accompanied by tumor cell death indicated by the high lactate dehydrogenase (LDH) level. Where TLS is frequently seen following oncologic therapy, spontaneous tumor lysis syndrome can occur in aggressive hematologic malignancies, particularly Burkitt lymphoma. His initial presentation fit the definition of laboratory TLS by a uric acid ≥8 mg/dL and phosphorous ≥4.5 mg/dL (adults).

The patient's baseline creatinine is presumed to be normal; therefore a serum creatinine of 2.1 mg/dL would classify as AKI by a rise in creatinine >0.3 mg/dL. The high urine specific gravity, history of nausea and vomiting with weight loss, and tachycardia all point toward volume contraction, which acts synergistically with hyperuricemia and hyperphosphatemia to cause AKI.

Management for this patient would include strict intake and output monitoring with intravenous fluids infusing at greater than two times maintenance rate. If oliguria develops, nephrology should be consulted for fluid management. His diagnosis of Burkitt lymphoma places him in the high risk patient population for TLS and warrants initiation of rasburicase dosed at 0.20 mg/kg/d to be continued for up to 5 days. He should be placed on a phosphorous restricted diet and if phosphorous levels remain high, oral phosphorous binders started. Serum electrolytes should be checked at least daily and his potassium level kept below 6.0 mEq/L.

Key Points

- TLS is an oncologic and metabolic emergency with the known complication of AKI.
- AKI seen in TLS is primarily due to obstructive uropathy from uric acid and calcium-phosphate crystal precipitation; however, crystal-independent mechanisms for AKI from hyperuricemia have been identified and include renal vasoconstriction, alterations in renal autoregulation through inhibition of nitric oxide synthase 1, decrease in endothelial cell nitric oxide, and stimulation of the renin–angiotensin system.
- Maintaining adequate volume expansion is the first step in managing patients at risk for TLS.
- Rasburicase use may expand and potentially replace allopurinol for the prevention and treatment of TLS.
- Prior recommendations of urinary alkalinization have been abandoned due to the increase risk of calcium-phosphate crystal precipitation in the renal tubules.

Cardiorenal Syndrome

Case 5

A 65-year-old man with a history of heart failure, moderate tricuspid regurgitation, and normal renal function presents to the emergency room with 3 days of worsening dyspnea on exertion. He reports a 10 pound weight gain in the past week and a drop in urine output despite doubling his home furosemide dose to 40 mg twice a day. He denies fever, chills, vomiting, diarrhea, urinary urgency, exposure to over the counter pain medications, or recent hospitalizations. Physical exam reveals a chronically ill appearing man in mild respiratory distress. His vitals are normal except for a heart rate of 112 beats/min, respiratory rate of 24 breaths/min, and a blood pressure of 160/95 mm Hg. Neck veins are elevated with the presence of a hepatojugular reflex, a III/VI systolic murmur is present at the left lower sternal border, bilateral rales auscultated on lung exam, and 2 plus dependent edema to the waist palpated. Initial laboratory values include a serum sodium of 122 mEq/L, blood urea nitrogen 50 mg/dL, creatinine 1.7 mg/dL, albumin 3.9 g/dL, hemoglobin 8.5 g/dL, B-type natriuretic peptide (BNP) 1,020 pg/mL (BNP from 2 months ago was 300 pg/mL), troponin within normal limits. His urinalysis has a specific gravity of 1.024 and is without blood or protein. Electrocardiogram shows sinus tachycardia with a QRS interval of 130 ms and no ST segment or T wave changes. A portable chest x-ray is read as pulmonary edema.

Introduction

The heart and kidney interact to control blood pressure, extracellular fluid balance, and tissue perfusion. When one organ becomes dysfunctional the other organ may be affected. The term "cardiorenal syndrome" was introduced to define this interdependency of the kidney and the heart [214]. Cardiorenal dysregulation seen in the various forms of heart failure (HF) leads to cardiorenal syndrome (CRS) when therapy to relieve congestive symptoms of HF are limited by further decline in renal function [215]. A consensus conference of the Acute Dialysis Quality Initiative defined CRS as, "disorders of the heart and kidney whereby acute or chronic dysfunction in one organ may induce acute or chronic dysfunction of the other." [216]

Five subtypes of CRS have been described, and AKI is seen in types 1 and 3. While presenting a generalized overview of CRS, this section focuses on AKI injury from acute decompensated heart failure (ADHF), CRS type 1.

Epidemiology

The prevalence of symptomatic heart failure in the United States is estimated at 2% in those over 45 years of age with a lifetime risk of HF estimated at 20% [217, 218]. It is the leading cause of hospitalization in people over age 65 and accounts for one million hospitalizations annually [219]. Furthermore, kidney disease is common in this population. CKD stage III or worse exists in 40–50% of outpatients with HF and 60% of ADHF experience moderate renal insufficiency [220].

Pathophysiology

The CRS includes both kidney disease in HF and cardiovascular complications in the setting of CKD or AKI. The pathophysiology of these two broad categories is quite different and this review focuses on the mechanism of kidney injury seen in heart failure.

Kidney dysfunction in HF was originally thought to be due to impaired renal blood flow in the setting of depressed left ventricular systolic function or as a consequence of overdiuresis, yet recent investigations do not support decreased renal perfusion as the primary derangement in CRS [221]. Cardiac output did not correlate with baseline renal function in the ESCAPE (Evaluation Study of Congestive Heart Failure and Pulmonary Artery Catheterization Effectiveness) trial, a large trial of pulmonary artery catheter- guided management of 433 individuals admitted with ADHF [222]. Also, Gottlieb et al. have shown that 47% of patients admitted for ADHF had worsening renal function during the first 3 days of hospitalization, when patients were still hypervolemic [223]. Overdiuresis, therefore, cannot be implicated in the renal dysfunction seen in nearly half of ADHF admissions.

With a lack of data to support poor forward flow or reduced renal perfusion from diuresis as the primary determinant of the progressive renal failure in the HF population, interest has shifted toward venous congestion. Increased central venous pressures from sodium retention not only lead to symptoms of congested heart failure but also are likely an important cause of CRS. High renal venous pressure seen with congestion attenuates the gradient between afferent and efferent circulations which causes a decrease in renal blood flow. In fact, in a canine study by Winton, rising renal venous pressure limited urine formation and renal blood flow more than a reduction in arterial pressure [224]. A study by Mullens et al. of 145 patients with ADHF supports this finding. Patients who developed worsening renal function had significantly higher central venous pressures (18 vs. 12 mmHg; *P* 0.001) than those that did not, and venous congestion was a stronger predictor of worsening renal function than cardiac index [225]. Also, tricuspid regurgitation, as a marker of central venous pressure, has been correlated with renal dysfunction in HF patients. A linear relationship exists between the severity of tricuspid regurgitation and the degree of renal impairment [226]. In summary, these observations support increased renal venous pressure as one of the primary pathophysiological mechanism underlying CRS. Inflammatory mediators may also have important effects.

Clinical Features

CRS type 1 (for subtypes see Table 21.14) presents in patients with ADHF whose clinical presentation is dominated by symptoms of congestion and volume overload. Patients will complain of dyspnea on exertion, orthopnea, body swelling, weight gain, night time cough, fatigue, and decreased urine output or response to chronic diuretics. AKI in CRS type 1 is typically oliguric due not only to the sodium avid state of congestive heart failure but also to the decreased glomerular filtration rate (GFR) from high renal venous pressures.

Physical exam findings will also mirror signs of volume overload. Patients may have neck vein distention, rales, an S3 gallop, hepatojugular reflex, tachycardia, and hypertension. Although blood pressures in chronic HF patients are typically low, both registries of ADHERE (Acute Decompensated Heart Failure National Registry) and OPTIMIZE-HF (Organized Program to Initiate Lifesaving Treatment in Hospitalized Patients with Heart Failure) found mean arterial blood pressures ≥140 mmHg in patients with ADHF [227, 228]. Increased sympathetic stimulation and volume likely contribute to the hypertension.

Diagnosis

Variability in defining CRS as well as its broad inclusion of any disorder relating to the interdependence of the heart and kidney has prevented the development of established diagnostic criteria. To better define specific pathologic relationships between the heart and kidney, five subtypes have been described (see Table 21.14) [229]. AKI is seen in types 1 and 3. In type 1 CRS acute heart failure exacerbation causes AKI, while AKI leads to a cardiac disorder (arrhythmia, heart failure, or ischemia) in type 3 CRS.

The diagnosis of type 1 CRS requires that the AKI be caused by worsened heart function

Table 21.14 Definition of CRS [238]

CRS (general)	Pathophysiologic disorder of the heart and kidneys, whereby acute or chronic dysfunction in one organ induces acute or chronic dysfunction in the other
CRS Type 1 (acute CRS)	Abrupt worsening of cardiac function leading to acute kidney injury
CRS Type 2 (chronic CRS)	Chronic abnormalities in cardiac function (e.g., chronic congestive heart failure) causing progressive and permanent chronic kidney disease
CRS Type 3 (acute renocardiac syndrome)	Abrupt worsening of renal function (e.g., acute tubular necrosis or glomerulonephritis) causing acute cardiac disorders (e.g., heart failure, arrhythmia, and ischemia)
CRS Type 4 (chronic renocardiac syndrome)	Chronic kidney disease contributing to decreased cardiac function, cardiac hypertrophy, increased risk of adverse cardiovascular events, or all
CRS Type 5 (secondary CRS)	Systemic condition (e.g., diabetes mellitus and sepsis) causing both cardiac and renal dysfunction

(i.e., ADHF), and independent causes of AKI including obstruction, interstitial nephritis, tubular necrosis, and glomerular disease must be excluded. A correlation in the timing of the ADHF and AKI strongly supports the diagnosis. When the diagnosis of ADHF is in question, the B-type natriuretic peptide (BNP) can be a useful parameter to measure. Plasma BNP or pro-BNP levels increase with left ventricular mass, wall stress and filling pressure and are often elevated in ADHF; prior BNP values and trends are helpful when interpreting results.

There are currently no radiographic studies to assist in diagnosing CRS; however, quantification of renal vein blood flow by Doppler technique is a promising future modality.

Management

Management of CRS varies by type. AKI in the setting of ADHF, CRS type 1, will be discussed here. At present, no agents have been shown to directly improve renal function in patients with HF [227]. Management of ADHF in CRS type 1 presents some clinical challenges including avoiding further renal impairment and hypotension, achieving electrolyte balance, and managing diuretic resistance [214].

In CRS type 1 the main driver of the pathophysiology and symptomatology is congestion. The focus of treatment is relieving the congestion without perturbing the hemodynamics of the cardiorenal axis [230]. Current therapy includes diuretics, natriuretic hormones, aquaretics (arginine vasopressin antagonists), vasodilators, inotropes, and ultrafiltration.

Diuretics

Loop diuretics are the mainstay pharmacologic treatment for the management of ADHF and how they are administered does not appear to effect outcomes. A randomized controlled trial of 308 patients with ADHF, found no significant difference between route of administration (intravenous or oral) or dose (high or low) of loop diuretic in the change in renal function or patient symptoms [231]. Patients exhibiting diuretic resistance may benefit from co-administration of a thiazide diuretic 30–60 min before the loop diuretic.

Natriuretics

Nesiritide, a synthetic BNP, has been used and studied in ADHF patients during the last decade. It reduces cardiac filling pressure and improves dyspnea, yet there are safety concerns with its use related to worsened renal function [232]. Its effects as a potent vasodilator perhaps predispose it to renal injury from hypotension, especially in the setting of aggressive diuretic use. For this reason, its use has significantly decreased.

Inotropes

The use of inotropes like dobutamine or milrinone to improve hemodynamics and symptoms in ADHF remains controversial. For patients with ADHF who have evidence of end-organ hypoperfusion or diuretic resistance, but no frank hypotension, the use of inotropic agents is not well supported [214]. The largest registry of patients with ADHF to date demonstrated a higher mortality with intravenous inotrope therapy as compared with nitroglycerin or nesiritide therapy [233].

Aquaretics

As part of the pathologic state of congestion in heart failure, arginine vasopressin (AVP) is released nonosmotically and often leads to hyponatremia. In an effort to enhance fluid removal while correcting hyponatremia, V2 receptor antagonists have been used in ADHF patients. The Efficacy of Vasopressin Antagonism in Heart Failure Outcome Study with Tolvaptan (EVEREST) evaluated the efficacy and safety of tolvaptan added to optimal medical management in ADHF. There was no significant difference in all-cause mortality, cardiovascular death, hospitalization, or renal function between tolvaptan and placebo [234]. There was, however, a significant increase in urine output associated with the use of these drugs.

Ultrafiltration

Ultrafiltration, a dialysis modality to remove fluid, is often considered when patients remain volume overloaded despite maximal diuretic therapy. Its efficacy has been compared to loop diuretics in the UNLOAD trial. The ultrafiltration versus Intravenous Diuretics for Patients Hospitalized for Acute Decompensated Heart Failure (UNLOAD) trial involved 200 patients with ADHF and showed that ultrafiltration compared with diuretics alone improved weight loss at 48 h (5.0 vs. 3.1 kg, *P* 0.001) and reduced the rate of readmission to hospital at 90 days (18% vs. 32%, *P* 0.02) [235].

Prognosis

CKD represents one of the strongest predictors of morbidity and mortality in HF patients [236]. In their meta-analysis of HF studies with greater than or equal to 1 year follow up, Smith et al. reported a mortality rate of 51% in those with moderate to severe renal impairment versus 24% in those with normal renal function [237]. In-hospital mortality and length of stay increased with stage of CKD. Data from the ADHERE showed in-hospital mortality of 1.9% with a 5.3 day length of stay with normal renal function versus 7.6% and 7 days in CKD stage IV [228].

Case 5 Discussion

The presented patient fits the clinical picture of a patient with ADHF. His renal function was reportedly normal; therefore with a creatinine of 1.6 mg/dL he can be diagnosed with AKI. The absence of obstructive symptoms, an active urinary sediment, exposure to nephrotoxins (no hospitalizations or reported over the counter medication use), or a prerenal history, makes causes of AKI independent of ADHF less likely. His reported oliguria and lack of diuretic response fits well with CRS. AKI in the setting of ADHF is consistent with CRS type 1. His history of moderate tricuspid regurgitation perhaps increases the likelihood of CRS due to increased renal venous pressure.

Despite an elevated creatinine from baseline, management of this patient still targets relief of congestion with fluid removal using loop diuretics. If he fails to diurese with loop diuretics alone, then a thiazide should be added before considering ultrafiltration. Trials to date have not shown a benefit using aquaretics in patients like him, but may benefit the subset of patients with serum sodium levels below 120 mEq/L. Given this patient's hypertension an inotrope is not indicated.

Key Points

- CRS is a pathologic disorder arising from an interdependence between the heart and kidney.
- AKI is seen in CRS types 1 and 3, with type 1 resulting from ADHF.
- Decreased renal perfusion from low cardiac output or overdiuresis does not appear to cause CRS.
- CRS is thought to be caused by increased renal venous pressure as a result of worsened sodium retention and high intra-abdominal pressures.

References

1. Mehta RL, et al. Spectrum of acute renal failure in the intensive care unit: the PICARD experience. Kidney Int. 2004;66(4):1613–21.
2. Rybak MJ, et al. Prospective evaluation of the effect of an aminoglycoside dosing regimen on rates of observed nephrotoxicity and ototoxicity. Antimicrob Agents Chemother. 1999;43(7):1549–55.
3. Hatala R, Dinh T, Cook DJ. Once-daily aminoglycoside dosing in immunocompetent adults: a meta-analysis. Ann Intern Med. 1996;124(8):717–25.
4. Ford DM, et al. Apically and basolaterally internalized aminoglycosides colocalize in LLC-PK1 lysosomes and alter cell function. Am J Physiol. 1994;266(1 Pt 1):C52–7.
5. Schwertz DW, Kreisberg JI, Venkatachalam MA. Effects of aminoglycosides on proximal tubule brush border membrane phosphatidylinositol-specific phospholipase C. J Pharmacol Exp Ther. 1984;231(1):48–55.
6. Lopez-Novoa JM, et al. New insights into the mechanism of aminoglycoside nephrotoxicity: an integrative point of view. Kidney Int. 2011;79(1):33–45.
7. Hsu CH, Kurtz TW, Weller JM. In vitro uptake of gentamicin by rat renal cortical tissue. Antimicrob Agents Chemother. 1977;12(2):192–4.
8. Hammond TG, et al. Gentamicin inhibits rat renal cortical homotypic endosomal fusion: role of megalin. Am J Physiol. 1997;272(1 Pt 2):F117–23.

9. Zager RA, Bredl CR, Schimpf BA. Direct amphotericin B-mediated tubular toxicity: assessments of selected cytoprotective agents. Kidney Int. 1992;41(6):1588–94.
10. Burgess JL, Birchall R. Nephrotoxicity of amphotericin B, with emphasis on changes in tubular function. Am J Med. 1972;53(1):77–84.
11. Cheng JT, et al. Amphotericin B nephrotoxicity: increased renal resistance and tubule permeability. Kidney Int. 1982;22(6):626–33.
12. Heyman SN, et al. Chronic amphotericin nephropathy: morphometric, electron microscopic, and functional studies. J Am Soc Nephrol. 1993;4(1):69–80.
13. Llinas MT, et al. Role of angiotensin II in the renal effects induced by nitric oxide and prostaglandin synthesis inhibition. J Am Soc Nephrol. 1997;8(4): 543–50.
14. Lopez R, et al. Role of nitric oxide and cyclooxygenase-2 in regulating the renal hemodynamic response to norepinephrine. Am J Physiol Regul Integr Comp Physiol. 2003;284(2):R488–93.
15. Dunn MJ. Nonsteroidal antiinflammatory drugs and renal function. Annu Rev Med. 1984;35:411–28.
16. Rodriguez F, et al. Renal changes induced by a cyclooxygenase-2 inhibitor during normal and low sodium intake. Hypertension. 2000;36(2):276–81.
17. Perico N, Dadan J, Remuzzi G. Endothelin mediates the renal vasoconstriction induced by cyclosporine in the rat. J Am Soc Nephrol. 1990;1(1):76–83.
18. Lanese DM, Conger JD. Effects of endothelin receptor antagonist on cyclosporine-induced vasoconstriction in isolated rat renal arterioles. J Clin Invest. 1993;91(5):2144–9.
19. Scherrer U, et al. Cyclosporine-induced sympathetic activation and hypertension after heart transplantation. N Engl J Med. 1990;323(11):693–9.
20. Novick AC, et al. Detrimental effect of cyclosporine on initial function of cadaver renal allografts following extended preservation. Results of a randomized prospective study. Transplantation. 1986;42(2): 154–8.
21. Stirling C, et al. Diarrhoea, vomiting and ACE inhibitors:an important cause of acute renal failure. J Hum Hypertens. 2003;17(6):419–23.
22. Toto RD, et al. Reversible renal insufficiency due to angiotensin converting enzyme inhibitors in hypertensive nephrosclerosis. Ann Intern Med. 1991; 115(7):513–9.
23. Huerta C, et al. Nonsteroidal anti-inflammatory drugs and risk of ARF in the general population. Am J Kidney Dis. 2005;45(3):531–9.
24. Cantu TG, et al. Acute renal failure associated with immunoglobulin therapy. Am J Kidney Dis. 1995;25(2):228–34.
25. Ahsan N, et al. Intravenous immunoglobulin-induced osmotic nephrosis. Arch Intern Med. 1994; 154(17):1985–7.
26. Dickenmann M, Oettl T, Mihatsch MJ. Osmotic nephrosis: acute kidney injury with accumulation of proximal tubular lysosomes due to administration of exogenous solutes. Am J Kidney Dis. 2008;51(3): 491–503.
27. Zager RA. Rhabdomyolysis and myohemoglobinuric acute renal failure. Kidney Int. 1996;49(2):314–26.
28. Heyman SN, et al. Myoglobinuric acute renal failure in the rat: a role for medullary hypoperfusion, hypoxia, and tubular obstruction. J Am Soc Nephrol. 1996;7(7):1066–74.
29. Holt S, Moore K. Pathogenesis of renal failure in rhabdomyolysis: the role of myoglobin. Exp Nephrol. 2000;8(2):72–6.
30. Rossert J. Drug-induced acute interstitial nephritis. Kidney Int. 2001;60(2):804–17.
31. Baldwin DS, et al. Renal failure and interstitial nephritis due to penicillin and methicillin. N Engl J Med. 1968;279(23):1245–52.
32. Abraham PA, Keane WF. Glomerular and interstitial disease induced by nonsteroidal anti-inflammatory drugs. Am J Nephrol. 1984;4(1):1–6.
33. Clive DM, Stoff JS. Renal syndromes associated with nonsteroidal antiinflammatory drugs. N Engl J Med. 1984;310(9):563–72.
34. Warren GV, et al. Minimal change glomerulopathy associated with nonsteroidal antiinflammatory drugs. Am J Kidney Dis. 1989;13(2):127–30.
35. Tam VK, et al. Nephrotic syndrome and renal insufficiency associated with lithium therapy. Am J Kidney Dis. 1996;27(5):715–20.
36. Wood IK, Parmelee DX, Foreman JW. Lithium-induced nephrotic syndrome. Am J Psychiatry. 1989;146(1):84–7.
37. Richman AV, et al. Minimal-change disease and the nephrotic syndrome associated with lithium therapy. Ann Intern Med. 1980;92(1):70–2.
38. Sartelet H, et al. Sirolimus-induced thrombotic microangiopathy is associated with decreased expression of vascular endothelial growth factor in kidneys. Am J Transplant. 2005;5(10):2441–7.
39. Myers BD. Cyclosporine nephrotoxicity. Kidney Int. 1986;30(6):964–74.
40. Pham PT, et al. Cyclosporine and tacrolimus-associated thrombotic microangiopathy. Am J Kidney Dis. 2000;36(4):844–50.
41. Bennett CL, et al. Thrombotic thrombocytopenic purpura associated with clopidogrel. N Engl J Med. 2000;342(24):1773–7.
42. Medina PJ, Sipols JM, George JN. Drug-associated thrombotic thrombocytopenic purpura-hemolytic uremic syndrome. Curr Opin Hematol. 2001;8(5): 286–93.
43. Perazella MA, Moeckel GW. Nephrotoxicity from chemotherapeutic agents: clinical manifestations, pathobiology, and prevention/therapy. Semin Nephrol. 2010;30(6):570–81.
44. Perazella MA. Crystal-induced acute renal failure. Am J Med. 1999;106(4):459–65.
45. Chen SC, Nankivell BJ, Dwyer DE. Indinavir-induced renal failure. AIDS. 1998;12(4):440–1.
46. Jones PG, Beier-Hanratty SA. Acyclovir: neurologic and renal toxicity. Ann Intern Med. 1986;104(6):892.

47. Markowitz GS, Perazella MA. Acute phosphate nephropathy. Kidney Int. 2009;76(10):1027–34.
48. Sedlacek M, et al. Ciprofloxacin crystal nephropathy-a 'new' cause of acute renal failure. Nephrol Dial Transplant. 2006;21(8):2339–40.
49. Perazella MA, Markowitz GS. Bisphosphonate nephrotoxicity. Kidney Int. 2008;74(11):1385–93.
50. Markowitz GS, Fine PL, D'Agati VD. Nephrotic syndrome after treatment with pamidronate. Am J Kidney Dis. 2002;39(5):1118–22.
51. Barri YM, et al. Podocyte injury associated glomerulopathies induced by pamidronate. Kidney Int. 2004;65(2):634–41.
52. Letavernier E, et al. Sirolimus interacts with pathways essential for podocyte integrity. Nephrol Dial Transplant. 2009;24(2):630–8.
53. Gonzalez E, et al. Early steroid treatment improves the recovery of renal function in patients with drug-induced acute interstitial nephritis. Kidney Int. 2008;73(8):940–6.
54. Buysen JG, et al. Acute interstitial nephritis: a clinical and morphological study in 27 patients. Nephrol Dial Transplant. 1990;5(2):94–9.
55. Nash K, Hafeez A, Hou S. Hospital-acquired renal insufficiency. Am J Kidney Dis. 2002;39(5):930–6.
56. Hou SH, et al. Hospital-acquired renal insufficiency: a prospective study. Am J Med. 1983;74(2):243–8.
57. Guitterez NV, et al. Determinants of serum creatinine trajectory in acute contrast nephropathy. J Interv Cardiol. 2002;15(5):349–54.
58. Bellomo R, et al. Acute renal failure—definition, outcome measures, animal models, fluid therapy and information technology needs: the Second International Consensus Conference of the Acute Dialysis Quality Initiative (ADQI) Group. Crit Care. 2004;8(4):R204–12.
59. Mehta RL, et al. Acute kidney injury network: report of an initiative to improve outcomes in acute kidney injury. Crit Care. 2007;11(2):R31.
60. McCullough PA, et al. Epidemiology and prognostic implications of contrast-induced nephropathy. Am J Cardiol. 2006;98(6A):5K–13.
61. Kuhns LR, et al. The predicted increased cancer risk associated with a single computed tomography examination for calculus detection in pediatric patients compared with the natural cancer incidence. Pediatr Emerg Care. 2011;27(4):345–50.
62. Weisbord SD, et al. Incidence and outcomes of contrast-induced AKI following computed tomography. Clin J Am Soc Nephrol. 2008;3(5):1274–81.
63. Murphy SW, Barrett BJ, Parfrey PS. Contrast nephropathy. J Am Soc Nephrol. 2000;11(1):177–82.
64. Rudnick MR, Goldfarb S. Pathogenesis of contrast-induced nephropathy: experimental and clinical observations with an emphasis on the role of osmolality. Rev Cardiovasc Med. 2003;4 Suppl 5:S28–33.
65. McCullough PA, et al. Risk prediction of contrast-induced nephropathy. Am J Cardiol. 2006;98(6A):27K–36.
66. Manske CL, et al. Contrast nephropathy in azotemic diabetic patients undergoing coronary angiography. Am J Med. 1990;89(5):615–20.
67. Parfrey PS, et al. Contrast material-induced renal failure in patients with diabetes mellitus, renal insufficiency, or both. A prospective controlled study. N Engl J Med. 1989;320(3):143–9.
68. Rudnick MR, et al. Nephrotoxicity of ionic and nonionic contrast media in 1196 patients: a randomized trial. The Iohexol Cooperative Study Kidney Int. 1995;47(1):254–61.
69. Schwab SJ, et al. Contrast nephrotoxicity: a randomized controlled trial of a nonionic and an ionic radiographic contrast agent. N Engl J Med. 1989;320(3):149–53.
70. Davidson CJ, et al. Cardiovascular and renal toxicity of a nonionic radiographic contrast agent after cardiac catheterization. A prospective trial. Ann Intern Med. 1989;110(2):119–24.
71. Cigarroa RG, et al. Dosing of contrast material to prevent contrast nephropathy in patients with renal disease. Am J Med. 1989;86(6 Pt 1):649–52.
72. Lautin EM, et al. Radiocontrast-associated renal dysfunction: a comparison of lower-osmolality and conventional high-osmolality contrast media. AJR Am J Roentgenol. 1991;157(1):59–65.
73. Lautin EM, et al. Radiocontrast-associated renal dysfunction: incidence and risk factors. AJR Am J Roentgenol. 1991;157(1):49–58.
74. Rihal CS, et al. Incidence and prognostic importance of acute renal failure after percutaneous coronary intervention. Circulation. 2002;105(19):2259–64.
75. Solomon RJ, et al. Cardiac Angiography in Renally Impaired Patients (CARE) study: a randomized double-blind trial of contrast-induced nephropathy in patients with chronic kidney disease. Circulation. 2007;115(25):3189–96.
76. Nikolsky E, et al. Low hematocrit predicts contrast-induced nephropathy after percutaneous coronary interventions. Kidney Int. 2005;67(2):706–13.
77. McCullough PA, et al. Acute renal failure after coronary intervention: incidence, risk factors, and relationship to mortality. Am J Med. 1997;103(5):368–75.
78. Stolker JM, et al. Pre-procedural glucose levels and the risk for contrast-induced acute kidney injury in patients undergoing coronary angiography. J Am Coll Cardiol. 2010;55(14):1433–40.
79. McCarthy CS, Becker JA. Multiple myeloma and contrast media. Radiology. 1992;183(2):519–21.
80. Mehran R, et al. A simple risk score for prediction of contrast-induced nephropathy after percutaneous coronary intervention: development and initial validation. J Am Coll Cardiol. 2004;44(7):1393–9.
81. Sgura FA, et al. Mehran contrast-induced nephropathy risk score predicts short- and long-term clinical outcomes in patients with ST-elevation-myocardial infarction. Circ Cardiovasc Interv. 2010;3(5):491–8.
82. Thomsen HS. European Society of Urogenital Radiology (ESUR) guidelines on the safe use of

iodinated contrast media. Eur J Radiol. 2006; 60(3):307–13.
83. Tumlin J, et al. Pathophysiology of contrast-induced nephropathy. Am J Cardiol. 2006;98(6A):14K–20.
84. Morris TW, Katzberg RW, Fischer HW. A comparison of the hemodynamic responses to metrizamide and meglumine/sodium diatrizoate in canine renal angiography. Invest Radiol. 1978;13(1):74–8.
85. Russo D, et al. Early effects of contrast media on renal hemodynamics and tubular function in chronic renal failure. J Am Soc Nephrol. 1995;6(5):1451–8.
86. Tumlin JA, et al. Fenoldopam mesylate blocks reductions in renal plasma flow after radiocontrast dye infusion: a pilot trial in the prevention of contrast nephropathy. Am Heart J. 2002;143(5):894–903.
87. Heyman SN, et al. Radiocontrast agents induce endothelin release in vivo and in vitro. J Am Soc Nephrol. 1992;3(1):58–65.
88. Margulies KB, et al. Radiocontrast increases plasma and urinary endothelin. J Am Soc Nephrol. 1991;2(5):1041–5.
89. Cantley LG, et al. Role of endothelin and prostaglandins in radiocontrast-induced renal artery constriction. Kidney Int. 1993;44(6):1217–23.
90. Deray G, et al. A role for adenosine calcium and ischemia in radiocontrast-induced intrarenal vasoconstriction. Am J Nephrol. 1990;10(4):316–22.
91. Lee HT, et al. A1 adenosine receptor knockout mice are protected against acute radiocontrast nephropathy in vivo. Am J Physiol Renal Physiol. 2006;290(6):F1367–75.
92. Ribeiro L, et al. Evaluation of the nitric oxide production in rat renal artery smooth muscle cells culture exposed to radiocontrast agents. Kidney Int. 2004;65(2):589–96.
93. Schwartz D, et al. Role of nitric oxide (EDRF) in radiocontrast acute renal failure in rats. Am J Physiol. 1994;267(3 Pt 2):F374–9.
94. Agmon Y, et al. Nitric oxide and prostanoids protect the renal outer medulla from radiocontrast toxicity in the rat. J Clin Invest. 1994;94(3):1069–75.
95. Bakris GL, Burnett Jr JC. A role for calcium in radiocontrast-induced reductions in renal hemodynamics. Kidney Int. 1985;27(2):465–8.
96. Liss P, et al. Injection of low and iso-osmolar contrast medium decreases oxygen tension in the renal medulla. Kidney Int. 1998;53(3):698–702.
97. Liss P, Nygren A, Hansell P. Hypoperfusion in the renal outer medulla after injection of contrast media in rats. Acta Radiol. 1999;40(5):521–7.
98. Heyman SN, et al. Early renal medullary hypoxic injury from radiocontrast and indomethacin. Kidney Int. 1991;40(4):632–42.
99. Bakris GL, et al. Radiocontrast medium-induced declines in renal function: a role for oxygen free radicals. Am J Physiol. 1990;258(1 Pt 2):F115–20.
100. Zager RA, Johnson AC, Hanson SY. Radiographic contrast media-induced tubular injury: evaluation of oxidant stress and plasma membrane integrity. Kidney Int. 2003;64(1):128–39.
101. Moreau JF, et al. Tubular nephrotoxicity of water-soluble iodinated contrast media. Invest Radiol. 1980;15(6 Suppl):S54–60.
102. Fang LS, et al. Low fractional excretion of sodium with contrast media-induced acute renal failure. Arch Intern Med. 1980;140(4):531–3.
103. Liu Y, et al. The contrast medium volume to estimated glomerular filtration rate ratio as a predictor of contrast-induced nephropathy after primary percutaneous coronary intervention. Int Urol Nephrol. 2012;44(1):221–9.
104. Marenzi G, et al. Contrast volume during primary percutaneous coronary intervention and subsequent contrast-induced nephropathy and mortality. Ann Intern Med. 2009;150(3):170–7.
105. Kian K, et al. Safety of low-dose radiocontrast for interventional AV fistula salvage in stage 4 chronic kidney disease patients. Kidney Int. 2006;69(8):1444–9.
106. Barrett BJ, Carlisle EJ. Metaanalysis of the relative nephrotoxicity of high- and low-osmolality iodinated contrast media. Radiology. 1993;188(1):171–8.
107. Aspelin P, et al. Nephrotoxic effects in high-risk patients undergoing angiography. N Engl J Med. 2003;348(6):491–9.
108. Solomon R. The role of osmolality in the incidence of contrast-induced nephropathy: a systematic review of angiographic contrast media in high risk patients. Kidney Int. 2005;68(5):2256–63.
109. Reed M, et al. The relative renal safety of iodixanol compared with low-osmolar contrast media: a meta-analysis of randomized controlled trials. JACC Cardiovasc Interv. 2009;2(7):645–54.
110. McCullough PA, et al. A meta-analysis of the renal safety of isosmolar iodixanol compared with low-osmolar contrast media. J Am Coll Cardiol. 2006; 48(4):692–9.
111. Solomon R. REMEDIAL: a role for sodium bicarbonate in the prevention of contrast-induced nephropathy. Nat Clin Pract Cardiovasc Med. 2007;4(9):474–5.
112. Merten GJ, et al. Prevention of contrast-induced nephropathy with sodium bicarbonate: a randomized controlled trial. JAMA. 2004;291(19):2328–34.
113. Motohiro M, et al. A New protocol using sodium bicarbonate for the prevention of contrast-induced nephropathy in patients undergoing coronary angiography. Am J Cardiol. 2012;107(11):1604–8.
114. Weisbord SD, Palevsky PM. Prevention of contrast-induced nephropathy with volume expansion. Clin J Am Soc Nephrol. 2008;3(1):273–80.
115. Hoste EA, et al. Sodium bicarbonate for prevention of contrast-induced acute kidney injury: a systematic review and meta-analysis. Nephrol Dial Transplant. 2010;25(3):747–58.
116. Ozcan EE, et al. Sodium bicarbonate, *N*-acetylcysteine, and saline for prevention of radiocontrast-induced nephropathy. A comparison of 3 regimens for protecting contrast-induced nephropathy in patients undergoing coronary procedures. A single-center

prospective controlled trial. Am Heart J. 2007; 154(3):539–44.
117. Zoungas S, et al. Systematic review: sodium bicarbonate treatment regimens for the prevention of contrast-induced nephropathy. Ann Intern Med. 2009;151(9):631–8.
118. Vasheghani-Farahani A, et al. Sodium bicarbonate plus isotonic saline versus saline for prevention of contrast-induced nephropathy in patients undergoing coronary angiography: a randomized controlled trial. Am J Kidney Dis. 2009;54(4):610–8.
119. Kim SM, et al. Incidence and outcomes of contrast-induced nephropathy after computed tomography in patients with CKD: a quality improvement report. Am J Kidney Dis. 2010;55(6):1018–25.
120. Maioli M, et al. Sodium bicarbonate versus saline for the prevention of contrast-induced nephropathy in patients with renal dysfunction undergoing coronary angiography or intervention. J Am Coll Cardiol. 2008;52(8):599–604.
121. Brar SS, et al. Sodium bicarbonate vs sodium chloride for the prevention of contrast medium-induced nephropathy in patients undergoing coronary angiography: a randomized trial. JAMA. 2008;300(9):1038–46.
122. Mitchell AM, et al. Incidence of contrast-induced nephropathy after contrast-enhanced computed tomography in the outpatient setting. Clin J Am Soc Nephrol. 2010;5(1):4–9.
123. Trivedi H, et al. High-dose *N*-acetylcysteine for the prevention of contrast-induced nephropathy. Am J Med. 2009;122(9):874. e9–15.
124. Marenzi G, et al. *N*-acetylcysteine and contrast-induced nephropathy in primary angioplasty. N Engl J Med. 2006;354(26):2773–82.
125. Koc F, et al. Intravenous *N*-acetylcysteine plus high-dose hydration versus high-dose hydration and standard hydration for the prevention of contrast-induced nephropathy: CASIS-A multicenter prospective controlled trial. Int J Cardiol. 2012;155(3):418–23.
126. Tepel M, et al. Prevention of radiographic-contrast-agent-induced reductions in renal function by acetylcysteine. N Engl J Med. 2000;343(3):180–4.
127. Thiele H, et al. Impact of high-dose *N*-acetylcysteine versus placebo on contrast-induced nephropathy and myocardial reperfusion injury in unselected patients with ST-segment elevation myocardial infarction undergoing primary percutaneous coronary intervention. The LIPSIA-N-ACC (Prospective, Single-Blind, Placebo-Controlled, Randomized Leipzig Immediate PercutaneouS Coronary Intervention Acute Myocardial Infarction N-ACC) Trial. J Am Coll Cardiol. 2010;55(20):2201–9.
128. Ferrario F, et al. Acetylcysteine and non-ionic isosmolar contrast-induced nephropathy-a randomized controlled study. Nephrol Dial Transplant. 2009; 24(10):3103–7.
129. Durham JD, et al. A randomized controlled trial of *N*-acetylcysteine to prevent contrast nephropathy in cardiac angiography. Kidney Int. 2002;62(6): 2202–7.
130. Amini M, et al. *N*-acetylcysteine does not prevent contrast-induced nephropathy after cardiac catheterization in patients with diabetes mellitus and chronic kidney disease: a randomized clinical trial. Trials. 2009;10:45.
131. Kelly AM, et al. Meta-analysis: effectiveness of drugs for preventing contrast-induced nephropathy. Ann Intern Med. 2008;148(4):284–94.
132. ACT Investigators. Acetylcysteine for prevention of renal outcomes in patients undergoing coronary and peripheral vascular angiography: main results from the randomized Acetylcysteine for Contrast-induced nephropathy Trial (ACT). Circulation. 2011; 124(11):1250–9.
133. Moon SS, et al. Hemodialysis for elimination of the nonionic contrast medium iohexol after angiography in patients with impaired renal function. Nephron. 1995;70(4):430–7.
134. Baars HG, Schabel J, Weiss M. Contrast medium elimination by hemodialysis. Z Urol Nephrol. 1984;77(8):473–81.
135. Cruz DN, et al. Extracorporeal blood purification therapies for prevention of radiocontrast-induced nephropathy: a systematic review. Am J Kidney Dis. 2006;48(3):361–71.
136. Kawashima S, et al. Prophylactic hemodialysis does not prevent contrast-induced nephropathy after cardiac catheterization in patients with chronic renal insufficiency. Circ J. 2006;70(5):553–8.
137. Reinecke H, et al. A randomized controlled trial comparing hydration therapy to additional hemodialysis or *N*-acetylcysteine for the prevention of contrast medium-induced nephropathy: the Dialysis-versus-Diuresis (DVD) Trial. Clin Res Cardiol. 2007;96(3):130–9.
138. Bagshaw SM, Ghali WA. Theophylline for prevention of contrast-induced nephropathy: a systematic review and meta-analysis. Arch Intern Med. 2005; 165(10):1087–93.
139. Stone GW, et al. Fenoldopam mesylate for the prevention of contrast-induced nephropathy: a randomized controlled trial. JAMA. 2003;290(17): 2284–91.
140. Spargias K, et al. Iloprost prevents contrast-induced nephropathy in patients with renal dysfunction undergoing coronary angiography or intervention. Circulation. 2009;120(18):1793–9.
141. Wang A, et al. Exacerbation of radiocontrast nephrotoxicity by endothelin receptor antagonism. Kidney Int. 2000;57(4):1675–80.
142. Spargias K, et al. Ascorbic acid prevents contrast-mediated nephropathy in patients with renal dysfunction undergoing coronary angiography or intervention. Circulation. 2004;110(18):2837–42.
143. Jo SH, et al. *N*-acetylcysteine versus AScorbic acid for preventing contrast-Induced nephropathy in patients with renal insufficiency undergoing coronary angiography NASPI study-a prospective randomized controlled trial. Am Heart J. 2009;157(3): 576–83.

144. Boscheri A, et al. Failure of ascorbic acid to prevent contrast-media induced nephropathy in patients with renal dysfunction. Clin Nephrol. 2007;68(5):279–86.
145. Zhang T, et al. Statins for the Prevention of Contrast-Induced Nephropathy: A Systematic Review and Meta-Analysis. Am J Nephrol. 2011;33(4):344–51.
146. Morikawa S, et al. Renal protective effects and the prevention of contrast-induced nephropathy by atrial natriuretic peptide. J Am Coll Cardiol. 2009;53(12):1040–6.
147. Dangas G, et al. Contrast-induced nephropathy after percutaneous coronary interventions in relation to chronic kidney disease and hemodynamic variables. Am J Cardiol. 2005;95(1):13–9.
148. Levy EM, Viscoli CM, Horwitz RI. The effect of acute renal failure on mortality. A cohort analysis. JAMA. 1996;275(19):1489–94.
149. Gruberg L, et al. The prognostic implications of further renal function deterioration within 48 h of interventional coronary procedures in patients with pre-existent chronic renal insufficiency. J Am Coll Cardiol. 2000;36(5):1542–8.
150. Gruberg L, et al. Acute renal failure requiring dialysis after percutaneous coronary interventions. Catheter Cardiovasc Interv. 2001;52(4):409–16.
151. Solomon RJ, et al. Contrast-induced nephropathy and long-term adverse events: cause and effect? Clin J Am Soc Nephrol. 2009;4(7):1162–9.
152. Subramanian S, et al. Economic burden of contrast-induced nephropathy: implications for prevention strategies. J Med Econ. 2007;10(2):119–34.
153. Gines A, Escorsell A, Gines P, Salo J, Jimenez W, Inglada L, Navasa M, Claria J, Rimola A, Arroyo V, et al. Incidence, predictive factors, and prognosis of the hepatorenal syndrome in cirrhosis with ascites. Gastroenterology. 1993;105:229–36.
154. Arroyo V, Gines P, Gerbes AL, Dudley FJ, Gentilini P, Laffi G, Reynolds TB, Ring-Larsen H, Scholmerich J. Definition and diagnostic criteria of refractory ascites and Hepatorenal syndrome in cirrhosis. International Ascites Club. Hepatology. 1996;23:164–76.
155. Moreau R, Durand F, Poynard T, Duhamel C, Cervoni JP, Ichai P, Abergel A, Halimi C, Pauwels M, Bronowicki JP, et al. Terlipressin in patients with cirrhosis and type 1 hepatorenal syndrome: A retrospective multicenter study. Gastroenterology. 2002;122:923–30.
156. Wadei H, Mai M, Ahsan N, Gonwa T. Hepatorenal syndrome: pathophysiology and management. Clin J Am Soc Nephrol. 2006;1:1066–79.
157. Salerno F, Gerbes A, Gines P, et al. Diagnosis, prevention, and treatment of hepatorenal syndrome in cirrhosis. Gut. 2007;56:1310–8.
158. Epstein M, Berk DP, Hollenberg NK, Adams DF, Chalmers TC, Abrams HL, Merrill JP. Renal failure in the patient with cirrhosis. The role of active vasoconstriction. Am J Med. 1970;49:175–85.
159. Kostreva DR, Castaner A, Kampine JP. Reflex effects of hepatic baroreceptors on renal and cardiac sympathetic nerve activity. Am J Physiol. 1980;238: R390–234.
160. Levy M, Wexler MJ. Hepatic denervation alters first-phase urinary sodium excretion in dogs with cirrhosis. Am J Physiol. 1987;253:F664–71.
161. Martin PY, Gines P, Schrier RW. Nitric oxide as a mediator of hemodynamic abnormalities and sodium and water retention in cirrhosis. N Engl J Med. 1998;339:533–41.
162. Mitchell JA, Kohlhaas KL, Sorrentino R, Warner TD, Murad F, Vane JR. Induction by endotoxin of nitric oxide synthase in the rat mesentery: Lack of effect on action of vasoconstrictors. Br J Pharmacol. 1993;109:265–70.
163. Schrier RW, Arroyo V, Bernardi M, Epstein M, Henriksen JH, Rodes J. Peripheral arterial vasodilatation hypothesis: a proposal for the initiation of renal sodium and water retention in cirrhosis. Hepatology. 1988;8:1151–7.
164. Martin PY, Gines P, Schrier RW. Nitric oxide as a mediator of hemodynamic abnormalities and sodium and water retention in cirrhosis. N Engl J Med. 1998;339:533–41.
165. Bosch J, Abraldes JG, Berzigotti A, Garcia-Pagan JC. Portal hypertension and gastrointestinal bleeding. Semin Liver Dis. 2008;28:3–25.
166. Ros J, Claria J, To-Figueras J, et al. Endogenous cannabinoids: a new system involved in the homeostasis of arterial pressure in experimental cirrhosis in the rat. Gastroenterology. 2002;122:85–93.
167. Gines P, Schrier R. Renal failure in cirrhosis. NEJM. 2009;361:1279–90.
168. Follo A, Llovet JM, Navasa M, Planas R, Forns X, Francitorra A, Rimola A, Gassull MA, Arroyo V, Rodes J. Renal impairment after spontaneous bacterial peritonitis in cirrhosis: Incidence, clinical course, predictive factors and prognosis. Hepatology. 1994;20:1495–501.
169. Sort P, Navasa M, Arroyo V, Aldeguer X, Planas R, Ruizdel-Arbol L, Castells L, Vargas V, Soriano G, Guevara M, Gines P, Rodes J. Effect of intravenous albumin on renal impairment and mortality in patients with cirrhosis and spontaneous bacterial peritonitis. N Engl J Med. 1999;341:403–9.
170. De Waele J, DeLaet I, Kirkpatrick A, et al. Intra-abdominal hypertension and abdominal compartment syndrome. Am J Kidney Dis. 2011;57: 159–69.
171. De Keulenaer BL, De Waele JJ, Powell B, Malbrain ML. What is normal intra-abdominal pressure and how is it affected by positioning, body mass and positive end-expiratory pressure? Intensive Care Med. 2009;35:969–76.
172. Magan A, Khalil A, Ahmed M. Terlipressin and Hepatorenal syndrome: What is important for nephrologists and hepatologists. World J Gastroenterol. 2010;16:5139–47.
173. Gludd L, Kjaer M, Christensen E. Terlipressin for Hepatorenal syndrome. Cochrane Database Syst Rev. 2006;4:CD005162.

174. Martín-Llahí M, Pépin MN, Guevara M, Díaz F, Torre A, Monescillo A, Soriano G, Terra C, Fábrega E, Arroyo V, Rodés J, Ginès P. Terlipressin and albumin vs. albumin in patients with cirrhosis and hepatorenal syndrome: a randomized study. Gastroenterology. 2008;134:1352–9.
175. Esrailian E, Pantangco E, Kyulo N, et al. Octreotide/midodrine therapy significantly improves renal function and 30-day survival in patients with Type 1 hepatorenal syndrome. Dig Dis Sci. 2007;57:742–8.
176. Fabrizi F, Dixit V, Martin P. Metaanalysis: terlipressin therapy for hepatorenal syndrome. Aliment Pharmacol Ther. 2006;24:935–44.
177. Sanyal AJ, Boyer T, Garcia-Tsao G, et al. A randomized, prospective, doubleblind, placebo-controlled study of terlipressin for type 1 hepatorenal syndrome. Gastroenterology. 2008;134:1360–8.
178. Angeli P, Volpin R, Gerunda G, et al. Reversal of type 1 hepatorenal syndrome with the administration of midodrine and octreotide. Hepatology. 1999;29:1690–7.
179. Duvoux C, Zanditenas D, et al. Effects of noradrenalin and albumin in patients with type I hepatorenal syndrome: a pilot study. Hepatology. 2002;36:374–80.
180. Wong F, Pantea L, Sniderman K. Midodrine, octreotide, albumin and TIPS in selected patients with cirrhosis and type 1 hepatorenal syndrome. Hepatology. 2004;40:55–64.
181. Ng C, Chan M, Tai M, Lam C. Hepatorenal syndrome. Clin Biochem Rev. 2007;28:11–7.
182. Guevara M, Gines P, Bandi JC, Gilabert R, Sort P, Jimenez W, Garcia-Pagan JC, Bosch J, Arroyo V, Rodes J. Transjugular intrahepatic portosystemic shunt in Hepatorenal syndrome: Effects on renal function and vasoactive systems. Hepatology. 1998;28:416–22.
183. Brensing KA, Textor J, Perz J, Schiedermaier P, Raab P, Strunk H, Klehr HU, Kramer HJ, Spengler U, Schild H, Sauerbruch T. Long term outcome after transjugular intrahepatic portosystemic stent-shunt in non-transplant cirrhotics with hepatorenal syndrome: A phase II study. Gut. 2000;47:288–95.
184. Keller F, Heinze H, Jochimsen F, Passfall J, Schuppan D, Buttner P. Risk factors and outcome of 107 patients with decompensated liver disease and acute renal failure (including 26 patients with hepatorenal syndrome): the role of hemodialysis. Ren Fail. 1995;17:135–46.
185. Capling RK, Bastani B. The clinical course of patients with type 1 hepatorenal syndrome maintained on hemodialysis. Ren Fail. 2004;26:563–8.
186. Navasa M, Feu F, Garcia-Pagan JC, Jimenez W, Llach J, Rimola A, Bosch J, Rodes J. Hemodynamic and humoral changes after liver transplantation in patients with cirrhosis. Hepatology. 1193;17:355–60.
187. Piscaglia F, Zironi G, Gaiani S, Mazziotti A, Cavallari A, Gramantieri L, Valgimigli M, Bolondi L. Systemic and splanchnic hemodynamic changes after liver transplantation for cirrhosis: a long-term prospective study. Hepatology. 1999;30:58–64.
188. Gonwa TA, Klintmalm GB, Levy M, Jennings LS, Goldstein RM, Husberg BS. Impact of pretransplant renal function on survival after liver transplantation. Transplantation. 1995;59:361–5.
189. Gines P, Guevara M, Arroyo V, Rodes J. Hepatorenal syndrome. Lancet. 2003;362:1819–27.
190. Chin-Dusting JP, Rasaratnam B, Jennings GL, Dudley FJ. Effect of fluoroquinolone on the enhanced nitric oxide-induced peripheral vasodilation seen in cirrhosis. Ann Intern Med. 1997;127:985–8.
191. Rasaratnam B, Kaye D, Jennings G, Dudley F, Chin-Dusting J. The effect of selective intestinal decontamination on the hyperdynamic circulatory state in cirrhosis: a randomized trial. Ann Intern Med. 2003;139:186–93.
192. Fernandez J, Navasa M, Planas R, et al. Primary prophylaxis of spontaneous bacterial peritonitis delays Hepatorenal syndrome and improves survival in cirrhosis. Gastroenterology. 2007;133:818–24.
193. Alessandria C, Ozdogan O, Guevara M, et al. MELD score and clinical type predict prognosis in hepatorenal syndrome: relevance to liver transplantation. Hepatology. 2005;41:1282–9.
194. Coiffier B, Altman A, Pui C, Younes A, Cairo M. Guidelines for the management of pediatric and adult tumor lysis syndrome: an evidence-based review. J Clin Oncol. 2008;26:2767–78.
195. Annemans L, Moeremans K, Lamotte M, et al. Incidence, medical resource utilisation and costs of hyperuricemia and tumour lysis syndrome in patients with acute leukaemia and non-Hodgkin's lymphoma in four European countries. Leuk Lymphoma. 2002;44:77–83.
196. Abu-Alfa A, Younes A. Tumor lysis syndrome and acute kidney injury: evaluation, prevention, and management. Am J Kid Dis. 2010;55:S1–13.
197. Jeha S, Kantarjian H, Irwin D, et al. Efficacy and safety of rasburicase, a recombinant urate oxidase (Elitek), in the management of malignancy-associated hyperuricemia in pediatric and adult patients: final results of a multicenter compassionate use trial. Leukemia. 2005;19:34–8.
198. Wossmann W, Schrappe M, Meyer U, et al. Incidence of tumor lysis syndrome in children with advanced stage Burkitt's lymphoma/leukemia before and after introduction of prophylactic use of urate oxidase. Ann Hematol. 2003;82:160–5.
199. Cairo MS, Bishop M. Tumour lysis syndrome: new therapeutic strategies and classification. Br J Haematol. 2004;127:3–11.
200. Roncal CA, Mu W, Croker B, et al. Effect of elevated serum uric acid on cisplatin-induced acute renal failure. Am J Physiol Renal Physiol. 2007;292:F116–22.
201. Nomdedeu J, Martino R, Sureda A, et al. Acute tumor lysis syndrome complicating conditioning therapy for bone marrow transplantation in a patient with chronic lymphocytic leukemia. Bone Marrow Transplant. 1994;13:659–60.
202. Markowitz GS, Stokes MB, Radhakrishnan J, D'Agati VD. Acute phosphate nephropathy follow-

ing oral sodium phosphate bowel purgative: an underrecognized cause of chronic renal failure. J Am Soc Nephrol. 2005;16:3389–96.
203. Davidson MB, Thakkar S, Hix JK, Bhandarkar ND, Wong A, Schreiber MJ. Pathophysiology, clinical consequences, and treatment of tumor lysis syndrome. Am J Med. 2004;116:546–54.
204. Conger JD, Falk SA. Intrarenal dynamics in the pathogenesis and prevention of acute urate nephropathy. J Clin Invest. 1977;59:786–93.
205. Coiffier B, Mounier N, Bologna S, et al. Groupe d'Etude des Lymphomes de l'Adulte Trial on Rasburicase Activity in Adult Lymphoma. Efficacy and safety of rasburicase (recombinant urate oxidase) for the prevention and treatment of hyperuricemia during induction chemotherapy of aggressive non-Hodgkin's lymphoma: results of the GRAAL1 (Groupe d'Etude des Lymphomes de l'Adulte Trial on Rasburicase Activity in Adult Lymphoma) study. J Clin Oncol. 2003;21:4402–6.
206. DeConti RC, Calabresi P. Use of allopurinol for prevention and control of hyperuricemia in patients with neoplastic disease. N Engl J Med. 1966;274:481–6.
207. Smalley RV, Guaspari A, Haase-Statz S, et al. Allopurinol: Intravenous use for prevention and treatment of hyperuricemia. J Clin Oncol. 2000;18:1758–63.
208. Pui C-H, Mahmoud HH, Wiley JM, et al. Recombinant urate oxidase for the prophylaxis or treatment of Hyperuricemia in patients with leukemia or lymphoma. J Clin Oncol. 2001;19:697–704.
209. Cortes J, Moore J, Maziarz R, Wetzler M, Craig M, et al. Control of plasma uric acid in adults at risk for tumor lysis syndrome: efficacy and saftey of rasburicase alone and rasburicase followed by allopurinol compared with allopurinol alone—results of a multicenter phase III study. J Clin Oncol. 2010;28: 4207–13.
210. Browning LA, Kruse JA. Hemolysis and methemoglobinemia secondary to rasburicase administration. Ann Pharmacother. 2005;39:1932–5.
211. Borinstein SC, Xu M, Hawkins DS. Methemoglobinemia and hemolytic anemia caused by rasburicase administration in a newly diagnosed child with Burkitt lymphoma/leukemia [letter]. Pediatr Blood Cancer. 2008;50:189.
212. Ducros J, Saingra S, Rampal M, et al. Hemolytic anemia due to G6PD deficiency and urate oxidase in a kidney-transplant patient. Clin Nephrol. 1991;35:89–90.
213. Coca SG, Peixoto AJ, Garg AX, Krumholz HM, Parikh CR. The prognostic importance of a small acute decrement in kidney function in hospitalized patients: a systematic review and meta-analysis. Am J Kidney Dis. 2007;50:712–20.
214. Sarraf M, Masoumi A, Schrier R. Cardiorenal syndrome in acute decompensated heart failure. Clin J Am Soc Nephrol. 2009;4:2013–26.
215. NHLBI Working Group: Cardio-Renal Connections in Heart Failure and Cardiovascular Disease. Available at http://www.nhlbi.nih.gov/meetings/workshops/cardiorenal-hf-hd.htm. Accessed August 2004
216. Ronco C, McCullough P, Anker SD, et al. Cardiorenal syndromes: report from the consensus conference of the acute dialysis quality initiative. Eur Heart J. 2010;31:703–11.
217. Redfield MM, Jacobsen SJ, Burnett JC, et al. Burden of systolic and diastolic ventricular dysfunction in the community: appreciating the scope of the heart failure epidemic. JAMA. 2003;289:194–202.
218. Lloyd-Jones DM, Larson MG, Leip EP, et al. Lifetime risk for developing congestive heart failure: the Framingham heart study. Circulation. 2002; 106:3068–72.
219. Smith GL, Lichtman JH, Bracken MB, et al. Renal impairment and outcomes in heart failure. Systematic review and meta-analysis. J Am Coll Cardiol. 2006;47:1987–96.
220. Mentz R, Lewis E. Epidemiology of cardiorenal syndrome. Cardiol Clin. 2011;29:301–14.
221. Bock J, Gottlieb S. Cardiorenal syndrome new perspectives. Circulation. 2010;21:2592–600.
222. Nohria A, Hasselblad V, Stebbins A, Pauly DF, Fonarow GC, Shah M, Yancy CW, Califf RM, Stevenson LW, Hill JA. Cardiorenal interactions: insights from the ESCAPE trial. J Am Coll Cardiol. 2008;51:1268–74.
223. Gottlieb Gottlieb SS, Abraham W, Butler J, Forman DE, Loh E, Massie BM, O'Connor CM, Rich MW, Stevenson LW, Young J, Krumholz HM. The prognostic importance of different definitions of worsening renal function in congestive heart failure. Card Fail. 2002;8:136–41.
224. Winton FR. The influence of venous pressure on the isolated mammalian kidney. J Physiol. 1931; 72:49–61.
225. Mullens W, Abrahams Z, Francis GS, Sokos G, Taylor DO, Starling RC, Young JB, Tang WH. Importance of venous congestion for worsening of renal function in advanced decompensated heart failure. J Am Coll Cardiol. 2009;53:589–96.
226. Maeder MT, Holst DP, Kaye DM. Tricuspid regurgitation contributes to renal dysfunction in patients with heart failure. J Card Fail. 2008;10:824–30.
227. Fonarow GC, Stough WG, Abraham WT, Albert NM, Gheorghiade M, Greenberg BH, O'Connor CM, Sun JL, Yancy CW, Young JB. Characteristics, treatments, and outcomes of patients with preserved systolic function hospitalized for heart failure: a report from the OPTIMIZE-HF registry. JACC. 2007;50:768–77.
228. Heywood JT, Fonarow GC, Costanzo MR, et al. High prevalence of renal dysfunction and its impact on outcome in 118,465 patients hospitalized with acute decompensated heart failure: a report from the ADHERE database. J Card Fail. 2007;13: 422–30.
229. Ronco C, Cruz D, Ronco F. Cardiorenal syndromes. Curr Opin Crit Care. 2009;15:384–91.

230. Sarraf M, Schrier R. Cardiorenal syndrome in acute heart failure syndromes. Int J Nephrol. 2011; 2:293938.
231. Felker M, Lee K, Bull D, Redfield M, et al. Diuretic strategies in patients with acute decompensated heart failure. N Engl J Med. 2011;364:797–805.
232. Sackner-Bernstein JD, Skopicki HA, Aaronson KD. Risk of worsening renal function with nesiritide in patient with acutely decompensated heart failure [published erratum in. Circulation. 2005;111: 1487–91.
233. Abraham WT, Adams KF, Fonarow GC, Costanzo MR, Berkowitz RL, LeJemtel TH, Cheng ML, Wynne J. ADHERE Scientific Advisory Committee and Investigators; ADHERE Study Group: In-hospital mortality in patients with acute decompensated heart failure requiring intravenous vasoactive medications: An analysis from the Acute Decompensated Heart Failure National Registry (ADHERE). J Am Coll Cardiol. 2005;46:57–64.
234. Konstam MA, Gheorghiade M, Burnett Jr JC, Grinfeld L, Maggioni AP, Swedberg K, Udelson JE, Zannad F, Cook T, Ouyang J, Zimmer C, Orlandi C. Efficacy of Vasopressin Antagonism in Heart Failure Outcome Study With Tolvaptan (EVEREST) Investigators: Effects of oral tolvaptan in patients hospitalized for worsening heart failure: The EVEREST Outcome Trial. JAMA. 2007;297: 1319–31.
235. Costanzo MR, Guglin ME, Saltzberg MT, Jessup ML, Bart BA, Teerlink JR, Jaski BE, Fang JC, Feller ED, Haas GJ, Anderson AS, Schollmeyer MP, Sobotka PA. UNLOAD Trial Investigators: Ultrafiltration versus intravenous diuretics for patients hospitalized for acute decompensated heart failure. J Am Coll Cardiol. 2007;49:675–83.
236. Shlipak MG, Smith GL, Rathore SS. Renal function, digoxin therapy, and heart failure outcomes: evidence from the digoxin intervention group trial. J Am Soc Nephrol. 2004;15:2195–203.
237. Smith GL, Lichtman JH, Bracken MB, et al. Renal impairment and outcomes in heart failure: systematic review and meta-analysis. J Am Coll Cardiol. 2006;47:1987–96.
238. Ronco C, Haapio M, House AA, et al. Cardiorenal syndrome. J Am Coll Cardiol. 2008;52:1527–39.

Management of Acute Kidney Injury 22

Jorge Cerdá and Shamik Shah

Case

A 55-year-old woman known to have diabetes mellitus for 10 years and baseline creatinine of 1.5 mg/dL was transferred to a tertiary care hospital from a community hospital. She initially presented with a history of high grade fever for 1 week, decreased urine output for 3 days, and a 1-day history of altered sensorium. She had been treated at the community hospital for 2 days with intravenous crystalloids and antibiotics but showed continued deterioration.

Upon arrival to the tertiary hospital, she was drowsy and only arousable to painful stimuli. The respiratory rate was 42 breaths/min; heart rate, 115 beats/min; blood pressure, 80/54 mmHg; and she was afebrile. She weighed 45 kg and was 5 ft tall. The physical examination was remarkable for anicteric sclera; equal reacting pupils; no lymphadenopathy; normal heart sounds with no murmur or rub; clear lung fields with occasional basilar rales; and a soft, non-tender abdomen. Laboratory studies were as follows: BUN 58 mg/dL; serum creatinine 3.7 mg/dL; white blood cell count 33.8×10^3 mL; hemoglobin 6.6 mg/dL; hematocrit 21.4%; platelet count 264×10^3 μL; and INR 1.6. Urinalysis demonstrated 1+ protein, specific gravity 1.010; several scattered muddy-brown granular casts; urine sodium (spot sample), 47 mEq/L; and urine osmolality, 290 mOsm/kg. The arterial blood gas demonstrated pH 7.36; PCO_2, 45 mmHg; bicarbonate 24 mEq/L; and PO_2, 117 mmHg with FIO_2 of 0.54 on a high-flow face mask.

Blood cultures and urine cultures obtained at the community hospital resulted in *Escherichia coli*. A bedside renal ultrasound showed mildly enlarged kidneys with a mild increase in parenchymal echogenicity, minimal left hydroureteronephrosis, and mild hepatomegaly.

Norepinephrine was added when blood pressure failed to stabilize with intravenous fluids. Within the next 24 h, the patient's respiratory status deteriorated and she was intubated and mechanically ventilated on 80% FIO_2. She became oliguric with a positive fluid balance of 6 L since admission to the tertiary hospital. Blood gas analysis showed metabolic acidosis and hyperkalemia with serum potassium 5.6 mEq/L.

For the case above, what is the next step in management of this patient's AKI?

J. Cerdá, M.D., F.A.C.P., F.A.S.N. (✉)
Division of Nephrology, Department of Medicine, Albany Medical College, Capital District Renal Physicians, 62 Hackett Blvd., Albany, NY 12209, USA
e-mail: cerda@nycap.rr.com, cerdaj@mail.amc.edu

S. Shah, M.B.B.S., M.D., D.N.B. (Nephrology)
Department of Nephrology, Apollo Hospitals, Gandhinagar, Gujarat 380054, India

E.V. Lerma and M. Rosner (eds.), *Clinical Decisions in Nephrology, Hypertension and Kidney Transplantation*,
DOI 10.1007/978-1-4614-4454-1_22, © Springer Science+Business Media New York 2013

General Approach

Conservative Management

In the majority of cases AKI can be effectively treated and resolved by adequate volume replacement, treatment of the underlying medical condition (e.g., sepsis, hemorrhage), and avoidance of nephrotoxic medications. An important goal of early management of AKI is to prevent further injury and to facilitate recovery of renal function. These goals can often best be achieved by strict attention to supportive therapy. Patients with AKI require careful attention to their hemodynamic status. Hypotension results in decreased renal perfusion. Management of blood pressure and cardiac output require careful titration of fluids and vasoactive medication. Vasopressors can further reduce tissue blood flow if there is insufficient circulating blood volume, but patients with AKI are also at increased risk of fluid overload due to continued fluid resuscitation despite increased intravascular volume. Fluids and vasoactive medications should be managed carefully and in conjunction with hemodynamic monitoring. The following series of questions and decisions can direct management of AKI:

Should We Expand This Patient's Extracellular Volume?

Is This Patient "Prerenal" and What Does Prerenal Mean?

In the natural history of AKI, the development of renal injury is a progressive process from risk to damage to functional failure [1–3]. In volume-contracted patients, re-expansion of the intravascular volume may translate in improvement in renal perfusion and avoidance of renal parenchymal injury. This situation was previously called "prerenal azotemia" but since the implication of absence of renal injury is not always correct, the condition has been re-designated "volume-responsive AKI" [4]. Conditions where "prerenal markers" (such as a low fractional excretion of sodium) are present include:

Volume-responsive ("prerenal") azotemia
Sepsis (early phase)
Contrast-induced AKI
Acute glomerulonephritis
Acute interstitial nephritis induced by non-steroidal anti-inflammatory drugs

The case in context. The patient might have been volume-responsive initially, when she was in the early phase of sepsis. By the time the patient arrived at the tertiary hospital, the urine showed abundant brown granular casts which, although not pathognomonic, are highly suggestive of tubular damage. Laboratory studies demonstrated worsening AKI with urinalysis and urine indices suggestive of acute tubular necrosis (ATN), including dipstick-positive proteinuria, muddy-brown granular casts on urinalysis, and an elevated urine sodium concentration (>20 mEq/L). The urine-specific gravity and osmolality are also consistent with the concentrating defect that occurs in patients with ATN. See Chap. 20 for discussion of this condition.

How Do We Assess Volume?

The purpose of assessing volume status is to predict whether volume expansion will result in improved cardiac output (CO), and hence improve peripheral tissue and organ perfusion. Static measures of volume status such as central venous pressure (CVP) or pulmonary capillary wedge pressure, or pulmonary occlusion pressure (PWP) measured with a Swan–Ganz catheter, have been repeatedly shown to be poor predictors of response to volume expansion [5]. Dynamic measures of the response of the cardiovascular system to increased preload appear to be better predictors [6]. Noninvasive measures of hemodynamics are generally considered inexact. Use of clinical assessment or imaging including chest X-rays is notoriously unreliable, especially in patients with concomitant lung injury, pneumonia, or chronic congestive heart failure. Other imaging methods including inferior vena cava ultrasound are valuable in the hands of especially trained practitioners. Adequately recorded intake and output and daily accurate weights are usually the best simple measures to estimate the volume status of the patient who has been hospitalized for a few days.

Volume Resuscitation: What Are the Goals?

In the past, studies suggested that supranormal delivery of oxygen to tissues would result in more effective resuscitation. Later studies failed to demonstrate benefit from such approach. On the basis of the work of Rivers et al. [7], current practice includes optimization of cardiac preload, afterload, and contractility, to balance oxygen delivery and demand within the first 6 h post-admission. This is achieved with a "bundle" of specific measures that may include intravenous fluids and inotropic support [8]. Application of such practice has demonstrated benefit, but those results will have to be confirmed in currently ongoing, larger multicentric studies [9]. However, given that these early trials of "goal-directed therapy" did not include renal outcomes it is currently unknown , whether such protocols actually decrease the risk of AKI.

Early resuscitation (defined as resuscitation within the first 3–6 h of presentation) has been shown to be beneficial [8]. Once past that initial time window, subsequent attempts at resuscitation with aggressive volume expansion may result in increased injury and adverse consequences Once organ injury (especially pulmonary and renal) has developed aggressive "resuscitation" can be hazardous [10–12, 17, 18, 32]. This is valid for the critically ill patient who, in the context of long-standing (>48 h) multiple organ failure, develops a de novo episode of sepsis. Evidence from a randomized controlled trial (RCT) [13] and retrospective studies [10] demonstrates that septic patients develop early lung injury and are therefore much more prone to pulmonary edema than normal subjects [14]. Lactate-base strategies may also be helpful in conjunction with clinical judgment in assessing response to volume loading [7, 8, 19, 20, 21].

The case in context. Our patient received aggressive resuscitation upon arrival to the tertiary care center. She is currently volume overloaded and oliguric with compromised pulmonary oxygenation. Giving more fluids will only lead to fluid overload and worsening pulmonary status.

If We Expand Volume: What should we use? Crystalloid vs. Colloid

Currently, there is an ongoing debate on the respective benefits of different products for volume expansion. There is currently no evidence of superiority of colloids over crystalloids [22]. As shown by the SAFE study, albumin is equivalent to crystalloids in a well-designed RCT [23]. Earlier reports regarding the use of high molecular weight hydroxy ethyl starch showed an increased risk of AKI [22].

Use of Transfusion to Raise Hgb and O_2 Transport

The initial Rivers et al. study [7] utilized blood transfusion whenever volume expansion and pressors/vasodilators did not result in improvement in SvO_2. Although apparently beneficial in this study, such a strategy is associated with risk. Recent studies have discouraged the use of blood transfusion for patient with a Hbg >7 g/dl given the risk of transfusional reaction and acute lung injury [24].

The case in context. In our patient, early transfusion might have been of marginal benefit. The rapidly worsening pulmonary edema, Caused by to septic end-organ injury plus fluid overload, could have worsened with the acute intravascular expansion caused by blood transfusion. As discussed, transfusion would have exposed the patient to higher risk of transfusion-related acute lung injury. Finally, this patient's hyperkalemia may have worsened due to the high concentration of K^+ in the serum of chilled blood.

Acid–Base Implications of the Fluids Chosen

Massive infusion of 0.9% NaCl solution (154 mEq/L of sodium chloride concentration) has been shown to be associated with the induction of hyperchloremic metabolic acidosis [22]. Balanced solutions such as Lactated Ringer's or 0.45% NaCl plus 75 mEq/L of $NaHCO_3$ may be better options for volume expansion, depending of the circumstances. Patients with volume contraction or chloride depletion-induced metabolic alkalosis may benefit from 0.9% NaCl solutions [21].

Should We Use Vasopressors? When?

As discussed above, in the septic patient hemodynamic resuscitation with exclusive use of volume re-expansion creates the risk of worsening pulmonary edema. In this situation, early use of vasoconstrictors (vasopressors) avoids the use of excessive volume and ensures adequate perfusion. Previous concerns that the use of norepinephrine (NE) leads to worsening renal ischemia have been proven baseless; on the contrary, NE has been shown to improve renal blood flow in animal models of sepsis.

What Is the Goal?

As discussed above, the usual goal is MAP 65 mmHg or better, but such goal is often unnecessary as long as other physiological markers indicate improved perfusion [15].

Which Pressors to Use?

It is not known which vasopressor agent is most effective for prevention and treatment of patients with AKI and septic shock. Most studies have focused on norepinephrine, dopamine, or vasopressin [30–31]. Norepinephrine has been shown to be beneficial in septic shock [25–27]. The previous claims of benefit of "renal dose" dopamine have been proven baseless. Moreover, the use of dopamine for patients with evolving AKI probably worsens intrarenal (medullary) ischemia and hence leads to injury to the most vulnerable regions of the ischemic kidney [26]. At high doses, Epinephrine (EN) is probably as effective as NE [28]. Previous concerns with possible induction of lactic acidosis are unfounded. In patients with severe shock, vasopressin (VP) has been shown to be beneficial especially when maximal doses of norepinephrine have been reached [29]. The expectation that VP can be used as an NE-sparing vasopressor has not been substantiated [29]. Doses of VP greater than 0.04 mg/kg/min have been associated with severe ischemic complications including the induction of intestinal ischemia and should therefore be avoided.

What Other Pharmacologic Agents Should We Consider?

There is currently no evidence to support the use of a specific pharmacological therapy in the treatment of AKI secondary to hypoperfusion injury and/or sepsis.

Should We Use Diuretics?

The rationale behind the use of loop diuretics was based on their putative ability to reduce the energy requirements of the cells of the ascending limb of Henle and therefore to ameliorate the resultant ischemic damage. Loop diuretics have also been used to convert patients with oliguric AKI to non-oliguric AKI, to facilitate the management of fluid and electrolyte disturbances and reduce the requirement for renal replacement therapy (RRT). Administration of diuretics to patients with AKI does not shorten the duration nor improve the outcome of renal dysfunction [32, 35]. Repeated attempts to use diuretics at increasing, inefficacious, and toxic doses often delay the initiation of necessary RRT [36]. RCTs and meta-analyses have demonstrated lack of benefit or in some cases adverse effects, including direct toxicity (such as ototoxicity) [37].

In patients with established AKI only loop diuretics are effective; occasionally, the addition of thiazides helps overcome tubular adaptation to the effects of loop diuretics. To be effective, loop diuretics often need to be administered in high doses or in continuous infusion to avoid a rebound in tubular sodium resorption during periods when blood levels are subtherapeutic. Coadministration of albumin in patients with hypoalbuminemia has not been proven to be effective. Lack of responsiveness to diuretics and increasing fluid overload are clear indications for initiation of RRT [12].

While numerous other drugs have been studied, RRT is still the only FDA-approved therapy for AKI. There is currently no strong evidence by RCTs to use mannitol, fenoldopam, atrial natriuretic peptides, adenosine receptor antagonists, or growth factors for the treatment of AKI.

Nutritional Considerations

Protein-calorie malnutrition is an important independent predictor of in-hospital mortality in patients with AKI.

What Are the Nutritional Goals in Patients with AKI?

When?

It is currently debated how early should patients be started on nutritional supplementation [39]. While in Europe nutrition is initiated very early (within 24–48) hours of the onset of shock, in the US nutrition is initiated later, generally after 48 h, due to concerns that in the early phases of shock, patients are unable to benefit from nutrition, given their hypercatabolic state. Moreover, early nutrition leads to complications including hyperglycemia, osmotic and volume load, and acidosis. A recent RCT demonstrates lack of benefit of early nutrition [40].

What Route: Enteral vs. Parenteral?

There is consensus that whenever possible, enteral nutrition is superior to parenteral nutrition [41–44].

With What?

The goal of nutrition should be to provide adequate composition and amounts of nutrients. In patients with sepsis and multiple organ failure including renal failure, normal or higher than normal nutritional requirements should be satisfied. The practice of limiting nutrition in patients with renal failure "to avoid dialysis" is inappropriate and should be avoided. One of the goals to initiate dialysis is to *allow adequate nutrition*. RRT should permit provision of all the nutrients the patient needs, and therefore the use of "renal" formulas may be inadequate in the setting of AKI.

The typical metabolic needs of the critically ill patient are not above baseline (25–30 kcal/kg/day); there is no clinically demonstrated evidence of benefit (and some suggestion of harm) in the administration of higher caloric loads. Recently, the concept of "permissive underfeeding" has arisen, (providing 10–15 kcal/kg/day), understanding that higher caloric feeding will be wasted and will potentially increase side effects. Protein requirements in critically ill patients are 1.5–2 g/kg/day (20–30% total caloric intake). Parenteral lipid formulations are the most concentrated form of nutrition. The minimal amount should be 2–4% of caloric goals; usual amounts are widely variable, traditionally 30% caloric intake. Short chain fatty acids are essential for intestinal nutrition; medium chain fatty acids can be used for energy storage. Long chain fatty acids (omega-6 fatty acids) are the traditional source of lipids in parenteral and enteral formulae.

The case in context. This tiny 45 kg female with a 5 ft height had a calculated BMI of 8.8 kg/m^2, clearly in the underweight category. Malnutrition and diabetes have certainly contributed to her decreased immune defenses. Initiation of nutritional intervention providing normal caloric requirements is needed, either by spontaneous oral nutrition or enteral nutrition via nasogastric tube while the patient is on the ventilator.

What About Glycemic Control?

While initial data from a single center showed the benefits of tight (normalization) glycemic control among critically ill surgical patients, such results could not be reproduced for critically ill medical patients. Subsequent multicenter studies did not find benefit in tight glycemic control and demonstrated significantly increased risks of hypoglycemia with such strategy. Discrepancy in these results is probably due to different populations and differences in the actual implementation of glucose monitoring and management [45]. Currently, a glucose range of 120–180 mg/dl is considered an adequate goal. Persistent hyperglycemia per se has been shown associated with increased risk of acute renal dysfunction and failure [46].

The case in context. This patient is a diabetic and therefore, glycemic control and monitoring will acquire even more relevance. While avoiding hypoglycemia, adequate glycemic control is warranted.

Renal Replacement Therapy

Choosing a Renal Replacement Therapy in AKI: Introduction

There is limited evidence on the optimal time to initiate RRT. In most instances, clinicians base RRT initiation on standard life-threatening indications, including drug intoxications, symptomatic uremia, volume overload, acidosis, and hyperkalemia that prove refractory to medical management.

RRTs rely on the principle of allowing water and solute transport through a semipermeable membrane and then discarding the waste products [49, 50]. Ultrafiltration is the process by which water is transported by a transmembrane pressure gradient across a semipermeable membrane. Diffusion and convection are the two processes by which solutes are transported across the membrane. Diffusion occurs by movement of solutes from an area of higher solute concentration to an area of lower concentration across a semipermeable membrane. The concentration gradient is maximized and maintained throughout the length of the membrane by running the dialysate (an electrolyte solution usually containing sodium, bicarbonate, chloride, magnesium, and calcium) countercurrent to the blood flow. Small-molecular-weight solutes, such as urea, are cleared efficiently by diffusion, but medium and large molecular-weight solutes are not. Convection occurs when the transmembrane pressure gradient drives water across a semipermeable membrane and "drags" with both small-molecular-weight (blood urea nitrogen, creatinine, potassium) and medium-molecular-weight (inulin, beta-2-microglobulin, tumor necrosis factor, vitamin B12) solutes. Membrane pore diameter limits the size of the solutes cleared.

Available RRT modalities use ultrafiltration for fluid removal and diffusion, convection, or a combination of the two to achieve solute clearance. RRT options include intermittent hemodialysis (IHD), peritoneal dialysis (PD), various forms of continuous renal replacement therapy (CRRT), and newer "hybrid" therapies, collectively known as extended duration dialysis (EDD) or sustained low-efficiency dialysis (SLED).

Most hospital-acquired AKI occurs in the ICU and is associated with elevated morbidity and mortality [2, 16]. While 80% of patients with AKI in the ICU are treated with CRRT, 17% are managed with IHD and 3% with peritoneal dialysis or SLED [47]. The ideal modality of RRT should fulfill multiple characteristics listed in Table 22.1 [48]. Hemodynamic stability of the critically ill patient determines the most appropriate dialysis modality (see Table 22.2).

When choosing the modality of RRT most appropriate for each patient, multiple other considerations must be kept in mind (see Table 22.3). In addition to the patient's hemodynamic stability, the choice between the various renal replacement modalities rests on solute clearance goals, volume control, and need for anticoagulation needs (see Table 22.4).

Intermittent Hemodialysis

IHD is usually delivered 3–6 times a week, 3–4 h per session, with a blood flow rate of 300–500 mL/min and a dialysate flow rate of 500–800 mL/min. In IHD, solute clearance occurs mainly by diffusion, whereas volume is removed by ultrafiltration. Advantages of IHD include rapid solute and volume removal. This results in rapid correction of electrolyte disturbances, such as hyperkalemia, and rapid removal of drugs or other substances in potentially fatal intoxications, in a matter of hours. IHD usually requires less anticoagulation as compared with other types of RRT, because of the faster blood flow rate and the shorter duration of treatment. The main disadvantage of IHD is the risk of systemic hypotension caused by rapid solute and fluid removal. Rapid solute clearance from the intravascular space can cause fluid shifts to the interstitial and intracellular compartments, causing cerebral edema and increased intracranial pressure this limits the usefulness of IHD in patients with head trauma or hepatic encephalopathy.

Table 22.1 Characteristics of the "ideal" treatment modality of AKI in the ICU

Characteristic
Preserves homeostasis
Does not increase co-morbidity
Does not worsen patient's underlying condition
Is inexpensive
Is simple to manage
Is not burdensome to the ICU staff

From Lameire et al. [71]

Table 22.2 Indications for specific renal replacement therapies

Therapeutic goal	Hemodynamics	Preferred therapy
Fluid removal	Stable	Intermittent isolated UF
	Unstable	Slow UF
Urea clearance	Stable	Intermittent hemodialysis
	Unstable	CRRT
		Convection: CAVH, CVVH
		Diffusion: CAVHD, CVVHD
		Both: CAVHDF, CVVHDF
Severe hyperkalemia	Stable/unstable	Intermittent hemodialysis
Severe metabolic acidosis	Stable	Intermittent hemodialysis
	Unstable	CRRT
Severe hyperphosphoremia	Stable/unstable	CRRT
Brain edema	Unstable	CRRT

HDF hemodiafiltration, *CVVH* continuous hemofiltration, *CVVHD* continuous hemodialysis, *CVVHDF* continuous hemodiafiltration, *IHD* intermittent hemodialysis, *IHF* intermittent hemofiltration, *UF* ultrafiltration (from Murray et al. [72])

Table 22.3 Considerations in renal replacement therapy for AKI

Consideration	Components	Varieties
Dialysis modality		
	Intermittent hemodialysis	Daily, every other day, SLED
	Continuous renal replacement therapies	AV, VV
	Peritoneal dialysis	
Dialysis biocompatibility	Membrane characteristics	
Dialyzer performance		
	Efficiency	
	Flux	
Dialysis delivery		
	Timing of initiation	Early, late
	Intensity of dialysis	Prescription vs. delivery
	Adequacy of dialysis	Dialysis dose

Table 22.4 Advantages and disadvantages of various renal replacement modalities

Modality	Use in hemodynamically unstable patients	Solute clearance	Volume control	Anticoagulation
PD	Yes	++	++	No
IHD	Possible	++++	+++	Yes/no
IHF	Possible	+++	+++	Yes/no
Intermittent IHF	Possible	++++	+++	Yes/no
Hybrid techniques	Possible	++++	++++	Yes/no
CVVH	Yes	+++/++++	++++	Yes/no
CVVHD	Yes	+++/++++	++++	Yes/no
CVVHDF	Yes	++++	++++	Yes/no

HDF hemodiafiltration, *CVVH* continuous hemofiltration, *CVVHD* continuous hemodialysis, *CVVHDF* continuous hemodiafiltration, *IHD* intermittent hemodialysis, *IHF* intermittent hemofiltration, *PD* peritoneal dialysis (modified from Davenport [73])

Peritoneal Dialysis

In PD, the peritoneum is used as a semipermeable membrane for diffusive removal of solutes. A dialysate solution is administered into the peritoneal cavity through a catheter, where it stays for a prescribed period of time and is then drained. The use of PD is limited by practical considerations. Acute PD requires the surgical insertion of a peritoneal dialysis catheter and is often complicated by catheter leakage and malfunction. The use of PD is limited by low solute clearance in hypercatabolic patients and pulmonary restriction due to increased intrabdominal pressure and diaphragm elevation. PD is contraindicated in patients who need abdominal surgery or have surgical drains. Because fluid and solute removal are less predictable PD continues to be less widely used than other therapies.

Continuous Renal Replacement Therapy

Over the past decade, CRRT has emerged as a viable modality for the management of hemodynamically unstable patients with AKI. The different modalities of CRRT [51] are defined by the main mechanism with which clearance is achieved: simple diffusion (continuous hemodialysis, CVVHD), convection (continuous hemofiltration, CVVH), or a combination of both (continuous hemodiafiltration, CVVHDF) [52]. These modalities differ in the magnitude of the clearance achieved by convection or diffusion, the vascular access, and the need for fluid replacement (hemofiltration) (see Table 22.5). Given the absence of evidence of superiority among the different CRRT modalities, the choice rests on the available equipment (membranes, pump systems), appropriate dialysate, and cost and conceptual considerations [53, 54–65]. The advantages of CRRT include hemodynamic tolerance caused by slower ultrafiltration [52, 66]. The gradual continuous volume removal makes control of volume status easier and allows administration of medications and nutrition with less concern for volume overload. Because it is a continuous modality, there is less fluctuation of solute concentrations over time and better control of azotemia, electrolytes, and acid–base status. With CRRT, the slower rate of urea clearance allows for equalization of solute concentrations between compartments and therefore, lessened water shifts and cell edema. This is particularly important in patients with intracranial hypertension, such as head trauma and severe liver failure [32, 66–68]. Lower core temperature and consequent peripheral vasoconstriction decrease hypotensive episodes and may play a role in hemodynamic stability [69, 70]. The main disadvantages of CRRT include access and filter clotting and the consequent need for long-term anticoagulation Use of citrate anticoagulation usually solves this problem and adds additional benefits.

Recent RCTs have established a dose of [20–25] ml/kg/hour as the minimum adequate delivered CRRT dose. Achieving that dose usually requires a prescription of [25–30] ml/kg/hour, taking into account down time and usual technical limitations. [54–65].

Sustained Low-Efficiency Dialysis or Extended Daily Dialysis

SLED and EDD are slower dialytic modalities run for prolonged periods using conventional hemodialysis machines with modification of blood and dialysate flows. Typically, they use low blood-pump speeds of 200 mL/min and low dialysate flow rates of 300 mL/min for 6–12 h daily. SLED and EDD combine the advantages of CRRT and IHD. They allow for improved hemodynamic stability through gradual solute and volume removal as in CRRT. At the same time, they are able to provide high solute clearances as in IHD and remove the need for expensive CRRT machines, costly customized solutions, and trained staff. Because they can be performed intermittently based on the needs of the patient, they also avoid the interruption of therapy for various diagnostic and therapeutic procedures that may be required in such patients.

The case in context. Given the high ventilator requirements, oliguria, electrolyte, and acid–base abnormalities, our patient was started on RRT. CRRT was initially chosen because of her hemodynamic instability and need for volume removal. Within 3 days, her metabolic acidosis was corrected, electrolyte levels normalized, and

Table 22.5 Modalities of continuous renal replacement therapy

	Clearance mechanism			
Technique	Convection	Diffusion	Vascular access	Fluid replacement
SCUF	+	–	Large vein	0
CAVH	++++	–	Artery and vein	+++
CVVH	++++	–	Large vein	+++
CAVHD	+	++++	Artery and vein	+++
CVVHD	+	++++	Large vein	+/0
CAVHDF	+++	+++	Artery and vein	++
CVVHDF	+++	+++	Large vein	++
CAVHFD	++	++++	Artery and vein	+/0
CVVHFD	++	++++	Large vein	+/0

CAVH continuous arteriovenous hemofiltration, *CAVHD* continuous arteriovenous hemodialysis, *CAVHDF* continuous arteriovenous hemodiafiltration, *CAVHFD* continuous arteriovenous high-flux hemodialysis, *CVVH* continuous venovenous hemofiltration, *CVVHD* continuous venovenous hemodialysis, *CVVHDF* continuous venovenous hemodiafiltration, *CVVHFD* continuous venovenous high-flux hemodialysis, *SCUF* slow continuous ultrafiltration; 0=not required, +=negligible, ++=some, +++=marked, ++++=major

blood pressure stabilized. After 6 days, vasopressors were stopped and she was successfully weaned off the ventilator. She was transferred to the floor and treated with IHD. On the 13th day after hospitalization, her urine output improved and increased to 3 L/day in the next few days. She was discharged home off hemodialysis 3 weeks after her initial hospital admission.

Conclusion

This section focused on the different modalities of RRT and briefly reviewed the basic concepts and the newest approaches to the management of the critically ill patient with AKI. There are no evidence-based guidelines for the selection of RRT modality for the treatment of AKI. The modality choice should therefore be guided by the individual patient's clinical status, local medical and nursing expertise, and equipment availability. It is now recognized that throughout the clinical course, more than one therapy can be utilized. Transitions in therapy are common and reflect the changing patient needs. In the case presented, the initial hemodynamic instability made CRRT preferable. Switching to IHD as soon as the patient becomes hemodynamically stable is consistent with general practice; it allows discharge from the ICU, and permits greater efforts at rehabilitation and ambulation, thus hastening overall patient recovery. Adjustments of RRT techniques to avoid exacerbation of hemodynamic instability and to decrease further renal injury, illustrate the importance of choosing the right RRT modality, to ensure patient survival and renal functional recovery.

References

1. Sharfuddin AA, Molitoris BA. Pathophysiology of ischemic acute kidney injury. Nat Rev Nephrol. 2011;7:189–200.
2. Cerda J, Lameire N, Eggers P, et al. Epidemiology of acute kidney injury. Clin J Am Soc Nephrol. 2008; 3:881–6.
3. Zarjou A, Agarwal A. Sepsis and acute kidney injury. J Am Soc Nephrol. 2011;22(6):999–1006.
4. Kellum JA. Acute kidney injury. Crit Care Med. 2008;36:S141–5.
5. Marik PE, Baram M, Vahid B. Does central venous pressure predict fluid responsiveness? A systematic review of the literature and the tale of seven mares. Chest. 2008;134:172–8.
6. Pinsky MR, Brophy P, Padilla J, Paganini E, Pannu N. Fluid and volume monitoring. Int J Artif Organs. 2008;31:111–26.
7. Rivers E, Nguyen B, Havstad S, et al. Early goal-directed therapy in the treatment of severe sepsis and septic shock. N Engl J Med. 2001;345: 1368–77.

8. Dellinger RP, Levy MM, Carlet JM, et al. Surviving Sepsis Campaign: international guidelines for management of severe sepsis and septic shock: 2008. Crit Care Med. 2008;36:296–327.
9. Maitland K, Kiguli S, Opoka RO, et al. Mortality after fluid bolus in African children with severe infection. N Engl J Med. 2011;364(26):2483–95.
10. Murphy CV, Schramm GE, Doherty JA, et al. The importance of fluid management in acute lung injury secondary to septic shock. Chest. 2009;136:102–9.
11. Payen D, de Pont AC, Sakr Y, et al. A positive fluid balance is associated with a worse outcome in patients with acute renal failure. Crit Care. 2008;12:R74.
12. Cerda J, Sheinfeld G, Ronco C. Fluid overload in critically ill patients with acute kidney injury. Blood Purif. 2010;29:11–8.
13. National Heart, Lung, and Blood Institute Acute Respiratory Distress Syndrome (ARDS) Clinical Trials Network, Wiedemann HP, et al. Comparison of two fluid-management strategies in acute lung injury. N Engl J Med. 2006;354:2564–75.
14. Van Biesen W, Yegenaga I, Vanholder R, et al. Relationship between fluid status and its management on acute renal failure (ARF) in intensive care unit (ICU) patients with sepsis: a prospective analysis. J Nephrol. 2005;18:54–60.
15. Kellum JA, Pinsky MR. Use of vasopressor agents in critically ill patients. Curr Opin Crit Care. 2002;8: 236–41.
16. Cerda J, Bagga A, Kher V, Chakravarthi RM. The contrasting characteristics of acute kidney injury in developed and developing countries. Nat Clin Pract Nephrol. 2008;4:138–53.
17. Schrier RW, Wang W. Acute renal failure and sepsis. N Engl J Med. 2004;351:159–69.
18. Liu KD, Matthay MA. Advances in critical care for the nephrologist: acute lung injury/ARDS. Clin J Am Soc Nephrol. 2008;3:578–86.
19. Nguyen HB, Rivers EP, Knoblich BP, et al. Early lactate clearance is associated with improved outcome in severe sepsis and septic shock. Crit Care Med. 2004;32:1637–42.
20. Lewis RJ. Disassembling goal-directed therapy for sepsis: a first step. JAMA. 2010;303:777–9.
21. Cerda J, Tolwani AJ, Warnock DG. Critical care nephrology: Management of acid-base disorders with CRRT. Kidney Int 2012;82(1):9–18.
22. Kellum JA, Cerda J, Kaplan LJ, Nadim MK, Palevsky PM. Fluids for prevention and management of acute kidney injury. Int J Artif Organs. 2008;31:96–110.
23. Finfer S, McEvoy S, Bellomo R, McArthur C, Myburgh J, Norton R. Impact of albumin compared to saline on organ function and mortality of patients with severe sepsis. Intensive Care Med. 2011;37:86–96.
24. Juffermans NP. Transfusion-related acute lung injury: emerging importance of host factors and implications for management. Expert Rev Hematol. 2010;3:459–67.
25. Russell JA, Walley KR, Singer J, et al. Vasopressin versus norepinephrine infusion in patients with septic shock. N Engl J Med. 2008;358:877–87.
26. De Backer D, Biston P, Devriendt J, et al. Comparison of dopamine and norepinephrine in the treatment of shock. N Engl J Med. 2010;362:779–89.
27. Kellum JA, Decker MJ. Use of dopamine in acute renal failure: a meta-analysis. Crit Care Med. 2001;29:1526–31.
28. Myburgh JA, Higgins A, Jovanovska A, Lipman J, Ramakrishnan N, Santamaria J. A comparison of epinephrine and norepinephrine in critically ill patients. Intensive Care Med. 2008;34:2226–34.
29. Gordon AC, Russell JA, Walley KR, et al. The effects of vasopressin on acute kidney injury in septic shock. Intensive Care Med. 2010;36:83–91.
30. Annane D, Cariou A, Maxime V, et al. Corticosteroid treatment and intensive insulin therapy for septic shock in adults: a randomized controlled trial. JAMA. 2010;303:341–8.
31. Russell JA, Walley KR, Gordon AC, et al. Interaction of vasopressin infusion, corticosteroid treatment, and mortality of septic shock. Crit Care Med. 2009;37: 811–8.
32. Cerda J. Oliguria: an earlier and accurate biomarker of acute kidney injury? Kidney Int. 2011;80: 699–701.
33. Kellum JA, Bellomo R, Ronco C. The concept of acute kidney injury and the RIFLE criteria. Contrib Nephrol. 2007;156:10–6.
34. Kellum JA, Mehta RL, Levin A, et al. Development of a clinical research agenda for acute kidney injury using an international, interdisciplinary, three-step modified Delphi process. Clin J Am Soc Nephrol. 2008;3:887–94.
35. Bagshaw SM, Delaney A, Jones D, Ronco C, Bellomo R. Diuretics in the management of acute kidney injury: a multinational survey. Contrib Nephrol. 2007; 156:236–49.
36. Mehta RL, Pascual MT, Soroko S, Chertow GM. Diuretics, mortality, and nonrecovery of renal function in acute renal failure. JAMA. 2002;288:2547–53.
37. Mehta RL, Cantarovich F, Shaw A, Hoste E, Murray P. Pharmacologic approaches for volume excess in acute kidney injury (AKI). Int J Artif Organs. 2008;31: 127–44.
38. Grams ME, Estrella MM, Coresh J, Brower RG, Liu KD. Fluid balance, diuretic use, and mortality in acute kidney injury. Clin J Am Soc Nephrol. 2011;6:966–73.
39. Meyfroidt G, Ingels C, Van den Berghe G. Glycemic control in the ICU. N Engl J Med. 2011;364:1280. author reply 1.
40. Casaer MP, Mesotten D, Hermans G, et al. Early versus late parenteral nutrition in critically Ill adults. N Engl J Med. 2011;365:506–17.
41. Brown RO, Compher C. A.S.P.E.N. clinical guidelines: nutrition support in adult acute and chronic renal failure. JPEN J Parenter Enteral Nutr. 2010;34:366–77.
42. Fiaccadori E, Cremaschi E, Regolisti G. Nutritional assessment and delivery in renal replacement therapy patients. Semin Dial. 2011;24:169–75.
43. Martin K, DeLegge M, Nichols M, Chapman E, Sollid R, Grych C. Assessing appropriate parenteral nutrition

ordering practices in tertiary care medical centers. JPEN J Parenter Enteral Nutr. 2011;35:122–30.
44. Mueller C, Compher C, Ellen DM. A.S.P.E.N. clinical guidelines: nutrition screening, assessment, and intervention in adults. JPEN J Parenter Enteral Nutr. 2011;35:16–24.
45. Gunst J, Van den Berghe G. Blood glucose control in the intensive care unit: benefits and risks. Semin Dial. 2010;23:157–62.
46. Gunst J, Schetz M. Clinical benefits of tight glycaemic control: effect on the kidney. Best Pract Res Clin Anaesthesiol. 2009;23:431–9.
47. Uchino S, Bellomo R, Morimatsu H, et al. Continuous renal replacement therapy: a worldwide practice survey. The beginning and ending supportive therapy for the kidney (B.E.S.T. kidney) investigators. Intensive Care Med. 2007;33:1563–70.
48. Mehta RL. Indications for dialysis in the ICU: renal replacement vs. renal support. Blood Purif. 2001;19: 227–32.
49. Palevsky PM, Bunchman T, Tetta C. The Acute Dialysis Quality Initiative—part V: operational characteristics of CRRT. Adv Ren Replace Ther. 2002;9:268–72.
50. Gibney N, Cerda J, Davenport A, et al. Volume management by renal replacement therapy in acute kidney injury. Int J Artif Organs. 2008;31:145–55.
51. Cerda J, Ronco C. Modalities of continuous renal replacement therapy: technical and clinical considerations. Semin Dial. 2009;22:114–22.
52. Ronco C. Recent evolution of renal replacement therapy in the critically ill patient. Crit Care. 2006;10:123.
53. Ricci Z, Ronco C, Bachetoni A, et al. Solute removal during continuous renal replacement therapy in critically ill patients: convection versus diffusion. Crit Care. 2006;10:R67.
54. Locatelli F, Manzoni C, Di Filippo S. The importance of convective transport. Kidney Int Suppl. 2002: (80):115–20.
55. Liao Z, Zhang W, Hardy PA, et al. Kinetic comparison of different acute dialysis therapies. Artif Organs. 2003;27:802–7.
56. Ronco C, Bellomo R, Homel P, et al. Effects of different doses in continuous veno-venous haemofiltration on outcomes of acute renal failure: a prospective randomised trial. Lancet. 2000;356:26–30.
57. Saudan P, Niederberger M, De Seigneux S, et al. Adding a dialysis dose to continuous hemofiltration increases survival in patients with acute renal failure. Kidney Int. 2006;70:1312–7.
58. Clark WR, Ronco C. CRRT efficiency and efficacy in relation to solute size. Kidney Int Suppl. 1999: (72): S3–7.
59. Brunet S, Leblanc M, Geadah D, Parent D, Courteau S, Cardinal J. Diffusive and convective solute clearances during continuous renal replacement therapy at various dialysate and ultrafiltration flow rates. Am J Kidney Dis. 1999;34:486–92.
60. Palevsky PM, Zhang JH, O'Connor TZ, et al. Intensity of renal support in critically ill patients with acute kidney injury. N Engl J Med. 2008;359:7–20.
61. Bellomo R. Do we know the optimal dose for renal replacement therapy in the intensive care unit? Kidney Int. 2006;70:1202–4.
62. Bellomo R, Cass A, Cole L, et al. Intensity of continuous renal-replacement therapy in critically ill patients. N Engl J Med. 2009;361:1627–38.
63. Clark WR, Turk JE, Kraus MA, Gao D. Dose determinants in continuous renal replacement therapy. Artif Organs. 2003;27:815–20.
64. Cerda J. Low serum creatinine is associated with higher mortality among critically ill patients. Crit Care Med. 2008;36:658–9. author reply 9.
65. Cerda J, Cerda M, Kilcullen P, Prendergast J. In severe acute kidney injury, a higher serum creatinine is paradoxically associated with better patient survival. Nephrol Dial Transplant. 2007;22:2781–4.
66. Davenport A, Will EJ, Davidson AM. Improved cardiovascular stability during continuous modes of renal replacement therapy in critically ill patients with acute hepatic and renal failure. Crit Care Med. 1993;21:328–38.
67. Davenport A, Will EJ, Davison AM, et al. Changes in intracranial pressure during machine and continuous haemofiltration. Int J Artif Organs. 1989;12: 439–44.
68. Ronco C, Bellomo R, Brendolan A, Pinna V, La Greca G. Brain density changes during renal replacement in critically ill patients with acute renal failure. Continuous hemofiltration versus intermittent hemodialysis. J Nephrol. 1999;12:173–8.
69. Santoro A, Mancini E, Canova C, Mambelli E. Thermal balance in convective therapies. Nephrol Dial Transplant. 2003;18 Suppl 7:vii41–5. discussion vii57.
70. Di Filippo S, Manzoni C, Andrulli S, Tentori F, Locatelli F. Sodium removal during pre-dilution haemofiltration. Nephrol Dial Transplant. 2003;18 Suppl 7:vii31–6. discussion vii57–8.
71. Lameire N, Van Biesen W, Vanholder R. Dialysing the patient with acute renal failure in the ICU: the emperor's clothes? Nephrol Dial Transplant. 1999;14:2570–3.
72. Murray P, Hall J. Renal replacement therapy for acute renal failure. Am J Respir Crit Care Med. 2000;162: 777–81.
73. Davenport A. Renal replacement therapy in acute kidney injury: which method to use in the intensive care unit? Saudi J Kidney Dis Transpl. 2008;19:529–36.

Part VI

Chronic Kidney Disease

Part VI

Chronic Kidney Disease

23 Chronic Kidney Disease: Definitions and General Approach

M. Rashid Ishaque and James L. Bailey

Case

A 59-year-old lady is seen by her family practitioner for a routine health evaluation. She has a history of hypertension, diabetes mellitus type 2, and gout of more than 10 years duration. She reports fatigue, decrease appetite, and lower extremity edema for the last few months. The patient's current medications include atenolol 50 mg daily, Hydrochlorothiazide 25 mg daily, and metformin 1,000 mg twice daily. She smokes one pack of cigarettes daily. Examination: Weight—60 kg, pulse—78, and BP—176/96 mmHg. She has no periorbital edema. Fundoscopic exam reveals arterio-venous nicking and scattered cotton wool exudates. JVD is 8 cm at 30°, lungs are clear to auscultation, and heart sounds regular. There are no abdominal masses, and lower extremities show diminished peripheral pulses and trace pedal edema. Current labs are normal except for a serum creatinine of 2.0 mg/dl.

How is renal function measured and assessed? What are some of the consequences of chronic kidney disease (CKD)? What is the optimal medical regimen for a patient with CKD? Finally, when should a patient be referred to nephrologist or CKD clinic?

M.R. Ishaque, M.D. (✉)
Department of Nephrology, Harbin Clinic,
1158 Monte Dr, Marietta, GA 30062, USA
e-mail: rashid292@gmail.com

J.L. Bailey, M.D.
Renal Division, Medicine, Emory University,
Atlanta, GA 30322, USA

Introduction

CKD, previously known as chronic renal failure, has become a critical health care concern over the course of the last few decades because of its inexorable rise and the large number of patients with this disease entity. Because it is poorly recognized by the medical community, a growing number of CKD patients progress to end stage renal disease (ESRD) without proper medical intervention. According to 1999–2004 National Health and Nutrition Examination Survey (NHANES) data, an estimated 16.8% of the US population aged 20 years or greater had CKD, compared with 14.5% from the 1988 to 1994 NHANES data [1]. Nevertheless, there has been a dramatic change in the past decade in the understanding and awareness of CKD, following publication of the National Kidney Foundation's (NKF's) Kidney Disease Outcomes Quality Initiative (KDOQI) CKD guidelines [2]. These were reinforced in a position statement from the NKF in 2007 [3].

Definitions

Over the past decade, CKD has become an area of increasing interest from an epidemiological, basic, and clinical science point of view and has required clarity in terms of definition. As per

E.V. Lerma and M. Rosner (eds.), *Clinical Decisions in Nephrology, Hypertension and Kidney Transplantation*, DOI 10.1007/978-1-4614-4454-1_23, © Springer Science+Business Media New York 2013

(KDOQI) guidelines [2], CKD is defined as kidney damage or a glomerular filtration rate (GFR) <60 ml/min/1.73 m^2 for 3 months or more, with or without any identifiable cause [1]. Some within the nephrology community have argued that this time interval is too short and have suggested that a time interval of 6, 9, or 12 months be used [4]. Despite these arguments, some of the largest research studies and databases including the NHANES have chosen to use only one serum creatinine reading to define CKD [5, 6]. A GFR of less than 60 ml/min/1.73 m^2 indicates that there has been a loss of half or more of normal kidney function. The normal GFR varies by gender, age, and body size [7]. Normal GFR is 120 ml/min/1.73 m^2 in young adult and generally declines with age by approximately 1 ml/min/1.73 m^2 per year after the third decade, but this does not occur in all populations [8].

There have been many methods, equations, and formulas to measure or estimate renal function. These include the Modified Diet in Renal Disease (MDRD) Study equation for estimating GFR [7], the Cockcroft–Gault equation for determining creatinine clearance (CrCl) [9], and recently the new CKD-EPI (Chronic Kidney Disease Epidemiology Collaboration) equation which reportedly allows for a better estimation of measured GFR [10]. There are pitfalls in using any of these equations. For example, the MDRD underestimates GFR in young adults and women, and the original cohort lacked individuals with diabetes or the very elderly (age >70). [18]. The Cockcroft–Gault equation has been historically used for calculation of medication dosages [9], but the normal ranges of creatinine in the laboratory do not take into account factors such as age, gender, muscle mass, diet, and body size [7]. As an example, two subjects with the same creatinine of 1.3 mg/dl are compared by using Cockcraft–Gault equation. Subject A is a 21-year-old man who weighs 176 lbs while subject B is an 81-year-old woman who weighs 132 lbs. Subject A has an estimated GFR of 102 ml/min/1.73 m^2 while subject B has an estimated GFR of 31 ml/min/1.73 m^2. This illustrates that care must be taken in interpreting the "creatinine" and "GFR" on routine laboratory data.

Newer equations have been proposed to overcome the limitations of the MDRD and Cockcroft–Gault equations. The CKD-EPI formula [10], Mayo quadratic equation [11], and cystatin C-based equations [12, 13] claim to be more accurate, reliable, and superior [14, 15] to both the MDRD and Cockcroft–Gault equations, especially in patients with higher GFR levels [16]. Regardless, it is important for the clinician to recognize when a patient has had a decrement in renal function and accurately stage the disease for appropriate follow-up and intervention.

Stages of CKD

There are six stages of CKD based on the level of kidney function as measured by GFR (see Table 23.1). This staging system has increased the recognition of CKD by clinicians and has improved communication between family physicians and nephrologists [19]. The addition of eGFR in routine in-patient and out-patient laboratory data with reference values has increased awareness in the medical community of the necessity of screening and managing efficiently the epidemic of CKD. High risk patients are identified early and management is directed to delay the progression of CKD (see Fig. 23.1).

Screening for CKD

There are more than 26 million Americans who have CKD; millions more are at risk. Unfortunately, the majority of them do not know that they have or are at increased risk of CKD [18]. As a consequence, CKD is a challenging health care problem, but it can be tackled through readily available diagnostic tools and knowledge of its natural history. A population-based screening program should be implemented for high risk groups such as patients with advanced age, diabetes, and hypertension [20]. It will also increase awareness in the general population since analysis of The National Kidney Foundation's Kidney Early Evaluation Program (KEEP®) from 2000 through 2005 [21] showed that the awareness of CKD among the public is

Table 23.1 Stages of chronic kidney disease: a clinical action plan

Stage	Description	GFR (ml/min/1.73 m^2)	Action[a]
1	Kidney damage with normal or ↑ GFR	≥90	Diagnosis and treatment, treatment of comorbid conditions, slowing progression, CVD risk reduction
2	Kidney damage with mild ↓ GFR	60–89	Estimating progression
3	Moderate ↓ GFR	30–59	Evaluating and treating complications
4	Severe ↓ GFR	15–29	Preparation for kidney replacement therapy
5	Kidney failure	<15 (or dialysis)	Replacement (if uremia present)

Reprinted from Am J Kidney Dis Suppl 1, 39, K/DOQI clinical practice guidelines for chronic kidney disease: Evaluation, classification, and stratification, S19, Copyright 2002, with permission from Elsevier

Chronic kidney disease is defined as either kidney damage or GFR <60 ml/min/1.73 m^2 for ≥3 months. Kidney damage is defined as pathologic abnormalities or markers of damage, including abnormalities in blood or urine tests or imaging studies; *CVD* cardiovascular disease

[a]Includes actions from preceding stages

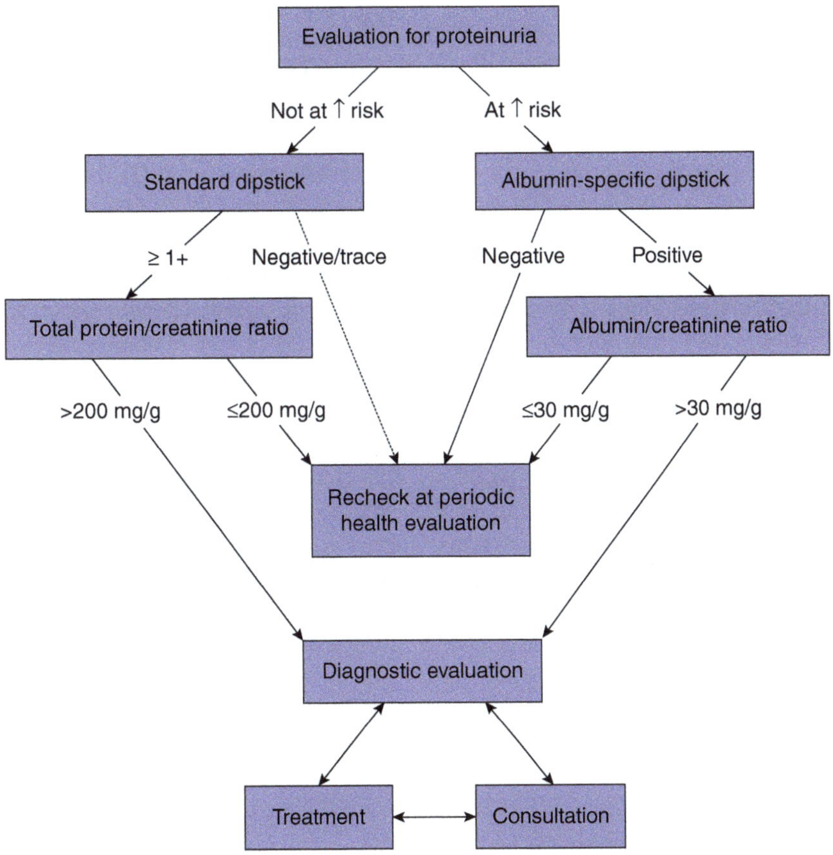

Fig. 23.1 A schematic presentation for evaluation of proteinuria. Reprinted from Am J Kidney Dis, 33, Keane WF, Eknoyan G, Proteinuria, albuminuria, risk assessment, detection, elimination (Parade): A position paper of the National Kidney Foundation, pp. 1004–1010, Copyright 1999, with permission from Elsevier

very low. Among those diagnosed with CKD, 90% of them had seen a physician within a year, but only 3–5% of patients with CKD stage 1 through 3 were aware that they had CKD.

The NKF's KEEP® offers free screening for those at risk—anyone 18 years and older with high blood pressure, diabetes, or a family history of kidney disease. It is designed to raise awareness about kidney disease among high risk individuals and provide free testing and educational information, so that kidney disease and its complications can be prevented or delayed.

Table 23.2 Signs and symptoms of chronic kidney disease

General: fatigue, malaise, edema, nocturia, decrease urine output, erectile dysfunction, insomnia
Cardiovascular: hypertension, chest pain, pericarditis, heart failure, fluid overload
Gastro intestinal: anorexia, nausea, vomiting, constipation, bleeding, dysgeusia (metallic taste)
Eye: fundoscopic evidence of hypertension (AV nicking, etc.) and DM (cotton wool spots, etc.)
Skin: pruruitis, easy bruising, pallor, echymosis
Neuromuscular: altered mental status, muscle cramps, bone pain, protein-energy malnutrition, loss of lean body mass, peripheral neuropathy, restless leg syndrome, impaired cognition, seizures, insomnia, decrease sexual drive, infertility

General Approach for Evaluation and Management of CKD

History and Physical Exam

The proper management of any disease starts with a well-rounded history and physical exam. This would include careful attention to any history of first degree family members with high blood pressure, diabetes mellitus, or kidney disease. Blood pressure and any signs of edema should be identified and all patients should be screened with a urinalysis looking for protein or blood. A urinalysis with careful review of the urine sediment should also be part of the complete work-up for any patient who has high blood pressure. If the patient has proteinuria, further work-up is outlined in Fig. 23.1. Most patients remain asymptomatic even in advance stages of kidney disease. If they do develop symptoms they are often nonspecific. Table 23.2 lists the most common signs and symptoms of CKD.

It would seem that the evaluation and management of CKD patients is best addressed through multidisciplinary CKD clinics (MDC) that include nephrologists, nurses, registered dieticians, and social workers. The advantages of early referral to a nephrologist for care of CKD patients in reducing adverse outcomes have been well documented [22–24], but the impact of multidisciplinary CKD clinics (MDC) on patient outcomes is uncertain [25, 26]. A recent study from Canada by Hammelgarn et al. [27] concluded that MDC for elderly CKD patients compared with routine care is associated with improved survival. However, the effectiveness of MDC on patient outcomes awaits confirmation through large randomized clinical trials such as Canadian Prevention of Renal and Cardiovascular Endpoints Trial (CANPREVENT) [28]

Birth Weight and CKD Risk

Low birth weight is associated with an increased risk for CKD, diabetic nephropathy, hypertension, proteinuria, and cardiovascular disease (CVD) [29, 32]. It has been hypothesized that lower birth weight is associated with smaller kidney volume, size, and lower number of nephrons [33, 34]. Vikse et al. [30] studied the records of more than two million children who were born in Norway between 1967 and 2004 and showed that low birth weight was associated with an increased risk of ESRD.

Overweight, Obesity, and CKD Risk

Obesity is defined as a BMI greater than 30. In the United States, obesity is the second leading cause of preventable diseases, behind only smoking; it is also associated with proteinuria and CKD [36].

Non-modifiable Risk Factors for CKD

Age

CKD progression correlates with aging. Elderly patients affected by glomerulonephritis generally

Table 23.3 Risk factors of chronic kidney disease

Risk factors
Hypertension and large vessel disease
Diabetes mellitus, type 1 or type 2
Glomerulonephritis, primary and secondary
Hereditary cystic and congenital renal disease
Interstitial nephritis and pyelonephritis
Malignant disease—solid tumors and multiple myeloma and lymphoma
Miscellaneous below
Collagen vascular disease—SLE, Sjogren syndrome, rheumatoid arthritis, scleroderma, vascultitis
Medications—NSAID, lithium, cisplatin
Chronic infections—Hepatitis B, C, HIV, endocarditis
Smoking
Periodontal disease

Table 23.4 Metabolic abnormalities associated with chronic kidney disease

Sodium ↑ or ↓ (hypernatremia or hyponatremia)
Potassium ↑ (hyperkalemia)
Bicarbonate ↓ (metabolic acidosis)
Phosphorus ↑ (hyperphosphatemia)
Calcium ↓ (hypocalcemia)
Parathyroid hormone (secondary hyperparathyroidism) ↑
Triglyceride ↑ (hypertriglyceridemia)
High density lipoprotein ↓
Albumin ↓ hypoalbuminemia
Uric acid ↑ hyperuricemia
Anemia ↓ normocytic anemia
Iron ↓ iron deficiency anemia
Vitamin D deficiency

have a faster decline in GFR. An exception is in individuals with type 1 insulin-dependent diabetes mellitus, in which a young age at diagnosis is associated with a faster decline in GFR. In the normal population, GFR declines with age by approximately 1 ml/min/1.73 m^2 per year after the third decade. Male gender is also associated with a faster decline in GFR [35] while the incidence and prevalence of diabetes and hypertension is higher among African American and Hispanic Americans [36].

Table 23.3 lists risk factors for CKD, and Table 23.4 lists metabolic abnormalities associated with CKD.

Modifiable Risk Factors for CKD

Cardiovascular Disease

CKD patients are at high risk for having CVD, and there is a greater likelihood that patients with CKD will die due to CVD rather than reaching ESRD [38]. Recent studies have shown that the risk of death was 83% higher for patients with CKD than age-matched controls and that the risk of dying from CVD was almost double that of age-matched controls [38]. Most patients with CKD die of heart disease rather than reaching ESRD [37]. This topic is discussed in other chapters in this section.

Hypertension

Hypertension is present in approximately 80–85% of patients with CKD independent of the primary cause of CKD. Numerous randomized control trials as well as prospective observational studies have shown that control of systemic hypertension slows the rate of progression of CKD in patients with or without diabetes [39–43]. Consequently, NKF (KDOQI) guidelines recommend a target BP less than 130/80 in CKD patients [39, 44]. To date, there have been at least three prospective randomized multicenter trials, which have specifically examined how far BP should be lowered among patients with CKD. These included the MDRD [45], the African American Study of Kidney Disease (AASK) [46], and the BP control for Renoprotection in Patients with Nondiabetic Chronic Renal Disease (REIN-2) trial [47]. It appears that lower blood pressure control results in improved outcomes. Nevertheless, Agarwal [48] questioned whether targeting a BP less than 130/80 was appropriate in the elderly, arguing that more aggressive control of BP could lead to a rapid decline in GFR in this population. He advocated that the target blood pressure in the elderly should be less than 140/90 especially as these trials demonstrated little evidence of improved survival or delay of CKD progression or a reduction of cardiovascular events below this threshold. Despite currently available antihypertensive medications, the cornerstone for BP control hinges on dietary salt restriction because a high salt intake blunts the effects of antihypertensive medications and the antiproteinuric effects of angiotensin converting enzyme inhibitors (ACEI) and ACE receptor blockers (ARB) [49].

ACEI and ARB are the first-line antihypertensive agents in CKD especially if the patients have any proteinuria. A number of large clinical trials have shown the renal protective effects of ACEI or ARB in lowering proteinuria and slowing the rate of progression of CKD [39–43]. Whether or not to combine an ACEI and ARB for management of BP was answered by the Telmisartan Alone and in Combination with Ramipril Global End Point Trial (ONTARGET) study, which showed that there is an increased risk of dialysis or doubling of the serum creatinine with combined ACEI and ARB therapy compared with a single agent [50].

The use of Dihydropyridine Calcium Channel Blockers (DHP-CCBs) versus non-Dihydropyridine Calcium Channel Blockers (non-DHP-CCBs) in slowing the rate of progression of CKD has been debated but not extensively studied. There are multiple trials which studied CCB alone or in combination of ACEI/ARB. The African American Study of Kidney Disease and Hypertension (AASK) trial, which compared amlodipine with ramipril, showed that DHP-CCB worsened proteinuria [51]. It has been shown in clinical studies that non-DHP-CCB reduce proteinuria comparable to ACEI, and DHP-CCB, particularly nifedipine, can worsen albuminuria [52]. Presently, KDOQI suggest that either a DHP-CCB or a non-DHP-CCB can be used for additional blood pressure control as long as the patient is on an ACEI or ARB.

Dyslipedemia

CKD patients frequently have dyslipidemia, predominately hypertryglyceredemia. Total cholesterol and HDL (high density lipoprotein) are reduced while the LDL (low density lipoprotein) is elevated. Total cholesterol is often low due to malnutrition and chronic inflammation. The KDOQI guidelines recommend goal LDL less than 100 mg/dl. This will be further discussed in other chapters in this section.

Proteinuria

Reduction of proteinuria is an integral component of the treatment of CKD and is associated with a slower rate of progression of CKD. Based on various studies, an ACEI or an ARB is considered first-line agent in achieving this goal. The African American Study of Kidney Disease and Hypertension (AASK) trial showed that an ACEI reduced the risk of adverse renal outcomes by 50% compared with amlodipine and 22% compared with metoprolol but a low BP goal (mean arterial pressure < 92 mmHg) conferred no additional benefit over the usual BP goal (mean arterial pressure 102–107 mmHg) [53, 54]. As noted, use of both an ACEI and ARB in combination showed no additional benefit than either alone [55]. There remains some uncertainty as to the optimal dose of an ACEI or ARB for slowing CKD progression. The ROAD (Renoprotection of Optimal Antiproteinuric Doses) study [56] has looked at conventional doses of ACEI, with higher than maximum FDA approved dosing of an ARB in nondiabetic CKD with proteinuria. This trial showed that higher than the maximum recommended doses of ARB reduced proteinuria and was associated with additional renoprotective benefits. Triple renin–angiotensin–aldosterone system (RAAS) blockade has also been a subject of interest. Clinical studies suggest that triple RAS Blockade therapy may reduce proteinuria more than dual RAS Blockade drug therapy or monotherapy using an ACEI and ARB, but the studies are small [57], and there is no conclusive study which proves it delays CKD progression. The newest RAAS-blocking agent is aliskiren, a direct renin inhibitor. This agent was studied in patients who had type 2 diabetes, hypertension, and proteinuria [58] and showed a reduction in albuminuria.

A reduction in urinary protein excretion to less than (300–500 mg/day) is associated with a slower rate of progression of CKD [59]. Moreover, clinical trials have shown that protein restriction also reduces proteinuria and the rate of progression of CKD [60]. It is recommended that dietary protein should be restricted to (0.8–1.0 g/kg IBW/day). See Chap. 27 in this section.

Uric Acid

The relationship with uric acid and risk of CKD and its progression was assessed in a study from the Atherosclerosis Risks in Communities (ARIC) and the Cardiovascular Health Study (CHS) [61]. These authors concluded that an elevated serum uric acid level is an independent risk factor, albeit modest, for incident kidney disease in the general population. Obermayer et al. [62] suggested that elevated uric acid levels are associated with higher incident of CKD. This is based on a study of more than 21,000 volunteers who were followed for a median of 7 years. After adjustment for baseline GFR, even a slight elevation of uric acid level (7.0–8.9 mg/dl) was associated with an almost twofold higher risk of incident of kidney disease; a uric acid level of more than 9.0 mg/dl was associated with a threefold risk of kidney disease. In a recent prospective, randomized, controlled trial, treatment with allopurinol 100–300 mg/day for 12 months showed a significant reduction in the level of uric acid and a reduced rate of CKD progression as compared with the control group [63].

Glycemic Control

Hyperglycemia contributes to the development of glomerular hyperfiltration and subsequently the development of glomerular sclerosis. Poor blood glucose control was associated with an increased risk of nephropathy and cardiovascular complications [64]. Currently there are no randomized clinical trials which have assessed the effect of glycemic control on CKD progression [65]. However, the United Kingdom Prospective Diabetes Study showed that intensive glucose control in patients with Diabetes mellitus type 2 could retard the progression from microalbuminuria to macroalbuminuria and could prevent the development of diabetic nephropathy [65, 66].

Anemia of CKD

Anemia is common in patient with CKD and diabetes [66]. Iron deficiency, blood loss, and decreased erythrocyte half-life are the major causes of anemia [67]. Typically, the anemia of chronic disease develops when GFR falls below 30 ml/min/1.73 m^2, but it can develop early in the course of CKD. An anemia work-up should include iron studies, reticulocyte count, red blood indices, Hgb/Hct, and stool for occult blood. Serum erythropoietin levels are not helpful in the work-up. Iron deficiency is present in almost one-third of the patients. This topic is further discussed in Chap. 25.

Mineral and Bone Disorders

CKD is characterized by decreased renal phosphate excretion, with resultant increases in serum phosphate levels. Furthermore, there is decreased conversion of vitamin D to its active form, 1, 25-dihydroxy vitamin D (1, 25(OH) D3), resulting in decreased levels of both circulating 1, 25(OH) D3 and serum calcium. Intestinal calcium absorption is also decreased. The hyperphosphatemia, hypocalcemia, and decreased levels of active vitamin D result in increased synthesis and secretion of parathyroid hormone. Hyperparathyroidism is present in more than half the patients who have a GFR of less than 60 ml/min/1.73 m^2 and is independently associated with increased mortality and an increased prevalence of CVD [68, 69]. Current guidelines recommend monitoring of serum calcium and phosphate levels (every 3–6 months), parathyroid hormone levels (every 6–12 months), and bone-specific alkaline phosphatase activity (every 6–12 months) in patients with stage IV CKD [68]. More importantly, dietary phosphorus should be restricted. For more information, see the chapters on renal bone disease and nutrition in this section.

Electrolyte and Acid–Base Disturbances

The kidney is generally able to compensate for a loss of functioning nephrons and maintain euvolemia, electrolyte balance, and acid–base balance until the GFR falls below 30 ml/min/1.73 m^2 [70]. When GFR falls below that level, renal sodium handling is impaired. In the setting of excessive dietary sodium intake, hypertension results [70]. Because of loss of the ability to form concentrated urine, patients with CKD are more prone to water disorders including hypo and hypernatremia. CKD patients can have other complex electrolyte and acid–base disorders including hyperkalemia and non-anion gap

Table 23.5 Suggestions for screening intervals and management of progression

CKD	Screening	Interval	Progression
Stage 3	PTH, Ca, Phos, Vit D, Hgb	Q 6–12 months	ACEI and ARB—diabetic, Statins
	Microalbuminuria, electrolytes		Diuretics, beta blocker—nondiabetic
			ESA, Biacarb supp, Phos binders, Vit D
Stage 4	PTH, Ca, Phos, Vit D, Hgb	Q 3 months	All of above with addition of loop diuretic
	Macroalbuminuria, electrolytes		Dietary restrictions 2/2/800 (na/k/phos)
	Dialysis access and education		0.6 g/kg protein
Stage 5	PTH, Ca, Phos, Vit D, Hgb	Q 3 months and PRN	All of above with frequent monitoring of electrolytes, acidosis, and uremic syndrome
	Proteinuria, electrolytes		
	Dialysis access and education		Timing of initiation of dialysis

Table 23.6 Target and goals for advanced stages of CKD

CKD	Targets and goals								
Stage	Diet	BP	A1C	Anemia	PT	Phos	25 OHD	LDL	HCO_3
3	Na/K/Phos	<130/80	<7%	10–12 mg/dl	35–70	<4.6	>30	<100	>22
	2/2/800								
	pro 0.6 g/kg								
4	As above	<130/80	<7%	10–12 mg/dl	70–110	<4.6	>30	<100	>22
5	As above	<130/80	<7%	10–12 mg/dl	150–300	<5.5		<100	

metabolic acidosis. This is particularly common in patients with diabetes and hypoaldosteroism. Hyperkalemia can develop in patients with CKD if they receive aldosterone antagonist, ACE Inhibitors, or ARB or if they have excessive dietary intake of potassium [71].

In patients with advanced CKD, there is a reduction in renal ammonia synthesis and a decrease excretion of titrable acids (phosphate) [72]. A recent randomized clinical trial demonstrated that bicarbonate supplementation slowed the rate of progression of CKD to ESRD and improved the nutritional status among patients with CKD [73]. It is strongly encouraged that sufficient sodium bicarbonate be given to any patient with CKD to maintain the serum bicarbonate between 22 and 25 mmol. Additional studies have shown that the risk of volume overload is minimal in that subjects utilized the bicarbonate and lost the excess sodium in the urine even with advanced CKD (see Tables 23.5 and 23.6) [74].

Case Revisited

Because of the elevated creatinine, the patient was referred to a nephrologist. After careful review of the history and physical exam, a urine dip stick was positive for trace albumin.

A renal ultrasound showed the right kidney to be 8.5 cm while the left kidney measured 8.7 cm. Both kidneys were echogenic. No hydronephrosis or renal stones were noted. Additional lab work was done (see Table 23.7).

The patient's medications were reviewed. Metformin was discontinued and insulin therapy was initiated with better glycemic control; the HCTZ was switched to furosemide. An ACE Inhibitor was added with close monitoring of both serum potassium and creatinine levels, and a non-DHP-CCB diltiazem was necessary to reach optimal blood pressure control. Because of iron deficiency, a gastroenterology work-up was done which was negative. The patient was started on

Table 23.7 Laboratory data

Laboratory data	(Reference values)
Hemoglobin: 9.6 g/dl	13.2–16.2 g/dl (male) 12.0–15.2 g/dl (female)
Platelets: 195 mmol/L	(140–440 mmol/L)
White blood cell count: 6.83 mmol/L with normal differential	(3.6–11.2 mmol/L)
Sodium: 135 mmol/L	(136–144 mmol/L)
Potassium: 5.2 mmol/L	(3.7–5.2 mmol/L)
Chloride: 105 mmol/L	(101–111 mmol/L)
Bicarbonate (HCO_3): 24 mmol/L	(20–29 mmol/L)
BUN: 32 mg/dl	(7–20 mg/dl)
Creatinine: 2.0 mg/dl	(0.7–1.4 mg/dl)
Calcium 8.4 mg/dl	(8.4–10.2 mg/dl)
Phosphorus 5.2 mg/dl	(2.6–4.5 mg/dl)
PTH (intact) 146 pg/ml	(10–60 pg/ml)
Hemoglobin A1C: 7.6%	(4.1–6.5%)
Urine Dip: 2+ protein	(Negative)
Urine 24 h protein excretion is 2.7 g	(Negative)

iron and ESA (erythropoeisis stimulating agent) and a hemoglobin of (11–12 mg/dl) was targeted. Following a dietary consult, the patient was started on a renal diet with phosphate binders added to each meal. Ergocalciferol supplementation was initiated. Statin therapy was started.

A discussion with the patient and family ensued regarding possible future renal replacement therapies including living and deceased renal transplantation. They were also provided information on peritoneal and hemodialysis in center and at home. Finally, timing of placement of a dialysis access was also discussed.

References

1. Prevalence of chronic kidney disease and associated risk factors—United States, 1999—2004. http://www.cdc.gov/mmwr/preview/mmwrhtml/mm5608a2.htm. Accessed 17 Feb 2011.
2. K/DOQI clinical practice guidelines for chronic kidney disease. Evaluation, classification, and stratification. Am J Kidney Dis. 2002;39:S1–266.
3. Vassalotti JA, Stevens LA, Levey AS. Testing for chronic kidney disease: a position statement from the National Kidney Foundation. Am J Kidney Dis. 2007;50:169–80.
4. Eriksen BO, Ingebretsen OC. In chronic kidney disease staging the use of the chronicity criterion affects prognosis and the rate of progression. Kidney Int. 2007;72:1242–8.
5. Coresh J, Astor BC, Greene T, et al. Prevalence of chronic kidney disease and decreased kidney function in the adult US population: third National Health and Nutrition Examination Survey. Am J Kidney Dis. 2003;41:1–12.
6. Weiner DE, Krassilnikova M, Tighiouart H, et al. CKD classification based on estimated GFR over three years and subsequent cardiac and mortality outcomes: a cohort study. BMC Nephrol. 2009;10:26.
7. Levey AS, Bosch JP, Lewis JB, et al. A more accurate method to estimate glomerular filtration rate from serum creatinine: a new prediction equation. Modification of Diet in Renal Disease Study Group. Ann Intern Med. 1999;130:461–70.
8. Lindeman RD, Tobin J, Shock NW. Longitudinal studies on the rate of decline in renal function with age. Baltimore Longitudinal Study—Johns Hopkins. J Am Geriatr Soc. 1985;33:278–85.
9. Cockcroft DW, Gault MH. Prediction of creatinine clearance from serum creatinine. Nephron. 1976;16:31–41.
10. Levey AS, Stevens LA, Schmid CH, et al. A new equation to estimate glomerular filtration rate. Ann Intern Med. 2009;150:604–12.
11. Rule AD, Larson TS, Bergstralh EJ, et al. Using serum creatinine to estimate glomerular filtration rate: accuracy in good health and in chronic kidney disease. Ann Intern Med. 2004;141:929–37.
12. Hoek FJ, Kemperman FA, Krediet RT. A comparison between cystatin C, plasma creatinine and the Cockcroft and Gault formula for the estimation of glomerular filtration rate. Nephrol Dial Transpl. 2003;18:2024–31.
13. Stevens LA, Coresh J, Schmid CH, et al. Estimating GFR using serum cystatin C alone and in combination with serum creatinine: a pooled analysis of 3,418 individuals with CKD. Am J Kidney Dis. 2008;51:395–406.
14. Marsik C, Endler G, Gulesserian T, et al. Classification of chronic kidney disease by estimated glomerular filtration rate. Eur J Clin Invest. 2008;38:253–9.
15. Fontsere N, Esteve V, Saurina A, et al. The search for a new marker of renal function in older patients with chronic kidney disease stages 3-4: usefulness of cystatin C-based equations. Nephron Clin Pract. 2009;112:c164–70.
16. Anderson J, Glynn LG. Definition of chronic kidney disease and measurement of kidney function in original research papers: a review of the literature. Nephrol Dial Transplant. 2011;0:1–6.
17. Levey AS, Coresh J, Greene T, Stevens LA, Zhang YL, Hendriksen S, Kusek JW, Van Lente F. Using standardized serum creatinine values in the modification of diet in renal disease study equation for estimating glomerular filtration rate. Ann Intern Med. 2006;145:247–54.
18. http://www.kidney.org/news/keep/index.cfm Accessed 12 Feb 2011.

19. Johnson CA, Levey AS, Coresh J, Levin A, Lau J, Eknoyan G. Practice guidelines for chronic kidney disease in adults: part I. Definition, disease stages, evaluation, treatment, and risk factors. Am Fam Physician. 2004;70(5):869–76.
20. Jaar BG, Khatib R, Plantinga L, Boulware LE, Powe NR. Principles of screening for chronic kidney disease. Clin J Am Soc Nephrol. 2008;3:601–9.
21. Saab G, Whaley-Connell AT, McCullough PA, Bakris GL. CKD awareness in the United States: the Kidney Early Evaluation Program (KEEP). Am J Kidney Dis. 2008;52:382–3.
22. Kazmi WH, Obrador GT, Khan SS, Pereira BJ, Kausz AT. Late nephrology referral and mortality among patients with end-stage renal disease: a propensity score analysis. Nephrol Dial Transplant. 2004;19:1808–14.
23. Khan SS, Xue JL, Kazmi WH, Gilbertson DT, Obrador GT, Pereira BJ, Collins AJ. Does predialysis nephrology care influence patient survival after initiation of dialysis? Kidney Int. 2005;67:1038–46.
24. Kinchen KS, Sadler J, Fink N, Brookmeyer R, Klag MJ, Levey AS, Powe NR. The timing of specialist evaluation in chronic kidney disease and mortality. Ann Intern Med. 2002;137:479–86.
25. Goldstein M, Yassa T, Dacouris N, McFarlane P. Multidisciplinary predialysis care and morbidity and mortality of patients on dialysis. Am J Kidney Dis. 2004;44:706–14.
26. Harris LE, Luft FC, Rudy DW, Kesterson JG, Tierney WM. Effects of multidisciplinary case management in patients with chronic renal insufficiency. Am J Med. 1998;105:464–71.
27. Hemmelgarn BR, Manns BJ, Zhang J, Tonell M, Klarenbach S, Walsh M. Bruce F. Culleton for the Alberta Kidney Disease Network. Association between multidisciplinary care and survival for elderly patients with chronic kidney disease. J Am Soc Nephrol. 2007;18:993–9.
28. Parfrey P, Barrett B, Levin A, Churchill D, Goeree R, Singer J, Molzahn A, Djurdjev O. The Canadian Prevention of Renal and Cardiovascular Endpoints Trial. 2006. http://clinicaltrials.gov. Accessed 1 Mar 2011.
29. Brenner BM, Mackenzie HS. Nephron mass as a risk factor for progression of renal disease. Kidney Int Suppl. 1997;63:S124–7.
30. Vikse BE, Irgens LM, Leivestad T, Hallan S, Iversen BM. Low birth weight increases risk for end-stage renal disease. J Am Soc Nephrol. 2008;19:151–7.
31. Al Salmi I, Hoy WE, Kondalsamy-Chennakes S, Wang Z, Healy H, Shaw JE. Birth weight and stages of CKD: a case-control study in an Australian population. Am J Kidney Dis. 2008;52:1070–8.
32. Li S, Chen SC, Shlipak M, Bakris G, McCullough PA, Sowers J, Stevens L, Jurkovitz C, McFarlane S, Norris K, Vassalotti J, Klag MJ, Brown WW, Narva A, Calhoun D, Johnson B, Obialo C, Whaley-Connell A, Becker B, Collins AJ. Low birth weight is associated with chronic kidney disease only in men. Kidney Int. 2008;73:637–42.
33. Foster MC, Hwang SJ, Larson MG, Lichtman JH, Parikh NI, Vasan RS, Levy D, Fox CS. Overweight, obesity, and the development of stage 3 CKD: the Framingham Heart Study. Am J Kidney Dis. 2008;52:39–48.
34. Young JA, Hwang SJ, Sarnak MJ, Hoffmann U, Massaro JM, Levy D, Benjamin EJ, Larson MG, Vasan RS, O'Donnell CJ, Fox CS. Association of visceral and subcutaneous adiposity with kidney function. Clin J Am Soc Nephrol. 2008;3:1786–91.
35. Berns JS, Fishbane S. Chronic kidney disease and progression. NephSAP. 2009;8(4):252–3.
36. Tarver-Carr ME, Powe NR, Eberhardt MS, LaVeist TA, Kington RS, Coresh J, Brancati FL. Excess risk of chronic kidney disease among African-American versus White subjects in the United States: a population-based study of potential explanatory factors. J Am Soc Nephrol. 2002;13:2363–70.
37. Foley RN, Parfrey PS, Sarnak MJ. Epidemiology of cardiovascular disease in chronic renal disease. J Am Soc Nephrol. 1998;9(12 suppl):S16–23.
38. Wen CP, Cheng TY, Tsai MK, Chang YC, Chan HT, Tsai SP, Chiang PH, Hsu CC, Sung PK, Hsu YH, Wen SF. All-cause mortality attributable to chronic kidney disease: a prospective cohort study based on 462 293 adults in Taiwan. Lancet. 2008;371:2173–82.
39. National Kidney Foundation. K/DOQI clinical practice guideline and clinical practice recommendations for diabetes and chronic kidney disease. Am J Kidney Dis. 2007;49 Suppl 2:S12–154.
40. Barnett AH, Bain SC, Bouter P, et al. Angiotensin-receptor blockade versus converting-enzyme inhibition in type 2 diabetes and nephropathy. N Engl J Med. 2004;351:1952–61.
41. Jafar TH, Stark PC, Schmid CH, et al. Progression of chronic kidney disease: the role of blood pressure control, proteinuria, and angiotensin-converting enzyme inhibition: a patient-level meta-analysis. Ann Intern Med. 2003;139:244–52.
42. Lewis EJ, Hunsicker LG, Clarke WR, et al. Renoprotective effect of the angiotensin-receptor antagonist irbesartan in patients with nephropathy due to type 2 diabetes. N Engl J Med. 2001;345:851–60.
43. Brenner BM, Cooper ME, de Zeeuw D, et al. Effects of losartan on renal and cardiovascular outcomes in patients with type 2 diabetes and nephropathy. N Engl J Med. 2001;345:861–9.
44. National Kidney Foundation. K/DOQI clinical practice guidelines on hypertension and antihypertensive agents in chronic kidney disease. Am J Kidney Dis. 2004;43 Suppl 1:S1–290.
45. Klahr S, Levey AS, Beck GJ, et al. The effects of dietary protein restriction and blood-pressure control on the progression of chronic renal disease. Modification of Diet in Renal Disease Study Group. N Engl J Med. 1994;330:877–84.
46. Wright Jr JT, Bakris G, Greene T, et al. Effect of blood pressure lowering and antihypertensive drug class on progression of hypertensive kidney disease: results from the AASK trial. JAMA. 2002;288:2421–31.

47. Ruggenenti P, Perna A, Loriga G, et al. Blood-pressure control for renoprotection in patients with nondiabetic chronic renal disease (REIN-2): multicentre, randomised controlled trial. Lancet. 2005;365:939–46.
48. Agarwal R. Blood pressure goal in chronic kidney disease: what is the evidence? Curr Opin Nephrol Hypertens. 2011;20(3):229–32.
49. Esnault VLM, Ekhlas AMR, Delcroix C, Moutel MG, Nguyen JM. Diuretic and enhanced sodium restriction results in improved antiproteinuric response to RAS blocking agents. J Am Soc Nephrol. 2005;16:474–81.
50. Mann JF, Schmieder RE, McQueen M, Dyal L, Schumacher H, Pogue J, Wang X, Maggioni A, Budaj A, Chaithiraphan S, Dickstein K, Keltai M, Metsarinne K, Oto A, Parkhomenko A, Piegas LS, Svendsen TL, Teo KK, Yusuf S. Renal outcomes with telmisartan, ramipril, or both, in people at high vascular risk (the ONTARGET study): a multicentre, randomized, double-blind, controlled trial. Lancet. 2008;372:547–53.
51. Agodoa LY, Appel L, Bakris GL, et al. Effect of ramipril vs amlodipine on renal outcomes in hypertensive nephrosclerosis. A randomized controlled trial. JAMA. 2001;285:2719–28.
52. Kloke HJ, Branten AJ, Huysmans FT, Wetzels JE. Antihypertensive treatment of patients with proteinuric renal disease: risks or benefits of calcium channel blockers. Kidney Int. 1998;53:1559–73.
53. Wright Jr JT, Bakris G, Greene T, Agodoa LY, Appel LJ, Charleston J, Cheek D, Douglas-Baltimore JG, Gassman J, Glassock R, Hebert L, Jamerson K, Lewis J, Phillips RA, Toto RD, Middleton JP, Rostand SG. Effect of blood pressure lowering and antihypertensive drug class on progression of hypertensive kidney disease: Results from the AASK trial. JAMA. 2002;288:2421–31.
54. Agodoa LY, Appel L, Bakris GL, Beck G, Bourgoignie J, Briggs JP, Charleston J, Cheek D, Cleveland W, Douglas JG, Douglas M, Dowie D, Faulkner M, Gabriel A, Gassman J, Greene T, Hall Y, Hebert L, Hiremath L, Jamerson K, Johnson CJ, Kopple J, Kusek J, Lash J, Lea J, Lewis JB, Lipkowitz M, Massry S, Middleton J, Miller III ER, Norris K, O'Connor D, Ojo A, Phillips RA, Pogue V, Rahman M, Randall OS, Rostand S, Schulman G, Smith W, Thornley-Brown D, Tisher CC, Toto RD, Wright Jr JT, Xu S. Effect of ramipril vs amlodipine on renal outcomes in hypertensive nephrosclerosis: a randomized controlled trial. JAMA. 2001;285:2719–28.
55. Yusuf S, Teo KK, Pogue J, Dyal L, Copland I, Schumacher H, Dagenais G, Sleight P, Anderson C. Telmisartan, ramipril, or both in patients at high risk for vascular events. N Engl J Med. 2008;358:1547–59.
56. Hou FF, Xie D, Zhang X, Chen PY, Zhang WR, Liang M, Guo ZJ, Jiang JP. Renoprotection of Optimal Antiproteinuric Doses (ROAD) Study: a randomized controlled study of benazepril and losartan in chronic renal insufficiency. J Am Soc Nephrol. 2007;18:1889–98.
57. Tylicki L, Rutkowski P, Renke M, Larczynski W, Aleksandrowicz E, Lysiak-Szydlowska W, Rutkowski B. Triple pharmacological blockade of the renin-angiotensin-aldosterone system in nondiabetic CKD: an open-label crossover randomized controlled trial. Am J Kidney Dis. 2008;52:486–93.
58. Parving HH, Persson F, Lewis JB, Lewis EJ, Hollenberg NK. Aliskiren combined with losartan in type 2 diabetes and nephropathy. N Engl J Med. 2008;358:2433–46.
59. Ruggenenti P, Cravedi P, Remuzzi G. Proteinuria: increased angiotensin-receptor blocking is not the first option. Nat Rev Nephrol. 2009;5:367–8.
60. Pedrini MT, Levey AS, Lau J, Chalmers TC, Wang PH. The effect of dietary protein restriction on the progression of diabetic and nondiabetic renal diseases: a meta-analysis. Ann Intern Med. 1996;124:627–32.
61. Weiner DE, Tighiouart H, Elsayed EF, Griffith JL, Salem DN, Levey AS. Uric acid and incident kidney disease in the community. J Am Soc Nephrol. 2008;19:1204–11.
62. Obermayr RP, Temml C, Gutjahr G, Knechtelsdorfer M, Oberbauer R, Klauser-Braun R. Elevated uric acid increases the risk for kidney disease. J Am Soc Nephrol. 2008;19:2407–13.
63. Siu YP, Leung KT, Tong MK, Kwan TH. Use of allopurinol in slowing the progression of renal disease through its ability to lower serum uric acid level. Am J Kidney Dis. 2006;47:51–9.
64. The Diabetes Control and Complications Trial Research Group. The effect of intensive treatment of diabetes on the development and progression of long-term complications in insulin-dependent diabetes mellitus. N Engl J Med. 1993;329:977–86.
65. UK Prospective Diabetes Study (UKPDS) Group. Intensive blood-glucose control with sulphonylureas or insulin compared with conventional treatment and risk of complications in patients with type 2 diabetes (UKPDS 33). Lancet. 1998;352:837–53 [Erratum, Lancet 1999;354:602].
66. El-Achkar TM, Ohmit SE, McCullough PA, et al. Higher prevalence of anemia with diabetes mellitus in moderate kidney insufficiency: the Kidney Early Evaluation Program. Kidney Int. 2005;67:1483–8.
67. KDOQI. KDOQI clinical practice guideline and clinical practice recommendations for anemia in chronic kidney disease: 2007 update of hemoglobin target. Am J Kidney Dis. 2007;50:471–530.
68. Kidney Disease: Improving Global Outcomes (KDIGO) CKD-MBD Working Group. KDIGO clinical practice guideline for diagnosis, evaluation, prevention, and treatment of chronic kidney disease-mineral and bone disorder (CKD-MBD). Kidney Int Suppl. 2009;113:S1–130.
69. Kestenbaum B, Sampson JN, Rudser KD, et al. Serum phosphate levels and mortality risk among people with chronic kidney disease. J Am Soc Nephrol. 2005;16:520–8.
70. Mitch WE, Wilcox CS. Disorders of body fluids, sodium and potassium in chronic renal failure. Am J Med. 1982;72:536–50.

71. Maddirala S, Khan A, Vincent A, Lau K. Effect of angiotensin converting enzyme inhibitors and angiotensin receptor blockers on serum potassium levels and renal function in ambulatory outpatients: risk factors analysis. Am J Med Sci. 2008;336:330–5.
72. Kraut JA, Kurtz I. Metabolic acidosis of CKD: diagnosis, clinical characteristics, and treatment. Am J Kidney Dis. 2005;45:978–93.
73. de Brito-Ashurst I, Varagunam M, Raftery MJ, Yaqoob MM. Bicarbonate supplementation slows progression of CKD and improves nutritional status. J Am Soc Nephrol. 2009;20:2075–84.
74. Papadoyannakis NJ, Stefanidis CJ, McGeown M. The effect of the correction of metabolis acidosis on nitrogen and potassium balance of patients with chronic renal failure. Am J Clin Nutr. 1984;40:623–7.

24 Mineral and Bone Disorders in Chronic Kidney Disease

Lynn E. Schlanger and James L. Bailey

Case

A 64-year-old woman with a history of chronic kidney disease (CKD) Stage 4 [estimated glomerular filtration rate (eGFR) of 17 cc/min/1.73 mm^2] is referred for evaluation of "poor kidney function." Over the last month she has complained of itching, skin eruptions on her arms and back, and nonspecific bone pain. She has been unable to sleep at night and denies changes in soap, laundry detergent, or perfume. She has never been prescribed a phosphate binder or vitamin D, has no dietary restrictions, and dines out a few times per week. She usually consumes bacon and eggs for breakfast, a sandwich with cheese and cold cuts for lunch, and beans and chicken or fish for dinner. She has never been to see a nutritionist but feels her dietary intake is adequate. Physical exam is remarkable for diffuse areas of excoriation on her arms and back with raised hard central pustules. Pertinent laboratory values: phosphorous—7.5 mg/dL, calcium—7.9 g/dL, albumin—4 g/dL, creatinine—3.5 mg/dL, urea—50 mg/dL, alkaline phosphatase—180 mg/dL, bicarbonate—20 mEq/L. Intact PTH and vitamin D 25 are pending at the end of her visit.

L.E. Schlanger, M.D. (✉)
Department of Nephrology, Veteran Affairs Medical Center at Atlanta, Decatur, Dekalb, GA 30033, USA
e-mail: lynn.schlanger@va.gov

J.L. Bailey, M.D.
Renal Division, Medicine, Emory University, Atlanta, GA 30322, USA

Introduction

The prevalence of CKD in the United States has risen from 10.3 to 13.1% and accounts for more than 25 million people [1]. Associated with a decline in kidney function are common metabolic derangements which include: mineral and bone disturbances; anemia; acid–base imbalance; and dyslipidemia. Anemia and dyslipidemia of CKD will be discussed in the other sections, and this chapter will focus upon mineral and bone disorder (MBD) commonly found in mild, moderate, and severe kidney disease.

By CKD stage 3 there is evidence of bone remodeling which progresses with advance kidney disease and is referred to as renal osteodystrophy. Interestingly, these changes may occur earlier [2, 3]. In a large cross-sectional study of the MBD biochemical markers, an elevated serum PTH was observed in 12% with an eGFR of >80 cc/min/1/73 mm^2 while the other biochemical bone parameters, serum phosphorous (Pi) and calcium (Ca), remained within the normal range until an eGFR of <40 cc/min/1.73 mm^2 [3]. These renal bone changes are responsible for fractures, bone pain, immobility, and weakness [2, 4, 5], and the associated MBD biochemical abnormalities have been shown to be associated with an increase in cardiovascular disease events, all-cause mortality, and sudden death [6–12].

E.V. Lerma and M. Rosner (eds.), *Clinical Decisions in Nephrology, Hypertension and Kidney Transplantation*, DOI 10.1007/978-1-4614-4454-1_24, © Springer Science+Business Media New York 2013

In observational studies in hemodialysis patients, the cardiovascular events correlated with the serum Pi, serum Ca and Pi product, and PTH level [6–9], and a few observational studies in pre-dialysis patients showed a similar correlation with elevated serum Pi and PTH levels [12, 13]. The elevated PTH in CKD is an adaptive response to the increase in the serum Pi from a decline in kidney function, a low serum Ca^{2+} from a decrease in 1,25 dihydroxyvitamin D (calcitriol), an increase in fibroblast growth factor (FGF-23), and a decrease in calcitriol from a decline in 1-α-hydroxylase production which is responsible for both renal osteodystrophy and the adverse clinical outcomes.

To develop more cohesive guidelines for the management of MBD in CKD, two work groups have been established: the Kidney Dialysis Outcomes Quality Initiative (KDOQI) in 2003 [14] and the Kidney Disease International Global Outcomes (KDIGO) in 2009 [4]. Although there are some differences between these two groups with regard to the definition of renal bone disease and treatment and monitoring, they have a common purpose to improve communications, facilitate decision making, and promote evidence-based clinical practice guidelines [11]. The newer KDIGO guidelines permit countries to adapt these specific guidelines to their own clinical practices [8]. KDIGO views MBD-CKD as a systemic disorder manifested by one or more of the following: (1) abnormalities of calcium, phosphorous, parathyroid hormone, or vitamin D metabolism, (2) abnormalities in bone pathology and histomorphometry marked by changes in bone turnover, mineralization, volume, linear growth, or strength (TMV system), and (3) the presence of vascular or other soft tissue calcification [4].

Soft tissue calcification is associated with a very high morbidity and mortality [15–17]. This is known as calciphylaxis or calcific uremic arteriolopathy (CUA). Fortunately, it is rare (1–4%) and more commonly found in advanced stages of CKD [15–17]. It is a vasculopathy characterized by extraosseous calcification of soft tissue and medial calcification of the arteries accompanied by necrosis of the skin and subcutaneous fat [15–18]. These areas can become painful ulcerative plaques and tend to be more pronounced in the lower extremities, but they are also found on the abdomen, breast, and buttocks [16]. Risk factors found to be associated with calciphylaxis in 18 hemodialysis patients include: female gender, low albumin, and elevated serum phosphorous and alkaline phosphatase. Calciphylaxis is associated with an eightfold increase in death [15, 17]. Other proposed risk factors are diabetes, race, obesity, trauma, hypotension, a high serum calcium and phosphate product, protein C deficiency, coumadin, and steroids [15–17].

Previously, renal osteodystrophy included both bone histology and biochemistry. Now, it is defined only by histology and histomorphometry obtained by a bone biopsy at an ideal location such as the iliac crest [2, 4]. There are four types of renal osteodystrophy: osteitis fibrosis (high turnover disease) related to elevated serum PTH, adynamic bone disease (low turnover), osteomalacia (low turnover), and mixed uremic osteodystrophy [2, 4, 14, 19, 20]. A bone biopsy should be considered in advanced renal disease for those with unexplained fractures, persistent bone pain, unexplained hypercalcemia, unexplained hypophosphatemia, possible aluminum toxicity, and prior to therapy with bisphosphonates [4].

To further complicate MBD, there is an increase in prevalence rates for both CKD and osteoporosis, especially in the elderly population in which they commonly coexist [21, 22]. Osteoporosis is an absorptive process while MBD-CKD is an imbalance of bone formation, mineralization, and volume; both can result in fractures. The treatment options differ for these two disorders and correct diagnosis is important in order to avoid inappropriate treatment. The dual-energy X-ray absorptiometry, a two-dimensional bone density scan used to diagnose osteoporosis, may not be helpful in differentiating between these two disorders and in fact may overestimate bone mineral density (BMD) in moderate CKD [21]. The quantitative computerized tomography and micro-magnetic resonance imaging better discriminate between the changes in the cortical and trabecular bone and on changes in bone volume [21] and aid in the correct diagnosis. However,

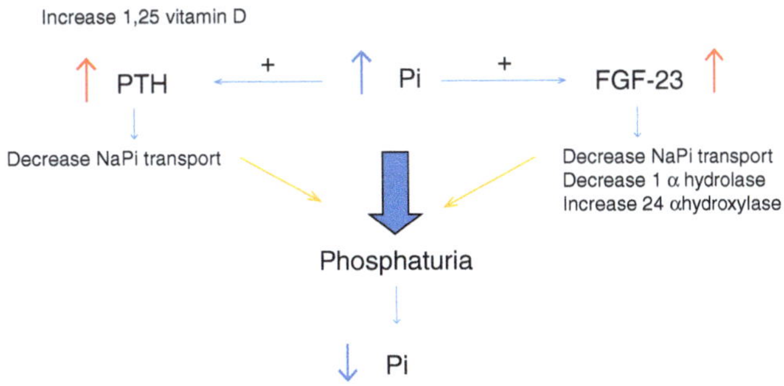

Fig. 24.1 Hyperphosphaturia. Increase in the serum Pi results in an increase of FGF-23 and PTH and decline in 1,25-dihydroxyvitamin D and an increase in urinary Pi to maintain normal serum Pi

the gold standard to differentiate between these two disorders is the two-phase tetracycline labeling bone biopsy [21, 22].

MBD: Biochemistry

Hyperphosphatemia, hypocalcemia, low calcitriol, elevated FGF-23, and serum PTH, all play a role at different times in MBD-CKD. Interestingly, the serum Pi is at the center of the new paradigm (Fig. 24.1). As kidney function declines, the serum Pi rises, the secretion of FGF-23 from the osteocytes is stimulated, there is a decline in the availability of the 1-α-hydroxylase in the proximal convoluting tubule, and an inactivity of the Na Pi transporter, resulting in phosphaturia. The low levels of calcitriol commonly seen in kidney failure may be secondary to inhibition from FGF-23 rather than from a decline in renal mass [24–26]. The components of the mineral bone abnormalities and their contribution to MBD will be discussed individually.

Calcium

Calcium is one of the major divalent cations in the body and contributes to skeletal structure and regulation of cellular function. 99% of the body's calcium is contained in the intracellular compartment, bone, and only 1% is available for calcium homeostasis [27, 28]. The normal range of calcium is 8.4–10.4 mg/dL. 50% circulates freely while the remainder is bound to albumin or anions. The maintenance of serum calcium is determined by various hormones, PTH, calcitonin, and calcitriol, which in turn regulate gut, kidney, and bone [27] to maintain the serum calcium level.

In advancing CKD there is a decreased calcium absorption in the small bowel secondary to a decline in calcitriol and dietary intake. An elevated Pi and a low serum Ca^{2+} increase PTH secretion via the Ca^{2+} sensing receptor [27, 28]. This rise in serum PTH results in an increase in Ca^{2+} reabsorption in renal distal tubules and increase resorption of bone in an attempt to maintain normal or near normal serum Ca^{2+}.

Parathyroid Hormone

PTH is a cleaved 1–84 amino acid protein with the first 6 amino acids accounting for its activity while the 7–84 amino acid fragment protein is inactive [4]. It is a major regulator of bone turnover and acts directly on osteoblasts and indirectly on osteoclasts [27] and is used as a marker for bone turnover [20]. There have been many different PTH assays [29]. The first generation assay is obsolete since it measured both PTH 1–84 and its numerous fragments [29]. A "second generation" assay, known as the "intact" PTH [4] measures both active and inactive PTH forms by binding with the amino acid and carboxy terminus and is the most commonly used. A "third generation" assay detects only the 1–84 amino acid hormone and is less available [4]. Although the intact second generation assay is currently recommended, therapy should be guided by trends in the serum PTH level rather than isolated laboratory values [4].

The serum PTH level is influenced by calcitriol [29–31], serum ionized Ca^{2+} [32], serum Pi [28], and possibly FGF-23 [28]. A low serum ionized Ca^{2+} level stimulates the parathyroid gland through a G protein-coupled calcium-sensing receptor [31]. PTH secretion is followed by a release of Ca^{2+} from bone [27]. In the kidney, the PTH influences both the proximal and distal tubules. In the PCT, the binding of PTH to PTH type 1 receptor down regulates the expression of the NaPi 2a co-transporter in the apical membrane [31]. An increase in phosphaturia normalizes the serum Pi [27, 31]. In the distal tubule, PTH increases Ca^{2+} reabsorption through the TPVR Ca^{2+} channels [27]. The proximal tubule is also the site for calcitriol production via 1-α-hydroxylase. Calcitriol binds to the vitamin D receptors (VDRs) and inhibits PTH gene transcription [33]; parathyroid gland hyperplasia and osteitis fibrosis is avoided. The VDR function is impaired by hypocalcemia and hyperphosphatemia [33].

In CKD, increased serum PTH values have been reported in African Americans, the obese, and nondiabetics [13]. Although the initial evaluation for MBD is recommended for patients with CKD stage 3, some observational studies suggest that secondary hyperparathyroidism occurs earlier [3, 13]. In one study, elevated PTH values were found in 50.1% of participants with CKD stage 3 and appeared to increase the risk for cardiovascular disease. This is interesting because there may be an association with elevated PTH and left ventricular hypertrophy, impaired glucose intolerance, and arterial stiffness [12]. Therefore, close surveillance for hyperparathyroidism is indicated in patients with CKD.

Phosphate

Phosphorus (Pi) plays a major role in bone formation, skeletal stability, cellular function, and cell membrane structure and exists mainly in the organic form [27, 31]. Eighty to eighty-five percentage of body Pi is located in the mineral phase of bone [27]; 1% of Pi is in the serum in an inorganic form [31], and the remainder is in other intracellular and extracellular compartments.

The normal serum Pi is largely unbound [27], ranges from 2.5 to 4.5 mg/dL and is maintained by the kidney and gastrointestinal tract. Under the influence of calcitriol, Pi is absorbed in the small intestine. In the kidney, unbound Pi is free across the glomerulus and 80–90% is reabsorbed in the PCT (60–70%) and distal nephron (20–30%) [27]. In early CKD, the serum Pi is maintained by decreased absorption in the GI tract from a decrease in calcitriol [27] and increased Pi excretion through decreased expression of the Na Pi 2a co-transporter in the PCT by PTH [27, 31] and FGF-23 [24, 34].

An increase of serum Pi by 1 mg/dL is associated with an increased prevalence of calcification of coronary arteries, descending aorta, aortic valve, and mitral valve [7]. Besides skeletal and extra-skeletal calcification, Pi may be responsible for other adverse outcomes. CKD rats on a high phosphate diet had higher heart weights than corresponding control rats [35].

Fibroblast Growth Factor 23

FGF-23, a 32 kDa protein secreted by osteocytes [24, 25, 36], induces renal phosphaturia by inhibiting renal production of calcitriol through enhanced expression of 24-hydroxylase. An increase in PTH follows [24, 25, 34]. Healthy medical students had an increase in FGF-23 16 h after being placed on a high Pi diet [36]. Calcitriol levels declined and urinary Pi excretion rose. No changes in these parameters were seen in the control group [36]. A rise in FGF-23 levels may be a mechanism of maintaining Pi homeostasis [32, 36] in early CKD.

Vitamin D

Vitamin D is involved in regulation of bone metabolism, skeletal muscle, and maintenance of calcium and phosphate homeostasis [37, 38]. Observational studies link vitamin D with extraosseous function involving the heart, immune system, renin hypertension, diabetes [37–40], and improved outcomes [41–43]. Only a small amount of 25-hydroxyvitamin D (calcidiol)

(5%) is converted by the kidney to calcitriol; the remainder is converted in other tissues [37, 38].

A large percentage of the population, particularly the elderly and the chronically ill, is vitamin D deficient or insufficient [37], where deficiency is defined as a calcidiol level less than 10 ng/mL [37, 38] and insufficient as a calcidiol level between 20 and 30 ng/mL [37]. There are two sources of calcidiol: the skin or food. Calcidiol levels will vary with the seasons, latitude, race, gender, and dietary intake [37]. Upon exposure to ultraviolet light, the pre-vitamin D3, 7- and 8-dehydrocholesterol, is non-enzymatically converted in the skin to Vitamin D3, cholecalciferol [37, 38]. The vitamin D3, prohormone, is then converted by the liver via 25-hydroxylase (CYP2R1) to calcidiol [37]. Around 40–50% of the circulating calcidiol is from sun exposure [37]. The remainder is from dietary supplementation with vitamin D2 (ergocalciferol) and vitamin D3 (cholecalciferol) [37]. Both can be converted by the liver to calcidiol. Serum calcidiol reflects total body vitamin D from dietary intake, skin, and liver stores [37]. Circulating calcidiol is bound to a vitamin D-binding protein (VDBP), is taken up by megalin-mediated endocytosis in the PCT, and converted to calcitriol, the active form, by 1-α-hydroxylase (CYP2B1) [38]. Production of the active form, calcitriol, is under the control of phosphorous, FGF-23, PTH, and calcitriol (negative feedback) [24, 25, 37, 38]. Chronic kidney patients may differ from the general population with vitamin D stores and treatment goals. Fifty to eighty percent of persons with CKD are profoundly deficient in calcidiol and calcitriol [41, 42]. This may be due to decreased sunlight exposure, restricted intake of vitamin D rich foods, decreased synthesis of cholecalciferol in response to sunlight, loss of VDBP with proteinuria, loss of renal mass of megalin, and 1-α-hydroxylase [37, 38].

Monitoring

The high morbidity and mortality associated with MBD makes early detection and the need for randomized control studies comparing different treatments and outcomes important. With slight differences, KDOQI and KDIGO recommend monitoring serum PTH, Pi, Ca^{2+}, and alkaline phosphatase beginning at CKD stage 3 (eGFR < 60 cc/min/1.73 mm^2) in adults and CKD stage 2 (eGFR 60–89 cc/min/1.73 mm^2) in children (see Tables 24.1 and 24.2). The United States KDOQI commentary to the KDIGO guidelines was in agreement with many of the guidelines but left it up to the discretion of the physician which guidelines to follow. Many of the hemodialysis

Table 24.1 Recommendation of KDIGO and KDOQI guidelines [4, 13]

Biochemical parameters	KDOQI	KDIGO
PTH (pg/mL)		
CKD 3 (30–59 cc/min/1.73 mm^2)	35–70	No descriptive target
CKD 4 (15–29 cc/min/1.73 mm^2)	70–110	No descriptive target
CKD 5/5D (<15 cc/min/1.73 mm^2)	150–300	130–600
Ca (mg/dL)		
CKD 3–4	Corrected total calcium	Reference range
CKD 5/5D	8.4–9.5	Reference range
PO_4 (mg/dL)		
CKD 3–4	≥2.7 to ≤4.6	Reference range
CKD 5/5D	≥3.5 to ≤5.5	Reference range
Ca × PO_4 (mg^2/dL^2)		
CKD 3–5	≤55	NA
Vit D 25 (ng/mL)		
CKD 3–5	>30, if PTH above target	Measure

Table 24.2 Monitoring recommendations of KDOQI and KDIGO [4, 13]

	CKD stages	
Biochemistry	KDOQI	KDIGO
Calcium	3-q 12 months 4-q 3 months 5-q 1 months	3-q 6–12 months 4- q 3–6 months 5-q 1–3 months
PO_4	3-q 12 months 4-q 3 months 5-q 1 months	3-q 6–12 months 4-q 3–6 months 5-q 1–3 months
Vitamin D 25	Measure if PTH above target	3/4/5-once then based on level and treatment
Intact PTH (variable assays)	3-q 12 months 4-q 3 months 5-q 3 months	3-once then based on level and CKD 4-q 6–12 months 5-q 3–6 months
Alkaline phosphatase	No recommendation	3-once 4/5-q 12 months

units have reviewed and adopted the KDIGO guidelines including maintenance of serum PTH levels between 130 and 600 pg/mL for CKD stage 5D.

Treatment

The purpose of treatment is to prevent adverse outcomes related to MBD [44]. Many of the articles in the treatment of MBD are non-randomized studies in dialysis patients; only a few studies pertain to CKD stages 3 and 4. Because of the increased occurrence of extra-skeletal calcifications in CKD, non-calcium containing Pi binders, paricalcitol rather than calcitriol, and newer calcimimetic agents are favored.

Dietary Restriction

Nutritional adjustments with a phosphate restriction in CKD stage 2 may prevent more advanced MBDs associated with severe kidney failure [45, 46] by preventing increases of FGF-23 and intact PTH (see Table 24.3). Caution is warranted since most of the ingested phosphate is from protein and an excessive protein restriction can cause malnutrition which is a risk factor for mortality. A dietary protein restriction is recommended in CKD stages 3–5, but they require careful dietary monitoring, especially a low protein (0.58 g/kg) [46] and a very low protein diet (0.28 g/kg/day) that is supplemented with a mixture of essential keto-acids and amino acids [47]. In CKD 4 and 5, the renal diet consists of a 0.6 g protein/kg, IBW, 2 g sodium, 2 g potassium, 1,000 mg Pi diet. Adjustments in the diet depend on laboratory values and physical findings (Table 24.3). With worsening renal function, it is more difficult to maintain serum Pi in the range of 2.7-4.6 mg/dL without the use of phosphate binders.

Vitamin D 25

In studies of CKD 2 through 5 [41–43] all cause mortality increased with calcidiol deficiency and serum level directly correlated to the GFR and inversely to the CVD. KDOQI and KDIGO recommend repleting calcidiol insufficiency (<20 ng/

Table 24.3 A list of phosphate-containing food that should be avoided or limited intake in CKD

Dairy products
Legumes
Chocolate
Nuts
Dark cola
Baking products with baking powder and preservatives
Meat—processed and organ meats
Soybean and products
Baking powder
Cereals—wheat based
Egg yolk

Table 24.4 The ergocalciferol dose repletion in vitamin D 25 deficiency or insufficiency at various CKD stagesa [4, 13]

Vitamin D 25 repletion	
CKD 3—PTH if >70 check vitamin D 25 if <30 ng/dL	Vitamin D 25: <5 ng/dL replete 50,000 IU of vitamin D2 weekly for 12 weeks then every month × 3 months
CKD 4—PTH >110 check vitamin D 25 if <30 ng/dL	Vitamin D 25: 5–15 ng/dL replete 50,000 IU of vitamin D2 weekly for 8 weeks then every month × 4 months
CKD V—PTH >300 treat with vitamin D analogue	Vitamin D 25: >15–30 ng/dL replete 50,000 IU of vitamin D2 every month × 6 months

[a]In CKD 3—if vitamin D 25 is less than 30 ng/dL and intact PTH is greater than 70 pg/dL; CKD stage 4—if vitamin D 25 is less than 30 ng/dL and intact PTH is greater than 110 pg/dL replete with ergocalciferol. For vitamin D 25 less than 5 ng/dL, then 50,000 IU of ergocalciferol is given weekly for 12 weeks then monthly for 3 additional months. For a serum vitamin D 25 level between 5 and 15 ng/mL, then 50,000 IU of ergocalciferol is given weekly for 8 weeks then monthly for 4 months. For a serum vitamin D 25 level between 15 and 30 ng/dL, then 50,000 IU of ergocalciferol is given monthly for 6 months. KDIGO recommend the use of cholecalciferol instead of ergocalciferol

dL) and depletion (<10 ng/dL) in CKD stages 3 and 4 [13] (Table 24.4).

Al-Alay and colleagues [48] studied ergocalciferol treatment on intact PTH in CKD stages 3 and 4. Calcidiol levels rose in 54% from 16 ± 0.7 to 27.2 ± 1.8 ng/dL ($p<0.05$) while the intact PTH declined from 231 ± 26 pg/mL to 193 ± 25 pg/mL ($p<0.005$). However, there was only a significant decline in intact PTH in CKD stage 3 [48]. In a large multicenter, randomized control trial, elderly ladies with CKD received 1,200 mg of Ca^{2+} and 800 IU of cholecalciferol for 2 years [49]. At baseline, over 86% of the participants had a serum cholecalciferol < 15 ng/mL. By 24 months, at least 65% had achieved the recommended serum calcidiol level of > 30 ng/mL while 42% showed a 30% decline in serum PTH levels as compared to placebo ($p<0.001$) [49]. This supports the recommendation of KDOQI for supplementing with ergocalciferol in CKD stages 3 and 4 for secondary hyperparathyroidism if there is a calcidiol deficiency or insufficiency.

Repletion of calcidiol is controversial. Following the review of literature, the Institute of Medicine suggested that the supplemental goal for calcidiol be 20 ng/mL in order to avoid complications such as hypercalcemia. However, CKD was not addressed and the goal per KDOQI guidelines remains >30 ng/dL [14].

Table 24.5 The different names of the vitamin D analogues

Calcitriol	Calcijex®
Paricalcitol	ZEMPLAR®
Doxercalciferol	Hectorol®
Vitamin D2	Ergocalciferol
Vitamin D3	Cholecalciferol
Vitamin D 25	Calcidiol

Vitamin D Analogues

In the last decade, the introduction of active vitamin D analogues, calcimimetic agents, and non-calcium binders was heralded as a medical advancement that precluded the need for surgical parathyroidectomy [50]. With the increase in extra-skeletal calcification and rise in CVD in those with CKD, there has been controversy over which vitamin D analogue to use [51–53]. Three different analogues are available in the Unites States: calcitriol, paricalcitol, doxercalciferol, while maxacalcitol is only available in Europe (Table 24.5). In a double-blinded randomized multicenter study, 476 hemodialysis patients received either calcitriol or paricalcitol for control of PTH. There were fewer episodes of hypercalcemia and elevated Pi × Ca^{2+} product in the paricalcitol group and the primary endpoint of a 50% reduction in PTH was met by 15 weeks for the paricalcitol group versus 23 weeks for the calcitriol group [52].

In a comparison study of the vitamin D analogues, calcitriol versus doxercalciferol, no differences in the serum Ca^{2+} and Pi level were found [26]. Changes in the serum Ca^{2+} and Pi level were more dependent on the type of binder used than the type of vitamin D analogue. Although there was a significant decline in the serum PTH over baseline for both analogues ($p<0.01$), intra-drug variation was not significant [26]. In a retrospective study evaluating vitamin

D analogues on mortality [53], no difference in death rates (15%) was found between the two vitamin D2 analogues, paricalcitol and doxercalciferol, while use of the vitamin D3 analogue, calcitriol, was associated with a statistically higher death rate (19.6%) ($p<0.0001$) [53]. However, no significant difference in the adjusted hazard ratio between these three vitamin D analogues was found [53].

Phosphate Restriction and Binders

Although the serum Pi level does not rise in CKD 3 until the eGFR falls below 40 cc/min/1.73 mm^2 [3], the intact PTH rises at this stage or earlier as a response to maintain serum Pi. FGF-23 acts similarly. When the dietary intake of Pi in dogs was titrated to the decline in kidney function, serum PTH, serum Pi, and excretion of Pi remained unchanged [45]. This study highlights the importance of dietary phosphate restriction in patients with CKD. High phosphorus foods are highlighted in Table 24.5.

With advanced kidney disease it becomes more difficult for the PTH and FGF-23 to maintain the serum Pi within the normal range without causing damage to other organs [2, 7, 35, 54]. The predialysis serum Pi goal is less than 4.6 mg/dL, and phosphate binders are prescribed if this goal is not achieved by diet alone. The available Pi binders are divided into calcium based and non-calcium based [55–57] (Table 24.6). The former include calcium carbonate and calcium acetate while the latter include the resin exchanger sevelamer carbonate, lanthanum-based binder, and aluminum-based binders. The long-term use of aluminum-based phosphate binders is contraindicated in patients with severe renal dysfunction[58, 59] because of the extra renal side effects which include low turnover bone decrease, fractures, encephalopathy, muscle weakness, and microcytic anemia with normal iron stores [19, 60, 61].

The association between calcium Pi binders and extra-skeletal calcifications has led to prescribing non-calcium-based Pi binders. If calcium-based Pi binders are prescribed, they should be limited to 1.5 g of elemental calcium per day [14, 62–65]. The calcium-based Pi binder, calcium acetate, was compared with the non-calcium Pi binders, sevelamer, in rates of calcification of both coronary arteries and aorta using electron beam technique (EBT) in dialysis patients [63]. At baseline, the EBT revealed that both groups had severe extensive vascular calcifications. At the end of the 2-year study there was no further progression of disease in the sevelamer group but a significant increase in the calcification in coronary arteries and aorta in the calcium acetate group [63]. The authors concluded that the use of non-calcium-based Pi binders might improve the long-term outcomes in patients with CKD.

Cinacalcet

Calcimimetic agents bind to the calcium sensor in many organs including the parathyroid gland chief cells which release intracellular calcium and decrease PTH secretion into the circulation [27, 32]. The only one available in the United States is cinacalcet which comes in dosages of 30, 60, and 90 mg tablets. It has FDA approval for patients on chronic renal replacement therapy but not for predialysis patients. It has been prescribed in those patients with elevated serum levels of Ca^{2+} and Pi with limited room to titrate the vitamin D analogues. Serum Ca^{2+} levels must be monitored weekly in order to avoid hypocalcemia while the dose is titrated monthly to achieve a serum PTH within an acceptable range [32]. Calcimimetic agents can cause an increase in calcium secretion by binding to the calcium sensor receptors located in the distal nephron in those with CKD [27, 32]. PTH secretion decreases within 1–2 h after receiving the drug [32] and a greater percentage reach a PTH<300 pg/dL than those receiving conventional treatment [32]. The major side effects are nausea, vomiting, and diarrhea [32].

Parathyroidectomy

In tertiary hypoparathyroidism the parathyroid gland becomes autonomous, nodular in composition, and unresponsive to feedback inhibition by

Table 24.6 Commonly used lowering agents in CKD [55, 56]

Phosphate lower agents	Action	Brand names	Advantages	Disadvantages	Costs[a]
Calcium carbonate 500 or 1,250 mg (<2,000 mg/day of elemental Ca^{2+})	Bind with Pi in the GI tract	Tums, Oscal, Calcichew, Titralac	Effective and inexpensive	Hypercalcemia	$20.99 for 1,250 mg (500 tablets) $13.99 for Oyst-cal 500 mg (120 tablets)
Calcium acetate 667 mg (<2,000 mg elemental Ca^{2+}/day)	Bind with Pi in the GI tract	Phoslo, Phosex	Effective, inexpensive and less calcium content than $CaCO_3$	Hypercalcemia; pH dependent	$197.99 for 667 mg (200 tablets)
Sevelamer hydrogen chloride or sevelamer carbonate 400 or 800 mg	Bind with Pi in the GI tract	Renagel, Renvela	Contains no aluminum or calcium, less acidosis then hydrogen chloride form, less hypercalcemia, decrease LDL and total cholesterol, slower progression of vascular calcification	Expensive; GI side effects: abdominal cramping, diarrhea, bloating, constipation	Renagel—$ 305.76 for 800 mg (90 tablets) Renvela—242.97 (90 tablets)
Lanthanum carbonate 500–1,000 mg	Bind with Pi in the GI tract	Fosrenol	Effective, contains no calcium or aluminum, less hypercalcemia	Expensive; pH dependent; accumulation in tissue	$728.91 for 1,000 mg (90 tablets)
Aluminum hydroxide 15–45 cc	Bind with Pi in the GI tract	Amphogel	Inexpensive and effective; no calcium	Al^{3+} accumulation with complication of encephalopathy, osteomalacia, fractures, anemia	$ 10–15 for 350 cc
Magnesium and Ca carbonate 300 mg	Bind with Pi in the GI tract	MagneBind	Inexpensive and effective; decrease calcium content	Accumulation of Mg^{2+} with a decrease of GFR < 30 cc/min/1.73 mm^2; GI side effects: diarrhea; hypercalcemia	$15.75 for 150 tablets
Nicotinamide 500–1,000 mg	Na^+ depend Pi co-transport in the small intestine	Slo-Niacin/Niacin SR	Inexpensive and effective, once daily, lowers LDL and increases HDL	Flushing; GI side effects: cramping, diarrhea; pruritus; increase uric acid	Slo-Niacin $25.99 for 500 mg (100 tablets) Niaspan $89.99 500 mg (30 tablets)

[a]From www.drugstore.com

vitamin D analogues due to a decline in VRD. Complications ensue related to deposition of calcium and phosphate in soft tissues. Tendons rupture; bones fracture. For these complications, a partial parathyroidectomy, where most of the parathyroid gland is removed and a small remnant left, is indicated [2].

Thiosulfate

There have been case reports using intravenous sodium thiosulfate, inorganic salt, for CUA with good results [66–68]. The primary treatment for CUA is to correct the metabolic derangements found in MBD such as elevated Pi, Ca^{2+} and Pi product, and PTH, in conjunction with aggressive local wound care, antibiotics, and pain management [68]. Thiosulfate appears to have an acute anti-oxidant/inflammatory action resulting in a rapid decrease in pain and chelating property with Ca^{2+} forming a soluble component removed by dialysis abilities or excreted dependent on the degree of kidney function [67]. Other possible therapeutic options for CUA are bisphosphonates, hyperbaric oxygen therapy, and cinacalcet [66, 69].

Case Revisited

This elderly lady has severe CKD; renal replacement therapy looms. Her symptoms and laboratory values are consistent with MBD-CKD. The pruritus is most likely secondary to poorly controlled serum phosphate. Nutritional counseling is indicated in order to decrease her Pi intake to 1,000 mg per day. A Pi binder is probably needed in order to achieve a serum Pi goal of 4.7 mg/dL. Non-Ca^{2+}-based Pi binders, either lanthanum or sevelamer is preferred. Following improvement in her serum Pi, vitamin D 25 or the active vitamin D analogue can be added, depending on the serum PTH. The elevated alkaline phosphatase suggests high bone turnover from an elevated PTH level. In fact, it was 600 pg/dL. Follow-up labs were scheduled within 1 month.

References

1. Coresh J, Selvin E, Stevens LA, Manzi J, Kusek JW, Eggers P, et al. Prevalence of chronic kidney disease in the United States. JAMA. 2007;298(17):2038–47.
2. Martin KJ, Olgaard K, Coburn JW, Coen GM, Fukagawa M, Langman C, et al. Diagnosis, assessment and treatment of bone turnover abnormalities in renal osteodystrophy. Am J Kidney Dis. 2004;43(3):558–65.
3. Levin A, Bakris GL, Molitch M, Smulders M, Tian J, Williams LA, Andress DL. Prevalence of abnormal serum vitamin D, PTH, calcium, and phosphorous in patients with chronic kidney disease: results of the study to evaluate early kidney disease. Kidney Int. 2007;71:31–8.
4. Kidney Disease: Improving Global Outcome (KDIGO) CKD-MBD Work group. KDIGO clinical practice guidelines for diagnosis, evaluation, prevention, and treatment of chronic kidney disease-mineral and bone disorder (CKD-MBD). Kidney Int Suppl. 2009;113:S1–S130.
5. Danese MD, Kim J, Doan QV, Dylan M, Griffths R, Chertow GM. PTH and the risks for hip, vertebral and pelvis fractures among patients on Dialysis. Am J Kidney Dis. 2008;47(1):149–58.
6. Block GA, Hulbert-Shearon T, Levin NW, Port FK. Association of serum phosphorous and calcium × phosphate product with mortality risk in chronic hemodialysis patients: a national study. Am J Kidney Dis. 1998;31(4):607–17.
7. Adeney KL, Siscovick DS, Ix JH, Seliger SL, Shlipak MG, Jenny NS, Kestenbaum BR. Association of serum phosphate with vascular and valvular calcification in moderate CKD. J Am Soc Nephrol. 2009;20(2):381–7.
8. Uhlig K, Berns J, Kestenbaum B, Kumar R, Leonard MB, Martin KJ, et al. KDOQI US commentary on 2009 KDIGO clinical practice guideline for diagnosis, evaluation, and treatment of CKD-mineral and bone disorder (CKD-MBD). Am J Kidney Dis. 2010;55(5):773–99.
9. Ganesh S, Stack AG, Levin NW, Hulbert-Shearon T, Port FK. Association of elevated serum Po_4, Ca × Po_4 product, and parathyroid hormone in cardiac mortality risk in chronic hemodialysis patients. J Am Soc Nephrol. 2001;12(10):2131–8.
10. Mathew S, Tustison KS, Sugatani T, Chaudhary LR, Rifas L, Hruska KA. The mechanism of phosphorous as a cardiovascular risk factor in CKD. J Am Soc Nephrol. 2008;19(6):1092–105.
11. Moe S, Drueke T, Cunningham J, Goodman W, Martin K, Olgaard K, et al. Definition, evaluation, and classification of renal osteodystrophy: a position statement from Kidney Disease: Improving Global Outcome (KDIGO). Kidney Int. 2006;69:1945–53.
12. Bhuriya R, Li S, Chen S-C, McCullough PA, Bakris GL. Plasma parathyroid hormone level and prevalent cardiovascular disease stage 3 and 4: an analysis from

the keep early evaluation program (KEEP). Am J Kidney Dis. 2009;53(4):S3–S10.
13. Vassalotti JA, Uribarri J, Chen S-C, Li S, Wang C, Collins AJ, et al. Trends in mineral metabolism: Kidney Early Evaluation Program (KEEP) and the National Health and Nutrition Examination Survey (NHANES) 1999–2004. Am J Kidney Dis. 2008;51(4):S56–68.
14. NKF/KDIQO. KDOQI clinical practice guidelines for bone metabolism and disease in chronic kidney disease. http://www.kidney.org/professionals/KDOQI/guidelines_bone/index.htm. Accessed 22 Mar 2011.
15. Angelis M, Wong L, Myers SA, Wong LM. Calciphylaxis in patients on hemodialysis: A prevalence study. Surgery. 1997;122:1083–90.
16. Fine A, Zacharias J. Calciphylaxis is usually non-ulcerating: risk factors, outcome and therapy. Kidney Int. 2002;61:2210–7.
17. Mazhar AR, Johnson RJ, Gillen D, Stivelman JC, Ryan MJ, et al. Risk factors and mortality associated with calciphylaxis in end-stage renal disease. Kidney Int. 2001;60:324–32.
18. Castro H, Cabeza-Rivera F, Green D. Combined therapy with sodium thiosulfate and parathyroidectomy in a patient with calciphylaxis. Dial Transplant. 2011;40:264–6.
19. Pierides AM, Edwards WG, Cullum UX, McCall JT, Ellis HA. Hemodialysis encephalopathy with osteomalacia fractures and muscle weakness. Kidney Int. 1980;18:115–24.
20. Islam MZ. Overview of renal osteodystrophy and current therapeutic approach. J Medicine. 2011;12:45–9.
21. Gordon PL, Fresetto LA. Management of osteoporosis in CKD stages 3 to 5. Am J Kidney Dis. 2010;55(5):941–56.
22. Miller PD, Roux C, Boonen S, Barton IP, Dunlap LE, Burgio DE. Safety and efficiency of risedronate in patients with age-related reduced renal function as estimated by Cockcroft and Gault method: a pooled analysis of nine clinical trials. J Bone Miner Res. 2005;20:2015–115.
23. Miller PD. The role of bone biopsy in patients with chronic renal failure. Clin J Am Soc Nephrol. 2008;3:S140–50.
24. Danziger J. The bone-renal axis in early chronic kidney disease: an emerging paradigm. Nephrol Dial Transplant. 2008;23(9):2733–7.
25. Lui S, Quarles LD. How fibroblast growth factor 23 works? J Am Soc Nephrol. 2007;18:1637–47.
26. Wesseling-Perry K, Pereira RC, Sahney S, Gales B, Wang H-J, Elashoff R, et al. Calcitriol and doxercalciferol are equivalent in controlling bone turnover, suppressing parathyroid hormone, and increasing fibroblast growth factor-23 in secondary hyperparathyroidism. Kidney Int. 2010;79:112–9.
27. Magyar CE, Friedman PA. Chapter 25. Renal regulation of calcium, phosphate, and magnesium. In: Dubose TD, Hamm LL, editors. Acid-base and electrolyte disorders. Philadelphia: Elsevier Saunders Copyright; 2002. p. 435–52.
28. Peacock M. Calcium metabolism in health and disease. Clin J Am Soc Nephrol. 2010;5(1):S23–30.
29. Souberbielle JC, Roth H, Fouque DP. Parathyroid hormone measurement in CKD. Kidney Int. 2010;77:93–100.
30. Cozzolino M, Gallieni M, Brancaccio D, Arcidiacono T, Bianchi G, Vezzoli G. Vitamin D retains an important role in the pathogenesis and management of secondary hyperparathyroidism. J Nephrol. 2006;19(5):566–77.
31. Foutounas C. Phosphorous metabolism in chronic kidney disease. Hippokratia. 2011;15:S50–52.
32. Messa P, Macário F, Yaqoob M, Bowman K, Braun J, Von Albertini B, et al. The OPTIMA Study: assessing a new cinacalcet (Sensipar/Mimpara) treatment algorithm for secondary hyperparathyroidism. Clin J Am Soc Nephrol. 2008;3(1):36–45.
33. Martin KJ, Gonzalez EA. Vitamin D analogs: action and role in the treatment of secondary hyperparathyroidism. Semin Nephrol. 2004;24(5):456–9.
34. Juppner H, Wolf M, Salusky IB. FGF-23: more than a regulator of renal phosphate handling? J Bone Miner Res. 2010;25(10):2091–7.
35. Neves KR, Graciolli FG, dos Reis LM, Pasqalucci CA, Moysés RM, Jorgetti V. Adverse effects of hyperphosphatemia on myocardial hypertrophy, renal function, and bone in rats with renal failure. Kidney Int. 2004;66:2237–44.
36. Vervloet MC, Ittersum FJ, Büttler RM, Heijboer AC, Blankenstein MA, Ter Wee PM. Effects of dietary phosphate and calcium intake on fibroblast growth factor-23. Clin J Am Soc Nephrol. 2011;6(2):383–9.
37. Rosen CJ. Vitamin D insufficiency. New Engl J Med. 2011;364:248–54.
38. Rojas-Rivera J, De La Piedra C, Ramos A, Ortiz A, Egido J. The expanding spectrum of biological actions of vitamin D. Nephrol Dial Transplant. 2010;25(9):1850–2865.
39. Zhou C, Lu F, Coa K, Xu D, Goltzman D, Miao D. Calcium-independent and 1,25(OH)2D3-dependent regulation of rennin-angiotensin system in 1alpha hydroxylase knockout mice. Kidney Int. 2008;74:170–9.
40. Zehnder D, Quinkler M, Eardley KS, Bland R, Lepenies J, Hughes SV, et al. Reduction of vitamin D hormonal system in kidney disease associated with increased renal inflammation. Kidney Int. 2008;74:1343–2353.
41. Thadhani R. Is calcitriol life-protective for patients with chronic kidney disease? J Am Soc Nephrol. 2009;20(11):2285–90.
42. Kandula P, Dobre M, Schold JD, Schrieber Jr MJ, Mehrotra R, Navaneethan SD. Vitamin D supplementation in chronic kidney disease: systemic review and meta-analysis of observational studies and randomized controlled trials. Clin J Am Soc Nephrol. 2011;6(6):50–62.
43. Ravani P, Malberti F, Tripepi G, Pecchini P, Cutrupi S, Pizzini P, et al. Vitamin D levels and patient

outcome in chronic kidney disease. Kidney Int. 2007;75:88–95.
44. Tentori F, Blayney MJ, Albert JM, Gillespsie BW, Kerr PG, Bommer J, et al. Mortality risk of dialysis patients with different levels of serum calcium, phosphorous and PTH: the Dialysis Outcomes and Practice Patterns study (DOPPS). Am J Kidney Dis. 2008;52(3):519–30.
45. Slatopolsky E, Caglar S, Gradowska L, Canterbury J, Reiss E, Bricker NS. On prevention of secondary hyperparathyroidism in experimental chronic renal disease using 'proportional reduction' of dietary phosphorous intake. Kidney Int. 1972;2:147–51.
46. Levey AS, Greene T, Sarnak MJ, Wang X, Beck GJ, Kusek JW, et al. Effect of dietary protein restriction on the progression of kidney disease: long-term follow-up of the modification of diet in renal disease (MDRD) study. Am J Kidney Dis. 2006;48(6):879–88.
47. Menon V, Kopple JD, Wang X, Beck GJ, Collins AJ, Kusek JW, et al. Effect of a very low-protein diet on outcome: long-term follow-up of the Modification of Diet in Renal Disease (MDRD) Study. Am J Kidney Dis. 2009;53(2):208–17.
48. Al-Aly Z, Qazi RA, González EA, Zeringue A, Martin KJ. Changes, in 25-hydroxyvitamin D 25 and plasma intact PTH levels following treatment with ergocalciferol in patients with CKD. Am J Kidney Dis. 2007;50(1):59–68.
49. Kooienga L, Fried L, Scragg R, Kendrick J, Smits G, Chonchol M. Effect of combined calcium and vitamin D3 supplementation on serum intact parathyroid hormone in moderate CKD. Am J Kidney Dis. 2009;53(3):408–16.
50. Schnieder R, Kolios G, Koch BM, Fernǻndez ED, Bartsch DF, Schlosser K. An economic comparison of surgical and medical therapy in patients with secondary hyperparathyroidism—German perspective. Surgery. 2010;148(6):1091–9.
51. Kovesdy CP, Ahmadzadch S, Anderson JE, Kalantar-Zadeh K. Association of activated vitamin D treatment and mortality in chronic kidney disease. Arch Intern Med. 2008;168(4):397–403.
52. Sprague SM, Llach F, Amdahl M, Taccetta C, Batille D. Paricacitol versus calcitriol in the treatment of secondary hyperparathyroidism. Kidney Int. 2003;63: 1483–90.
53. Tentori F, Hunt WE, Stidley CA, Rohrscheib MR, Bedrick EJ, Meyer KB, et al. Mortality risk among hemodialysis patients receiving different vitamin D analogs. Kidney Int. 2006;70:1858–65.
54. Gutiérrez OM, Januzzi JL, Isakova T, Laliberte K, Smith K, Collerone G. Fibroblast growth factor 23 and left ventricular hypertrophy in chronic kidney disease. Circulation. 2009;119:2545–52.
55. Tonelli M, Pannu N, Manns B. Oral phosphate binders in patients with kidney failure. New Eng J Med. 2010;362:1312–24.
56. Navaneethan SD, Palmer SC, Craig JC, Elder GJ, Strippoli GFM. Benefits and harms of phosphate binders in CKD: a systemic review of randomized controlled trial. Am J Kidney Dis. 2009;54(4):619–37.
57. Hutchison A. Oral phosphate binders. Kidney Int. 2009;75:906–14.
58. Nolan CR, Califano JR, Butzin CA. Influence of calcium acetate or calcium citrate on intestinal aluminum absorption. Kidney Int. 1990;38:937–41.
59. Froment DPH, Molitoris BA, Buddington B, Miller N, Alfrey AC. Site and mechanism of enhanced gastrointestinal absorption of aluminum by citrate. Kidney Int. 1989;36:978–84.
60. Alfrey AC. Dialysis encephalopathy. Kidney Int. 1986;29:S53–7.
61. Hodsman AB, Sherrard DJ, Alfrey AC, Ott S, Brickman AS, Miller NL, et al. Bone aluminum and histomorphometric features of renal osteodystrophy. Clin Endocrinol Metab. 1982;54(3):539–46.
62. Cozzolino M, Mazzaferro S, Brandenburg V. The treatment of hyperphosphatemia in CKD: calcium-based or calcium-free phosphate binders? Nephrol Dial Transplant. 2011;26:402–7.
63. Chertow GM, Raggi P, McCarthy JT, Schulman G, Silberzweig J, Kuhlik A, et al. Effect of sevelamer and calcium acetate on proxies of atherosclerotic and atherosclerotic vascular disease in hemodialysis patients. J Nephrol. 2003;23(5):307–14.
64. Chertow GM, Burke SK, Lazarus JM, Stenzel KH, Wombolt D, Goldberg D, et al. Poly[allylamine hydrochloride] (RenaGel): a noncalcemic phosphate binder for the treatment of hyperphosphatemia in chronic renal failure. Am J Kidney Dis. 1997;29(1):66–71.
65. Qunibi W, Moustafa M, Muenz LR, He DY, Kessler PD, Diaz-Buxo JA, et al. 1-year randomized trial of calcium acetate versus sevelamer on progression of coronary artery calcification in hemodialysis patients with comparable lipid control: The Calcium Acetate Renagel Evaluation-2 (CARE-2) Study. Am J Kidney Dis. 2008;51(6):952–65.
66. Raymond CB, Wanzy LD. Sodium thiosulfate, bisphosphonates, cinacalcet for treatment of calciphylaxis. Am J Health Syst Pharm. 2008;65:1419–29.
67. Hayden MR, Goldsmith DJA. Sodium thiosulfate: new hope for treatment of calciphylaxis. Semin Dial. 2010;23:258–62.
68. Baldwin C, Farah M, Leung M, Taylor P, Werb R, Kiaii M, et al. Multi-intervention management of calciphylaxis: a report of 7 cases. Am J Kidney Dis. 2011;58(6):988–91.
69. Shiraishi N, Kitamura K, Miyoshi T, Adachi M, Kohda Y, Nonoguchi H, et al. Successful treatment of patient with severe calcific uremic arteriolopathy (calciphylaxis) by etidronate disodium. Am J Kidney Dis. 2006;48(1):151–4.

25 Anemia

Jason Cobb and Tahsin Masud

Case 1

A 32-year-old man with a history of diabetes mellitus type I and chronic kidney disease (CKD) stage V presents to the nephrology clinic after 1 year of being lost to follow-up, complaining of increasing edema of 1 month duration. His past medical history includes diabetes mellitus type I for 12 years, diabetic retinopathy, hypertension, and anemia. Medications include insulin, furosemide, and amlodipine. The patient reports rare alcohol use and no smoking or drug use. His family history includes diabetes mellitus and hypertension. Physical exam includes a blood pressure of 150/90. There is 2+ bilateral lower extremity edema extending to his knees. His creatinine is 10.6 mg/dL with an eGFR (estimated glomerular filtration rate) of 7 mL/min. His eGFR was below 15 mL/min 1 year ago. His hemoglobin a year ago was 10.6 g/dL; currently, the hemoglobin is 7.6 g/dL and hematocrit of 23. Other labs include a serum iron level of 76 mcg/dL, total iron binding capacity (TIBC) of 217 mcg/dL, iron saturation of 35%, total serum ferritin level of 207 ng/mL, a reticulocyte production index of 0.7, a parathyroid hormone level of 220 pg/mL, and a hemoglobin A1C of 7.3%. What should be included in the work-up for patients with CKD who present with anemia? What are possible causes for the anemia?

J. Cobb, M.D. (✉) • T. Masud, M.D.
Renal Division, Emory University School of Medicine, 1639 Pierce Dr. WMB Room 338, Atlanta, GA 30322, USA
e-mail: jcobb2@emory.edu

Diagnosis of Anemia

In the United States there are an estimated 525,000 patients with end-stage renal disease (ESRD) and an estimated 11.5% of the adult population with CKD [1]. A major comorbid condition in this population is anemia, and its prevalence increases as renal function declines. It is often multifactorial with uremia, iron deficiency, vitamin deficiencies, blood loss, chronic inflammation, and other comorbid conditions such as human immunodeficiency virus (HIV) infection listed as possible causes. CKD patients with anemia have increased rates of cardiovascular disease, increased rates of transfusion requirements, a decreased quality of life, and increased mortality [2]. The 2006/2007 KDOQI (Kidney Disease Outcomes Quality Initiative) guidelines suggest screening for anemia once the hemoglobin drops below 13.5 g/dL in adult men and below 12 g/dL in women [2]. The World Health Organization (WHO) defines anemia as a hemoglobin less than 13 g/dL in men and a hemoglobin less than 12 g/dL in nonpregnant women [3]. Patients below these targets warrant a work-up for their anemia. Studies have shown that the prevalence of anemia increases to 20% for CKD stage III, 65% for CKD stage IV, and 75% for CKD stage V [4]. Although all stages of kidney disease show

E.V. Lerma and M. Rosner (eds.), *Clinical Decisions in Nephrology, Hypertension and Kidney Transplantation*, DOI 10.1007/978-1-4614-4454-1_25, © Springer Science+Business Media New York 2013

a significant increase in the rates of anemia, it is most marked when the eGFR falls below 60 mL/min.

The initial work-up for anemia should include a complete history. The clinical manifestations of weakness, fatigue, decreased exercise tolerance, and shortness of breath require special attention. Follow-up questions should rule out other causes such as acute blood loss (melena, hematemesis, bright red blood per rectum, menses) and chronic comorbid conditions (such as HIV, diabetes). Also, a detailed review of medications including ace inhibitors (ACEi) and angiotensin receptor blockers should be done, which were reported to be associated with impaired erythropoiesis and anemia in hemodialysis patients [5]. However, many subsequent studies, including a prospective crossover study where ACEi were given for 4 months and then switched to other antihypertensives, were not associated with any difference in hemoglobin or erythropoietin stimulating agent (ESA) doses [6]. Nutritional deficiencies such as vitamin B12 and folate deficiencies (possible causes: alcoholism, malnutrition, antiretroviral medications) should be excluded. If hemolysis is present, conditions such as sickle cell anemia, sepsis, and TTP should be considered. If other blood cell lines are affected, aplastic anemia, leukemia, and medications are in the differential diagnosis. On the physical exam, special attention should be made to evaluate for pallor, jaundice (hemolysis), mucosal bleeding (platelet involvement), vitiligo (vitamin B12 deficiency), tachycardia, heart murmur (usually systolic ejection murmur), hepatomegaly (liver disease), and splenomegaly (liver disease, splenic sequestration).

The typical anemia of CKD is normochromic (normal color and hemoglobinization) and normocytic (normal red blood cell size) with a hypoproliferative bone marrow. It is further characterized by a normal MCV (mean cell volume) and a low erythropoietin level [7].

For the initial work-up, a complete blood cell count should be ordered with special attention to red blood cell indices such as the MCV level. A reticulocyte count, percent, and index should also be ordered. The hemoglobin level is the preferred method of diagnosing anemia since the hematocrit is a derived value that can be affected by storage techniques and instrumentation [2]. In the non-dialysis CKD patient, the time of blood testing is not important. In the ESRD population, the labs are affected by volume status, so the labs are usually drawn mid-week pre-dialysis (on Wednesday or Thursday according to dialysis schedule) and are less influenced by long interdialytic weight gains or hemoconcentration post-dialysis. A reticulocyte index of less than 2.5 is indicative of a hypoproliferative bone marrow [7]. The erythropoietin level is generally not checked as part of the routine work-up of anemia in CKD; it is assumed to be low in the CKD population. The work-up of iron deficiency is discussed under the section "Iron Deficiency Anemia."

The KDOQI working group suggests that a hemoglobin level should be checked at least annually in patients with CKD and monthly if a patient requires erythropoietin supplementation. The frequency of testing increases if clinical conditions warrant it such as hospitalization, increased requirements for erythropoietin, and an inability to achieve target hemoglobin levels. The iron panel should be checked every month during initial ESA treatment and at least every 3 months if chronically on ESA therapy [2]. A diagnostic approach to the anemia of CKD is provided (Fig. 25.1).

Treatment of Anemia: ESAs

Epoetin and darbepoetin are approved by the FDA (US Food and Drug Administration) for the correction of anemia in CKD, for HIV patients treated with zidovudine, and for postoperative patients to reduce the need for red blood cell transfusions [8].

The potential benefits for kidney disease patients in maintaining the hemoglobin concentration at least 11 g/dL include the following: a decrease in all-cause mortality [9], a decrease in nonfatal cardiovascular (CV) events [10], a reduction in the progression of left ventricular hypertrophy [11–13], an increased quality of life [14, 15], decreased transfusion requirements

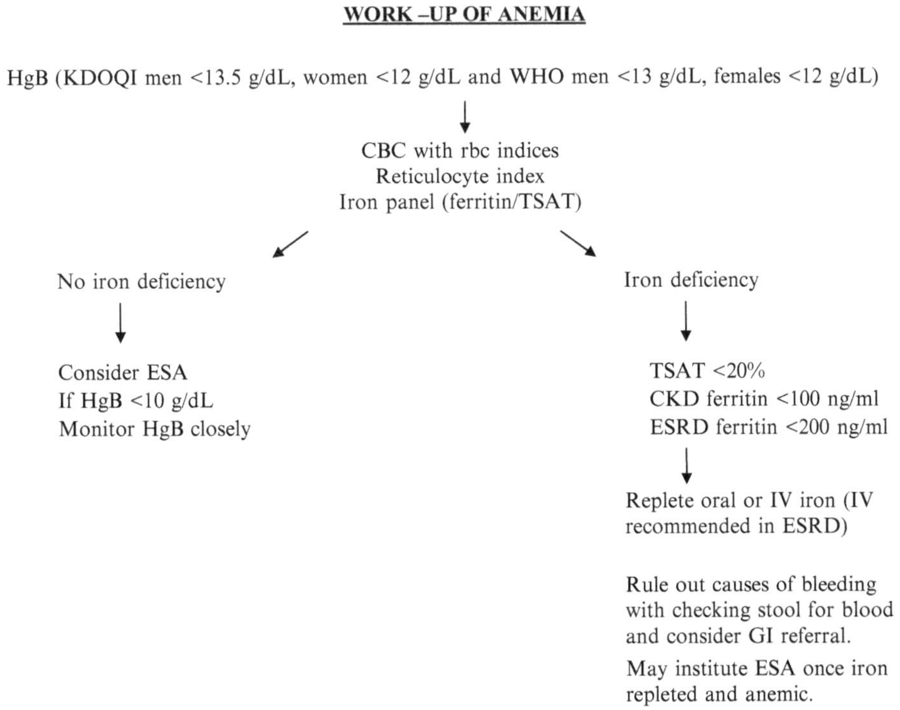

Fig. 25.1 Anemia work-up summary

[16], and a decrease in kidney disease progression [17]. Potential harmful side effects in kidney disease patients include the following: thromboembolic events [18, 19], access thrombosis [8, 19], seizures [8], and aggravation of hypertension [8, 19].

The target hemoglobin level for anemic kidney disease patients treated with ESAs has been the subject of considerable controversy. This issue was the subject of four recent outcome studies in patients with CKD and ESRD being treated with ESAs.

The Normal Hematocrit Study examined the effects of normalizing the hematocrit to 42% versus 30% in 1,233 hemodialysis patients with established cardiac disease (heart failure or ischemic heart disease). The primary end points of the study were length of time to death or first nonfatal myocardial infarction (MI). There were 183 deaths and 19 myocardial infarctions in the normal hematocrit group and 150 deaths and 14 myocardial infarctions in the lower hematocrit group. The study was stopped secondary to a statistically significant increase in deaths in the normal hematocrit group and a non-statistically significant increase in nonfatal MI [20].

The CHOIR (Correction of Hemoglobin and Outcomes in Renal Insufficiency) Study examined the optimal level of hemoglobin correction in 1,432 subjects not yet on dialysis with an eGFR 15–50 mL/min and no previous ESA usage. In this study 715 patients were enrolled in the higher hemoglobin group with an average hemoglobin of 13.5 g/dL, while 717 patients were enrolled in the lower hemoglobin group with an average hemoglobin of 11.3 g/dL. Primary end points were death, MI, hospitalization for congestive heart failure (CHF), and cerebrovascular accident (CVA). The primary end points were observed in 125 patients in the higher hemoglobin group and 97 patients in the lower hemoglobin patients with a hazard ratio of 1.34. In summary, a higher hemoglobin target of 13.5 g/dL was associated with increased adverse events with no statistically significant improvement in other parameters such as quality of life [21].

The CREATE (Cardiovascular Risk Reduction by Early Anemia Treatment with Epoetin Beta)

Study examined non-dialysis patients with severe kidney dysfunction (eGFR of 15–35 mL/min) to ascertain if correction of anemia would improve cardiovascular outcomes. In this study, 603 patients with hemoglobin ranging from 11 to 12.5 g/dL were assigned to a target hemoglobin of 13–15 g/dL versus a subnormal target of 10.5–11.5 g/dL. Subcutaneous epoetin was initiated in the higher hemoglobin target group at randomization while administration of epoetin was delayed in the lower hemoglobin target group until a hemoglobin target of less than 10.5 g/dL was reached. Primary end points were time to first event in eight cardiovascular events including sudden death, MI, CVA, and CHF. Secondary end points included left ventricular mass index, quality of life scores, and progression of CKD. In the 3-year study, there were 58 cardiovascular events in the higher hemoglobin group and 47 cardiovascular events with a hazard ration of 0.78. The authors concluded that correction of anemia to a target of 13–15 g/dL did not reduce the risk of cardiovascular events [14].

In the TREAT (Trial to Reduce Cardiovascular Events with Aranesp Therapy) Study, 4,038 CKD patients not on dialysis with diabetes mellitus and anemia were randomized to treatment with darbepoetin to a hemoglobin target of 13 g/dL or to placebo. The latter group received darbepoetin as a rescue drug if their hemoglobin became less than 9 g/dL. Primary end points included death or cardiovascular events (MI, CHF, and CVA) and occurred in 632 patients in the darbepoetin group and in 602 patients in the placebo group. The hazard ratio was 1.06. An adverse event, CVA, occurred in 101 patients in darbepoetin group and 53 patients in placebo group with a hazard ratio of 1.92. The TREAT study found that increasing the hemoglobin to a higher target was associated with a modest increase in quality of life scores, but there was a higher likelihood of CVA [18].

A large meta-analysis of 10,452 patients from 27 clinical trials including some of the above studies did not find any statistically significant improvement in all-cause mortality or rates of progression to ESRD in the CKD population with higher hemoglobin targets. Instead, there was a higher likelihood for CVA, hypertension, and vascular access thrombosis [19].

The 2006/2007 KDOQI guidelines recommend that the hemoglobin concentration be maintained between 11 and 12 g/dL; there is insufficient evidence to keep the hemoglobin at 13 g/dL or greater with an ESA [2]. There has been a change of opinion on target hemoglobin levels as new data is presented. New updates from nephrology national and international work groups are pending. The FDA released an update in June 2011 on dosing guidelines for ESA use to treat anemia in patients with CKD (Fig. 25.2). According to the FDA, patients with CKD should be considered for starting ESA treatment when hemoglobin level <10 g/dL. Further, if hemoglobin level exceeds 10 g/dL, reduce or interrupt the dose of ESA. The practitioner should individualize dosing and use the lowest dose of ESA sufficient to reduce the need for red blood cell transfusions. The target hemoglobin range of 10–12 g/dL on the labels has been removed for ESAs [8]. There will be a need for long-term studies to see if patients have any deleterious effects from these lower hemoglobin levels.

Also, increased mortality has been seen in patients with large hemoglobin fluctuations and it demonstrates the difficulty of keeping patients within narrow hemoglobin target levels [22]. There is a need for improvement in defining targets and establishing clinic and dialysis facility anemia management protocols to avoid these hemoglobin fluctuations in patients.

The Use of ESAs

The two current options for treatment of anemia in the United States are epoetin alpha and darbepoetin alfa which are available for subcutaneous and intravenous (IV) usage. In other countries, biosimilar agents, epoetin beta, and CERA (continuous erythropoietin receptor activators) are available. Because the half-life of darbepoetin alfa is prolonged, less frequent dosing is required. The ESA doses are usually administered more frequently with the shorter half-life ESA such as epoetin alpha and epoetin beta, and they are

CKD

The ESA labels now warn:

- In controlled trials with CKD patients, patients experienced greater risks for death, serious adverse cardiovascular reactions, and stroke when administered ESAs to target a emoglobin level of greater than 11 g/dL.
- No trial has identified a hemoglobin target level, ESA dose, or dosing strategy that does not increase these risks.

ESA labels now recommend:

- For patients with CKD, consider starting ESA treatment when the hemoglobin level is less than 10 g/dL. This advice does not define how far below 10 g/dL is appropriate for an individual to initiate. This advice also does not recommend that the goal is to achieve a hemoglobin of 10 g/dL or a hemoglobin above 10 g/dL. Individualize dosing and use the lowest dose of ESA sufficient to reduce the need for red blood cell transfusions.

  Adjust dosing as appropriate.

The drug label previously recommended that ESAs should be dosed to achieve and maintain hemoglobin levels within the target range of 10 to 12 g/dL in CKD patients. This target concept has been removed from the label.[8]

Fig. 25.2 FDA modified dosing recommendations to improve the safe use of ESAs in CKD

usually given every 1–2 weeks to non-dialysis CKD patients and three times a week to ESRD patients. The manufacturer recommends that the starting dose for epoetin alpha be between 50 and 100 U/kg three times per week. A dose such as 4,000 U is a reasonable starting dose. Darbepoetin alfa is typically dosed in clinical practice every 1–2 weeks in ESRD patients and every 2–4 weeks in non-dialysis CKD patients since it has a longer half-life. The recommended starting dose is 0.45 mcg/kg weekly; a dose of darbepoetin 40 mcg every 2 weeks is a reasonable starting dose. If the patient responds to the ESA with a brisk increase in the hemoglobin of more than 2.5 g/dL per month, the dose should be decreased by 25%. There is data showing that there is less variability in dosing and a decrease in the total dose of ESA used when the medication is titrated downward, instead of completely withholding it If the hemoglobin continues to rise you may need to hold the medication. If there is no response to treatment in 1 month, the dose should be increased by 25% [8]. A poor response to ESAs may have prognostic value as an analysis of the TREAT study showed that patients with a poor initial response to ESA had higher mortality rates [23].

Table 25.1 ESA hyporesponsiveness

Chronic inflammation: infections (such as HIV and HCV)
Hematologic: multiple myeloma, myelodysplastic syndrome, solid organ tumors, sickle cell disease
Medications: ace inhibitors, angiotensin receptor blockers
Miscellaneous: iron deficiency (likely most common) and secondary hyperparathyroidism

The mechanism of this finding is unknown. Potential causes of ESA hyporesponsiveness are provided (Table 25.1).

Studies have examined less frequent dosing with both the shorter half-life epoetin and the longer half-life darbepoetin. In a study that randomized 262 patients to receive epoetin alpha 40,000 IU every 4 weeks versus every week or every 2 weeks, there were similar rates of hemoglobin increase in all groups [24]. Currently, the CERA, which is an extended-dosing longer half-life ESA, is not available in the United States. In a study of 324 patients with CKD, CERA administered once every 2 weeks was just as effective as darbepoetin administration every week in maintaining a target hemoglobin of 11–13 g/dL

Table 25.2 ESAs [8, 24, 30, 31]

Formulation	Dose	Route	Side effects
Epoetin alfa (EPO)	50–100 U/kg 3 times a week. IV or SC. Also, can be given qweek, q2weeks or qmonth. May take 2–6 weeks for effect, recommend not changing dose earlier than 4 weeks	SC routes shown to need less total dose. Hemodialysis IV usually given for patient comfort. Non-dialysis usually SC route	Hypertension, cardiovascular events, stroke, edema, headache, dialysis access clotting, seizures, fever, dizziness, insomnia, nausea, vomiting, arthralgias. Pure red cell aplasia (seen more SC route)
Darbepoetin alfa (Aranesp)	Hemodialysis: 0.45 mcg/kg qweek. Non-dialysis CKD: 0.75 mcg/kg q2weeks. May take 2–6 weeks for effect, recommend not changing dose earlier than 4 weeks	SC routes shown to need less total dose. Hemodialysis IV usually given for patient comfort. Non-dialysis usually SC route	Edema, stroke, cardiovascular events, hypertension, hypotension, headache, fever, nausea, vomiting, diarrhea, arthralgia, upper respiratory infection. Pure red cell aplasia (seen more SC route)

[25]. A novel product peginesatide (Hematide) is an ESA which has proved to be noninferior to epoetin in non-dialysis and dialysis CKD patients, which has the advantage of once a month dosing [26, 27]. Another novel product includes FG-4592 which is an oral drug that elevates EPO levels in CKD patients [28, 29]. Both peginesatide (Hematide) and FG-4592 are under investigation.

A number of studies have shown a lower dose of total erythropoietin needed with subcutaneous form in comparison to IV formulation [30, 31]. In most facilities non-dialysis CKD and peritoneal dialysis patients receive ESA by subcutaneous route. Most hemodialysis patients are given ESA by IV route for patient comfort by removing the need for subcutaneous injection. The frequency and dosing route may change in hemodialysis patients with the institution of the bundling payment system that includes ESA in the total patient care payment. A summary of ESA dosing, routes, and potential side effects are listed in Table 25.2.

A side effect that is infrequently seen but well documented is pure red blood cell aplasia which is characterized by decrease in hemoglobin level with normal white blood cells and platelets. Usually seen in subcutaneous epoetin formulations, and the Eprex subcutaneous formulation removed because of it. It is due to the formation of anti-EPO antibodies [32, 33]. Peginesatide is a synthetic peptide and may be useful in patients with antibodies to other ESAs [26].

Recently, the FDA has issued warnings of an increase in mortality and risk of tumor progression for patients treated with ESAs who have certain types of cancers (breast, non-small cell lung, head and neck, lymphoid, and cervical cancers). It is recommended that the lowest possible dose of ESAs be used to minimize the risk and also avoid red blood cell transfusions. Because of these risks, all prescribers of ESAs in cancer patients must enroll in the ESA Apprise Oncology Program with the prescriber and patient signing documentation that they understand the risks and benefits with ESA usage. The FDA also advises preoperative deep vein thrombosis prophylaxis for surgical patients using ESAs since there is an increased rate of deep venous thrombosis in this group [8].

Case 2

A 64-year-old lady with a history of CHF and CKD stage IV presents to the hospital with a CHF exacerbation and worsening renal function. The past medical history includes atrial fibrillation, hypertension, anemia, and dyslipidemia. Medications include carvedilol, warfarin, aspirin, zolpidem, pravastatin, amiodarone, furosemide, and a multivitamin. Her family history is concerning for coronary artery disease and hypertension; she denies any alcohol, smoking, or drug usage. Physical exam is significant for a blood pressure of 130/81, jugular venous distension at 5–6 cm at 30°, a 2/6 holosystolic heart murmur, and 3+ pitting lower extremity edema extending to the thighs bilaterally. Labs: creatinine 2.61 mg/dL (eGFR of 18 mL/min), white blood cell count: 9,000/mm^3, hemoglobin: 9 g/dL, hematocrit: 28%, platelets: 273,000/mm^3, parathyroid hormone: 169 pg/mL, vitamin D 25: 29 ng/mL, albumin: 3.5 g/dL, INR: 2.40, blood urea nitrogen: 91 mg/dL, iron: 14 mcg/dL, TIBC: 372 mcg/dL, iron saturation: 4%, ferritin: 50 ng/mL, and reticulocyte production index: 0.8. What is iron deficiency anemia and how should you treat iron deficiency anemia?

Iron Deficiency Anemia

Iron deficiency anemia in CKD patients stems from multiple causes including chronic inflammation from renal disease, other comorbidities and reduced gastrointestinal absorption of iron. Dialysis specific causes of blood loss related to the procedure include aberrant needle sticks, thrombotic events, and blood loss in the tubing system. Other non-renal causes include gastrointestinal and menstrual bleeding. The source of the loss may not be readily apparent despite a detailed history from the patient. Iron homeostasis is maintained by a complex system regulating iron balance in response to iron deficiency, anemia, and hypoxia. The system includes gastrointestinal absorption of dietary iron by enterocytes in the duodenum, the recycling of iron from senescent erythrocytes by macrophages, and the flux of iron from intracellular spaces to the plasma. The iron absorption, storage, and transportation to plasma are mainly regulated by hepcidin, a 25 amino acid peptide, synthesized in the liver. Hepcidin binds to ferroportin, a cellular iron export channel, leading to its internalization and degradation, and results in the cessation of iron release [34]. During anemic states and hypoxemia, hepcidin synthesis is decreased, and during inflammatory states hepcidin production increases. The normal response to infection is to decrease iron availability in order to decrease the available iron for the pathogen's cellular processes. It seems that chronic inflammatory states and CKD have excess hepcidin, and anemia develops despite adequate iron stores [35].

Diagnosis of iron deficiency in patients with renal disease and on dialysis is complex. Serum iron concentration, TIBC, transferrin saturation (TSAT), and serum ferritin level are routinely checked as part of the work-up for the anemia of CKD. The serum iron concentration, TIBC, and MCV have extremely poor sensitivity for diagnosing iron deficiency anemia. TSAT, a calculated value from serum iron and TIBC, is more reliable test for diagnosing iron deficiency. It measures the circulating iron available for erythropoiesis, is a faster more reliable test for iron deficiency than the MCV which may take weeks before iron deficiency becomes apparent. However, its limitations are that like serum ferritin it has some acute-phase reactivity, as serum transferrin may be elevated in the setting of inflammation, which would lower TSAT if circulating iron is constant. Malnutrition and chronic diseases decrease synthesis of transferrin, which would raise TSAT if circulating iron is constant. There are also significant diurnal fluctuations in TSAT, mainly due to fluctuating serum iron levels [36]. The goal should be to keep the TSAT at least 20% which gives a sensitivity of 88% and specificity of 63% for diagnosing iron deficiency comparable to gold standard of bone marrow staining [37]. The serum ferritin level is indicative of iron storage and is typically normal or elevated in the anemia of CKD. Many patients with CKD will have a component of chronic inflammation contributing to their anemia. Ferritin, an acute-phase reactant, increases with infection/inflammatory states, malignancies, alcohol consumption, and with oral contraceptives without reflecting change in iron stores. The desired serum ferritin level should be >100 ng/mL in non-dialysis CKD and >200 ng/mL in the dialysis-dependent patient [2]. These patients may have high serum ferritin levels but may not have enough available iron to be mobilized especially if on ESA, referred to as functional iron deficiency. This situation is often encountered in hemodialysis patients who are resistant to high doses of ESA but still respond with improvement in hemoglobin with intravenous iron in spite of serum ferritin values in the 200–1,000 ng/mL range. Whether or not to give intravenous iron in cases of a low TSAT and a ferritin greater than 500 ng/mL must be handled on an individual basis. Some clinicians may use higher TSAT goals and administer IV iron in patients with normal TSAT and high serum ferritin levels (even above 500 ng/mL) in an attempt to decrease total ESA dose (possibly to protect patients from some of the previously mentioned side effects of ESAs). That approach may be supported by the DRIVE and DRIVE II studies, but consideration must be given to possible side effects of IV iron such as hypotension, anaphylaxis, and iron overload [38, 39].

If diagnosis of iron deficiency is established, its etiology should be evaluated. Patients on hemodialysis are most likely to be iron deficient from chronic residual blood loss in blood lines with each session of dialysis. If these patients exhibit frequent need for iron administration and those not on hemodialysis, a work-up includes gastrointestinal endoscopy and addressing other reasons for bleeding such as menorrhagia and epistaxis. If other blood cell lines are affected (leukopenia and thrombocytopenia), a peripheral smear evaluation and other appropriate studies should be ordered.

For dialysis patients the preferred method to treat iron deficiency is through IV iron administration. A recent meta-analysis of 13 trials with 6 of these including non-dialysis CKD patients and 7 trials with dialysis patients showed a better response with IV iron in dialysis patients with only a marginal effect in non-dialysis CKD patients [40]. Advantages of IV iron use in hemodialysis patients are that it is easier to administer with the treatment, certainty that the patient has received it, and evidence showing a greater response to this route of administration. Current KDOQI guidelines recommend intravenous iron as the treatment of choice in the dialysis CKD patient [2].

With the non-dialysis CKD patient, oral iron is recommended as first line therapy because of minimal differences in response between the oral and IV routes. In non-dialysis CKD patients with more severe iron deficiency anemia, the administration of IV iron is preferred in order to avoid transfusion. The clinician must weigh the inconvenience of placing an IV and possible adverse reactions with each treatment. Oral iron is associated with gastrointestinal discomfort including constipation while intravenous iron is associated with an increased risk of infection, hypotension, and anaphylaxis. The latter is rarely reported now as most centers are using ferric gluconate and iron sucrose formulations. The KDOQI guidelines recommend that resuscitative medications and personnel be available for the treatment of anaphylaxis if intravenous iron dextran is administered [2]. The recommended dose for oral iron supplementation is 200 mg of elemental iron each day. To maximize absorption, oral iron should be taken between meals (empty stomach) and not simultaneously with calcium-based phosphate binders, antacids, proton pump inhibitors, tetracyclines, and other things that may inhibit its absorption. Absorption is best in an acidic environment and taking ascorbic acid 150–200 mg tablet or with orange juice [2, 41]. In choosing the appropriate method of iron replacement (IV or oral), some consideration must be given to the costs. The oral formulations are definitely less expensive in comparison to the IV formulations, and IV formulations are usually less expensive than admitting patients for red blood cell transfusions. A summary on iron deficiency anemia (Table 25.3), along with information on IV iron formulations (Table 25.4) and oral iron preparations (Table 25.5), is provided.

Adjuvant Therapy

There is inconclusive evidence to promote the use of adjuvant therapy for anemia of CKD such as L-carninite, vitamin C, and androgens. There may be a niche for pentoxifylline and statins because

Table 25.3 Summary on iron deficiency anemia

Iron panel should be checked in all patients with anemia of CKD
If the ferritin level <200 ng/mL and <100 ng/mL in the dialysis and non-dialysis patients, respectively, or if the iron saturation (TSAT) <20% the patient should receive iron replacement. If ferritin 500 ng/mL and TSAT <20% the clinician must use discretion as there are no current recommendations to keep ferritin >500 ng/mL
IV or oral route depends on ease of administration (current KDOQI guidelines recommend IV iron in ESRD); there is no strong evidence favoring one route over the other
IV dextran should be avoided due to a higher side effect profile such as anaphylaxis

Table 25.4 IV iron formulations [41–46]

Formulation[a]	Dose[b] (mg IV/IM)	Frequency	Side effects	Test dose	Efficacy
Iron dextran (Dexferrum)	100	Limit 100 mg/day	Anaphylaxis (common and severe), angioedema, arrhythmia, bronchospasm, hypotension, nausea, vomiting	25 mg IV	Effective in increasing hemoglobin and ferritin Decreases total ESA dose
Iron sucrose (Venofer)	100, 200, 500	Hemodialysis: 100 mg, max 3 times a week. Non-dialysis CKD: 200 mg × 5 doses in 14 days. 500 mg used in much 4 h infusion	Hypotension, generalized skin reactions (flushing, urticaria), edema, nausea, vomiting, diarrhea, dyspnea, pruritis. Rare anaphylaxis	Not recommended	Effective in increasing hemoglobin and ferritin. Decreases total ESA dose. As effective as ferric gluconate
Ferric gluconate (Ferrlecit)	125	Hemodialysis: 125 mg in 8 sequential treatments. Non-dialysis CKD: up to 250 mg × 4 doses in 14 days	Hypotension, malaise, fever, chills, nausea, vomiting, pruritis, paresthesias, rash. Rare anaphylaxis	Label recommends 25 mg IV	Effective in increasing hemoglobin and ferritin levels. Decreases total ESA dose. As effective as iron sucrose
Ferumoxytol (Feraheme)	510	Hemodialysis: 510 mg IV Non-dialysis CKD: 510 mg IV followed by second dose in 3–8 days	Hypotension, edema, hypertension, nausea, vomiting, diarrhea, pruritis, dyspnea. Rare anaphylaxis	No test dose but on dialysis to give after 1 h on dialysis to monitor for hypotension	Effective in increasing hemoglobin level in comparison to oral iron

[a]Numerous studies have shown that IV iron therapy in the treatment of anemia of CKD is not associated with causing infections[45]
[b]Usual goal 1,000 mg total dose

Table 25.5 Oral iron preparations

Iron formulation	Elemental iron content (mg)
Ferrous fumarate 100 mg tablet	33
Ferrous gluconate 300 mg tablet	36
Ferrous sulfate 325 mg tablet	65
Ferrous sulfate elixir 10 mL	88

Recommended 200 mg of elemental iron each day in oral iron repletion
Common side effects: Gastrointestinal related such as constipation, nausea
May inhibit iron absorption: Coffee, tea, milk, cereals, sodas with phosphorous, enteric coated iron tablets, antacids, H2 blockers, proton pump inhibitors, and antibiotics such as tetracyclines
May facilitate absorption: Acidic stomach environment such as ascorbic acid or vitamin c containing juices such as orange juice, and taking tablets while fasting. Also, using non-enteric coated formulations [41, 47]

of their anti-oxidant and anti-inflammatory properties but more evidence is needed before widespread use is encouraged for the treatment of the anemia of CKD.

Case 1 Revisited

For the 32-year-old man with diabetes mellitus type I, CKD stage V, and anemia, there were no signs of active bleeding on physical examination. Iron studies were consistent with anemia of chronic disease. Iron, TIBC, and reticulocyte index were low while the ferritin and iron saturation were normal. Risk factors for the anemia included CKD, diabetes mellitus, and the presence of fluid overload. He was initiated weekly on darbepoetin 60 mcg subcutaneously and peritoneal dialysis for uremic symptoms and fluid overload.

Case 2 Revisited

For the 64-year-old lady with CHF, CKD stage IV, and anemia, her history and physical exam do not suggest active blood loss. Although the normal TIBC, low reticulocyte percent, and low reticulocyte production index suggest anemia of CKD, the low iron level, very low iron saturation, and a low ferritin level are also consistent with iron deficiency anemia. An esophagogastroduodenoscopy and colonoscopy showed no signs of bleeding. The patient's iron stores were repleted with IV iron sucrose and darbepoetin was initiated subcutaneously at 2 week intervals.

References

1. The United States Renal Data System. http://www.usrds.org/. Accessed 1 Mar 2011.
2. National Kidney Foundation. KDOQI clinical practice guidelines and clinical practice recommendations for anemia in chronic kidney disease. Am J Kidney Dis. 2006;47 Suppl 3:S1–146.
3. de Benoist B, McLean E, Egli I, Cogswell M, editors. Worldwide prevalence of anaemia 1993–2005. WHO global database on anaemia. WHO: Geneva; 2008. p. 1–51.
4. McFarlane SI, Chen SC, Whaley-Connell AT, et al. Prevalence and associations of anemia of CKD: Kidney Early Evaluation Program (KEEP) and National Health and Nutrition Examination Survey (NHANES) 1999–2004. Am J Kidney Dis. 2008;51:S46–55.
5. Thervet E, Legendre C, Debure A, et al. Angiotensin-converting enzyme (ACE) inhibitors have been reported to induce or worsen anemia in patients on hemodialysis. Am J Kidney Dis. 1991;18:282–3.
6. Abu-Alfa AK, Cruz D, Perazella MA, et al. ACE inhibitors do not induce recombinant human erythropoietin resistance in hemodialysis patients. Am J Kidney Dis. 2000;35:1076–82.
7. Adamson JW, Longo DL. Anemia and polycythemia. In: Kasper DL, Braunwald E, Fauci AS, Hauser SL, Longo DL, Jameson JL, editors. Harrison's principles of internal medicine. 16th ed. New York: McGraw-Hill Medical Publishing Division; 2005. p. 329–36.
8. U.S. Food and Drug Administration. http://www.fda.gov/. Accessed 1 Mar 2011.
9. McClellan WM, Flanders WD, Langston RD, et al. Anemia and renal insufficiency are independent risk factors for death among patients with congestive heart failure admitted to community hospitals: a population-based study. J Am Soc Nephrol. 2002;13:1928–36.
10. Jurkovitz CT, Abramson JL, McClellan WM, et al. Association of high serum creatinine and anemia increases the risk of coronary events: results from the prospective community-based atherosclerosis risk in communities (ARIC) study. J Am Soc Nephrol. 2003;14:2919–25.
11. Ayus JC, Alan SG, Fernando V, et al. Effects of erythropoietin on left ventricular hypertrophy in adults with severe chronic renal failure and hemoglobin <10 g/dL. Kidney Int. 2005;68:788–95.
12. Frank H, Heusser K, Hoffken B, et al. Effect of erythropoietin on cardiovascular prognosis parameters in hemodialysis patients. Kidney Int. 2004;66:832–40.

13. Hampl H, Rosenberger C, Amirkhalily M, et al. Effects of optimized heart failure therapy and anemia correction with epoetin beta on left ventricular mass in hemodialysis patients. Am J Nephrol. 2005;25:211–20.
14. Drueke TB, Locatelli F, Clyne N, et al. Normalization of hemoglobin level in patients with chronic kidney disease and anemia. N Engl J Med. 2006;355:2071–84.
15. Gandra SR. Impact of erythropoiesis-stimulating agents on energy and physical function in nondialysis CKD patients with anemia: a systematic review. Am J Kidney Dis. 2010;55:519–34.
16. Nissenson AR, Korbet S, Faber M, et al. Multicenter trial of erythropoietin in patients on peritoneal dialysis. J Am Soc Nephrol. 1995;5:1517–29.
17. Locatelli F, Aljama P, Barany P, et al. Revised European best practice guidelines for the management of anaemia in patients with chronic renal failure. Nephrol Dial Transplant. 2004;19:S1–47.
18. Pfeffer MA, Burdmann EA, Chen C, et al. A trial of darbepoetin alfa in type 2 diabetes and chronic kidney disease. N Engl J Med. 2009;361:2019–32.
19. Palmer SC, Navaneethan SD, Craig JC, et al. Meta-analysis: erythropoiesis-stimulating agents in patients with chronic kidney disease. Ann Intern Med. 2010;153:23–33.
20. Besarab A, Bolton WK, Browne JK, et al. The effects of normal as compared with low hematocrit values in patients with cardiac disease who are receiving hemodialysis and epoetin. N Engl J Med. 1998;339:584–90.
21. Singh AK, Szczech L, Tang KL, et al. Correction of anemia with epoetin alfa in chronic kidney disease. N Engl J Med. 2006;355:2085–98.
22. Pisoni RL, Bragg-Gresham JL, Fuller D, et al. Facility-level interpatient hemoglobin variability in hemodialysis centers participating in the dialysis outcomes and practice patterns study (DOPPS): associations with mortality, patient characteristics and facility practices. Am J Kidney Dis. 2011;57:266–75.
23. Solomon SD, Uno H, Lewis EF, et al. Erythropoietic response and outcomes in kidney disease and type 2 diabetes. N Engl J Med. 2010;363:1146–55.
24. Spinowitz B, Germain M, Benz R, et al. A randomized study of extended dosing regimens for initiation of epoetin alfa treatment for anemia of chronic kidney disease. Clin J Am Soc Nephrol. 2008;3:1015–21.
25. Macdougall IC, Walker R, Provenzano R, et al. C.E.R.A. corrects anemia in patients with chronic kidney disease not on dialysis: results of a randomized clinical trial. Clin J Am Soc Nephrol. 2008;3:337–47.
26. Macdougall I, Rossert J, Casadevall N, et al. A peptide-based erythropoietin-receptor agonist for pure red-cell aplasia. N Engl J Med. 2009;361:1848–55.
27. Schiller B, Zeig S, Hura C, et al. Safety and efficacy of peginesatide for treatment of anemia in hemodialysis patients previously on epoetin alfa. Am J Kidney Dis. 2011;57:A1–108.
28. Provenzano R, Goodkin D, Klaus S, et al. Evaluation of FG-4592, a novel oral hypoxia-inducible factor prolyl hydroxylase inhibitor, to treat anemia in hemodialysis patients. Am J Kidney Dis. 2011;57:A108.
29. Provenzano R, Tumlin J, Zabaneh R, et al. Pharmacokinetics of oral FG-4592 to treat anemia in hemodialysis patients. Am J Kidney Dis. 2011;57: A1–108.
30. Kaufman J, Reda D, Fye C, et al. Subcutaneous compared with intravenous epoetin in patients receiving hemodialysis. N Engl J Med. 1998;339:578–83.
31. Paganini E, Eschbach J, Lazarus J, et al. Intravenous versus subcutaneous dosing of epoetin alpha in hemodialysis patients. Am J Kidney Dis. 1995;26:331–40.
32. Casadevall N, Nataf J, Viron B, et al. Pure red-cell aplasia and antierythropoietin antibodies in patients treated with recombinant erythropoietin. N Engl J Med. 2002;346:469–75.
33. Guest S, Levitt L. Pure red-cell aplasia secondary to antierythropoietin antibodies. N Engl J Med. 2003; 349(26):2572–3.
34. Li H, Ginzburg YZ. Cross talk between iron metabolism and erythropoesis. Adv Hematol. 2010;2010:605435.
35. Nemeth E, Ganz T. Regulation of iron metabolism by hepcidin. Annu Rev Nutr. 2006;26:323–42.
36. Wish J. Assessing iron status: beyond serum ferritin and transferring saturation. Clin J Am Soc Nephrol. 2006;1:S4–8.
37. Kalantar-zadeh K, Hoffken B, Wunsch H, et al. Diagnosis of iron deficiency anemia in renal failure patients during the post-erythropoietin era. Am J Kidney Dis. 1995;26:292–9.
38. Coyne D, Kapoian T, Suki W, DRIVE Study Group, et al. Ferric gluconate is highly efficacious in anemic hemodialysis patients with high serum ferritin and low transferrin saturation: results of the dialysis patients response to IV iron with elevated ferritin (DRIVE) study. J Am Soc Nephrol. 2007;18:975–84.
39. Kapoian T, O'Mara NB, Singh AK, et al. Ferric gluconate reduces epoetin requirements in hemodialysis patients with elevated ferritin. J Am Soc Nephrol. 2008;19:372–9.
40. Rozen-Zvi B, Gafter-Gvili A, Paul M, et al. Intravenous versus oral iron supplementation for the treatment of anemia in CKD: systematic review and meta-analysis. Am J Kidney Dis. 2008;52:897–906.
41. Horl W. Clinical aspects of iron use in the anemia of kidney disease. J Am Soc Nephrol. 2007;18:382–93.
42. Spinowitz B, Kausz A, Baptista J, et al. Ferumoxytol for treating iron deficiency anemia in CKD. J Am Soc Nephrol. 2008;19:1599–605.
43. Asma S, Boga C, Ozdogu H. Safety, therapeutic effectiveness, and cost of parenteral iron therapy. Int J Hematol. 2009;90:24–7.
44. Bailie G, Johnson C, Mason N. Parenteral iron use in the management of anemia in end-stage renal disease patients. Am J Kidney Dis. 2000;35:1–12.
45. Aronoff G. Safety of intravenous iron in clinical practice implications for anemia management protocols. J Am Soc Nephrol. 2004;15:S99–106.
46. Provenzano R, Schiller B, Rao M, et al. Ferumoxytol as an intravenous iron replacement therapy in hemodialysis patients. Clin J Am Soc Nephrol. 2009;4:386–93.
47. Alleyne M, Horne M, Miller J, et al. Individualized treatment for iron-deficiency anemia in adults. Am J Med. 2008;121:943–8.

26 Goals of Therapy: Slowing Progression and Dyslipidemias

M. Salman Singapuri and Janice P. Lea

Case 1

A 47-year-old man with type 2 diabetes mellitus with no evidence of retinopathy, hypertension, chronic kidney disease (CKD) stage 3, and congestive heart failure (CHF) presents for a follow-up visit at the clinic. Recently, he developed fatigue and shortness of breath with effort. He takes lisinopril 20 mg daily, metoprolol 50 mg twice a day, and a nightly subcutaneous shot of 30 U of insulin glargine. On physical examination, he is afebrile, heart rate is 83 bpm, and BP is 163/89 mmHg. His physical examination is normal other than a S4 and a displaced PMI. His serum creatinine is 1.8 mg/dl (6 months ago it was noted to be 1.5 mg/dl); a hemoglobin A1C is 8.8%. The rest of his chemistries are within normal range. His hemoglobin is 8.9 g/dl. Both platelet and white cell counts are normal. His urinanalysis reveals 2+ protein with a urine protein:creatinine ratio of 1.8 g/g of creatinine. On ECG, voltage criteria for LVH are met. What are the risk factors for progression of CKD in this patient? How can these risk factors be controlled and what other agents may be added to his medication regimen? What is the optimal blood pressure goal?

Case 2

A 56-year-old man with a history of diet-controlled diabetes mellitus type 2, CKD stage 3, COPD, dyslipidemia, and obesity presents for a follow-up visit with his primary care physician. He admits to smoking two packs per day for the past 20 years, but recently noticed foamy urine. On exam he is afebrile, heart rate is 87 bpm, BP is 142/79 mmHg, and weight is 295 pounds with a body mass index (BMI) of 38.89 kg/m^2. His most recent chemistry shows a creatinine 1.5 mg/dl (7 months ago, it was 1.1 mg/dl), serum bicarbonate of 22 mEq/L, and uric acid level of 9.6 mg/dl with the remainder chemistries being normal. His CBC reveals a Hg of 14.7 mg/dl, normal platelet counts and white blood cells with differentials. Lipid profile shows an low-density lipoprotein (LDL) of 129 mg/dl, high-density lipoprotein (HDL) of 37 mg/dl, TG of 243 mg/dl, and a total cholesterol of 203 mg/dl. His urinanalysis reveals trace proteinuria. What are his risk factors for progression of kidney disease? How should this case be managed?

CKD is usually an irreversible, progressive disease which over time can lead to end-stage renal disease (ESRD). It is a significant and growing problem worldwide. In the USA, more than 20 million people have CKD [1], and it is estimated that by 2030, more than two million people in the USA will need either dialysis or transplantation for ESRD [2]. Despite these high numbers, less than 2% of patients with

M.S. Singapuri, M.D. (✉) • J.P. Lea, M.D., M.Sc.
Division of Nephrology, Department of Medicine, Emory University of Medicine, Atlanta, GA 30324, USA
e-mail: mohammed.singapuri@emoryhealthcare.org

E.V. Lerma and M. Rosner (eds.), *Clinical Decisions in Nephrology, Hypertension and Kidney Transplantation*,
DOI 10.1007/978-1-4614-4454-1_26, © Springer Science+Business Media New York 2013

CKD will require renal replacement therapy (RRT) [3], mainly because most individuals with CKD die from cardiovascular disease before they reach ESRD [4]. Over the past decade, there has been a growing awareness of CKD and the implications for provision of RRT [5]. The incidence of recognized CKD among Medicare patients aged 65 and older reached 4.3% in 2008, 3.7 times greater than the rate of 1.2 seen in 1995 [6]. It is more prevalent in women with 35% and 20% of people aged 20 years or more having diabetes and hypertension, respectively. The rate of progression of CKD is highest in African Americans. Unfortunately, the diagnosis of CKD is often delayed, largely because of its indolent course but also because the serum creatinine (an insensitive marker of kidney function) is often used to gauge kidney function [7].

Slowing the progression of CKD has always been a challenge for both the internist and the nephrologist. Recently, much attention has focused on the important observation that CKD is associated with markedly increased cardiovascular risk [4] and it is therefore not surprising that cardiovascular disease is also associated with an increased risk of CKD.

CKD is associated with a two- to threefold higher risk of death. In addition, there is a higher risk of requiring dialysis and developing CHF or other cardiovascular event [8]. Despite this higher risk, preventative care that included both lipid and glycemic monitoring among individuals with diabetes was no higher among Medicare patients with CKD than in patients without CKD [8, 9]. In 2006, the cost to the federal government for the treatment of ESRD was $23 billion, and the corresponding treatment cost for CKD was $49 billion [6, 10].

Considering that a CKD patient is more likely to have a cardiovascular event and die than to reach ESRD, it is imperative that this high-risk population be identified and further scrutinized for risk factors for cardiovascular events and death, and kidney disease progression. Table 26.1 illustrates the potential causes of CKD.

Table 26.1 Major causes of CKDa

Cause	%
• Diabetes type 1	3.9%
• Diabetes type 2	41%
• Hypertension	27.2%
• Glomerulonephritis	8.2%
• Chronic interstitial nephritis	3.6%
• Hereditary or cystic disease	3.1%

[a]Data from the USRDS 2006

Diabetes Mellitus

Diabetes is a major health issue in the USA with nearly 26 million people ages 20 years or older having the disease [11]. It is the leading cause of kidney failure, accounting for 44% of all new cases of ESRD in 2008 [11]. Obesity is a major risk factor for type 2 diabetes mellitus [12]. Insulin-dependent diabetes mellitus is associated with long-term micro- and macrovascular and neurologic sequelae leading to diabetic nephropathy (DN). The pathogenesis of DN is complex. In its early phase, the key change at a molecular level is hyperfiltration within the glomerulus. This is thought to be secondary to chronic hyperglycemia [13] and leads to an increased glomerular filtration rate (GFR) [14]. The earliest marker for DN is the appearance of low but abnormal levels (≥30 mg/day or 20 μg/min) of microalbuminuria [15]. If left untreated, overt nephropathy develops after 10–15 years. Table 26.2 illustrates clinical features characteristic of type 2 DN.

Strict glycemic control is imperative and of paramount importance. This was demonstrated in the Diabetes Control and Complication Trial (DCCT) in which intensive glucose control prevented the development of diabetic nephropathy and retarded the progression from microalbuminuria to overt proteinuria in patients with type 1 diabetes mellitus [16]. Similar findings were reported in patients with type 2 diabetes mellitus from the UK Prospective Diabetes Study (UKPDS) Group [17]. There are many agents available for the treatment of diabetes mellitus, but special consideration has to be given to the

Table 26.2 Clinical features of type 2 diabetic nephropathy

• Most common after age 40 years
• Abdominal obesity present in 90%
• Insulin resistance/hyperinsulinemia
• Hypertension is common
• ↑ VLDL and ↓ HDL cholesterol
• Accelerated atherosclerosis
• Increased prevalence in AA, MA, and NAI

AA African Americans, *MA* Mexican Americans, *NAI* Native American Indians, *VLDL* very low-density lipoprotein, *HDL* high-density lipoprotein

CKD population. Exogenous insulin is mainly renally cleared by way of filtration, extensive tubular secretion, and cellular catabolism in the kidney. As renal failure progresses, insulin clearance declines; the half-life of insulin increases, and requirements for insulin diminish [18]. Metformin, another commonly used medication for diabetes, is contraindicated in men with creatinine values more than 1.5 mg/dl and in women with creatinine values of more than 1.4 mg/dl [19, 20]. First-generation sulfonylureas are associated with prolonged hypoglycemia which is related to parent drug and/or active metabolite accumulation [21]. Glipizide and gliclazide are metabolized by the liver to several inactive metabolites and are considered safe for use in patients with reduced renal function [22].

Hypertension

Hypertension has long been recognized as a consequence of renal impairment and an important factor in the progression of CKD. It is the second leading cause of CKD. Patients with hypertension typically require multiple agents to control BP [23]. Table 26.3 illustrates key features of CKD patients with hypertensive nephrosclerosis.

According to Retnakaran et al., an elevated systolic blood pressure was an independent risk factor for the development of albuminuria or renal impairment among patients with type II diabetes mellitus [24]. Several studies have found a close association between the magnitude of increased risk and the level of blood pressure such that even modest elevations in blood pressure, below the threshold for a diagnosis of hypertension, are associated with an increased risk of ESRD. Although the major importance of BP as an independent risk factor for renal disease progression has also been emphasized by recent meta-analyses, rennin–angiotensin–aldosterone system (RAAS) blockade is strongly recommended as the initial regimen of choice for renoprotection [25]. In the past two decades, RAAS inhibitors have become a mainstay for the treatment of hypertension [26]. Therapies that target the RAAS offer particular benefit to hypertensive, proteinuric patients with kidney disease because these agents reduce proteinuria as well as BP [27, 28]. A baseline reduction of proteinuria by more than 30% within the first 6–12 months of treatment in patients with kidney disease has favorable long-term renal [29] and cardiovascular (CV) outcomes [30]. The African American Study of Kidney Disease and Hypertension (AASK) Trial [31] supported the use of ACE inhibitors over beta and calcium channel blockers (CCB) in hypertensive renal disease patients. A long-term follow-up subgroup analysis suggested that a mean arterial pressure goal of 92 mm Hg or lower retarded disease progression in African Americans with hypertensive renal disease with a urinary protein to creatinine ratio of more than 0.22.

Table 26.3 Clinical features of hypertensive nephrosclerosis

• Proteinuria
• No other etiology for kidney disease
• Onset of HTN at 25–45 years of age
• Increased prevalence in AA
• Family history of HTN
• Long standing or severe HTN with an onset of HTN prior to the development of proteinuria or an increase in serum creatinine
• Evidence of other target organ damage such as retinopathy and/or LVH
• Renal biopsy demonstrating hyalinization of arterioles and fibroplastic intimal thickening of small arteries, glomerular ischemia, and interstitial fibrosis

HTN hypertension, *LVH* left ventricular hypertrophy, *AA* African Americans

The optimal BP for adults to safeguard and sustain optimal cardiac and renal protection is unknown, but it is widely accepted that a systolic BP goal of less than 130 mmHg is best [22]. In many cases, multiple antihypertensive agents in different combinations are required to attain this goal. In addition, salt intake should be minimized as a high salt intake blunts the effect of antihypertensive agents and also the antiproteinuric effects of ACE inhibitors and ARBs [32]. ACE inhibitors and ARBs are recommended as first line agents for hypertensive patients with CKD and proteinuria with or without diabetes. Diuretics are useful in patients with volume overload; type is dictated by the GFR. In patients with a GFR less than 50 ml/min, loop diuretics should be administered while patients with a higher GFR may just require a thiazide diuretic [33]. Non-dihydropyridines (DHP) CCBs are recommended over DHP-CCB as the former reduces proteinuria and slows progression of diabetic nephropathy [34, 35].

When combination therapies are needed, the Joint National Committee on Prevention, Detection, Evaluation, and Treatment of High Blood Pressure (JNC 7) [36] indicate a strong predilection for thiazide diuretics (see Table 26.4). However, combinations that do not include thiazide diuretics should also be considered. The Avoiding Cardiovascular Events through Combination Therapy in Patients Living with Systolic Hypertension (ACCOMPLISH) trial [37] showed that initial treatment for high blood pressure with benazepril plus amlodipine was superior to benazepril plus hydrochlorothiazide in reducing cardiovascular disease and mortality. In addition, the renal outcomes of the ACCOMPLISH trial by Bakris and colleagues [38] favor the combination of benazepril plus amlodipine over the combination of benazepril plus hydrochlorothiazide since it helps to slow nephropathy to a greater extent.

Anemia

According to the data from National Health and Nutrition Examination Survey (NHANES), the prevalence of anemia, as defined as a hemoglobin concentration of less than 11 g/dl, in CKD stages 3, 4, and 5 is 1.3%, 5.2%, and 44.1%, respectively [39]. It may be an independent predictor of adverse cardiovascular events [40] and its occurrence with CKD may result in a milieu that adversely promotes cardiac ischemia and left ventricular hypertrophy [41]. Major causes of anemia in CKD are erythropoietin insufficiency, blood loss, iron deficiency, and shortened half-life of erythrocytes [42]. Anemia correction has been variably associated with good outcomes. In a recent study by Alexander et al. [43], anemia correction led to improvements in physical activity, vitality, and fatigue. Anemia develops earlier and more severely in patients with diabetic nephropathy than in CKD patients without diabetes [44]. As anemia decreases tissue oxygenation, the cardiovascular system compensates with tachycardia, vasodilation, and increased cardiac work, leading over time to left ventricular hypertrophy [45]. If anemia is left untreated, an accelerated progression to ESRD can be expected but is abrogated with initiation of erythropoietin therapy [46, 47]. Treating anemia with erythropoietin stimulating agents (ESAs) augments diminished renal erythropoietin production and alleviates tissue hypoxia, which in turn may prevent or reverse left ventricular hypertrophy.

Table 26.4 Recommendations for BP and RAAS management in CKD

Patient group	Goal BP (mmHg)	First line agent	Adjunctive agent
+ Diabetes + Proteinuria	<130/80	ACEI or ARB	CCB then BB or diuretics
– Diabetes + Proteinuria	<130/80	ACEI or ARB	Diuretics then CCB or BB
– Diabetes – Proteinuria	<130/80	No specific preference Diuretics then ACEI, ARB, CCB, or BB	

ACEI angiotensin converting enzyme inhibitor, *ARB* angiotensin II receptor blocker, *CCB* calcium channel blocker, *BB* beta blocker

Four clinical studies [48–51] have demonstrated that treatment of anemia with ESAs in CKD patients slows the progression of renal failure.

Recent guidelines suggest that Hg should be targeted for levels between 11 and 12 g/dl [42]. Iron and ESAs are the cornerstones of therapy in the management of anemia in this population. In general ESA therapy should be initiated when Hg levels fall below 10 g/dl and other reversible factors of anemia have been identified and corrected [52]. Treatment with ESAs has been shown to enhance quality of life [53]. More discussion and details can be found in the section on "Anemia."

Acidosis

Metabolic acidosis in CKD results from the reduced capacity of the kidneys to make ammonium and subsequently excrete H^+ [54]. It may also result from decreased production of new bicarbonate or to a lesser extent decreased bicarbonate reabsorption [55]. It results in many deleterious complications [56] including stunted growth in children, loss of bone and muscle mass, negative nitrogen balance, and acceleration of progression of CKD [57]. The KDOQI recommends a bicarbonate level above 22 mEq/mL in all patients [58]. In a recent study by de Brito-Ashurst et al. [59], bicarbonate supplementation slowed the rate of progression of renal failure to ESRD and improved nutritional status among patients with CKD.

Proteinuria

Proteinuria has long been recognized as an important risk factor for progression of renal disease as well as an independent risk factor for cardiovascular morbidity and mortality [60]. The magnitude of proteinuria is associated with a graded increase in the risk of progression to ESRD and cardiovascular events [61]. In individuals with hypertension and diabetes, proteinuria is a late sequelae of ischemic heart disease, stroke, CHF, and intermittent claudication [62, 63]. In the early stages of CKD, microalbuminuria is detectable and as disease progresses to clinical or overt nephropathy, macroalbuminuria becomes a prominent feature. Hemodynamic injury to the vascular endothelium and glomerulus can be induced by both systemic and glomerular hypertension, which, in turn, is promoted by an activated RAAS. Overactivity of the RAAS has been implicated in the deterioration of renal function in patients with diabetic nephropathy and in patients who have stage 3 or 4 CKD with micro- or macroalbuminuria [64]. Angiotensin II, the primary mediator of this system, is the common denominator in all stages of renal pathophysiology [65].

In the Bergamo Nephrologic Diabetes Complications (BENDCIT) Trial [66] ACE inhibition with trandolapril was associated with a 53% decrease in the rate of microalbuminuria in patients with hypertension and type 2 diabetes mellitus. In a post hoc analysis of the BENDCIT trial, Ruggenenti et al. [67] noted that the greater treatment effect in the study was probably due to higher baseline and follow-up blood pressures. In the Angiotensin-Converting Enzyme Inhibition in Progressive Renal Insufficiency (AIPRI) trial, Maschio et al. [68] randomly assigned 583 patients with renal disease of diverse etiologies to treatment with benazepril or placebo. After 3 years of follow-up, there was a 53% reduction with ACE inhibitor treatment, in the combined risk of doubling of the baseline serum creatinine or need for dialysis. In the Randomized Olmesartan and Diabetes Microalbuminuria Prevention (ROADMAP) study [69], olmesartan increased the time to the onset of microalbuminuria in patients with type 2 diabetes, even when BP control was less than 130/80 mmHg in both treatment arms. In the African American Study of Kidney Disease and Hypertension (AASK) study trial, 1,094 hypertensive African American were randomized to either a β-blocker, an ACE inhibitor, or a DHP-CCB, and found that changes in low levels of proteinuria, in nondiabetic kidney disease, were predictive of the annual rate of decline in the GFR and the development of ESRD [61]. Direct Renin Inhibitors have proven useful in combination with ACE inhibitors or ARBs for superior RAAS blockade, but special attention has to be given for development of hyperkalemia and renal failure.

Obesity

Obesity is defined as a BMI of 30 or greater. It is a growing problem globally with the estimated prevalence in the USA being 32.2% among adult men and 35.5% among adult women [70]. Obesity is a risk factor for a variety of chronic conditions including diabetes, hypertension, high cholesterol, stroke, heart disease, certain cancers, and arthritis [71]. Higher grades of obesity are associated with excess mortality, primarily from cardiovascular disease, diabetes, and certain cancers [72]. In a study by Tozawa et al. [73], obesity correlated with urinary albumin excretion in men not known to be diabetic, hypertensive, lipidemic, or proteinuric. In a study by Sietsma et al. [74], in lean individuals, there was an association between central body fat distribution and reduced kidney function. Moreover, in a study by Praga et al. [75], a correlation was noticed between weight loss and reduction in proteinuria.

Adiponectin is a protein hormone that modulates a number of metabolic processes, including glucose regulation and fatty acid catabolism [76] and is exclusively secreted from adipose tissue. It is a novel predictor of CKD progression in men but not in women [77]. In an observational study of patients with type 1 diabetes mellitus and overt diabetic nephropathy, higher serum adiponectin levels predicted ESRD progression [78]. Weight loss should be endorsed and reinforced for all patients with CKD, not only as part of their health maintenance but also as part of their routine nephrology follow-up.

Smoking

In developed countries, cigarette smoking is considered to be the most common cause of death in adults [79]. Among diabetic patients, smoking seems to be an independent risk factor for nephropathy and appears to accelerate the rate of progression of renal disease [80]. In hypertensive patients, smoking independently increases the risk for albuminuria and may contribute to a decline of renal function [81]. Nicotine, present in cigarette smoke, increases BP and heart rate [82]. Because increased BP is one of the most important factors promoting progression of CKD, it is likely to play an important role in mediating smoking-induced renal damage.

Regarding smoking cessation strategies in renal patients, there are no randomized controlled trials and reliance on the data from the general population has to be taken into consideration for guidance [83]. Weaning smokers from their habit is a challenging task and should start by interrogation of their habits. It cannot be stressed enough that physician advice per se is an effective, evidence-based strategy [84]. As a second line, nicotine replacement therapy (NRT), in the form of gum, patch, or spray may be used. Because nicotine accumulates in patients with impaired renal function [85], a reduction of NRT dosage should be undertaken. As smoking is an important risk factor for progression of renal disease, nephrologists have to invest additional efforts to motivate patients to stop smoking [83].

Gout/Uric Acid

The role of uric acid in CKD progression has been under study but the results are inconsistent. The Atherosclerosis Risks in Communities (ARIC) and the Cardiovascular Health Study (CHS) [86] trials reported that there was a 7–11% higher risk for a decline in kidney function for each 1 mg/dl increase in baseline uric acid level. It was also a significant risk factor for death or incident kidney disease. Moreover, Obermayer et al. studied 17,000 Vietnamese adults without known kidney disease and identified a high serum uric acid level as a risk factor for new-onset CKD [87]. In contrast, the Mild to Moderate Kidney Disease (MMKD) Study [88] concluded that uric acid levels were not an independent predictor for CKD progression. Despite these results, a recent prospective, randomized, controlled trial of 54 patients who had CKD and hyperuricemia and were randomly assigned to treatment with allopurinol 100–300 mg daily or usual therapy for 12 months found that treatment with allopurinol reduced CKD progression [89]. In conclusion, uric acid may contribute towards progression of CKD and uric acid lowering agents may help retard progression of renal disease; however, larger trials are needed to ascertain their benefit.

Dyslipidemia

That lipids might contribute to the progression of CKD was first proposed in 1982 by Moorhead et al. [90]. Moreover, modifying them may delay the progression of CKD [91]. In the Atherosclerosis Risk in Communities (ARC) study, high triglyceride and low HDL cholesterol levels were associated with an increased risk for developing renal dysfunction [92]. Low HDL cholesterol levels were also an independent risk factor for the development of incident CKD in the Framingham Offspring study [93]. In the Modification of Diet in Renal Disease (MDRD) study, which included patients with moderate-to-severe renal disease of various etiologies, low HDL independently predicted a faster decline in GFR [94]. The mechanism by which lipids cause kidney damage is most likely complex and intricate, but hypercholesterolemia and hypertriglyceridemia are associated with podocyte injury, which secondarily leads to mesangial sclerosis [95]. Lipid abnormalities were originally considered a complication of ESRD, but these changes can be present in early stages of CKD and may contribute in the accelerated pathogenesis of atherosclerotic vascular disease. Premature CVD extends from mild to moderate stages of CKD. In a pooled analysis of four community-based studies, moderate renal insufficiency carried a 19% excess risk of cardiovascular complication [96].

Dyslipidemia is a well-known risk factor for CVD in the general population and large-scale observational studies have shown that total and LDL-cholesterol values are two of the most important independent predictors of cardiovascular morbidity and mortality [97]. Hypertriglyceridemia is an early feature of renal failure [98] and secondary hyperparathyroidism may contribute to its development [99]. The most common quantitative lipid abnormalities in CKD patients are hypertriglyceridemia, increased concentrations of triglyceride-rich lipoprotein remnants, reduced HDL cholesterol levels, as well as increased concentrations of lipoprotein(a) [100]. Notably, total and LDL cholesterol levels are usually within normal limits or slightly reduced in these individuals [101]. Despite their low or normal levels, this small dense atherogenic particle contributes to atherosclerosis [102].

Statins are by far the most commonly prescribed hypolipidemic drugs in the general population, and numerous large, randomized, prospective studies have shown that their use is accompanied by a remarkable diminution in the incidence of cardiovascular events [103]. In patients with mild to moderate renal failure, post hoc analysis of several large, prospective, placebo-controlled trials of statins revealed a significant reduction in cardiovascular morbidity and mortality [104–107]. In a 1-year prospective, placebo-controlled, open-label study on patients with CKD, proteinuria, and hypercholesterolemia, patients receiving atorvastatin had a small, insignificant decline in CrCl, whereas those receiving placebo showed a significant decrease in renal function [108]. In the same study, there was also evidence of a synergistic effect between statins and RAAS inhibitors on renal protection.

In 2003, the National Cholesterol Education Program Adult Treatment Panel (ATP III) guidelines for treatment of dyslipidemia in the general population were adopted by the National Kidney Foundation Kidney Disease Outcomes Quality Initiative (K/DOQI) for application to patients with stages 1–4 CKD. Accordingly, the target LDL level should be less than 100 mg/dl for people with stages 1–4 CKD and less than 70 mg/dl for patients who also have diabetes [109]. Aggressive reduction in lipid levels can also be achieved by adding ezetimibe. The second United Kingdom Heart and Renal protection study (UKHARP-II) [110] showed that the addition of ezetimibe to simvastatin was safe and effective in treating dyslipidemia in CKD. In the recent double-blinded, placebo-controlled Study of Heart and Renal Protection (SHARP) trial, administration of ezetimibe 10 mg and simvastatin 20 mg daily in patients with CKD was associated with one-sixth fewer MIs, strokes, or major atherosclerotic events [111]. There are virtually no data showing a benefit of raising HDL cholesterol levels and lowering triglyceride levels in CKD patients [112] in slowing the progression of CKD. Although fibrates may be used as a lipid lowering therapy, it is associated with an extremely high risk of muscular toxicity in individuals with impaired renal function [113]. In summary, the primary goal should be lowering LDL cholesterol levels primarily with statins.

Case 1 Revisited

According to the MDRD calculator the patient has a GFR of 49 ml/min/1.73 m^2 placing him at stage 3 CKD. His BP regimen was intensified by increasing lisinopril to 40 mg/day (with appropriate and serial monitoring of serum creatinine and electrolyte levels) and adding a thiazide diuretic. The patient also admitted that he was not compliant with a dietary sodium restriction; at times he skipped his insulin. Following intense nutritional counseling and adherence to his medical regimen, his BP declined to 138/78 mmHg, HgA1C dropped to 7.5%, and urinary protein excretion was 678 mg/g of creatinine. Appropriate counseling and referral to multidisciplinary clinics can assist patients in delaying the progression of kidney disease.

Case 2 Revisited

This patient has CKD stage 3 secondary to diabetic nephropathy, but his disease is complicated by other factors including HTN and obesity. Upon further investigation, the patient was consuming a high protein diet and had gouty attacks. He was referred to a weight loss clinic and nutritional counselor. In the interim he was initiated on allopurinol, low dose transdermal nicotine patch, and atorvastatin 10 mg/day. A decision was made to hold off on the bicarbonate repletion. He was followed up in the nephrology clinic monthly to monitor his renal function and progress with smoking cessation. At the end of 5 months, his BMI dropped to 31 kg/m^2, bicarbonate levels rose to 23 mEq/L, and both serum creatinine and LDL trended downwards to 1.3 mg/dl and 95 mg/dl, respectively. With strong encouragement and reinforcement from his primary physician, he was weaned from his smoking habits. In general, the patient admitted to feeling better. On subsequent visits his decline in kidney function stabilized.

References

1. Centers for Disease Control and Prevention. National Chronic Kidney Disease Fact Sheet: general information and national estimates on chronic kidney disease in the United States, 2010. Atlanta, GA: U.S. Department of Health and Human Services, Centers for Disease Control and Prevention; 2010 [cited 31 Mar 2011]. http://www.cdc.gov/diabetes/pubs/factsheets/kidney.htm.
2. U.S. Renal Data System Annual report: atlas of end stage renal disease in the United States National Institutes of Health And National Institute of Diabetes and Digestive and Kidney Diseases; 2005. Bethesda, MD.
3. Keith DS, et al. Longitudinal follow-up and outcomes among a population with chronic kidney disease in a large managed care organization. Arch Intern Med. 2004;164(6):659–63.
4. Go AS, et al. Chronic kidney disease and the risks of death, cardiovascular events, and hospitalization. N Engl J Med. 2004;351(13):1296–305.
5. Taal MW, Brenner BM. Predicting initiation and progression of chronic kidney disease: developing renal risk scores. Kidney Int. 2006;70(10):1694–705.
6. U.S. Renal Data System, USRDS 2008 Annual Data Report: atlas of chronic kidney disease and end-stage renal disease in the United States, National Institutes of Health, National Institute of Diabetes and Digestive and Kidney Diseases.
7. Stigant C, Stevens L, Levin A. Nephrology: 4. Strategies for the care of adults with chronic kidney disease. CMAJ. 2003;168(12):1553–60.
8. Collins AJ, et al. Chronic kidney disease and cardiovascular disease in the Medicare population. Kidney Int Suppl. 2003;87:S24–31.
9. U.S. Renal Data System Annual Data Report: atlas of end-stage renal disease in the United States. National Institutes of Health, National Institute of Diabetes and Digestive and Kidney Diseases: Bethesda, MD; 2003.
10. National Institute of Diabetes and Digestive and Kidney Diseases (U.S.) and USRDS Coordinating Center., U.S. renal data system … annual data report, researcher's guide, reference tables, ADR slides, in U.S. Renal Data System. Atlas of chronic kidney disease and end-stage renal disease in the United States.

National Institute of Diabetes and Digestive and Kidney Diseases: Bethesda, MD; 2008. p. CD-ROMs.
11. Centers for Disease Control and Prevention. National diabetes fact sheet: national estimates and general information on diabetes and prediabetes in the United States, 2011. Atlanta, GA: U.S. Department of Health and Human Services, Centers for Disease Control and Prevention; 2011.
12. Mokdad AH, et al. Diabetes trends in the U.S.: 1990–1998. Diabetes Care. 2000;23(9):1278–83.
13. Zatz R, et al. Prevention of diabetic glomerulopathy by pharmacological amelioration of glomerular capillary hypertension. J Clin Invest. 1986;77(6):1925–30.
14. Lea JP, Nicholas SB. Diabetes mellitus and hypertension: key risk factors for kidney disease. J Natl Med Assoc. 2002;94(8 Suppl):7S–15.
15. Molitch ME, et al. Nephropathy in diabetes. Diabetes Care. 2004;27 Suppl 1:S79–83.
16. Reichard P, Nilsson B-Y, Rosenqvist U. The effect of intensive treatment of diabetes on the development and progression of long-term complications in insulin-dependent diabetes mellitus. The Diabetes Control and Complications Trial Research Group. N Engl J Med. 1993;329(14):977–86.
17. Unnikrishnan AG, et al. Intensive blood-glucose control with sulphonylureas or insulin compared with conventional treatment and risk of complications in patients with type 2 diabetes (UKPDS 33). UK Prospective Diabetes Study (UKPDS) Group. Lancet. 1998;352(9131):837–53.
18. Biesenbach G, et al. Decreased insulin requirement in relation to GFR in nephropathic type 1 and insulin-treated type 2 diabetic patients. Diabet Med. 2003;20(8):642–5.
19. Haneda M, Morikawa A. Which hypoglycaemic agents to use in type 2 diabetic subjects with CKD and how? Nephrol Dial Transplant. 2009; 24(2):338–41.
20. Mani MK. Metformin in renal failure—weigh the evidence. Nephrol Dial Transplant. 2009;24(7):2287–8.
21. Krepinsky J, Ingram AJ, Clase CM. Prolonged sulfonylurea-induced hypoglycemia in diabetic patients with end-stage renal disease. Am J Kidney Dis. 2000;35(3):500–5.
22. KDOQI. KDOQI clinical practice guidelines and clinical practice recommendations for diabetes and chronic kidney disease. Am J Kidney Dis. 2007;49(2 Suppl 2):S12–154.
23. Bakris GL. Slowing nephropathy progression: focus on proteinuria reduction. Clin J Am Soc Nephrol. 2008;3 Suppl 1:S3–10.
24. Retnakaran R, et al. Risk factors for renal dysfunction in type 2 diabetes: U.K. Prospective Diabetes Study 74. Diabetes. 2006;55(6):1832–9.
25. Griffin KA, Bidani AK. Progression of renal disease: renoprotective specificity of renin-angiotensin system blockade. Clin J Am Soc Nephrol. 2006;1(5):1054–65.
26. Berl T. Review: renal protection by inhibition of the renin-angiotensin-aldosterone system. J Renin Angiotensin Aldosterone Syst. 2009;10(1):1–8.
27. Palmer BF. Proteinuria as a therapeutic target in patients with chronic kidney disease. Am J Nephrol. 2007;27(3):287–93.
28. Williams ME. Diabetic nephropathy: the proteinuria hypothesis. Am J Nephrol. 2005;25(2):77–94.
29. de Zeeuw D, et al. Proteinuria, a target for renoprotection in patients with type 2 diabetic nephropathy: lessons from RENAAL. Kidney Int. 2004;65(6):2309–20.
30. de Zeeuw D, et al. Albuminuria, a therapeutic target for cardiovascular protection in type 2 diabetic patients with nephropathy. Circulation. 2004;110(8):921–7.
31. Wright Jr JT, et al. Effect of blood pressure lowering and antihypertensive drug class on progression of hypertensive kidney disease: results from the AASK trial. JAMA. 2002;288(19):2421–31.
32. Esnault VL, et al. Diuretic and enhanced sodium restriction results in improved antiproteinuric response to RAS blocking agents. J Am Soc Nephrol. 2005;16(2):474–81.
33. Bakris GL, et al. Preserving renal function in adults with hypertension and diabetes: a consensus approach. National Kidney Foundation Hypertension and Diabetes Executive Committees Working Group. Am J Kidney Dis. 2000;36(3):646–61.
34. Effect of verapamil on mortality and major events after acute myocardial infarction (the Danish Verapamil Infarction Trial II—DAVIT II). Am J Cardiol. 1990;66(10):779–85.
35. Bakris GL, et al. Calcium channel blockers versus other antihypertensive therapies on progression of NIDDM associated nephropathy. Kidney Int. 1996;50(5):1641–50.
36. Chobanian AV, et al. The Seventh Report of the Joint National Committee on Prevention, Detection, Evaluation, and Treatment of High Blood Pressure: the JNC 7 report. JAMA. 2003;289(19):2560–72.
37. Jamerson K, et al. Benazepril plus amlodipine or hydrochlorothiazide for hypertension in high-risk patients. N Engl J Med. 2008;359(23):2417–28.
38. Bakris GL, et al. Renal outcomes with different fixed-dose combination therapies in patients with hypertension at high risk for cardiovascular events (ACCOMPLISH): a prespecified secondary analysis of a randomised controlled trial. Lancet. 2010;375(9721):1173–81.
39. Astor BC, et al. Association of kidney function with anemia: the Third National Health and Nutrition Examination Survey (1988–1994). Arch Intern Med. 2002;162(12):1401–8.
40. Sabatine MS, et al. Association of hemoglobin levels with clinical outcomes in acute coronary syndromes. Circulation. 2005;111(16):2042–9.
41. Abramson JL, et al. Chronic kidney disease, anemia, and incident stroke in a middle-aged, community-based population: the ARIC Study. Kidney Int. 2003;64(2):610–5.
42. KDOQI. KDOQI clinical practice guideline and clinical practice recommendations for anemia in chronic kidney disease: 2007 update of hemoglobin target. Am J Kidney Dis. 2007;50(3):471–530.
43. Alexander M, et al. Association of anemia correction with health related quality of life in patients not on dialysis. Curr Med Res Opin. 2007;23(12):2997–3008.

44. Lea JP, Norris K, Agodoa L. The role of anemia management in improving outcomes for African-Americans with chronic kidney disease. Am J Nephrol. 2008;28(5):732–43.
45. McCullough PA, Lepor NE. The deadly triangle of anemia, renal insufficiency, and cardiovascular disease: implications for prognosis and treatment. Rev Cardiovasc Med. 2005;6(1):1–10.
46. Silverberg D. Outcomes of anaemia management in renal insufficiency and cardiac disease. Nephrol Dial Transplant. 2003;18 Suppl 2:ii7–12.
47. Lefebvre P, et al. The economic impact of epoetin alfa therapy on delaying time to dialysis in elderly patients with chronic kidney disease. Dis Manag. 2007;10(1):37–45.
48. Jungers P, et al. Beneficial influence of recombinant human erythropoietin therapy on the rate of progression of chronic renal failure in predialysis patients. Nephrol Dial Transplant. 2001;16(2):307–12.
49. Kuriyama S, et al. Reversal of anemia by erythropoietin therapy retards the progression of chronic renal failure, especially in nondiabetic patients. Nephron. 1997;77(2):176–85.
50. Tapolyai M, Kadomatsu S, Perera-Chong M. r.hu-erythropoietin (EPO) treatment of pre-ESRD patients slows the rate of progression of renal decline. BMC Nephrol. 2003;4:3.
51. Gouva C, et al. Treating anemia early in renal failure patients slows the decline of renal function: a randomized controlled trial. Kidney Int. 2004;66(2):753–60.
52. KDOQI, National Kidney Foundation. II. Clinical practice guidelines and clinical practice recommendations for anemia in chronic kidney disease in adults. Am J Kidney Dis. 2006;47(5 Suppl 3):S16–85.
53. Jones M, et al. Impact of epoetin alfa on clinical end points in patients with chronic renal failure: a meta-analysis. Kidney Int. 2004;65(3):757–67.
54. Kalantar-Zadeh K, et al. Metabolic acidosis and malnutrition-inflammation complex syndrome in chronic renal failure. Semin Dial. 2004;17(6):455–65.
55. Dass PD, Kurtz I. Renal ammonia and bicarbonate production in chronic renal failure. Miner Electrolyte Metab. 1990;16(5):308–14.
56. Mitch WE. Metabolic and clinical consequences of metabolic acidosis. J Nephrol. 2006;19 Suppl 9:S70–5.
57. Mitch WE. Influence of metabolic acidosis on nutrition. Am J Kidney Dis. 1997;29(5):xlvi–xlviii.
58. KDOQI, National Kidney Foundation. Clinical practice guidelines for nutrition in chronic kidney disease; 2000 [cited 1 Mar 2011]. http://www.kidney.org/professionals/kdoqi/pdf/KDOQI2000NutritionGL.pdf.
59. de Brito-Ashurst I, et al. Bicarbonate supplementation slows progression of CKD and improves nutritional status. J Am Soc Nephrol. 2009;20(9):2075–84.
60. Venkat KK. Proteinuria and microalbuminuria in adults: significance, evaluation, and treatment. South Med J. 2004;97(10):969–79.
61. Lea J, et al. The relationship between magnitude of proteinuria reduction and risk of end-stage renal disease: results of the African American study of kidney disease and hypertension. Arch Intern Med. 2005;165(8):947–53.
62. Schmieder RE, et al. Low-grade albuminuria and cardiovascular risk: what is the evidence? Clin Res Cardiol. 2007;96(5):247–57.
63. Arnlov J, et al. Low-grade albuminuria and incidence of cardiovascular disease events in nonhypertensive and nondiabetic individuals: the Framingham Heart Study. Circulation. 2005;112(7):969–75.
64. Lewis EJ, et al. Renoprotective effect of the angiotensin-receptor antagonist irbesartan in patients with nephropathy due to type 2 diabetes. N Engl J Med. 2001;345(12):851–60.
65. Brewster UC, Perazella MA. The renin-angiotensin-aldosterone system and the kidney: effects on kidney disease. Am J Med. 2004;116(4):263–72.
66. Ruggenenti P, et al. Preventing microalbuminuria in type 2 diabetes. N Engl J Med. 2004;351(19):1941–51.
67. Ruggenenti P, et al. Impact of blood pressure control and angiotensin-converting enzyme inhibitor therapy on new-onset microalbuminuria in type 2 diabetes: a post hoc analysis of the BENEDICT trial. J Am Soc Nephrol. 2006;17(12):3472–81.
68. Maschio G, et al. Angiotensin-converting enzyme inhibitors and kidney protection: the AIPRI trial. The ACE Inhibition in Progressive Renal Insufficiency (AIPRI) Study Group. J Cardiovasc Pharmacol. 1999;33 Suppl 1:S16–20. discussion S41–3.
69. Haller H, et al. Olmesartan for the delay or prevention of microalbuminuria in type 2 diabetes. N Engl J Med. 2010;364(10):907–17.
70. Flegal KM, et al. Prevalence and trends in obesity among US adults, 1999–2008. JAMA. 2010;303(3):235–41.
71. Malnick SD, Knobler H. The medical complications of obesity. QJM. 2006;99(9):565–79.
72. Flegal KM, et al. Cause-specific excess deaths associated with underweight, overweight, and obesity. JAMA. 2007;298(17):2028–37.
73. Tozawa M, et al. Influence of smoking and obesity on the development of proteinuria. Kidney Int. 2002;62(3):956–62.
74. Pinto-Sietsma SJ, et al. A central body fat distribution is related to renal function impairment, even in lean subjects. Am J Kidney Dis. 2003;41(4):733–41.
75. Praga M, et al. Effects of body-weight loss and captopril treatment on proteinuria associated with obesity. Nephron. 1995;70(1):35–41.
76. Diez JJ, Iglesias P. The role of the novel adipocyte-derived hormone adiponectin in human disease. Eur J Endocrinol. 2003;148(3):293–300.
77. Kollerits B, et al. Gender-specific association of adiponectin as a predictor of progression of chronic kidney disease: the Mild to Moderate Kidney Disease Study. Kidney Int. 2007;71(12):1279–86.
78. Jorsal A, et al. Serum adiponectin predicts all-cause mortality and end stage renal disease in patients with type I diabetes and diabetic nephropathy. Kidney Int. 2008;74(5):649–54.
79. Ejerblad E, et al. Association between smoking and chronic renal failure in a nationwide population-based

case-control study. J Am Soc Nephrol. 2004;15(8): 2178–85.
80. Orth SR. Smoking—a renal risk factor. Nephron. 2000;86(1):12–26.
81. Regalado M, Yang S, Wesson DE. Cigarette smoking is associated with augmented progression of renal insufficiency in severe essential hypertension. Am J Kidney Dis. 2000;35(4):687–94.
82. Orth SR. Effects of smoking on systemic and intrarenal hemodynamics: influence on renal function. J Am Soc Nephrol. 2004;15 Suppl 1:S58–63.
83. Orth SR, Hallan SI. Smoking: a risk factor for progression of chronic kidney disease and for cardiovascular morbidity and mortality in renal patients—absence of evidence or evidence of absence? Clin J Am Soc Nephrol. 2008;3(1):226–36.
84. Hobbs SD, Bradbury AW. Smoking cessation strategies in patients with peripheral arterial disease: an evidence-based approach. Eur J Vasc Endovasc Surg. 2003;26(4):341–7.
85. Molander L, et al. Pharmacokinetics of nicotine in kidney failure. Clin Pharmacol Ther. 2000;68(3):250–60.
86. Weiner DE, et al. Uric acid and incident kidney disease in the community. J Am Soc Nephrol. 2008;19(6): 1204–11.
87. Obermayr RP, et al. Predictors of new-onset decline in kidney function in a general middle-European population. Nephrol Dial Transplant. 2008;23(4):1265–73.
88. Sturm G, et al. Uric acid as a risk factor for progression of non-diabetic chronic kidney disease? The Mild to Moderate Kidney Disease (MMKD) Study. Exp Gerontol. 2008;43(4):347–52.
89. Siu YP, et al. Use of allopurinol in slowing the progression of renal disease through its ability to lower serum uric acid level. Am J Kidney Dis. 2006;47(1): 51–9.
90. Moorhead JF, et al. Lipid nephrotoxicity in chronic progressive glomerular and tubulo-interstitial disease. Lancet. 1982;2(8311):1309–11.
91. Lewis D, Haynes R, Landray MJ. Lipids in chronic kidney disease. J Ren Care. 2010;36 Suppl 1:27–33.
92. Muntner P, et al. Plasma lipids and risk of developing renal dysfunction: the atherosclerosis risk in communities study. Kidney Int. 2000;58(1):293–301.
93. Fox CS, et al. Predictors of new-onset kidney disease in a community-based population. JAMA. 2004; 291(7):844–50.
94. Hunsicker LG, et al. Predictors of the progression of renal disease in the Modification of Diet in Renal Disease Study. Kidney Int. 1997;51(6):1908–19.
95. Joles JA, et al. Early mechanisms of renal injury in hypercholesterolemic or hypertriglyceridemic rats. J Am Soc Nephrol. 2000;11(4):669–83.
96. Weiner DE, et al. Chronic kidney disease as a risk factor for cardiovascular disease and all-cause mortality: a pooled analysis of community-based studies. J Am Soc Nephrol. 2004;15(5):1307–15.
97. Lewington S, et al. Blood cholesterol and vascular mortality by age, sex, and blood pressure: a meta-analysis of individual data from 61 prospective studies with 55,000 vascular deaths. Lancet. 2007;370(9602):1829–39.
98. Tsimihodimos V, Dounousi E, Siamopoulos KC. Dyslipidemia in chronic kidney disease: an approach to pathogenesis and treatment. Am J Nephrol. 2008;28(6):958–73.
99. Vaziri ND, Wang XQ, Liang K. Secondary hyperparathyroidism downregulates lipoprotein lipase expression in chronic renal failure. Am J Physiol. 1997;273(6 Pt 2):F925–30.
100. Vaziri ND, Moradi H. Mechanisms of dyslipidemia of chronic renal failure. Hemodial Int. 2006;10(1):1–7.
101. Vaziri ND. Dyslipidemia of chronic renal failure: the nature, mechanisms, and potential consequences. Am J Physiol Renal Physiol. 2006;290(2):F262–72.
102. Deighan CJ, et al. Atherogenic lipoprotein phenotype in end-stage renal failure: origin and extent of small dense low-density lipoprotein formation. Am J Kidney Dis. 2000;35(5):852–62.
103. Baigent C, et al. Efficacy and safety of cholesterol-lowering treatment: prospective meta-analysis of data from 90,056 participants in 14 randomised trials of statins. Lancet. 2005;366(9493):1267–78.
104. Lemos PA, et al. Long-term fluvastatin reduces the hazardous effect of renal impairment on four-year atherosclerotic outcomes (a LIPS substudy). Am J Cardiol. 2005;95(4):445–51.
105. Tonelli M, et al. Pravastatin for secondary prevention of cardiovascular events in persons with mild chronic renal insufficiency. Ann Intern Med. 2003;138(2):98–104.
106. Tonelli M, et al. Effect of pravastatin on cardiovascular events in people with chronic kidney disease. Circulation. 2004;110(12):1557–63.
107. Holdaas H, et al. The effect of fluvastatin on cardiac outcomes in patients with moderate to severe renal insufficiency: a pooled analysis of double-blind, randomized trials. Int J Cardiol. 2007;117(1):64–74.
108. Bianchi S, et al. A controlled, prospective study of the effects of atorvastatin on proteinuria and progression of kidney disease. Am J Kidney Dis. 2003;41(3):565–70.
109. National Kidney Foundation. KDOQI clinical practice guidelines for managing dyslipidemias in chronic kidney disease. Am J Kidney Dis. 2003;41 suppl 3:S1–92.
110. Landray M, et al. The second United Kingdom Heart and Renal Protection (UK-HARP-II) Study: a randomized controlled study of the biochemical safety and efficacy of adding ezetimibe to simvastatin as initial therapy among patients with CKD. Am J Kidney Dis. 2006;47(3):385–95.
111. The SHARP Collaborative Group. LB-FC6. Presented at: Renal Week 2010. Denver, CO; 16–21 Nov 2010.
112. Molitch ME. Management of dyslipidemias in patients with diabetes and chronic kidney disease. Clin J Am Soc Nephrol. 2006;1(5):1090–9.
113. Brown WV. Expert commentary: the safety of fibrates in lipid-lowering therapy. Am J Cardiol. 2007;99(6A):19C–21.

27 Nutrition

Sejal P. Sarolia and Harold A. Franch

Case 1

Mr. N is a 54-year-old man with a history of hypertension, coronary disease, peripheral vascular disease, gout, dyslipidemia, and chronic kidney disease (CKD) Stage III (MDRD eGFR 35 mL/min) who presents with a 10 kg weight gain over the last 2 months. The patient reports that he has not been very compliant with his diet or exercise program. Gout attacks have been frequent. Physical exam: Height 5′9″; Weight 97 kg, 213 lb; BMI 31. The patient has 7 cm JVD at 30° and 1+ bilateral lower extremity edema. The exam is otherwise unremarkable. Significant labs: creatinine 2.3 mg/dL, triglycerides: 346 mg/dL, serum bicarbonate: 19 mEq/L, potassium: 5.7 mEq/L, phosphorus: 5.5 mg/dL, and PTH: 220 pg/dL. Despite the presence of volume overload, his blood urea nitrogen (BUN) to Cr ratio is 20:1. The patient also has proteinuria (albumin to creatinine ratio: 830 μg/mg).

How does his diet influence his presentation? What dietary instructions should be given to him?

Case 2

Mr. N, now a 59-year-old gentleman with CKD Stage IV (MDRD eGFR 19 ml/min), presents to you complaining of progressive weakness. He was hospitalized 3 months ago for osteomyelitis and is undergoing physical therapy. The patient is a thin gentleman with a 30 kg weight loss in the last year with 20 kg of that loss occurring since his hospitalization (now 67 kg; 147 lb with BMI 22). He is now noticeably frail. He reports that he has been compliant with his renal diet; however, he does not seem to have any energy. On exam, he has no edema, rub, or asterixis, but has a non-healing wound on his right second toe. He has temporal muscle wasting; his tricep skin fold is loose, and his midarm muscle circumference is 5% less than 3 months ago. Labs show no change in serum creatinine, but the BUN to creatinine ratio has decreased to 5:1, total cholesterol is 87 mg/dL (high-density lipoprotein (HDL) 23 mg/dL), and he has a mild metabolic acidosis (bicarbonate 20 mEq/L) following discontinuation of sodium bicarbonate in the hospital. His serum albumin is 2.7 mg/dL. A 24 h urine urea nitrogen is 3.1 g.

S.P. Sarolia, M.D. (✉)
14615 Lindale Rose Lane, Humble, TX 77396, USA
e-mail: ssarolia@emory.edu

H.A. Franch, M.D.
Renal Division, Atlanta Veterans Affairs Medical Center and Emory University School of Medicine, Decatur, GA 30033, USA

E.V. Lerma and M. Rosner (eds.), *Clinical Decisions in Nephrology, Hypertension and Kidney Transplantation*,
DOI 10.1007/978-1-4614-4454-1_27,

What type of nutritional process is responsible for his loss of muscle mass? How do you determine adequate protein and calorie nutrition?

Introduction

Because the kidney excretes salts and metabolites derived from the diet, nutrition has a central role in the management of all stages of CKD. Dietary changes affect not only the progression of CKD but also mortality and comorbidities, especially cardiovascular disease. As renal function declines, retention of sodium, phosphorous, and nitrogenous waste products, along with decreased compensation for dietary electrolytes and water intake, leads to complications. More recently, it has become clear that development of insulin resistance and inefficient energy utilization, abnormal lipid metabolism, failure to activate vitamin D, hormonal changes, and muscle wasting contribute to increased cardiovascular mortality. Over-consumption of food (the 54-year-old Mr. N) can lead to obesity, gout, metabolic syndrome, diabetes, hypertension, dyslipidemia, and excess protein intake that are associated with HTN, increased proteinuria, disability, CVD risk, and a more rapid decline in glomerular filtration rate. When comorbidities are present, under consumption of food (Mr. N at 59) is now recognized as equally dangerous in CKD, particularly in end-stage renal disease. Protein energy wasting (PEW) as manifested by loss of body weight and muscle mass, inflammation, and low serum albumin is highly associated with cardiovascular death. Thus, PEW is considered a nontraditional risk factor for cardiovascular events.

Whether the patient has pre-dialysis CKD, currently undergoing renal replacement therapy, or has received a kidney transplant, timely and appropriate nutritional intervention can optimize patient care and outcomes [1]. Nutritional counseling is essential in CKD and is covered by the US Medicare program for CKD stage 3 and greater. The most important step in nutritional management remains recognition that a patient has CKD [2]. Studies suggest that early knowledge of CKD leads to management changes (including diet) that improve the rate of loss of kidney function, survival, and transplant rates.

Assessment of Nutritional Status

Evaluation of nutritional status should be used to determine protein and caloric intake and to diagnosis PEW. Longitudinal evaluation over 6 months to a year is superior to a single assessment. Table 27.1 summarizes some of the methods used for assessing nutritional status. Excess intake of protein and calories and consumption of electrolytes and minerals can be estimated based

Table 27.1 Nutritional assessment methods for screening

Type	Factor (desirable values)
Food intake	Dietary history (protein intake/calorie intake at goal)[a]
	24 h urine urea (calculated protein intake at goal)[b]
	Calculated nPCR from dialysis data (calculated protein intake at goal)[b]
Biochemical	Serum albumin (≥3.8)[b]
	CRP (normal range for lab for CKD 1–4)[b]
	HDL cholesterol (>40 with total cholesterol >100)[b]
	Non-HDL cholesterol (<130)[b]
	Triglycerides (normal range for lab)[b]
Body weight	BMI (20–25 for CKD 1–4, >23 for CKD 5, ESRD)
	Change in body weight (no unintentional weight loss <5% of body weight)
Body composition	Bioelectrical impedance
	Ultrasonography
	Dual-energy X-ray absorptiometry
	Grip strength
	Skin fold thickness[b]
	Midarm muscle circumference[b]
Other useful clues	Activities of daily living[b]
	Dentition[b]
	Behavioral (psychological or cognitive impairment)[b]
	Comorbid conditions (see Table 27.3)[b]

[a]Easily performed with nutrition consult
[b]Easily performed in primary care office or in dialysis unit

on dietary history and following trends in BUN, phosphorus, and potassium levels. Additionally, protein consumption can be estimated using a 24-h urine collection. Estimated protein intake (g protein/kg/day) = 6.25 × [UUN + (0.031 × weigh t in kg)], where UUN is urine urea nitrogen excretion in grams of nitrogen per kilogram per day. The same formula can be used to estimate non-dialysis clearance from residual kidney function [1]. Biophysical assessment from anthropometric measurements (BMI), in addition to waist circumference or waste to hip ratio, can be used as markers of the metabolic syndrome. Worsening microalbuminuria suggests excess protein intake. Total body sodium is estimated from volume status on physical exam. Elevated low-density lipoprotein (LDL), triglycerides, non-HDL cholesterol, CRP, and fasting blood glucose are used to further estimate metabolic syndrome and CVD risk.

To assess for PEW, estimation of dietary protein and calorie intake by history and urinary urea nitrogen is extremely useful. Unintentional weight loss and/or low BMI are powerful predictors of CV mortality in the presence of advanced CKD and its comorbidities. Declines in the BUN, serum phosphate and potassium, and cholesterol suggest PEW. Physical exam demonstrates muscle wasting and volume depletion. Measurement of skin fold thickness and midarm muscle circumference, which are low in PEW, provides quantitative assessments of nutritional status. Lastly, serum proteins are extremely important index of nutritional status. In many studies, a low serum albumin is the best single predictor of cardiovascular risk, but serial measurements of albumin are much more useful than a single level, as illness, transient inflammatory state, or volume overload (diluting albumin) may confound results. Radiological evaluation and bioimpedance can aid in determining the level of nutritional pathology, but these techniques are often restricted to research centers and are not needed when the other markers of PEW are present. In general, a low albumin or a high CRP combined with markers of body mass, protein intake, or muscle mass predicts mortality much more strongly than single markers alone.

Nutrients

Specific dietary parameters for each stage of CKD are listed in Table 27.2. Because of individual differences in dietary habits, underlying comorbidities, and baseline nutritional status the recommendations should be tailored to each patient.

Calories

In the general population obesity is associated with higher levels of cardiovascular mortality and in CKD patients with higher levels of proteinuria and disease progression. In the absence of comorbidities associated with PEW, overall caloric balance is maintained to prevent obesity. However, in a patient with multiple comorbidities, a higher BMI is associated with increased survival [3]. Although the data on causality are not clear, it appears that the greater muscle mass associated with a higher BMI is protective against the development of PEW. Thus, there are concerns that caloric restriction may lead to PEW. At all stages of CKD, there are concerns that a strict calorie reduction will lead to an intolerance of a protein restriction.

In the absence of PEW, obtaining a normal weight in pre-dialysis CKD appears highly desirable. Intentional weight loss by diet and exercise programs appears to be as safe and effective in pre-dialysis CKD as in the general population and reduces proteinuria and rate of loss of renal function in short-term studies [4, 5]. Rapid weight loss by diet alone, without exercise, should be avoided to conserve muscle mass and the protein content of the diet has to be raised during weight loss to protect muscle mass. Bariatric surgery seems to have similar short-term benefits in individuals with obesity-related proteinuria, but may carry long-term nutritional problems [5]. In ESRD, reduced calorie, but not protein, diets combined with exercise can be used to lose weight as needed prior to transplant [4]. Long-term outcomes and incidence of PEW are not known.

Table 27.2 Dietary recommendations for chronic kidney disease

Factor	Normal renal function	CKD stages 1–2	CKD stages 3–5	Hemodialysis	Peritoneal dialysis	Transplant
Protein (g/kg/IBW/day) (atleast 50% high biological value)	0.8–1.4	0.6–1.0 (depends on dietary supervision and comorbidities)	0.6–1.0 (depends on dietary supervision and comorbidities)	1.0–1.2	1.2–1.4	1.3–1.5 initial 1.0 for maintenance
Energy (kcal/kg)	To maintain a healthy weight	To maintain a healthy weight	35 (<60 year) 30–35 (>60 year)	35 (<60 year) 30–35 (>60 year)	35 (<60 year including dialysate calories) 30–35 (>60 year including dialysate calories)	30–35 initial 25–30 for maintenance
Fat	Fat content of the diet may vary as long as polyunsaturated and monounsaturated fats predominate. Adequate omega 3 fatty acid should be consumed					
	Less than 10% of energy as saturated fat, <1% of energy as *trans* fat. Except in patients with PEW, consume <300 mg cholesterol/day					
Sodium (mg/day)	1,500–4,000 (depending on BP and sweat losses)	1,500–2,000	2,000	2,000	2,000	5,000–6,000
Potassium (mg/day)	Unrestricted	Unrestricted	Reduce if hyperkalemic	2,000–3,000	Unrestricted	Reduce if hyperkalemic
Calcium (mg/day)	1,000–1,500	1,000–1,500	Not to exceed 2,000	Not to exceed 2,000	Not to exceed 2,000	1,200
Phosphorus	Unrestricted	Unrestricted	Reduce, level dependent	Reduce, level dependent	Reduce, level dependent	Unrestricted (reduce if advanced stage)
Fluid (mL/day)	Unrestricted	Unrestricted	Reduce if hyponatremic	2,000	2,000	Unrestricted

Data from sources: [1, 10, 13, 19, 21, 32]

In stages 4 and 5 CKD and in ESRD, patients tend to lose muscle mass over time making them vulnerable to PEW. Basal metabolic rate is increased in advanced CKD, and caloric requirements increase. Adequate calorie intake is considered essential for preventing PEW by making protein metabolism more efficient. However, calorie intake can be excessive, particularly in peritoneal dialysis patients. Exercise and carefully designed diets may be required. Similarly, the glucocorticoids used in transplantation often lead to overeating, so calorie restriction is frequently required.

Protein

Providing adequate, but not excessive dietary protein has been the cornerstone of all renal diets. Protein in excess of daily requirements is degraded to urea, other nitrogenous waste, acid, and sulfates. In addition, protein rich foods are also rich in phosphate and purines, the uric acid precursor. These waste products accumulate in patients with uremia, leading to muscle catabolism, bone loss, gout, and vascular calcification. Protein restriction slows the progression of CKD and minimizes bone loss and gout [6, 7]. Diets with a protein goal of 0.8 g protein/kg/day can reduce renal death in patients with CKD, particularly if the GFR is more than 15 mL/min. Since mortality was included as an end point in these studies, good patient survival suggests that such diets also meet nutritional requirements [8]. Studies in humans indicate that glomerular hyperfiltration, a cause of glomerular damage, can be induced by diets high in animal protein, whereas complete vegetable protein has less of an adverse effect [9]. Dietary Approaches to Stop Hypertension (DASH) or American Diabetes Association (ADA) style diets, which contain ample sources of vegetable protein, are frequently recommended for CKD stages 1 and 2.

The use of low protein diets is limited by difficulty with compliance and the need to assure safe levels of protein intake [10, 11]. Dietitian involvement is mandatory: Even in randomized trials, patients typically consume 0.1–0.2 g/kg/day more protein than prescribed. Although lower protein diets have been used experimentally, diets below 0.6 g protein/kg/day (with frequent dietitian supervision) or 0.75 g/kg/day (without frequent supervision) are not recommended in CKD patients. In patients with PEW or who have significant comorbidities that are frequently associated with PEW (see Table 27.3), low protein diets are not tolerated and 0.9–1.0 g/kg/day protein is required. Inflammation, acidosis, and glucocorticoids prevent the adaptations needed to use dietary protein efficiently. Similarly, acutely ill CKD patients need a more liberalized protein intake until they recover.

Hemodialysis and peritoneal dialysis cause inflammation and the loss of amino acids. In hemodialysis patients, the recommended dietary protein intake is 1.0–1.2 g/kg IBW/day; whereas

Table 27.3 Common comorbid conditions causing protein energy wasting

Factor	Causative etiology
Chronic illness	Underlying disease
	– Diabetes mellitus
	– COPD
	– Congestive heart failure
	– SLE
	– Malignancy
Anorexia	Uremic toxins
	Mechanical
	– Dentition
	– Ambulation
	Financial
Acute illness	Superimposed illness
Maintenance dialysis	Nutrient loss
Medical therapy	Medications
	Radiation
	Surgery
Blood loss	GI bleed
	Phlebotomy
Gastrointestinal-renal disorders	ESRD related GI disorders
	Transplant associated GI illness
	CKD related symptoms
	GI-renal systemic illness

Modified from Kopple JD. Pathophysiology of protein-energy wasting in chronic renal failure. J Nutr. 1999;129(1S Suppl):247S–51S in peritoneal dialysis (where the patient loses albumin as well), it is 1.2–1.4 g/kg IBW/day. In both cases, 50% of the protein should be of high biological value. Transplant patients need a liberalized protein diet immediately after surgery. Subsequently, protein intake is determined by renal function and is slightly higher than a non-transplant patient because steroids are a usual part of immunosuppressive regimen. Although diets must be individualized, protein intake should be kept above 0.8 g/kg IBW/day protein.

Carbohydrates

In patients with CKD, carbohydrate metabolism is impaired, leading to glucose intolerance, insulin resistance, and impaired insulin secretion [1]. Resistance to the action of insulin and its decreased sensitivity occurs primarily in skeletal muscle. These effects are somewhat offset by the longer half-life of insulin due to decreased renal catabolism of insulin. The increased half-life can lead to hypoglycemic episodes in diabetics on insulin or oral hypoglycemic agents.

Generally, an ample intake of carbohydrates is needed in CKD to provide sufficient caloric intake when protein is restricted. A diet moderate to rich (depending on caloric needs) in complex carbohydrates is advised to minimize insulin resistance. In stages 1–2 CKD, complex carbohydrates can easily make up the bulk of carbohydrates. However, the phosphorous and potassium content of legumes, whole grains, fruit, and starchy vegetables will gradually lead to a restriction of these sources of complex carbohydrates in CKD 3–5 and hemodialysis leaving a preponderance of simple starch. Among the less complex carbohydrates, added sugars (sucrose and high fructose corn syrup) create an additional concern: their high fructose content predisposes to hypertriglyceridemia (especially in obese individuals), insulin resistance, and increased uric acid production. In patients with PEW simple sugars are useful to provide calories, but promote obesity and can cause hyperglycemia due to insulin resistance. Little is known about the safety of artificial sweeteners in CKD.

Lipids

The risk of cardiovascular events and mortality increases as renal function declines although the relative risk of mortality contributed by the standard Framingham risk factors declines as renal function falls. LDL cholesterol does not predict mortality as well as low HDL, cholesterol, and triglycerides in patients with CKD 5 and ESRD [12]. Thus in stages 1–3 of CKD, lipids are managed just as they are in general population with similar dietary advice. This would include choosing polyunsaturated and monounsaturated fats, ample omega 3 fatty acids, <10% of calories from saturated fat, with approximately 250–300 mg cholesterol/day restriction [13]. Although there is no evidence of effectiveness, the latter two restrictions are sometimes lifted in patients with PEW. In stages 4 and 5 of CKD and dialysis patients, current data support a modest increase in dietary fat intake, especially the healthy fats mentioned above, to compensate for reduced energy intake in protein-restricted diets and to minimize the use of simple carbohydrates. However, patients who are obese should be encouraged to lose weight while maintaining or, preferably, increasing muscle mass [14]. Statins, while effective in the early stages of CKD, do not appear to reduce cardiovascular mortality from PEW.

Minerals and Electrolytes

Phosphorous/Calcium/Vitamin D

While this area is covered in the separate chapter 24 on calcium/phosphorous metabolism, it is worth noting that retention of phosphorous is inversely dependent on GFR, but directly related to dietary consumption. Elevated serum phosphorus levels are associated with the risk of developing CKD and ESRD in the general population, increased mortality in the CKD population, metabolic bone disease, and vascular calcification [15]. Numerous studies have shown that reducing protein, particularly foods such as dairy and legumes, reduces dietary phosphorus and serum phosphorous levels in CKD stages 4 and 5 [16]. Dietary phosphorus should be restricted to 800–1,000 mg/

day (adjusted for dietary protein needs) when the serum phosphorus levels are elevated (>4.6 mg/dL [1.49 mmol/L]) in stages 3 and 4 of CKD and >5.5 mg/dL (1.78 mmol/L) in those with kidney failure (stage 5). Processed foods, especially colas, baking powder, and cured meat, may contain large amounts of phosphorus. To allow adequate protein intake, oral phosphate binders (calcium, lanthanum, and polymers) are taken with meals to lower gut absorption of phosphorus [13].

The total daily intake of elemental calcium (dietary plus calcium phosphate binders) in CKD patients should not exceed 2,000 mg/day and may need to be lower in patients treated with high dose activated vitamin D analogs [17, 18].

Sodium

Sodium excretion is directly proportional to GFR in CKD except in rare cases of tubular dysfunction. Thus, reducing dietary sodium or using diuretics is necessary in almost all CKD patients in order to control hypertension or volume overload. However, most dietary sodium is added in the processing of food. To reduce salt intake, intake of processed foods must be reduced. This can be difficult in Western societies [19]. In the USA, the sodium content of food is reported in milligrams. By reading food labels, patients can adhere to the recommended dietary sodium restriction of 2,000 mg/day [20, 21]. Foods that are high in sodium, protein, phosphate, and saturated fat such as cured meats are best avoided altogether, and thus, low protein and phosphorous diets tend to be lower in sodium. Transplanted kidneys may show some sodium wasting during the first year, and low sodium diets are generally avoided until the renal function has stabilized.

Potassium

In the presence of normal renal and adrenal function, it is difficult to ingest enough potassium (K^+) to become hyperkalemic. Dietary intake only contributes to hyperkalemia when there is impaired kidney function. Potassium excretion does not decline linearly with GFR, but rather depends on sodium intake, alkalosis, and adrenal and distal tubular function. In the presence of a type 4 RTA or in advanced renal disease (stages 4 or 5), dietary potassium restriction is often required. Restricting dietary potassium is not without cost. A high potassium diet helps excrete sodium and lower blood pressure; potassium rich vegetables contain compounds that lower oxidative stress and reduce cancer risk.

On the other hand, spontaneous decreases in potassium intake that lower serum K^+ below 4.0 mmol/L in ESRD predict increased mortality, because they may mark decreased food intake and the onset of PEW. Recent evidence shows that the levels of serum K^+ that are associated with lowest risk for mortality are between 4.1 and 5.5 mmol/L. Maintaining serum K^+ in this range may optimize survival in patients with CKD [22, 23]. Empiric potassium restriction should not be implemented in CKD patients unless indicated. In peritoneal dialysis, patients are usually hypokalemic and a potassium rich diet is emphasized. No restrictions are placed on transplant patient unless a type 4 RTA is present. In hemodialysis patients, potassium is restricted to 2,000–3,000 mg/day.

Magnesium

Other than iatrogenic administration, sustained hypermagnesemia only occurs in end-stage kidney disease. Fortunately dietary potassium restriction reduces magnesium intake while magnesium containing laxatives should be avoided in advanced CKD. CKD patients generally have high normal levels of magnesium unless PEW is present and food intake is low. Low magnesium levels in PEW may increase the risk of cardiac complications, but no adequately powered study confirms the benefit of raising magnesium levels in these patients [24].

Trace Elements

Trace elements are generally retained in CKD, but are variably cleared by dialysis. However, zinc deficiency is prevalent in CKD and ESRD patients either from inanition or from removal during the dialysis process [25]. Furthermore, zinc deficiency is common in human inflammatory disease, such as PEW. Unfortunately, plasma levels of zinc do not reliably identify individuals with zinc deficiency. Erythrocyte concentrations of zinc may provide a more useful measure of zinc status during acute or chronic inflammation [26]. Zinc supplements may be used to meet daily recommendations if zinc rich diets (nuts, lentils, and whole grains) are not tolerated due to potassium or phosphorous content. Chronic dialysis patients have significantly lower concentrations of selenium and manganese, but a significantly higher concentration of nickel. Copper levels do not change [27].

Vitamins

Vitamins may be retained with loss of renal function, removed by dialysis, or deficient in restricted diets or from increased demand due to altered metabolism. Vitamins A (on a binding protein) and vitamin C are renally excreted; excessive supplementation may cause toxicity in advanced CKD and ESRD. Because vitamin C is cleared by dialysis, supplementation at 100 mg/day is required. All B vitamins are cleared by dialysis and must be supplemented. Moreover, the requirements for certain B vitamins, especially folic acid, are increased under inflammatory conditions in advanced CKD. Although Vitamin E supplementation is not toxic, benefits remain unproven in ESRD patients. Most renal vitamins contain only B vitamins, vitamin C, and folic acid and can be used in both advanced stage CKD and ESRD, but multivitamins low in A and rich in folate (such as prenatal vitamins) may be used as a substitute [28]. In dialysis patients, there is a strong positive effect on survival associated with vitamin usage [28, 29].

Vitamin D is activated by 1 hydroxylation in the kidney and active vitamin D levels are low in most patients with stage 3 CKD and below. These low levels contribute to hyperparathyroidism. Supplementation to a 25 vitamin D level of 30 or above may be helpful to control PTH in stage 3 CKD, but active vitamin D is required in most patients starting from the later stages of CKD to ESRD (see chapter 24 on bone).

Treatment of Protein Energy Wasting

As discussed above, PEW is characterized by corporal losses of protein and fat stores associated with an increase in cardiovascular mortality. Protein or energy depletion can result from an inadequate diet (for example, anorexia nervosa), but in kidney disease, there are usually conditions resulting in loss of lean body mass not related to reduced nutrient intake. Stressors initiating this cascade of nutritional decline include comorbidities (see Table 27.3), nonspecific inflammatory processes (inflammation from dialysis, dialysis catheters); transient, intercurrent catabolic illnesses; nutrient losses during dialysis; acidemia; and endocrine disorders (especially high glucocorticoids and hyperparathyroidism) [3]. Patients with PEW should be carefully examined for undiagnosed comorbidities and known comorbidities should be intensively treated. Nutritional intervention and dietary supplements are often needed to assure adequate protein and calorie intake until the underlying disorder is diagnosed and corrected. In some patients the cause is elusive; nutrition may be therapeutic. The anorexia of CKD is further compounded by underlying illness, taste abnormalities, loss of dentures, gastropathy, enteropathy, medications, psychosocial conditions, aging, and HD-related factors [30]. In addition to managing these underlying factors, aggressive nutritional counseling has helped in ESRD patients in improving nutritional status [31]. No appetite stimulant has been shown to be both safe and effective [30]. Randomized trials show that megesterol acetate increases appetite in ESRD patients, but severe side effects and continued loss of muscle mass make this therapy unattractive. Physical therapy or exercise programs help relieve debility and allow muscle to recover. In patients with CKD, a restricted diet can be resumed, once the patient's nutritional status improves [8].

Conclusion

Nutrition is an important aspect of the overall care of kidney patients and is an important indicator of mortality. Appropriate counseling, dietary restrictions, nutritional supplementations, and monitoring for nutritional pathology can assist in delaying CKD progression and improving mortality.

Mr. N at 54 has excessive protein, calorie, potassium, sodium and phosphorous intake, causing weight gain, gout, metabolic acidosis, hyperlipidemia, and hyperkalemia. His lipid profile suggests that he consumes excessive amounts of saturated fats and simple carbohydrates. Nutritional counseling is indicated. The choice between a 0.6 and 0.75 g/kg protein restriction will depend on his willingness, reliability, and availability of regular dietary supervision. Dietary potassium and possibly sodium and phosphorous may need to be restricted beyond that achieved with protein restriction. He may also need sodium bicarbonate for acidosis and a phosphorous binder. He needs to consume more polyunsaturated fats and omega 3 fatty acids.

Mr. N, at 59, is suffering from PEW which is probably related to his recent illness, but osteomyelitis must be investigated. His estimated protein intake, using the urine urea nitrogen, is approximately 0.47 g/kg and his low potassium and cholesterol suggest low calorie intake. A careful history of his eating habits may reveal dysphagia, depression, or an unfortunate change in his social situation. CKD related anorexia (esp. since the MDRD prediction equation may underestimate GFR in wasted individuals) must also be considered. He will need to increase his protein (1.0 g/kg/day) and calorie intake (>30 kcal/kg) as part of a liberalized diet with or without supplements to improve his lean muscle mass. Sodium bicarbonate therapy for acidosis is indicated. The increased nutrition may require adjustment of his phosphate binder and his potassium will have to be monitored closely. He may need physical therapy to help with his frailty to reduce the risk of falls. A protein-restricted diet may be resumed after comorbidities improve and he regains weight, normalizes his albumin, and returns to his baseline functional status.

References

1. Bailey JL, Franch H. Nutritional considerations in kidney disease: core curriculum 2010. Am J Kidney Dis. 2010;55(6):1146–61.
2. Saab G, Whaley-Connell AT, McCullough PA, Bakris GL. CKD awareness in the United States: the kidney early evaluation. Program (KEEP). Am J Kidney Dis. 2008;52:382–3.
3. Fouque D, Kalantar-Zadeh K, Kopple J, et al. A proposed nomenclature and diagnostic criteria for protein-energy wasting in acute and chronic kidney disease. Kidney Int. 2008;73(4):391–8.
4. Teta D. Weight loss in obese patients with chronic kidney disease: who and how? J Ren Care. 2010;36 Suppl 1:163–71.
5. Navaneethan SD, Yehnert H, Moustarah F, Schreiber MJ, Schauer PR, Beddhu S. Weight loss interventions in chronic kidney disease: a systematic review and meta-analysis. Clin J Am Soc Nephrol. 2009;4(10):1565–74.
6. Chanutin A, Ferris EB. Experimental renal insufficiency produced by partial nephrectomy I. Control diet. Arch Intern Med. 1932;49:767–87.
7. Chanutin A, Ludewig S. Experimental renal insufficiency produced by partial nephrectomy. V. Diets containing whole dried meat. Arch Intern Med. 1936;58:60–80.
8. Franch HA, Mitch WE. Navigating between the Scylla and Charybdis of prescribing dietary protein for chronic kidney diseases. Annu Rev Nutr. 2009;29:341–64.
9. Kontessis P, Jones S, Dodds R, et al. Renal, metabolic and hormonal responses to ingestion of animal and vegetable proteins. Kidney Int. 1990;38:136.
10. Kopple JD. National kidney foundation K/DOQI clinical practice guidelines for nutrition in chronic renal failure. Am J Kidney Dis. 2001;37(1 Suppl 2): S66–70.
11. Kopple JD. Pathophysiology of protein-energy wasting in chronic renal failure. J Nutr. 1999;129(1S Suppl):247–51.
12. Kaysen GA. Lipid and lipoprotein metabolism in chronic kidney disease. J Ren Nutr. 2009;19(1):73–7.
13. Beto JA, Bansal VK. Medical nutrition therapy in chronic kidney failure: integrating clinical practice guidelines. J Am Diet Assoc. 2004;104(3):404–9.
14. Axelsson TG, Irving GF, Axelsson J. To eat or not to eat: dietary fat in uremia is the question. Semin Dial. 2010;23(4):383–8.
15. O'Seaghdha CM, Hwang SJ, Muntner P, et al. Serum phosphorus predicts incident chronic kidney disease and end-stage renal disease. Nephrol Dial Transplant. 2011;26(9):2885–90. doi:10.1093/ndt/gfq808.
16. Martin KJ, Gonzalez EA. Prevention and control of phosphate retention/hyperphosphatemia in CKD-MBD: what is normal, when to start, and how to treat? Clin J Am Soc Nephrol. 2011;6(2):440–6.
17. Eknoyan G, Levin A, Levin NW. Bone metabolism and disease in chronic kidney disease. Am J Kidney Dis. 2003;42 Suppl 3:1–201.

18. Peacock M. Calcium metabolism in health and disease. Clin J Am Soc Nephrol. 2010;5 Suppl 1:S23–30.
19. Krikken JA, Laverman GD, Navis G. Benefits of dietary sodium restriction in the management of chronic kidney disease. Curr Opin Nephrol Hypertens. 2009;18(6):531–8.
20. World Health Organization. Reducing salt intake in populations: report of a WHO forum and technical meeting. 2006; Paris, France.
21. Klaus D, Hoyer J, Middeke M. Salt restriction for the prevention of cardiovascular disease. Dtsch Arztebl Int. 2010;107(26):457–62.
22. Palmer BF. A physiologic-based approach to the evaluation of a patient with hyperkalemia. Am J Kidney Dis. 2010;56(2):387–93.
23. Korgaonkar S, Tilea A, Gillespie BW, et al. Serum potassium and outcomes in CKD: insights from the RRI-CKD cohort study. Clin J Am Soc Nephrol. 2010;5(5):762–9.
24. Spiegel D. Magnesium in chronic kidney disease: unanswered questions. Blood Purif. 2011;31:172–6.
25. Lobo JC, Torres JPM, Fouque D, et al. Zinc deficiency in chronic kidney disease: a relationship with adipose tissue and atherosclerosis? Biol Trace Elem Res. 2010;135:16–21.
26. Oakes EJ, Lyon TD, Duncan A, et al. Acute inflammatory response does not affect erythrocyte concentrations of copper, zinc and selenium. Clin Nutr. 2008;27:115.
27. Hsieh YY, Shen WS, Lee LY, et al. Long-term changes in trace elements in patients undergoing chronic hemodialysis. Biol Trace Elem Res. 2006;109(2): 115–21.
28. Handelman GJ, Levin NW. Guidelines for vitamin supplements in chronic kidney disease patients: what is the evidence? J Ren Nutr. 2011;21(1):117–9.
29. Fissell RB, Bragg-Gresham JL, Gillespie BW, et al. International variation in vitamin prescription and association with mortality in the dialysis outcomes and practice patterns study (DOPPS). Am J Kidney Dis. 2004;44:293–9.
30. Bossola M, Tazza L, Giungi S, et al. Anorexia in hemodialysis patients: an update. Kidney Int. 2006;70: 417–22.
31. Akpele L, Bailey JL. Nutrition counseling impacts serum albumin levels. J Ren Nutr. 2004;14:143–8.
32. American Heart Association Nutrition Committee, Lichtenstein AH, Appel LJ, et al. Diet and lifestyle recommendations revision 2006: a scientific statement from the American Heart Association Nutrition Committee. Circulation. 2006;114(1):82–96.

Ethics in Chronic Kidney Disease

28

Shaun D. Conlon, Hussain A. Gilani, and James L. Bailey

Case 1

Mr. Smith, a 76-year-old man with a history of hypertension, type 2 diabetes mellitus, and coronary artery disease with three-vessel bypass grafting, presents to you for routine follow-up for his stage 5 chronic kidney disease. He lives alone and has difficulty affording his medications and making it to his appointments due to lack of transportation. Today, he reports a decreased appetite and a 5 lb weight loss since his last visit 2 months ago. He denies headaches, chest pain, shortness of breath, confusion, pruritis, or a metallic taste to his foods. His medications include metoprolol, lisinopril, insulin, sevelemer, erythropoietin, and calcitriol. His exam today is notable for blood pressure of 156/94 and trace ankle edema. He has no asterixis. His labs are notable for an estimated glomerular filtration rate (eGFR) of 13 mL/min. He asks you for more information about his eventual need for dialysis.

What should the clinician consider in advising a patient about options for renal replacement therapy? Should the patient be concerned that his choice of dialysis modality is irreversible? Is it appropriate to discuss end-of-life care?

S.D. Conlon, M.D. (✉) • H.A. Gilani, M.D.
Nephrology, Emory University,1639 Pierce Drive, WMB 338, Atlanta, GA 30322, USA
e-mail: shaun.conlon@emory.edu

J.L. Bailey, M.D.
Medicine, Renal Division, Emory University, Atlanta, GA 30322, USA

Case 2

Mr. Rodriguez, a 46-year-old Hispanic man with no documented past medical history, is admitted to the emergency room for altered mental status, hyperkalemia, and volume overload. Prior to this he had never seen a physician, but his brother died of “kidney failure” 3 years ago. He is an undocumented worker originally from El Salvador. He has no social security card and does not have private insurance. For the past 2 months, his family reports that the patient has been “swollen all over” and his mental status has gradually worsened. He does not drink or smoke and lives with his wife and four children. He has not worked for the past 2 months, but prior to this, he had been working as a painter for a construction company. His vital signs are notable for a blood pressure of 184/105 and an oxygen saturation of 94% on 2 L nasal canula. His physical exam shows anasarca and bilateral rhonchi. A summation gallop is auscultated on cardiac exam. He receives emergent dialysis through a temporary vascular catheter. Subsequent work-up reveals small echogenic kidneys on renal ultrasound. The patient is now lucid and without respiratory distress. The patient says he needs to return to work, and he is anxious to leave the hospital, but expresses concern over how he will manage his condition.

E.V. Lerma and M. Rosner (eds.), *Clinical Decisions in Nephrology, Hypertension and Kidney Transplantation*, DOI 10.1007/978-1-4614-4454-1_28, © Springer Science+Business Media New York 2013

What are some of the barriers to care for this patient? What considerations should be made for this patient? What should you advise the patient to do?

There are several ethical issues that are specific to chronic kidney disease. The majority of these issues involve various forms of renal replacement therapy (dialysis and transplantation). They can be quite complex and they may not have any readily discernable answers.

Initiation of Dialysis

Ever since Clyde Shields became the first patient to start chronic hemodialysis, patients with advanced chronic kidney disease have enjoyed greatly increased life expectancy as exemplified by Mr. Shields who lived for 11 years after starting dialysis [1]. Initially, dialysis was only utilized in younger patients who had less comorbidity. Dialysis was provided with the intention of allowing the patient to remain a productive member of society. If the patient was unable to work, then the patient was not considered to be a suitable dialysis candidate. Obviously, these patients derived substantial benefit from the initiation of dialysis, as it was a life saving treatment. In 1972, congress passed a bill entitling most Americans to chronic dialysis treatment [2]. This action was in response to a congressional member's child being denied access to dialysis, because of an inability to work. For those who are eligible and have paid into social security for six quarters, the program is fully funded by Medicare. For those patients who have never worked and are American citizens, state run Medicaid programs cover the cost of dialysis. Today, there are few reasons that preclude a patient from being initiated on dialysis. As a consequence, the dialysis population has grown substantially and many older patients with more comorbid conditions are started on dialysis.

A recent study looked back at patients aged 80 or older who started dialysis in the USA between 1996 and 2003 [3]. The number of patients in this age group starting dialysis increased from 7,054 in 1996 to 13,577 in 2003, and the overall 1-year mortality was 46%. In contrast, the 1-year mortality for all patients newly started on dialysis is less than 25% [4]. Although life expectancy worsens with aging, the median survival for those aged 80–84 newly started on dialysis is just 15.6 months and further decreases to 8.4 months for those aged 90 and older.

Because of these dismal survival rates for the elderly starting on dialysis, it was hypothesized that these individuals might live as long off dialysis if they were treated conservatively with a low protein diet, addition of sodium bicarbonate for correction of metabolic acidosis, vigorous blood pressure control, and careful laboratory monitoring. This question was studied in 129 patients older than 75 who were either started on dialysis or managed conservatively [5]. Although both groups had higher than expected survival rates, those patients starting dialysis had a higher 1-year survival (84%) than those patients not initiated on dialysis (68%). That survival advantage was lost in patients with significant comorbidities, especially ischemic heart disease. The study underscores how difficult it is for patients to decide whether or not to proceed with dialysis, especially if they have multiple medical problems.

Dialysis is a therapy that carries a substantial burden. Most patients in the USA undergo intermittent hemodialysis at a dialysis center. This involves traveling to and from a center 3 days/week for treatments that last for 3–4 h. In addition, considerable time is spent in both the preparation and termination of the procedure, especially if there are complications such as hypotension during the treatment. The total time spent in dialysis can approach 5 h or more. Depending upon weight gains and fluid shifts, the patients may experience fatigue, muscle cramps, or even exhaustion. As a consequence, patients may necessarily require a nap as soon as they arrive at home. This also has its untoward consequences as usual sleep patterns are disrupted, meals missed, and the usual interactions with friends and others are disrupted.

Withdrawal from Dialysis

Another issue that faces nephrologists is the deceleration of care for patients on dialysis. This is difficult subject to broach with patients but it is important because almost 80,000 chronic dialysis patients die each year in the USA and withdrawal from dialysis represents the second leading cause of death [4]. It occurs in up to 30% of chronic dialysis patients. When surveyed, nephrologists report that the most common reason they withdraw dialysis is neurological impairment [6].

Nephrologists must necessarily engage patients and their families in end-of-life discussions when they present with terminal illness. When surveyed, the majority of nephrologists (61%) reported not being well prepared to discuss end-of-life issues with their patients [7]. The Renal Physicians Association published guidelines in 2000 that were recently updated to help guide nephrologists through the process of initiation and withdrawal of dialysis [8, 9]. There are ten specific recommendations to help guide the clinician. Not surprisingly, Davison et al. noted that the nephrologists who perceived themselves as being well prepared to make end-of-life decisions were older, had been in practice longer, had withdrawn more patients from dialysis in the preceding year, were more likely to use time-limited trials of dialysis, and were more aware of the RPA/ASN clinical practice guidelines [7]. There is also guidance from the literature to guide advance care planning in a patient centered manner [10, 11].

Advanced care planning (ACP) does not occur routinely in dialysis units [12]. Most patients fail to complete any advance directives and relatively few choose to implement a "do not resuscitate" order despite their poor chance of survival [13]. Moreover, most patients are unaware that they have the option to withdraw from dialysis [14]. If a patient does implement an advance care directive, they often do not address withdrawal of dialysis. As a result, advance directives fail to improve end-of-life care. The role of the physician in this process is to provide information about the disease process and prognosis early around the time of initiation of dialysis and provide information about the impact of treatment on daily life. As an empathetic listener, the physician can affirm the self-worth of patients. In many instances, patients may wish to enlist the family in these discussions and even designate a family member as a spokesperson. Through shared decision-making, patients likely will feel less uncertainty and isolation regarding their decision. It also helps them to feel relief that they are not burdening family and loved ones with end-of-life decision-making as they have affirmed their wishes with the support of their loved ones [10]. The interdisciplinary renal care team can also encourage patient–family discussion and ACP and include advance care planning in the overall plan of care for each individual patient.

For any discussion on renal replacement therapies, the physician must fully inform the patient about various dialysis treatments. The discussion should include information about the risks and benefits of the treatments with full consideration for the patient's values and preferences. The discussion should involve at a minimum the patient and the physician, and the patient should be encouraged to identify and include another person who could serve as the patient's decision-maker in the case that the patient was unable to do so. Shared decision-making options include: (1) Available dialysis modalities. Renal transplantation is considered a dialysis modality. This option along with other dialysis modalities should be discussed and the suitability of the patient for each modality fully considered. (2) Not starting dialysis and continuing medical management. (3) Initiating a time-limited trial of dialysis. The patient should be informed that he always has the option of discontinuing dialysis at any time and that his participation in dialysis is completely voluntary. Besides treatment options, the patient should be informed of his diagnosis and be aware that his prognosis may be limited by other comorbidities such as hypertension, diabetes, and coronary artery disease. Of course, the physician should make clear that his or her ability to predict survival is limited.

Asking clinicians, a simple question—"Would you be surprised if this patient died in the next year?" was informative. Patients in whom the answer was "no" were 3.5 times more likely to die in the next year as compared with patients in whom the answer was "yes" [15]. For patients with end-stage renal disease, the above "surprise" question can be used together with known risk factors to assess prognosis. Factors that are associated with poor prognosis are as follows: age older than 75, comorbid conditions such as hypertension, diabetes mellitus, coronary artery disease and peripheral vascular disease, severe malnutrition with a serum albumin less than 2.5 g/dL, and poor functional status as measured by a Karnofsky Performance score of less than 40.

In many instances, forgoing dialysis is appropriate. Patients with full decision-making capacity, who have been fully informed, may refuse dialysis or request that dialysis be discontinued. Patients who no longer have decision-making capacity or who may have profound neurological impairment may have dialysis discontinued. In these cases, palliative care is an integral part of the decision to forgo dialysis. Other indications for forgoing dialysis include terminal illness such as cancer or because the patient's condition is too unstable during the dialysis treatment. Profound hypotension is one example.

In some instances, the clinician may be uncertain about the prognosis or there is no consensus from the patient or family members on what is the best option. In these instances, consideration can be made for a time-limited trial of dialysis. All parties including the patient, the nephrologist, the patient's legal agent, and the patient's family agree in advance on the length of the trial and parameters to be assessed during and at the completion of the trial to determine whether dialysis has benefited the patient and whether the dialysis should be continued.

Dialysis in Unfunded Patients

The USA has provided automatic insurance coverage to individuals with ESRD (either on dialysis or having received a transplant) since 1972 [2]. However, there are caveats to this coverage. Coverage is granted to individuals who have paid Social Security and Medicare taxes—thus individuals who have not worked or have worked and not paid into Medicare are not eligible for coverage. However, these individuals can receive coverage through state directed Medicaid programs if they are US citizens. Additionally, patients from other countries who are undocumented are not eligible for coverage. The care of these undocumented patients is a substantial problem. This problem has worsened in recent years following a federal court ruling in 2001, which declared that dialysis and chemotherapy were chronic, nonemergent therapies, and thus were excluded from funding through Medicaid. This left the onus of providing funding to local government and charitable organizations. As a result, several county hospitals have responded by closing entire dialysis units for these unfunded patients in an effort to cut costs and balance budgets. The Emergency Medical Treatment and Active Labor Act dictates that hospitals must provide emergency health care treatment regardless of citizenship, legal status, or ability to pay. This provides a safety net for dialysis on an emergent basis only. A recent survey of nephrologists indicated that 91% of undocumented individuals had access to emergent dialysis but only 51% had access to maintenance dialysis [16].

The prognosis of patients who have been started on dialysis but who cannot receive maintenance dialysis is poor. Historical studies have shown that mortality is higher in patients who receive less dialysis [17]. Patients with access only to emergency dialysis will receive less dialysis than those on scheduled maintenance hemodialysis. Moreover, the care of these patients becomes fragmented and is often limited to numerous short hospitalizations.

Financial decisions about providing dialysis to this population are often left to local governments and hospitals. Some choose to provide dialysis on a scheduled basis at no cost while others force undocumented individuals to obtain dialysis only on an emergent basis. One study compared the two approaches and found that providing dialysis only on an emergent basis was almost four times as expensive as providing it on a regularly scheduled basis [18].

Several local health departments have investigated the option of repatriation, that is having undocumented workers return to their home country. This option is appealing for many local health departments; however, it may force patients away from their families in the USA, and the care they will receive in their home country is uncertain [19].

Social and political stigma exists towards this population because the general public erroneously assumes that these individuals have immigrated here specifically for access to health care. The available evidence suggests, otherwise. Patients within this cohort usually have higher employment rates and do not generally receive medical care before they begin dialysis [18]. Moreover, this lack of predialysis care makes it more likely that these patients will suffer more complications and suffer higher mortality rates as a consequence of this lack of intervention.

Renal Transplantation

Despite the financial burden dialysis imparts upon society, its relative availability to most persons allows practitioners' freedom in administrating it to their patients. In contrast, the relative scarcity of renal allografts raises several ethical considerations in how this therapy is distributed. Determination of transplant candidacy is center specific and factors that are considered in this evaluation include sources of funding, family and social support, comorbidities, and age.

Although the cost benefits of renal transplantation over renal replacement therapy are well documented, the funding can be challenging. Medicare will cover the costs of transplantation and anti-rejection medications for up to 3 years; however, it will not cover medications that are not transplant related. Patients will need supplemental sources of funding to fill in the gaps. Screenings are also performed to determine if patients have the appropriate social structure to maintain their renal allografts.

Allocation of allografts to patients with advanced age and comorbidities has also been considered; it is also cite specific. Age alone is generally not considered a contraindication to transplantation. From the Transplant Registry, patients aged 70 or older had a 41% lower risk of death compared to age-matched wait-listed candidates [20]. Patient cohorts with significant comorbidity or advanced age have the option of accepting extended criteria allografts.

Studies have shown that race plays a factor in renal allograft distribution as well. Ethnic minorities have significantly lower rates of kidney transplantation compared with whites. This discrepancy is even worse in living donor transplants. Surveys have shown that blacks are less likely to discuss organ donation with family, are less likely to sign donor cards, and have a higher level of mistrust of the health care system [21,22]. Outreach programs have been established in minority communities to tackle this discrepancy.

Case 1 Revisited

The subject of dialysis and renal replacement therapies should have been broached with Mr. Smith by his nephrologist when his chronic kidney disease was in stage 4. This would allow adequate planning for placement of an arteriovenous fistula if the patient chose to do hemodialysis or allow time for a transplant evaluation. Planning for peritoneal dialysis requires less time and can take place at very advanced stages of chronic kidney disease. Given his multiple comorbid conditions, it is readily understandable why his nephrologist may have delayed the discussion. However, explaining to the patient that his age, diabetes, hypertension, and coronary disease decreases his chances for survival is part of the informed consent and allows for joint decision-making. Following initial discussions, the patient enlisted his niece to join him. Following additional discussion on advance directives, the patient decided against resuscitation efforts and elected to forgo placement of an arteriovenous fistula, stating that he wanted to think about his options a little more. Two months later, he was found dead in bed by his niece. By not electing to begin the process of dialysis, the patient chose to continue medical management. The case further underscores that very few patients with chronic kidney disease ever make it to dialysis. The vast majority succumb to heart disease.

Case 2 Revisited

Mr. Rodriguez is rightfully concerned about his ability to receive dialysis. He is not eligible for Medicare based on his undocumented status. Some states may provide funding for dialysis but many do not. Fortunately for Mr. Rodriguez, his nephrologist decided to assume his long-term care. He prevailed on the vascular surgeon to place an arteriovenous fistula and placed the patient in his own dialysis unit. Unfortunately, nearly half of all indigent patients will not be so lucky. For these patients, dialysis care is done semi-emergently. This results in suboptimal dialysis and generally bad outcomes. In these cases, patients need to be aware that care will be suboptimal if they are unable to receive maintenance hemodialysis. In the latter cases, alternative options should be discussed including repatriation.

References

1. Drukker W. Haemodialysis: a historical review. In: Maher JF, editor. Replacement of renal function by dialysis: a textbook of dialysis. 3rd ed. Dordrect, Holland: Kluwer Academic Publishers; 1989. p. 20–86.
2. Schreiner GE. How end-stage renal disease (ESRD)-medicare developed. Am J Kidney Dis. 2000;35(4 Suppl 1):S37–44.
3. Kurella M, Covinsky KE, Collins AJ, Chertow GM. Octogenarians and nonagenarians starting dialysis in the United States. Ann Intern Med. 2007;146(3):177–83.
4. U.S. Renal Data System. USRDS 2010 annual data report: atlas of end-stage renal disease in the United States. Bethesda, MD: National Institutes of Health, National Institute of Diabetes and Digestive and Kidney Diseases; 2009.
5. Murtagh FEM, Marsh JE, Donohoe P, et al. Dialysis or not? A comparative survival study of patients over 75 years with chronic kidney disease stage 5. Nephrol Dial Transplant. 2007;22(7):1955–62.
6. Holley JL. Palliative care in end-stage renal disease: focus on advance care planning, hospice referral, and bereavement. Semin Dial. 2005;18(2):154–6.
7. Holley JL, Foulks CJ, Moss AH. Nephrologists' reported attitudes about factors influencing recommendations to initiate or withdraw dialysis. J Am Soc Nephrol. 1991;1(12):1284–8.
8. Davison SN, Jhangri GS, Holley JL, Moss AH. Nephrologists' reported preparedness for end-of-life decision-making. Clin J Am Soc Nephrol. 2006;1(6): 1256–62.
9. Galla JH. Clinical practice guideline on shared decision-making in the appropriate initiation of and withdrawal from dialysis. The Renal Physicians Association and the American Society of Nephrology. J Am Soc Nephrol. 2000;11(7):1340–2.
10. Anon. Shared decision-making in the appropriate initiation of and withdrawal from dialysis: clinical practice guidelines. 2010
11. Davison SN. Facilitating advance care planning for patients with end-stage renal disease: the patient perspective. Clin J Am Soc Nephrol. 2006;1(5):1023–8.
12. Davison SN, Torgunrud C. The creation of an advance care planning process for patients with ESRD. Am J Kidney Dis. 2007;49(1):27–36.
13. Holley JL, Stackiewicz L, Dacko C, Rault R. Factors influencing dialysis patients' completion of advance directives. Am J Kidney Dis. 1997;30(3):356–60.
14. Moss AH, Holley JL, Upton MB. Outcomes of cardiopulmonary resuscitation in dialysis patients. J Am Soc Nephrol. 1992;3(6):1238–43.
15. Hines SC, Glover JJ, Babrow AS, et al. Improving advance care planning by accommodating family preferences. J Palliat Med. 2001;4(4):481–9.
16. Moss AH, Ganjoo J, Sharma S, et al. Utility of the "surprise" question to identify dialysis patients with high mortality. Clin J Am Soc Nephrol. 2008;3(5): 1379–84.
17. Hurley L, Kempe A, Crane LA, et al. Care of undocumented individuals with ESRD: a national survey of US nephrologists. Am J Kidney Dis. 2009;53(6): 940–9.
18. Owen Jr WF, Lew NL, Liu Y, Lowrie EG, Lazarus JM. The urea reduction ratio and serum albumin concentration as predictors of mortality in patients undergoing hemodialysis. N Engl J Med. 1993;329(14): 1001–6.
19. Landers M. Illegal immigrant sent home to Mexico, still seeking care. Savannah Morning News. 2007.
20. Coritsidis GN, Khamash H, Ahmed SI, et al. The initiation of dialysis in undocumented aliens: the impact on a public hospital system. Am J Kidney Dis. 2004;43(3):424–32.
21. Rao PS, Merion RM, Ashby VB, et al. Renal transplantation in elderly patients older than 70 years of age: results from the Scientific Registry of Transplant Recipients. Transplantation. 2007;83(8):1069–74.
22. Siminoff LA, Lawrence RH, Arnold RM. Comparison of black and white families' experiences and perceptions regarding organ donation requests. Crit Care Med. 2003;31(1):146–51.

29 Chronic Kidney Disease in the Aging

Lynn E. Schlanger

Case

An 81-year-old man with a history of hypertension and severe peripheral vascular disease from many years of tobacco use is told by his primary care physician that he has chronic kidney disease (CKD) and that his kidneys are functioning approximately 56% of normal. He stopped smoking 10 years ago and is compliant with his medications. Although he remains quite active and exercises three times a week, he is concerned that he will require hemodialysis therapy in the next year or so. After leaving his doctor's office he is unable to sleep secondary to his concerns of starting dialysis and knowing that one of his friends did poorly on hemodialysis. The following day he calls his doctor to discuss the possibility of requiring dialysis in the future. He is referred to a local nephrologist to discuss his kidney function.

Introduction

In 2006, the first of the "baby boomers" joined the aging population. By 2030, it is estimated that one-fifth, 71 million, of the US population will be composed of the elderly (>65 years of age) and very elderly (>80 years of age) [1, 2]. This growth parallels the rise in CKD. In 2004, an estimated 26 million persons were diagnosed with CKD, of which 47% were 70 years of age or older and largely in CKD stages 3 and 4 [3]. The high prevalence of CKD is from diabetes mellitus, hypertension, and obesity as well as aging [3]. These findings were confirmed by the Kidney Early Evaluation Program (KEEP), the National Health and Nutrition Examination Survey (NHANES) 1999–2006, and the Medicare 5% Sample which looked at the prevalence of CKD in the elderly and associated age-specific comorbidities [4]. Forty-four percent of those with CKD were 65 years old or greater in the KEEP and NHANES, and the greater decline in kidney disease in elderly patients was associated with hypertension, coronary artery disease, diabetes, elevated cholesterol, cancer, and cerebrovascular disease [4].

In 2002, the Kidney Disease Outcome Quality Initiative (K/DOQI) published 15 clinical practice guidelines on CKD based on system-evidence review of the literature [5]. The elderly were considered at high risk for developing CKD and screening for evidence of CKD was recommended, using laboratory measurements of markers of kidney disease, abnormal radiologic findings, and pathological abnormalities (see Table 29.1). This was highlighted by a 5-year observational study of CKD in a cohort with an estimated glomerular filtration rate (eGFR) <90 ml/min/1.73 m^2 [6]. Although the likelihood of requiring renal placement therapy was 1.1%, 1.3%, and 19.9% for CKD stage 2, 3, and 4,

L.E. Schlanger, M.D. (✉)
Department of Nephrology, Veteran Affairs Medical Center at Atlanta,1670 Clairmont Road, Decatur, Dekalb, GA 30033, USA
e-mail: lynn.schlanger@va.gov

E.V. Lerma and M. Rosner (eds.), *Clinical Decisions in Nephrology, Hypertension and Kidney Transplantation*, DOI 10.1007/978-1-4614-4454-1_29, © Springer Science+Business Media New York 2013

Table 29.1 NKF/KDOQI definition of CKD

CKD stage ≥3 months[a]	Definition
CKD 1	GFR >90 ml/min/1.73 m^2 and pathological abnormalities or marker of kidney damage—blood or urine or imaging
CKD 2	GFR 60–89 ml/min/1.73 m^2 and pathological abnormalities or marker of kidney damage—blood or urine or imaging
CKD 3	GFR 30–59 ml/min/1.73 m^2
CKD 4	GFR 15–29 ml/min/1.73 m^2
CKD 5	GFR <15 ml/min/1.73 m^2

[a]The definition of CKD stages 1 and 2 requires both the GFR and evidence of kidney damage. The definition of CKD 3, 4, 5 does not require evidence of kidney disease to establish the diagnosis [5]

respectively; the associated mortality was 19.5%, 24.3%, and 45.7%. The authors concluded that the elderly with CKD were more likely to die from other causes than progress to requiring dialysis and end-stage renal disease [6].

With aging, there is a decline in glomerular filtration rate (GFR). Cross-sectional studies and a few but not all longitudinal studies have observed a decline in renal function beginning at age 40 [7–10]. The longest study, the Baltimore Longitudinal Study of Aging, spanned more than 23 years [8–10]. The overall decline in creatinine clearance was 0.87 ml/min/year and a lesser decline of 0.75 ml/min/year was noted in those with no underlying hypertension or renal disease. The greater decline in renal function correlated with aging and mean arterial pressure ≥107 [8]. Remarkably, a third of the participants' renal function remained stable or improved; they had no underlying hypertension or renal disease [10]. In a large elderly community [7], the rate of decline of GFR was slow over 2 years of follow-up. The rate of decline of eGFR was 0.8 ml/min/1.73 m^2/year in women and 1.4 ml/min/1.73 m^2/year in men. Those with diabetes mellitus, severe kidney disease, and hypertension had the greatest decline. These studies suggest that in the absence of superimposed illness, there is a minimal loss of renal function [10].

Senescence Kidney

As we age there are histological, functional, and molecular changes that are part of "the normal aging process." The structural and histological changes that occur have been studied in both animals and humans [11–13]. In humans, the histological changes have been obtained from medical examiner reports, nephrectomies, and renal donor transplant kidneys [11, 12, 14, 15] (see Table 29.2). Grossly, there is a 30% loss in length by 80 years of age and a decrease in weight from 400 to 300 g by 90 years of age [11, 16, 17]. In the cortex, the percentage of global glomerulosclerosis increases with age from 5% or less at 40 years of age [18] to 10–30% in those 80 years of age [11, 18]. Interestingly, the medulla is spared. The renal arterioles also undergo changes. Two types of changes are noted: (1) Obliteration of the glomeruli and arterioles with loss of nephron function and (2) "Aglomerulus" in which an anastomosis is formed between the afferent and efferent arterioles and blood is diverted to the juxtamedullary area [19]. In the interstitium there is tubular atrophy, interstitial fibrosis, and mononuclear infiltrates [20]. These structural and histological changes are accompanied by a 50% decrease in renal plasma flow and a 20% decline in GFR [11, 12, 14, 15] with the greatest decline in measured GFR in the very elderly [21].

Table 29.2 Kidney senescence

Attributes of the senescent kidney
Increase glomerulosclerosis in cortex
Thickening of basement membrane
Podocyte fusion and vacuolization
Arteriole hyalinosis
Aglomerular afferent and efferent arterioles
Loss of the afferent–glomerulus–efferent arteriole unit in the cortex
Increase atrophy and fibrosis in the interstitium
Mononuclear infiltrate in the interstitium
Diverticulum of the distal tubules

Measurement of GFR in the Elderly

In general, the serum creatinine is not a good marker for screening of kidney disease in the elderly because of its variability and dependence on meat intake, medications, age, muscle mass, and ethnicity [22, 23]. The decrease in muscle mass in the elderly results in a decline in the generation of creatinine and therefore a lower serum creatinine level. As a result, the serum creatinine may overestimate the GFR.

The gold standard for measuring the GFR is inulin or alternative exogenous markers such as I^{125} iothalamate or iohexol [22, 23], but these markers are too expensive and time consuming for routine testing. Therefore, two creatinine-based equations are recommended by the National Kidney Foundation/Kidney Disease Outcome Quality Initiative (NKF/KDOQI). These include the abbreviated Modified Diet in Renal Disease estimate glomerular filtration rate (MDRD eGFR) or Cockcroft–Gault (C–G) equation [5]. Each formula has its shortcomings and has not been validated in the elderly [24]. The C–G formula was derived from hospitalized men. Compared with the creatinine clearance [25], it underestimates GFR in the elderly [21, 24]. In contrast, the MDRD eGFR was developed by stepwise regression and compared with I^{125} iothalamate GFR in a selected population with moderate CKD and validated in smaller groups [5, 22]. The MDRD eGFR has been shown to overestimate GFR in the elderly [24]. This could impact therapy especially antibiotic dosing [24]. The MDRD eGFR is not recommend in pregnant women, vegetarians, individuals with extreme body habitus, quadriplegics, and individuals with severe muscle loss [22]. In these groups, a 24-h urine collection is advised.

More recently, a new equation, Chronic Kidney Disease Epidemiology Collaboration (CKD-EPI), was formulated to improve the accuracy and avoid bias for GFR >60 cm^3/min/1.73 mm^2 since the MDRD eGFR is underestimated for a GFR >60 ml/min/1.73 mm^2 [23]. The CKD-EPI was shown to be more accurate than the MDRD eGFR formula compared with the measured GFR [23].

Cystatin C, a cysteine protease inhibitor with a molecular weight of 13 kDa, is produced by most nucleated cells and excreted into the bloodstream [22, 26–28]. It has been touted as a new marker for kidney function since it is less dependent on muscle mass, gender, or age and is freely filtered by the kidney and reabsorbed and metabolized by the proximal tubules [22, 26, 28]. It is a more sensitive marker for early decline in the renal function. In the elderly this is especially important since the serum cystatin C will increase with less variability than the serum creatinine as renal function declines [28]. However, cystatin C is elevated in the setting of excessive cortisol, thyroid disease, and malignancy and observed to be an independent risk factor for all-cause mortality and cardiovascular events in the elderly [26–28]. Shlipak et al. [27] observed a greater decline in renal function in the elderly using cystatin C (1.6 ± 2.6 ml/min/1.73m^2/year) versus creatinine (0.4 ± 3.6 ml/min/1.73 m^2/year) [27]. Age was the strongest predictor for a rapid decline in kidney function and cystatin C is a better estimate of that decline than creatinine eGFR [27].

Peralta and colleagues [26] evaluated the CKD classification using the eGFR based on creatinine versus the eGFR based on cystatin C in 11,909 adults from the Multi-ethnic study of Atherosclerosis (MESA) and the Cardiovascular Health Study (CHS). The prevalence of CKD (eGFR less than 60 cm^3/min/1.73 m^2) was threefold higher in measurements using creatinine than in measurements using cystatin C. The overall clinical outcome was worse with the cystatin-based formula than the creatinine-based formula. Compared with cohorts with no CKD, the adjusted hazard ratio for mortality was 0.8 for creatinine versus 3.32 for cystatin-based formula and 1.93 using both formulas [26]. The outcomes were similar in heart failure (HF), cardiovascular disease (CVD), and kidney failure [26]. Although the use of cystatin C may identify those at risk of adverse outcomes in the early stages of CKD [26], it is costlier than creatinine and not routinely incorporated into labs. Presently, the MDRD or CKD-EPI formulas are recommended for use in CKD measurements.

Morbidity and Mortality of CKD in Aging

CKD in the elderly is associated with an increase in cardiovascular events, all-cause mortality, sudden death, infections, and hospitalizations [29–36]. Diabetes mellitus and hypertension are the most common causes of CKD and are associated with the high incidence of CVD which occurs more frequently with advanced stages of CKD. Both traditional and non-traditional risk factors contribute to all-cause mortality and cardiovascular events [33], and a rapid decline in kidney function is associated with a significant risk for CVD in older patients [35].

Age appears to affect the clinical outcome in CKD stage 3 or higher. The elderly with CKD have a higher mortality rate at an eGFR of <45 ml/min/1.73 mm^2 compared with younger cohorts, elderly with CKD ≥50 ml/min/1.73 mm^2, or elderly without CKD [31, 32]. The likelihood of reaching end-stage kidney failure (ESKF) differs greatly with age; in the elderly with an eGFR of <15 ml/min/1.73 m^2 there is a greater risk of progressing to ESKF than death while in younger cohorts (<45 years of age) this trend is seen at a GFR <45 ml/min/1.73 m^2 [31]. Therefore, the elderly in CKD stage 3 are more likely to succumb to death and less likely to progress to ESKD while younger individuals are more likely to progress to ESKD [30–32]. Because of the effect of age on outcome in CKD, treatment plans must be individualized in the elderly [31].

In the very elderly (75 years of age or older) with CKD, 58% died during a median follow-up of 7.3 years; 42% of those deaths were from CVD [34]. As in previous studies, there was an increase in crude mortality rate with worsening kidney function in men with a eGFR <60 ml/min/1.73 m^2), but this only became apparent in women when the eGFR fell below 45 ml/min/1.73 m^2. Proteinuria increased as renal function declined and was independently associated with all-cause mortality in both elderly men and women [34].

In the Cardiovascular Health Study, 4,380 older adults were followed for a median of 9.9 years. A rapid decline of both eGFR creatinine and cystatin C (>3 cm^3/min/1.73 mm/year) was associated with an increase in all-cause mortality [35]. Those with a more rapid decline were more likely to have more comorbid conditions and older at baseline [35]. A follow-up study looked at the primary cardiovascular end points: heart failure, myocardial infarction, stroke, and peripheral arterial disease [37]. Those with rapid decline in eGFR were older, black, diabetic, and hypertensive and had higher baseline eGFR. There was an increased risk of heart failure, myocardial infarction, and stroke with rapid decline using eGFR$_{\text{cystatin}}$ and of heart failure with eGFR$_{\text{creatinine}}$ with an adjusted hazard ratio of 1.33, 1.35, 1.16, and 2.93, respectively [37]. Following multivariate analysis, rapid decline in kidney function was associated with a 30% risk of heart failure, a 48% risk for myocardial infarction, and a 67% risk for peripheral artery disease [37]. The prevention of a rapid decline in GFR may alter the high incidence of cardiovascular events seen in the elderly [37].

Multidisciplinary care (MDC) exists for dialysis patients but not for those patients with CKD stages 3 and 4 [38]. This is important because the establishment of MDC may have a greater impact on outcomes and death in the elderly. In a recent study, the effect of a MDC team on survival and hospitalizations was compared with usual care in the elderly with CKD over a 3-year period. All-cause mortality was greater in the non-MDC group compared with the MDC group, 41.2% versus 32.6% [38]. Moreover, there was a 50% reduction in the risk of death in the MDC group which was not influenced by age, hemoglobin, serum albumin, gender, baseline eGFR, diabetes, and other comorbidities [38]. Overall hospitalizations were reduced by 17% in the MDC group with a 24% reduction in hospitalizations for cardiovascular events [38].

Functional Status

In the elderly, cognitive ability declines and both the incidence and prevalence of orthostasis, fragility, and dementia increase as renal function worsens [39–44]. Although these changes in functional capacity have been evaluated in those with CKD nearing the need for dialysis or those already on renal replacement [39–44], there have been few studies in the elderly with CKD stages 3 and 4.

Tomlinson and colleagues [41] evaluated the prevalence of hypotension in the elderly with mild to moderate CKD using a 24-h ambulatory blood pressure monitor. The results were compared with a younger cohort. There was a higher prevalence of lower diastolic pressures, higher pulse pressures, and an increased frequency of systolic pressures less than 100 mmHg in the elderly cohort. Unfortunately, hypotension was common among elderly participants. The authors concluded that tight blood pressure control with a goal of less than 130/80 might not be ideal in the older population because of its unintended consequences which included increases in mortality, pre-syncopal episodes, acute kidney injury, and inability to perform daily activities [45, 46].

The Health ABC Study evaluated the changes in body composition and clinical conditions affecting the physical and functional status of the elderly with CKD over time [39]. Participants were recruited from eligibility lists provided by Medicare from two states. Ages ranged from 70 to 79 years old. Initially, participants had no functional impairment. The primary outcome was persistent functional impairment. By the end of the study, 36.3% of participants had developed persistent functional limitations and 62.2% of these individuals witnessed a functional decline in an eGFR <60 ml/min/1.73 mm^2 [39]. Functional limitations were more pronounced in those with severe CKD and independent of comorbidities, body composition, tests of strength, and physical performance [39]. Similarly, the National Nursing Home Registry identified 3,702 nursing home residents newly initiated on dialysis from 1998 until 2000 in order to assess their functional status pre-dialysis and at 3 and 12 months after dialysis initiation. Functional capacity and ability to perform ADLs declined in most individuals during the 12-month observation period. Only 13% maintained their functional status [47]. This decline in functional status was independent of age, sex, race, and functional trajectory before initiation of dialysis [47].

In the Rush Memory and Aging Project, 886 elderly participants without dementia were evaluated for the effect of decline in eGFR on cognitive function [42]. A greater rate of cognitive decline was associated with a lower eGFR at baseline and included a decline in semantic memory, episodic memory, and working memory [42]. This decline was seen in individuals with both moderate and severely impaired renal function. The functional and cognitive decline associated with CKD in the elderly requires redirection of medical treatment to avoid adverse effects and mobilize other disciplines to care for these patients as a whole.

Renal Replacement Therapy

Although most of the elderly and very elderly with CKD stage 3 will die before reaching CKD stage 5D, the highest incident rate in need for dialysis is seen in the very elderly. By 2010 it was predicted that over 600,000 people in the United States would be on renal replacement therapy (RRT). Prior to 1972, dialysis therapy was rationed in the United States. Persons over 45 years of age and diabetics were excluded. With the change in the Social Security Act of 1972, anyone in need could be considered for RRTs. Today, the elderly and very elderly are offered RRTs, including hemodialysis, peritoneal dialysis, or renal transplantation. With the introduction of extended donor criteria for renal transplantation, age is not a deterrent to receiving a kidney. Is there a benefit in initiating RRT in the very elderly?

From 1990 until 1999, the number of those >75 years of age or older initiating dialysis increased from 32.7% in the period from 1990 to 1994 to 40.0% in the period from 1995 to 1999 in the Canadian Organ Replacement Registry [48]. Survival increased from 25.8 to 33.5% in those aged 65–74 years old and increased from 14.2 to 20.3% in those >75 years or older despite an increase in comorbid conditions [48]. Estimated life expectancy was shortened in those requiring dialysis as compared to matched controls with the number of years depending upon the age at the time of initiation which ranged from 2.59 to

4.62 years [48]. Causes of death were largely attributed to cardiac or vascular events even though many were unknown.

The survival benefit of initiating dialysis in the very elderly was evaluated in a 12-year observational study in octogenarians [49]. The median survival on RRT was 28.9 months compared to 8.9 months on medical therapy alone [49]. In the group initiated on dialysis, late referral, poor nutritional status, and poor functional status were independent predictors of death within the first year of dialysis. After 1 year, the comorbid condition associated with death on dialysis was peripheral vascular disease [49]. Other factors influencing outcome were cardiac function and serum phosphate [50]. Those not placed on dialysis were more likely to be women, late referrals, diabetics, and individuals lacking social support [49].

Retrospective case-note and computer-based analysis looked at the outcome on RRT in the very elderly in the United Kingdom [51] compared with younger age groups: <65 years old versus 65–74 years old versus ≥75 years old. One-year survival, ranging from youngest to oldest age group, was 90.6, 72.6, and 53.5% while the 5-year survival was 61.4, 18.8, and 2.4%. The common causes of death were withdrawal from dialysis (38%), CVD (28%), and infections (22%). The median survival was 16, 29, and 86 months from the oldest to youngest age groups. When compared with similar age groups without CKD the life expectancy was greatly shortened for each age group [51].

Early referral to a nephrologist prior to initiation of RRT has been shown to have a positive effect on survival in some studies because of a favorable impact on kidney disease symptoms, metabolic abnormalities, and psychological profile [28, 43, 51]. Nevertheless, a higher number of older patients and women are referred later to the nephrologist. In one study, only 27.3% of elderly persons with severe renal failure were referred to nephrologist while those with a serum creatinine of ≤1.7 mg/dl were less likely to be referred [52]. Men and diabetics were more likely to be referred than women [52].

Not surprisingly, there is a relatively poor outcome associated with the initiation of dialysis in the very elderly with many coexisting comorbidities and a decrease in functional status. However, the decision to initiate RRT should be individualized with consideration of various factors including the overall health and socioeconomic status of the individual.

Case Revisited

There is little likelihood that this 81-year-old man will progress to end-stage kidney disease requiring RRT unless there is an intervening event that results in acute kidney injury. More likely, the patient will die from a cardiovascular event. Factors that would forestall RRT would be blood pressure control, addressing both the traditional and the non-traditional risk factors for CVD, and avoiding medications which could be damaging to his kidney function.

References

1. Centers for Disease Control and Prevention. Public health and aging: trend in aging-United States and worldwide. MMWR Morbidity Mortal Weekly Rep. 52:101–106; 2003, http://www.census.gov/hhes/www/laborfor/Working-Beyond-Retirement-Age.pdf viewed 1/2011.
2. http://www.census.gov/prod/2001pubs/c2kbr01-10.pdf viewed 1/2011 viewed 1/2011
3. Coresh J, Selvin E, Stevens LA, Manzi J, Kusek JW, Eggers P, et al. Prevalence of chronic kidney disease in the United States. JAMA. 2007;298(17):2038–47.
4. Stevens LA, Li S, Wang C, Huang C, Becker BN, Bomback AS, et al. Prevalence of CKD and comorbid illness in elderly patients in United States: results from kidney early evaluation prevention. Am J Kidney Dis. 2010;55(3):S23–33.
5. Levey AS, Coresh J, Balk E, Kausz AT, Levin A, Steffes MW, et al. National kidney foundation practice guidelines for chronic kidney disease: evaluation, classification, and stratification. Ann Intern Med. 2003;139(2):137–47.
6. Keith DS, Nichols GA, Gullion CM, Brown JB, Smith DH. Longitudinal follow-up and outcomes among a population with chronic kidney disease in a large managed care organization. Arch Intern Med. 2004;164:659–63.
7. Hemmelgarn R, Zhang J, Manns BJ, Tonelli M, Larsen E, Ghali WA, et al. Progression of kidney dysfunction in the community –dwelling elderly. Kidney Int. 2006;69:2155–61.

8. Lindeman RD, Tobin JD, Shock NW. Association between blood pressure and the rate of decline in the renal function with age. Kidney Int. 1984;26(6):861–8.
9. Lindeman RD, Tobin J, Shock NW. Longitudinal studies on the rate of decline in renal function with age. J Am Geriatr Soc. 1985;33(4):278–85.
10. Rowe JW, Andres R, Tobin JD, Norris AH, Shock NW. The effect of age on creatinine clearance in men: A cross-sectional and longitudinal study. J Gerontol. 1976;31(2):155–63.
11. Anderson S, Brenner BM. Effect of aging on the renal glomerulus. Am J Med. 1986;80:436–42.
12. Hollenberg NK, Adams DF, Solomon HJ, Rashid A, Abrams HL, Merrill JP, et al. Senescence in the renal vasculature in normal man. Circ Res. 1974;34:309–16.
13. Baylis C, Corman B. The aging kidney: insights from experimental studies. J Am Soc Nephrol. 1998;9(4):699–709.
14. Rule AD, Amer H, Cornell LD, Taler SJ, Cosio FG, Kremers WK, et al. The age association between age and nephrosclerosis on renal biopsy. Ann Intern Med. 2010;152:561–7.
15. Kasiske BL. Relationship between vascular disease and age-associated changes in the human kidney. Kidney Int. 1987;31:1153–9.
16. Emamian SA, Nielsen MB, Pedersen JF, Ytte L. Kidney dimensions at sonography: correlation with age, sex, and habitus in 655 adult volunteers. Am J Roentgenol. 1993;160:83–6.
17. Gourtsoyiannis N, Prassopoulos P, Cavouras D, Pantelidis N. The thickness of the renal parenchyma decreases with age: a CT study of 360 patients. Am J Roentgenol. 1990;155:541–4.
18. Kaplan C, Pasternack B, Shah H, Gallo G. Age-related incidence of sclerotic glomeruli in human kidneys. J Pathol. 1975;80(2):227–34.
19. Takazakura E, Sawabu N, Handa A, Takada A, Shinoda A, Takeachi J, et al. Intrarenal vascular changes with age and disease. Kidney Int. 1972;2:224–30.
20. Thomas SE, Anderson S, Gordon K, Oyama TT, Shankland SJ, Johnson RJ. Tubulointerstitial disease in aging: evidence for underlying peritubular capillary damage, a potential role for renal ischemia. J Am Soc Nephrol. 1998;9(2):231–42.
21. Christensson A, Elmståhl S. Estimation of the age-dependent decline of glomerular filtration rate from formulas based on creatinine and cystatin C in the general elderly population. Nephron Clin Pract. 2011;117:c40–50.
22. Stevens LA, Coresh J, Greene T, Levey AS. Assessing kidney function- measured and estimate glomerular filtration rate. N Engl J Med. 2006;354:2473–83.
23. Levey AS, Stevens LA, Schmidt CH, Zhang Y, Castro III AF, Feldman HI, et al. A new equation to estimate glomerular filtration rate. Ann Intern Med. 2009;150(9):604–12.
24. Roberts GW, Isben PM, Schiøler CT. Modified diet in renal disease method overestimates renal function in selected elderly patients. Age Ageing. 2009;38:698–703.
25. Cockcroft DW, Gault MH. Prediction of creatinine clearance from serum creatinine. Nephron. 1976;16:31–41.
26. Peralta CA, Katz R, Sarnak MJ, Ix J, Fried LF, De Boer I, Palmas W, Siscovick D, Levey AS, Shlipak MG. Cystatin C identifies chronic kidney disease patients at higher risk for complications. J Am Soc Nephrol. 2011;22:147–55.
27. Shlipak MG, Katz R, Kestenbaum B, Fried LF, Newman AB, Siscovick DS, et al. Rate of kidney function decline in older adults: A comparison using creatinine and cystatin C. Am J Nephrol. 2009;30(3):171–8.
28. de Jong PE, Ganesvoort NT. Is cystatin C the answer to detecting progression in CKD? J Am Soc Nephrol. 2001;22(1):1–13.
29. Nitsch D, Nonvane BAS, Smeeth L, Bulpitt CJ, Roderick PJ, Fletcher A. CKD and hospitalization in the elderly: a community-based cohort study in the United Kingdom. Am J Kidney Dis. 2011;57(5):664–72.
30. Fried LF, Shlipak MG, Crump CC, Bleyer AJ, Gottdiener JS, Kronmal RA, et al. Renal insufficiency as a predictor of cardiovascular outcomes and mortality in the elderly individuals. J Am Coll Cardiol. 2002;14(8):1364–72.
31. O'Hare AM, Cho AI, Bertenthal P, Bachetti P, Garg AX, Kaufman JS, Walter LC, Mehta MA, Steinman MA, Allon M, McClellan W, Landefeld M. Age affects outcomes in chronic kidney disease. J Am Soc Nephrol. 2007;18:2758–65.
32. O'Hare AM, Bertenthal D, Covinsky KE, Landefeld CS, Sen S, Mehta S, et al. Mortality risk stratification in chronic kidney disease: one size for all ages? J Am Soc Nephrol. 2006;17:846–53.
33. Munter P, He J, Astor BC, Folsom AR, Coresh J. Traditional and nontraditional risk factors predict coronary heart disease in chronic kidney disease: results from the atherosclerosis risk in communities study. J Am Soc Nephrol. 2005;16:529–38.
34. Roderick PJ, Atkins RJ, Smeeth L, Mylne A, Nitsch DDM, Hubbard RB, et al. CKD and mortality risk in older people: a community- based population study in the United Kingdom. Am J Kidney Dis. 2009;53:950–60.
35. Rifkin DE, Shlipak MG, Katz R, Fried LF, Siscovick D, Chonchol M, et al. Rapid kidney function decline and mortality risk in older adults. Arch Intern Med. 2008;168(20):2212–8.
36. Shlipak MG, Sarnak MJ, Katz R, Fried LF, Seliger SL, Newman AB, et al. Cystatin C and the risk of death and cardiovascular events among elderly persons. N Engl J Med. 2005;352:2049–60.
37. Shlipak MG, Katz R, Kestenbaum B, Siscovick D, Fried L, Newman A, Rifkin D, et al. Rapid decline of kidney function increases cardiovascular risk in the elderly. J Am Soc Nephrol. 2009;20:2625–30.
38. Hemmelgran BR, Manns BJ, Zhang J, Tonneli M, Klarenbach S, Walsh M, et al. Association between multidisciplinary care and survival for elderly patients with chronic kidney disease. J Am Soc Nephrol. 2007;18:993–9.

39. Fried LF, Lee JS, Shlipak M, Chertow GA, Green C, Ding J, et al. Chronic kidney disease and functional limitation in older people: health, aging and body composition study. J Am Geriatr Soc. 2006;54:750–6.
40. Kurella M, Chertow GM, Fried LF, Cummings SR, Harris T, Simonsick E, et al. Chronic kidney disease and cognitive impairment in the elderly: the health, aging, and body composition study. J Am Soc Nephrol. 2005;16(5):2127–33.
41. Tomlinson LA, Holt SG, Leslie AR, Rajkumar C. Prevalence of ambulatory hypotension in elderly patients with CKD stages 3 and 4. Nephrol Dial Transplant. 2009;24(12):3751–5.
42. Buchman AS, Tanne D, Boyle PA, Shah RC, Leurgans SE, Bennett DA. Kidney function is associated with the rate of cognitive decline in the elderly. Neurology. 2009;73(12):920–7.
43. Boini S, Frimat L, Kessler M, Briançon S, Thilly N. Predialysis therapeutic care and health-related quality of life at dialysis onset (The pharmacoepidemiologic AVENIR study). Health Qual Life Outcomes. 2011;9:7.
44. Cook WL, Jassal SV. Prevalence of falls among seniors maintained on hemodialysis. Int Urol Nephrol. 2005;37:649–52.
45. Mann JFE, Schmieder RE, McQueen M, Dyal L, Schumacher H, Pogue J, et al. Renal outcomes with telmisartan, ramipril, or both, in people at high vascular risk (the ONTARGET study): a multicentre, randomized, double-blind, controlled trial. Lancet. 2008;372:547–53.
46. Weiss JW, Johnson ES, Petrik A, Smith DH, Yang X, Thorp ML. Systolic blood pressure and mortality among older community-dwelling adults with CKD. Am J Kidney Dis. 2010;56(6):1062–71.
47. Tamura MK, Covinsky KE, Chertow GM, Yaffe K, Landefeld CS, McCulloh CE. Functional status of elderly adults before and after initiation of dialysis. N Engl J Med. 2009;361:1539–47.
48. Jassal SV, Trpeski L, Zhu N, Fenton S, Hemmelgram B. Changes in survival among elderly patients initiating dialysis from 1990 to 1999. CMAJ. 2007;177(9):1033–8.
49. Joly D, Anglicheau D, Alberti C, Ngyen A-T, Touam M, Grunfeld J-P. Octogenarians reaching end-stage renal disease: cohort study of decision-making and clinical outcomes. J Am Soc Nephrol. 2003;14:1012–21.
50. Jassal SV, Douglas JF, Stout RW. Prognostic markers in older patients starting renal replacement therapy. Nephrol Dial Transplant. 1996;11(6):1052–7.
51. Munshi SK, Vijayakumar N, Taub NA, Bhullar H, Lo TCN, Warwick G. Outcome of renal replacement therapy in the very elderly. Nephrol Dial Transplant. 2001;16:128–33.
52. Swedko PJ, Clark HD, Paramsothy K, Akbari A. Serum creatinine is an inadequate screening test for renal failure in elderly patients. Arch Intern Med. 2003;163:356–60.

Part VII

Dialysis Therapies

Counseling Patients for Renal Replacement Therapy Based on Outcomes

30

Mark G. Parker

Case 1

A 52-year-old woman with autosomal dominant polycystic kidney disease (ADPKD) presents for nephrology follow-up. Her most recent serum creatinine is 2.9 mg/dl and estimated glomerular filtration rate (eGFR) is 28 ml/min/1.73m^2. She is married, has no children, and works full-time as a health care administrator. She feels well except that she finds herself more fatigued at the end of each workday than at previous visits. She denies nausea, anorexia, edema, or pruritis. She has not required erythropoietic stimulating agents to date. One sister with ADPKD has received a transplant from a brother. One other sister, age 54, has had a normal renal ultrasound and is interested in donating a kidney to the patient. The patient wishes to discuss her future renal replacement therapy (RRT) options.

What are her RRT options? When is the best time to initiate this discussion and begin preparation? What is the role of team-based education in this process? What is the influence of preparation on outcomes?

Case 2

An 80-year-old man presents for his third visit to the nephrology clinic. He first visit was 2 months ago when he was referred with a serum creatinine of 3.2 mg/dl and an eGFR of 14 ml/min/1.73m^2. His medical history includes adult onset diabetes mellitus for 18 years—poorly controlled on oral agents, continued cigarette smoking with a 60-pack-year history, a five-vessel coronary artery bypass graft surgery 10 years ago, cardiomyopathy with left ventricular ejection fraction of 25% and a history of non-sustained ventricular tachycardia, and a lower extremity bypass graft 5 years ago. He lives alone, has limited social contact, and rarely leaves home. He has a niece who shops for him, prepares his medication tray, and checks on him daily. He is weak, tired, and has lost 10 lb over 8 weeks. He is finding it harder to bath, dress, and prepare his meals. The topic of dialysis was introduced at his last visit, but he is ambivalent about preparing for such therapy.

What are his options for therapy? Is dialysis an appropriate choice and, if so, what form of dialysis is most suitable? What is the role of palliative care as a management choice?

Introduction

Patients with advanced chronic kidney disease face a complex series of decisions about treatment options for end-stage renal disease

M.G. Parker, M.D. (✉)
Division of Nephrology and Transplantation, Maine Medical Center, 22 Bramhall Street, Portland, ME 04102, USA
e-mail: parkem@mmc.org

E.V. Lerma and M. Rosner (eds.), *Clinical Decisions in Nephrology, Hypertension and Kidney Transplantation*, DOI 10.1007/978-1-4614-4454-1_30, © Springer Science+Business Media New York 2013

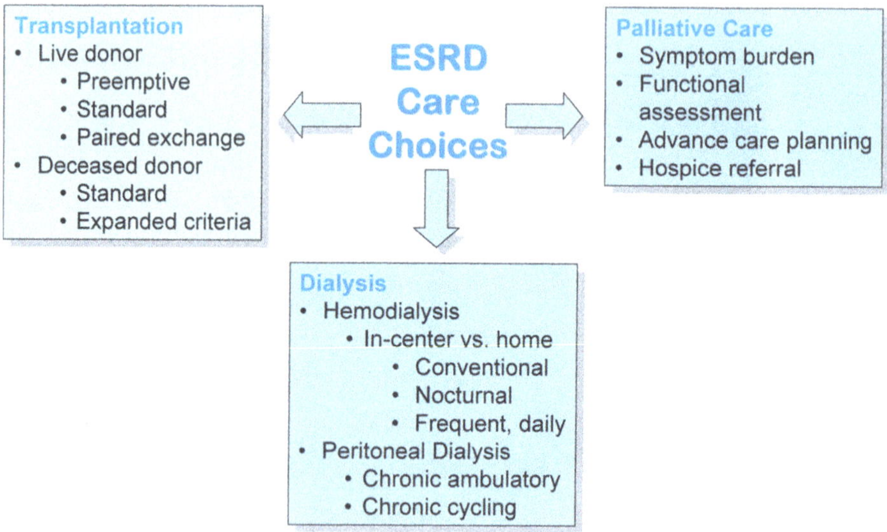

Fig. 30.1 End-stage renal disease options

(ESRD). Sufficient lead time is necessary to provide education, share decision-making, and allow preparation for kidney transplantation, dialysis, or palliative care services (Fig. 30.1). For those individuals with live donors and ample preparatory time, preemptive transplantation confers an allograft survival benefit. Some investigators have demonstrated that a systematic process of patient education in late stage CKD improves outcomes in dialysis care as well. Palliative care is a reasonable treatment choice that has been overlooked, in some ways, for many years in the ESRD realm. However, recent advances in our understanding of dialysis outcomes, particularly in the very elderly and infirm, have renewed interest in educating appropriate individuals about this option and providing services that maintain a sense of well-being.

NKF-DOQI and others designate chronic kidney disease stage IV as the best time to prepare for RRT [1]. Patients with an eGFR of 15–30 ml/min/1.73m^2 exhibit many metabolic derangements of severe impairment of renal function, yet usually retain the physical and cognitive capacity to maintain their daily activities. They are capable of participating in classes and other activities organized around preparation for ESRD. Successful preparation for ESRD involves a variety of interdisciplinary personnel, regardless of treatment choice. For all treatment choices, the nephrologist is central to the commencement and orchestration of this care process. Timely referral to the nephrologist in order to facilitate ongoing clinical care, provide patient education, and allow preparation for renal replacement modalities has been associated with best ESRD outcomes [2, 3].

Consideration of Transplantation

Specific considerations for kidney transplant recipient evaluation will be addressed in Chap. 34. All patients with advanced CKD or ESRD on dialysis should be provided with information about kidney transplantation. Indeed, current federal guidelines in the United States mandate transplant consideration for all ESRD patients [4]. If a patient declines transplantation or is deemed unacceptable due to medical contraindications, documentation of this discussion is required.

Patients without clear contraindications to kidney transplantation should be informed of this treatment option and referred for formal transplant evaluation. Although there is an increased mortality risk in the early months after kidney transplantation, the long-term relative risk of death for transplant recipients is 48–82% lower than for matched patients on the transplant waiting list who are receiving dialysis [5]. The benefit appears to be most substantial among young adults in general, white patients, and young diabetics. Further, nonuse of dialysis or minimized dialysis exposure enhances allograft survival. Preemptive transplantation reduces the risk of allograft failure by 52% in the first year after transplant and by 86% after 2 years [6]. Longer waiting times on dialysis have a negative impact on survival [7], so advance planning is advantageous for the CKD patient. Unfortunately, only 2.5% of incident patients receive kidney transplants preemptively [7, 8].

The transplant multidisciplinary team typically includes nephrologists, transplant surgeons, coordinators, nurses, social workers, and nutritionists. Individuals from many other disciplines, such as cardiology or psychiatry, are often consulted in the course of the process. Preemptive transplant education by members of the transplant team may have the advantage of increasing living donation rates, providing benefit both to the individual and to the CKD and ESRD communities at large [9]. In addition, the use of formal, comprehensive education in a chronic kidney disease clinic has been shown to improve the rate of preemptive transplantation to as much as 24% and reduce transplant wait times [10].

Dialysis Preparation

Regardless of potential for transplantation or consideration of palliative care, advanced CKD patients should be educated about dialysis modalities. For potential kidney transplant recipients, education about dialysis often occurs in parallel with transplant evaluation. It is particularly important if there is uncertainty about the prospect for live donor renal transplant. With sufficient advance information, patients may make reasoned care choices and allow time for dialysis access preparation. Home therapy is more difficult to prepare when time is limited, yet may be a preferred treatment option for many patients. It offers elements of patient autonomy and comfort, reduced exposure to certain infections encountered in health care environments, favorable costs compared with in-center therapies, and possibly, outcome advantages. As with transplantation, dialysis education is facilitated best by a multidisciplinary team. The team often includes nephrologists, nurses, social workers, and nutritionists.

Five randomized controlled trials have been performed to assess the impact of predialysis educational interventions on dialysis choice and clinical outcomes, such as time to dialysis initiation and survival [11–15]. In one study, subjects who received educational manuals and a video on self-care and home dialysis, followed 2 weeks later by a group problem-solving discussion, were more likely (adjusted odds ratio, 10.2) to state an intention for self-care than subjects who had usual clinic instruction [11]. All patients who had initiated dialysis by 11 months followed through on their stated choice. The intervention group also exhibited increased knowledge about self-care and better training self-efficacy ($p=0.02$). Long-term follow-up—even up to 20 years—in another investigation has demonstrated that other educational strategies, including slide lectures with booklets, are associated with delayed time to dialysis initiation as well as improved median survival after starting dialysis (relative risk, 1.32) [13].

Despite their potential advantages, home therapy options tend to get the least mention, particularly when kidney disease awareness is poor or nephrology referral occurs late. Investigators of ESRD Network 18 conducted a survey prior to initiation of a quality improvement initiative around RRT [16]. Prior to intervention, 36% of patients were aware of their kidney disease or first saw a nephrologist <4 months before beginning dialysis. In this cohort, 66% of patients stated that they were not offered peritoneal dialysis as a treatment option and 88% replied that they were not told about home hemodialysis. Eighty-seven percent of this cohort responded that RRT was not presented as a set of options at all.

Most recently, a cohort from the United States Renal Data System (USRDS) Comprehensive Dialysis Study was analyzed and demonstrated that among 631 patients who were not educated initially about peritoneal dialysis as a therapy option, only 1.9% eventually used this modality [17]. Among 1,621 patients who did receive education about peritoneal dialysis, 10.9% chose this therapy. Even the latter remains a disappointingly low number for advocates of peritoneal dialysis. The numbers are even lower for home hemodialysis. Only 1% of the dialysis population currently utilizes this form of therapy [18].

Modality Selection and Outcome

Several studies have demonstrated that peritoneal dialysis conveys a potential early survival advantage for the incident RRT population, perhaps due to preservation of residual renal function, though the survival benefit appears to wane with time [19–22]. Such studies have been criticized for selection bias, poor study design, and differences in comorbid disease burden. To overcome some of these limitations, propensity analysis was applied to a retrospective cohort of nearly 99,000 patients who initiated dialysis in the United States in 2003 [23]. This study reported an 8% reduction in mortality risk for peritoneal dialysis patients compared to hemodialysis patients at initiation. The mortality difference disappeared after 24 months. Long-term patients appear to do equally as well with hemodialysis as peritoneal dialysis.

In the realm of hemodialysis, home therapy appears to offer advantages over conventional thrice-weekly in-center therapy, but a true difference in survival remains to be definitely demonstrated. In addition, intensive variants of both home and in-center therapy have garnered recent attention. Both in-center nocturnal hemodialysis (INHD) and nocturnal home dialysis (NHHD) have been studied, as well as short daily dialysis, in part based on the observation that low rates of ultrafiltration may improve survival. INHD is associated with improved calcium–phosphorus and blood pressure control, reduced erythropoietin-stimulating agent use, and improved quality of life scores [24–26]. Similar results are seen with NHHD as well as reduction in left ventricular mass (LVM) [27]. The investigators of the Frequent Hemodialysis Network reported that short in-center daily dialysis reduces the risk of the composite end point of mortality or increase in LVM compared to conventional hemodialysis (12-month observation: hazard ratio 0.061, confidence interval 0.46–0.82), but was associated with a need for more frequent vascular access interventions [28]. The outcomes associated with these variations on hemodialysis therapy support the need for patient education about these options and encouragement to give strong consideration to their use.

Dialysis Access Preparation

One of the advantages of timely and comprehensive predialysis education is the ability to provide dialysis access well in advance of dialysis therapy. For patients choosing hemodialysis therapy, vascular access preparation has a direct impact on outcome.

The ideal vascular access is a native arteriovenous fistula (AVF) of an upper extremity. Inability to establish a mature AVF in advance of dialysis initiation often results in the use of central venous catheter (CVC) access for therapy. Numerous studies have correlated dialysis initiation by CVC with poor outcomes. Despite the success of the Fistula First Breakthrough Initiative, which has increased the prevalence of AVF use in the United States from 27% in 1998 to 55.5% in 2010 [29], 82% of hemodialysis patients still initiate therapy with a CVC [30]. In 2008, a CVC was used for dialysis treatments in the United States for an estimated 26% of patient-days [31]. Bloodstream infections associated with tunneled CVCs occur at a rate of 4.2 events/100 patient-months as compared to rates of 0.5/100 patient-months with AVF [32]. Indeed, CVC access for hemodialysis has been identified as an independent risk factor for death (adjusted hazard ratio 1.71) in the first 120 days of dialysis [2]. The CHOICE investigators also found a graded risk of annual mortality from AVF (11.7%) to arteriovenous grafts (14.2%) to CVC (16.1%) [33]. Early education, referral for AVF creation, and then careful monitoring of fistula maturation or referral for salvage, when necessary, are the best practices for hemodialysis access preparation.

Peritoneal dialysis catheter referral is typically done much closer to the time of anticipated dialysis initiation. There are no published studies addressing the ideal timing of catheter placement or correlations with dialysis outcomes. In practice, the catheter is placed at least 2 weeks before dialysis initiation, and embedding the catheter to prevent infection is an option for those patients who may have a delayed start to therapy. Details of placing peritoneal dialysis access are addressed in Chap. 32.

Palliative Care

In recent years, palliative care has evolved as a specialized area of medicine. Historically, there has been little emphasis on palliative care as a treatment option for ESRD. Considerable interest has been generated from positive associations between frank end-of-life discussions and patient mental outlook, supportive care near death, caregiver bereavement adjustment, and overall health care costs in the final weeks of life [34, 35].

As a consequence of end-of-life observations in other areas of medicine and decades of dialysis experience in the nephrology community, palliative care has gained traction in the nephrology community as a reasonable treatment option [36]. Indeed, an entire textbook about palliative support for renal patients is now in its second edition [37]. Fueling attention to this care option, there have been several publications emphasizing the reduced life expectancy and burden of limited functional status for subsets of ESRD patients. Tamura et al. studied a cohort of 3,702 United States nursing home patients who started dialysis during a 2-year interval. They found that 58% of these patients died within 12 months of starting dialysis and only 13% maintained predialysis functional status [38]. Other investigators have found no significant survival advantage to dialysis therapy for elderly patients with ischemic heart disease [39] or who are referred to nephrology in a late or emergent fashion for consideration of dialysis [40]. Clinical prediction tools have been developed and validated to provide prognostic information for care providers and patients in shared decision-making about initiation or withholding of dialysis [41, 42]. One such tool assigns points for nine risk factors and scores correlate well with 6-month mortality, ranging from 8% in the lowest risk group to 70% in the highest risk group [42]. The introduction of these tools into the discussion of RRT preparation gives the provider a quantitative methodology to assist the patient's decision.

Chapter 33 explores palliative care for ESRD in more depth.

Case 1 Revisited

This middle age woman with polycystic kidney disease and no major coincident illnesses is likely to be a good candidate for transplantation. As she is in early stage IV CKD, the time is appropriate to initiate team-based education about both transplantation and dialysis. In view of the fact that she has a healthy sibling who is willing to be her kidney donor, a preemptive kidney transplant would be the most desirable goal. In the event that her sister has a contraindication to donation or there is incompatibility (e.g., blood type), then additional options for donors should be explored, such as other relatives, friends, or even paired organ exchange involving the sister. In parallel with transplant evaluation, she should learn about dialysis options and her provider should develop a plan with her for possible dialysis preparation in case preemptive transplantation is untenable. If a suitable donor and the recipient successfully complete the evaluation process and are approved for transplantation, it is reasonable to forego dialysis access preparation. If there are barriers (e.g., donor contraindications) to preemptive transplantation, then dialysis modality selection and satisfactory preparatory time for access are necessary while the transplant evaluation continues and deceased organ donor wait listing subsequently occurs. In particular, if she plans hemodialysis therapy, creation of a native AVF with sufficient time for maturation will reduce her odds of a poor dialysis outcome.

Case 2 Revisited

This elderly man has several reasons to give strong consideration to a palliative care plan. He has marked cumulative cardiovascular morbidity, including peripheral vascular disease, advanced cardiomyopathy, uncontrolled diabetes, and ongoing tobacco use. His life expectancy is limited. In addition, he has been referred to nephrology care relatively late in his CKD course, further increasing the chance of a poor dialysis outcome. Finally, he exhibits ambivalence towards dialysis therapy. An attempt should be made to fully inform him about his options. If he is willing, team-based dialysis education should be offered. However, he should also be advised that dialysis is not likely to enhance his life expectancy nor will it necessarily improve his quality of life. Quantitative prediction of his life expectancy might be used to guide counseling. The scoring tool of Couchoud et al. would yield 6 of 16 possible points based upon risk factors and therefore predict 6-month mortality of 35%. A choice of palliative care should be supplemented by a discussion of plans for symptom assessment and management, resources for home care, hospice and bereavement needs, and assurance that the provider team will provide ongoing support.

Key Points

1. Timely referral to a nephrologist and multidisciplinary education of patients in early stage IV chronic kidney disease confers the best RRT outcome. The care algorithm is complex (Fig. 30.2) and guided by the nephrologist. Decision-making should be a shared process with the patient.
2. Consideration of preemptive transplantation for potential recipients with suitable living donors helps avoid dialysis therapy and provides a survival advantage.
3. For patients selecting or requiring dialysis therapy, a broad range of options should be

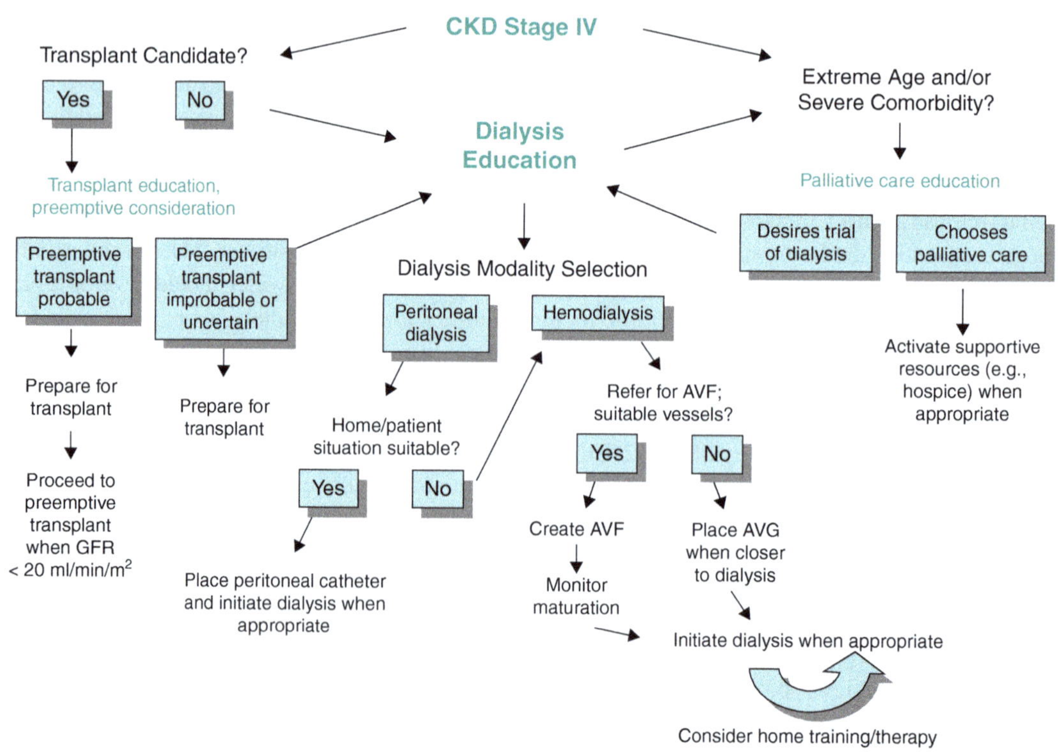

Fig. 30.2 Preparation for renal replacement therapy in late stage kidney disease

discussed. Patients should be informed about all in-center and home therapy modalities, including variations which alter the intensity of therapy and may convey additional health and life quality advantages.

4. While no form of dialysis therapy has clearly been proven superior to all others, there may be an early survival benefit for patients initiating RRT with peritoneal dialysis compared with hemodialysis. This difference in mortality outcome is not durable over the long term, however.
5. Palliative care is a very reasonable form of management for appropriate patients with advanced age or severe burden of coexistent illness, particularly if life expectancy is limited. Comprehensive care of this type is becoming more common in nephrology.

References

1. National Kidney Foundation. National Kidney Foundation K/DOQI clinical practice guidelines. National Kidney Foundation 2011; Available at: URL: http://www.kidney.org/professionals/kdoqi/guidelines/. Accessed 20 Jun, 2011.
2. Bradbury BD, Fissell RB, Albert JM, et al. Predictors of early mortality among incident US hemodialysis patients in the dialysis outcomes and practice patterns study (DOPPS). Clin J Am Soc Nephrol. 2007;2(1):89–99.
3. Kinchen KS, Sadler J, Fink N, et al. The timing of specialist evaluation in chronic kidney disease and mortality. Ann Intern Med. 2002;137(6):479–86.
4. Medicare. Medicare program: hospital conditions of participation: requirements for approval and re-approval of transplant centers to perform organ transplants. Final rule. Fed Regist. 2007;72(61):15197–280.
5. Wolfe RA, Ashby VB, Milford EL, et al. Comparison of mortality in all patients on dialysis, patients on dialysis awaiting transplantation, and recipients of a first cadaveric transplant. N Engl J Med. 1999;341(23):1725–30.
6. Mange KC, Joffe MM, Feldman HI. Effect of the use or nonuse of long-term dialysis on the subsequent survival of renal transplants from living donors. N Engl J Med. 2001;344(10):726–31.
7. Meier-Kriesche HU, Port FK, Ojo AO, et al. Effect of waiting time on renal transplant outcome. Kidney Int. 2000;58(3):1311–7.
8. Abecassis M, Bartlett ST, Collins AJ, et al. Kidney transplantation as primary therapy for end-stage renal disease: a national kidney foundation/kidney disease outcomes quality initiative (NKF/KDOQITM) conference. Clin J Am Soc Nephrol. 2008;3(2):471–80.
9. Hays R, Waterman AD. Improving preemptive transplant education to increase living donation rates: reaching patients earlier in their disease adjustment process. Prog Transplant. 2008;18(4):251–6.
10. Khosla N, Gordon E, Nishi L, Ghossein C. Impact of a chronic kidney disease clinic on preemptive kidney transplantation and transplant wait times. Prog Transplant. 2010;20(3):216–20.
11. Manns BJ, Taub K, Vanderstraeten C, et al. The impact of education on chronic kidney disease patients' plans to initiate dialysis with self-care dialysis: a randomized trial. Kidney Int. 2005;68(4):1777–83.
12. Binik YM, Devins GM, Barre PE, et al. Live and learn: patient education delays the need to initiate renal replacement therapy in end-stage renal disease. J Nerv Ment Dis. 1993;181(6):371–6.
13. Devins GM, Mendelssohn DC, Barre PE, Taub K, Binik YM. Predialysis psychoeducational intervention extends survival in CKD: a 20-year follow-up. Am J Kidney Dis. 2005;46(6):1088–98.
14. Devins GM, Mendelssohn DC, Barre PE, Binik YM. Predialysis psychoeducational intervention and coping styles influence time to dialysis in chronic kidney disease. Am J Kidney Dis. 2003;42(4):693–703.
15. Devins GM, Hollomby DJ, Barre PE, et al. Long-term knowledge retention following predialysis psychoeducational intervention. Nephron. 2000;86(2):129–34.
16. Mehrotra R, Marsh D, Vonesh E, Peters V, Nissenson A. Patient education and access of ESRD patients to renal replacement therapies beyond in-center hemodialysis. Kidney Int. 2005;68(1):378–90.
17. Kutner NG, Zhang R, Huang Y, Wasse H. Patient awareness and initiation of peritoneal dialysis. Arch Intern Med. 2011;171(2):119–24.
18. National Institutes of Health N. USRDS 2010 Annual data report: atlas of chronic kidney disease and end-stage renal disease in the United States. United States Renal Data System 2011; Available at: URL: http://www.usrds.org/adr.htm. Accessed 20 Jun 2011.
19. Chaudhary K, Sangha H, Khanna R. Peritoneal dialysis first: rationale. Clin J Am Soc Nephrol. 2011;6(2): 447–56.
20. Khawar O, Kalantar-Zadeh K, Lo WK, Johnson D, Mehrotra R. Is the declining use of long-term peritoneal dialysis justified by outcome data? Clin J Am Soc Nephrol. 2007;2(6):1317–28.
21. McDonald SP, Marshall MR, Johnson DW, Polkinghorne KR. Relationship between dialysis modality and mortality. J Am Soc Nephrol. 2009;20(1):155–63.
22. Mehrotra R, Chiu YW, Kalantar-Zadeh K, Bargman J, Vonesh E. Similar outcomes with hemodialysis and peritoneal dialysis in patients with end-stage renal disease. Arch Intern Med. 2011;171(2):110–8.
23. Weinhandl ED, Foley RN, Gilbertson DT, Arneson TJ, Snyder JJ, Collins AJ. Propensity-matched mortality comparison of incident hemodialysis and peritoneal dialysis patients. J Am Soc Nephrol. 2010;21(3):499–506.
24. Bugeja A, Dacouris N, Thomas A, et al. In-center nocturnal hemodialysis: another option in the management

of chronic kidney disease. Clin J Am Soc Nephrol. 2009;4(4):778–83.
25. Troidle L, Hotchkiss M, Finkelstein F. A thrice weekly in-center nocturnal hemodialysis program. Adv Chronic Kidney Dis. 2007;14(3):244–8.
26. Saran R, Bragg-Gresham JL, Levin NW, et al. Longer treatment time and slower ultrafiltration in hemodialysis: associations with reduced mortality in the DOPPS. Kidney Int. 2006;69(7):1222–8.
27. Culleton BF, Walsh M, Klarenbach SW, et al. Effect of frequent nocturnal hemodialysis vs conventional hemodialysis on left ventricular mass and quality of life: a randomized controlled trial. JAMA. 2007;298(11):1291–9.
28. Chertow GM, Levin NW, Beck GJ, et al. In-center hemodialysis six times per week versus three times per week. N Engl J Med. 2010;363(24):2287–300.
29. Lynch JR, Wasse H, Armistead NC, McClellan WM. Achieving the goal of the fistula first breakthrough initiative for prevalent maintenance hemodialysis patients. Am J Kidney Dis. 2011;57(1):78–89.
30. Collins AJ, Foley RN, Gilbertson DT, Chen SC. The state of chronic kidney disease, ESRD, and morbidity and mortality in the first year of dialysis. Clin J Am Soc Nephrol. 2009;4 Suppl 1:S5–11.
31. Centers for Disease Control. Vital signs: central line-associated blood streem infections–United States, 2001, 2008, and 2009. MMWR Morb Mortal Wkly Rep. 2010;60:1–6.
32. Klevens RM, Edwards JR, Andrus ML, Peterson KD, Dudeck MA, Horan TC. Dialysis surveillance report: national healthcare safety network (NHSN)-data summary for 2006. Semin Dial. 2008;21(1):24–8.
33. Astor BC, Eustace JA, Powe NR, Klag MJ, Fink NE, Coresh J. Type of vascular access and survival among incident hemodialysis patients: the choices for healthy outcomes in caring for ESRD (CHOICE) study. J Am Soc Nephrol. 2005;16(5):1449–55.
34. Wright AA, Zhang B, Ray A, et al. Associations between end-of-life discussions, patient mental health, medical care near death, and caregiver bereavement adjustment. JAMA. 2008;300(14):1665–73.
35. Zhang B, Wright AA, Huskamp HA, et al. Health care costs in the last week of life: associations with end-of-life conversations. Arch Intern Med. 2009;169(5): 480–8.
36. Kurella TM, Cohen LM. Should there be an expanded role for palliative care in end-stage renal disease? Curr Opin Nephrol Hypertens. 2010;19(6): 556–60.
37. Chambers E, Gemain M, Brown E. Supportive and palliative care for renal patients. 2nd ed. Oxford: Oxford University Press; 2010.
38. Kurella TM, Covinsky KE, Chertow GM, Yaffe K, Landefeld CS, McCulloch CE. Functional status of elderly adults before and after initiation of dialysis. N Engl J Med. 2009;361(16):1539–47.
39. Murtagh FE, Marsh JE, Donohoe P, Ekbal NJ, Sheerin NS, Harris FE. Dialysis or not? A comparative survival study of patients over 75 years with chronic kidney disease stage 5. Nephrol Dial Transplant. 2007;22(7):1955–62.
40. Carson RC, Juszczak M, Davenport A, Burns A. Is maximum conservative management an equivalent treatment option to dialysis for elderly patients with significant comorbid disease? Clin J Am Soc Nephrol. 2009;4(10):1611–9.
41. Cohen LM, Ruthazer R, Moss AH, Germain MJ. Predicting six-month mortality for patients who are on maintenance hemodialysis. Clin J Am Soc Nephrol. 2010;5(1):72–9.
42. Couchoud C, Labeeuw M, Moranne O, et al. A clinical score to predict 6-month prognosis in elderly patients starting dialysis for end-stage renal disease. Nephrol Dial Transplant. 2009;24(5):1553–61.

31 Hemodialysis: Initiation and Complications

C. John Sperati

Case 1

A 60-year-old man with Stage V chronic kidney disease due to biopsy-proven diabetic and hypertensive nephropathy presents to clinic for a routine visit. His estimated glomerular filtration rate is 10 ml/min/1.73 m^2 and his blood pressure is 145/80 mmHg. Laboratory studies demonstrate potassium 4.9 mEq/L, total CO_2 19 mEq/L, phosphorus 5.0 mg/dL, and hemoglobin 10.5 g/dL. He feels well without weight loss, anorexia, or nausea. He is reluctant to have an arteriovenous fistula placed, and he does not wish to initiate hemodialysis. The patient desires to know the optimal time to initiate dialysis. If he requires dialysis initiation through a tunneled dialysis catheter, what measures can be taken to reduce his risk for catheter infection?

Case 2

A 24-year-old woman is intubated and mechanically ventilated for acute respiratory distress syndrome in the setting of ethylene glycol ingestion. She is hypotensive despite crystalloid resuscitation and the use of three intravenous vasopressors. Laboratory studies demonstrate acute kidney injury with serum creatinine 3.2 mg/dL, BUN 56 mg/dL, potassium 4.5 mEq/L, total CO_2 8 mEq/L, arterial pH 7.05, and her urine output has been 5 ml/h for the past 6 h. What is the optimal use of dialysis in the management of poisonings? Does dialysis dose impact patient outcome in acute kidney injury?

Overview

The principle of dialysis is attributed to the laboratory work of Scottish scientist Thomas Graham in 1861. Research over the ensuing years led to Georg Haas performing the first human hemodialysis (HD) in 1924 and culminated in the first clinically feasible human HD utilizing a rotating drum dialyzer by Willem Kolff in Nazi occupied Netherlands in 1943. Dr. Kolff's first patient, 29-year-old Janny Schrijver, was dialyzed 12 times, and in Dr. Kolff's words, "the last time I had to give up because there was no good vascular access anymore and she died." The ensuing 70 years have seen the development of compact portable dialysis machines and vascular access devices that permit the continuation of life-sustaining HD for many years. While the technology has matured, the principles and indications for dialysis remain fundamentally unchanged. Major challenges today focus on timing of initiation, optimal dosing, and further reducing the rate of complications.

C.J. Sperati, M.D., M.H.S. (✉)
Department of Medicine, Division of Nephrology, Johns Hopkins University School of Medicine,
1830 East Monument Street, Room 416, Baltimore, MD 21205, USA
e-mail: jsperati@jhmi.edu

E.V. Lerma and M. Rosner (eds.), *Clinical Decisions in Nephrology, Hypertension and Kidney Transplantation*,
DOI 10.1007/978-1-4614-4454-1_31, © Springer Science+Business Media New York 2013

Epidemiology

The incidence of acute kidney injury (AKI) is estimated at 200–500 per 100,000 persons annually, and approximately 20–30 per 100,000 cases of AKI require dialysis [1–3]. A large multinational observational study suggested approximately 13% of individuals with AKI requiring dialysis remained dialysis-dependent at hospital discharge [4]. In the USA, 379 per million men (58,130) developed end-stage renal disease (ESRD) and initiated long-term HD in 2008, as did 285 per million women (44,742) [5]. Hemodialysis is the most common modality, representing 94% of new dialysis starts as compared to 6% employing peritoneal dialysis. Annual mortality in patients with ESRD receiving HD remains high at 18.7% (20.3% in Whites versus 16.6% in African-Americans). Older individuals and those with diabetes have higher rates of death, and HD services for the ESRD population total $77,506 per person per year contributing to a total expenditure of 23 billion dollars per year for the US ESRD program. Presently, 99.5% of HD is provided thrice weekly in-center, with the remaining small proportion delivered via home HD. Home HD options include thrice weekly HD, short daily HD, and nocturnal HD via a small, portable machine operated by the patient. Despite numerous small studies suggesting clinical and psychosocial advantages to home HD, a mortality advantage of this modality has yet to be conclusively demonstrated [6]. Presently, bioartificial and wearable artificial kidneys for the real-time, ambulatory provision of HD are an area of active research. While proof-of-concept trials have demonstrated small-scale feasibility of the technologies, they are unlikely to be a clinical option in the care of ESRD patients for many more years [7].

Physiology and Technology of Hemodialysis

Hemodialysis technology has progressed from the original rotating drum dialyzers utilizing cellophane tubing to modern machines employing hollow fiber biocompatible synthetic membranes. Operating on the principle of countercurrent flow, blood moves through hollow fiber channels while fresh dialysate (Table 31.1) flows in the opposing direction along the outside of the fibers (Fig. 31.1). High efficiency (i.e., large surface area, defined by term *KoA* >700 ml/min) filters permit rapid dialysis of small molecules, while high flux filters (i.e., large pore filters, defined by term K_{UF} > 10–20 ml/min/mmHg) enable larger molecular weight molecules to be cleared via solvent drag during ultrafiltration (UF). The application of a pressure across the dialysis membrane from the blood to the dialysate compartment permits UF—the removal of water and isotonic solute. The rate of UF (ml/min) is determined by the K_{UF} × transmembrane pressure. As noted, larger molecules will be cleared via solvent drag, and smaller solutes will be cleared at an amount approximately equal to the concentration in plasma. Isolated UF can be performed by simply not perfusing the filter with dialysate.

Table 31.1 Typical dialysate composition for intermittent HD (IHD) and continuous venovenous HD (CVVHD)

Solute	IHD (mEq/L)	CVVHD (mEq/L)
Na	130–145	140
K	0–4	0–4
Cl	105	109.5
HCO_3	20–45	32
Acetate	4	–
Lactate	–	3
Ca	0–3	0 or 3.5
Mg	0.75	1
Glucose	200 mg/dL	0

For IHD, [Na], [K], and [Ca] can be adjusted according to the clinical requirements. Typical concentrations for a stable patient would be [Na] 138 mEq/L, [K] 2 mEq/L, and [Ca] 2.25 mEq/L. For CVVHD, [K] and [Ca] can be adjusted

The most common measure of dialysis adequacy is the dimensionless term *Kt*/*V*, where *K* = dialyzer urea clearance (ml/min), *t* = time, and *V* = urea volume of distribution. This term represents the number of times the urea volume of distribution has been processed through the dialyzer, and a minimum achieved value of 1.2 three times a week is the standard for outpatient in-center

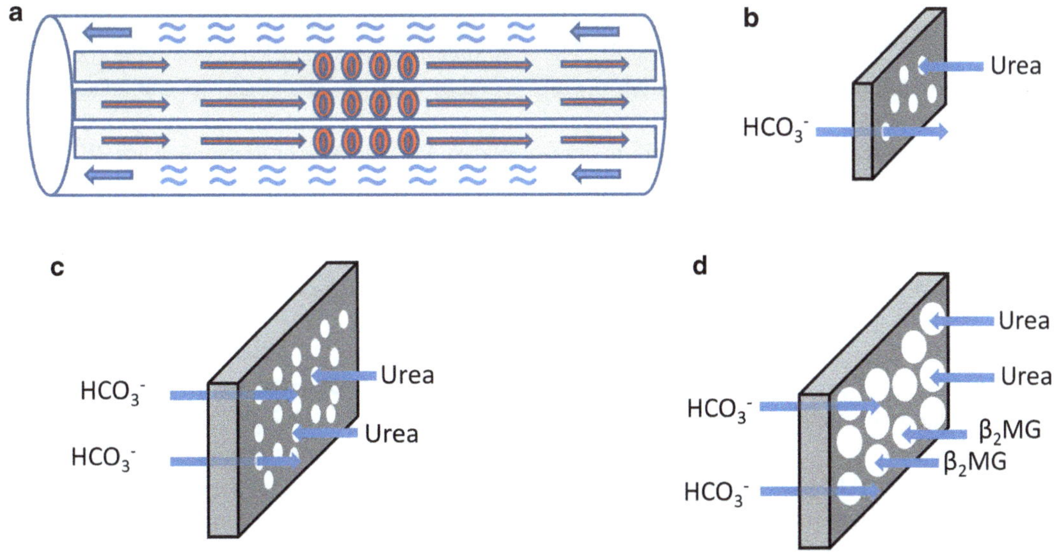

Fig. 31.1 Dialysis membrane surface area and flux. (**a**) Fresh dialysate flows in a countercurrent direction to blood to maximize the dialytic gradient. (**b**) Low efficiency membranes have less surface area for small molecule diffusion and lower urea clearance (K) as compared to larger surface area, high efficiency membranes (**c**). High efficiency high flux (**d**) membranes have larger pores to facilitate clearance of larger molecular weight molecules such as β_2-microglobulin (β2MG)

HD. As *Kt*/*V* can be greater than 1 yet post-dialysis BUN is never 0, there is inherently recirculation of previously "cleaned" blood through the circuit. Dialysis adequacy can also be quickly estimated via the urea reduction ratio (URR). URR = 1–PostBUN/PreBUN. The relationship between *Kt*/*V* and URR is represented by *Kt*/*V*=−ln(1−URR). Thus, a URR of 0.63 equals a *Kt*/*V* of 1.0, and 0.70 approaches a *Kt*/*V* of 1.2. Urea is generated and subsequently cleared while the patient is on dialysis, and a quantity of urea is removed without a change in blood concentration when UF is performed. As such, a more accurate bedside estimation of *Kt*/*V* requires accounting for this intradialytic urea generation and additional removal via UF. In this regard, *Kt*/*V* can be better estimated by

$$\frac{Kt}{V} = -\ln\left(\frac{\text{postBUN}}{\text{preBUN}} - 0.008t\right) + \left(4 - 3.5\frac{\text{postBUN}}{\text{preBUN}}\right) \times \left(0.55\frac{\text{UF}}{V}\right), \text{ where}$$

$$t = \text{length in hours, UF} = \text{ ultrafiltration volume, } V = \text{ post - HD urea distribution volume}$$

Lastly, the use of even more precise yet computationally more complex urea kinetic modeling is feasible for automated, outpatient monitoring systems but is rarely used at the bedside.

Faster blood flow (e.g., >350 ml/min) and high efficiency filters permit greater urea and small molecule clearance, while longer duration sessions enable better clearance of larger molecular weight molecules and substances largely restricted to the intracellular space. As hemoglobin increases and relative proportion of blood water decreases, intracellular substances such as phosphorus and creatinine experience a greater drop in clearance per time than urea. Longer treatment sessions may be required to achieve required metabolic control, despite otherwise seemingly adequate *Kt*/*V*. Dialysate flow rate also enhances clearance, although the incremental benefit is small at rates >600 ml/min. Residual renal function (K_{ru}) is often small in patients on HD, but it will nonetheless contribute to adequacy goals in patients with ≥2 ml/min/1.73 m^2, and this can be quantitated via timed urine collection [8]. The use of high efficiency, high flux filters with blood flow rates of 350–500 ml/min and dialysate flow rates of 600–800 ml/min is commonplace in most modern dialysis prescriptions. Treatment length must be individualized to the patient, although sessions shorter than 3.5 h thrice weekly are unlikely to achieve adequate solute control. Obese patients will typically require sessions ≥4 h for adequate clearance, as will patients with β_2-microglobulin amyloidosis or inadequate phosphate control.

In patients with AKI or ESRD without a permanent arteriovenous (AV) access, initiation of timely dialysis requires the use of tunneled or non-tunneled catheters. Only tunneled catheters should be used in the outpatient setting due to the lower risk of infection as compared to non-tunneled devices. The internal jugular veins are the preferred access site, followed by femoral veins. The subclavian veins and peripherally inserted central catheters should be avoided due to a higher incidence of vascular stenosis that may preclude future AV access creation. In patients with CKD, consideration to permanent AV access creation in the nondominant arm should be made at eGFR <20 ml/min/1.73 m^2. The exact timing of surgery is dependent upon the rate at which kidney function is declining. At that time, the nondominant arm should no longer be used for blood pressure measurements or phlebotomy to minimize the risk for venous injury. Arteriovenous fistulas (AVF) are the preferred access, due to higher patency and lower infection rates than arteriovenous grafts (AVG). An AVF should be created at least 3–4 months prior to intended use, as maturation of the access often requires 8–12 weeks. Initial cannulation attempts of an AVF in a patient with a dialysis catheter typically involve arterial cannulation only, with venous return via the catheter for the first several treatments. Should an arterial needle become dislodged, the resultant hematoma will be smaller than that resulting from dislodgement of a venous needle returning blood under positive pressure. Initial cannulation should utilize 17 gauge needles until adequacy of the AVF is demonstrated, with arterial pump pressure maintained above −250 mmHg. A graft utilizing a tunneled polytetrafluoroethylene conduit is acceptable when vascular anatomy will not permit AVF creation, and an AVG should be placed 4–6 weeks prior to intended use. With good surgical healing and resolution of edema, an AVG can potentially be cannulated in as little as 2 weeks. Unfortunately, approximately 50% of AVG are no longer patent at 2 years.

Indications for Hemodialysis

Hemodialysis is most commonly initiated for the management of acid–base disorders, electrolyte abnormalities, poisoning by dialyzable substances, volume overload, and uremia. While generally accurate, these simplified indications fail to identify which patients actually require renal replacement therapy and provide no guidance on how best to deliver it. To lower the risk for acute complications with dialysis initiation, three sessions are typically performed on consecutive days, with the first two sessions utilizing low efficiency filters and/or slower blood flows for shorter treatment times. A representative dialysis prescription is shown in Fig. 31.2.

Acid–Base Disturbance

Metabolic acidemia is the most common acid–base disturbance resulting in HD initiation, although no solid data exist identifying an absolute pH at which HD is indicated. As HD corrects acidemia predominately through the delivery of bicarbonate, its use is fundamentally similar to an intravenous infusion of alkali. Many authorities would administer alkali or consider HD, if otherwise indicated, for arterial pH <7.2, although significant controversy exists. A recent survey indicated 35% of intensivists required pH <7.0 prior to administering alkali, as compared to only 6% of nephrologists [9]. While correction of non-anion gap acidosis is less contentious, the use of sodium bicarbonate in the management of lactic acidosis is associated with poorer outcomes [10–12]. The effect of dialysis on patient mortality initiated solely for pH management in association

HD Session	*Dialyzer*	*Blood Flow Rate (ml/min)*	*Dialysate Flow Rate (ml/min)*	*Dialysis Time (hours)*	*Frequency*
First	*Low efficiency*	*200*	*≥ 600*	*2*	
Second	*High efficiency*	*250*	*≥ 600*	*2.5*	*Performed over 3 consecutive days*
Third	*High efficiency*	*300*	*≥ 600*	*3*	
Fourth +	*High efficiency*	*350 - 500*	*≥ 600*	*3.5 +*	*Thrice weekly or as indicated*

Plasma (mEq/L)	*Dialysate (mEq/L)*
Sodium	*138* or *within 10 – 15 mEq if plasma <128*
*Potassium**	
≥6	*1* or 0 *with caution*
4 - 6	*2*
3.5 – 3.9	*3*
≤3.4	*4*
Bicarbonate	*20 – 45 based on total CO_2 and pH (if known)*

UF: *Volume should be based on interdialytic weight gain and fluid removal goals. UF rates should typically be kept <1400 ml/min to minimize risk of hypotension and muscle cramping. Treatment times can be extended, either with or without dialysis, to maintain acceptable UF rates.*

Hypotension: *Decrease or stop UF. Evaluate for medical emergency or dialysis-associated complication. Normal saline bolus 250cc can be administered if no contraindication. Consider cooling dialysate (35°C) or use of sodium modeling.*

Filter clotting: *If no contraindication to use of heparin, administer 30 units/kg bolus into the venous limb of the access 5 minutes prior to start of treatment. Another 20 units/kg should then be infused over the course of the treatment, divided into an equal hourly rate. The heparin infusion should be discontinued 30 minutes prior to the end of the HD session.*

AV fistula cannulation: *The first several cannulation attempts should utilize 17 gauge needles by an experienced provider. If a catheter is present, arterial cannulation can be performed with venous return via the catheter until the suitability of the access has been demonstrated. Blood flow should be limited to 200 – 250 ml/m in through small needles with arterial pump pressure maintained above -250 mmHg. Needle size should be progressively increased to 14 – 15 gauge as permitted by the access. An AV fistula often requires 8 – 12 weeks for full maturation, while an AVG can typically be cannulated in 2 – 4 weeks.*

Fig. 31.2 Typical intermittent HD prescription

with lactic acidosis is unknown. Caution is warranted in this setting, although HD can be preferable to a continuous bicarbonate infusion to minimize the potential complications of hypernatremia and volume overload. Nevertheless, most authorities would not initiate HD solely for acidemia unless respiratory fatigue is impending or other indications for acute HD exist.

Electrolyte Disorders

Electrolyte disorders—in particular hyperkalemia—are common indications for HD. The decision to initiate HD must include consideration of the severity of hyperkalemia, feasibility of medical management, and presence of other indications for dialysis. Severe hyperkalemia >6.9 mEq/L is an indication for HD if timely pharmacologic control is not

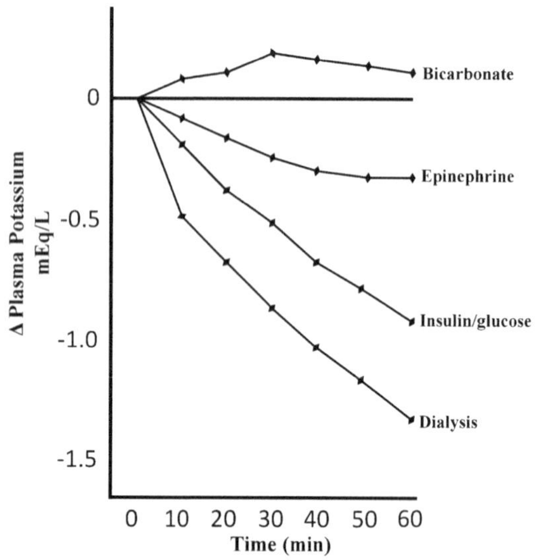

Fig. 31.3 Changes in plasma potassium (mEq/L) during intravenous infusion of 8.4% bicarbonate, epinephrine, insulin + glucose, and HD. Reprinted from Am J Med, 85(4), Blumberg A, et al. Effect of various therapeutic approaches on plasma potassium and major regulating factors in terminal renal failure, 507–512, Copyright 1988, with permission from Elsevier

possible or if QRS prolongation is present. Less severe hyperkalemia is also an indication for HD in the presence of ECG changes, and HD is the preferred intervention for hyperkalemia in the ESRD patient with a functioning HD access. In patients with nonoliguric AKI and hyperkalemia <7.0 without ECG changes, medical management may be feasible if other indications for HD are not present. HD is the most effective intervention for hyperkalemia, typically lowering potassium approximately 1 mEq/L in an hour (Fig. 31.3). The actual quantity removed, however, is highly dependent upon blood flow, dialyzer surface area, and dialysate potassium concentration. Dialysate potassium <2 mEq/L is a risk factor for fatal arrhythmia, particularly in patients on digoxin, and low potassium dialysate should be used only for life-threatening hyperkalemia. When utilizing low potassium dialysate, plasma potassium should be measured every 30 min until <5.0 mEq/L, at which time dialysate potassium should be increased to 2–3 mEq/L. Dialysis against a relatively hypernatremic dialysate will worsen hyperkalemia due to transcellular shifting of potassium into blood, while higher bicarbonate dialysate will result in hypokalemia due to alkalosis-induced uptake of potassium into cells [13, 14]. As the gradient for dialysis is greatest in the first hour, the hypokalemic effects of progressive alkalinization do not markedly lower the total quantity of potassium removed. It does, however, contribute to the rebound in blood potassium concentration that develops in the hours following HD. This rebound hyperkalemia may warrant additional medical and/or dialytic therapy, and follow-up blood work should be obtained 4 h after dialysis. In the management of life-threatening hyperkalemia, dialysis utilizing a large surface area filter, maximized blood flow rate, and an isonatremic dialysate with bicarbonate concentration 25 mEq/L is a reasonable prescription.

In addition, HD is commonly used to manage hyperphosphatemia of ESRD, and acute hyperphosphatemia with neuromuscular compromise is an indication for emergent HD. Phosphorus is predominately restricted to the intracellular and bony compartments, with <1% of total body phosphorus present in plasma. Thus, while phosphorus is easily dialyzable, long or frequent HD sessions are required to remove a substantial quantity of phosphorus. Approximately 800–1,000 mg of phosphorus is removed with a 3–4 h HD session, representing the approximate daily intake and roughly 10–12% of total body phosphorus. Severe hyperphosphatemia >14 mg/dL can result in respiratory paralysis and is an indication for renal replacement therapy in the presence of symptoms. Since blood phosphorus is lowered more rapidly by HD, it is appropriate to first initiate HD in the hemodynamically stable patient with life-threatening hyperphosphatemia and to then switch to continuous renal replacement therapy (CRRT) for ongoing removal of total body phosphorus to minimize rebound.

Less commonly, HD may be utilized in the management of hypercalcemia, hypermagnesemia, and marked hypo- or hypernatremia associated with volume overload. For dysnatremias, attention to the dialysate sodium concentration is necessary to avoid overly rapid correction of the sodium concentration. Calculating the necessary dialysate sodium concentration, however, is rather difficult due to constant changes in plasma water concentration as dialysis progresses. Roughly, a dialysate sodium concentration 1.02 times greater than plasma sodium concentration is at equilibrium with plasma [15, 16]. The dialysate sodium ideally should be adjusted within 10 mEq/L of this equilibrium for a typical 4 h treatment. In the setting of normal renal function, hypercalcemia and hypermagnesemia can often be managed with medical interventions. With impaired renal function and cardiovascular instability, HD with real-time electrocardiographic monitoring is an effective intervention. Low calcium dialysate containing 0, 1, or 2 mmol/L of calcium can be used with measurement of ionized calcium every 30–60 min. In one study, zero calcium dialysate lowered ionized calcium from approximately 1.44 to 0.99 mmol/L over 3 h [17]. In patients with combined hyperkalemia and hypercalcemia, the potassium should be addressed first to minimize potential myocardial instability from a rapidly falling calcium.

Poisoning

Since its introduction, HD has been a valuable although rarely needed tool in the management of poisoning. Of 2,479,355 poisonings reported to the American Association of Poison Control Centers in 2009, only 2,210 were treated with HD or hemoperfusion [18]. HD effectively removes organic acids and water soluble toxins <500 Da that have a small volume of distribution (<1 L/kg) and little protein binding. If kidney function is normal and severe metabolic consequences (e.g., pH<7.2) are not present, appropriate medical therapy is generally sufficient. In the setting of impaired renal function or significant end-organ toxicity, HD utilizing a high-efficiency, high-flux filter and blood flow >400 ml/min is appropriate for dialyzable toxins (Table 31.2) [19]. For some substances such as lithium, blood levels can rebound after HD into the toxic range as diffusion from the intracellular to the extracellular space occurs. For this, CRRT is a useful adjunct following initial stabilization by HD [20]. HD has also proven quite effective in the management of hyperammonemia due to inborn errors of metabolism, hepatic failure, and valproic acid poisoning. For poisoning by highly protein bound substances (e.g., digoxin, acetaminophen), hemoperfusion offers a theoretical advantage over supportive care, although the technology is not commonly available and no strong data exist to demonstrate clinical superiority [21].

Table 31.2 Commonly encountered dialyzable toxins

Lithium	Valproic acid
Ethylene glycol	Metformin
Methanol	Theophylline
Isopropanol	Carbamazepine
Ethanol	Barbiturates
Salicylates	

Volume Overload

As diuretics are potent activators of the renin–angiotensin–aldosterone system (RAAS), there is strong interest in the use of extracorporeal therapies in the management of cardiorenal syndromes. Heart failure is characterized by combined sodium and water overload, although loop diuretics generate a hypotonic fluid loss. Ultrafiltration removes sodium at an isotonic concentration, thereby avoiding complications of hypernatremia and pharmacologic activation of the RAAS. Although preliminary data support the use of ultrafiltration in the management of cardiorenal syndromes, data from high quality randomized trials demonstrating superiority to the use of diuretics and inotropic agents do not exist [22]. It is reasonable to initiate isolated ultrafiltration (or dialysis if electrolyte abnormalities or uremia coexist) in the management of decompensated heart failure in patients with oliguria. In patients with end-stage liver disease, approximately 1 L of ascites can be mobilized into the plasma space daily [23]. As such, ultrafiltration is more successful at limiting the formation of new ascites than at reducing the volume of existing peritoneal fluid. The use of HD in addition to ultrafiltration is appropriate in the management of hypo- or hypernatremia coexistent with volume overload.

Uremia

The most common indication for HD in the acute and chronic setting is management of the uremic milieu. The presence of uremic pericarditis is a clear indication and typically warrants 14 days of daily HD [24, 25]. For most patients, however, HD is initiated for the constellation of metabolic issues and volume overload typical at low eGFR, without a specific imminently life-threatening abnormality. The major challenges today surround optimal dosing and timing of initiation. Timing of initiation in ESRD has undergone fundamental shifts over the past two decades. From 1996 to 2006, the proportion of individuals initiating HD with an eGFR >10 ml/min/1.73 m^2 increased from 20 to 52%, and the proportion with an eGFR >15 ml/min/1.73 m^2 increased from 4 to 17% [26]. Predicated on the assumption that earlier correction of uremia would lessen complications of chronic kidney disease, earlier initiation of HD gained popularity. Recent studies, however, have questioned this practice. Data from the Initiating Dialysis Early and Late (IDEAL) study demonstrated no survival benefit to initiating dialysis with an eGFR >10–14 ml/min/1.73 m^2. Additionally, observational studies have suggested that mortality may actually be increased with dialysis initiation at higher eGFR, although concerns for residual confounding in these cohorts exist [26–28]. At a minimum, the costs of earlier initiation may be greater than delaying until eGFR is <10 ml/min/1.73 m^2 [29]. While the optimal eGFR at which to initiate dialysis is not known, it is reasonable to delay initiation until eGFR is <10 ml/min/1.73 m^2 provided effective medical management of the complications of CKD is feasible.

Similarly, the trend toward earlier initiation of outpatient HD has been mirrored by many authorities advocating early (BUN <76 mg/dL generally considered "early") initiation of HD for inpatients with AKI. Numerous studies of dialysis in AKI have failed to identify an optimal indicator for initiation, although avoiding complications of AKI such as volume overload may portend a survival advantage [30–33]. The advantages and disadvantages of timing of initiation need to be weighed carefully given the absence of outcome data, although if recovery of renal function is deemed unlikely, it may be preferable to initiate HD earlier and in a non-emergent fashion. The use of CRRT vs. HD is guided by the hemodynamics and clearance needs of the patient, as there are no data to support superiority of one modality over the other. In both chronic and acute HD, conflicting evidence exists as to the benefit of biocompatible membranes versus older generation cellulose-based filters. As outcomes may be superior and the likelihood of dialyzer reactions are less with biocompatible synthetic membranes, the use of biocompatible filters is generally preferred.

Once initiated, the delivered dose of dialysis does impact outcome. Based on data from multiple randomized controlled trials, patients dialyzed for AKI on a typical schedule of three sessions per week should receive a minimum *Kt/V* of 1.2 per session. As clinical circumstances may dictate changes to the dialysis schedule, the concept of a standard weekly *Kt/V* can be used to ensure adequate dialysis delivery in the course of a week (Fig. 31.4). A standard weekly *Kt/V* of 2.0 should be targeted through the proper combination of dialysis frequency and duration. For patients receiving CRRT the minimum delivered dose is 20 ml per kg body weight per hour, with little evidence that more intensive dialysis is beneficial [34–38]. For outpatient ESRD therapy, the minimum delivered *Kt/V* is 1.2 three times a week, with evidence that women may have even lower mortality when dialyzed to a minimum *Kt/V* 1.65 (Table 31.3) [39–42]. Patients on dialysis for more than 3 years and those with dialysis-associated amyloidosis may have additional benefit from high flux filters. Similarly, filters with hydrophobic domains adsorb plasma proteins and may contribute to increased clearance of larger molecular weight proteins.

Complications of Hemodialysis

Hemodialysis is a remarkably well-tolerated procedure, although complications are common and potentially fatal (Table 31.4). Most patients on HD report quality of life limitations, with over 80% reporting fatigue [43]. Muscle cramping is

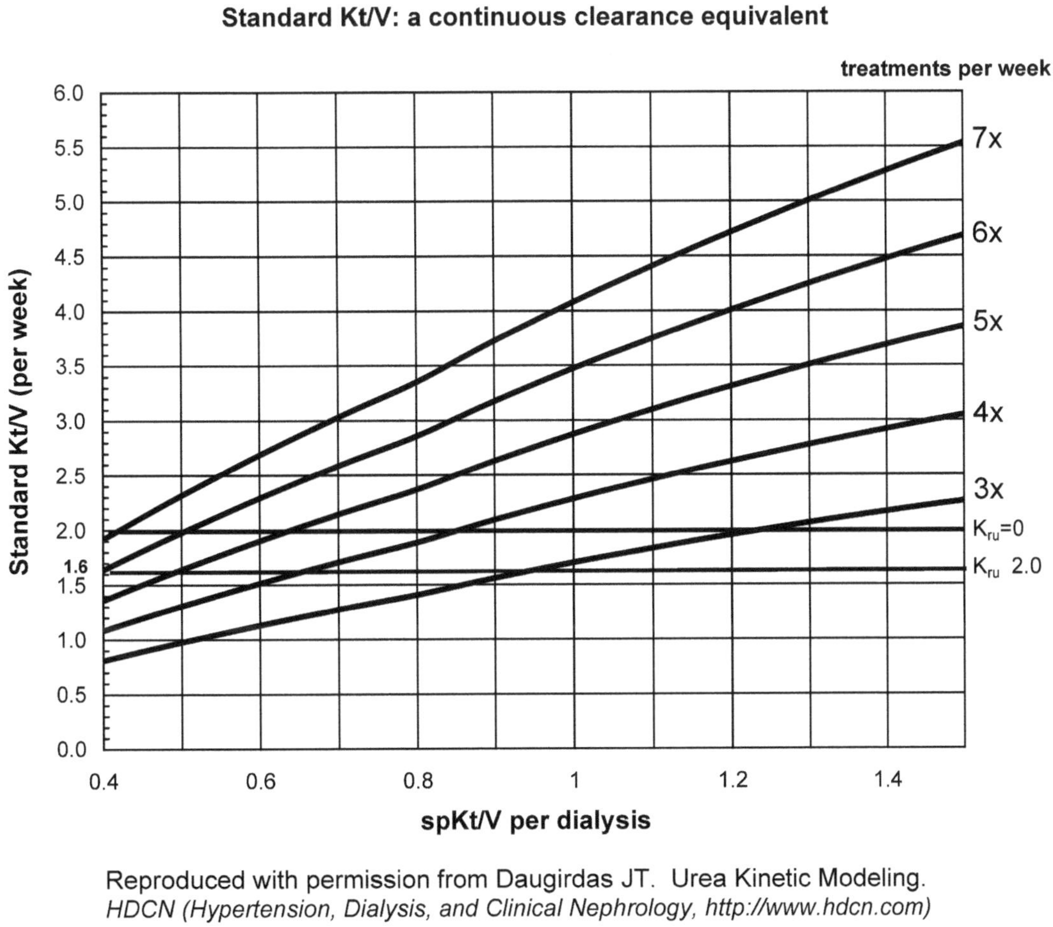

Fig. 31.4 The weekly standard *Kt*/*V* can be determined by plotting the per treatment single pool *Kt*/*V* along the curve representing the number of treatments per week. A standard *Kt*/*V* of 2.0 can be obtained through various combinations of HD frequency and intensity. A standard *Kt*/*V* of 2.0 can be achieved in a patient with residual urea clearance (Kru) of 2 ml/min by plotting the intersection of desired treatment curve with Kru = 2.0. Reproduced with permission from Daugirdas JT. Urea Kinetic Modeling. http://www.hdcn.com

frequent and improves with saline bolus and higher calcium dialysate.

Dialysis Disequilibrium Syndrome and Dialyzer Reactions

Dialysis disequilibrium syndrome (DES) is a morbid and potentially fatal complication resulting in acute cerebral edema and characterized by nausea, vomiting, headache, confusion, and seizure. DES is believed to result from the rapid drop in blood osmolality with dialysis initiation, resulting in intracellular movement of water along osmolal gradients. Changes in intracellular brain pH and rapid decline in blood sodium concentration have also been implicated [44, 45]. This syndrome is most common in patients with high solute burden (e.g., acute kidney failure) dialyzed for the first time. DES can be avoided through the use of small surface area filters (i.e., low efficiency filters), short treatment times, and slow blood flow rates for the first several HD sessions (Fig. 31.2). A common starting prescription is dialysis utilizing a low efficiency filter for 2 h at blood flow 200 ml/min. Mild symptoms can be managed with a further reduction in blood flow. For more severely symptomatic patients, dialysis

Table 31.3 Strategies to increase *Kt*/*V*

• Use higher efficiency filter
• Minimize dialyzer reuse
• Preferentially utilize AV fistula or graft rather than double-lumen HD catheters
• Ensure tips of cannulation needles are at least 3 in. apart to minimize recirculation
• Achieve minimum blood flows of 350 ml/min and preferably 400–500 ml/min
– Utilize 14–15 gauge needles
– Assess for access stenosis, catheter thrombosis, and/or central stenosis if blood flow target unobtainable
• Evaluate for access dysfunction
– Measure access recirculation (>10% via urea-based method is abnormal)
– Replace or repair HD catheters running "in reverse"
• Utilize anticoagulation if necessary to prevent filter clotting
• Maintain dialysate flow rates of 600–800 ml/min
• Increase treatment time
– Ensure treatment starts and ends on time
– Assess for treatment interruptions (e.g., clotted circuit)
– Increase length of treatment

Table 31.4 Complications of hemodialysis

Dialysis disequilibrium syndrome	Catheter-associated clot
Hypotension	Bleeding/Heparin-induced thrombocytopenia
Infection	Dialyzer reaction
Muscle cramping	Arrhythmia/sudden cardiac death
Fatigue	Electrolyte imbalance
Nausea and vomiting	Hypertension due to removal of dialyzable anti-hypertensives
Headache	Air embolism
AV fistula/graft hematoma or thrombosis	Hemolysis
Filter clotting	Pruritus
Restless legs syndrome	Nutritional deficiencies

should be terminated and hypertonic saline administered for seizures or obtundation. Similarly, cerebral edema is more likely to occur in patients undergoing HD within the first 24 h of stroke or cerebral hemorrhage. These patients should undergo CRRT until the mild increase in intracranial pressure that occurs with intermittent HD is deemed safe.

Allergic reactions to dialysis filters are now uncommon with the use of biocompatible synthetic membranes. The classically described Type A and B reactions are now exceedingly uncommon. Older cellulose and substituted cellulose membranes resulted in Type A reactions in less than 1% of treatments, characterized by onset within minutes of constitutional symptoms, back pain, dyspnea, hypotension, and possibly death. In many cases, these were anaphylactoid reactions to ethylene oxide used for sterilization or to contaminating bacterial peptides. Type B reactions occurred in <5% of treatments and are notable for more mild symptoms within 30 min of dialysis that generally did not require dialysis cessation. For Type A reactions, HD should be terminated and the blood not returned to the patient. For more mild Type B reactions, symptomatic management is usually sufficient. Dialyzer reactions to current generation biocompatible membranes are quite uncommon. Mild Type B reactions are possible, and angiotensin-converting enzyme inhibitors should be avoided with polyacrylonitrile (AN-69) membranes used in some CRRT circuits due to risk for bradykinin-induced hypotension. Thrombocytopenia has also been infrequently reported with modern filters.

Machine-Related Complications

Modern volumetrically controlled HD machines have numerous safety mechanisms to prevent patient injury due to equipment malfunction. Failure of these devices can result in air embolism, inappropriate ultrafiltration resulting in hypotension (risk greater with high flux filters), as well as excessive pump pressures resulting in hemolysis and injury to the AV access.

Failure of the water purification system, the presence of copper, chlorine, or chloramine in the water, and overheating of the dialysate can result in infection or hemolysis (pink tinted effluent). Multiple patients affected simultaneously should prompt immediate concern for water contamination or air embolism from air in the dialysate. The more common etiology of air embolism is a leak in the venous circuit resulting in a foamy appearance to the venous blood. Failure to properly cap a catheter port or the utilization of poor technique when inserting and removing central venous catheters can also lead to air embolism. If a patient should develop chest discomfort, dyspnea, or hypotension suspicious for hemolysis or air embolism, HD should be terminated immediately and blood not returned to the patient. For air embolism, the patient should be positioned supine and slightly on the left side while being administered 100% oxygen. The presence of a right-to-left shunt may result in paradoxical air emboli to the brain with resultant stroke. Patients with large emboli that are not immediately fatal may benefit from hyperbaric oxygen therapy.

Structural defects in the filter can permit direct mixing of dialysate and blood. Filter thrombosis may require the use of unfractionated heparin, and the minimum necessary dose should be used to lessen the bleeding and osteoporosis risk. In patients on CRRT at high risk for bleeding, regional citrate anticoagulation can be used to limit anticoagulation only to the filter. Antibodies to platelet factor 4 may be more common in patients with recurrent filter clotting, and the use of direct thrombin inhibitors may be of utility in this setting [46].

Infection

Access-associated infection remains a major cause of morbidity and mortality in the ESRD population, with catheters posing the greatest risk. Although the proportion of patients receiving an AV fistula as first access is increasing, in 2008 there were 429 per 1,000 HD patients receiving a tunneled dialysis catheter versus 253 receiving an AV fistula or graft [5]. The Centers for Disease Control estimated 37,000 catheter-associated infections occurred in 2008 in outpatient ESRD patients [47]. Incident dialysis patients with catheters are more likely to be admitted to the hospital and to have access-related infections [48]. Strategies to reduce the risk of catheter infection include aggressive efforts to place a permanent access, strict site hygiene, and use of intraluminal antimicrobial lock solutions [49]. Uncomplicated catheter infections can often be managed with antibiotics and catheter exchange over a wire, although more serious infections and those involving *S. aureus* or fungus often warrant catheter removal [50]. Infection of the catheter tunnel generally requires catheter removal in addition to antibiotic therapy.

Hypotension and Arrhythmia

Dialysis-associated hypotension is a multifactorial problem. Proposed etiologies include temporary loss of blood to the extracorporeal circuit, induced intracellular water shifts due to falling blood osmolality, ultrafiltration below dry weight or more rapidly than plasma volume can be refilled, autonomic instability, relative vasopressin deficiency, and mesenteric blood pooling. Provided infection or arrhythmia is not the etiology, the hypotensive patient should be evaluated for hypovolemia and evidence of cardiac tamponade. Slower blood flow rates may contribute to improved hemodynamic stability in some patients. Dialysate can be cooled to 35 °C to increase peripheral vasoconstriction, and sodium modeling can be used to lessen the drop in blood osmolality to minimize intracellular fluid shifts. Dialysate cooling may be contraindicated in patients with markedly impaired cardiac function, and sodium modeling should be avoided in patients with intravascular volume overload due to heart or liver failure. Sodium modeling induces thirst, and limiting the removal of total body sodium is often counterproductive to the management of decompensated heart and liver failure [51, 52]. Newer technologies to limit hypotension include the use of blood temperature monitoring, relative blood volume monitoring, and ultrafiltration profiling, although the efficacy of these techniques remains to be proven on a larger scale. In select patients, the use of midodrine may be beneficial [53]. Albumin administered shortly before HD can sometimes facilitate ultrafiltration in the hospitalized, hypotensive, volume-overloaded patient, although its use is largely nonevidence based.

Furthermore, arrhythmias are common complications of the dialysis treatment. The most common arrhythmia is sinus tachycardia, and while the differential diagnosis is similar to that in nondialyzed patients, it is a common indication of excessive UF or infection. Atrial fibrillation may occur in the absence of demonstrable electrolyte abnormalities and is likely due to an irritable myocardium in the setting of solute and fluid shifts. Ventricular tachycardia and fibrillation are life-threatening, and pre-HD hyperkalemia and the use of low potassium dialysate (<2 mEq/L) and/or low calcium dialysate (<2 mEq/L) are likely risk factors for intradialytic sudden cardiac death. Small intradialytic fluid gains, moderate UF rates, optimal management of interdialytic potassium balance, and avoidance of low potassium and calcium dialysates help ensure hemodynamic stability during HD.

Mechanical Complication of the Dialysis Access

Mechanical complications including thrombosis, aneurysm/pseudoaneurysm formation of the permanent access, and hematoma are unfortunately common. Hypotension, prolonged compression (e.g., body position during surgery, large hematoma), slow blood flow, central stenosis, and hypercoagulable states are risk factors for AVF and AVG thrombosis. AV grafts are particularly prone to thrombosis, with approximately 50% of AVG patent at 2 years. Percutaneous or surgical thrombectomy should be attempted within 24–48 h of AVF thrombosis, while AVG can often be salvaged several weeks after clotting.

Aneurysms of the AVF develop from repeated needle punctures at the same site, and these aneurysms are often more prominent in patients who have lost subcutaneous adipose tissue in the setting of weight loss. Pseudoaneurysms of the AVG develop via a similar mechanism, as repeated needle punctures without adequate site rotation ultimately lead to destruction of the synthetic material. Accesses that have spontaneous or difficult to control bleeding, taut shiny skin with slow to heal puncture scabs, rapid enlargement of the size of the aneurysm/pseudoaneurysm, or a pseudoaneurysm larger than twice the size of the graft should prompt immediate surgical evaluation. Aneurysms of AVF that are larger than twice the size of the fistula typically do not require further evaluation provided additional worrisome signs noted above are absent.

In addition, hematoma formation due to improper cannulation can lead to temporary inability to use the access, as well as pain and discoloring of the skin. Ice packs can be applied in the immediate setting, although quality data support neither ice nor heat in the longer-term management. As noted previously, initial cannulation of AVF should utilize small (17 gauge) needles at slow blood flows to minimize risk for hematoma formation. During HD, the extremity containing the access should remain uncovered at all times to permit rapid detection of accidental needle dislodgement and subsequent hemorrhage.

Quality of Life and Nutrition

Although life sustaining, HD is associated with numerous and potentially debilitating symptoms that impair patients' quality of life. Insomnia, sleep-disordered breathing, and fatigue are present in most patients, and many HD patients spend the interdialytic day recovering from the prior therapy. Uremic pruritus affects approximately 80% of HD patients, and despite the name, it is not limited to patients with inadequate dialysis [54]. Effective therapy is limited by a poor understanding of the mechanisms, although histamine release in the skin, increased interleukin-2 production, and neurotransmission via opioid receptors are believed to be involved [55]. Itching is commonly symmetrical bilaterally, often involves the back, and may progress to visible lesions such as prurigo nodularis. Numerous clinical factors such as failure to achieve adequate Kt/V, increased β_2-microglobulin level, hyperphosphatemia, calcium × phosphorus product >55, increased aluminum levels, hyperparathyroidism, and xerosis have been associated with uremic pruritus. A number of interventions have demonstrated variable efficacy. Careful control of mineral metabolism is mandatory but often fails to fully resolve pruritus, and the use of high flux dialysis membranes and longer treatment times may be helpful. Topical lubricating emollients are safe and may benefit approximately 40–75% of patients, and capsaicin cream 0.025% may be of particular value in patients with prurigo nodularis [56]. Gabapentin administered thrice weekly shows promise, and while ultraviolet-B phototherapy and opioid antagonists may relieve symptoms in a proportion of patients, these interventions are limited by lack of wide-spread availability and difficulty of administration [57].

In addition, a mixed sensorimotor peripheral neuropathy is common in patients with ESRD, although severe motor manifestations are rare. The most common symptom is restless legs syndrome (RLS), with upwards of 50% of HD patients in some studies experiencing lower limb discomfort at rest that is relieved only with movement of the extremities [58]. It may be more common in women, and RLS potentially associates with an increased risk for cardiovascular events. Similar to non-ESRD patients with RLS, correction of iron deficiency may ameliorate symptoms. Moreover, ESRD patients with functional iron deficiency and normal or elevated ferritin levels may benefit from additional intravenous iron administration, although there is a risk for iron overload and the duration of symptom relief may be less than 4 weeks. The use of tricyclic antidepressants, selective serotonin reuptake inhibitors, lithium, and dopamine antagonists may aggravate symptoms, while the use of dopamine agonists may provide some relief. In general, however, the success of pharmacologic therapy is often disappointing [59]. Intensification of the traditional dialysis prescription does not necessarily alleviate symptoms of RLS, but short daily hemodialysis may hold promise and renal transplantation can be an effective intervention for many, but not all, patients [60].

Lastly, water soluble vitamins are lost during dialysis, plasma proteins can adsorb to the filter, and proteins are lost to the effluent with high flux filters. For example, the loss of thiamine may contribute to the development of heart failure and peripheral neuropathy. Patients should take a daily multivitamin (after HD on dialysis days) enriched for water soluble vitamins and ingest adequate daily protein (1.0–1.2 g/kg) to lessen these complications.

Cases Revisited

In past years, many authorities would have recommended dialysis initiation in the patient from Case 1 with diabetes and an eGFR <15 ml/min/1.73 m^2. Given current evidence, however, there is no apparent benefit to initiating HD at an eGFR of 10 ml/min/1.73 m^2 in the absence of medically unmanageable conditions or uremic signs and symptoms. The patient's hyperphosphatemia and metabolic acidosis can be addressed through dietary and pharmacologic intervention. Whether there exists a subset of patients (e.g., persistent hyperphosphatemia despite therapy, declining albumin) that would benefit from earlier dialysis initiation remains to be determined. The most important strategy to limiting catheter infection is the avoidance of catheter use. With meticulous care, catheter infections can be limited to approximately 1 per 1,000 catheter days. The use of antimicrobial lock solutions may further lower this risk.

The patient in Case 2 warrants initiation of CRRT for management of ethylene glycol poisoning complicated by AKI and hemodynamic instability. The presence of impaired kidney function with marked acidemia is an indication for dialysis and removal of ethylene glycol metabolites. Lesser affected patients with preserved kidney function may be successfully treated with fomepizole. The optimal dose of dialysis in organic acid poisonings has not been defined, but based on studies of patients with other etiologies of AKI, the delivered dose should be at least 20 ml/kg/h. As delivered dose is often less than prescribed, a higher prescribed dose with further adjustment based on metabolic need is usually required [61].

References

1. Centers for Disease Control and Prevention (CDC). Hospitalization discharge diagnoses for kidney disease-United States, 1980–2005. MMWR Morb Mortal Wkly Rep. 2005;57:309–12.

2. Waikar SS, Curhan GC, Wald R, McCarthy EP, Chertow GM. Declining mortality in patients with acute renal failure, 1988 to 2002. J Am Soc Nephrol. 2006;17(4):1143–50.
3. Hsu CY, McCulloch CE, Fan D, Ordonez JD, Chertow GM, Go AS. Community-based incidence of acute renal failure. Kidney Int. 2007;72(2):208–12.
4. Uchino S, Kellum JA, Bellomo R, Doig GS, Morimatsu H, Morgera S, Schetz M, Tan I, Bouman C, Macedo E, Gibney N, Tolwani A, Ronco C, Beginning and Ending Supportive Therapy for the Kidney (BEST Kidney) Investigators. Acute renal failure in critically ill patients: a multinational, multicenter study. JAMA. 2005;294(7):813–8.
5. U.S. Renal Data System. USRDS 2010 Annual Data Report: Atlas of Chronic Kidney Disease and End-Stage Renal Disease in the United States, National Institutes of Health, National Institute of Diabetes and Digestive and Kidney Diseases, Bethesda, MD, 2010.
6. The Frequent Hemodialysis Network (FHN) Trial Group, Rocco MV, Lockridge Jr RS, Beck GJ, Eggers PW, Gassman JJ, Greene T, Larive B, Chan CT, Chertow GM, Copland M, Hoy CD, Lindsay RM, Levin NW, Ornt DB, Pierratos A, Pipkin MF, Rajagopalan S, Stokes JB, Unruh ML, Star RA, Kliger AS, Kliger A, Eggers P, Briggs J, Hostetter T, Narva A, Star R, Augustine B, Mohr P, Beck G, Fu Z, Gassman J, Greene T, Daugirdas J, Hunsicker L, Larive B, Li M, Mackrell J, Wiggins K, Sherer S, Weiss B, Rajagopalan S, Sanz J, Dellagrottaglie S, Kariisa M, Tran T, West J, Unruh M, Keene R, Schlarb J, Chan C, McGrath-Chong M, Frome R, Higgins H, Ke S, Mandaci O, Owens C, Snell C, Eknoyan G, Appel L, Cheung A, Derse A, Kramer C, Geller N, Grimm R, Henderson L, Prichard S, Roecker E, Rocco M, Miller B, Riley J, Schuessler R, Lockridge R, Pipkin M, Peterson C, Hoy C, Fensterer A, Steigerwald D, Stokes J, Somers D, Hilkin A, Lilli K, Wallace W, Franzwa B, Waterman E, Chan C, McGrath-Chong M, Copland M, Levin A, Sioson L, Cabezon E, Kwan S, Roger D, Lindsay R, Suri R, Champagne J, Bullas R, Garg A, Mazzorato A, Spanner E, Rocco M, Burkart J, Moossavi S, Mauck V, Kaufman T, Pierratos A, Chan W, Regozo K, Kwok S. The effects of frequent nocturnal home hemodialysis: the Frequent Hemodialysis Network Nocturnal Trial. Kidney Int. 2011;80(10):1080–91.
7. Kim JC, Ronco C. Current technological approaches for a wearable artificial kidney. Contrib Nephrol. 2011;171:231–6.
8. Vilar E, Wellsted D, Chandna SM, Greenwood RN, Farrington K. Residual renal function improves outcome in incremental haemodialysis despite reduced dialysis dose. Nephrol Dial Transplant. 2009;24(8):2502–10.
9. Kraut JA, Kurtz I. Use of base in the treatment of acute severe organic acidosis by nephrologists and critical care physicians: results of an online survey. Clin Exp Nephrol. 2006;10(2):111–7.
10. Graf H, Leach W, Arieff AI. Evidence for a detrimental effect of bicarbonate therapy in hypoxic lactic acidosis. Science. 1985;227(4688):754–6.
11. Sabatini S, Kurtzman NA. Bicarbonate therapy in severe metabolic acidosis. J Am Soc Nephrol. 2009;20(4):692–5.
12. Aschner JL, Poland RL. Sodium bicarbonate: basically useless therapy. Pediatrics. 2008;122(4):831–5.
13. Capdevila M, Ruiz IM, Ferrer C, Monllor F, Ludjvick C, Garcia NH, Juncos LI. The efficiency of potassium removal during bicarbonate hemodialysis. Hemodial Int. 2005;9(3):296–302.
14. Heguilen RM, Sciurano C, Bellusci AD, Fried P, Mittelman G, Rosa Diez G, Bernasconi AR. The faster potassium-lowering effect of high dialysate bicarbonate concentrations in chronic haemodialysis patients. Nephrol Dial Transplant. 2005;20(3):591–7.
15. Nissenson AR, Fine RN, editors. Clinical dialysis. 4th ed. USA: McGraw-Hill Companies, Inc.; 2005.
16. Mann H, Stiller S. Sodium modeling. Kidney Int Suppl. 2000;76:S79–88.
17. Koo WS, Jeon DS, Ahn SJ, Kim YS, Yoon YS, Bang BK. Calcium-free hemodialysis for the management of hypercalcemia. Nephron. 1996;72(3):424–8.
18. Bronstein AC, Spyker DA, Cantilena Jr LR, Green JL, Rumack BH, Giffin SL. 2009 Annual Report of the American Association of Poison Control Centers' National Poison Data System (NPDS): 27th Annual Report. Clin Toxicol (Phila). 2010;48(10):979–1178.
19. Bayliss G. Dialysis in the poisoned patient. Hemodial Int. 2010;14(2):158–67.
20. Meertens JH, Jagernath DR, Eleveld DJ, Zijlstra JG, Franssen CF. Haemodialysis followed by continuous veno-venous haemodiafiltration in lithium intoxication; a model and a case. Eur J Intern Med. 2009;20(3):e70–3.
21. Bismuth C, Conso F, Wattel F, Gosselin B, Lambert H, Genestal M. Coated activated charcoal hemoperfusion: experience of French anti-poison centers about 60 cases. Vet Hum Toxicol. 1979;21(Suppl):2–4.
22. Costanzo MR, Guglin ME, Saltzberg MT, Jessup ML, Bart BA, Teerlink JR, Jaski BE, Fang JC, Feller ED, Haas GJ, Anderson AS, Schollmeyer MP, Sobotka PA, UNLOAD Trial Investigators. Ultrafiltration versus intravenous diuretics for patients hospitalized for acute decompensated heart failure. J Am Coll Cardiol. 2007;49(6):675–83.
23. Pockros PJ, Reynolds TB. Rapid diuresis in patients with ascites from chronic liver disease: the importance of peripheral edema. Gastroenterology. 1986;90(6):1827–33.
24. Alpert MA, Ravenscraft MD. Pericardial involvement in end-stage renal disease. Am J Med Sci. 2003;325(4):228–36.
25. Tseng JR, Lee MJ, Yen KC, Weng CH, Liang CC, Wang IK, Chang CT, Lin-Tan DT, Lin JL, Yen TH. Course and outcome of dialysis pericarditis in diabetic patients treated with maintenance hemodialysis. Kidney Blood Press Res. 2009;32(1):17–23.
26. Rosansky SJ, Eggers P, Jackson K, Glassock R, Clark WF. Early start of hemodialysis may be harmful. Arch Intern Med. 2011;171(5):396–403.
27. Hwang SJ, Yang WC, Lin MY, Mau LW, Chen HC, Taiwan Society of Nephrology. Impact of the clinical

conditions at dialysis initiation on mortality in incident haemodialysis patients: a national cohort study in Taiwan. Nephrol Dial Transplant. 2010;25(8):2616–24.
28. Evans M, Tettamanti G, Nyren O, Bellocco R, Fored CM, Elinder CG. No survival benefit from early-start dialysis in a population-based, inception cohort study of Swedish patients with chronic kidney disease. J Intern Med. 2011;269(3):289–98.
29. Harris A, Cooper BA, Jing J, Bulfone L, Branley P, Collins JF, Craig JC, Fraenkel MB, Johnson DW, Kesselhut J, Luxton G, Pilmore A, Rosevear M, Tiller DJ, Pollock CA, Harris DC. Cost-effectiveness of initiating dialysis early: a randomized controlled trial. Am J Kidney Dis. 2011;57(5):707–15.
30. Bouman CS, Oudemans-Van Straaten HM, Tijssen JG, Zandstra DF, Kesecioglu J. Effects of early high-volume continuous venovenous hemofiltration on survival and recovery of renal function in intensive care patients with acute renal failure: a prospective, randomized trial. Crit Care Med. 2002;30(10):2205–11.
31. Liu KD, Himmelfarb J, Paganini E, Ikizler TA, Soroko SH, Mehta RL, Chertow GM. Timing of initiation of dialysis in critically ill patients with acute kidney injury. Clin J Am Soc Nephrol. 2006;1(5):915–9.
32. Bouchard J, Soroko SB, Chertow GM, Himmelfarb J, Ikizler TA, Paganini EP, Mehta RL, Program to Improve Care in Acute Renal Disease (PICARD) Study Group. Fluid accumulation, survival and recovery of kidney function in critically ill patients with acute kidney injury. Kidney Int. 2009;76(4):422–7.
33. Payen D, de Pont AC, Sakr Y, Spies C, Reinhart K, Vincent JL, Sepsis Occurrence in Acutely Ill Patients (SOAP) Investigators. A positive fluid balance is associated with a worse outcome in patients with acute renal failure. Crit Care. 2008;12(3):R74.
34. Ronco C, Bellomo R, Homel P, Brendolan A, Dan M, Piccinni P, La Greca G. Effects of different doses in continuous veno-venous haemofiltration on outcomes of acute renal failure: a prospective randomised trial. Lancet. 2000;356(9223):26–30.
35. Schiffl H, Lang SM, Fischer R. Daily hemodialysis and the outcome of acute renal failure. N Engl J Med. 2002;346(5):305–10.
36. VA/NIH Acute Renal Failure Trial Network, Palevsky PM, Zhang JH, O'Connor TZ, Chertow GM, Crowley ST, Choudhury D, Finkel K, Kellum JA, Paganini E, Schein RM, Smith MW, Swanson KM, Thompson BT, Vijayan A, Watnick S, Star RA, Peduzzi P. Intensity of renal support in critically ill patients with acute kidney injury. N Engl J Med. 2008;359(1):7–20.
37. Tolwani AJ, Campbell RC, Stofan BS, Lai KR, Oster RA, Wille KM. Standard versus high-dose CVVHDF for ICU-related acute renal failure. J Am Soc Nephrol. 2008;19(6):1233–8.
38. RENAL Replacement Therapy Study Investigators, Bellomo R, Cass A, Cole L, Finfer S, Gallagher M, Lo S, McArthur C, McGuinness S, Myburgh J, Norton R, Scheinkestel C, Su S. Intensity of continuous renal-replacement therapy in critically ill patients. N Engl J Med. 2009;361(17):1627–38.
39. Hemodialysis (HEMO) Study Group, Eknoyan G, Beck GJ, Cheung AK, Daugirdas JT, Greene T, Kusek JW, Allon M, Bailey J, Delmez JA, Depner TA, Dwyer JT, Levey AS, Levin NW, Milford E, Ornt DB, Rocco MV, Schulman G, Schwab SJ, Teehan BP, Toto R. Effect of dialysis dose and membrane flux in maintenance hemodialysis. N Engl J Med. 2002;347(25):2010–9.
40. Depner T, Daugirdas J, Greene T, Allon M, Beck G, Chumlea C, Delmez J, Gotch F, Kusek J, Levin N, Macon E, Milford E, Owen W, Star R, Toto R, Eknoyan G, Hemodialysis Study Group. Dialysis dose and the effect of gender and body size on outcome in the HEMO Study. Kidney Int. 2004;65(4):1386–94.
41. Port FK, Wolfe RA, Hulbert-Shearon TE, McCullough KP, Ashby VB, Held PJ. High dialysis dose is associated with lower mortality among women but not among men. Am J Kidney Dis. 2004;43(6):1014–23.
42. Hemodialysis Adequacy 2006 Work Group. Clinical practice guidelines for hemodialysis adequacy, update 2006. Am J Kidney Dis. 2006;48 Suppl 1:S2–90.
43. Caplin B, Kumar S, Davenport A. Patients' perspective of haemodialysis-associated symptoms. Nephrol Dial Transplant. 2011;26(8):2656–63.
44. Arieff AI. Dialysis disequilibrium syndrome: current concepts on pathogenesis and prevention. Kidney Int. 1994;45(3):629–35.
45. Silver SM, Sterns RH, Halperin ML. Brain swelling after dialysis: old urea or new osmoles? Am J Kidney Dis. 1996;28(1):1–13.
46. Lasocki S, Piednoir P, Ajzenberg N, Geffroy A, Benbara A, Montravers P. Anti-PF4/heparin antibodies associated with repeated hemofiltration-filter clotting: a retrospective study. Crit Care. 2008;12(3):R84.
47. Centers for Disease Control and Prevention (CDC). Vital signs: central line—associated blood stream infections—United States, 2001, 2008, and 2009. MMWR Morb Mortal Wkly Rep. 2011;60(8): 243--248.
48. Ng LJ, Chen F, Pisoni RL, Krishnan M, Mapes D, Keen M, Bradbury BD. Hospitalization risks related to vascular access type among incident US hemodialysis patients. Nephrol Dial Transplant. 2011;26(11):3659–66.
49. Betjes MG. Medscape. Prevention of catheter-related bloodstream infection in patients on hemodialysis. Nat Rev Nephrol. 2011;7(5):257–65.
50. Mermel LA, Allon M, Bouza E, Craven DE, Flynn P, O'Grady NP, Raad II, Rijnders BJ, Sherertz RJ, Warren DK. Clinical practice guidelines for the diagnosis and management of intravascular catheter-related infection: 2009 Update by the Infectious Diseases Society of America. Clin Infect Dis. 2009;49(1):1–45.
51. Dheenan S, Henrich WL. Preventing dialysis hypotension: a comparison of usual protective maneuvers. Kidney Int. 2001;59(3):1175–81.
52. Selby NM, McIntyre CW. A systematic review of the clinical effects of reducing dialysate fluid temperature. Nephrol Dial Transplant. 2006;21(7):1883–98.

53. Prakash S, Garg AX, Heidenheim AP, House AA. Midodrine appears to be safe and effective for dialysis-induced hypotension: a systematic review. Nephrol Dial Transplant. 2004;19(10):2553–8.
54. Mathur VS, Lindberg J, Germain M, Block G, Tumlin J, Smith M, Grewal M, McGuire D, ITCH National Registry Investigators. A longitudinal study of uremic pruritus in hemodialysis patients. Clin J Am Soc Nephrol. 2010;5(8):1410–9.
55. Kuypers DR. Skin problems in chronic kidney disease. Nat Clin Pract Nephrol. 2009;5(3):157–70.
56. Balaskas E, Szepietowski JC, Bessis D, Ioannides D, Ponticelli C, Ghienne C, Taberly A, Dupuy P. Randomized, double-blind study with glycerol and paraffin in uremic xerosis. Clin J Am Soc Nephrol. 2011;6(4):748–52.
57. Gunal AI, Ozalp G, Yoldas TK, Gunal SY, Kirciman E, Celiker H. Gabapentin therapy for pruritus in haemodialysis patients: a randomized, placebo-controlled, double-blind trial. Nephrol Dial Transplant. 2004;19(12):3137–9.
58. Kavanagh D, Siddiqui S, Geddes CC. Restless legs syndrome in patients on dialysis. Am J Kidney Dis. 2004;43(5):763–71.
59. de Oliveira MM, Conti CF, Valbuza JS, de Carvalho LB, do Prado GF. The pharmacological treatment for uremic restless legs syndrome: evidence-based review. Mov Disord. 2010;25(10):1335–42.
60. Jaber BL, Schiller B, Burkart JM, Daoui R, Kraus MA, Lee Y, Miller BW, Teitelbaum I, Williams AW, Finkelstein FO, FREEDOM Study Group. Impact of short daily hemodialysis on restless legs symptoms and sleep disturbances. Clin J Am Soc Nephrol. 2011;6(5):1049–56.
61. Granado RC, Macedo E, Chertow GM, Soroko S, Himmelfarb J, Ikizler TA, Paganini EP, Mehta RL. Effluent volume in continuous renal replacement therapy overestimates the delivered dose of dialysis. Clin J Am Soc Nephrol. 2011;6(3):467–75.

Peritoneal Dialysis: Initiation and Complications

32

Joni H. Hansson

Ca se 1

Mr. S. is a 30-year-old man who has developed end-stage renal disease (ESRD) secondary to FSGS. After education concerning modality options, he selected peritoneal dialysis (PD) as a bridge until he receives a kidney transplant. A Tenckhoff catheter (brand of PD catheter) was placed and 2 weeks later he started PD training first with manual exchanges. Two days after performing manual exchanges at home, he developed problems with ultrafiltration and then presented with scrotal swelling. He was diagnosed with an inguinal hernia. PD was held and he underwent a hernia repair. PD was resumed 24 h after his surgery. He then was trained on the cycler. His PD prescription was 8 h on the cycler with a total of 11 L of 1.5% low calcium dextrose dialysate. His cycler fill volumes were 2 L with a last fill of 1 L. He noted that his initial drains were only 2–300 ml. A peritoneal equilibration test (PET) was performed and revealed that he was a "high" transporter. His prescription was modified. His *Kt*/*V* revealed that he was obtaining adequate dialysis on this new regimen, but 40% of his clearance is from his endogenous renal function. After 1 year on dialysis he developed nausea, vomiting, abdominal pain, and cloudy fluid. He was diagnosed with peritonitis and was started on empiric antibiotics. His PD fluid grew *Staphylococcus epidermidis* and he completed a 2-week course of intraperitoneal vancomycin. Six months later he underwent a successful kidney transplant.

1. *What are the early and late non-infections complications of PD?*
2. *What are the different modalities of PD?*
3. *How and why is the PD prescription modified?*
4. *How is peritonitis diagnosed and treated?*

Case 2

Ms. N. is a 51-year-old woman with ESRD secondary to hypertension who has been on in-center hemodialysis for the last 3 years. She refused AVF placement and was dialyzed through a central venous catheter (CVC). She was admitted to the hospital with a cough and a low-grade fever. It was noted that she had a new diastolic murmur. Her blood cultures grew coagulase negative *Staphylococcus*. An echocardiogram revealed a large aortic valve vegetation, severe aortic insufficiency as well as an abnormal mitral valve. Her tunneled hemodialysis catheter was removed. It was felt that she required urgent surgical intervention, but the cardiothoracic surgeon was concerned about the need for a CVC for hemodialysis. After discussion with the patient and her family, a Tenckhoff catheter was

J.H. Hansson, M.D. (✉)
Department of Medicine, Section of Nephrology, Hospital of Saint Raphael,1450 Chapel Street, New Haven, CT 06511, USA
e-mail: ahansson@comcast.net

E.V. Lerma and M. Rosner (eds.), *Clinical Decisions in Nephrology, Hypertension and Kidney Transplantation*, DOI 10.1007/978-1-4614-4454-1_32, © Springer Science+Business Media New York 2013

placed and peritoneal dialysis was initiated the next day. The patient underwent a successful aortic valve replacement and mitral valve repair. Postoperatively her filling pressures were elevated and her dialysis prescription was modified.

1. *Is there a role for PD in acute settings where CVCs can be avoided?*
2. *How is the PD prescription modified to optimize the patient's fluid status?*

Introduction

Peritoneal dialysis is one of the modality options for chronic renal replacement therapy. There have been tremendous advances in the technology of peritoneal dialysis over the past few decades. With these advances there has been a dramatic rise in the use of PD worldwide. However, although there has been an increase in the number of ESRD patients in the USA, patients on PD now account for only 6% of all new dialysis patients [1]. The etiology for the underutilization of PD is multifactorial [2, 3], and inadequate predialysis education about renal replacement therapies is one of these factors. It has been shown, that when patients receive unbiased education about dialysis modalities a much larger percentage will choose PD [4–6]. Therefore, it is important that patients are educated about PD as an effective home modality of renal replacement therapy that offers the patient flexibility, self-autonomy and promotes optimal quality of life. It is also essential that patients be educated that there is a survival benefit of PD compared to hemodialysis (HD) for incident ESRD patients [7–10], and a similar long-term survival [1, 11].

This chapter focuses on the basics of PD, how to initiate PD and the factors that are considered in managing the PD prescription. In addition, a discussion of both the infectious and noninfectious complications of PD is reviewed.

Peritoneal Dialysis Basics

In peritoneal dialysis, fluid (dialysate) is placed in the peritoneal cavity. Movement of solutes and fluid occurs across the "dialyzer" that separates the blood compartment from the fluid in the peritoneal cavity. This fluid is left in the peritoneal cavity for a period of time (dwell time) to allow this transfer of solutes and fluid to occur, and then is drained and discarded. Fresh dialysate is then instilled. This cycle of instilling dialysate, allowing the fluid to dwell for a period of time and then draining the fluid, is referred to as an exchange (see Fig. 32.1), and is the basic procedure in PD. The PD dialyzer is the peritoneal membrane, which includes the mesothelial layer, the interstitium, and the peritoneal capillaries, but it is the capillary vascular surface area that is the most important determinant of solute transport [12]. The anatomy, physiology, and models of solute transport in PD are complex and are reviewed in detail elsewhere [13–16]. Solute transport occurs primarily by diffusion, although some are removed by convection (solvent drag). For small solutes diffusive flux is highest in the first hour of the dwell, where the concentration gradient is largest and then both decrease with time. Ultrafiltration, or fluid movement across the peritoneal membrane, occurs as a result of an osmotic gradient. Approximately 40–50% of the fluid movement across the capillary wall occurs through water (aquaporin) channels [13]. Different concentrations of dextrose in the dialysate are used primarily as the osmotic agent. The permeability of the peritoneal membrane to glucose can affect ultrafiltration, since varying amounts of glucose can be absorbed. Table 32.1 outlines factors that can influence diffusion and ultrafiltration [13]. The highlighted factors are those that can be adjusted when prescribing PD and will be discussed later.

Initiating Peritoneal Dialysis

The ultimate goals of PD therapy are listed in Table 32.2. In order to prescribe PD a fundamental knowledge of peritoneal access, dialysis solutions, peritoneal membrane transport function, and PD modalities is required. In the following section, these items and how to initiate and modify the PD prescription will be discussed.

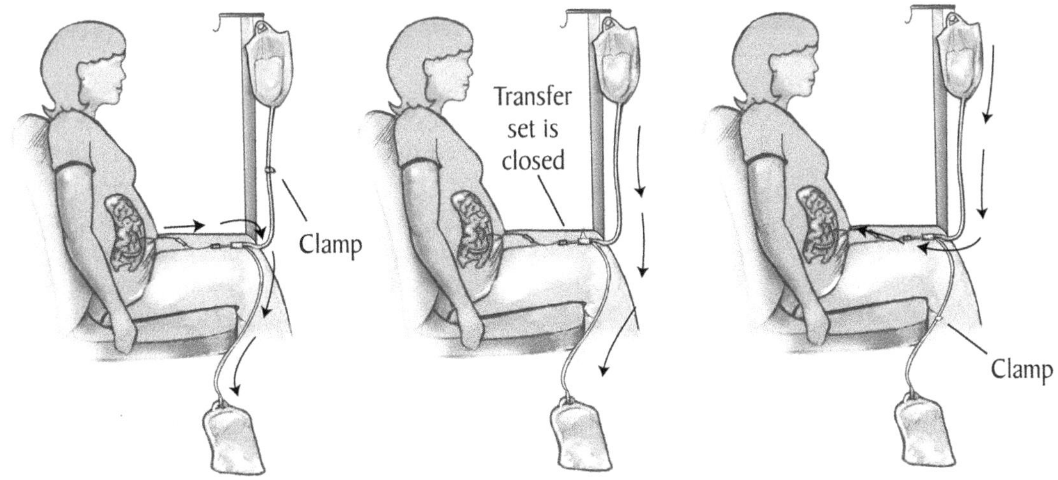

Fig. 32.1 The PD exchange. Reproduced with permission from NIDDK

Table 32.1 Factors that influence diffusion and ultrafiltration in peritoneal dialysis

Diffusion	Ultrafiltration
Peritoneal surface area	Peritoneal surface area
Peritoneal membrane permeability	Peritoneal membrane permeability
Concentration gradient of the solute	Net pressure gradient of the following forces:
Characteristics of the solute	Hydrostatic
Temperature of dialysis solution	Oncotic
Blood flow	**Osmotic**
Total 24 h dialysate volumes	
Dwell time	

Factors in **bold** are those that can be adjusted in the PD prescription

Table 32.2 Goals of peritoneal dialysis therapy

Optimal solute clearance
Optimal control of electrolytes
Optimal control of acid–base status
Optimal control of extracellular volume
Maintain residual renal function
Prevent short- and long-term complications
Optimize quality of life

Peritoneal Dialysis Access

Once a patient has chosen PD as their choice for renal replacement therapy, a peritoneal dialysis catheter will need to be inserted before PD can be initiated. Appropriate peritoneal access is crucial to minimize catheter-related problems and should be performed by an operator with expertise in placing peritoneal access [17–20]. There are multiple catheter designs, each having an intra-peritoneal, a transmural, a subcutaneous tunneled, and an external segment [18]. Most catheters also have two cuffs: one deep and one superficial (see Fig. 32.2). The deep cuff is usually placed in the rectus muscle and the superficial cuff approximately 2–3 cm from the exit site. The choice of the catheter will depend upon where it will be placed in the abdomen along with operator preference. Appropriate preoperative marking and planning of the exit-site placement is critical to minimize complications [19, 20]. The PD catheter can be inserted by a variety of techniques [19, 20]. Any abdominal/inguinal hernias present should be repaired during the same surgical procedure. Potential catheter-related complications will be discussed later. It has been recommended that catheter insertion should be performed at least 2 weeks before initiating peritoneal dialysis [17]. However, PD may be started earlier if needed using low volume exchanges while the

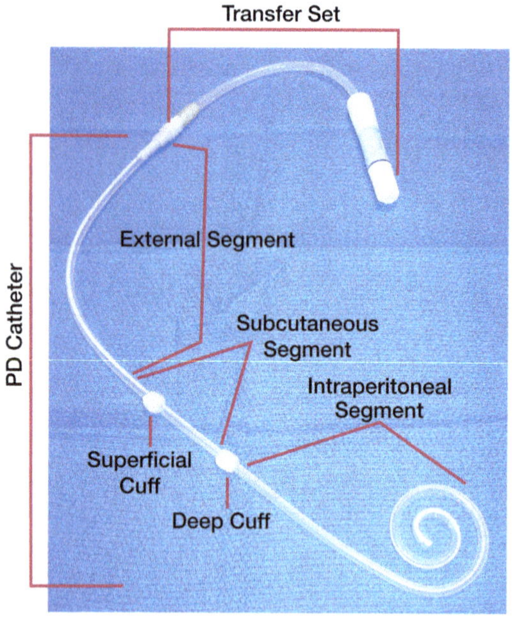

Fig. 32.2 The PD catheter and transfer set

patient is in the supine position [21]. If it is unclear when the patient will need to initiate PD, the PD catheter can be placed with the external limb embedded in the subcutaneous tissue [19]. When the patient needs to start dialysis, the catheter can be exteriorized in the office setting and PD initiated that day. Embedding the catheter is recommended in individuals who will not be starting PD for at least 6 weeks up to 6 months. This can help avoid temporary hemodialysis with vascular catheters.

Case 1 illustrates the most common planning for PD where the catheter is placed and used after a 2-week period of time to allow healing. On the other hand, Case 2 demonstrates that PD can be commenced shortly after the PD catheter is placed. This may minimize the need for temporary hemodialysis and a CVC, which was important in this patient. The use of low volume exchanges in the supine position will help minimize the increase in intra-abdominal pressures and reduce the risk for leaks. There is now renewed interest in the use of PD in AKI [22–24]. PD should be considered to reduce the use of CVC, which is associated with increased mortality [25, 26].

Exit-Site Care

Education on exit-site care is crucial after PD catheter placement. This will include how to care for the exit site, identify an exit-site infection and how to immobilize the catheter to avoid trauma [18, 27] Exit-site application of antibiotic creams as part of routine care has decreased both exit-site infections and peritonitis. While mupirocin and gentamicin cream have both been used, gentamicin cream was as effective as mupirocin in preventing *S. aureus* infections, and also reduced *Psuedomonas aeruginosa* and other gram-negative catheter-related infections and peritonitis [28, 29].

Peritoneal Dialysis Solutions

A variety of PD solutions are available for clinical use. The composition of the most common peritoneal dialysis solutions available in the USA are shown in Table 32.3. The electrolyte concentrations vary slightly by manufacturer [30]. When prescribing PD, the choice of calcium concentration and type of osmotic agent will need to be specified. Traditionally, the "regular" calcium solutions that are used have 3.5 mEq/L of calcium which is higher than normal serum calcium levels. This may result in a positive calcium balance. With the increased use of calcium-based phosphate binders and vitamin D analogues, and

Table 32.3 Composition of common peritoneal dialysis solutions

	Dextrose based	Icodextrin
Sodium (mEq/L)	132–134	132
Chloride (mEq/L)	96–102	96
Potassium (mEq/L)	0	0
Calcium (mEq/L)	2.5 or 3.5	3.5
Magnesium (mEq/L)	0.5–1.5	0.5
Lactate (mEq/L)	35, 40	40
Bicarbonate (mEq/L)	0	0
Glucose (g/dL)	1.5, 2.5, 4.25	0
Icodextrin (g/dL)	0	7.5
Osm (mOsmol/kg)	346, 396, 485	282
pH	5.2	5.2

the concerns of positive calcium balance on vascular and soft tissue calcification, there has been increased use of the low-calcium dialysate. These solutions contain 2.5 mEq/L of calcium. Lactate is used as the buffer, since the low pH of the solution prevents caramelization of the glucose during the autoclaving process and also decreases the generation of glucose degradation products (which is toxic to the peritoneal membrane) [30]. The use of bicarbonate has been limited due to concerns of precipitation of calcium with bicarbonate if they are present in the same solution. Glucose is the most common osmotic agent utilized in PD and is available in three different concentrations: 1.5, 2.5, and 4.25%. The higher the dextrose concentration used, the higher the osmotic gradient, and therefore the more ultrafiltration that will be expected. The dextrose concentration used can be adjusted daily to fit the volume management needs of the patient on that day. Dextrose is not the ideal osmotic agent since it is absorbed, which can limit ultrafiltration and also result in hyperglycemia, hyperinsulinemia, hyperlipidemia, weight gain and may contribute to loss of peritoneal membrane function. A glucose polymer-containing solution (icodextrin) is now available to replace some of the glucose-containing solutions. Although this solution is isosmolar, it exerts a colloid-like oncotic force since it is a large molecule which has limited absorption [13, 30]. Ultrafiltration with icodextrin increases throughout the length of exposure. Therefore, it is useful for a long dwell (especially in rapid transporters—see below) and in diabetics to limit glucose exposure. The use of icodextrin is associated with increased levels of maltose, maltotriose, and other oligopolysaccharides [31] and has been associated with an increased incidence of cutaneous reactions. Icodextrin and maltose can interfere or cause false elevated glucose results. One needs to ensure that the patient is using a glucometer that is compatible with icodextrin use [32]. There continues to be intensive research to design PD solutions that limit toxicity to the peritoneal membrane, offer predictable solute clearance, and correct acidosis in a cost-effective manner.

The Peritoneal Equilibration Test

Since the peritoneal membrane is unique to each individual, understanding the transport characteristics of each patient is important in designing a PD prescription. The standard PET [33] is a reproducible procedure used to assess peritoneal transport of small solutes and ultrafiltration capacity. After a long overnight dwell, 2 L of a 2.5% dextrose dialysate are infused with the patient supine and allowed to dwell for 4 h. Dialysate samples are taken immediately after the infusion and then again at 2 and 4 h into the dwell. Each sample is measured for urea, creatinine, and glucose. After the initial sample is obtained the patient is encouraged to ambulate. A blood sample testing for glucose, urea, and creatinine is drawn at 120 min. The patient is drained upright after 4 h and the drain volume is then recorded. The Dt/D0 (dextrose concentration at time *t*/dextrose concentration at time 0) and the *D*/*P* (dialysate/plasma) ratios for creatinine and urea are calculated for each time point and compared with standard PET curves [33]. Patients are classified into one of four categories based on their 4-h *D*/*P* creatinine ratio: high, high-average, low-average, and low transporter. The transport status based on the *D*/*P* ratio at 4 h for creatinine is illustrated in Table 32.4. If a patient is a "slow or low" transporter, glucose diffuses out of the peritoneal cavity more slowly, maintaining the osmotic gradient longer resulting in more ultrafiltration. In addition, solute clearance takes longer. This patient may benefit from longer dwell times. On the other hand, if a patient is a "rapid or high" transporter, he/she can achieve rapid equilibration for small solutes in the dialysate. Glucose diffuses out of the peritoneal cavity more rapidly, dissipating the osmotic gra-

Table 32.4 Transport status by 4 h *D*/*P* creatinine ratio using the standard PET

Transport status	Creatinine 4 h *D*/*P*
High	0.82–1.03
High-average	0.66–0.81
Low-average	0.50–0.65
Low	0.34–0.49

D/*P* dialysate/plasma

dient faster resulting in less ultrafiltration. To minimize the loss of the osmotic gradient, this patient may benefit from shorter dwell times. It is generally recommended that the PET be done 4 weeks after starting PD as a baseline [34]. This can be repeated if there is a concern for alterations in membrane transport characteristics. Modifications of the standard PET do exist [35, 36].

A PET was performed on the patient in Case 1. He was found to be a high transporter and this would explain why he absorbed most of his last fill. His prescription was modified as explained below.

Peritoneal Modalities

There have been many different modalities of chronic PD developed since PD was first introduced (Fig. 32.3) [37, 38]. The ultimate modality choice takes into consideration several factors

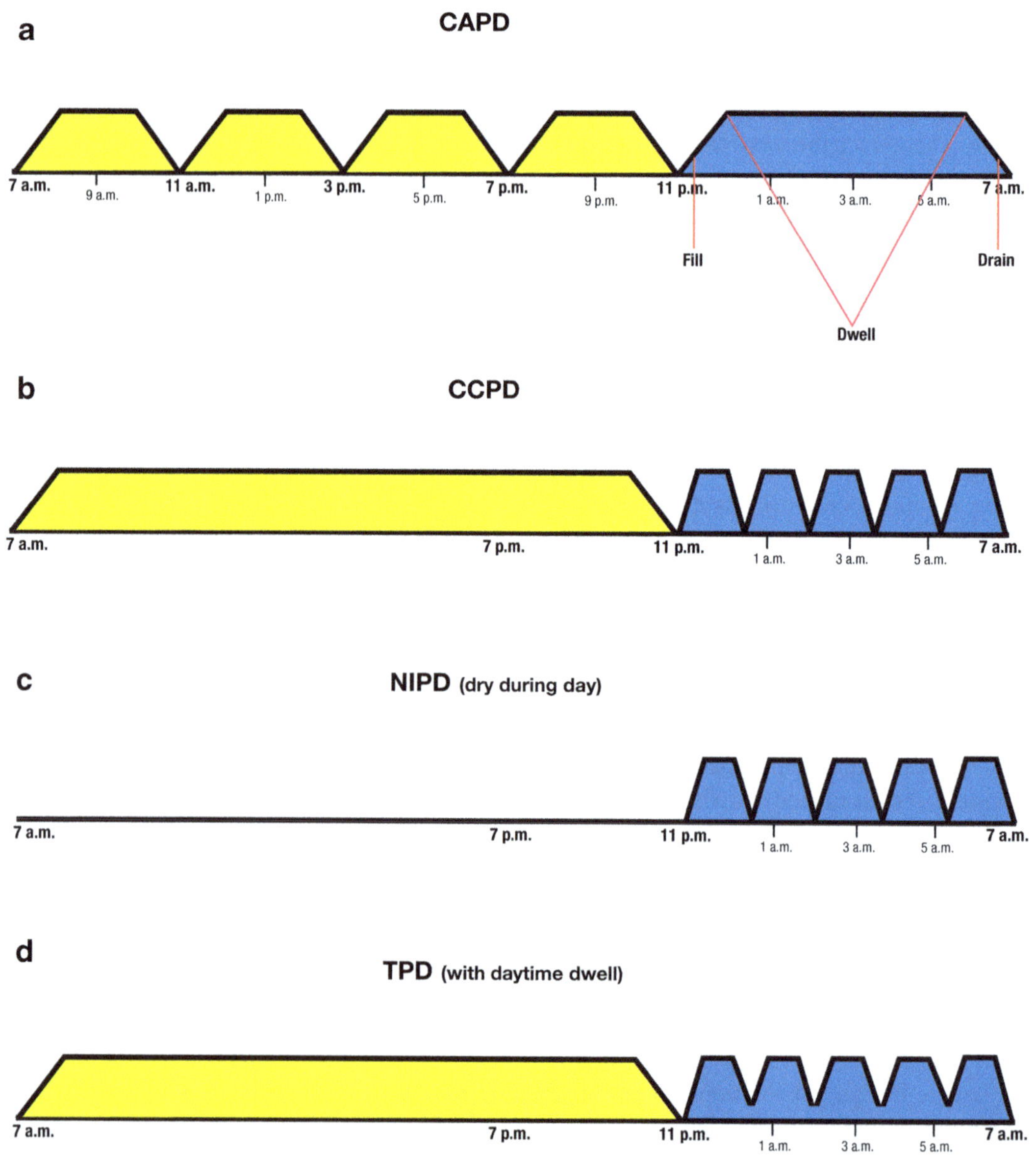

Fig. 32.3 Pictorial representation of the basic PD modalities

which include residual renal function (RRF), transport status, and lifestyle issues of the patient. There are two broad categories of PD: continuous ambulatory PD (CAPD) and automated PD (APD). Patient outcomes are similar with CAPD and APD [39, 40].

CAPD (Fig. 32.3a) usually involves 3–5 exchanges a day with a set volume of dialysate instilled with each exchange. Most commonly, a long overnight dwell is used, so the patient's sleep is not interrupted. Figure 32.1 displays the steps in an exchange using a double bag system. Once the patient has filled, they would carefully disconnect from this system, until they are ready for their next exchange with fresh dialysate.

APD uses a cycler (machine) to perform the exchanges. This allows PD to be performed at night and frees the patient up during the day. When the cycler therapy is complete, the patient can be left with or without fluid in their abdomen. There are several different types of cycler-based therapy. CCPD, continuous cycling PD (Fig. 32.3b), involves exchanges being done by the cycler at night and the patient is left with fluid in them during the day. In nocturnal intermitted PD (NIPD), exchanges are done by the cycler at night, but the patient remains dry during the day (Fig. 32.3c). The use of tidal peritoneal dialysis (TPD) involves only a portion of the intraperitoneal fluid volume be replaced with each exchange (% tidal), so that there is continuous fluid–membrane contact which can improve efficiency (Fig. 32.3d). TPD is also used in patients who develop abdominal pain when their peritoneal cavity is drained of fluid. Hybrids of the above modalities can also be prescribed.

Peritoneal Dialysis Prescription

The PD prescription must take many factors into account. These include transport status, RRF, diabetes status, clearance targets, size of patient, and lifestyle issues. Initially, when patients have significant RRF, any PD modality can be used and usually achieve adequate clearance and volume control. However, as a person's RRF declines, their PD prescription may need to be modified to ensure adequate clearance. Adequacy for small solute removal is measured by total (renal and peritoneal) clearance of urea termed, *Kt*/*V* urea [41]. This is an index of urea clearance (*K*) per unit time (*t*) related to total body water (*V*). The minimal target for weekly *Kt*/*V* is 1.7 [42, 43].

Patients are initially trained in the performance of manual exchanges. Once this is mastered, the patient is started on CAPD or a form of APD. The prescription can be based on an incremental versus a maximal approach [38]. In the incremental approach PD is used to make up the differences between residual renal clearance and targeted clearance. This approach is less costly and may decrease total glucose exposure and risk of peritonitis. It does require frequent monitoring of RRF, to ensure adequate total clearance is being delivered. In the maximal approach a sufficient prescription of PD is provided to reach clearance targets with PD alone.

The initial prescription of CAPD or APD must specify the factors that are listed in Table 32.5. A typical starting CAPD regimen would be four exchanges a day with 2 L fill volumes. An example of an initial cycler prescription is 10 L total volume, 7 h on the cycler, 2 L fill volumes, 4 cycles, with a 2 L last fill. The type of solutions would be based on the patient's volume and transport status (see below). After approximately a month on the original PD prescription a formal clearance study (*Kt*/*V*) should be obtained. Based on these results further modifications of the prescription can be made. Table 32.6 illustrates certain features that should be considered when modifying a patient's dialysis prescription.

Table 32.5 Prescription details for CAPD and APD

CAPD	APD
Number of exchanges/24 h	Time on the cycler
Dwell volume	Number of cycles
Type of dialysate	Cycler dwell volume
	Type of dialysate—cycler
	For TPD—% tidal
	Number of daytime dwells
	Volume of daytime dwells
	Type of dialysate—daytime

Table 32.6 Variables to consider when modifying PD prescriptions

Variable	Consideration
Rapid transport status	NIPD with short dwell times
Rapid transport status with inadequate dialysis	NIPD with increased length of therapy NIPD with increased volume of exchange CCPD with short dwell times on the cycler and icodextrin as last fill
Slow transport status	CAPD CCPD with fewer cycles and longer dwell times
Slow transport status with inadequate dialysis	Increase number of CAPD exchanges Increase volume of exchange CCPD with daytime manual exchange
Diabetic patient	Loop diuretic if still makes urine CCPD with icodextrin for last fill CAPD with icodextrin for overnight dwell Goal—limit glucose exposure
Large patient	Higher fill volumes CCPD with daytime dwell and manual exchange if needed
Small patient	Lower fill volumes Potentially dry during the day if symptoms of abdominal bloating
Drain pain	TPD
Icodextrin use	Diabetics Rapid transporters –overnight dwell on CAPD –last fill on CCPD
Volume overload/ excess	Ensure patient on sodium and fluid restriction Adjust diuretics if still urinates Increase use of higher % dextrose solutions Icodexdrin for day time dwell
Volume depletion	Decrease use of higher % dextrose solutions Hold icodextrin Hold diuretics

Case 1 was found to be a high transporter and absorbed most of his daytime dwell. Since he had significant RRF changing his prescription to NIPD was appropriate. By doing this, the patient was prescribed several frequent exchanges on the cycler to allow for optimal dialysis clearance.

In this case it is important to monitor for loss of RRF and repeat total *Kt*/*V* on a regular basis. If he lost RRF, the total time or the number of cycles could be increased in his NIPD regimen in order to increase solute clearance by PD. If he required a daytime dwell to achieve adequate solute clearance, he could be changed to CCPD using icodextrin as his last fill.

Case 2 had an early start to PD. Initially, her prescription should use low volume exchanges when she is supine. NIPD with 1 L exchanges with a longer time on the cycler was prescribed. She was left dry during the day, since intra-abdominal pressures are higher in the seated and standing positions compared with being supine. This will help minimize the risk of a leak.

Volume Management in PD

Volume assessment and maintaining euvolemia is important in PD patients. By adjusting the type of dialysis solution used, ultrafiltration can be modified. Current available dextrose containing dialysate comes in 1.5, 2.5, or 4.25% solutions. Increasing the strength of the dextrose solution used can increase ultrafiltration due to an increased osmotic gradient and be useful in a patient who is volume overloaded. If a patient is hypotensive, decreasing the strength of the dextrose solution is indicated. The chronic use of high dextrose containing solutions can lead to both damage to the peritoneal membrane long term and ultrafiltration failure (UF) (see below). Icodextrin can be used to help with volume management especially in diabetics and rapid transporters.

In addition to adjusting the types of solutions used, attention needs to be given to non-dialysis factors that can help with volume management.

Patients should be counseled about salt and fluid restrictions. Compliance with the PD regimen should be confirmed and appropriateness of the PD prescription reviewed. RRF plays a role important in solute clearance and volume control. Diuretic use in patients with RR may help limit the use of high dextrose containing solutions. In addition to contributing to solute and volume control, the presence of RRF is associated with better patient and technique survival [44]. PD is associated with a slower decrease in RRF compared to hemodialysis. Therefore, careful attention should also be given to maintaining RRF. Potential nephrotoxins should be avoided, if possible. The use of angiotensin receptor blockers (ARB) or angiotensin-converting enzyme inhibitors (ACEI) has been associated with a reduced risk for loss of RRF [45].

When Case 2 was initiated on PD, twelve 1-L exchanges using 1.5% dextrose solutions were prescribed. Her hemodynamic measurements were tenuous preoperatively. Post-op, her blood pressure was much improved and her filling pressures were found to be elevated. Her prescription was modified by changing to all 2.5% dialysate. Her nightly net ultrafiltration increased from 500 to 1,800 ml with improvement in her filling pressures

Case 1 has significant RRF. Diuretic use should be considered first, before increasing the % dextrose solution used, if the patient becomes volume expanded. Nephrotoxins should be avoided. If he were hypertensive, he should be on either an ACEI or ARB, assuming no contraindication, to potentially help reduce the rate of decline of his RRF.

Complications of PD

A variety of infectious and noninfectious complications can occur during PD therapy (Table 32.7). Knowledge of these complications will aid in early recognition and treatment, which will help reduce patient morbidity. A discussion of the more common or serious complications of PD will be discussed below

Table 32.7 Complications of peritoneal dialysis

Noninfectious	Infectious
Catheter dysfunction	Peritonitis
Constipation	
Catheter malposition	
Catheter occlusion	
Intraluminal	
Extraluminal	
Kinked catheter	
Leaks	Exit-site infections
Hernias	
Abdominal wall leaks	
Pericatheter leaks	
Hydrothorax	
Hemoperitoneum	Tunnel infections
Pain	
Metabolic	
Hyperglycemia/hyperinsulinemia	
Hyperlipidemia	
Weight gain	
hypoalbuminemia	
Peritoneal membrane failure	
Encapsulating peritoneal sclerosis	

Noninfectious Complications of PD

Catheter Dysfunction

Catheter dysfunction is present when there is inadequate filling or draining of the dialysate. This usually occurs after the catheter is placed but may occur at any time during the life of the catheter. This most commonly occurs due to one of the following: kinking of the catheter, catheter malposition, constipation, intraluminal catheter occlusion, or extraluminal catheter occlusion [46, 47]. Kinking of the catheter usually is noted early and may be associated with both inflow and outflow problems. Treatment usually involves catheter replacement or removal of the superficial cuff. Catheter malposition is usually associated with an outflow problem. Repositioning of the catheter can sometimes be managed under fluoroscopy using a stiff wire to reposition the catheter, however, recurrences are not uncommon. This may require surgical redirection. Catheter migration resulting in malpositioning, may occur due to omental attachments to the catheter. The patient will then require surgery for omentectomy and repositioning of the catheter. Intra-abdominal adhesions may also result in outflow failure and require adhesiolysis to help salvage the catheter [48]. Constipation is a common cause of outflow obstruction. Constipation can cause catheter migration or external compression of the lumen by bowel. Liberal use of laxatives is important to promote and maintain good catheter function. Obstruction to inflow of PD fluid suggests intraluminal blockage. This usually occurs secondary to fibrin or blood. Heparin should be added to the PD fluid (250–500 U/L) when fibrin is seen in the effluent to help prevent outflow obstruction. However, if obstruction is present, the catheter should be flushed. Instillation of intraluminal thrombolytics may be necessary if flushing is ineffective [46].

When faced with a patient with inadequate drainage of dialysate, one should assess the patient for kinking of the catheter in the tunnel track, for the presence of fibrin in recent exchanges and recent history of bowel movements. If the patient is noted to have fibrin, heparin should be added to the dialysate. Moving the position of the patient may facilitate drainage by moving the catheter to a dependent position. If the problem persists an abdominal X-ray should be ordered. If the film reveals constipation a bowel regimen should be prescribed. If the catheter is malpositioned, kinked, or problems with drainage persist, a surgical consult should be obtained.

Leaks

The intra-abdominal pressure increases with instillation of dialysis fluid into the peritoneal cavity. Not only does this pressure increase with increasing dialysate volume [49], but the position of the patient affects this pressure [50] The intra-abdominal pressure is lowest with the patient supine, compared with standing, and is highest with the patient sitting. Straining, coughing, or bending can transiently increase the intra-abdominal pressure to very high levels. This increased pressure in patients on PD, may result in a variety of mechanical complications, as will be described in the following sections.

Hernias

Hernia formation is a common complication of PD with an incidence that ranges between 2 and 37% [50, 51]. Potential risk factors for hernia formation include large dialysate volume, sitting position, isometric exercise, valsalva maneuver, recent abdominal surgery, increasing age, increased body mass index, mutiparity, congenital anatomical defects, and polycystic kidney disease [52, 53]. Sites of anatomic weakness predispose to hernia formation. Many different types of hernias have been described but inguinal, exit site and umbilical are the most common. Once formed these hernias may enlarge and lead to local swelling, problems with ultrafiltration, to intestinal incarceration and/or strangulation. The diagnosis of a hernia often is clinically apparent, but if not, CT peritoneography or peritoneal scintigraphy may be utilized to detect leaks from the peritoneal cavity [54, 55]. Elective surgical repair is recommended. For uncomplicated hernia repairs, PD may be resumed within a few days without interim HD [51, 56, 57]. The dialysis regimen should be modified to decrease intra-abdominal pressures (low volume use of cycler at night and dry during the day) for the next few weeks following surgical repair. For individuals with significant RRF, PD may be held for several days and then resumed with low volume exchanges.

Case 1 developed a leak of dialysate into his processus vaginalis which resulted in a large inguinal hernia. He underwent hernia repair. Since he had significant RRF, PD was held for a week. When PD was resumed, low volume exchanges were used to minimize the increase in intra-abdominal pressure.

Abdominal Wall Leaks

Abdominal wall leaks may be difficult to diagnose and can occur at any time. Patients may present with problems with ultrafiltration, weight gain, or abdominal wall asymmetry with focal or diffuse fullness/edema. The diagnosis can be made using the same imaging techniques as described above in the hernia section. The dialysis regimen should be changed to decrease intra-abdominal pressures. If this is not successful, temporary discontinuation of PD may be necessary. If a hernia is identified, it should then be repaired.

Pericatheter Leak

A pericatheter leak is a postoperative complication of PD catheter placement [46]. It usually presents as wetness on the exit-site dressing as PD is being initiated. If checked, the fluid will be positive for glucose. The risk for a leak is increased if the catheter is used soon after it is placed. The patient should be drained and PD discontinued for several days to allow the leak to seal. With time, the leak will usually seal spontaneously, but the patient may require temporary hemodialysis. If the leak persists, the PD catheter will need to be removed and reinserted at another site.

If Case 2 developed moistness at her exit site, one should be concerned about a pericatheter leak. A high glucose content of the fluid around the catheter exit site would confirm this diagnosis. PD would need to be discontinued for at least several days to allow the leak to seal. She may then require temporary HD. A recent study demonstrated that immediate initiation of PD after percutaneous catheter placement had a very low rate of pericatheter leakage [21]. Again, low volume exchanges should be used, when the patient is in the supine position to decrease intra-abdominal pressures.

Hydrothorax

Hydrothorax is a serious complication of PD, which can occur at any time during its course. The incidence of hydrothorax ranges between 1.6 and 10% of PD patients [58–60] and most commonly presents on the right side. It results most often due to a pleuroperitoneal communication (congenital or acquired). The presentation may range from being asymptomatic, having ultrafiltration problems, or progressive or acute dyspnea. The diagnosis can be made from analysis of the pleural fluid which will reveal a high glucose level (higher than serum glucose) ergo, this has been termed "sweet" hydrothorax [61]. Peritoneal scintigraphy can be used to noninvasively confirm this pleuroperitoneal communication. Cessation of PD is the initial management. This conservative management is effective in approximately half of the patients. When PD is resumed, low volume exchanges with the patient supine should be initiated. For patients who fail conservative management, chemical pleurodesis or video-assisted thorascopic pleurodesis and/or diaphragmatic repair can be pursued, if they wish to return to PD [58, 59].

Hemoperitoneum

Hemoperitoneum, bloody peritoneal effluent, is an uncommon event that can cause significant alarm. Most commonly, it is due to benign etiologies such as menstruation, ovulation, trauma, coagulopathy, or ruptured renal/ovarian cysts [50, 62, 63]. However, it may be associated with more serious etiologies such as encapsulating peritoneal sclerosis (EPS) or other intra-abdominal pathologies which could occur in non-dialysis patients (e.g., cancer, pancreatitis, ischemic bowel, splenic rupture). A careful history and physical exam should be obtained. If the bleeding is heavy, prolonged or associated with pain and/or fever an urgent evaluation is indicated to exclude intra-abdominal pathology that may require prompt surgical intervention. In general, hemoperitoneum is not a common presenting sign of peritonitis. Treatment of the underlying cause is important. Supportive measures may be indicated for idiopathic or benign etiologies. This can include the instillation of heparin (500 U/L) in the dialysate to prevent clotting of the catheter and frequent exchanges. Some have advocated the use of room temperature dialysate to cause vasoconstriction which may decrease bleeding [64]. The risk/benefit of continuation of anticoagulants or antiplatelet agents will need to be assessed on an individual basis.

Pain

Patients may complain about pain or discomfort while performing PD [65, 66]. This may be related to the low pH of the dialysis solutions, omental attachment to the catheter, pressure created in a neighboring structure, abdominal distention from fluid in the abdomen (more pronounced during the day in the upright posture). Certainly peritonitis should be considered and excluded. Treatment will depend on the cause. Omental attachment to the catheter may require surgical revision. For individuals with pain when the abdomen is drained, TPD may alleviate this symptom. Abdominal distention from fluid in the abdomen during the day may be treated by decreasing the fill volumes for daytime exchanges or switching the patient to NIPD. Back pain may occur is some patients who carry a daytime dwell. The presence of this fluid may affect posture by increasing the tendency of the spine into a more lordotic position [66]. This may increase pain in an individual with a preexisting back condition. Minimizing the daytime fill volume or NIPD may be useful in this setting.

Metabolic

A detailed discussion of the metabolic and nutritional complications of PD is beyond the scope of this chapter, but they are important to be mentioned. Many of the metabolic complications of PD are secondary to systemic glucose absorption [67]. This may contribute to hyperinsulinemia, hyperglycemia, and hyperlipidemia. Glucose levels need to be closely monitored and diabetic regimens adjusted accordingly. In addition, glucose absorption contributes to the patient's caloric intake and may cause weight gain [68]. In some patients, this can be significant. The use of nonglucose solutions (icodexdrin) may help limit this weight gain. Hypoalbuminemia is common in PD patients, with typical albumin levels being 3.3–3.6 mg/dL. This is in part due to significant protein loss across the peritoneum, which is more pronounced in rapid transporters. Acute inflammation, such as peritonitis, can also exacerbate protein losses. Close attention to the nutritional status of patients on PD is crucial.

Ultrafiltration Failure

Ultrafiltration failure is clinically manifested by progressive fluid overload and is one potential reason for patients to transfer to hemodialysis. This loss of function is felt to be secondary to structural changes of the peritoneal membrane (fibrosis and angiogenesis) that occurs over time [69–71]. The etiology of these changes is likely multifactorial (includes low pH of dialysate, glucose exposure, hyperosmolality, glucose degradation products, lactate, inflammation to list a few) and is an active area of basic research. The initial evaluation will include a detailed history and physical to identify treatable causes of volume overload (see Table 32.8) [72]. Once completed, the next step would be a reevaluation of peritoneal membrane function using a modified PET [73]. This is similar to the standard PET, except it is performed using a 4.25% dextrose exchange, to create a greater osmotic gradient. UF failure is defined as less than 400 ml net ultrafiltration at 4 h. Small solute transport should also be determined. If this reveals high transport status, it may be due to three scenarios [72]: no change from baseline testing, recent peritonitis, or peritoneal membrane changes associated with long-term PD. APD and icodextrin for the daytime dwell are recommended for patients with UF failure and high transport status. For individuals with UF failure and low transport status transfer to hemodialysis may be required for adequate patient management. This type of failure usually results from adhesions and reduced peritoneal surface area. For patients with intermediate solute transport, treatment will be focused on general measures to improve volume control, the use of icodextrin or adjusting the PD prescription for net negative fluid balance.

Table 32.8 Approach to the patient with volume overload

Contributing factor	Potential treatment
Diet noncompliance	Dietary education: low sodium diet and fluid restriction
PD prescription compliance	Patient education
Residual renal function (RRF)	If present consider diuretic use If recent loss of RRF—adjust dialysate
Evaluate appropriateness of PD Rx	Adjust for transport status (see Table 32.6)
Appropriate use of osmotic agent	Adjust tonicity of dialysate used
Poor drainage	Treat constipation Evaluate for catheter dysfunction Evaluate for leaks (see text)
Change in membrane function	Based on modified PET

Encapsulating Peritoneal Sclerosis

EPS is a rare but serious complication of PD [74–76]. The incidence varies between 0.5 and 4.4%. Clinical manifestations include symptoms of bowel obstruction, the presence of an abdominal mass, hemoperitoneum, malnutrition, failure to thrive, and ultrafiltration problems. A change in membrane transport status to a high transporter is not diagnostic of EPS, but may indicate membrane failure. Findings on CT may reveal a constellation of abnormalities: peritoneal thickening and calcification, bowel wall thickening, bowel tethering, bowel dilation, and loculated fluid collections [77, 78]. Pathologic findings can range from the formation of a thin membrane on the visceral and/or parietal peritoneum to cocoon-like encapsulation of the entire intestine found with advanced cases. Various degrees of peritoneal thickening and calcification may be present. The diagnosis requires the presence of both, clinical features of intestinal obstruction or disturbed gastrointestinal motility, plus evidence of bowel encapsulation either radiographically or pathologically. EPS is associated with significant morbidity and mortality. The pathogenesis of EPS is a subject of intense research [79–81]. Although many potential factors have been described, the only consistent risk factor is the duration of being on peritoneal dialysis. Of interest, EPS may present after PD has been discontinued. Treatment includes aggressive nutritional support. In most cases, PD should be discontinued. Although many drugs have been used to treat EPS, there is no clear evidence-based data for drug therapy [76, 82]. For refractory bowel obstruction, surgical intervention should be considered, but the patient should be referred to a center with experience in surgery for EPS [82]. There is a 26–58% mortality associated with EPS.

Infectious Complications of PD

Peritonitis

Peritonitis is a serious complication of PD, which is associated with significant morbidity and increased mortality risk [83–86]. It is also a major cause of technique failure resulting in transfer to hemodialysis. Therefore, once peritonitis is suspected or diagnosed, prompt treatment with empiric antibiotics is imperative. Table 32.9 outlines the basic approach for a patient with peritonitis. The

Table 32.9 Peritonitis: nuts and bolts

Peritonitis
Symptoms: Nausea, vomiting, abdominal pain, change in bowel pattern
Findings: Abdominal pain (mild to severe), fever, cloudy fluid, print not easily read through the effluent bag
Evaluation: Send PD fluid for cell count, gram stain, and culture
Detailed history and physical including careful exam of exit site
Abdominal imaging in selected cases
Diagnosis: PD wbc count >100 cells/μl with >50% PMNs
Initial Rx: Immediate empiric antibiotics to cover both gram-positive and gram-negative organisms
Intraperitoneal administration preferred
Final Rx: Antibiotic treatment modified by final culture results

diagnosis of peritonitis should be suspected in any patient who develops abdominal pain or cloudy fluid. The differential for a patient that presents with cloudy fluid includes culture positive infectious peritonitis; infectious peritonitis with sterile cultures; chemical peritonitis, eosinophilia of the effluent; hemoperitoneum, malignancy, chylous effluent, and a specimen taken from a dry abdomen [87]. A sample of dialysate should be sent for cell count, gram stain, and culture. The diagnosis of peritonitis is made by the presence of >100 white blood cells/μl, with at least 50% polymorphonuclear neutrophilic cells [87, 88]. Most cases of peritonitis are due to skin bacteria from touch contamination or a catheter-related infection. Other sources of the bacteria are from transvisceral migration from intra-abdominal pathology, hematogenous route, vaginal leak, and bacterial biofilm along the PD catheter. Therefore, a careful history should be obtained with attention to any breaks in technique, recent endoscopic or gynecologic procedures, gastrointestinal illness, urinary tract infections, or recent antibiotic therapy. Careful inspection of the exit site is important to exclude a concomitant exit-site infection.

The microbiology and epidemiology of peritonitis in PD patients has varied by location and over time [83, 85, 89–95]. Overall the incidence of peritonitis has decreased over time but the emergence of resistant organisms has increased [89, 90]. Table 32.10 outlines broadly, the causative organisms of peritonitis from several studies. International Society for Peritoneal Dialysis (ISPD) guidelines recommends that empiric antibiotics cover both gram-positive and gram-negative organisms [87]. Gram-positive organisms should be covered with vancomycin or a cephalosporin, and gram-negative organisms with a third generation cephalosporin or aminoglycoside. Intraperitoneal administration of antibiotics is superior to IV dosing, and intermittent and continuous dosing are equally efficacious [87]. The choice of which antibiotic to initiate will depend on several factors. Patient-related factors will include medication allergies and ability to administer intraperitoneal antibiotics. Center-related factors will largely be determined by local antibiotic sensitivities of various common organisms in the community. Antibiotic therapy should then be adjusted based on final culture results and sensitivities. Algorithms for antibiotic dosing and length of therapy for specific organisms are outlined in detail in the ISPD guidelines ([87]. Antibiotic dosing may need to be increased in patients with RRF. Removal of the PD catheter is sometimes indicated for infection related indications as summarized in Table 32.11 [87]. Catheter removal is required in 16–18% of episodes of peritonitis [85, 96]. Unfortunately, less than 50% of these patients are able to successfully return to PD [96].

Case 1 presented with nausea, vomiting, abdominal pain, and cloudy fluid. His fluid was sent for a cell count and culture. Empiric intraperitoneal antibiotics were initiated with vancomycin

Table 32.10 Organisms causing peritonitis

Organism		Percentage (%)
Gram positive		48–80
	Staphylococcus epidermidis	13–40
	Staphylococcus aureus	8–22
Gram negative		16–29
Yeast		1–6
Culture negative		15–20

Table 32.11 Infectious-related indications for PD catheter removal

Infectious indications for PD catheter removal
Fungal peritonitis
Refractory exit-site and tunnel infection
Refractory Peritonitis (failure to respond to appropriate therapy within 5 days)
Relapsing peritonitis (episode of peritonitis within 4 weeks of completion of antibiotics)
Pseudomonas peritonitis with exit-site infection
Consider catheter removal for: Repeat peritonitis (peritonitis that occurs > 4 weeks of completion of antibiotics with the same organism) Mycobacterial peritonitis Pseudomonal peritonitis VRE peritonitis Multiple enteric organisms

and ceftazidime. His cell count was 1,500 wbc/μl with 80% being polymorphonuclear leukocytes, meeting the definition of peritonitis. The culture grew methicillin resistant *Staphylococcus epidermidis* and his antibiotics were changed to intermitted IP vancomycin. Two grams of vancomycin (15–30 mg/kg) was put into a 2 L bag of dialysate. This was instilled into the patient and let dwell for 6 h. Since he had significant RRF, his vancomycin levels were monitored, so as not to become subtherapeutic and would be able to be appropriately redosed. His vancomycin level was 15 mg/ml after 4 days of his load. He then received a vancomycin IP load every 4 days to complete a 2-week course of therapy. With each episode of peritonitis the PD staff should take the opportunity to reeducate the patient on sterile techniques and exit-site care.

Exit-Site and Tunnel Infections

The presence of purulent drainage at the catheter-skin interface is by definition an exit-site infection. This may or may not be associated with erythema [87, 88]. Erythema without purulent drainage may not be an infection and represent a skin reaction. A tunnel infection is an infection in the subcutaneous tract of the catheter. This may present with pain, erythema, and edema over the subcutaneous path of the catheter, however it may not be clinically apparent. Usually a tunnel infection occurs with a coexistent exit-site infection. *Staphylococcus aureus* and *Pseudomonas aeruginosa* are the most common and serious exit-site pathogens. Since these infections can lead to peritonitis prompt initiation of empiric antibiotics are indicated. A culture of the exit-site drainage should be obtained and sent to the microbiology lab for gram stain and culture. Empiric antibiotic therapy should cover *S aureus*. Anti-pseudomonal coverage should be included if the patient has a history of pseudomonas exit-site infections. Antibiotic therapy can then be adjusted based on the culture result. Oral antibiotics are generally used (with the exception of MRSA) and the length of therapy is usually 2–3 weeks until the exit site appears normal. If the exit-site infection fails to resolve, recurs, or progresses to peritonitis, catheter removal may be necessary. Exit-site infections, especially with a tunnel infection, caused by *P. aeruginosa* are often difficult to eradicate and catheter removal should be considered early. In addition to antibiotic therapy, local exit-site care should also be reviewed with the patient and intensified.

Erosion of the superficial cuff through the skin may occur because of an exit-site infection or because of placement too close to the exit site [46]. The superficial cuff should then be surgically released/removed from the subcutaneous position. If there is a coexisting tunnel infection the catheter may need to be removed.

Summary

Peritoneal dialysis is an effective “bloodless” form of renal replacement therapy. It offers patient autonomy and flexibility. Patient satisfaction is high and is associated with better preservation of RRF. There is a survival benefit of PD compared to HD for new ESRD patients and should be considered in every patient approaching ESRD.

Acknowledgments I wish to acknowledge Patricia Mich for her assistance with the graphic designs of the figures in this chapter.

References

1. U.S. Rental Data System: USRDS 2010 Annual Data Report: Atlas of Chronic Kidney Disease and End-Stage Renal Disease in the United States, Bethesda, MD. National Institute of Health, National Institute of Diabetes and Digestive and Kidney Disease, 2010.
2. Chaudhary K, Sangha H, Khanna R. Peritoneal dialysis first: rationale. Clin J Am Soc Nephrol. 2011;6: 447–56.
3. Blake PG, Finkelstein FO. Why is the proportion of patients doing peritoneal dialysis declining in North America? Perit Dial Int. 2001;21:107–14.
4. Mehrotra R, Marsh D, Vonesh E, Peters V, Nissenson A. Patient education and access of ESRD patients to renal replacement therapies beyond in-center hemodialysis. Kidney Int. 2005;68:378–90.
5. Golper T. Patient education: can it maximize the success of therapy? Nephrol Dial Transplant. 2001;16 Suppl 7:20–4.
6. Goovaerts T, Jadoul M, Goffin E. Influence of Pre-Dialysis Education Programme (PDEP) on the mode of

renal replacement therapy. Nephrol Dial Transplant. 2005;20:1842–7.

7. Khawar O, Kalantar-Zadeh K, Lo WK, Johnson D, Mehrotra R. Is the declining Use of long-term peritoneal dialysis justified by outcome data? Clin J Am Soc Nephrol. 2007;2:1317–28.
8. Weinhandl ED, Foley RN, Gilbertson DT, Arneson TJ, Snyder JJ, Collins AJ. Propensity-matched mortality comparison of incident hemodialysis and peritoneal dialysis patients. J Am Soc Nephrol. 2010;21: 499–506.
9. Vonesh EF, Snyder JJ, Foley RN, Collins AJ. The differential impact of risk factors on mortality in hemodialysis and peritoneal dialysis. Kidney Int. 2004;55:2389–401.
10. McDonald SP, Marshall MR, Johnson DW, Polkinghorne KR. Relationship between dialysis modality and mortality. J Am Soc Nephrol. 2009;20:155–63.
11. Mehrotra R, Chiu Y, Kalantar-Zadeh K, Bargman J, Vonesh E. Similar outcomes with hemodialysis and peritoneal dialysis in patients with end-stage renal disease. Arch Intern Med. 2011;171:110–8.
12. Blake PG, Daugirdas JT. Physiology of peritoneal dialysis. In: Daugirdas JT, Blake PG, Ing TS, editors. Handbook of dialysis. 4th ed. Philadelphia, PA: Lippincott Williams & Wilkins; 2007. p. 323–38.
13. Teitelbaum I. Anatomy and Physiology of Peritoneal Dialysis. 2011. http://ispd.org/NAC/education/pd-curriculum/. Accessed May 2011.
14. Devuyst O, Goffin E. Water and solute transport in peritoneal dialysis: models and clinical application. Nephrol Dial Transplant. 2008;23:2120–3.
15. Flessner MF. Distributed model of peritoneal transport: implications of the endothelial glycocalyx. Nephrol Dial Transplant. 2008;23:2142–6.
16. Rippe G. Free water transport, small pore transport and the osmotic pressure gradient three-pore model of peritoneal transport. Nephrol Dial Transplant. 2008;23:2147–53.
17. Figueiredo A, Goh B, Jenkins S, Johnson DW, Mactier R, Ramalakshmi S, Shrestha B, Struijk D, Wilkie M. Clinical practice guidelines of peritoneal access. Perit Dial Int. 2010;30:424–9.
18. Gokal R, Alexander S, Ash S, Chen TW, Danielson A, Holmes C, Joffe P, Moncrief J, Nichols K, Piraino B, Prowant B, Slingeneyer A, Stegmayr B, Twardowski Z, Vas S. Peritoneal catheters and exit-site practices toward optimum peritoneal access: 1998 update. Perit Dial Int. 1998;18:11–33.
19. Crabtree JH. Selected best demonstrated practices in peritoneal dialysis access. Kidney Int. 2006;70:S27–37.
20. Mehrotra R, Crabtree J. PD Catheter Placement and Management. 2011. http://ispd.org/NAC/education/pd-curriculum/. Accessed May 2011.
21. Jo Y, Shin SK, Lee J, Song J, Park J. Immediate initiation of CAPD following percutaneous catheter placement without break-in procedure. Perit Dial Int. 2007;27: 179–83.
22. Gabriel DP, Caramori JT, Martin LC, Barretti P, Balbi AL. Continuous peritoneal dialysis compared with daily hemodialysis in patients with acute kidney injury. Perit Dial Int. 2009;29 suppl 2:S62–71.
23. George J, Varma S, Kumar S, Thomas J, Gopi S, Pisharody R. Comparing continuous venovenous hemodiafiltration and peritoneal dialysis in critically Ill patients with acute kidney injury: a pilot study. Perit Dial Int. 2011;31(4):422–9.
24. Chionh CY, Soni S, Cruz DN, Ronco C. Peritoneal dialysis for acute kidney injury: techniques and dose. Contrib Nephrol. 2009;163:278–84.
25. Allon M, Daugirdas J, Depner TA, Greene T, Ornt D, Schwab SJ. Effect of change in vascular access on patient mortality in hemodialysis patients. Am J Kidney Dis. 2006;47:469–77.
26. Polkinghorne KR, McDonald SP, Atkins RC, Kerr PG. Vascular access and All-cause mortality: a propensity score analysis. J Am Soc Nephrol. 2004;15: 477–86.
27. Peritoneal access—Guidelines. Nephrol Dial Transplant. 2005; 20 (suppl 9):ix8–ix12.
28. Keane WF, Bailie GR, Boeschoten E, Gokal R, Golper TA, Holmes CJ, Kawaguchi Y, Piraino B, Riella M, Vas S. Adult peritoneal dialysis-related peritonitis treatment recommendations: 2000 update. Perit Dial Int. 2000;20:396–411.
29. Bernardini J, Bender F, Florio T, Sloand J, PalmMontalbano L, Fried L, Piraino B. Randomized, double-blind trial of antibiotic exit site cream for prevention of exit site infection in peritoneal dialysis patients. J Am Soc Nephrol. 2005;26:539–45.
30. Heimburger O, Blake PG. Apparatus for peritoneal dialysis. In: Daugirdas JT, Blake PG, Ing TS, editors. Handbook of dialysis. 4th ed. Philadelphia, PA: Lippincott Williams & Wilkins; 2007. p. 339–55.
31. Garcia-Lopez E, Lindholm B. Icodextrin metabolites in peritoneal dialysis. Perit Dial Int. 2009;29:370–6.
32. Flore KMJ, Delanghe JR. Analytical interfereneces in point-of-care testing glucometers by icodextrin and its metabolites: an overview. Perit Dial Int. 2009;29: 377–83.
33. Twardowski ZJ, Nolph KO, Khanna R, Prowant BF, Leonor P, Ryan P, Moore HL, Nielsen MP. Peritoneal equilibration test. Perit Dial Bull. 1987;7:138–47.
34. Johnson DW, Mudge DW, Blizzard S, Arndt M, O'Shea A, Watt R, Hamilton J, Cottingham S, Isbel NM, Hawley CM. A comparison of peritoneal equilibration tests performed 1 and 4 weeks after PD commencement. Perit Dial Int. 2004;24:460–5.
35. La Milla V, DiFilippo S, Crepaldi M, Del Vecchio C, Dell'Oro C, Andrulli S, Locatelli F. Mini-peritoneal equilibration test: a simple and fast method to assess free water and small solute transport across the peritoneal membrane. Kidney Int. 2003;68:840–6.
36. Pride ET, Gustafson J, Graham A, Spainhour L, Mauck V, Brown P, Burkart JM. Comparison of a 2.5% and a 4.25% Dextrose Peritoneal Equilibration Test. Perit Dial Int. 2002;22:365–70.
37. Blake PG. Adequacy of peritoneal dialysis and chronic peritoneal dialysis prescription. In: Daugirdas JT, Blake PG, Ing TS, editors. Handbook of dialysis. 4th

ed. Philadelphia, PA: Lippincott Williams & Wilkins; 2007. p. 387–409.

38. DeVita MV, Gaiki M, Gilles E. Peritoneal Dialysis Prescription and Modalities. 2011 http://ispd.org/NAC/education/pd-curriculum/. Accessed May 2011
39. Mehrotra R, Chiu Y, Kalantar-Zadeh K, Vonesh E. The outcomes of continuous ambulatory and automated peritoneal dialysis are similar. Kidney Int. 2009;76:97–107.
40. Michels WM, Verduijn M, Boeschoten EW, Dekker FW, Krediet RT. Similar survival on automated peritoneal dialysis and continuous ambulatory peritoneal dialysis in a large prospective cohort. Clin J Am Soc Nephrol. 2009;4:943–9.
41. Watnick S. Peritoneal Dialysis Adequacy. 2011. http://ispd.org/NAC/education/pd-curriculum/. Accessed May 2011
42. Lo W, Bargman JM, Burkart J, Krediet RT, Pollock C, Kawanishi H, Blake PG. Guideline on targets for solute and fluid removal in adult patients on chronic peritoneal dialysis. Perit Dial Int. 2006;26:520–2.
43. K/DOQI Clinical Practice Guidelines for Peritoneal Dialysis Adequacy. Am J Kidney Dis. 2006;48 (suppl 1):S99-S129.
44. Marron B, Remon C, Perez-fontan MP, Quiros P, Ortiz A. Benefits of preserving residual renal function in peritoneal dialysis. Kidney Int. 2008;73:S42–51.
45. Li PK, Chow K, Wang TY, Leung C, Szeto C. Effects of an angiotensin-converting enzyme inhibitor on residual renal function in patients receiving peritoneal dialysis. A randomized, controlled study. Ann Intern Med. 2003;139:105–12.
46. Ash SR, Daugirdas JT. Peritoneal access devices. In: Daugirdas JT, Glake PG, Ing TS, editors. Handbook of dialysis. 4th ed. Philadelphia, PA: Lippincott Williams & Wilkins; 2007. p. 356–75.
47. McCormick BB, Bargman JM. Noninfectious complications of peritoneal dialysis: implications for patient and technique survival. J Am Soc Nephrol. 2007;18: 3023–5.
48. Yilmazlar T, Kirdak T, Bilgin S, Yavuz M, Yurtkuran M. Laparoscopic findings of peritoneal dialysis catheter malfunction and management outcomes. Perit Dial Int. 2006;26:374–9.
49. Dejardin A, Robert A, Goffin E. Intraperitoneal pressure in PD patients: relationship to intraperitoneal volume, body size and PD-related complications. Nephrol Dial Transplant. 2007;22:1437–44.
50. Bargman JM. Non-Infectious Complications of Peritoneal Dialysis. 2011. http://ispd.org/NAC/education/pd-curriculum/. Accessed May 2011.
51. Martinez-Mier G, Garcia-Almazan E, Reyes-Devesa HE, Garcia-Garcia V, Cano-Gutierrez S, Fermin RM, Estrada-Oros J, Budar-Fernandez LF, Avila-Pardo SF, Mendez-Machado GF. Abdominal wall hernias in end-stage renal disease patients on peritoneal dialysis. Perit Dial Int. 2008;28:391–6.
52. Bargman JM. Hernias in peritoneal dialysis patients: limiting occurrence and recurrence. Perit Dial Int. 2008;28:349–51.
53. Del Peso G, Bajo MA, Costero O, Hevia C, Fernando G, Diaz C, Aguilera A, Selgas R. Risk factors for abdominal wall complications in peritoneal dialysis patients. Perit Dial Int. 2003;23:249–54.
54. Juergensen PH, Rizvi H, Caride VJ, Kliger AS, Finkelstein FO. Value of scintigraphy in chronic peritoneal dialysis patients. Kidney Int. 1999;55:1111–9.
55. Hollett MD, Marn CS, Ellis JH, Francis IR, Swartz RD. Complications of continuous ambulatory peritoneal dialysis: evaluation with CT peritoneography. Am J Roentgenol. 1992;159:983–9.
56. Garcia-Urena MA, Rodrigues CR, Ruiz VV, Hernandez FJC, Fernandez-Ruiz E, Gallego JMV, Garcia MV. Prevalence and management of hernias in peritoneal dialysis patients. Perit Dial Int. 2006;26:198–202.
57. Shah H, Chu M, Bargman JM. Perioperative management of peritoneal dialysis patients undergoing hernia surgery without the use of interim hemodialysis. Perit Dial Int. 2006;26:684–7.
58. Szeto CC, Chow KM. Pathogenesis and management of hydrothorax complicating peritoneal dialysis. Curr Opin Pulm Med. 2004;10:315–9.
59. Lew SQ. Hydrothorax: pleural effusion associated with peritoneal dialysis. Perit Dial Int. 2010;30:13–8.
60. Mancebo RD, Bilsanz DP, Rodriguez M, Fernandez B, Gonzalez MO, Rubio MAB, Gutierrez RS. Pleuroperitoneal communication in patients on peritoneal dialysis. One hospital's experience and a review of the literature. Nefrologia. 2011;31:213–7.
61. Yang P, Kiu T. Massive "sweet" hydrothorax. CMAJ. 2010;182:1883.
62. Lew SQ. Hemoperitoneaum: bloody peritoneal dialysate in ESRD patients receiving peritoneal dialysis. Perit Dial Int. 2007;27:226–33.
63. Tse K, Yip P, Lam M, Li F, Choy B, Chan T, Lai K. Recurrent hemoperitoneum complicating continuous ambulatory peritoneal dialysis. Perit Dial Int. 2002;22:488–91.
64. Goodkin DA, Benning MG. An Outpatient Maneuver to Treat Bloody Effluent during Continuous Ambulatory Peritoneal Dialysis (CAPD). Perit Dial Int. 1990;10: 227–9.
65. Mahael AS, Katyal A, Khanna R. Complications of peritoneal dialysis related to increased intra-abdominal pressure. Adv Perit Dial. 2003;19:130–5.
66. Bargman JM. Mechanical complications of peritoneal dialysis. In: Daugirdas JT, Blake PG, Ing TS, editors. Handbook of dialysis. 4th ed. Philadelphia, PA: Lippincott Williams & Wilkins; 2007. p. 440–5.
67. Prichard SS. Metabolic complications of peritoneal dialysis. In: Daugirdas JT, Blake PG, Ing TS, editors. Handbook of dialysis. 4th ed. Philadelphia, PA: Lippincott Williams & Wilkins; 2007. p. 446–52.
68. Burkart J. Metabolic consequences of peritoneal dialysis. Semin Dial. 2004;17:498503.
69. Goffin E. Peritoneal membrane structural and functional changes during peritoneal dialysis. Semin Dial. 2008;21:258–65.
70. Williams JD, Craig KJ, Topley N, Von Ruhland C, Fallon M, Newman GR, Mackenzie RK, Williams GT.

Morphologic changes in the peritoneal membrane of patients with renal disease. J Am Soc Nephrol. 2002;13:470–9.
71. Devuyst O, Margetts PJ, Topley N. The pathophysiology of the peritoneal membrane. J Am Soc Nephrol. 2010;21:1077–85.
72. Mujais S, Nolph K, Gokal R, Blake P, Burkart J, Coles G, Kawaguchi Y, Kawanishi H, Korbet S, Krediet R, Lindholm B, Oreopoulos D, Rippe B, Selgas R. Evaluation and management of ultrafiltration problems in peritoneal dialysis. Perit Dial Int. 2000;20 suppl 4:S5–21.
73. Ho-dac-Pannekeet MM, Atasever B, Struijk DG, Krediet RT. Analysis of ultrafiltration failure in peritoneal dialysis patients by means of standard peritoneal permeability analysis. Perit Dial Int. 1997;17: 144–50.
74. Kawaguchi Y, Kawanishi H, Mujais S, Topley N, Oreopoulos DG. Encapsulating peritoneal sclerosis: definition, etiology, diagnosis, and treatment. Perit Dial Int. 2000;20 suppl 4:S43–55.
75. Brown EA, Viesen WV, Finkelstein FO, Hurst H, Johnson DW, Kawanishi H, Pecoits-Filho R, Woodrow G. Length of time on peritoneal dialysis and encapsulating peritoneal sclerosis: position paper for ISPD. Perit Dial Int. 2009;29:595–600.
76. Hansson JH, Cameron SF, Protopapas Z, Mehrotra R. Encapsulating Peritoneal Sclerosis (EPS). 2011. http://ispd.org/NAC/education/pd-curriculum/. Accessed May 2011
77. Tarzi RM, Lim A, Moser S, Ahmad S, George A, Balasubramaniam G, Clutterbuck EJ, Gedroyc W, Brown EA. Assessing the validity of an abdominal CT scoring system in the diagnosis of encapsulating peritoneal sclerosis. Clin J Am Soc Nephrol. 2008;3: 1702–10.
78. Vlijm A, Stoker J, Bipata S, Spijkerboer AM, Saffire Phoa S, Maes R, Struijk DG, Krediet RT. Computed Tomographic Findings Characteristic for Encapsulating Peritoneal Sclerosis: A Case-Control Study. Perit Dial Int. 2009;29:517–22.
79. Honda K, Oda H. Pathology of encapsulating peritoneal sclerosis. Perit Dial Int. 2005;25 suppl 4:S19–29.
80. Schmidt DW, Flessner MF. Pathogenesis and treatment of encapsulating peritoneal sclerosis: basic and translational research. Perit Dail Int. 2008;28 suppl 5:S10–5.
81. Park S, Kim Y, Lindholm B. Experimental encapsulating peritoneal sclerosis models: pathogenesis and treatment. Perit Dial Int. 2008;28 suppl 5:S21–8.
82. Lo WK, Kawanishi H. Encapsulating peritoneal sclerosis: medical and surgical treatment. Perit Dial Int. 2009;29(suppl2):S211–4.
83. Bunke CM, Brier ME, Golper TA. Outcomes of single organism peritonitis in peritoneal dialysis: Gram negatives versus gram positives in the Network 9 Peritonitis Study. Kidney Int. 1997;52:524–9.
84. Fontan MP, Rodriguez-Carmona A, Garcia-Naveiro R, Rosales M, Villaverde P, Valdes F. Peritonitis-related mortality in patients undergoing chronic peritoneal dialysis. Perit Dial Int. 2005;25:274–84.
85. Mujais S. Microbiology and outcomes of peritonitis in North America. Kidney Int. 2006;70:S55–62.
86. Piraino B. Peritoneal infections. Adv Ren Replace Ther. 2000;7:280–8.
87. Li PK, Szeto CC, Piraino B, Bernardini J, Figueiredo AE, Gupta A, Johnson DW, Kuijper EJ, Lye W, Salzer W, Schaefer F, Struijk DG. Peritoneal dialysis-related infections recommendations: 2010 update. Perit Dial Int. 2010;30:393–423.
88. Piraino B. PD-Related Infections Recommendation. 2011. http://ispd.org/NAC/education/pd-curriculum/. Accessed May 2011.
89. Wong SSY, Ho P, Yuen K. Evolution of antibiotic resistance mechanisms and their relevance to dialysis-related infections. Perit Dial Int. 2007;27 suppl 2:S272–80.
90. Furgeson SB, Teitelbaum I. New treatment options and protocols for peritoneal dialysis-related peritonitis. Contrib Nephrol. 2009;163:169–76.
91. Zelenitsky S, Barns L, Findlay I, Alfa M, et al. Analysis of microbiological trends in peritoneal dialysis-related peritonitis from 1991 to 1998. Am J Kidney Dis. 2000;36:1009–13.
92. Kavanagh D, Prescott GJ, Mactier RA. Peritoneal dialysis-associated peritonitis in Scotland (1999-2002). Nephrol Dial Transplant. 2004;19:2584–91.
93. Kim DK, Yoo T, Ryu D, Xu Z, Kim HJ, Choi KH, Lee HY, Han D, Kang S. Changes in causative organisms and their antimicrobial susceptibilities in CAPD peritonitis: a single Center's experience over One decade. Perit Dial Int. 2004;24:424–32.
94. Oo TH, Roberts T, Collins AJ. A comparison of peritonitis rates from the United States Renal Data System Database: CAPD versus continuous cycling peritoneal dialysis patients. Am J Kidney Dis. 2005;45: 372–80.
95. Port FK, Held PJ, Nolph KD, Turenne MN, Wolfe RA. Risk of peritonitis and technique failure by CAPD connection technique: a national study. Kidney Int. 1992;42:967–74.
96. Troidle L, Gorban-Brennan N, Finkelstein FO. Outcome of patients on chronic peritoneal dialysis undergoing peritoneal catheter removal because of peritonitis. Adv Perit Dail. 2005;21:98–101.

Additional Resources

PD Curriculum. North American Chapter of the International Society of Peritoneal Dialysis. (2011) http://ispd.org/NAC/education/pd-curriculum/. (Accessed May 2011).

Palliative Care in Renal Disease

33

James C. Wasserman

Case

Mr. Mario I. was 86-year-old man returning to nephrology clinic for follow-up of chronic kidney disease (CKD) stage IV/V in the setting of hypertension and presumed hypertensive nephrosclerosis. He had a history of uremia over the past 8 months with increased fatigue, somnolence, and anorexia; observed decreased attentiveness and increased need for assistance with activities of daily living (ADL) concerning to his wife; and it was increasing difficulty to control his edema and maintain euvolemia.

Mr. I. had been referred to the dialysis clinic 5 years earlier after having initiated hemodialysis at an out-of-state clinic where he had been diagnosed with end-stage renal disease (ESRD). However, additional assessment after his referral had shown a creatinine clearance of 14 mL per minute and so a trial off dialysis was begun. Mr. I. did well without dialysis for more than 4 years. He maintained an active family and social life. He exercised regularly, walked the beach, remained out of the hospital, and was overjoyed about life without renal replacement therapy.

Over the past year, Mr. I. had become more symptomatic and his creatinine clearance fell to 8 mL per minute. At this visit, the nephrologist discussed options for ESRD management, including peritoneal dialysis, in-center hemodialysis, home hemodialysis, and in-center nocturnal dialysis, as well as conservative management without dialysis therapy. Estimations of prognosis, life expectancy, and likely quality of life with and without renal replacement therapy were discussed, as was the role of hospice in conservative management and dialysis care.

Mr. and Ms. I. thought that they would like to proceed without dialysis but they wanted to talk it over with their children. They "didn't see the point" of restarting dialysis, as it was not the type of life Mr. I. wanted. All agreed that conservative management to optimize quality of life and the use of hospice care at the appropriate time were rational and "good choices" for Mr. I.

At follow-up 1 week later, Mr. and Ms. I. informed the nephrologist that their children had convinced them to try dialysis again with the hope that it would increase Mr. I.'s life expectancy and quality of life. With Mr. I.'s permission, the nephrologist also spoke with the children, reviewing their father's prognosis, life expectancy, and quality of life with and without dialysis. They were surprised and taken aback by how little renal replacement therapy might offer him, but still thought it was reasonable to proceed with a trial period of dialysis.

1. What principals and paradigms of care did the nephrologist use in discussions of treatment options with Mr. and Ms I. and their children?

J.C. Wasserman, M.D., B.A. (✉)
Division of Nephrology and Transplantation, Main Medical Center, Bramhall Street, Portland, Cumberland County, ME 04102, USA
e-mail: wassej@mmc.org

E.V. Lerma and M. Rosner (eds.), *Clinical Decisions in Nephrology, Hypertension and Kidney Transplantation*, DOI 10.1007/978-1-4614-4454-1_33, © Springer Science+Business Media New York 2013

2. Do you think this was time well spent? Are you able to find enough time in your practice to have discussions like this?
3. Do you feel well trained to provide prognosis and life expectancies to your patients? Do you believe there is sufficient information to provide an accurate assessment? Does this information extinguish patient's hopes?
4. Do you think the timing of discussions with Mr. and Mrs. I. about end-of-life care was appropriate? Should they have begun sooner in this doctor–patient relationship and been part of a larger discussion of advanced care planning?
5. When and under what circumstances do you begin end-of-life discussions? Do you include family members and primary care physicians? Do you feel comfortable and capable when conducting end-of-life discussions?
6. Is shared-decision-making between caregivers, patients, and patient families always the best method in choosing treatment options? Is it ever appropriate to tell patients and families that dialysis care is of no value?
7. What provisions and resources do you have in your practice for patients who choose conservative therapy? Are you familiar and comfortable with providing palliative care? Do you believe palliative care should be part of standard CKD and ESRD care?

Practicum for Starting a Palliative-Care Dialogue in ESRD

Dr. N: Thanks for coming in today, Mr. I. and Ms. I. What brings you back earlier than planned?

Mrs. I: I'm just so concerned about Mario, doctor. He's not himself. He has no interest in anything. He doesn't want to eat or even get out of bed. I practically have to drag him out to help him wash up and get dressed. That's just not him. I increased the water pill like you told me, but his feet and legs are still as swollen as before, and he has to go to the bathroom all the time.

Dr. N: I see. What do you think, Mario?

Mr. I: I don't know… you're the doctor. I feel fine. I don't feel any different. [Addressing his wife:] What do you want me to do?

Mrs. I: I want you to do something. You just sit there. I want you to be Mario.

Dr. N: Well, Mario, your wife may be onto something. You've lost weight and you certainly walked more slowly to and from the waiting room today.

Mr. I: Doc, I'm 86 years old. We all slow down after a while.

Dr. N: That's true, but I think some of your symptoms and what your wife sees at home may be from low kidney function. By your last blood tests, your kidneys are only working at 7–8% of normal. The way you're feeling—no ambition, tired all the time, no appetite—and the increased leg swelling are caused by this low kidney function.

Mr. I: Geez, what should we do? Is there anything that can make my kidneys better?

Dr. N: Mario, you've had decreased kidney function for a long time now. This is probably due to years of high blood pressure and your increased age, and it's not likely to get better. I know that you were able to stop dialysis and feel better after we first met. But I was never quite sure of the circumstances or why you had started dialysis before then. Maybe you had an acute injury to your kidneys 5 years ago and you were able to recover from it. But over the past 4 years, you haven't had any acute illnesses or events affecting that slow downward trend we've been following in your kidney function. I think it's just the natural progression of chronic kidney disease. Unfortunately, I know of no treatments that can reverse or cure it. But we still need to decide on the best treatment for you.

Mr. I: If you're talking about dialysis, I don't know.

Dr. N: Dialysis is one option.

Mr. I: Yeah, and what's the other—dying?

Dr. N: Not dying, but living without dialysis. You'll go on living but probably for a shorter period of time than if you restarted dialysis.

Mr. I: What sort of time period are we talking about—days…weeks?

Dr. N: No, without dialysis I think you will live another year to year-and-a-half. If you decided to receive dialysis treatments, I think you would live another two to two-and-a-half years.

But much of that extra time would be spent in the dialysis clinic or possibly in the hospital tending to illnesses that arise while you're receiving dialysis.

Mr. I: What if I don't choose dialysis? What kind of life will I have? . . .

Historical Perspective: Creation of a Technology-Centered ESRD Program

Ever since the invention of the Scribner shunt brought about the inception and creation of chronic intermittent dialysis care, the issue of patient selection for this life-saving treatment has loomed large and created controversy [1]. When the first ESRD program was started in Seattle in 1962, the primary issue was of patient selection for renal replacement therapy. Huge costs and lack of trained personnel and machines necessitated rationing of the limited number of hemodialysis spots for a growing population in need. Patient selection criteria became paramount. Potential candidates for dialysis at the Seattle Artificial Kidney Center were first screened and evaluated for physical and psychological fitness to receive renal replacement therapy, then adjudicated by what came to be known as the "God Committee," lay members of the Seattle community who chose the final candidates for dialysis based on their assessment of an individual's worth to society [1–4].

As chronic dialysis spread to other cities throughout the USA, news of this life-saving therapy and the ramifications of its rationing became known to the public, triggering a strong response to the workings of patient selection committees in the lay and medical press [1]. The visceral reaction to rationing of life-saving therapy found its way to political leaders, and in 1972 Section 2991 of the Social Security Amendments was enacted [5]. It established almost universal coverage for treatment of ESRD under Medicare, thereby eliminating the need for rationing and patient selection based on financial stresses. One rationale for providing universal insurance coverage for ESRD was the expectation that dialysis therapy would not only extend life but also enable many patients disabled by ESRD to return to work and their normal life activities [6–8]. Initially, patient selection was not completely eliminated from the bill; a provision stipulated that all patients referred for renal replacement therapy be screened for the appropriateness of intervention. However, with no legislative precedent to clarify a review, no additional governmental codification to implement screening, and the newly created ESRD Networks dealing with other matters, this requirement was removed in 1978.

The US nephrology community was ready to serve an ever-increasing patient population, one rapidly changing in size and characteristics from the 1960s. Indeed, the ESRD community was becoming increasingly older and populated primarily by patients with diabetes mellitus and hypertension as the primary cause of kidney disease—conditions that had previously been contraindications for the treatment of ESRD.

Dialysis Without Selection: Maturation of the USRDS Population

The overall incidence and prevalence of ESRD appears to have reached a plateau [9–13], except for people over the age of 65 (Fig. 33.1) [13]. Increased longevity, availability of dialysis technology, and broadened public and medical expectations have led to a marked growth in the elderly ESRD population [11], such that patients over the age of 75 are now the fastest growing segment of the US ESRD population in the USA [14].

Comorbid conditions occur more frequently in this age group and lead to increased symptom burden, shortened survival, often poor quality of life, and increased withdrawal from dialysis [15–20]. People over the age of 70 comprised half of all dialysis deaths—37,000 out of 74,000—in 2005 [21]. Those over the age of 75 starting dialysis have an annualized mortality rate of approximately 50% in the initial 6 months of renal replacement therapy (Fig. 33.2) [21]. This extraordinary rate reflects the general health and well-being of patients with CKD. An analysis of 209,622 veterans showed that all patients with CKD over 65 years were more

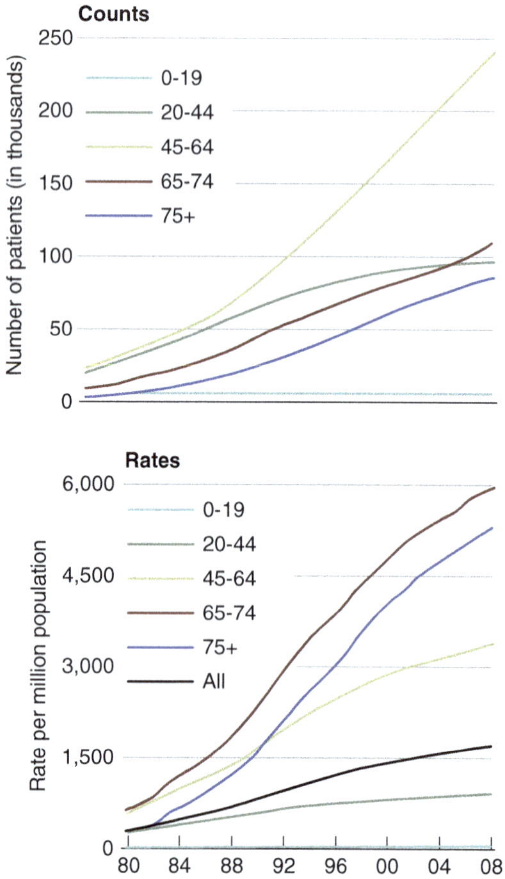

Fig. 33.1 Emergence of an aging population of patients with ESRD: incidence and prevalence in the USA in 2010. December 31 point prevalent ESRD patients; adjusted for gender and race. USRDS 2010. Adapted from the US Renal Data System, USRDS 2010 Annual Data Report: Atlas of End-Stage Renal Disease in the United States, National Institutes of Health, National Institute of Diabetes and Digestive and Kidney Diseases, Bethesda, MD, 2010. The data reported here have been supplied by the United States Renal Data System (USRDS). The interpretation and reporting of these data are the responsibility of the author(s) and in no way should be seen as an official policy or interpretation of the US government

likely to die than start dialysis [22], and as patients become older, death becomes increasingly more likely than dialysis [16, 22]. This high risk of death prior to the initiation of dialysis is probably related to the tremendous cardiovascular comorbid conditions found in the older CKD population.

In patients with such a limited life expectancy, one might propose that dialysis be started to alleviate the symptoms of uremia and to improve quality of life and functional status. This includes the ability to perform ADL such as arising from bed, toileting, dressing, bathing, and feeding. Even so, high rates of functional impairment are reported in the ESRD population [23–25]. Among US nursing home residents starting dialysis, a marked decline in functional status has been observed during the period surrounding the initiation of dialysis. One year after the start of dialysis, only one of eight residents was found to have functional capacity maintained at predialysis levels (Fig. 33.3) [23]. This decline can also be attributed to the high degree of disability in these patients, including impairment related to coexisting conditions such as cardiovascular disease, cerebrovascular disease and dementia, which are not improved by dialysis.

Dialysis carries with it attendant burdens such as excessive travel, vascular access, a reduction in time for meals and physical activity, depression, fatigue, and pain. These hardships interfere with rehabilitation and stabilization of functional status. Patients with ESRD are among the most symptomatic of any chronic disease groups. Pain is a common symptom and has an impact on virtually every aspect of health-related quality of life [19, 26–32] (Table 33.1) [29]. Davison and others have shown that 37–50% of hemodialysis patients experience chronic pain, most of it moderate to severe in intensity [26, 32–34] and similar to that of cancer patients hospitalized in palliative care settings [26, 27, 35]. Additional symptoms such as fatigue, insomnia, depression, anorexia, and lack of well-being all lead to depression, anxiety, and low mental and physical quality of life [27–29]. The extraordinary risk of dying, loss of bodily function, pain, depression, and other symptoms has led 20–30% of patients with ESRD to withdraw from dialysis by choice [36, 37]—the second-leading cause of death in this population.

The Rise of Technology and Fall of Patient-Centered Care

How did this happen? How did this life-saving and life-extending therapy originally rationed and limited to individuals of the "highest social worth" become a technological treatment in

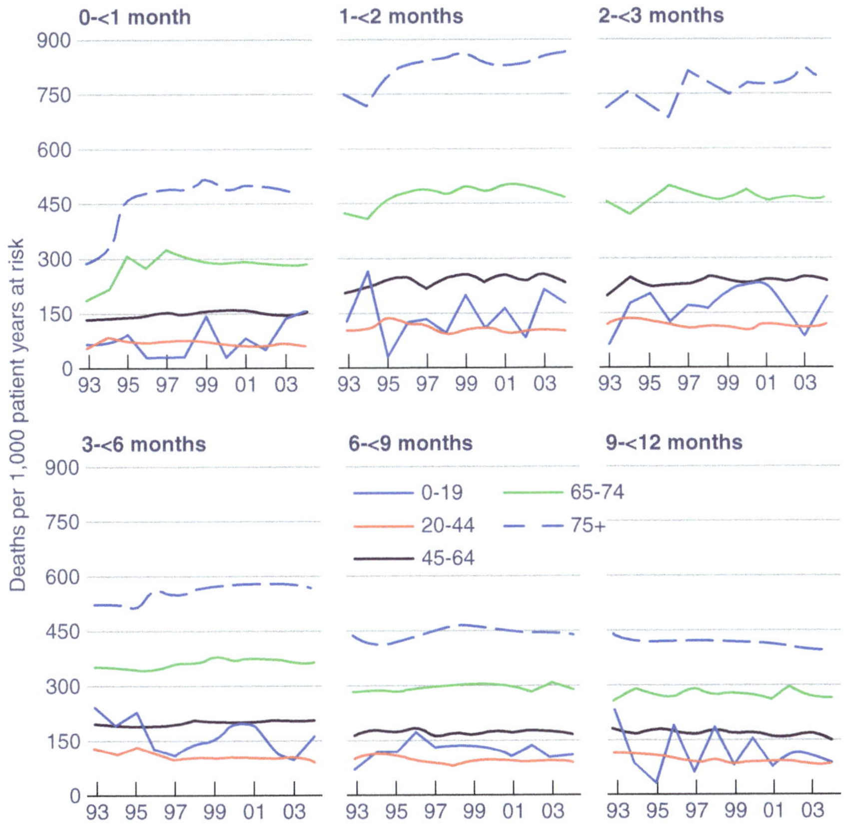

Fig. 33.2 Pronounced annualized mortality among older patients with ESRD in the USA within 6 months of initiation of dialysis. Incident dialysis patients; adjusted for age, gender, race, and primary diagnosis. Incident ESRD patients, 1993, used as reference cohort. USRDS 2007. Adapted from the US Renal Data System, USRDS 2007 Annual Data Report: Atlas of End-Stage Renal Disease in the USA, National Institutes of Health, National Institute of Diabetes and Digestive and Kidney Diseases, Bethesda, MD, 2007 [21]. The data reported here have been supplied by the United States Renal Data System (USRDS). The interpretation and reporting of these data are the responsibility of the author(s) and in no way should be seen as an official policy or interpretation of the US government

which the burdens of therapy frequently outweigh the benefits [38]? How have nephrologists allowed themselves to become providers of dialysis therapy to a growing population for whom they perceive it to be of marginal benefit?

Perhaps it occurred because the nephrology community was scarred by its rationing experience of the 1960s. Removal of this barrier was followed shortly by the industrialization of dialysis services and overreliance on technology to ensure ESRD therapy to an ever-increasing patient population, without our stopping to examine the short-term and long- term outcomes and the cost–benefit ratios for patients being treating. We have come to deny the nephrologist's role as a primary-care geriatrician to an aging and ill population of patients receiving dialysis. It begins in nephrology fellowship training, where end-of-life care is not well addressed [39–41]. Second-year fellows report feeling uncomfortable discussing prognosis and end-of-life issues with patients and unprepared to care for them (Figs. 33.4, 33.5, 33.6) [39]. This has produced clinicians who are not trained to assist patients in the complex end-of-life decision-making required when caring for those with CKD and ESRD [41].

Communication of prognosis and discussions related to planning for morbid and mortal events are, therefore, lacking in the routine care of patients with CKD. Most patients starting dialysis

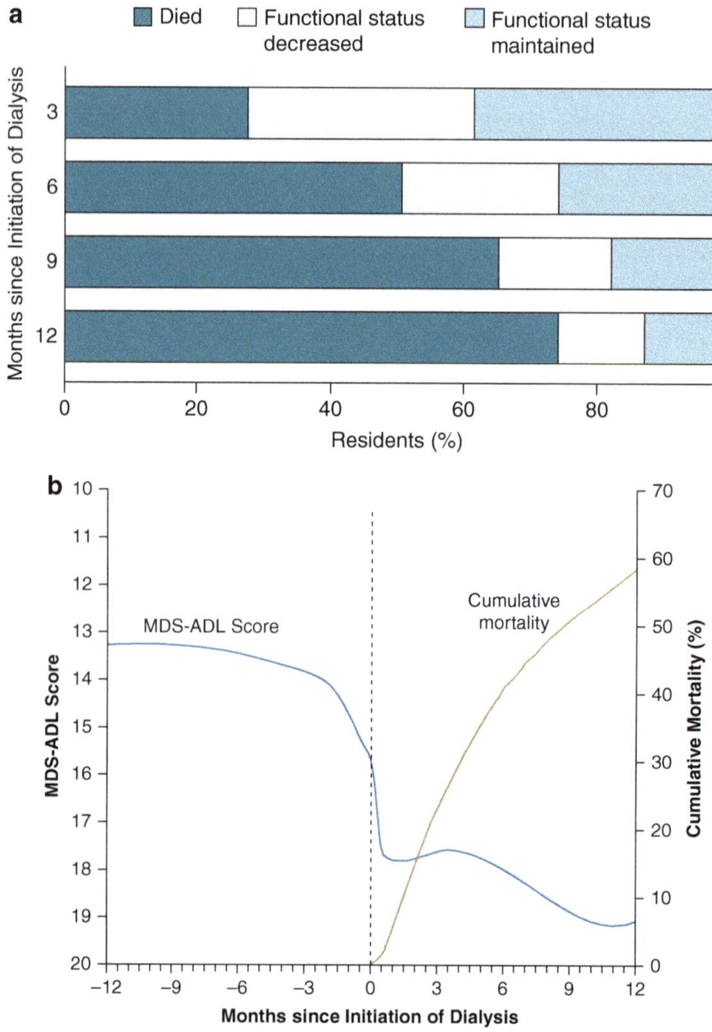

Fig. 33.3 Mortality and change in functional status among 3,702 elderly persons in nursing homes in the US starting dialysis. (**a**) Percent of residents who died or experienced a decrease or maintained functional status within 3 months of starting dialysis. (**b**) Trajectory of functional status before and after the initiation of dialysis and cumulative mortality rate. Reproduced with permission from Kurella Tamura et al. [23]

do not appreciate the likelihood of clinical deterioration over the first year of treatment [1]. Over 90% of patients in one study reported having had no discussion about prognosis with a doctor and as few as 10% in other studies have engaged in any form of end-of-life decisions [1, 29, 42–44]. Lack of training and a greater commitment to technology are now coupled unfortunately with a focus on serving a growing population of older patients, such that significant barriers against advance care planning exist within the dialysis community [41, 43, 44]. Neglect of advance care planning in the ESRD population naturally leads to an underutilization of palliative and hospice care and a caregiver–patient relationship where end-of-life needs are unlikely to be met. More than 20% of patients receiving dialysis terminate therapy before death. Most of these patients will die within 8–14 days of stopping treatment [45], yet few are enroll in hospice (Fig. 33.7) [46]. Murray et al. found 42% of patients who stopped dialysis between January

Table 33.1 Prevalence and severity of common symptoms among 591 hemodialysis patients (average age 61.3 years)

mESAS Symptoms[a]			
	Percent of patients		
	Symptom	Moderate/ severe	
Symptom	Present	Symptoms	Mean (SD)
Tired	92.2	73.1	5.1 (2.7)
Lack of well-being	90.9	59.1	4.2 (2.5)
Appetite	82.1	47.0	3.6 (2.7)
Drowsy	77.0	45.7	3.4 (2.8)
Itching	75.8	44.5	3.6 (3.1)
Pain	72.4	46.5	3.5 (3.0)
Anxious	65.7	39.1	2.8 (2.9)
Depressed	64.6	37.7	2.8 (2.9)
Shortness of breath	61.9	32.7	2.6 (2.8)
Nauseated	54.3	24.2	2.0 (2.5)
Total Symptom Distress Score			33.4 (18.3)

[a]*mESAS* modified Edmonton Symptom Assessment System. Reproduced with permission from Davison and Jhangri [29]

2001 and December 2002 used hospice [46]—a less than satisfactory percentage in and of itself—and overall, it is estimated that only 13.5% of dialysis patients are enrolled in hospice before death. The large majority of patients with CKD die in acute care facilities not having utilized palliative care services [46–48]. It is unclear why the majority of patients who withdraw from dialysis are not enrolled in hospice, but a lack of focus on patient's wishes and symptoms and an inability and discomfort of caregivers to discuss end-of-life issues must play a large role [46].

Palliative Care: A Model of Humanistic and Supportive Care in CKD and ESRD

The dearth of clinical research in symptom management and lack of training in this area within nephrology have led to under-recognition and undertreatment of pain in ESRD [26]. Inadequate pain management leads to poor health-related quality of life in all measured domains [19, 30, 49] and needless suffering in patients who are dying [31]. Symptom management and end-of-life care are clear priorities for patients and they believe this is a responsibility of their renal care team [48]. The nephrologist and nephrology nurses are also perceived as important potential resources for emotional, social, and spiritual support. However, current paradigms of patient care established in the US ESRD program engender caregivers departing from this role. Fortunately, a large and active movement within the nephrology community is beginning to arise, aimed at restoring sensible, supportive, and humanistic care for our patients with CKD and ESRD [1, 49, 50].

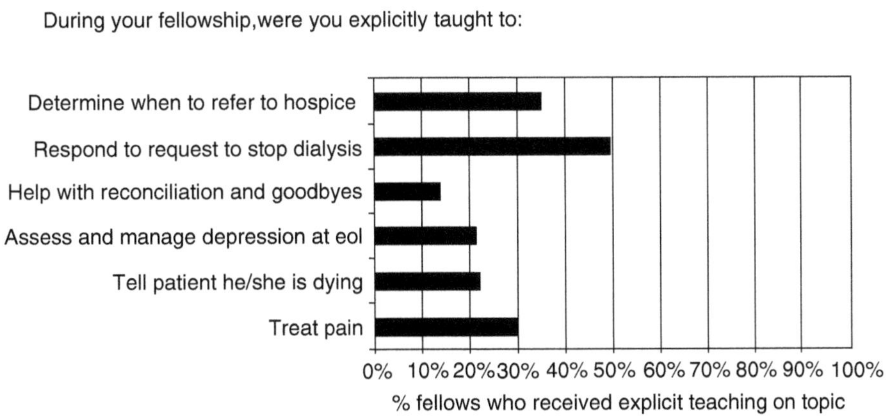

Fig. 33.4 Palliative care training among 173 second-year renal fellows: Reported content area taught explicitly during renal fellowship concerning end-of-life care (national survey). Adapted with permission from Holley et al. [39]

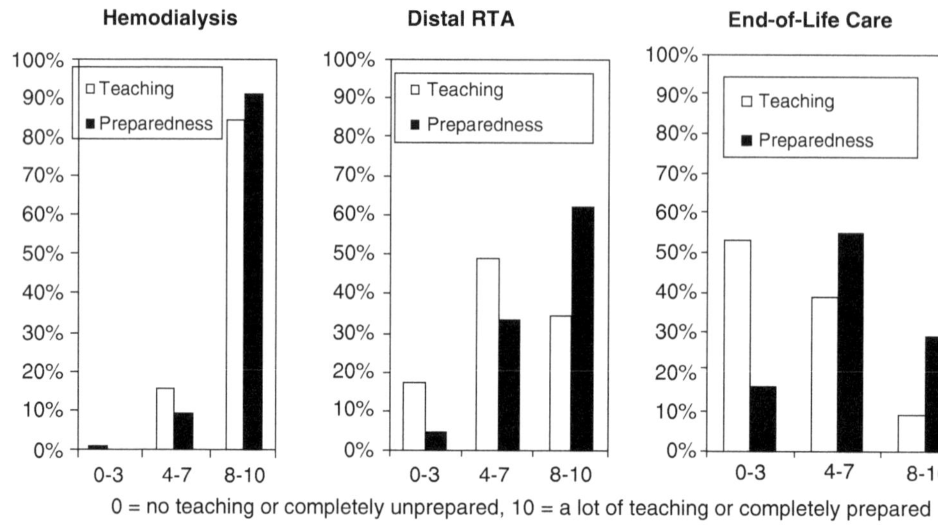

Fig. 33.5 Palliative care training among 173 second-year renal fellows: Perceived preparedness, compared with teaching during training for hemodialysis, distal RTA, or end-of-life care (national survey). Scale: 0 = no teaching or completely unprepared; 10 = a lot of teaching or completely prepared. Adapted with permission from Holley et al. [39]

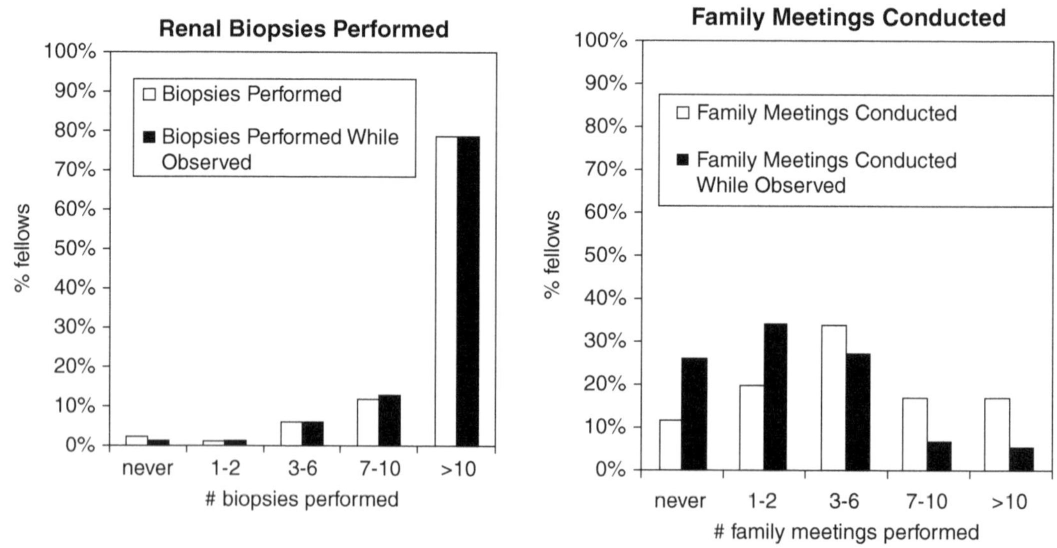

Fig. 33.6 Palliative care training among 173 second-year renal fellows: Skill development during training for renal biopsy compared with family meetings conducted (national survey). Adapted with permission from Holley et al. [39]

This care model ideally begins with the diagnosis of CKD because it is at this point in time that care shifts from a curative to a supportive—or palliative—focus. Supportive care becomes paramount and the well-being and quality of life of the patient and his or her family resides at the center of care [6, 51–54]. Because the symptom burden of dialysis patients is high, this population is aging, and these patients with ESRD have a markedly shortened life expectancy, palliative care is appropriate for them and their families. Components of palliative care in ESRD include

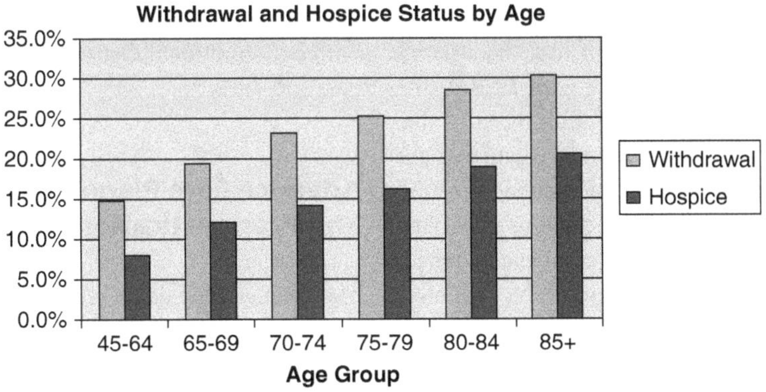

Fig. 33.7 Dialysis withdrawal and hospice status by age (USRDS 2001–2002 deceased cohort. Among the 115,239 deceased patients, 21.8% overall withdrew from dialysis and 13.5% used hospice. Withdrawal rates and hospice use increase with advancing age ($p<0.001$). Reproduced with permission from Murray et al. [46]

identification and management of pain and other symptoms, advance care planning and communication, psychosocial and spiritual support, and addressing ethical issues in dialysis decision-making [6, 51–54]. These components are also emphasized as guiding principals in the WHO definition of palliative care, a treatment that strives to improve quality of life and relieve suffering for patients with life-threatening illness and for their families [55], which is intended to relieve pain and other distressing symptoms rather than cure disease or delay progression. Other aspects include integration of psychosocial and spiritual needs with medical care, coordination of medical and social services, and creation of a support system to help the patient and family cope with illness and prepare for death [56]. Palliative care can be delivered at any point during the course of an illness and can be provided in conjunction with curative or life-saving therapy and hospice or non-hospice care.

Palliative and Advance Care Planning

How can we as practicing nephrologists incorporate palliative care into our CKD and ESRD practice so that the well-being and quality of life of our patients and their families become the center of our care? The Institute of Medicine first addressed this question in their 1991 report, *Kidney Failure and the Federal Government* [38], in a chapter on ethics. Their recommendation on acceptance and patient withdrawal from dialysis note that "patient acceptance criteria should be based on medical assessment of the benefits and burdens of treatment and on the best interest of individual patients, not on economic objectives or cost containment… Nephrologists have a professional responsibility to deal with issues of initiation and termination of treatment. Renal professionals should discuss with ESRD patients their wishes for dialysis, cardiopulmonary resuscitation, and other life sustaining treatments and encourage documented advanced directive" [38].

Building on this, the *End-Stage Renal Disease Workgroup on End-of-Life Care* recommends that dialysis clinics begin this process by facilitating advance care planning, open discussions, and a shared decision-making process. There is little evidence, however, that these guidelines have been widely implemented in clinical practice [43, 57, 58].

Advance care planning differs from traditional advance directives, which are legal documents that tend to outline limited treatment options and are only one optional component of a full plan, which helps to determine goals of care and sharpen the focus of present and future treatments. Advance care planning provides information early in a patient's illness that describes the impact of treatment and disease on daily life. It also provides information on prognosis and expected quality and quantity of life [59].

Many health professionals believe that including realistic prognosis and end-of-life discussions may destroy hope for patients with ESRD [40, 60, 61]. These beliefs are based on the idea that denial is a major coping mechanism patients use to adapt to a time-limited life on dialysis [62, 63]. Physicians often believe that patients receiving dialysis care do not view themselves as terminally ill and falsely assume they can be kept alive indefinitely with renal replacement therapy. Consistent with this belief is the finding that few patients choose "do-not—resuscitate" orders despite their very low chance of survival after cardiorespiratory arrest [64, 65].

These attitudes, an overreliance on laboratory monitoring as a substitute for patient care, and the commonly expressed idea that advanced care planning and end-of-life discussions may destroy hope for patients with ESRD lead to an avoidance of communicating prognosis to patients and what to expect during a life with renal replacement therapy [40, 60, 61]. This can result in unrealistic expectations of patients for their goals of care and survival, and it runs counter to the evidence recent studies reveal. Davidson et al. [59] found the process of advanced care planning more often serves as a means of enhancing hope. They determined that providing information early in ESRD on its impact on daily life empowered patients and enhanced their relationships with loved ones and staff. In this study, patients looked to physicians for assistance for making the necessary connections between their lives and the bewildering array of technology and information affecting treating them. Helping patients see future possibilities consistent with their values is what maintained their hope. Patients also changed as they learned more about their illness and who they are and what they can become in the context of a progressive disease. The researchers concluded that as illness progresses, health professionals, through advance care planning, play a critical role in patients' plans and hopes for the future. Patients given prognostic information reshaped their hopes, rather than remain anxious and fearful about an unknown future. These finding are consistent with the palliative care literature on hope in other patient groups, which have demonstrated that open discussion of prognosis is associated with less emotional distress during the dying process [66–68].

Advance Care Planning and Prognostication

The Renal Physician Association (RPA) and American Society of Nephrology (ASN) clinical practice guideline on shared decision-making when starting or stopping dialysis recommends that discussions contain an estimate of prognosis, life expectancy, and likely quality of life [1, 50]. Prognostic information is often the single most important item that patients need to make informed choices [69, 70]. Discussions regarding prognosis or end-of-life issues are often difficult for physicians, who can be uncomfortable about the uncertainty of clinical information provided to patients and families and the sensitive nature of the topic. There is not a single formula that combines all risk factors to provide a numerical estimate of life expectancy for patients with ESRD, but there are factors identified by multivariate analysis that are significant predictors of mortality. These include age, nutritional status, functional status, and comorbid illnesses [69, 71, 72]. Use of these factors as well as the Charleston Comorbidity Index of Coexistent Diseases [73] will greatly assist physicians in their ability to talk with patients and their families about realistic but uncertain prognosis in the setting of CKD and ESRD.

As little data support the notion that providing truthful information will destroy hope [70], physicians are obligated to provide their patients prognostic information. To withhold this information is to abrogate our professional responsibility and moral duty [68, 69]. Communication about prognosis associated with CKD and ESRD is of primary importance and a crucial contribution to the physician/patient relationship in shared decision-making. It is also a vital piece of information in the advanced care planning process. This is a learned process and there are many guidelines and position papers that instruct and illustrate methods to implement these practices in for our patients with CKD and ESRD and their families.

Symptom Control in Palliative Care

Symptom control is a central tenet of palliative care. The highly untreated symptom burden in patients with CKD and ESRD suggests that the nephrology community is not providing adequate palliative care [37, 52]. Even patients with early stages of CKD have many symptoms, yet most nephrologists would be surprised to learn that patients with stage 5 CKD not yet receiving dialysis have the same symptom burden as patients with cancer, HIV, and COPD [74, 75]. With the initiation of dialysis therapy, the majority of patients have five or more clinical symptoms [27]. However, relief of pain and other symptoms affecting quality of life are often not part of the care package delivered to or expected by patients with ESRD. This can be attributed in part to caregivers not asking about or discussing these issues with their patients with ESRD and to the emphasis on laboratory results and clinical guidelines rather than patient-centered care [41].

In one study by Davison and Jhangri in which 591 patients on hemodialysis were surveyed using the modified Edmonton Symptom Assessment System, the most frequently reported symptoms were tiredness (92%), decreased well-being, (91%) and anorexia (82%), and drowsiness, itchiness, and pain were reported in three quarters of the patients surveyed [29]. Tiredness or fatigue has been consistently shown to be one of the most prevalent symptoms in patients with ESRD [76, 77]. It has been associated with multiple causes including hypotension, rapid osmotic shifts with the dialysis procedure, depression, insomnia, carnitine deficiency, poor nutrition, medication side effects, and dialysis membrane blood interactions [78–81]. An initial investigation should include an evaluation of sleep habits, sleep apnea, restless leg syndrome, and dialysis dose.

Anorexia may be an indication of uremia, inadequate delivery of dialysis, or both [82]. It is very common in patients with diabetes and ESRD who suffer from autonomic dysfunction and gastric paresis. Anorexia may also be exacerbated by dry mouth due to side effects caused by many of the medications patients with ESRD take. Finally, anorexia may result from depression. Ensuring adequate dialysis dose, treating gastric paresis with pro-motility agents, relieving dry mouth by avoiding anti-cholinergic drugs, assessing for depression, and considering the appetite stimulants megase or marinol are all initial steps towards the treatment of anorexia [83, 84].

Davison and Jhangi reported that pain was experienced in 72% of patients receiving dialysis who they surveyed, and it was moderate to severe in intensity 46% [29]. The majority of pain reported is musculoskeletal in origin [32] and predominantly attributed to osteoarthritis and metabolic bone disease. There is also a significantly greater prevalence of neuropathic and ischemic pain in patients with ESRD compared with populations suffering from other chronic illness. Patients with ESRD patients usually experience more than one type of pain, and up to 75% of patients report that pain management is ineffective in controlling their symptoms [32].

The symptoms of pain, lack of well-being, and tiredness are all independent predictors in multivariate regression analysis of mental and physical health-related quality of life (HRQoL) [29]. Total symptom burden has been found to be highly predictive of HRQoL, but fatigue, pain, a lack of well-being, and anorexia have the greatest negative impact. In addition, the symptom of pain is significantly associated with an increased reporting of depression and insomnia when analyzed by multivariate analysis [27]. Insomnia has been reported by 50–90% of patients receiving dialysis [85–87]. It can be related to pain, but research has also demonstrated a high incidence of specific primary sleep disorders. These include sleep apnea, periodic leg movement disorders, and restless leg syndrome. Pain is also associated with anxiety and difficulty coping with stressful situations, as well as increased consideration of withdrawal from dialysis [27].

Depression, like pain, is a common but often undiagnosed and untreated syndrome in patients receiving dialysis. Depending on the depression-reporting tool, 20–50% of patients receiving dialysis are depressed [88]. Depression alters the presentations of chronic pain, complicates its treatment, and interferes with a patient's ability to cope with all of his or her infirmities [89].

The exact causative relationship between pain, insomnia, fatigue, and depression is often difficult to sort out and determine for both patient and clinician. However, no matter what the relationship, clinicians need to be mindful of all of these symptoms in order to improve the overall quality of life in the ESRD population. The initial steps in evaluation and management in these interrelated symptom complexes require communication with patients and their families. Listening to and acknowledging the adverse symptoms affecting patient quality of life will assist nephrology caregivers in their assessment of chronic illness and in their ability to design a comprehensive treatment plan that may allow a patient to live well with their chronic illness. The diagnoses and treatment of these syndromes are beyond the scope of this chapter. The reader is referred to many excellent reviews [26, 27, 32, 90–98]. However, attention to these syndromes and symptoms is central to the well-being of this patient population. As most decisions to withdraw from dialysis are associated with a decrease in HRQoL and pain syndrome [35], additional attention to palliative care may have an unexpected effect of decreasing both morbidity and mortality rates in the ESRD population. In contrast, studies show no association between the "key clinical indicators"—dialysis adequacy, serum albumin, hemoglobin, and bone metabolism—and chronic pain, symptom burden, and HRQoL [26].

Palliative Care and End-of-Life Care

A central tenet of palliative care is providing a good death when the end-of-life approaches. When a patient, or a family member making the decision for a patient, chooses to withhold the initiation of dialysis or to withdraw from ongoing dialysis treatment, nephrology caregivers should be able to provide a symptom-controlled death. As more than 20% of the US ESRD population withdraw from dialysis, end-of-life care should be considered an important part of the nephrology caregiving. Despite a predicted death within 1–2 weeks of terminating dialysis treatment, only 42% of these patients are enrolled in hospice programs [35, 46]. Furthermore, while more than 20% of all patients receiving dialysis care will die in a given year, only 13.5% of all patients in the ESRD program are enrolled in hospice [46]. Dying patients with ESRD use hospice approximately half as much as dying patients in the USA as a whole [35, 46, 99].

As this population remains burdened with many symptoms until the time of death, hospice care is particularly important. Hospice care is recognized for its ability to provide comfort care near the end of life. It stands to reason that the institution and increased use of hospice would relieve symptoms and improve the care of those patients with ESRD who have less than 6 months to live. Cohen et al. found that patients with ESRD experienced better pain control while dying with hospice at home than in the hospital [35]. Murray et al. reported that patients receiving dialysis care were more likely to die at home if they were enrolled in hospice care [46]. For these patients, the median number of days spent in hospital the last week of life was reduced from four to zero and the median care cost was reduced by 67%. Conditions associated with increased hospice use included failure to thrive and a gradual decline in health, increased age, Caucasian race, and availability of hospice services. Nephrology caregivers' lack of training and comfort in discussing and implementing hospice care remains a barrier for this therapy.

Patient receiving renal replacement therapy might be eligible for both ESRD and hospice benefits under Medicare coverage. To receive hospice care while continuing with dialysis, a patient must have a life expectancy of less than 6 months as determined by his or her physician and must have a terminal diagnosis other than ESRD [46, 100, 101].

It is most important to our patients that we provide the opportunity for a good death when end of life is approaching. When dialysis is withdrawn or withheld, we should be able to promise our patients a relatively brief and symptom-controlled death. Timely and appropriate use of hospice care has been recognized by the

RPA and ASN as a crucial aspect of ESRD care [1, 49, 102–104]. They have published and updated a clinical practice guideline and a position statement that directly endorses hospice care for patients with ESRD who are at the end of life.

Conclusion

Hospice care remains just one aspect of advanced care planning and shared decision-making between the patient with CKD and ESRD and the nephrology caregiver [105]. This should be part of an ongoing process and discussion that begins with the recognition of chronic disease and evolves through a period of life events, disease trajectories and the establishment of a trusting and confident patient-and-care-giver long-term relationship. Implementation of hospice and end-of-life care would follow a "natural" course already established by processes put in place in advance by a practice centered on palliative care.

It is now generally recognized by the nephrology community that patients with CKD and ESRD are an aging population with multiple comorbid conditions, symptoms, and a severely limited survival. In order to provide the best care for their patients, many nephrologists are beginning to address the need to improve their knowledge and skills in palliative care, including end-of-life care. Starting with the seminal paper by Neu and Kjellstrand in1986 [45], there has been a growing body of research, literature, and guidelines assembled to aid the practicing nephrologist in this area of patient care. The RPA and ASN have since developed the second edition of *Shared Decision-Making in the Appropriate Initiation of and Withdrawal from Dialysis* [50]. These guidelines provide clinicians, patients, and families with tools to make informed decisions about dialysis and proceed with advance care planning, and when indicated, end-of-life decision-making. This is the most recent addition to a large body of literature specific to CKD and ESRD that can assist nephrologists in their role as providers of palliative care. Web sites, text books, and a core body of research are now available to guide nephrologists in our efforts to integrate palliative care into our clinical practice.

References

1. Moss AH. Renal Physicians Association, American Society of Nephrology Working Group. A new clinical practice guideline on initiation and withdrawal of dialysis that makes explicit the role of palliative medicine. J Palliat Med. 2000;3:253–60.
2. Sand P, Livingston G, Wright RG. Psychological assessment of candidates for a Hemodialysis program. Ann Intern Med. 1966;64:602–10.
3. Murray JS, Tu WH, Albers JB, Burnell JM, Scribner BH. A community center for the treatment of chronic uremia. Trans Am Soc Artif Intern Organs. 1962;8:315.
4. Lindholm DD, Burnell JM, Murray JS. Experience in the treatment of chronic uremia in an outpatient community dialysis center. Trans Am Soc Artif Intern Organs. 1963;9:3–10.
5. Social Security Amendment of 1972. Public Law 92-603, Section 2991. 1972 Oct 31.
6. Kurella Tamura M, Cohen LM. Should there be an expanded role for palliative care in end-stage renal disease? Curr Opin Nephrol Hypertens. 2010;19:556–60.
7. Blagg CR. The early history of dialysis for chronic renal failure in the United States: a view from Seattle. Am J Kidney Dis. 2007;49:482–96.
8. Knauf F, Aronson PS. ESRD as a window into America's cost crisis in healthcare. J Am Soc Nephrol. 2009;20:2093–7.
9. Carson RC, Juszczak M, Davenport A, Burns A. Is maximum conservative management an equivalent treatment option to dialysis for elderly patients with significant comorbid disease? Clin J Am Soc Nephrol. 2009;4:1611–9. Epub 2009 Sep 24.
10. Farrington K, Rao R, Gilg J, Ansell D, Feest T. Chapter 3. New adult patients starting renal replacement therapy in the UK in 2005. In: Ansell D, Feest T, Hodsman R, Rao R, Tomson C, Udayaraj U, Williams A, Warwick G, editors. UK Renal Registry: The Ninth Annual Report. Bristol, United Kingdom: The Renal Association; 2006. p. 15–41.
11. Kurella M, Covinsky KE, Collins AJ, Chertow GM. Octogenarians and nonagenarians starting dialysis in the United States. Ann Intern Med. 2007;146:177–83.
12. Collins AJ, Foley R, Herzog C, et al. Excerpts from the United States Renal Data System 2007 annual report: ESRD incidence and prevalence. Am J Kidney Dis. 2008;51:S81–98.
13. US Renal Data System. *USRDS 2010 Annual Data Report: Atlas of End-Stage Renal Disease in the United States*. National Kidney and Urologic Disease Information Clearinghouse, 3 Information Way,

Bethesda, MD 20892-3560; 301.654.4415, nkudic@info.niddk.nih.gov.
14. Collins AJ, Kasiske B, Herzog C, et al. Excerpts from the United States Renal Data System 2006 annual data report. Am J Kidney Dis. 2007;49(A6–7):S1–296.
15. Krishnan M, Lok CE, Jassal SV. Epidemiology and demographic aspects of treated end-stage renal disease in the elderly. Semin Dial. 2002;15:79–83.
16. Germain MJ, Cohen LM. Maintaining quality of life at the end of life in the end-stage renal disease population. Adv Chronic Kidney Dis. 2008;15:133–9. Review.
17. US Renal Data System. USRDS 2005 Annual Data Report: Atlas of End-Stage Renal Disease in the united States, Bethesda, National Institutes of Health, National Institutes of Diabetes and Digestive and Kidney Diseases, 2005.
18. Davison SN. Chronic pain in end-stage renal disease. Adv Chronic Kidney Dis. 2005;12:326–34.
19. Davison SN, Jhangri GS, Johnson JA. Cross-sectional validity of a modified Edmonton Symptom Assessment System (ESAS) in dialysis patients: A simple method for the assessment of symptom burdens. Kidney Int. 2006;69:1621–5.
20. Register Canadian Organ Replacement. Dialysis and Renal Transplantation: Canadian Organ Replacement Register, 2001 Report. Canadian Institute for Health Information: Ottawa; 2002.
21. Renal Data US, System USRDS. Annual data report: Atlas of end-stage renal disease in the United States. National Institute of Diabetes and Digestive and Kidney Diseases, Bethesda, MD: National Institutes of Health; 2007. 2007.
22. O'Hare AM, Choi AI, Berenthal D. Age effects outcomes in chronic kidney disease. J Am Soc Nephrol. 2007;18:2758–65.
23. Kurella Tamura M, Covinsky KE, Chertow GM, Yaffe K, Landefeld S, McCulloch CE. Functional status of elderly adults before and after initiation of dialysis. N Engl J Med. 2009;361:1539–47.
24. Cook WL, Jassal SV. Functional dependencies among the elderly on hemodialysis. Kidney Int. 2008;73:1289–95.
25. DeOreo PB. Hemodialysis patient-assessed functional health status predicts continued survival, hospitalizations, and dialysis-attendance compliance. Am J Kidney Dis. 1997;30:204–12.
26. Davison SN. The prevalence and management of chronic pain in end-stage renal disease. J Palliat Med. 2007;10:1277–87.
27. Davison SN, Jhangri GS. The impact of chronic pain on depression, sleep, and the desire to withdraw from dialysis in hemodialysis patients. J Pain Symptom Manage. 2005;30:465–73.
28. Davison SN, Jhangri GS, Johnson JA. Longitudinal validation of a modified Edmonton symptom assessment system (ESAS) in haemodialysis patients. Nephrol Dial Transplant. 2006;21:3189–95.
29. Davison SN, Jhangri GS. Impact of pain and symptom burden on the health-related quality of life in hemodialysis patients. J Pain Symptom Manage. 2010;39:477–85.
30. Weisbord SD, Fried LF, Arnold RM, et al. Prevalence, severity, and importance of physical and emotional symptoms in chronic Hemodialysis patients. J Am Soc Nephrol. 2005;16:2487–94.
31. Chater S, Davison SN, Germain MJ, Cohn LM. Withdrawal from dialysis. A palliative care perspective. Clin Nephrol. 2006;66:364–72.
32. Davison SN. Pain in hemodialysis: prevalence, cause, severity, and management. Am J Kidney Dis. 2003;42:1239–47.
33. Fainsinger RL, Davison SN, Brenneis C. A supportive care model for dialysis patients. Palliat Med. 2003;17:81–2.
34. Fortina F, Agllata S, Ragazzoni E, et al. Chronic pain during dialysis. Pharmacologic therapy and its costs. Minerva Urol Nefrol. 1999;51:85–7.
35. Cohen LM, Germain M, Poppel DM, Woods A, Kjellstrand CM. Dialysis discontinuation and palliative care. Am J Kidney Dis. 2000;36:140–4.
36. United States Renal Data System: Causes of death. In: USRDS 1999 Annual Data Report. Bethesda, MD: National Institutes of Health, National Institute of Diabetes and Digestive and Kidney Diseases, 1999, pp 89-100.
37. Holley JL. Palliative care in end-stage renal disease: focus on advance care planning, hospice referral, and bereavement. Semin Dial. 2005;18:154–6.
38. Rettig RA, Levinsky NG, editors. Kidney Failure and the Federal Government Committee for the Study of the Medicare ESRDS Program, Division of Health Care Services. Washington, DC: Institute of Medicine, National Academy Press; 1991.
39. Holley JL, Carmody SS, Moss AH, Sullivan AM, Cohen LM, Bloack SD, Arnold RM. The need for end-of-life care training in nephrology: national survey results of nephrology fellows. Am J Kidney Dis. 2003;42:813–20.
40. Perry E, Schwartz R, Smith-Wheelock L, et al. Why is it difficult for staff to discuss advance directives with chronic dialysis patients? J Am Soc Nephrol. 1996;7:2160–8.
41. Davison SN, Jhangri GS, Holley JL, Moss AH. Nephrologists' reported preparedness for end-of-life decision-making. Clin J Am Soc Nephrol. 2006;1:1256–62. Epub 2006 Sep 13.
42. Hines SC, Glover JJ, Holley JL, et al. Dialysis patients' preferences for family-based advance care planning. Ann Intern Med. 1999;130:825–8.
43. Holley JL, Hines SC, Glover JJ, et al. Failure of advance care planning to elicit patents' preferences for withdrawal from dialysis. Am J Kidney Dis. 1999;33:688–93.
44. Singer PA. Advance care planning in dialysis. Am J Kidney Dis. 1999;33:980–91.
45. Neu S, Kjellstrand CM. Stopping long-term dialysis: An empirical study of withdrawal of life-supporting treatment. N Engl J Med. 1986;314:14–20.
46. Murray AM, Arko C, Chen SC, Gilbertson DT, Moss AH. Use of hospice in the United Stated dialysis population. Clin J Am Soc Nephrol. 2006;1:1248–55. Epub 2006 Sep 6.

47. Brown EA. Epidemiology of renal palliative care. J Palliative Med. 2007;10:1248–52.
48. Davison SN. End-of-life care preferences and needs: perceptions of patients with chronic kidney disease. Clin J Am Soc Nephrol. 2010;5:195–204. Epub 2010 Jan 14.
49. Kimmel PL, Emont SL, Newmann JM, Danko H, Moss AH. ESRD patient quality of life: symptoms, spiritual beliefs, psychosocial factors, and ethnicity. Am J Kidney Dis. 2003;42:713–21.
50. Renal Physicians Association. Shared decision-making in the appropriate initiation of and withdrawal from dialysis. Clinical practice guideline. 2nd ed. Rockville, Maryland: October 2010. Pp. 1-10.
51. Holley JL. Palliative care in end-stage renal disease: illness trajectories, communication, and hospice use. Adv Chronic Kidney Dis. 2007;14:402–8.
52. Moss AH, Holley JL, Davison SN, et al. Core curriculum in nephrology: Palliative care. Am J Kidney Dis. 2004;43:172–85.
53. Chambers EJ, Germain M, Brown E. Supportive Care for the Renal Patient. Oxford University Press: Oxford, England; 2004.
54. Berzoff J, Swantkowski J, Cohen LM. Developing a renal supportive care team from the voices of patients, families, and palliative care staff. Palliat Support Care. 2008;6:133–9.
55. WHO definition of palliative care. http://www.who.int/cancer/palliative/definition/en/. [Accessed May 25, 2011.
56. Morrison RS, Meier DE. Clinical practice: palliative care. N Engl J Med. 2004;350:2582–90.
57. Kandoian EA. Due process in the allocation of scarce lifesaving medical resources. Yale Law School J. 1975;84:1734–49.
58. Holley JL, Nespor S, Rault R. The effects of providing chronic hemodialysis patients with material on advance directives. Am J Kidney Dis. 1993;22:413–8.
59. Davison SN, Simpson C. Hope and advance care planning in patients with end stage renal disease: qualitative interview study. BMJ. 2006;333:886. Epub 2006 Sep 21. [doi:10:.1136/bmj:38965.626250.55].
60. Johnston SC, Pfeifer NP, McNutt R. for the End-of-Life Study Group. The discussion about advance directives. Patient and physician opinions regarding when and how it should be conducted. Arch Intern Med. 1995;155:1025–30.
61. Morrison RS, Morrison EW, Glickman DF. Physician reluctance to discuss advance directives. Arch Intern Med. 1994;154:2311–8.
62. Cohen LM, Germain M, Woods A, Gilman ED, McCue JD. Patient attitudes and psychological considerationsindialysisdiscontinuation.Psychosomatics. 1993;34:395–401.
63. Cohen LM, McCue JD, Germain M, Woods A. Denying the dying. Advance directives and dialysis discontinuation. Psychosomatics. 1997;38:27–34.
64. Moss AH, Hozayen O, King K, Holley JL, Schmidt RJ. Attitudes of patients toward cardiopulmonary resuscitation in the dialysis unit. Am J Kidney Dis. 2001;38:847–52.
65. Moss AH, Holley JL, Upton MB. Outcomes of cardiopulmonary resuscitation in dialysis patients. J Am Soc Nephrol. 1992;3:1238–43.
66. Carson V, Soeken K, Shanty J, Terry L. Hope and spiritual well-being: essentials for living with AIDS. Perspect Psychiatr Care. 1990;26:28–34.
67. Forbes M. Hope in older adults with illness. Appl Nurs Res. 1999;22:74–87.
68. Christakis NA. Death Foretold: Prophecy and Prognosis in Medical Care. Chicago: University of Chicago Press; 1999. p. 179.
69. Michel DM, Moss AH. Communicating prognosis in the dialysis consent process: a patient-centered guideline-supported approach. Adv Chronic Kidney Dis. 2005;12:196–201.
70. Weissman DE. Decision making at a time of crisis near the end of life. JAMA. 2004;292:1738–43.
71. Beddhu S, Bruns FJ, Saul M, et al. A simple comorbidity scale predicts clinical outcomes and costs in dialysis patients. Am J Med. 2000;108:609–13.
72. Miskulin DC, Martin AA, Brown R, et al. Predicting 1 year mortality in an outpatient haemodialysis population: a comparison of comorbidity instruments. Nephrol Dial Transplant. 2004;19:413–20.
73. Hudson M, Weisbord S, Arnold RM. Prognostication in patients receiving dialysis #191. J Palliat Med. 2007;10:1402–3.
74. Levinsky NG, Mesler DE. Measuring, managing, and improving the quality of end-stage renal disease. Am J Kidney Dis. 1994;24:235–46.
75. Solano JP, Gomes B, Higginson IJ. A comparison of symptom prevalence in far advanced cancer, AIDS, heart disease, chronic obstructive pulmonary disease and renal disease. J Pain Symptom Manage. 2006;31:58–69.
76. Merkus MP, Jager KJ, Dekker FW, de Haan RJ, Boeschoten EW, Krediet RT. Physical symptoms and quality of life in patients on chronic dialysis: Results of the Netherlands Cooperative Study on Adequacy of Dialysis (NECOSAD). Nephrol Dial Transplant. 1999;14:1163–70.
77. Curtin RB, Bultman DC, Thomas-Hawkins C, Walters BA, Schatell D. Hemodialysis patients' symptom experiences: effects on physical and mental functioning. Nephrol Nurse J. 2002;29(562):567–74.
78. Flynn 3rd JJ, Mitchell MC, Caruso FS, McElligott MA. Midodrine treatment for patients with hemodialysis hypotension. Clin Nephrol. 1996;45:261–7.
79. Sklar AH, Riesenberg LA, Silber AK, Ahmed W, Ali A. Postdialysis fatigue. Am J Kidney Dis. 1996;28:732–6.
80. Robertson HT, Haley NR, Guthrie M, Cardenas D, Eschbach JW, Adamson JW. Recombinant erythropoietin improves exercise capacity in anemic Hemodialysis patients. Am J Kidney Dis. 1990;15:325–32.
81. Wuerth D, Finkelstein SH, Ciarcia J, Peterson R, Kliger AS, Finkelstein FO. Identification and treatment of depression in a cohort of patients maintained on chronic peritoneal dialysis. Am J Kidney Dis. 2001;37:1011–7.
82. Lew SQ, Albertini B, Bosch JP. The digestive tract. In: Daugirdas JT, Blake PG, Ing TS, editors. Handbook

of Dialysis. 3rd ed. Philadelphia: Lippincott Williams & Wilkins; 2001. p. 601.
83. Boccanfuso JA, Hutton M, McAllister B. The effects of megestrol acetate on nutritional parameters in a dialysis population. J Ren Nutr. 2000;10(1):36–43.
84. Lien YH, Ruffenach SJ. Low dose megestrol increases serum albumin in malnourished dialysis patients. Int J Artif Organs. 1996;19:147–50.
85. Kimmel PL, Miller G, Mendelson WB. Sleep apnea syndrome in chronic renal disease. Am J Med. 1989;86:308–14.
86. Mendelson WB, Wadhwa NK, Greenberg HE, Gujavarty K, Bergofsky E. Effects of hemodialysis on sleep apnea syndrome in end-stage renal disease. Clin Nephrol. 1990;33:247–51.
87. Gigli GL, Adorati M, Dolso P, Piani A, Valente M, Brotini S, Budai R. Restless legs syndrome in end-stage renal disease. Sleep Med. 2004;5:309–15.
88. Smith MD, Hong BA. Diagnosis of depression in patients with end-stage renal disease. Comparative analysis. Am J Med. 1985;79:160–6.
89. Davison S. Chronic kidney disease: psychosocial impact of chronic pain. Geriatrics. 2007;62:17–23.
90. Murtagh FEM, Addington-Hall JM, Edmonds PM, Donohoe P, Carey I, Jenkins K, Higginson IJ. Symptoms in advanced renal disease: a cross-sectional survey of symptom prevalence in stage 5 chronic kidney disease managed without dialysis. J Palliat Med. 2007;10:1266–76.
91. Cohen LM, Moss AH, Weisbord SD, Germain MJ. Renal palliative care. J Palliative Med. 2006;9:977–92.
92. Douglas C, Murtagh FEM, Chambers EJ, Howse M, Ellershaw J. Symptom management for the adult patient dying with advanced kidney disease: a review of the literature and development of evidence-based guidelines by a United Kingdom Expert Consensus Group. Palliat Med. 2009;23:103–10.
93. Barakzoy AS, Moss AH. Efficacy of the World Health Organization analgesic ladder to treat pain in end-stage renal disease. J Am Soc Nephrol. 2006;17:3198–203.
94. Kurella M, Bennett WM, Chertow GM. Analgesia in patients with ESRD: a review of available evidence. Am J Kidney Dis. 2003;42:217–28.
95. Pham P-CT, Toscano E, Pham P-MT, Pham P-AT, Pham SV, Pham P-TT. Pain management in patients with chronic kidney disease. NDT Plus. 2009;2:111–8.
96. Dean M. Opioids in renal failure and dialysis patients. J Pain Symptom Manage. 2004;28:497–504.
97. Launay-Vacher V, Karie S, Fau J-B, Izzedine H, Deray G. Treatment of pain in patients with renal insufficiency: The World Health Organization three-step ladder adapted. J Pain. 2005;6:137–48.
98. Davison SN, Davison JS. Is there a legitimate role for the therapeutic role of cannaboids for symptom management in chronic kidney disease? J Pain Symptom Manage. 2011;41:768–78.
99. Deaths, Percent of Total Deaths, and Death Rates for the 15 Leading Causes of Death in Selected Age Groups, by Race and Sex: United States, 2000. Available: http://www. cdc.gov/nchs/data/dvs/LCWK3_2000.pdf.
100. Moss AH. Improving end-of-life care for dialysis. Editorial. Am J Kidney Dis. 2005;45:209–12.
101. Cohen LM, Ruthazer R, Moss AH, Germain MJ. Predicting six-month mortality for patients who are on maintenance Hemodialysis. Clin J Am Soc Nephrol. 2010;5:72–9. Epub 2009 Dec 3.
102. Renal Physicians Association, American Society of Nephrology: *Clinical Practice Guideline on Shared Decision-Making in the Appropriate Initiation of and Withdrawal from Dialysis*, Washington, DC, Renal Physicians Association, 2000.
103. Moss AH. Renal Physicians Association, American Society of Nephrology Working Group. Shared decision making in dialysis: a new clinical practice guideline to assist with dialysis-related ethics consultations. J Clin Ethics. 2001;12:406–14.
104. Renal Physicians Association, American Society of Nephrology: *Position Paper on Quality Care at the End of Life*, Rockville, Renal Physicians Association, 2002
105. Davison SN. Integrating palliative care for patients with advanced chronic kidney disease: recent advance, remaining challenges. J Palliat Care. 2011;27:53–61.

Part VIII

Kidney Transplantation

Donor and Recipient Evaluation

34

Elizabeth C. Lorenz and Suzanne M. Norby

Case 1

A 51-year-old man with stage 4 chronic kidney disease (CKD) is referred for kidney transplant evaluation. The patient has a history of type 2 diabetes mellitus, hypertension, hyperlipidemia, and coronary artery stenting.

Is he a kidney transplant candidate?

What testing should his evaluation include?

Case 2

A 24-year-old woman with a history of obesity (BMI 41 kg/m^2) is interested in donating a kidney to the patient in Case 1. Her mother has a history of kidney stones.

Is she a kidney donor candidate?

What testing should her evaluation include?

E.C. Lorenz, M.D. (✉)
Division of Nephrology and Hypertension, Mayo Clinic, Rochester, Minnesota,
Rochester, MN, USA
e-mail: lorenz.elizabeth@mayo.edu

S.M. Norby, M.D.
Division of Nephrology and Hypertension, Mayo Clinic, Rochester, MN, USA

Introduction

Kidney transplantation is the preferred form of renal replacement therapy for acceptable candidates, affording patients with end-stage renal disease (ESRD) longer survival and better quality of life compared to patients on the kidney transplant wait list [1]. Preemptive transplantation, performed prior to the initiation of dialysis, and living donor transplantation are associated with better patient and graft survival compared to deceased donor transplantation [1]. Patients with Stage 4 CKD, or an estimated glomerular filtration rate (eGFR) between 15 and 29 ml/min/1.73 m^2, should receive education about options for renal replacement therapy, including transplantation [2]. Typically, a transplant candidate is referred to a transplant center for kidney transplant evaluation when renal replacement therapy is expected to be needed within 12 months and/or when the eGFR is irreversibly reduced to less than 20–25 ml/min/1.73 m^2. This advanced planning allows for adequate time to perform the transplant evaluation, to address underlying medical issues, and to determine whether a suitable living donor exists, before initiation of dialysis is required. While preemptive transplantation is beneficial, it should not be performed earlier than necessary. Performing early preemptive transplantation at higher levels of GFR has not been associated with improved outcomes and may waste the native kidney function of the recipient [3, 4].

E.V. Lerma and M. Rosner (eds.), *Clinical Decisions in Nephrology, Hypertension and Kidney Transplantation*, DOI 10.1007/978-1-4614-4454-1_34,

Candidates approved for transplantation who do not have a living donor are placed on the deceased donor wait list. Waitlisted patients can receive an organ via either donation after brain death (DBD) or donation after cardiac death (DCD). In general, both groups of organs have similar graft survival rates but DCD kidneys are associated with an increased risk of delayed graft function [5, 6]. DBD donors can be further divided into two groups based on the quality of the donor organs: expanded-criteria donor (ECD) or standard-criteria donor (SCD). An ECD kidney refers to an organ from a donor aged ≥60 or aged 50–59 year with two of the following criteria: (1) death due to cerebrovascular accident, (2) history of hypertension, and (3) terminal serum creatinine >1.5 mg/dl [7]. All kidneys obtained via DBD that do not fulfill the criteria for ECD are considered SCD kidneys. While they do expand the donor pool, ECD kidneys have a 70% increased risk for graft loss compared to SCD kidneys [8]. Although ECD kidneys have worse graft survival rates compared to SCD kidneys, they still may afford a mortality benefit compared to remaining on dialysis depending on the candidate's age [9–11]. Therefore, an ECD kidney may be a reasonable option in an older transplant candidate who desires less waiting time.

In order to determine if a patient is a kidney transplant candidate, a thorough evaluation (Table 34.1) is conducted by a multidisciplinary transplant team, generally comprised of a transplant nephrologist, transplant surgeon, nurse transplant coordinator, nutritionist, and social worker. Providing patient-level education about kidney transplantation is crucial, and informed consent must be documented [12]. While specific aspects of the kidney transplant evaluation vary among centers, comprehensive general guidelines have been published by several international professional societies [3, 13–15].

Evaluation of the Potential Kidney Transplant Recipient

History and Physical Exam

A comprehensive history and physical exam aimed at detecting underlying conditions that may preclude kidney transplantation are necessary components of the transplant evaluation. The presence of psychiatric disease, nonadherence to prescribed therapy, and medical comorbidities including malignancies, infections, and morbid obesity should be assessed. For example, obesity increases the risk of surgical complications, delayed graft function, allograft loss, and post-transplant diabetes mellitus [16]. Weight loss with a BMI goal of <30 kg/m^2 is often recommended [3, 15].

Evaluation of Renal Disease

In order to be placed on the wait list for deceased donor kidney transplantation, glomerular filtration rate (GFR) must be ≤20 ml/min/1.73 m^2. In transplant candidates, GFR is most commonly determined by 24-h urine creatinine clearance, although radioisotope clearance and GFR estimating equations are used as well. Urinalysis, urine culture, and quantitation of urinary protein are performed. Native kidney proteinuria decreases after transplant, and a subsequent increase in proteinuria post-transplant heralds a poor graft outcome [17]. Whenever possible, the reason for ESRD should be determined, preferably via renal biopsy, in order to assess the risk of recurrent disease post-transplant.

Assessment of Operative Risk

Laboratory testing typically ordered during the pre-transplant evaluation, including complete blood count, basic metabolic profile, fasting glucose, and liver function tests (Table 34.1), is valuable in the assessment of overall operative risk. Electrocardiogram (ECG) and chest X-ray should be performed in all patients. Pulmonary function testing is indicated in patients with respiratory symptoms or a history of significant smoking [13].

Surgical Considerations

History of prior abdominal surgeries, peripheral vascular disease, and bladder dysfunction should

Table 34.1 Evaluation of the potential kidney transplant recipient[a]

Comprehensive history and physical exam, including:
• Etiology of kidney disease (cause of prior allograft loss when applicable)
• Urinary tract disorders
• Cardiovascular disease
• Obesity
• Malignancy
• Risks for sensitization (pregnancies, prior blood product administration)
• Infections and immunizations
• Prior abdominal surgeries
• Abnormal bleeding
• Thromboembolism
• Risk of anesthesia complications
• Formal psychosocial evaluation
Evaluation of renal disease
• Measurement or estimation of glomerular filtration rate (in patients not receiving dialysis) using 24-h urine creatinine clearance, radioisotope clearance, estimating equations
• Measurement of urinary protein by 24-h urine collection or random urine protein:creatinine ratio
• Urinalysis and urine culture
• Consider renal biopsy if cause of kidney disease is unknown
• Consider measurement of post-void residual, urodynamic studies, and/or cystoscopy in patients with a history of recurrent urinary tract infections and/or symptoms suggestive of bladder dysfunction
Laboratory testing
• Complete blood count, serum chemistry panel, fasting blood glucose, calcium, phosphorus, liver tests, prothrombin time (PT), activated partial thromboplastin time (aPTT)
• Pregnancy test in females
• Consider evaluation of CKD complications when indicated: phosphorus, albumin, parathyroid hormone, iron and total iron binding capacity, ferritin, lipid panel
Histocompatibility testing
• ABO blood group determination (performed twice)
• Human leukocyte antigen (HLA) typing
• Single antigen bead and crossmatch testing to identify the presence or specific type of anti-HLA antibodies
Screening for cardiovascular disease
• Electrocardiogram
• Chest X-ray
• Noninvasive cardiac stress test in patients at high risk for cardiovascular disease (indicated in patients with a history and/or symptoms of coronary artery disease; consider in asymptomatic high-risk patients)
• Consider imaging of iliac vessels in patients at high risk for cardiovascular disease and/or thromboembolic disease
• Pulmonary function testing when indicated
Screening for infectious diseases
• Antibodies to human immunodeficiency virus (HIV), hepatitis B and C viruses, Epstein–Barr virus (EBV), cytomegalovirus virus (CMV), varicella zoster virus (VZV)
• Syphilis screen
• Tuberculosis testing with PPD or interferon gamma release assay (Quantiferon)
• Urine culture
• Chest X-ray
Screening for malignancies
• Females: clinical breast exam, pelvic exam, PAP smear and mammogram based on risk factors and according to current guidelines
• Males: testicular exam, prostate-specific antigen (PSA) test, and digital-rectal exam based on risk factors and according to current guidelines
• Colonoscopy based on risk factors and according to current guidelines
• Urine cytology
• Renal imaging with ultrasound or CT in patients on dialysis for several years
• Consider serum protein electrophoresis based on risk factors and according to current guidelines in patients over age 50 or with unexplained kidney disease

[a]Additional testing may be indicated depending upon patient characteristics

be elicited. Patency of the iliac arteries and veins can be assessed using Doppler ultrasound, computed tomography (CT) angiography, or magnetic resonance (MR) angiography, avoiding the use of gadolinium in patients with advanced CKD due to the risk of developing nephrogenic systemic fibrosis [18]. Urologic evaluation is warranted in patients with a history of recurrent urinary tract infections (UTIs) or with symptoms suggesting neurogenic bladder or bladder outlet obstruction. Depending on the specific circumstances, measurement of post-void residuals, voiding cystourethrography (VCUG), urodynamic studies, and/or cystoscopy may be indicated [3, 13, 15].

Screening for Cardiovascular Disease

Since cardiovascular disease is the leading cause of death in kidney transplant recipients, the potential kidney transplant recipient's cardiovascular status is an important factor in determining eligibility for transplantation. Pre-transplant cardiac testing can identify coronary artery disease, valvular disease, congestive heart failure, and pulmonary arterial hypertension. Severe cardiac disease may preclude transplantation [13, 19]. While it is generally accepted that low-risk patients do not require noninvasive cardiac stress testing (NCST), high-risk patients generally undergo NCST during the pre-transplant evaluation. High-risk candidates may include patients with a history of coronary artery disease or active cardiac symptoms, older patients (≥45 years old for males and ≥55 years old for females, for example), and patients with a history of diabetes mellitus, hypertension, hyperlipidemia, >1 year on dialysis, or prior kidney transplant [3, 13]. No firm consensus has been established about how to evaluate high-risk candidates, particularly those who do not have cardiac symptoms [19, 20]. At many transplant centers, high-risk candidates routinely undergo NCST using stress echocardiography or radionuclide imaging [19]. If NCST is positive, patients are referred for formal cardiology evaluation and consideration of coronary angiography. Usually, revascularization is performed if significant coronary artery disease is discovered. However, the effect of these diagnostic and therapeutic procedures on mortality is not well defined, and work-up may lead to contrast nephropathy and delay in transplantation [3, 15, 19, 20].

Infectious Disease Screening

Pre-transplant infectious disease screening has multiple purposes, including identification of infections requiring treatment prior to kidney transplantation and ascertainment of risk of acquiring certain infections post-transplant [21]. Obtaining a complete history of travel and prior immunizations is important. The immunosuppressed recipient is more susceptible to common and atypical infections as well as to reactivation of prior or latent infections. As part of the evaluation, chest X-ray is performed to evaluate the presence of pulmonary infections, and urinalysis and urine culture are used to detect UTIs. In addition, tuberculosis testing with purified protein derivative (or more recently, interferon gamma release assays) is mandatory, as is serologic testing for multiple other pathogens, including human immunodeficiency virus (HIV), hepatitis B and C, varicella zoster virus, and syphilis [21, 22]. It is crucial to determine whether a potential kidney transplant candidate has been previously exposed to cytomegalovirus (CMV) and Epstein–Barr virus (EBV). De novo infection which develops in a seronegative recipient who received an organ from a seropositive donor can result in severe, multisystem infection with CMV or post-transplant lymphoproliferative disorder in the case of EBV [23, 24]. Knowledge of prior exposure to CMV, as well as to certain herpes simplex viruses, is important when determining the type and duration of post-transplant antiviral prophylaxis [25]. Screening for other infections, such as Strongyloides or Chagas disease, may be indicated in endemic areas. Finally, appropriate immunizations should be administered before transplantation. Live virus vaccines are contraindicated post-transplant; moreover, response to vaccination is lower post-transplant in the setting of immunosuppressive medication use [21, 26].

Psychosocial Evaluation

Psychosocial evaluation of transplant candidates is generally conducted by a social worker, adding formal psychiatric consultation when indicated. In addition to exploring potential psychiatric symptoms such as depression and the possibility of cognitive dysfunction [13], it is important to assess the patient's social support system, insurance coverage, and financial resources. The psychosocial evaluation also includes the candidate's use of tobacco, alcohol, and other recreational drugs, as well as the likelihood of adherence to the complex post-transplant therapeutic regimen.

Screening for Malignancies

Age-appropriate cancer screening is recommended for all potential renal transplant candidates, including screening for breast, cervical, prostate, and colon cancer. Urine cytology is routinely performed to screen for urinary tract malignancy, and imaging of the kidneys by ultrasound or CT can detect renal cell carcinoma, which is more prevalent among dialysis patients than in the general population [13]. Additional testing to evaluate for other malignancies may be indicated based on clinical characteristics as well as family history. For example, persistent microhematuria would prompt imaging of the upper urinary tract and cystoscopy. A current diagnosis of cancer, other than non-melanoma skin cancer, is a contraindication to kidney transplantation, and depending on the type of malignancy and potential for recurrence, a disease-free interval of 2–5 years is warranted in most cases (Table 34.2) [3, 13, 14].

Table 34.2 Suggested tumor-free time interval after successful treatment of malignancy before proceeding with kidney transplantation [3, 13, 14]

Time interval < 2 years (or interval not needed, depending on the clinical situation)
• Noninvasive, non-melanoma skin cancer
• In situ cancer or noninvasive papilloma of the bladder
• Cervical carcinoma in situ
• Focal, microscopic low-grade, low-risk prostate cancer
• Renal cell carcinoma (<5 cm, incidentally discovered)
Minimum 2-year time interval
• Bladder cancer (other than superficial)
• Early stage breast cancer, including ductal carcinoma in situ[a]
• Localized cervical cancer[b]
• Hodgkin's and non-Hodgkin's lymphoma
• Leukemia
• Post-transplant lymphoproliferative disorder
• Lung cancer
• Melanoma in situ
• Prostate cancer (other than above; transplantation not recommended for patients with advanced disease)
• Renal cell carcinoma (>5 cm, invasive, or symptomatic)
• Sarcomas, including Kaposi's sarcoma
• Testicular cancer
• Thyroid cancer
• Uterine cancer
• Wilm's tumor of the kidney[a]
Minimum 5-year time interval
• Breast cancer (stages I and II; transplantation not recommended for patients with stages III and IV)
• Colon cancer (Duke's stages A and B1 may require a shorter interval of 2–5 years)
• Melanoma

[a]Canadian guidelines recommend minimum 1-year interval [3]
[b]5-year interval recommended in some cases [13]

Histocompatibility Testing

Histocompatibility testing refers to the evaluation of donor and recipient compatibility and is based on the identification of major human leukocyte antigens (HLAs). A detailed discussion of histocompatibility testing is beyond the scope of this chapter. Briefly, HLAs play a key role in immune system activation by binding foreign peptides and displaying them to host lymphocytes. Antibodies directed against donor-derived HLA antigens contribute to both acute and chronic graft rejection. During transplant evaluation, both donor and recipient undergo HLA typing via DNA-based methods. In addition, a crossmatch is performed to determine whether the recipient has any circulating anti-HLA antibodies against their donor or donor-specific antibodies (DSA). DSA can be detected via either cell-based or solid-phase assays. Cell-based assays include the complement-dependent lymphocytotoxicity (CDC) assay and flow cytometry. In the CDC assay donor lymphocytes are incubated with recipient serum and complement is added. Cell lysis indicates the presence of DSA. A positive cytotoxicity crossmatch is a contraindication to transplantation due to the high risk of hyperacute rejection. Flow cytometry assays are more sensitive at detecting DSA than CDC assays. In flow cytometry, donor lymphocytes are incubated with recipient serum and a fluorescent secondary antibody targeting DSA in recipient serum is added and analyzed by flow cytometry. A negative cytotoxicity crossmatch with a positive flow cytometry crossmatch suggests lower levels of donor-specific antibody [27]. Solid-phase assays utilize solid surfaces such as flow beads coated with purified HLA antigens. Flow beads coated with one HLA antigen per bead are referred to as single antigen beads. Recipient serum is added to the beads and analysis is performed using flow cytometric techniques. Solid-phase assays allow for quantification of DSA activity. In addition, the reactivity of individual anti-HLA antibodies can be determined allowing for recognition of donor specificity [27].

Cell-based and solid-phase assays can also be used to assess recipient sensitization. Traditionally recipients were screened for HLA antibodies using a cell-based test called panel reactive antibody (PRA) in which lymphocytes from a panel of representative donors is incubated with recipient serum and cell lysis is detected [28]. Results are expressed as the percentage of panel cells lysed. PRA provides an estimate of the percentage of donors who would be unacceptable for a particular recipient. Due to inconsistencies in this technique, solid-phase assays are now used to generate a calculated PRA (cPRA). HLA antigens to which a candidate is known to be sensitized are listed as "unacceptable antigens" for that candidate. Using those antigens, a computer program calculates a cPRA which represents the percentage of donors that would be incompatible for that candidate. Unacceptable antigens can also be used to perform a "virtual crossmatch." Transplant programs can accept organs containing no unacceptable antigens knowing that the final cell-based crossmatch testing will likely be acceptable [27].

Case 1

In order to determine whether the patient in this case is a transplant candidate, he must undergo a thorough evaluation as outlined above. In this patient's case, consideration could be given to performing a native kidney biopsy since the etiology of his CKD is unclear. In addition, he should undergo NCST due to his history of coronary artery stenting.

Evaluation of the Potential Living Kidney Donor

Kidney donation is an altruistic act that confers low, but not negligible, short-term and long-term risks. Short-term risks are generally related to the risk of the surgical procedure itself. Long-term risks are more complex. Based on currently available evidence, kidney donation does not appear to increase the rate of ESRD or mortality in kidney donors [30–33]. Rates of ESRD for living kidney donors have been reported to range from 0.1 to 1.1% [34]. Data from follow-up studies of kidney donors suggest that blood pressure may increase slightly after donation but that rates of hypertension and albuminuria are similar to matched controls [30]. However, some studies suggest that female kidney donors who subsequently become pregnant have an increased risk of preeclampsia in post-donation pregnancies [35]. For these reasons, it is ethically mandated that potential kidney donors be fully informed of the risks of donation and provide informed consent [36]. Each transplant center in the United States is required to have a donor advocate to protect the interests of potential kidney donors [12]. Furthermore, details of the donor evaluation must be kept confidential. Consensus exists that potential kidney donors should have multiple opportunities to opt out of donation at any point during the process leading up to donor nephrectomy [37]. Similar to the evaluation of potential kidney transplant recipients, there is no uniform evaluation for kidney donors and transplant centers employ different donor selection criteria [38–40]. Multiple groups and professional societies internationally have published guidelines regarding the evaluation and selection of kidney donors [37, 41, 42]. Potential kidney donors must undergo a psychosocial evaluation that assesses motivation to donate, absence of coercion or financial gain, and presence of psychological illness or active substance abuse [32, 37]. They must also undergo a thorough medical evaluation that includes a complete history incorporating family history of kidney disease, physical exam, assessment of operative risk (laboratory screening, chest X-ray, ECG, NCST if indicated), screening for active infectious disease, and appropriate cancer screening (Table 34.3).

Potential kidney donors also undergo ABO blood typing and histocompatibility testing to determine compatibility with potential kidney transplant recipients. In most cases, a kidney donor donates a kidney to a particular recipient with whom they have a pre-existing familial or emotional relationship. However, in an effort to offer successful kidney transplantation to more patients, novel approaches such as paired donation and donor exchange have recently been used when incompatibility occurs between multiple potential kidney donor–recipient pairs. The living donors are matched to compatible recipients and the donor organs are exchanged so that all recipients receive a compatible kidney transplant [43]. Non-directed kidney donors, who are motivated for altruistic reasons to donate a kidney to an unknown recipient, may donate to the best matched recipient on the national deceased donor kidney transplant waiting list or as part of a paired exchange program.

Assessment of Renal Function

Most transplant centers measure donor GFR via 24-h urinary creatinine clearance or radioisotope clearance. Estimation equations are not reliable in the donor population [44]. In general, GFR ≥80 ml/min/1.73 m^2 or no more than two standard deviations below the mean GFR for age is considered to be an acceptable level of kidney function. Proteinuria >200–300 mg/day is generally considered unacceptable [41]. The presence of persistent microhematuria requires a complete urologic structural evaluation including urine cytology and cystoscopy; if structural evaluation is unrevealing, a kidney biopsy may be required to exclude the presence of significant glomerular disease [45]. Structural evaluation is reliably done with CT angiogram (which can also be configured to include a CT urogram), MR angiogram, or standard renal arteriogram plus spiral CT of the abdomen and pelvis [46].

Screening for Medical Comorbidities

It is important to identify conditions in potential donors that confer an increased risk of CKD. Significant hypertension is generally a contraindication to donation although some centers may accept potential donors with easily controlled hypertension, particularly older donors with no evidence of microalbuminuria [38, 41, 47]. Diabetes mellitus (defined as fasting blood glucose ≥126 mg/dl on two occasions or an abnormal oral glucose tolerance test) is an absolute contraindication to kidney donation [40, 41]. Obesity increases the risk of surgical complications and the risk of developing diabetes and hypertension. Most centers exclude potential donors with a BMI ≥35 kg/m^2. Nephrolithiasis may be considered a contraindication to donation if bilateral stones are present or if the potential donor is found to have underlying metabolic abnormalities predisposing to recurrent stone formation [41]. Contraindications to donation are summarized in Table 34.4.

Case 2

The patient's BMI currently would preclude her from donation at most transplant centers. She should be encouraged to lose weight and

Table 34.3 Evaluation of the potential kidney donor[a] [41]

Comprehensive history and physical exam, including:
• History of high blood pressure, elevated blood glucose, nephrolithiasis, urinary tract infections, hematuria, proteinuria
• Family history of kidney disease, nephrolithiasis, hypertension, diabetes, cardiovascular disease
• Cardiovascular disease
• Obesity
• Malignancy
• Infections
• Abnormal bleeding
• Thromboembolism
• Risk of anesthesia complications
• Psychosocial evaluation
Histocompatibility testing
• ABO blood group determination (performed twice)
• Human leukocyte antigen (HLA) typing
Basic evaluation
• Complete blood count, serum electrolytes, calcium, phosphorus, uric acid, liver tests, lipid screen, prothrombin time (PT), activated partial thromboplastin time (aPTT)
• Fasting blood glucose; consider oral glucose tolerance test
• Serologic testing for HIV, hepatitis B and C viruses, EBV, CMV
• Syphilis screen
• Pregnancy test in females
• Chest X-ray and electrocardiogram
• Noninvasive cardiac stress test when indicated
• Pulmonary function testing when indicated
Specific kidney evaluation
• Accurate blood pressure measurement, preferably using ambulatory monitoring
• Serum creatinine and blood urea nitrogen (BUN)
• Measurement or estimation of glomerular filtration rate using 24-h urine creatinine clearance or radioisotope clearance
• Measurement of urinary protein by 24-h urine collection (less commonly by random urine protein:creatinine ratio) [38]
• Urinalysis and urine culture
• Evaluation of renal anatomy, most commonly using computed tomography (CT) [38]
Screening for malignancies
• Females: clinical breast exam, pelvic exam, and PAP smear; mammogram based on risk factors and according to current guidelines
• Males: testicular exam, prostate-specific antigen (PSA) test, and digital rectal exam
• Colonoscopy based on risk factors and according to current guidelines
• Consider serum protein electrophoresis in patients over age 50

[a]Additional testing may be indicated depending upon patient characteristics

be re-evaluated for donation when her BMI is ≤35 kg/m^2. If she eventually proceeds with evaluation, she should undergo imaging to assess for kidney stones. If stones are apparent, a 24-h urine supersaturation should be obtained to help determine risk for subsequent stone formation.

Key Points

1. The evaluation of potential kidney transplant candidates should focus on identifying medical, psychiatric, and social conditions that could adversely affect the outcome of transplantation.

Table 34.4 Contraindications to kidney donation [41, 46]

• Renal function
GFR <80 ml/min/1.73 m^2 or lower than two standard deviations below the mean value for age
• Hypertension
Significant hypertension
• Urine studies
Proteinuria >200–300 mg/day
Persistent microhematuria
• Obesity
BMI ≥ 35 kg/m^2
• Diabetes mellitus
• Nephrolithiasis
Potential donors with bilateral stones or underlying metabolic abnormalities predisposing to recurrent stone formation
• Malignancy
Active malignancy or a history of malignancy that may place the potential donor at increased risk for chronic kidney disease
• Comorbidities
Chronic systemic illness
Significant cardiovascular or pulmonary disease
• Anatomy
Significant urologic or renal vascular anatomic abnormalities
• Infections
Active infection or history of chronic infections including HIV, hepatitis C, hepatitis B, recurrent urinary tract infections
• Psychosocial assessment
Active alcohol or chemical dependency
Active smoking
Active psychiatric condition
Questionable motivation

2. Evaluation for kidney transplantation should involve a multidisciplinary team approach.
3. High-risk candidates should undergo NCST with coronary angiography as needed to help delineate cardiac risk.
4. Potential kidney donors should be educated about the potential risks of donation and provide informed consent.
5. Potential donors should thoroughly be screened for the presence of underlying physical and psychological factors that may increase the risk associated with kidney donation.

References

1. Wolfe R, Ashby V, Milford E. Comparison of mortality in all patients on dialysis, patients on dialysis awaiting transplantation and recipients of a first cadaveric transplant. New Engl J Med. 1999;341:725–30.
2. K/DOQI Clinical Practice Guidelines on Chronic Kidney Disease Part 4. Definition and classification of stages of chronic kidney disease. Am J Kidney Dis. 2002;39(2):S46–75.
3. Knoll G, Cockfield S, Blydt-Hansen T, et al. Canadian Society of Transplantation consensus guidelines on eligibility for kidney transplantation. Can Med Assoc J. 2005;173(10):O1–25.
4. Grams ME, Massie AB, Coresh J, Segev DL. Trends in the timing of pre-emptive kidney transplantation. J Am Soc Nephrol. 2011;22(9):1615–20.
5. Doshi MD, Hunsicker LG. Short- and long-term outcomes with the use of kidneys and livers donated after cardiac death. Am J Transplant. 2007;7(1):122–9.
6. Gagandeep S, Matsuoka L, Mateo R, et al. Expanding the donor kidney pool: utility of renal allografts procured in a setting of uncontrolled cardiac death. Am J Transplant. 2006;6(7):1682–8.
7. Rao PS, Ojo A. The alphabet soup of kidney transplantation: SCD, DCD, ECD–fundamentals for the practicing nephrologist. Clin J Am Soc Nephrol. 2009;4(11):1827–31.
8. Metzger RA, Delmonico FL, Feng S, Port FK, Wynn JJ, Merion RM. Expanded criteria donors for kidney transplantation. Am J Transplant. 2003;3 Suppl 4:114–25.
9. Merion RM, Ashby VB, Wolfe RA, et al. Deceased-donor characteristics and the survival benefit of kidney transplantation. JAMA. 2005;294(21):2726–33.
10. Ojo AO, Hanson JA, Meier-Kriesche H, et al. Survival in recipients of marginal cadaveric donor kidneys compared with other recipients and wait-listed transplant candidates. J Am Soc Nephrol. 2001;12(3):589–97.
11. Pascual J, Zamora J, Pirsch JD. A systematic review of kidney transplantation from expanded criteria donors. Am J Kidney Dis. 2008;52(3):553–86.
12. Medicare program; hospital conditions of participation: requirements for approval and re-approval of transplant centers to perform organ transplants. Final rule. Fed Regist 722007:15198–280.
13. Kasiske B, Cangro C, Hariharan S, et al. The evaluation of renal transplantation candidates: clinical practice guidelines. Am J Transplant. 2001;1 Suppl 2:3–95.
14. Abbud-Filho M, Adams P, Alberu J, et al. A report of the Lisbon Conference on the care of the kidney transplant recipient. Transplantation. 2007;83(8):S1–22.
15. Dudley C, Harden P. Clinical Practice Guidelines: Assessment of the Potential Kidney Transplant Recipient. 2011; 5: http://www.renal.org/Libraries/Guidelines/Assessment_of_the_Potential_Kidney_Transplant_Recipient_-_Final_Version_12_January_2011.sflb.ashx. Accessed April 7, 2011.

16. Gore J, Pham P, Danovitch G. Obesity and outcome following renal transplantation. Am J Transplant. 2006;6:357–63.
17. Amer H, Fidler M, Myslak M, et al. Proteinuria after kidney transplantation, relationship to allograft histology and survival. Am J Transplant. 2007;7(12):2748–56.
18. US Food and Drug Administration Drug Safety Communication: New warnings for using gadolinium-based contrast agents in patients with kidney dysfunction. http://www.fda.gov/Drugs/DrugSafety/ucm223966.htm#sa. Accessed April 25, 2011.
19. Wang J, Kasiske B. Screening and management of pretransplant cardiovascular disease. Curr Opin Nephrol Hypertens. 2010;19(6):586–91.
20. Pilmore H. Cardiac assessment for renal transplantation. Am J Transplant. 2006;6:659.
21. Fischer S, Avery R. Screening of donor and recipient prior to solid organ transplantation. Am J Transplant. 2009;9 Suppl 4:S7–18.
22. Subramanian A, Dorman S. Mycobacterium tuberculosis in solid organ transplant recipients. Am J Transplant. 2009;9 Suppl 4:S57–62.
23. Humar A, Snydman D. Cytomegalovirus in solid organ transplant recipients. Am J Transplant. 2009;9 Suppl 4:S78–86.
24. Allen U, Preiksaitis J. Epstein-barr virus and post-transplant lymphoproliferative disorder in solid organ transplant recipients. Am J Transplant. 2009;9 Suppl 4:S87–96.
25. Kotton C, Kumar D, Caliendo A, et al. International consensus guidelines on the management of cytomegalovirus in solid organ transplantation. Transplantation. 2010;89(7):779–95.
26. Danzinger-Isakova L, Kumar D. Guidelines for vaccination of solid organ transplant candidates and recipients. Am J Transplant. 2009;9 Suppl 4:S258–62.
27. Gloor J, Stegall MD. Sensitized renal transplant recipients: current protocols and future directions. Nat Rev Nephrol. 2010;6(5):297–306.
28. Fuggle S, Martin S. Tools for human leukocyte antigen antibody detection and their application to transplanting sensitized patients. Transplantation. 2008;86(3):384–90.
29. Stegall MD, Diwan T, Raghavaiah S, et al. Terminal complement inhibition decreases antibody-mediated rejection in sensitized renal transplant recipients. Am J Transplant. 2011;11(11):2405–13.
30. Ibrahim H, Foley R, Tan L, et al. Long-term consequences of kidney donation. N Engl J Med. 2009;360(5):459–69.
31. Segev D, Muzaale A, Caffo B, et al. Perioperative mortatlity and long-term survival following live kidney donation. JAMA. 2010;303(10):959–66.
32. Gai M, Giunti S, Lanfranco G, Segoloni G. Potential risks of living kidney donation–a review. Nephrol Dial Transplant. 2007;22:3122–7.
33. Friedman A, Cheung K, Roman S, Sosa J. Early clinical and economic outcomes of patients undergoing living donor nephrectomy in the United States. Arch Surg. 2010;145(4):356–62.
34. Davis C. Living kidney donors: current state of affairs. Adv Chronic Kidney Dis. 2009;16(4):242–9.
35. Reisaeter AV, Roislien J, Henriksen T, Irgens LM, Hartmann A. Pregnancy and birth after kidney donation: the Norwegian experience. Am J Transplant. 2009;9(4):820–4.
36. Davis C, Cooper M. The state of living kidney donors. Clin J Am Soc Nephrol. 2010;5:1873–80.
37. Ethics Committee of the Transplantation Society. The consensus statement of the amsterdam forum on the care of the live kidney donor. Transplantation. 2004;78:491–2.
38. Mandelbrot D, Pavlakis M, Danovitch G, et al. The medical evaluation of living kidney donors: a survey of US transplant centers. Am J Transplant. 2007;7(10):2333–43.
39. Rodrigue J, Pavlakis M, Danovitch G, et al. Evaluating living kidney donors: relationship types, psychosocial criteria, and consent processes at US transplant programs. Am J Transplant. 2007;7(10):2326–32.
40. Pavlakis M. Live kidney donation: a 36-year-old woman hoping to donate a kidney to her mother. JAMA. 2011;305(6):592–9.
41. Delmonico F. Council of the Transplantation Society. A report of the Amsterdam forum on the care of the live kidney donor: data and medical guidelines. Transplantation. 2005;79(6):S53–66.
42. The Declaration of Istanbul on Organ Trafficking and Transplant Tourism. Clin J Am Soc Nephrol 2008;3:1227–31.
43. Gentry SE, Montgomery RA, Segev DL. Kidney paired donation: fundamentals, limitations, and expansions. Am J Kidney Dis. 2011;57(1):144–51.
44. Rule AD, Gussak HM, Pond GR, et al. Measured and estimated GFR in healthy potential kidney donors. Am J Kidney Dis. 2004;43(1):112–9.
45. Koushik R, Garvey C, Manivel J, Matas A, Kasiske B. Persistent, asymptomatic, microscopic hematuria in prospective kidney donors. Transplantation. 2005;80(10):1425–9.
46. Davis C, Delmonico F. Living-donor kidney transplantation: a review of the current practices for the live donor. J Am Soc Nephrol. 2005;16(7):2098–110.
47. Textor S, Taler S, Driscoll N, et al. Blood pressure and renal function after kidney donation from hypertensive living donors. Transplantation. 2004;78(2):276–82.

Immunosuppression in the Renal Transplant Recipient

35

Claire M. Kennedy and Colm C. Magee

Case 1

A 44-year-old man developed end-stage kidney disease (ESKD) due to IgA nephropathy. After 8 months of hemodialysis, he received a deceased donor kidney transplant. Cytomegalovirus (CMV) IgG serology was positive in the donor and negative in the recipient. The initial postoperative course was uncomplicated and the kidney functioned well; by day 14 the creatinine had fallen to 1.1 mg/dl. His medications included tacrolimus, mycophenolate mofetil (MMF) 750 mg bd, prednisolone 5 mg qd, co-trimoxazole 480 mg qd, valganciclovir 900 mg qd, and a calcium/vitamin D preparation.

He now attends for routine review 3 months after transplant. He is systemically well without fever, malaise, mouth ulcers, altered bowel habit, or dyspnea. His blood results are shown in Table 35.1.

What is the likely cause of the neutropenia? What tests should be performed? What medication changes, if any, should be made?

C.M. Kennedy, M.R.C.P.I. (✉)
Department of Nephrology, Beaumont Hospital, Beaumont Road, Dublin, Ireland
e-mail: kennedyclaire@gmail.com

C.C. Magee, M.D., M.P.H., F.R.C.P.I.
Beaumont Hospital, Dublin, Ireland

Case 2

A 73-year-old white farmer with diabetic nephropathy and hypertension received a deceased donor kidney transplant 14 years ago. Baseline creatinine was 1.4 mg/dl and proteinuria was 0.8 g/day. Regular medications were cyclosporine (last trough 72 ng/ml), azathioprine 100 mg qd, prednisone 5 mg qd, aspirin 75 mg qd, insulin, ramipril 10 mg qd, hydrochlorothiazide 12.5 mg qd, and labetalol 200 mg bd. He has had numerous small skin malignancies excised by his dermatologist.

He now attends for review with a red, swollen, tender big toe, clinically consistent with gout. He also reports a new skin lesion, close to his left eye, which has developed since his last visit. It is clinically suspicious for an ulcerated basal cell carcinoma and will require surgery.

What medications are contributing to the gout? Why is he having recurrent skin cancers? What medication changes would you consider? What is the best timing for these changes? What are the risks of making such changes?

Case 3

A 54-year-old woman developed severe chronic kidney disease from autosomal dominant polycystic kidney disease. She received a preemptive living unrelated kidney transplant (i.e., a transplant before starting dialysis). Immunological

E.V. Lerma and M. Rosner (eds.), *Clinical Decisions in Nephrology, Hypertension and Kidney Transplantation*, DOI 10.1007/978-1-4614-4454-1_35, © Springer Science+Business Media New York 2013

Table 35.1 Laboratory results in case 1

Creatinine (mg/dl)	1.1
Hematocrit (%)	45
Platelets ($\times10^9$/l)	226
White cell count ($\times10^9$/l)	1.36
Neutrophils ($\times10^9$/l)	0.25
Bilirubin (mg/dl)	0.8
AST (iU/l)	15
Alkaline phosphatase (iU/l)	52

risk (of rejection) was standard. CMV IgG serology was negative in both donor and recipient. The postoperative course was uncomplicated and the creatinine was 1.0 mg/dl by day 8. Regular medications were tacrolimus, MMF 750 mg bd, prednisolone 5 mg qd, co-trimoxazole 480 mg qd, labetalol 200 mg bd, and a calcium/vitamin D preparation.

Four months after transplant, she presents with headaches, nausea, and a symmetrical fine tremor. She reports full compliance with the above medications. She also reports a recent respiratory tract infection, for which she received a 1-week course of antibiotics. She also asks whether you recommend that she receive the seasonal influenza vaccine.

Examination showed a fine tremor, pulse 72/min regular, and 180/95 mmHg. Neurological examination was otherwise unremarkable. Her blood results showed hyperkalemia (6.2 mEq/l), hypomagnesemia (0.5 mEq/l), and creatinine 1.4 mg/dl. Urinalysis was normal.

What tests should be performed? What further history should be elicited? What is the management? What advice should you give her regarding the influenza vaccine?

The History of Renal Tra nsplant Immunosuppression

Following several unsuccessful renal transplant experiments in the first half of the twentieth century, the first real success was in 1954 at the Peter Bent Brigham Hospital in Boston. The recipient was 23-year-old Richard Herrick, who had glomerulonephritis, and the donor was his identical twin Ronald, who did not have the disease. The transplant team confirmed that the twins had shared a placenta in utero and shared identical fingerprints and all known blood groups as adults. The operation was a success and Richard lived for 8 years with a functioning transplant and without immunosuppression. Dr. Joseph Murray, the lead surgeon, went on to share the Nobel Prize in Physiology or Medicine in 1990 for his contribution to the field of transplant medicine [1].

Immunological barriers limited further developments in renal transplant medicine until the 1960s when new immunosuppressive agents were developed. By the 1970s, using a combination of azathioprine and corticosteroids, 2-year transplant kidney survival following living donation reached 50 %, albeit with high infection and malignancy rates. A publication in 1978, documenting improved transplant outcomes with cyclosporin A, represented a major breakthrough [2].

Since then, huge progress has been made in the field of renal transplantation. The short- and medium-term survival of kidneys transplanted from living (both related and unrelated) and deceased donors is now excellent. Much of this progress is due to an evolving understanding of the immune system and manipulation thereof.

Pathophysiology

The principal aim of renal transplant medicine is to prevent rejection, without over-immunosuppression. T-cells play a key role in mediating the rejection process and are the principal targets of current immunosuppressive drugs.

Antigen-presenting cells (APCs) present donor alloantigens (these are antigens that distinguish self from non-self) to host T-cells in the lymphoid tissues. Activated T-cells proliferate and differentiate into various effector cell subtypes. These cells return to the transplant, recruit other inflammatory cells, and cause inflammation and destruction of the transplant kidney. This process of T-cell-mediated rejection is summarized in Fig. 35.1.

T-cells are activated in a 3-signal process (see Fig. 35.2).

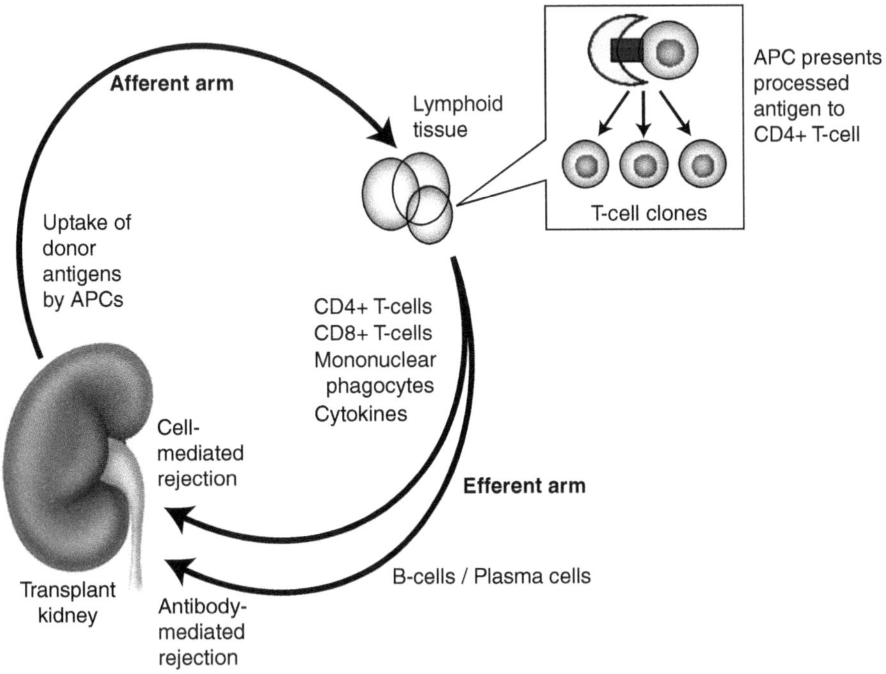

Fig. 35.1 Summary of (unchecked) immune response to the transplant kidney. In the afferent arm of the immune response, APCs of the donor and recipient take up and process donor antigens. These antigens are then presented to CD4+ T-cells, leading to activation of these cells. In the efferent arm, CD4+ cells activate various effector pathways (cell-mediated cytotoxicity, antibody-mediated damage, NK cell-mediated cytotoxicity, etc.), which ultimately lead to damage of the transplant kidney

Signal 1: APCs endocytose alloantigens and display them on the cell surface in an MHC–peptide complex. This complex binds the T-cell receptor, which activates the CD3 signaling complex. This results in increased cytosolic ionized calcium and ultimately leads to the transcription of genes for several cytokines, including IL-2.

Signal 2: Co-stimulatory signals, such as that between CD28 on the T-cell and CD80/86 on the APC, lead to amplified and prolonged cell signaling. In the absence of signal 2, there is anergy of the activated T-cell, preventing autoimmunity against host antigens.

Signal 3: A number of cell-signaling pathways are activated by signals 1 and 2 above. These pathways include the calcium–calcineurin pathway, the Ras–mitogen-activated protein (MAP) kinase pathway, and the nuclear factor kappa B (NF-κB) pathway. Together, these activate various transcription factors that lead to the production of IL-2 and other molecules. These molecules act in an autocrine and paracrine fashion to trigger entry into the cell cycle, clonal expansion, and differentiation into effector T-cells.

T-cells differentiate into either cytotoxic CD8 cells, helper CD4 cells, or inflammatory CD4 cells. These effector T-cells ultimately damage the transplanted kidney by various mechanisms including direct cytotoxicity, cytokine secretion, recruitment of other inflammatory cells, and stimulation of B-cell function (see below). The histological hallmarks of T-cell-mediated rejection are tubulitis and endothelialitis, where T-cells invade the tubules and arteriolar intima, respectively. Clinically, there is elevation in plasma creatinine; localizing symptoms/signs (such as pain) are actually quite rare today.

The role of B-cells in acute and chronic transplant rejection is increasingly recognized. B-cell receptors bind alloantigen and secrete immunoglobulin (antibody) of the same specificity. Antibody deposition in the transplant can activate

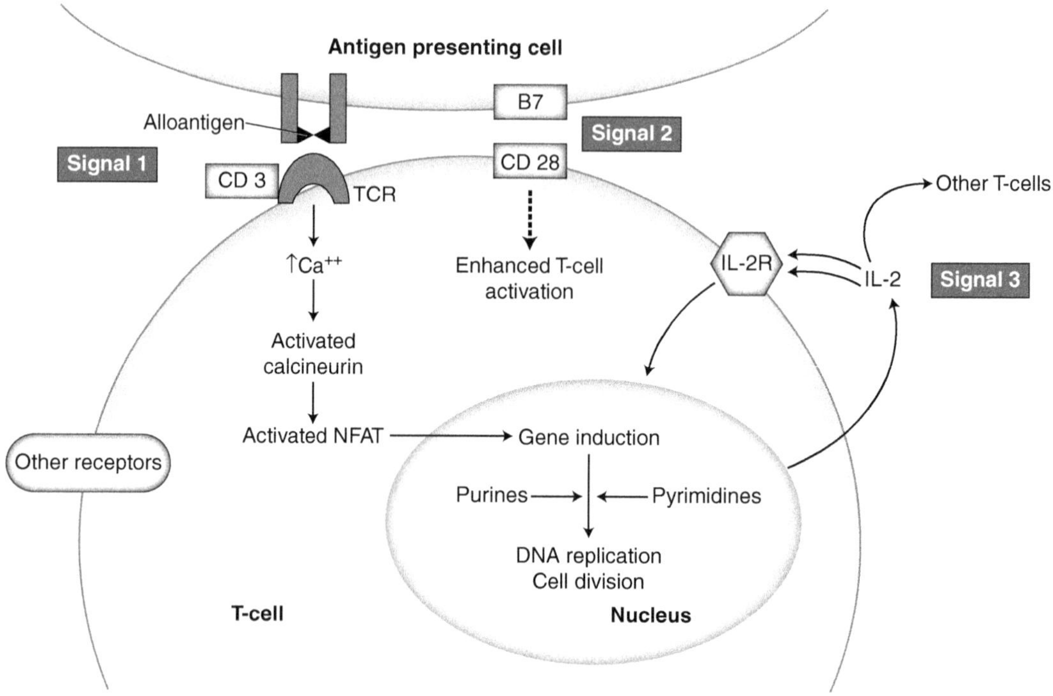

Fig. 35.2 T-cell activation

various effector mechanisms, including natural killer cells, phagocytes, and complement. Histologically, this is characterized by glomerulitis, peritubular capillaritis; antibody to donor HLA is usually detectable in the serum. This so-called antibody-mediated rejection is often difficult to treat.

Immunosuppressive Agents

Post-transplant immunosuppression is divided into two phases: induction and maintenance. *Induction* therapy is given in the perioperative period, when the risk of rejection is highest. In the setting of immunosuppression, host T-cells become less responsive to persistent alloantigens over time, a process termed "host–graft adaptation" [3]. Therefore, during the long-term *maintenance* phase of therapy, immunosuppression requirements fall, as the risk of rejection is lower. The agents used during both phases of treatment are described below. Their individual targets, in relation to T-cell function, can be visualized in Fig. 35.3 (see also Table 35.2).

Patient specific factors also influence immunosuppression choices. There is a spectrum of immunological risk ranging from monozygotic twin transplantation to ABO-incompatible transplantation (Table 35.3). Factors that confer a higher immunological risk are outlined below. A patient with none of these risk factors requires less total immunosuppression than a patient with some or all of these risk factors. Patients at either end of the spectrum are discussed later.

Induction Immunosuppression

Two approaches to induction phase immunosuppression exist. Conventional maintenance agents can be administered at high dose and, over time, tapered to standard doses. This approach is limited by the inherent nephrotoxicity of the calcineurin inhibitors (CNIs) (see later). To avoid this problem, an antibody induction agent, with

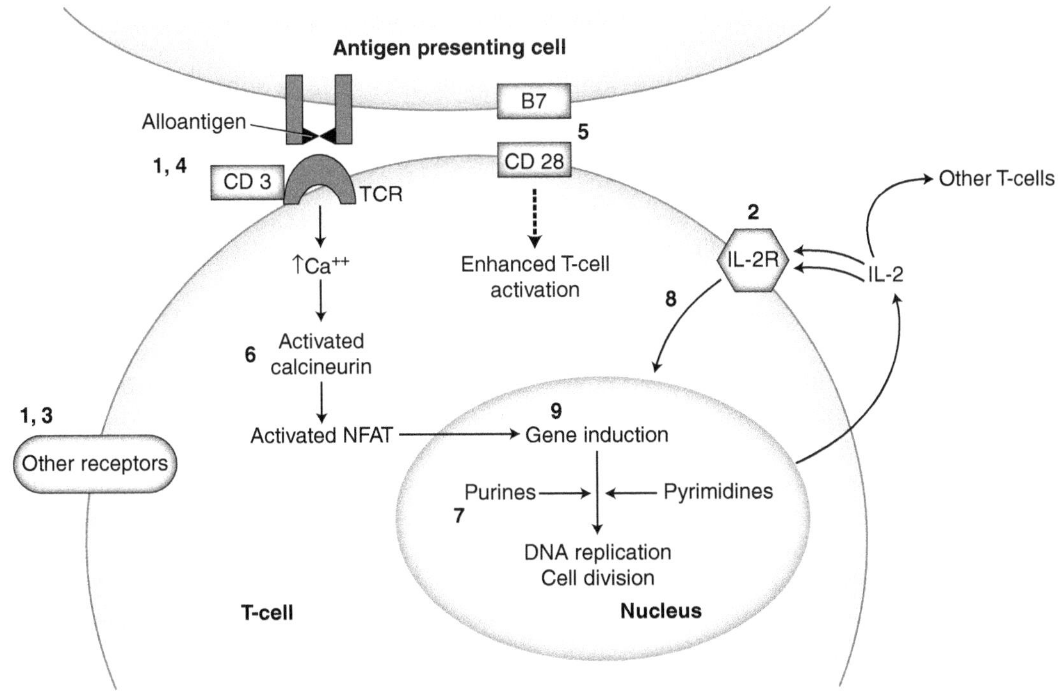

Fig. 35.3 Mechanism of action of commonly used immunosuppressive agents

Table 35.2 Mechanism of action of commonly used immunosuppressive agents

1	Thymoglobulin
2	Anti-IL2 receptor antibodies
3	Alemtuzumab
4	OKT3
5	Belatacept
6	CNI
7	Anti-metabolites
8	Sirolimus
9	Corticosteroids

potent anti-T-cell activity, can be administered perioperatively (see Table 35.4). This facilitates standard dosing of the maintenance agents.

Polyclonal Antibody Preparations

Thymoglobulin is produced by immunizing rabbits with human thymocytes and harvesting purified gamma globulin. The polyclonal product contains multiple antibodies directed against various leukocyte antigens. It has a prolonged and profound depleting effect on T-cells and other

Table 35.3 Factors that confer higher immunological risk of rejection

Previous transplant (especially if lost to rejection)[a]
High levels of antibodies to HLA proteins
Black ethnicity
Previous multiple pregnancies[a]
Multiple blood transfusions (especially if recent)[a]

[a]Due to previous exposure to human leucocyte antigens (HLA)

Table 35.4 Induction antibodies used in renal transplantation

Induction antibody agents	
Polyclonal antibody preparations	Thymoglobulin
Monoclonal antibody preparations	Basiliximab, daclizumab
	Alemtuzumab
	OKT3
	Belatacept

cell lines, leading to prolonged and marked immunosuppression.

Anti-thymocyte globulin (ATG) is a similar compound, used in Europe, derived from an activated Jurkat T-cell leukemia line.

Monoclonal Antibody Preparations

The anti-IL2 receptor antibodies, *daclizumab* and *basiliximab*, target the α (alpha) chain (CD25) of the IL2 receptor. This blocks rapid T-cell proliferation and, therefore, amplification of the immune response. As their target is expressed on activated T-cells only, these agents are much more selective in their mode of action than the polyclonal antibody preparations.

To prevent development of anti-mouse antibodies, daclizumab is a humanized murine monoclonal antibody, whereas basiliximab is chimeric. This also affects individual affinity for the IL2 receptor and, therefore, dosing regimens. These agents induce prolonged IL2 receptor blockade. However, as the immune system has several overlapping (redundant) mechanisms, the total immunosuppression conferred by IL2 receptor blockade is relatively mild.

Alemtuzumab (Campath 1H) is a humanized anti-CD52 monoclonal antibody that has rapid, profound, and prolonged T- and B-cell depleting effects. A recent randomized controlled trial compared alemtuzumab induction therapy to "conventional" induction therapy after renal transplantation [4]. All patients underwent early steroid withdrawal. In those of standard immunological risk, alemtuzumab was associated with less early rejection than basiliximab, but more late rejection and serious infections. In those of higher immunological risk, alemtuzumab was associated with similar outcomes but, again, more late rejection than thymoglobulin. Although used as a "first-line" induction agent in some centers, alemtuzumab is not yet FDA approved for this indication.

OKT3 is a murine monoclonal antibody that targets the CD3 complex; an intrinsic part of the T-cell receptor. Upon binding, OKT3 initially activates T-cells with massive release of numerous cytokines; the cells are then "cleared" from the peripheral circulation.

Although OKT3 is a powerful immunosuppressant, the potentially fatal cytokine release syndrome has limited its use. The declining use of the agent led to market withdrawal in 2009, with remaining stocks to be used up.

Belatacept (LEA29Y) is a competitive antagonist of CD28 in the binding of CD80/86 on the APC, thereby inhibiting "signal 2." Phase III trials demonstrated a potential role for belatacept as a co-induction agent [5, 6]. Initial reports suggested an increased rate of post-transplant lymphoproliferative disease (PTLD), specifically in those patients who were Epstein–Barr virus (EBV) naïve. However, FDA approval was granted for belatacept in 2011, for use as a co-stimulatory agent with basiliximab in the context of maintenance immunosuppression with corticosteroids and MMF (i.e., CNI free). A caveat exists; the FDA has approved its use in patients with IgG antibodies to EBV only (contraindicated if negative or unknown EBV serostatus). There is a paucity of long-term information regarding the adverse effects of belatacept administration. Rigorous registry maintenance and post-marketing research are planned in order to capture such data.

There is growing evidence to support induction therapy [7, 8]. In line with this, the use of induction agents in the USA has steadily increased over the last 10 years (Fig. 35.4). The specific choice of induction agent depends on local expertise, cost, ease of administration, and patient safety.

The 2009 KDIGO guideline on induction therapy in renal transplant recipients suggests that induction therapy be given to all recipients [10]. IL2 receptor blockers are recommended as the first-line agent. Thymoglobulin is preferred in those recipients at high immunological risk [11, 12].

Maintenance Immunosuppression

Over time, as the risk of rejection falls, the combined immunosuppression dose is lowered to minimize the risk of infections and malignancy. The maintenance agents used in clinical practice are outlined below (Table 35.5).

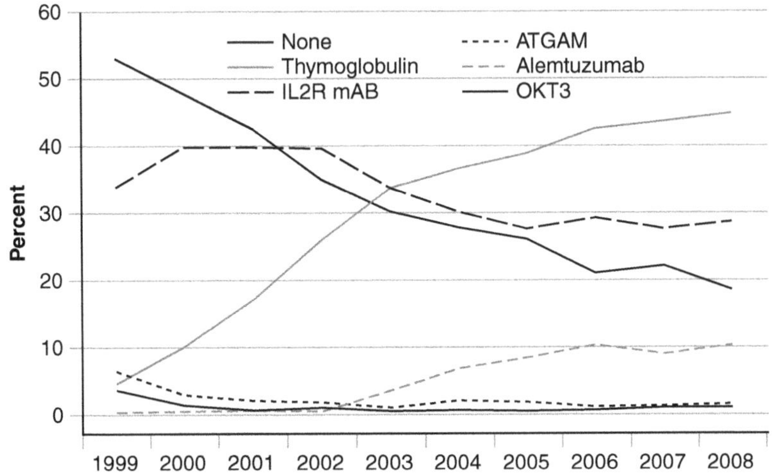

Fig. 35.4 The use of induction agents in the United States from 1999 to 2008 [9]

Table 35.5 Maintenance agents in renal transplantation

Maintenance agents	
Calcineurin inhibitors	Cyclosporine
	Tacrolimus
Anti-metabolites	Mycophenolate mofetil
	Azathioprine
mTOR inhibitors	Sirolimus
	Everolimus
Corticosteroids	

The 2009 KDIGO guideline on maintenance immunosuppression recommends that a CNI, an anti-metabolite, and corticosteroids be used in combination. Tacrolimus, MMF, and prednisone/prednisolone are the first-line agents [10]. The theoretical benefit of combining three classes of agents is to provide adequate immunosuppression without excess toxic effects of one particular agent.

Calcineurin Inhibitors

The discovery of *cyclosporine*, an 11 amino acid polypeptide, revolutionized renal transplant medicine. It binds cyclophylin, forming a complex that binds and inhibits calcineurin, a rate-limiting enzyme in T-cell activation.

The older "standard" preparations of cyclosporine had complex and variable pharmacokinetic properties. The newer microemulsion preparations have improved absorption and less inter-patient variability.

Tacrolimus (FK-506) is a macrolide antibiotic. It binds FK binding protein (FK-BP), a ubiquitous cytosolic protein. The complex binds calcineurin, resulting in reduced T-cell activation. Thus, although binding to a different intracellular receptor, its downstream effects are very similar to those of cyclosporine.

Many centers now use tacrolimus as the first-line CNI. The recent ELITE (Efficacy Limiting Toxicity Elimination)-Symphony trial [13] randomized 1,645 patients to MMF plus corticosteroids and one of the following: tacrolimus, sirolimus, standard cyclosporine, or low dose cyclosporine. The group assigned to tacrolimus achieved higher glomerular filtration rate (GFR), superior transplant kidney survival, and lower rates of rejection, all at 12 months.

An extensive meta-analysis of 30 randomized controlled trials [14] concluded that tacrolimus was superior to cyclosporine in terms of transplant survival and acute rejection at 3 years. Although there was no significant difference in rates of infections or malignancy, tacrolimus was associated with higher rates of post-transplant diabetes mellitus.

Both cyclosporine and tacrolimus are metabolized by the cytochrome P450 system. Therefore drugs that inhibit or induce these enzymes may interact with CNI levels and should be co-prescribed with caution.

Anti-metabolites

Azathioprine is a purine analogue that is metabolized to 6-mercaptopurine (6-MP) and 6-thiouric acid in the liver. These compounds halt replication of DNA and RNA, and therefore suppress the proliferation of activated B- and T-cells, amongst other cells. The metabolism of 6-MP to inactive compounds is catalyzed by xanthine oxidase.

The main adverse effect of azathioprine is bone marrow suppression, potentially leading to depletion of all three peripheral blood cell lines. Allopurinol, a xanthine oxidase inhibitor, leads to significantly higher 6-MP levels, if co-prescribed with azathioprine. This interaction can lead to profound—and potentially fatal—bone marrow suppression.

MMF is a pro-drug that is hydrolyzed to mycophenolic acid (MPA). MPA inhibits inosine monophosphate dehydrogenase (IMPDH), which is the rate-limiting enzyme in de novo purine biosynthesis. As T- and B-cells are dependent on this pathway for nucleotide synthesis, MMF, at least in theory, has a more selective T- and B-cell effect. Gastrointestinal adverse effects (nausea, abdominal discomfort, diarrhea) are common but usually respond to dose reduction. As it is a more powerful immunosuppressive agent than azathioprine, MMF has become the anti-metabolite of choice in recent years.

Mammalian Target of Rapamycin Inhibitors

Sirolimus (rapamycin) is a macrolide antibiotic derived from *Streptomyces hygroscopicus*. It also binds FK-BP, but has a different mechanism of action to tacrolimus. It leads to inhibition of a regulatory kinase called mammalian target of rapamycin (mTOR) and causes cell cycle arrest in the G1-S phase, leading to reduced proliferation of T-cells and other cells.

Sirolimus, in theory, lacks the nephrotoxic effects of CNIs but this has not necessarily lead to improved outcomes. In the ELITE-Symphony trial [13], those patients receiving sirolimus had a significantly higher rate of acute rejection, and a lower GFR, than those receiving tacrolimus.

There is emerging evidence that sirolimus has important anti-neoplastic effects in transplant recipients with skin or other malignancies. Several mechanisms of action have been identified, including decreased vascular endothelial growth factor (VEGF) production and inhibition of malignant cell growth in the G1-S phase. Conversely, the anti-proliferative effects of sirolimus can delay tissue and wound healing. Therefore, it should be avoided immediately post-transplant and in the setting of major non-transplant surgery.

Everolimus is a derivative of sirolimus with similar effects. Its role in renal transplantation, and indeed the management of certain malignancies, is at the center of several ongoing trials.

Corticosteroids

Corticosteroids have multiple immunosuppressive and anti-inflammatory effects. They inhibit the production of various cytokines, including TNF-α (alpha) and IL-2. They cause neutrophilia, but with inhibition of neutrophil chemotaxis. They also downregulate production of NF-κB (nuclear factor kappa B) and activator protein-1, which are potent transcription factors for a number of pro-inflammatory cytokines.

There is no consensus on the dosing of *corticosteroids* in renal transplantation. Typically, a large dose of intravenous corticosteroids is given peri-transplant as part of the induction schedule. An oral dose of prednisolone 20 mg/day is then tapered, over 1–3 months, to a maintenance dose of approximately 5 mg daily. Some centers now use very low dose corticosteroid protocols.

Table 35.6 Common/serious adverse effects of induction antibody agents

Induction agent	Adverse effect	Precautions/ monitoring
Thymoglobulin	First dose effects Leucopenia, thrombocytopenia	Slow infusion Monitor CBC; reduce dose
Basiliximab/ daclizumab	Similar rates to placebo	
Alemtuzumab	Potential increase in autoimmune disease	
Belatacept	PTLD (early reports)	Avoid if Epstein–Barr virus (EBV) IgG is negative (or unknown) prior to transplant

Table 35.7 Common/serious adverse effects of maintenance immunosuppressive agents

Maintenance agent	Adverse effect	Precautions/ monitoring
Cyclosporine	Nephrotoxicity* Hypertension Diabetes Cosmetic (hirsutism, gum hyperplasia) Hyperlipidemia	Monitor blood trough levels
Tacrolimus	Nephrotoxicity* Hypertension Diabetes Hyperlipidemia Headache/tremor Electrolyte abnormalities (↑K^+, ↓Mg^{2+})	Monitor blood trough levels
Azathioprine	Leucopenia Anemia Thrombocytopenia Abnormal liver function tests (LFTs)	Monitor CBC Monitor LFTs
Mycophenolate mofetil	Nausea/diarrhea/ abdominal discomfort Leucopenia Thrombocytopenia	Monitor CBC Reduce dose
Sirolimus/ everolimus	Impaired wound healing Acne Hyperlipidemia Mouth ulcers	Avoid if patient undergoing major surgery Avoid early post-transplant
Corticosteroids*	Osteoporosis Diabetes Hypertension Hyperlipidemia Cushingoid appearance Peptic ulcer disease Cataracts	Minimize dose

Adverse Effects of Immunosuppression

The most important adverse effects of generalized immunosuppression are malignancies and infections, including opportunistic infections. These will be discussed in more detail later.

Individual drugs have specific adverse effect profiles. The main adverse effects of the induction and maintenance agents are listed in Tables 35.6 and 35.7, respectively. Those marked * are described in more detail below.

CNI-Induced Nephrotoxicity

There are several mechanisms by which the CNIs may cause nephrotoxicity.

A reversible, dose-related, hemodynamic effect occurs, by which the afferent and efferent arterioles constrict, with intact tubular function. This causes a decrease in GFR, which can sometimes be difficult to distinguish from rejection. The urinalysis is bland, as there is no structural kidney damage.

It is thought that over time, prolonged renal vasoconstriction leads to ischemic structural changes in the kidney. Such changes include narrowing of arterioles and tubulo-interstitial fibrosis.

An idiosyncratic thrombotic microangiopathy may (rarely) occur giving rise to a hemolytic uremic syndrome (HUS) picture. This is probably due to CNI-induced endothelial injury.

To minimize CNI nephrotoxicity, most centers try to safely limit CNI doses by maximizing MMF doses and using induction antibody. Results from the ELITE-Symphony Study [13] support the notion that tacrolimus is less nephrotoxic than cyclosporine for a given level of protection against rejection.

Corticosteroid Minimization

There is increasing interest in minimizing corticosteroid exposure after renal transplantation, to avoid the many long-term adverse effects of corticosteroids. Various strategies, including "steroid-free" and "steroid withdrawal" protocols, have been described. Some single center reports are encouraging, but it must be remembered that the majority of patients in these studies are at low immunological risk and have received powerful induction therapy.

A well-designed trial randomized 386 renal transplant recipients to corticosteroid withdrawal at 7 days after renal transplantation or standard long-term prednisolone 5 mg daily. Early withdrawal was associated with an increase in acute rejection, without improved rates of fracture, blood pressure control, serum cholesterol, or new-onset diabetes mellitus [15].

Our belief is that *low dose* steroid protocols provide the best balance of efficacy and toxicity and that more data are required before steroid-free protocols can be routinely recommended.

Important Pharmacological Interactions

Common and/or serious drug interactions encountered post-transplant are outlined in Table 35.8. Any physician involved in the care of a transplant recipient should be aware of these potentially serious interactions. Table 35.8 is not exhaustive; a complete list of interactions can be found in the product literature.

Monitoring of Immunosuppressive Medications

The 2009 KDIGO guideline regarding monitoring of renal transplant function suggests the schedule outlined in Table 35.9 [10].

As the risk of rejection is highest immediately post-transplant, higher target drug levels are used during this time. If induction therapy is administered, lower drug levels may suffice.

The drug levels measured in clinic practice are CNI levels, mammalian target of rapamycin inhibitor (mTORi) levels, and, in certain centers, MMF/MPA levels. Routine monitoring for other adverse effects of immunosuppressive drugs (such as leucopenia and hepatitis) is also performed.

CNI Levels

Given the narrow therapeutic index of the CNIs, and the variable pharmacokinetics of cyclosporine, drug monitoring is routine.

Cyclosporine trough levels (C_0) are routinely measured (12 h post-dose). Target C_0 levels in the first 3 months are approximately 200–300 ng/ml, with the lower target C_0 of 50–150 ng/ml thereafter [16].

There has been interest in using a 2-h peak cyclosporine level (C_2) to guide dosing, as C_2 levels *may* correlate better with the area under the curve (AUC) and overall drug exposure. It is unclear whether such an approach leads to improved clinical outcomes [17].

Tacrolimus monitoring is less researched. C_0 levels correlate well with the AUC. Target tacrolimus levels, following induction therapy, are in the region of 5–10 ng/ml [16]. The recent ELITE-Symphony study [13] recruited relatively low immunological risk patients following daclizumab induction therapy and targeted the tacrolimus levels to 3–7 ng/ml, with good clinical outcomes.

The 2009 KDIGO guideline regarding monitoring of immunosuppressive medication suggests that CNI levels are checked as outlined in Table 35.10 [10].

mTORi Levels

In practice, C_0 levels are used to adjust sirolimus dosing [18]. As it has a long half-life, and takes several days to reach a steady state, C_0 levels

Table 35.8 Important pharmacological interactions with maintenance immunosuppressive agents

Drug	Interacting drug	Mechanism	Result
CNI	Ketoconazole, voriconazole, fluconazole	CYP3A4 inhibition	Increased CNI level with resultant nephrotoxicity
	Nondihydropyridine calcium channel blockers, e.g., diltiazem	CYP3A4 inhibition	As above
	Macrolide antibiotics, e.g., clarithromycin	CYP3A4 inhibition	As above
Azathioprine	Allopurinol	Xanthine oxidase inhibition	Bone marrow suppression
MMF	Antacids	Decreased absorption	Reduced MMF effect
	Cyclosporine	Decreased enterohepatic recirculation	MPA levels reduced

Table 35.9 Monitoring schedule of renal transplant recipient

Week 1	Weeks 2–4	Months 2–3	Months 4–6	Months 7–12	Year 2+
Daily	Twice/week	Weekly	Every 2 weeks	Monthly	Every 2–3 months

Table 35.10 Recommended monitoring of CNI levels

On alternate days immediately post-transplant
If medication changes are made
If patient clinical status changes
If there is a decline in renal function

taken within a week of dose adjustment are not very helpful. If sirolimus is used in conjunction with a CNI, low sirolimus levels are often targeted. If sirolimus is used in a CNI-free protocol, higher levels are targeted.

MMF/MPA Levels

The MPA trough level (C_0) correlates poorly with the AUC and is not routinely monitored in clinical practice. Instead, MMF is usually administered as a fixed dose between 500 and 1,500 mg bid. The dose is then adjusted based on immunological risk and adverse effects, especially gastrointestinal symptoms and the peripheral white cell count.

Special Considerations

Pregnancy

Successful renal transplantation rapidly restores female reproductive health. Pregnancy should be avoided, with appropriate contraception, for the first year, until renal function has stabilized on baseline immunosuppression [19].

The CNIs are considered relatively safe in pregnancy, although there is less long-term evidence for tacrolimus. Levels should be closely monitored, as pregnancy-related changes in the volume of distribution are often significant. Steroids are also relatively safe in pregnancy. Higher dose should be given temporarily in the peri-partum period. Although azathioprine crosses the placenta, the immature fetal liver does not convert it to its active metabolite, and so it too may be used in pregnancy.

MMF is contraindicated in pregnancy due to an increased risk of pregnancy loss and congenital malformations, including cleft lip and palate. Sirolimus is also contraindicated in pregnancy given its fetotoxic effects in animal studies.

Thus, at least 2 months prior to conception, female renal transplant recipients should be switched to a combination of CNI, azathioprine, and steroids.

High Immunological Risk Transplant Recipients

Complex induction immunosuppression protocols are required for recipients receiving ABO-incompatible or HLA-incompatible transplants. Higher total immunosuppression is required during the maintenance period. Corticosteroids should not be withdrawn.

Low Immunological Risk Transplant Recipients

Patients with a particularly low immunological risk include those in receipt of a renal transplant from a very closely matched sibling or a monozygotic twin. In this setting, immunosuppression is minimized.

Post-transplant Diabetes Mellitus

Unfortunately, corticosteroids, CNIs, and mTORi are diabetogenic, both individually and in combination. Post-transplant diabetes mellitus is associated with worse transplant kidney outcomes and increased rates of cardiovascular disease.

Manipulation of immunosuppression can sometimes improve glucose control, although consensus regarding the best approach is lacking. A transplant recipient at high risk of diabetes (e.g., obese, hepatitis C) should be on the lowest acceptable dose of corticosteroids and CNI. Cyclosporine causes less diabetes than tacrolimus and so conversion to cyclosporine may help, particularly if glycemic control is proving difficult. The above changes must be weighed against the risk of rejection on a case-by-case basis.

Malignancy

Renal transplant recipients are at an increased lifetime risk of developing cancer, including non-melanoma skin cancer and PTLD. Several factors increase this risk including impaired immune-mediated elimination of pre-cancer/cancer cells and uncontrolled proliferation of oncogenic viruses (such as human papilloma virus (HPV) and EBV). The risk of developing gynecological malignancy, which is often associated with HPV, is increased 18-fold after renal transplantation [20]. Interestingly, common cancers (in the general population), such as prostate, breast, and colorectal cancers, are not increased in incidence in renal transplant recipients [20].

Some cancers, such as PTLD, may respond to a reduction in immunosuppression. In selected patients with multiple or aggressive non-melanoma skin cancers, conversion from a CNI to sirolimus should be considered. Such conversion can, however, increase the risk of rejection, proteinuria, and decreased transplant kidney survival.

Cost

In some countries, drug costs are a limiting factor in renal transplantation. Certain cost-minimizing measures may be appropriate in such a setting [10]. Rigorously tested generic drug preparations can help to reduce cost. Azathioprine may be used instead of MMF (with comparable outcomes in some studies). Ketoconazole or diltiazem, via their interaction with the cytochrome P450 system, can facilitate administration of lower doses of CNIs.

Preventative Medicine

Long-term immunosuppression is associated with an increased risk of infections, including opportunistic infections. Various preventative measures should be taken prior to, and following, transplantation.

Live vaccines are contraindicated post-transplant due to a risk of disseminated infection.

Inactive or killed vaccines are safe and should be administered in accordance with Table 35.11. Travelers should seek advice from a travel clinic regarding appropriate vaccination.

Ideally, vaccines should be administered 6 weeks pre-transplant or 6 months post-transplant, when an optimal response is more likely. One exception is the seasonal influenza vaccine. This should be avoided in the first month post-transplant but thereafter should be administered prior to the influenza season in all renal transplant recipients. Household contacts should also receive annual influenza vaccination to protect themselves and, indirectly, the transplant recipient from seasonal influenza.

Further information regarding specific vaccines can be obtained at http://www.cdc.gov/vaccines.

In the post-transplant setting, prophylaxis against *Pneumocystis carinii* pneumonia and other bacterial infections is achieved by using co-trimoxazole for 6–12 months. Prophylaxis against CMV disease for 3–6 months is also required in those patients with donor or recipient seropositivity.

Cases Revisited

Case 1

The leucopenia and neutropenia are probably adverse effects of his medications, particularly the combination of MMF, valganciclovir, and co-trimoxazole. CMV disease can also cause neutropenia but is much less likely as he has no fever or systemic symptoms, his liver function tests are normal (mild hepatitis is often seen in CMV disease), and he has been taking anti-CMV prophylaxis. Nevertheless, CMV disease should be excluded, by means of serum CMV-PCR.

While CMV disease is being excluded, the following medication changes should be considered:

Reduction/temporary cessation of co-trimoxazole

Reduction/temporary cessation of valganciclovir

Reduction/temporary cessation of MMF; monitoring closely for evidence of rejection

Increasing steroid dose to increase peripheral neutrophil count and protect against rejection (if MMF is stopped)

In the absence of CMV disease, it is reasonable to make some or all of the above medication changes and follow the CBC closely. Typically, the WBC will improve within days. A bone marrow biopsy in this setting is rarely indicated. If the neutropenia is particularly severe or unresponsive to medication changes, G-CSF therapy can be considered, although experience with use of this agent in renal transplant recipients is limited.

In this case, CMV viremia was not detected. Co-trimoxazole and valganciclovir were discontinued, and the MMF dose was reduced to 250 mg bd. The neutrophil count improved daily and after

Table 35.11 Vaccination recommendations in renal transplant recipients

Vaccine	Live/inactive	Pre-transplant	Post-transplant	Comments
Influenza	Inactive	Y	Annual	Vaccinate household contacts
Hepatitis B	Inactive	Y	Per titers	Consider annual titer with booster if titer falls <10 iU/l
Pneumococcal	Inactive	Y	Every 3–5 years	
DTP	Inactive	Y	Every 10 years	
Meningococcus	Inactive	Y	Y	If high risk
Hemophilus influenza B	Inactive	Y	Y	As per regular age-appropriate schedule
Varicella zoster	Live	Y	N	
BCG	Live	Varies between countries	N	
MMR	Live	Y	N	
Oral polio	Live	Y	N	

1 week was within the normal range. At this point, MMF was cautiously increased to 500 mg bd. After 3 weeks, with close monitoring of renal function and white cell count throughout, the initial dose of MMF was tolerated (750 mg bd), along with low dose valganciclovir and low dose co-trimoxazole.

Case 2

Both cyclosporine and the thiazide diuretic may contribute to the development of gout. Several factors have contributed to his recurrent skin malignancies: white ethnicity, outdoor occupation (with exposure to UV light), and long-term immunosuppression.

The following medication changes should be considered for acute gout management and gout prophylaxis:

Colchicine or increased dose corticosteroids (with appropriate insulin adjustment) for acute gout management. NSAIDs are rarely used in renal transplant recipients because they may cause prerenal acute kidney injury.

Replacement of thiazide diuretic with another antihypertensive agent.

Switching cyclosporine to an alternative agent.

It must be remembered that azathioprine essentially precludes the use of allopurinol (see above). The two drugs can be used together in exceptional cases, but only with significant azathioprine dose reduction and close monitoring of the CBC. One potential solution is conversion of azathioprine to MMF, enabling safe co-prescription of allopurinol. Another is to use probenecid instead of allopurinol.

Febuxostat, also a xanthine oxidase inhibitor, was recently approved by the FDA for gout prophylaxis. It similarly interacts with azathioprine, and co-prescription should be avoided. Its use in patients with chronic kidney disease is currently being researched. There is no trial evidence regarding its use in renal transplant recipients and so routine use cannot be recommended.

The patient should be reminded about the need to use sunscreen with a high sun protection factor (SPF) and to wear appropriate clothing (long sleeved shirts, cap covering ears, etc.) whenever he is outdoors. A dermatologist should review his suspicious skin lesion. Conversion of cyclosporine to sirolimus should be considered as the latter has anti-neoplastic effects. This should be delayed, however, until after any surgery as sirolimus impairs wound healing. Other adverse effects of sirolimus include marrow suppression and increased proteinuria.

In this particular case, colchicine was used to treat the acute gout. The thiazide diuretic was discontinued, and the labetalol increased to 400 mg bd. A dermatologist reviewed his skin lesion and arranged excision by a plastic surgeon. Eight weeks after the operation, when the wound had fully healed, cyclosporine was converted to sirolimus, with close monitoring of transplant function. No new skin lesions have developed since this switch was made.

Case 3

An ultrasound of the transplant kidney should be considered to rule out an obstructive process. As her symptoms are the classic features of tacrolimus toxicity, a tacrolimus trough level should be checked. Her recent antibiotic may have interfered with tacrolimus metabolism via the cytochrome P450 mechanism.

Indeed, on further questioning, the patient confirmed that she had taken a course of clarithromycin, a macrolide antibiotic that interferes with tacrolimus metabolism and increases the circulating tacrolimus levels (see Table 35.8).

Her tacrolimus trough level was supratherapeutic at 17 ng/ml. The dose was temporarily reduced; her symptoms quickly resolved and her creatinine returned to baseline. She was reminded of the importance of checking carefully with her physicians and pharmacist before taking any new medications.

She should be educated regarding the importance of annual influenza vaccination. This should be administered prior to the influenza season each year, including the year of transplantation. Her household contacts should also be vaccinated on an annual basis.

Table 35.12 Key points regarding immunosuppression in the renal transplant recipient

Individual assessment of immunological risk is crucial
Risk of rejection must be balanced against risk of long-term adverse effects of immunosuppressive drugs
Appropriate preventative measures should be taken
Potential drug interactions must be considered prior to introduction of new drugs

Key Points

For the key points in this chapter please see Table 35.12.

Disclosures The data and analyses reported in the 2009 Annual Report of the US Organ Procurement and Transplantation Network and the Scientific Registry of Transplant Recipients have been supplied by UNOS and Arbor Research under contract with HHS/HRSA. The authors alone are responsible for reporting and interpreting these data; the views expressed herein are those of the authors and not necessarily those of the US Government.

References

1. Petechuk D. Organ transplantation. Westpost, CT: Greenwood; 2006.
2. Calne RY, White DJG, Thiru S, Evans DB, McMaster P, Dunn DC, et al. Cyclosporin A in patients receiving renal allografts from cadaver donors. Lancet. 1978;2:1323–7.
3. Halloran P. Immunosuppressive drugs for kidney transplantation. N Engl J Med. 2004;351:2715–29.
4. Hanaway MJ, Woodle ES, Mulgaonkar S, Peddi VR, Kaufman DB, First MR, Croy R, Holman J, INTAC Study Group. Alemtuzumab induction in renal transplantation. N Engl J Med. 2011;364:1909–19.
5. Vincenti F, Charpentier B, Vanrenterghem Y, Rostaing L, Bresnahan B, Darji P, Massari P, Mondragon-Ramirez GA, Agarwal M, Di Russo G, Lin CS, Garg P, Larsen CP. A phase III study of belatacept-based immunosuppression regimens versus cyclosporine in renal transplant recipients (BENEFIT study). Am J Transplant. 2010;10(3):535–46.
6. Durrbach A, Pestana JM, Pearson T, Vincenti F, Garcia VD, Campistol J, Rial Mdel C, Florman S, Block A, Di Russo G, Xing J, Garg P, Griny J. A phase III study of belatacept versus cyclosporine in kidney transplants from extended criteria donors (BENEFIT-EXT study). Am J Transplant. 2010;10(3): 547–57.
7. Szczech LA, Berlin JA, Aradhye S, Grossman RA, Feldman HI. Effect of anti-lymphocyte induction therapy on renal allograft survival: a meta-analysis. J Am Soc Nephrol. 1997;8(11):1771–7.
8. Webster AC, Playford EG, Higgins G, Chapman JR, Craig JC. Interleukin 2 receptor antagonists for renal transplant recipients: a meta-analysis of randomized trials. Transplantation. 2004;77(2):166–76.
9. 2009 OPTN/SRTR Annual report 1999–2008. HHS/HRSA/HSB/DOT (see disclosures).
10. Kidney Disease: Improving Global Outcomes (KDIGO) Transplant Work Group. KDIGO clinical practice guideline for the care of kidney transplant recipients. Am J Transplant. 2009;9 Suppl 3:S6–9.
11. Brennan DC, Daller JA, Lake KD, Cibrik D, Del Castillo D, Thymoglobulin Induction Study Group. Rabbit antithymocyte globulin versus basiliximab in renal transplantation. N Engl J Med. 2006;355(19):1967–77.
12. Noël C, Abramowicz D, Durand D, Mourad G, Lang P, Kessler M, Charpentier B, Touchard G, Berthoux F, Merville P, Ouali N, Squifflet JP, Bayle F, Wissing KM, Hazzan M. Daclizumab versus antithymocyte globulin in high- immunological-risk renal transplant recipients. J Am Soc Nephrol. 2009;20(6):1385–92.
13. Ekberg H, Tedesco-Silva H, Demirbas A, Vitko S, Nashan B, Grkan A, Margreiter R, Hugo C, Griny JM, Frei U, Vanrenterghem Y, Daloze P, Halloran PF, ELITE-Symphony Study. Reduced exposure to calcineurin inhibitors in renal transplantation. N Engl J Med. 2007;357(25):2562–75.
14. Webster AC, Woodroffe RC, Taylor RS, Chapman JR, Craig JC. Tacrolimus versus ciclosporin as primary immunosuppression for kidney transplant recipients: meta-analysis and meta-regression of randomised trial data. BMJ. 2005;331(7520):810.
15. Woodle ES, First MR, Pirsch J, Shihab F, Gaber AO, Van Veldhuisen P, Astellas Corticosteroid Withdrawal Study Group. A prospective, randomized, double-blind, placebo-controlled multicenter trial comparing early (7 day) corticosteroid cessation versus long-term, low-dose corticosteroid therapy. Ann Surg. 2008;248(4):564–77.
16. Schiff J, Cole E, Cantarovich M. Therapeutic monitoring of calcineurin inhibitors for the nephrologist. Clin J Am Soc Nephrol. 2007;2(2):374–84.
17. Knight SR, Morris PJ. The clinical benefits of cyclosporine C2-level monitoring: a systematic review. Transplantation. 2007;83(12):1525–35.
18. Kahan BD, Napoli KL, Kelly PA, Podbielski J, Hussein I, Urbauer DL, Katz SH, Van Buren CT. Therapeutic drug monitoring of sirolimus: correlations with efficacy and toxicity. Clin Transplant. 2000;14(2):97–109.
19. McKay DB, Josephson MA, Armenti VT, August P, Coscia LA, Davis CL, et al. Reproduction and transplantation: report on the AST Consensus Conference on Reproductive Issues and Transplantation. Am J Transplant. 2005;5:1592.
20. Chapter 10. ANZDATA Registry 2009 report. http://www.anzdata.org.au.

Complications of Kidney Transplantation

36

Hatem Amer, Lena Sibulesky and Hani M. Wadei

Case 1

A 65-year-old recipient of a deceased donor kidney transplant presents for a routine evaluation. End-stage renal disease (ESRD) was due to adult autosomal dominant polycystic kidney disease. She received her transplant 4 months previously. Induction was accomplished by anti-thymocyte globulin and has been maintained on tacrolimus, mycophenolate mofetil, and prednisone. Her baseline creatinine had been between 1.1 and 1.4 mg/dL. She reports noticing some ankle swelling, weight gain, and increased home blood pressure readings. On exam she has 1+ pitting ankle edema; lungs are clear; heart regular with no murmur. Routine chemistry reveals a creatinine of 1.8 mg/dL.

Case 2

A 55-year-old Caucasian patient received a deceased donor kidney transplant complicated by delayed graft function. He subsequently had a nadir creatinine of 1.6 mg/dL. Two weeks post-transplant he had swelling of his feet. Right greater than left and an increase in creatinine to 2.1. He was found to have a lymphocele and a peritoneal window was performed. Edema improved and creatinine returned to baseline. He presents to you 6 months after the transplant reporting that he has had malaise, low grade fevers, and night sweats.

Case 3

A 74-year-old female patient was the recipient of a living donor kidney transplant from her son 15 years previously. She has had excellent stable renal allograft function with no rejection episodes. Has had one to two urinary tract infections (UTIs) a year on average and has had recurrent squamous cell cancers of the skin requiring frequent resections. She is maintained on tacrolimus, mycophenolate mofetil, and prednisone.

It is increasingly likely to encounter kidney transplant recipients in various clinical settings. For the non-transplant physician is it important to be able to identify transplant related complications, and if need be refer to appropriate

H. Amer, M.D. (✉)
Division of Nephrology and Hypertension, Department of Medicine and the William J von Liebig Transplant Center, Mayo Clinic, 200 First Street SW, Rochester, MN 55905, USA
e-mail: amer.hatem@mayo.edu

L. Sibulesky, M.D. • H.M. Wadei, M.D.
Department of Transplantation, Mayo Clinic Florida, Jacksonville, FL 32224, USA

E.V. Lerma and M. Rosner (eds.), *Clinical Decisions in Nephrology, Hypertension and Kidney Transplantation*, DOI 10.1007/978-1-4614-4454-1_36, © Springer Science+Business Media New York 2013

specialists. In this chapter we will discuss several common and/or serious complications that can occur in these patients.

Surgical Complications

Renal allografts are usually placed extra- or intraperitoneal through a lower right or left abdominal quadrant incision. The ureter is anastomosed to the bladder and the renal artery and vein to the iliac vessels. Post-transplant fluid collections can occur around the transplanted kidney and, in some cases, result in decreased graft function.

Ultrasonography plays an important role in diagnosing postoperative allograft dysfunction [1]. Perinephric fluid collections seen on an ultrasound include urinoma, lymphocele, hematoma, and abscess.

Urinoma

The reported incidence of urinary leaks (urinoma) is approximately 1–5% [2, 3]. They commonly present with deteriorating allograft function, pain over the kidney site, fever, urine drainage from the wound, and perinephric fluid collection. The urine leak is confirmed by finding a higher creatinine in a sample of the fluid obtained under radiologic guidance than that in serum. Renal scintigraphy is another modality that is useful in confirming the diagnosis by showing the abnormal uptake of the radionuclide around the transplant [4].

Antegrade nephrostography can be both diagnostic and therapeutic [5]. It can diagnose the site of the leak. Percutaneous nephrostomy can divert the urine flow and thus promote the healing at the site of the leak [6]. If nonoperative route of treatment is undertaken, a Foley catheter is placed to decompress the bladder and the perinephric fluid collection is percutaneously drained. Alternatively, the surgical options include reimplantation of the transplant ureter to the bladder, ureteroneocystostomy, and anastomosing it to the native ureter—ureteroureterostomy.

Lymphocele

A lymphocele is a perinephric collection of lymphatic fluid. The incidence of lymphoceles after renal transplantation is up to 20% [7]. They usually occur within the first 3 months after transplantation [8]. The most common site of lymph leak arises from the lymphatics disrupted at the time of the dissection around the iliac vessels in preparation for the implantation of the renal allograft. It can also arise from the disrupted lymphatics in the donor kidney hilum.

Diagnosis of a lymphocele is made via ultrasound (Fig. 36.1) [3]. Aspiration of clear fluid with a creatinine level similar to the serum

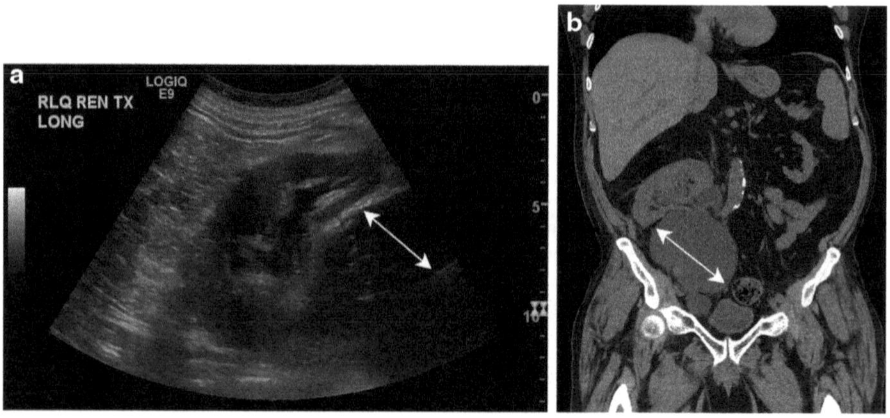

Fig. 36.1 (**a**) Ultrasound and (**b**) CT scan showing a lymphocele

creatinine level is also diagnostic of a lymphocele. Approximately 5% of lymphoceles are symptomatic. The most common presentations are pain over the graft due to increasing size of the collection, deterioration of the renal function as a result of ureteral compression, swollen extremity, and deep vein thrombosis due to compression of the recipient ipsilateral iliac vein [9].

While small asymptomatic collections can be managed conservatively, symptomatic ones require intervention. There are several modalities of treatment. Percutaneous aspiration alone carries a recurrence rate close to a 100% [10]. Percutaneous placement of a drainage catheter and installation of sclerosing agents, including povidone-iodine solution, alcohol, and fibrin sealant, are 70–100% successful [11–13]. Surgical intervention involves creating a peritoneal window to allow the fluid to drain into the peritoneum and thus be absorbed. Laparoscopic fenestration is safe and effective with recurrence rate of approximately 4% and is considered the first line of operative treatment [8, 14].

Incisional Hernia

Incisional hernia is defined as separation of muscle and fascia at the renal transplant wound site. It is reported in up to 4% of patients undergoing kidney transplantation [15]. Risk factors are older age, nutritional impairment, prolonged uremia, diabetes mellitus, obesity, infection of the wound, reoperation, lymphocele, urinoma, use of corticosteroids, and immunosuppressive therapy, including sirolimus and mycophenolate mofetil [16, 17]. They may present with a bulge at the wound, pain, or increased wound drainage. CT scans are useful in their identification (Fig. 36.2). Typically, sirolimus therapy is stopped and other agents, such as tacrolimus or cyclosporine, are used prior to herniorrhaphy to allow proper healing and mesh incorporation. The majority of hernias develop between 3 months and a year [18]. With any hernia a surgical consultation is recommended.

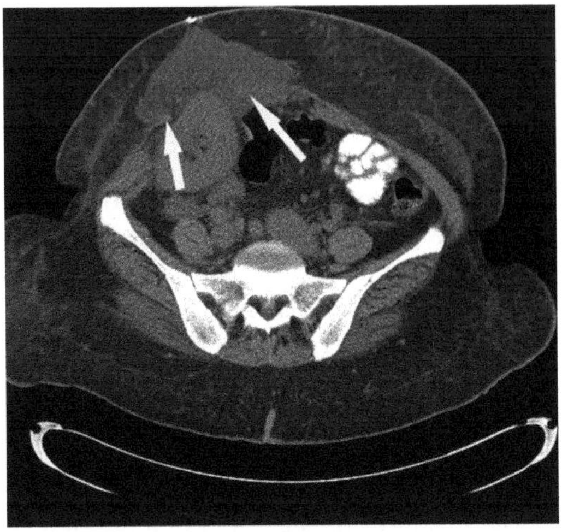

Fig. 36.2 CT scan of an incisional hernia. *Arrows* point to the ends of the fascia

Allograft Rejection

Being allografts (transplants between non-genetically identical members of the same species) kidney allografts are susceptible to rejection. This can be categorized into acute and chronic as well as cellular and humoral (antibody mediated). Acute rejection is an acute process in which there is inflammation and/or injury of the kidney. It can be cellular rejection where there is a cellular, mainly lymphocytic infiltrate of the kidney, or humoral (antibody) mediated. In this situation, which usually occurs if there are pre-formed antibodies directed against human leukocyte antigens (HLAs) present on the allograft, there is endothelial damage and renal allograft damage that can range from a picture of acute tubular injury to endovascular thrombosis and necrosis.

The Banff classification is commonly used to grade the histological findings [19, 20]. Acute rejections may be clinical with noticeable allograft dysfunction manifesting as an elevation of creatinine and may also present with increasing blood pressure, hyperkalemia, and volume expansion. It may also be subclinical discovered only on protocol biopsies [21]. Risk factors for an acute rejection include prior sensitization as can occur with previous transplants, blood transfusions or pregnancy, non-adherence to immunosuppressive medications, African American heritage, increased HLA mismatches between the donor and recipient, and younger recipient age [22, 23].

Chronic rejection is a term referring to a gradual decline in renal allograft function that may occur over many years due to a multitude of factors. Some of these are immune mediated and others are not [24]. Transplant glomerulopathy is a form of chronic antibody medicated damage to the renal allograft microvasculature that results in decreased renal function and is commonly associated with proteinuria [25].

The treatment of acute rejection depends on the type, degree, clinical presentation, and the particular circumstances of the patient.

Case 1 Revisited

The patient has allograft dysfunction evidenced by the increase in creatinine. The lower extremity edema may also be a result of kidney dysfunction resulting in fluid retention. Next steps in evaluating this patient would be an ultrasound of the kidney to exclude obstruction or transplant renal artery stenosis and renal allograft biopsy. Blood work should also include quantitative BK virus PCR and tacrolimus trough level.

Post-transplant Proteinuria

The prevalence of post-transplant proteinuria varies depending on the definition used. In one study of 613 patients with the strictest definition of >150 mg/day of protein, it was found in 45% of kidney transplant recipients at 1-year post-transplant [26]. High levels of proteinuria (>1,500 mg/day) related to renal allograft glomerular pathology such as recurrent membranous nephropathy or transplant glomerulopathy. Lower proteinuria levels did not correlate with a particular histology. Increasing levels of proteinuria correlate with increased risk of graft loss. This occurs even at very low levels of proteinuria. Compared to grafts with <150 mg/day of protein, those with 150–500 mg/day had a 4.1-fold increased risk of graft loss (Fig. 36.3) [27]. The

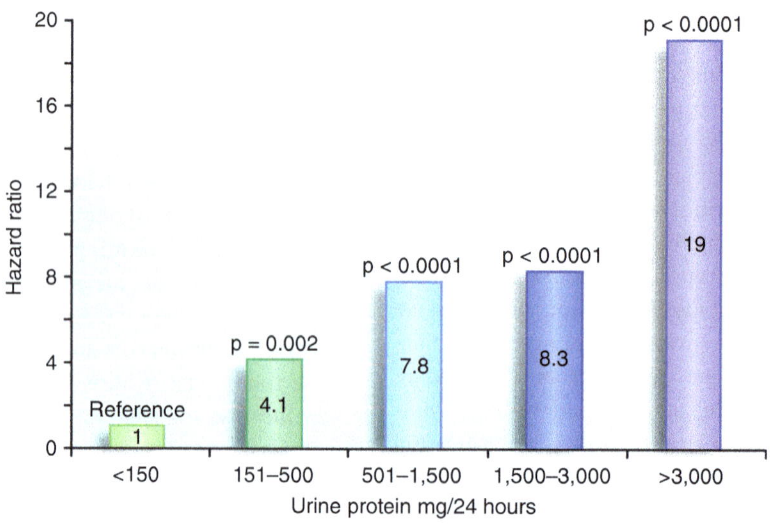

Fig. 36.3 Relationship between increasing levels of proteinuria at 1 year post-transplant and subsequent graft survival. In absolute terms, 3.9, 9.9, 20, 33.3, and 41.2% of kidney allografts were lost during a period of 46 ± 20 months of follow-up in patients who at 1 year had proteinuria <150 (n=337), 151–500 (n=182), 501–1,500 (n=50), 1,500–3,000 (n=27), and >3,000 (n=17) mg/day, respectively (From Amer H, Cosio FG, J Am Soc Nephrol. 2009;20:2490–2, with permission.)

relationship between graft survival and proteinuria remained statistically significant in a multivariable model containing graft histology. In cases of graft interstitial fibrosis and tubular atrophy the level of proteinuria was able to further risk stratify grafts. Increasing levels of albuminuria, in addition to be being related to graft loss, have also been correlated with increased risk of patient death [28].

Protein and albumin found in the urine post-transplant can be a consequence of injury to the graft at various levels encompassing both glomerular and tubular damage. Immunosuppressive medications can have a modulating effect on proteinuria post-transplant. Calcineurin inhibitors (tacrolimus and cyclosporine) can reduce the degree of proteinuria while mTOR inhibitors (sirolimus and everolimus) are associated with increased levels and have been implicated in some cases of focal segmental glomerulosclerosis (FSGS) [29, 30]. It is not recommended to use mTOR inhibitors in proteinuric patients when daily protein excretion is more than 500 mg/day [27].

The role of inhibiting the rennin angiotensin system in proteinuric renal transplant recipients remains to be elucidated [31]. Concerns revolve around decreased renal allograft function, risk of developing significant hyperkalemia or anemia. When used, these parameters should be followed carefully.

Viral Infections

Transplant patients are at increased risk for viral infections. These can be acquired from the community, transferred from the donor, or result from activation of latent viral infections in the setting of immunosuppression. These infections include: cytomegalovirus (CMV), Epstein–Barr virus (EBV), BK, HIV, Hepatitis B and C, herpes including herpes 8.

BK

BK virus is one of the polyoma viruses. It is named after the initials of the first patient in which it was identified [32]. BK virus is ubiquitous and series have shown that up to 83% of the population has been exposed [33]. Once infection occurs it remains latent and activates in the setting of suppressed T-cell immunity. In kidney transplant recipients it can cause interstitial nephritis with allograft dysfunction and subsequent loss (Fig. 36.4). It is usually preceded by asymptomatic viruria and viremia [34, 35]. With the use of potent immunosuppression regimens, the incidence of BK nephropathy has increased with rates reported around 2–10% [26, 36]. Most cases are identified in the first year post-transplant but delayed BK virus reactivation is known to occur.

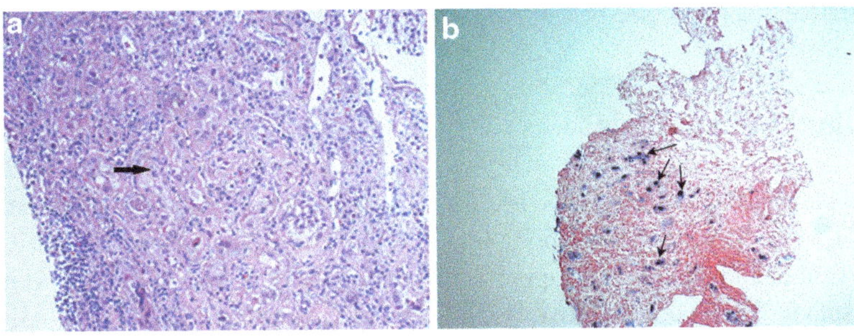

Fig. 36.4 BK virus associated nephropathy. (**a**) H&E 40× showing interstitial inflammation and nuclear cytopathic changes (*arrows*). (**b**) In situ hybridization for BK virus showing nuclear staining

Active surveillance by PCR testing of the urine or blood is recommended. The main stay of therapy is reduction of immunosuppression. No specific antivirals are approved for BK nephropathy but various groups have used agents such as cidofovir, leflunomide, and ciprofloxacin in conjunction with reduced immunosuppression [37–39].

Cytomegalovirus

CMV infection is usually acquired in childhood and remains latent in lymphoid cells. Post-transplant it may activate and manifest with a broad spectrum of clinical manifestations ranging from mild nonspecific constitutional symptoms to invasive tissue disease including hepatitis, pneumonitis, and colitis. Disease is more common as a primary infection following a mismatched transplant (donor positive/recipient negative). Ganciclovir and valganciclovir are available for treatment. Many centers routinely employ antiviral prophylaxis for 3–6 months post-transplant [40].

Epstein–Barr Virus

Similar to CMV, EBV infection is usually acquired early in life. It is the cause of infectious mononucleosis. Post-transplant it may re-activate or if there is a donor–recipient mismatch (donor positive/recipient negative) primary infection may occur.. Primary EBV infection or activation post-transplant is a risk factor for post-transplant lymphoproliferative disorders (see below).

Post-transplant Malignancies

Transplant recipients are at increased risk for malignancy [41, 42]. This is due to both pre-transplant risk factors and the immunosuppressed state post-transplant. The overall relative risk of malignancy in transplant recipients is 4.3-fold higher than the general population in one study. Not all cancers have the same increased risk. Some like breast, colorectal, and prostate have only minimally increased risk in this population while others such as skin cancer have reported 50–200-fold increased risk in transplant patients and warrant more than the standard recommendation for screening of the general population. The risk of skin cancer is increased with duration of immunosuppression and sun exposure. Recent studies from Spain and Australia have shown a decreased risk with the use of mTOR inhibitors [43, 44].

Returning to *case 3*, if there is no significant proteinuria or other contraindications she may benefit from substituting sirolimus for tacrolimus.

Post-transplant lymphoproliferative disorders are a heterogenous group of abnormal proliferation of lymphoid tissue. EBV is implicated in 60–70% of cases. Commonly they are associated with constitutional symptoms. Extranodal involvement occurs in 70–85% of cases, CNS involvement occurs in 10–15%. Treatment involves a reduction in immunosuppression in conjunction with rituximab and chemotherapy [45].

In regard to *Case 3* the work-up for these patients' symptoms should include checking blood PCR for CMV and EBV as well as CT scan of the thorax and abdomen to evaluate for lymphadenopathy.

Urinary Tract Infection

UTI is the most common bacterial infection following renal transplantation and is a major cause of morbidity and recurrent hospitalizations. In the immediate post-transplant period, 40–50% of the kidney transplant recipients will develop UTI [46, 47]. The incidence of UTI increases up to 70% in the first 6 months post-transplantation [48]. Recurrent UTI (three or more episodes in a 12-month period) and late UTI beyond the first post-transplant year are also common [49, 50]. UTI is also the principal cause of septicemia which occurs in 3–7% of kidney transplant recipients following UTI [51]. Allograft pyelonephritis is another serious complication from UTI and is detected in 9–16% of cases (Fig. 36.5) [48, 51, 52]. Gram-negative organisms and Enterococcus species are the most common

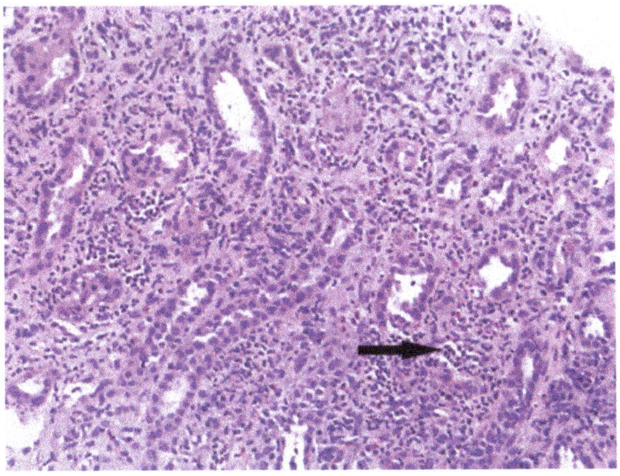

Fig. 36.5 Light microscopic picture showing evidence of interstitial inflammation and tubular injury and many interstitial neutrophils. Neutrophils are infiltrating the tubular epithelium with WBC cast consistent with allograft pyelonephritis (*arrow*)

pathogens with Enterococcal infection now becoming the predominant uropathogen under the current immunosuppression regimens [46, 51]. Precipitating factors for UTI varies between studies but UTI is more likely to occur in females, in older patients, following deceased donor kidney transplantation, following excessive immunosuppression medication, in those with complex urological anatomy, following urological instrumentations especially when prolonged, and in patients with partial or complete urinary retention due to either neurogenic bladder, bladder outlet obstruction from an enlarged prostate, or the presence of a cystocele [46, 51, 53]. Diagnosis of UTIs in the kidney transplant patient is similar to the general population and is based on detection of pyuria on urine analysis and bacteruria detected on urine culture [53]. The presence of dysuria, frequency, or fever is not essential for the diagnosis of post-transplant UTI as many cases are asymptomatic as a consequence of immunosuppression. Similarly, the presence of allograft tenderness is not essential for the diagnosis of allograft pyelonephritis as the transplanted kidney is denervated and in many cases pyelonephritis is detected on allograft biopsy. In most cases, the bacteria are sensitive to oral antibiotics but multidrug resistant organisms have been described [47]. In these cases, hospital admission and intravenous antibiotic treatment are needed. Uncomplicated UTI can be treated for 7–10 days while the presence of pyelonephritis requires more prolonged therapy for at least 14 days. Eradication of the organism should be confirmed with a follow-up urine analysis and culture. In patients with recurrent UTIs, urological evaluation with cystoscopy and urodynamic studies can identify a cause for the disease recurrence. In some cases, especially in those with residual native kidney function, the native kidneys are the source of the recurrent infections. In these cases, cystoscopy with selective urine sampling from the native ureters can identify the site of infection and native kidney nephrectomy might be needed to prevent further recurrence. Other strategies to prevent recurrence include chronic antibiotic therapy with either a single agent or with alternating antibiotics to avoid the emergence of bacterial resistance.

The role of prophylactic therapy to prevent UTI in the immediate post-transplant period is unclear and carries the risk of emergence of resistant bacterial strains but recent studies have shown that prophylactic antibiotic use reduces the risk of septicemia and symptomatic and asymptomatic UTI without affecting overall patient or allograft survival [54, 55]. Fortunately most transplant centers implement an antibiotic prophylaxis protocol for 3–6 months after transplantation against *Pneumocystis jiroveci* using trimethoprim–sulfamethoxazole which has been shown to reduce the risk of UTI including patients with double-J ureteric stents [56, 57].

Studies have reached conflicting results as to whether UTIs increase the risk of graft loss. In a retrospective cohort of almost 29,000 transplanted patients, Abbott et al. showed a significant association between UTI and graft loss and worse patient survival [49]. Other studies have also demonstrated increased mortality in kidney transplant patients with UTIs [50]. However, these studies do not establish whether UTIs are the primary cause of death or are a mere consequence of over immunosuppression. Allograft pyelonephritis has also been associated with deterioration in allograft function with no detectable effect on allograft or patient survivals [48, 52, 58].

Recurrent Glomerular Disease

Glomerulonephritis (GN) is the cause of ESRD in 30% of kidney transplant recipients [59] and glomerular disease does recur after kidney transplantation in a significant number of these cases. Although the prevalence of GN recurrence is estimated to be between 2 and 20%, the true prevalence of disease recurrence is unknown due to the different biopsy practice among transplant centers and the inability to differentiate between recurrent and de novo GN in the absence of native kidney biopsy [60–64]. The prevalence of disease recurrence also varies according to the type of GN and the duration of follow-up period after transplantation. For example, the recurrence risk of FSGS is around 30% in primary allografts and 80% of recurrent disease manifest in the first post-transplant year. On the other hand, the risk of recurrent IgA nephropathy progressively increases over time with almost 10% of the cases manifesting more than 10 years after transplantation [65]. Figure 36.6 depicts the expected time from transplant to allograft loss from recurrent disease in 1,505 primary renal allograft recipients with biopsy-proved glomerular disease [62].

GN with the highest risk of recurrence include: FSGS, atypical hemolytic uremic syndrome (HUS), and membranoproliferative glomerulonephritis (MPGN) (Table 36.1). Previous allograft loss from recurrent disease is a major risk factor for disease recurrence and subsequent allograft loss [64]. This is particularly notable in the case of FSGS and atypical HUS where the risk of

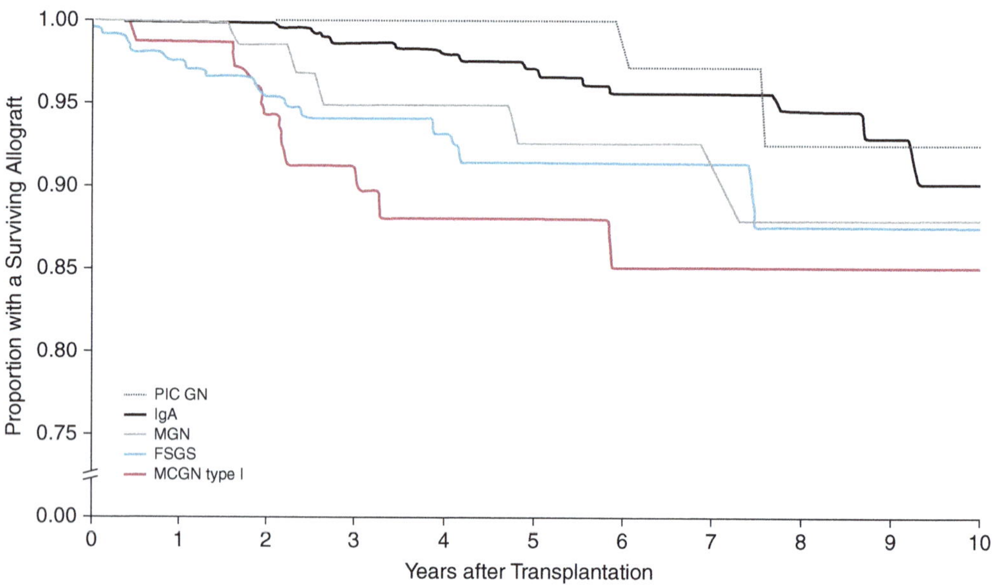

No, AT Risk											
PIC GN	102	90	74	62	56	48	36	26	16	5	2
IgA	532	462	398	312	253	217	153	119	87	47	15
MGN	81	70	60	49	44	40	31	20	15	9	5
FSGS	221	189	156	124	103	91	65	54	36	19	5
MCGN type I	88	75	64	57	48	40	28	25	16	12	4

Fig. 36.6 Time from transplant to allograft loss varies by the type of recurrent glomerular disease. The majority of losses from recurrent FSGS and MPGN occur early while allograft loss from recurrent IgAN is a late event. PIC GN denotes pauci-immune crescentic glomerulonephritis. *IgA* IgA nephropathy, *MGN* membranous glomerulonephropathy, *FSGS* focal segmental glomerulosclerosis, *MCGN* mesangiocapillary glomerulonephritis (From Briganti E et al. N Engl J Med 2002;347:103, with permission. Copyright © 2002 Massachusetts Medical Society. All rights reserved)

Table 36.1 Risk of recurrence and allograft loss from recurrent disease in different glomerulonephritides

Type of GN	Risk of recurrence (%)	Risk of allograft loss within 5–10 years from transplant (%)
FSGS	30	20
IgA nephropathy	15–50	10
Henoch-Schonlein purpura (HSP)	25–50	10
Atypical HUS	65	65
Membranous nephropathy	40	15
MPGN type I	30–50	15
MPGN type 2	80	30
ANCA related glomerulonephritis	10–15	5
Lupus nephritis	7	3
Anti-GBM	Rare	Rare

recurrence and allograft loss in the second transplant approaches 80–100% [66]. Another important risk factor for GN recurrence is the short duration from GN diagnosis to ESRD [67, 68]. Male gender, living donor transplantation, better HLA matching, high panel reactive antibody (PRA) have been reported as risk factors for GN recurrence [62, 63]. Choice of immunosuppressive regimen does not appear to impact the risk of renal allograft failure due to recurrent glomerulonephritis. Mulay et al. recently examined the United States Renal Data System (USRDS) database to look at the association between immunosuppressive medication and recurrent glomerulonephritis in over 40,000 patients between 1990 and 2003. After adjustment for many important covariates, there was no difference in graft loss in patients treated with cyclosporine, tacrolimus, azathioprine, mycophenolate mofetil, prednisone, or sirolimus [69]. Similarly, the 4-year actuarial risk of recurrence, graft, and patient survivals are comparable between those who did and those who did not receive maintenance steroids [70].

Recurrent disease carries the same pathological and clinical presentations as the primary lesion. Clinically manifesting recurrent disease is hallmarked by proteinuria, hematuria, and deteriorating allograft function. Recurrent glomerular disease is the third cause of renal allograft loss after death with functioning graft and chronic rejection (Fig. 36.7) but disease recurrence is not equivalent to allograft loss [60]. In fact allograft lossfrom recurrent GN occurs in only 8.4% of patients. with biopsy evidence of disease recurrence GN and varies according to the type of recurrent disease (delete underlined) [62]. However, with the increasing utilization of surveillance biopsies, more allograft losses are being attributed to recurrent disease [24, 71, 72]. Table 36.1 summarizes the expected rate of allograft loss in different types of recurrent GN. The distinction between recurrent GN and other causes of progressive decline in allograft function can be made on histopathological evaluation of the allograft. Other glomerular lesions that might affect the allograft include de novo glomerular diseases and transplant glomerulopathy (TGN). In the case of de novo disease, a native kidney disease other than GN or a glomerular lesion other than the incident one needs to be the cause of renal failure. In many cases, biopsy evidence of the original disease is lacking and this determination is hard to make. TGN is easier to separate from recurrent disease due to the lack of immune complex deposition in the former.

Prevention and treatment of recurrent disease remains to be a challenge. Plasmapheresis has been tried to prevent recurrence of FSGS, MPGN type I, anti-GBM disease, and HUS with variable success rates. Delaying transplantation to ensure complete resolution of the immunological insult may be helpful in anti-GBM in reducing the risk of recurrence but not in other types of GN.

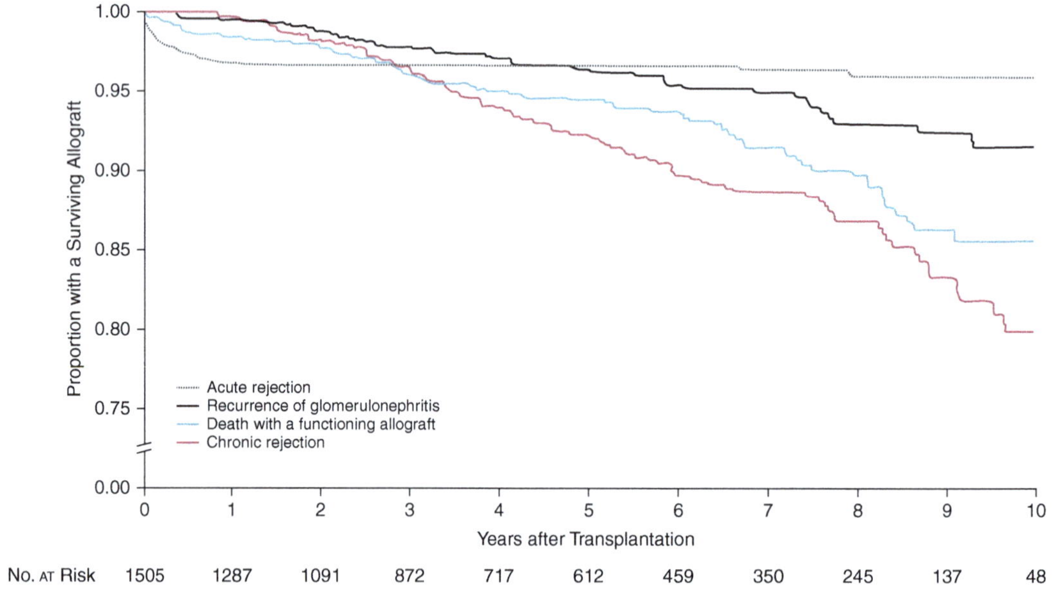

Fig. 36.7 Kaplan–Meier analysis of the different causes of allograft loss in 1,505 patients with biopsy-proved glomerulonephritis who received a primary renal transplant in Australia from 1988 through 1997. Recurrent disease was the third most common cause of allograft loss after 10 years of follow-up (From Briganti E et al. N Engl J Med 2002;347:103, with permission. Copyright © 2002 Massachusetts Medical Society. All rights reserved)

Table 36.2 Potential preventive and treatment options in patients with recurrent glomerulonephritis after transplantation

Type of GN	Potential options
IgA nephropathy	No prevention strategy. Proteinuria control with ACE-I and ARB. Cyclophosphamide in cases with crescentic IgA
FSGS	Proper counseling regarding recurrence risk especially in patients with previous allograft loss from recurrent disease
	Monitor closely for proteinuria and consider early plasmapheresis
	Rituximab in resistant cases
Membranous nephropathy	Monitor allograft function and protein excretion
	Consider rituximab in cases with worsening function and/or worsening proteinuria
MPGN	Plasmapheresis with limited success
ANCA related GN	Avoid transplantation in active disease
	Cyclophosphamide, rituximab in selected cases
Anti-GBM	Avoid transplantation in active disease
	Cyclophosphamide, rituximab in selected cases

The anti-CD20 rituximab has been successful in treating recurrent membranous GN and recurrent FSGS [71, 73–76]. Table 36.2 summarizes some of the prevention and treatment options of recurrent GN according to type of glomerular disease. Figures 36.8, 36.9, 36.10, and 36.11 show some examples of recurrent glomerular disease.

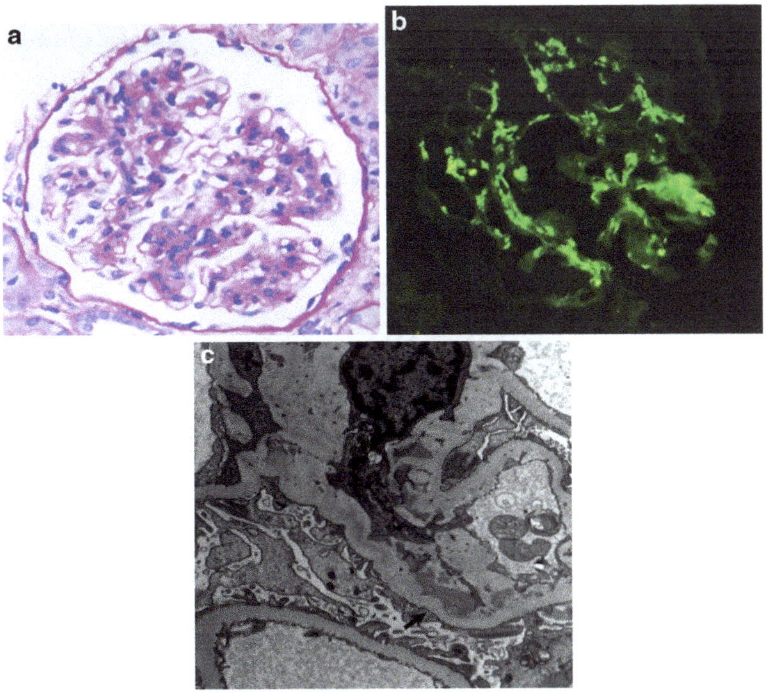

Fig. 36.8 Recurrent IgA nephropathy. (**a**) Light microscopic picture showing moderate mesangia expansion with both increased matrix and mesangial cells. The glomerular basement membrane is unremarkable (PAS, 40×). (**b**) Immunofluorescence picture showing characteristic dominant or co-dominant mesangial staining with IgA (anti-IgA immunofluorescence, 40×). (**c**) Electron microscopic picture showing immune complex deposits present within the mesangium, primarily underlying the paramesangial glomerular basement membrane (*arrow*). There are no glomerular basement membrane deposits (TEM, 5,800×)

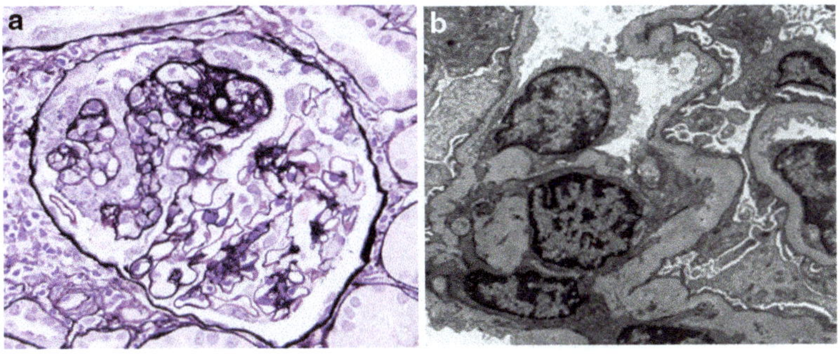

Fig. 36.9 Recurrent FSGS. (**a**) Light microscopic picture showing segmental sclerosis with tuft adhesion to adjacent Bowman's capsule. A few capillary loop foam cells are also seen. The uninvolved portion of the glomerulus shows minimal histologic changes (Jones' silver stain, 400×). (**b**) Electron microscopic picture showing mild mesangial matrix expansion with extensive foot process effacement. No immune complex deposits are present (TEM, 4,700×)

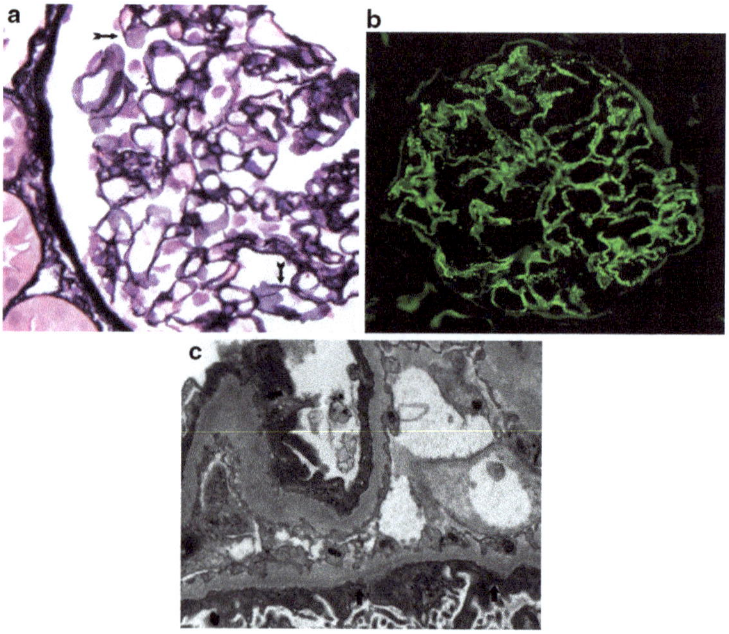

Fig. 36.10 Recurrent membranous nephropathy. (**a**) Light microscopic picture showing the glomerular basement membrane with rare, barely discernable pinholes without spike formation (*arrows*). The mesangium is unremarkable (Jones' silver stain, 400×). (**b**) Immunofluorescence picture showing a finely granular capillary loop staining with IgG without mesangial staining, characteristic of idiopathic membranous nephropathy (anti-IgG immunofluorescence, 400×). (**c**) Electron microscopic picture showing scattered small subepithelial immune complex-type deposits with minimal surrounding basement membrane reaction, as seen in early stage I membranous nephropathy (*arrows*). Overlying foot processes are moderately effaced (TEM, 5,800×)

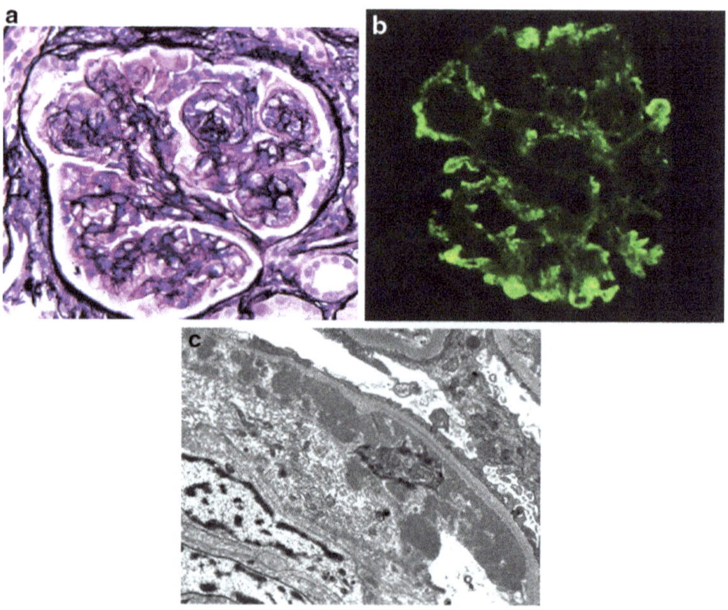

Fig. 36.11 Recurrent MPGN. (**a**) Light microscopic picture showing an enlarged glomerulus with mesangial expansion and endocapillary proliferation, imparting a lobular appearance. Segmental glomerular basement membrane splitting with subendothelial eosinophilic material corresponding to cryoglobulin deposits is present (Jones' silver stain, 400×). (**b**) Immunofluorescence picture showing segmental, irregular, and chunky capillary loop and mesangial staining with IgM. Similar staining with C3 and lesser IgG is also present (anti-IgM immunofluorescence, 400×). (**c**) Electron microscopic picture showing large subendothelial deposits with mesangial interposition and glomerular basement reduplication, imparting a split appearance. The deposits have vague substructure, frequently seen with cryoglobulin deposits (TEM, 7,400×)

References

1. Gottlieb RH, Voci SL, Cholewinski SP, et al. Sonography: a useful tool to detect the mechanical causes of renal transplant dysfunction. J Clin Ultrasound. 1999;27(6):325–33.
2. Englesbe MJ, Dubay DA, Gillespie BW, et al. Risk factors for urinary complications after renal transplantation. Am J Transplant. 2007;7(6):1536–41.
3. Kobayashi K, Censullo ML, Rossman LL, Kyriakides PN, Kahan BD, Cohen AM. Interventional radiologic management of renal transplant dysfunction: indications, limitations, and technical considerations. Radiographics. 2007;27(4):1109–30.
4. Rosenberg RJ, Schweizer RT, Spencer RP. Ureteral leak after renal transplantation. Clin Nucl Med. 1999;24(6):440–2.
5. Smith TP, Hunter DW, Letourneau JG, et al. Urine leaks after renal transplantation: value of percutaneous pyelography and drainage for diagnosis and treatment. AJR Am J Roentgenol. 1988;151(3):511–3.
6. Matalon TA, Thompson MJ, Patel SK, Ramos MV, Jensik SC, Merkel FK. Percutaneous treatment of urine leaks in renal transplantation patients. Radiology. 1990;174(3 Pt 2):1049–51.
7. Doehn C, Fornara P, Fricke L, Jocham D. Laparoscopic fenestration of posttransplant lymphoceles. Surg Endosc. 2002;16(4):690–5.
8. Bailey SH, Mone MC, Holman JM, Nelson EW. Laparoscopic treatment of post renal transplant lymphoceles. Surg Endosc. 2003;17(12):1896–9.
9. Zargar-Shoshtari MA, Soleimani M, Salimi H, Mehravaran K. Symptomatic lymphocele after kidney transplantation: a single-center experience. Urol J Winter. 2008;5(1):34–6.
10. Shaver TR, Swanson III SJ, Fernandez-Bueno C, Kocandrle V. The optimal treatment of lymphoceles following renal transplantation. Transpl Int. 1993;6(2):108–10.
11. Montalvo BM, Yrizarry JM, Casillas VJ, et al. Percutaneous sclerotherapy of lymphoceles related to renal transplantation. J Vasc Interv Radiol. 1996;7(1): 117–23.
12. Tasar M, Gulec B, Saglam M, Yavuz I, Bozlar U, Ugurel S. Posttransplant symptomatic lymphocele treatment with percutaneous drainage and ethanol sclerosis: long-term follow-up. Clin Imaging. 2005;29(2):109–16.
13. Chin A, Ragavendra N, Hilborne L, Gritsch HA. Fibrin sealant sclerotherapy for treatment of lymphoceles following renal transplantation. J Urol. 2003;170(2 Pt 1):380–3.
14. Garay JM, Alberu J, Angulo-Suarez M, Bezauri-Rivas P, Herrera MF. Laparoscopic drainage of lymphocele after kidney transplant. J Laparoendosc Adv Surg Tech A. 2003;13(2):127–9.
15. Yannam GR, Gutti TL, High R, Stevens RB, Thompson JS, Morris MC. Experience of laparoscopic incisional hernia repair in kidney and/or pancreas transplant recipients. Am J Transplant. 2011;11(2):279–86.
16. Laschke MW, Haufel JM, Roller J, Schorr H, Menger MD. Rapamycin, but not cyclosporine A, inhibits vascularization and incorporation of implanted surgical meshes. Transpl Int. 2009;22(6):654–62.
17. Humar A, Ramcharan T, Denny R, Gillingham KJ, Payne WD, Matas AJ. Are wound complications after a kidney transplant more common with modern immunosuppression? Transplantation. 2001;72(12):1920–3.
18. Antonopoulos IM, Nahas WC, Mazzucchi E, Piovesan AC, Birolini C, Lucon AM. Is polypropylene mesh safe and effective for repairing infected incisional hernia in renal transplant recipients? Urology. 2005;66(4):874–7.
19. Solez K, Colvin RB, Racusen LC, et al. Banff 07 classification of renal allograft pathology: updates and future directions. Am J Transplant. 2008;8(4):753–60.
20. Sis B, Mengel M, Haas M, et al. Banff '09 meeting report: antibody mediated graft deterioration and implementation of Banff working groups. Am J Transplant. 2010;10(3):464–71.
21. Rush D. Protocol biopsies for renal transplantation. Saudi J Kidney Dis Transpl. 2010;21(1):1–9.
22. Meier-Kriesche HU, Ojo A, Magee JC, et al. African-American renal transplant recipients experience decreased risk of death due to infection: possible implications for immunosuppressive strategies. Transplantation. 2000;70(2):375–9.
23. Meier-Kriesche HU, Scornik JC, Susskind B, Rehman S, Schold JD. A lifetime versus a graft life approach redefines the importance of HLA matching in kidney transplant patients. Transplantation. 2009;88(1):23–9.
24. El-Zoghby ZM, Stegall MD, Lager DJ, et al. Identifying specific causes of kidney allograft loss. Am J Transplant. 2009;9(3):527–35.
25. Cosio FG, Gloor JM, Sethi S, Stegall MD. Transplant glomerulopathy. Am J Transplant. 2008;8(3):492–6.
26. Amer H, Fidler ME, Myslak M, et al. Proteinuria after kidney transplantation, relationship to allograft histology and survival. Am J Transplant. 2007;7(12): 2748–56.
27. Amer H, Cosio FG. Significance and management of proteinuria in kidney transplant recipients. J Am Soc Nephrol. 2009;20(12):2490–2.
28. Halimi JM, Buchler M, Al-Najjar A, et al. Urinary albumin excretion and the risk of graft loss and death in proteinuric and non-proteinuric renal transplant recipients. Am J Transplant. 2007;7(3):618–25.
29. Letavernier E, Bruneval P, Mandet C, et al. High sirolimus levels may induce focal segmental glomerulosclerosis de novo. Clin J Am Soc Nephrol. 2007;2(2):326–33.
30. Bertoni E, Bruschi M, Candiano G, et al. Posttransplant proteinuria associated with everolimus. Transplant Proc. 2009;41(4):1216–7.
31. Knoll GA. Proteinuria in kidney transplant recipients: prevalence, prognosis, and evidence-based management. Am J Kidney Dis. 2009;54(6):1131–44.

32. Gardner SD, Field AM, Coleman DV, Hulme B. New human papovavirus (B.K.) isolated from urine after renal transplantation. Lancet. 1971;1(7712):1253–7.
33. Gardner SD. Prevalence in England of antibody to human polyomavirus (B.k.). Br Med J. 1973;1(5845): 77–8.
34. Funk GA, Hirsch HH. From plasma BK viral load to allograft damage: rule of thumb for estimating the intrarenal cytopathic wear. Clin Infect Dis. 2009;49(6): 989–90.
35. Hirsch HH, Suthanthiran M. The natural history, risk factors and outcomes of polyomavirus BK-associated nephropathy after renal transplantation. Nat Clin Pract Nephrol. 2006;2(5):240–1.
36. Boothpur R, Brennan DC. Human polyoma viruses and disease with emphasis on clinical BK and JC. J Clin Virol. 2010;47(4):306–12.
37. Bernhoff E, Gutteberg TJ, Sandvik K, Hirsch HH, Rinaldo CH. Cidofovir inhibits polyomavirus BK replication in human renal tubular cells downstream of viral early gene expression. Am J Transplant. 2008;8(7):1413–22.
38. Bernhoff E, Tylden GD, Kjerpeseth LJ, Gutteberg TJ, Hirsch HH, Rinaldo CH. Leflunomide inhibition of BK virus replication in renal tubular epithelial cells. J Virol. 2010;84(4):2150–6.
39. Gabardi S, Waikar SS, Martin S, et al. Evaluation of fluoroquinolones for the prevention of BK viremia after renal transplantation. Clin J Am Soc Nephrol. 2010;5(7):1298–304.
40. Eid AJ, Razonable RR. New developments in the management of cytomegalovirus infection after solid organ transplantation. Drugs. 2010;70(8):965–81.
41. Carroll RP, Ramsay HM, Fryer AA, Hawley CM, Nicol DL, Harden PN. Incidence and prediction of nonmelanoma skin cancer post-renal transplantation: a prospective study in Queensland, Australia. Am J Kidney Dis. 2003;41(3):676–83.
42. Wimmer CD, Rentsch M, Crispin A, et al. The Janus face of immunosuppression – de novo malignancy after renal transplantation: the experience of the transplantation center Munich. Kidney Int. 2007;71(12): 1271–8.
43. Campistol JM, Eris J, Oberbauer R, et al. Sirolimus therapy after early cyclosporine withdrawal reduces the risk for cancer in adult renal transplantation. J Am Soc Nephrol. 2006;17(2):581–9.
44. Salgo R, Gossmann J, Schofer H, et al. Switch to a sirolimus-based immunosuppression in long-term renal transplant recipients: reduced rate of (pre-) malignancies and nonmelanoma skin cancer in a prospective, randomized, assessor-blinded, controlled clinical trial. Am J Transplant. 2010;10(6):1385–93.
45. Evens AM, Roy R, Sterrenberg D, Moll MZ, Chadburn A, Gordon LI. Post-transplantation lymphoproliferative disorders: diagnosis, prognosis, and current approaches to therapy. Curr Oncol Rep. 2010;12(6):383–94.
46. Alangaden GJ, Thyagarajan R, Gruber SA, et al. Infectious complications after kidney transplantation: current epidemiology and associated risk factors. Clin Transplant. 2006;20(4):401–9.
47. Dantas SR, Kuboyama RH, Mazzali M, Moretti ML. Nosocomial infections in renal transplant patients: risk factors and treatment implications associated with urinary tract and surgical site infections. J Hosp Infect. 2006;63(2):117–23.
48. Pellé G, Vimont S, Levy PP, et al. Acute pyelonephritis represents a risk factor impairing long-term kidney graft function. Am J Transplant. 2007;7(4): 899–907.
49. Abbott KC, Swanson SJ, Richter ER, et al. Late urinary tract infection after renal transplantation in the United States. Am J Kidney Dis. 2004;44(2): 353–62.
50. Chuang P, Parikh CR, Langone A. Urinary tract infections after renal transplantation: a retrospective review at two US transplant centers. Clin Transplant. 2005;19(2):230–5.
51. Maraha B, Bonten H, Van Hooff H, Fiolet H, Buiting AG, Stobberingh EE. Infectious complications and antibiotic use in renal transplant recipients during a 1-year follow-up. Clin Microbiol Infect. 2001;7(11): 619–25.
52. Kamath NS, John GT, Neelakantan N, Kirubakaran MG, Jacob CK. Acute graft pyelonephritis following renal transplantation. Transpl Infect Dis. 2006;8(3):140–7.
53. de Souza RM, Olsburgh J. Urinary tract infection in the renal transplant patient. Nat Clin Pract Neph. 2008;4(5):252–64.
54. Green H, Rahamimov R, Gafter U, Leibovitci L, Paul M. Antibiotic prophylaxis for urinary tract infections in renal transplant recipients: a systematic review and meta-analysis. Transpl Infect Dis. 2011;13(5):441–7.
55. Rafat C, Vimont S, Ancel PY, et al. Ofloxacin: new applications for the prevention of urinary tract infections in renal graft recipients. Transpl Infect Dis. 2011;13(4):344–52.
56. Khosroshahi HT, Mogaddam AN, Shoja MM. Efficacy of high-dose trimethoprim-sulfamethoxazol prophylaxis on early urinary tract infection after renal transplantation. Transplant Proc. 2006;38(7): 2062–4.
57. Wilson CH, Bhatti AA, Rix DA, Manas DM. Routine intraoperative ureteric stenting for kidney transplant recipients. Cochrane Database Syst Rev. 2005;(4): CD004925.
58. Giral M, Pascuariello G, Karam G, et al. Acute graft pyelonephritis and long-term kidney allograft outcome. Kidney Int. 2002;61(5):1880–6.
59. Cohen DJ, St. Martin L, Christensen LL, Bloom RD, Sung RS. Kidney and pancreas transplantation in the United States, 1995–2004. Am J Transplant. 2006;6(5 Pt 2):1153–69.
60. Morzycka M, Croker Jr BP, Siegler HF, Tisher CC. Evaluation of recurrent glomerulonephritis in kidney allografts. Am J Med. 1982;72(4):588–98.
61. Kotanko P, Pusey CD, Levy JB. Recurrent glomerulonephritis following renal transplantation. Transplantation. 1997;63(8):1045–52.

62. Briganti EM, Russ GR, McNeil JJ, Atkins RC, Chadban SJ. Risk of renal allograft loss from recurrent glomerulonephritis. N Engl J Med. 2002;347(2):103–9.
63. Hariharan S, Adams MB, Brennan DC, et al. Recurrent and de novo glomerular disease after renal transplantation: a report from Renal Allograft Disease Registry (RADR). Transplantation. 1999;68(5):635–41.
64. Briggs JD, Jones E. Recurrence of glomerulonephritis following renal transplantation. Scientific Advisory Board of the ERA-EDTA Registry. European Renal Association-European Dialysis and Transplant Association. Nephrol Dial Transplant. 1999;14(3):564–5.
65. Ponticelli C, Traversi L, Feliciani A, Cesana BM, Banfi G, Tarantino A. Kidney transplantation in patients with IgA mesangial glomerulonephritis. Kidney Int. 2001;60(5):1948–54.
66. Dall'Amico R, Ghiggeri G, Carraro M, et al. Prediction and treatment of recurrent focal segmental glomerulosclerosis after renal transplantation in children. Am J Kidney Dis. 1999;34(6):1048–55.
67. Ingulli E, Tejani A. Incidence, treatment, and outcome of recurrent focal segmental glomerulosclerosis posttransplantation in 42 allografts in children–a single-center experience. Transplantation. 1991;51(2):401–5.
68. Ducloux D, Rebibou JM, Semhoun-Ducloux S, et al. Recurrence of hemolytic-uremic syndrome in renal transplant recipients: a meta-analysis. Transplantation. 1998;65(10):1405–7.
69. Mulay AV, van Walraven C, Knoll GA. Impact of immunosuppressive medication on the risk of renal allograft failure due to recurrent glomerulonephritis. Am J Transplant. 2009;9(4):804–11.
70. Ibrahim H, Rogers T, Casingal V, et al. Graft loss from recurrent glomerulonephritis is not increased with a rapid steroid discontinuation protocol. Transplantation. 2006;81(2):214–9.
71. El-Zoghby ZM, Grande JP, Fraile MG, Norby SM, Fervenza FC, Cosio FG. Recurrent idiopathic membranous nephropathy: early diagnosis by protocol biopsies and treatment with anti-CD20 monoclonal antibodies. Am J Transplant. 2009;9(12):2800–7.
72. Gourishankar S, Leduc R, Connett J, et al. Pathological and clinical characterization of the 'troubled transplant': data from the DeKAF study. Am J Transplant. 2010;10(2):324–30.
73. Fervenza FC, Abraham RS, Erickson SB, et al. Rituximab therapy in idiopathic membranous nephropathy: a 2-year study. Clin J Am Soc Nephrol. 2010;5(12):2188–98.
74. Hickson LJ, Gera M, Amer H, et al. Kidney transplantation for primary focal segmental glomerulosclerosis: outcomes and response to therapy for recurrence. Transplantation. 2009;87(8):1232–9.
75. Dello Strologo L, Guzzo I, Laurenzi C, et al. Use of rituximab in focal glomerulosclerosis relapses after renal transplantation. Transplantation. 2009;88(3):417–20.
76. Fornoni A, Sageshima J, Wei C, et al. Rituximab targets podocytes in recurrent focal segmental glomerulosclerosis. Sci Transl Med. 2011;3(85):85ra46.

Infectious Disease in Kidney Transplantation

37

Scott L. Sanoff

Introduction

Infection is a common and significant source of morbidity and mortality in the kidney transplant population. In a detailed review of Medicare claims data for 64,751 patients receiving kidney transplant between 1991 and 1998, 51% suffered some type of infection within their first year of transplant, 31% with bacterial and 23% with viral infections [1]. The United States Renal Data System (USRDS) reports that infection was the second most common cause of death with a functioning graft among kidney transplant recipients between 2004 and 2008, exceeded only by cardiovascular disease (21% vs. 30%), but that infection surpassed cardiac disease as a cause of hospitalization following transplant during this time, at approximately 33 admissions per 100 patient years in the first year, compared to approximately 15 per 100 patient years [2].

Most nephrologists provide some primary care for their patients with end-stage kidney disease [3] (ESKD), and most transplant patients see a nephrologist following transplant, a practice that varies between transplant centers [4]. In the immediate perioperative period, nephrologists are often part of a multidisciplinary care team that includes a transplant surgeon, clinical pharmacist, and in some instances, an infectious disease specialist. However, in the weeks and months following the transplant event, nephrologists often play a more prominent, independent role in patients' care, as transplanted patients return to their transplant centers less often, if at all [4].

Given the significance of infection in the renal transplant population, and the prominent role of nephrologists caring for both candidates and recipients, it is critical that practicing nephrologists possess a basic knowledge of risk factors for infection before and after the transplant event, and that they are capable of making timely diagnosis and initiating appropriate management for common infections. In the chapter that follows, real cases are used to illustrate important principles, as well as concrete guidelines regarding the screening, prevention, diagnosis, and management of common infections in the kidney transplant population. The reader is encouraged to proactively consider the differential diagnosis, and appropriate diagnostic and management strategies in each case, prior to reviewing the case discussion.

Case 1

A 46-year-old man with a 25-year history of type-1 diabetes status post kidney and pancreas transplants presents with generalized weakness for 6 weeks, and 3 weeks of increasing diarrhea. The patient had no detectable anti-CMV antibodies

S.L. Sanoff, M.D., M.P.H. (✉)
Division of Nephrology, Department of Medicine, University of Virginia, 5th Floor West Complex, Box 800133, Charlottesville, VA 22908, USA
e-mail: ssanoff@virginia.edu

E.V. Lerma and M. Rosner (eds.), *Clinical Decisions in Nephrology, Hypertension and Kidney Transplantation*, DOI 10.1007/978-1-4614-4454-1_37,

at the time of the first transplant (i.e., was CMV-IgG negative pre-transplant), but received his kidney 2 years prior to presentation from a living donor with evidence of past CMV exposure (i.e., was CMV-Ig G positive), and received thymoglobulin and steroids for induction. He went on to receive a bladder drained pancreas transplant more than a year later, just 10 months prior to presenting in clinic, receiving the same immune suppressant induction regimen a second time.

His clinical course following the kidney transplant was uneventful, but he has had several hospital admissions for dehydration and acute creatinine elevation since his pancreas transplant, each attributed to excessive pancreatic secretions. During a recent admission, he received three large doses of methylprednisolone intravenously as empiric treatment for pancreas rejection following a drop in urinary amylase. Also of note, the patient has an extended history of neurogenic bladder for which he performs self-catheterization three times per day.

In the office, this normally vibrant individual is ill appearing, with a blood pressure of 82/46, a heart rate of 116, and is orthostatic, though afebrile. His creatinine is elevated at 2.5 mg/dL, from a baseline of 1.4 mg/dL. His serum sodium is 127 mmol/L. He has a very mild elevation in his transaminases as well, but normal total-bilirubin. His admission chest X-ray reveals a nodule.

What are this patient's risk factors for infection and what additional historical information would be helpful to determine the current source of infection?

Important Risk Factors for Infection

Preventing and evaluating infection in kidney transplant recipients begins with an understanding of their risk factors for infection. The risks factors are defined by two characteristics of the transplant population—their unique *susceptibility* to infection and unique *exposures* to potential pathogens, each of which varies predictably with time from the initial transplant event. Immediately after surgery, the rate and identity of specific infections are driven by surgery related risk factors and the initial induction immune suppression. Meanwhile, later infections are less likely influenced by the initial surgical event, and more often attributable to accumulated exposure to chronic immune suppression, with a notable decline in the rate of infection moving out from the transplant event [5]. Figure 37.1 illustrates the relationship between these factors from the time of transplant providing a model for patient assessment. The relationship of these factors has been well summarized by experts in the field [6–8].

Unique Susceptibility to Infection

Recognizing transplant recipients' *unique susceptibility* to infection is key to preventing infection and to timely and accurate diagnosis of active infection. This susceptibility is derived from both pre-transplant and post-transplant factors including medical comorbidities, the presence of indwelling vascular and urinary catheters and stents, the unique anatomy of their new transplant organ, and immune-suppressive medications. This susceptibility may be mitigated in part by pre-transplant immunity/vaccination, and the use of prophylactic antibiotics.

Comorbidities

Comorbidities in the transplant recipient are often numerous, and are generally well known by practicing nephrologists who care for these patients prior to transplantation. Among Medicare beneficiaries receiving deceased donor kidney transplants (DDKTx) between 1992 and 2005, approximately 30% had diabetes, 15% had a history of congestive heart failure, 9% had peripheral vascular disease, and 8% had chronic obstructive pulmonary disease (COPD) [9]. These conditions are not unique to the chronic kidney disease, end-stage kidney disease, or the transplant populations, but it is important to recognize their relevance as risk factors for infection following transplant. For example, diabetes and vascular disease are described risk factors for wound infections following transplantation [10].

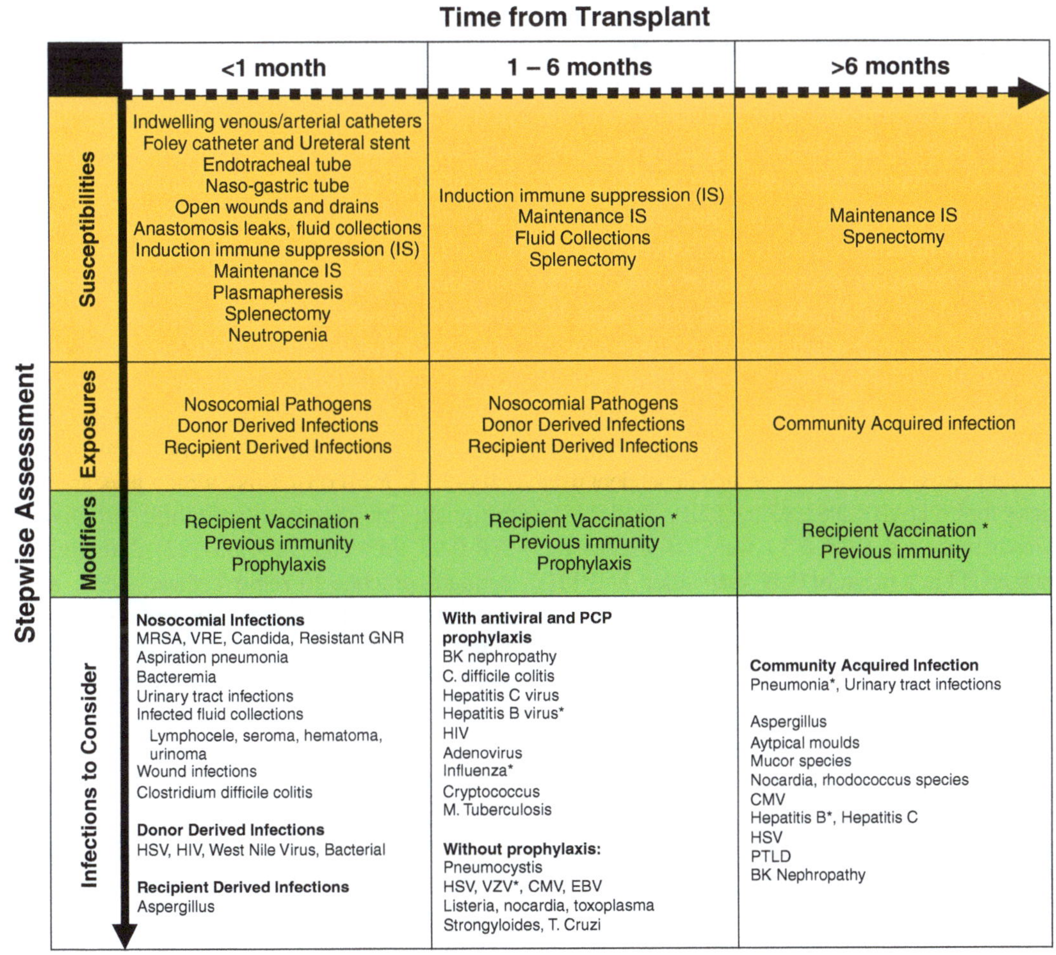

Fig. 37.1 Assessing infection in a kidney transplant recipient. Risk factors and common pathogens affecting the kidney transplant recipient change predictably from the initial transplant event. This figure offers a simplified integrated tool to guide the initial assessment of infection, based upon the work of others [6–8]. In the proposed model, the first step is to consider the timing of the patient's presentation relative to the transplant event, moving across the chart. Moving down the chart, one should then consider the patient's unique susceptibilities and exposures to infection, captured in the *orange boxes*. It is important to then consider mitigating factors for specific infections highlighted in the *green boxes*. These are generally well described in the donor and recipient pre-transplant evaluations. Common pathogens and sites of infection are listed in the final boxes, and should be considered on a case-by-case basis based upon the full history and physical exam. Modified from Fishman [6]

COPD has been associated with postoperative pneumonia following major noncardiac surgery [11]. Further, nearly 10% of kidney transplant recipients have polycystic kidney disease (PCKD) listed as the cause of their renal failure. Renal cysts may become infected following transplant with contamination of the urinary space and require special consideration for selection of antibiotics that penetrate cysts. Meanwhile, hepatic cysts, which are common in PCKD, are also potential sites of infection, though they typically harbor a different array of infectious organisms [12].

Many transplant recipients have preexisting dysfunction of the urinary tract that can predispose to urinary tract infections (UTI) and pyelonephritis. Common abnormalities include reduced bladder compliance and contractility, prostatic obstruction, vesicoureteral reflux, and urethral strictures [13, 14]. In a selected group of transplant recipients who underwent urologic testing prior to transplant, low bladder compliance (<20 mL/cm H_2O) was seen in 30% of those on dialysis less than 12 months, and was more common with increasing time on dialysis, reaching more than 60% after just a couple of years of renal replacement therapy. In cases where patients are oliguric or aneuric, many of these abnormalities may go undiscovered until after the transplant event. A large study using Medicare claims data reported that approximately 10% of kidney transplant recipients were newly diagnosed with BPH within 3 years following the transplant event, and that more than 50% of these diagnosis were made within the first year [15]. In this study BPH was found to be an independent risk factor for UTI (AHR 2.62; 95% CI 2.19–3.13) [15]. Among those with BPH, 6.5% were later diagnosed with a UTI at a mean of 0.39 years after the BPH diagnosis [15].

Indwelling Catheters

Indwelling central venous catheters, urinary catheters, and urinary stents are ubiquitous in the perioperative period, and each is considered a risk factor for infection as they breach natural protective barriers. Approximately 70% of incident dialysis patients in the United States start hemodialysis with central venous catheters, and most keep their catheters for more than 90 days following the start of dialysis [16]. Catheter-related bacteremia has been reported between 0.9 and 2.0 episodes/patient-year [17]. This means that many transplant recipients enter surgery with long standing central lines. And, as more than 20% of deceased donor kidney transplant recipients require some dialysis following the transplant event, many keep their dialysis catheters for some time following induction immune suppression [18]. Additionally, central venous access is also commonly used perioperatively for administration of induction therapy with anti-thymocyte globulin, though this has been given safely through peripheral access [19].

Foley catheters, which are often used to avoid urinary retention that could compromise the transplant ureter anastomosis, are also common following transplant. The increased risk of UTI from indwelling foley catheters is well described in the non-transplant population [20], and its augmented risk in the transplant population may be inferred from the observation that earlier removal is associated with a lower early rate of UTI [21]. More proximally in the urinary tract, temporary internal ureteral stents bridging the ureteral anastomosis have become standard practice at many centers. They have been shown to reduce the incidence of major urology complications (e.g., urinary leak), but are also associated with higher rates of UTI (RR 1.49 95% CI 1.04–2.15, $P=0.03$), a risk which appears to be mitigated by standard antibiotic prophylaxis (RR 0.97, 95% CI 0.71–1.33) [22]. Although it is standard practice to remove these stents in the weeks following transplant, recurrent sepsis syndrome has been associated with retained stents discovered years after their placement [23].

Anatomic Considerations

The risk of infection may be further compounded by the anatomy of the kidney transplant whose architecture is fundamentally altered during surgery, "short circuiting" natural defenses against infection. The transplant ureter lacks a natural valve to protect against vesicourteral reflux (VUR), and there is evidence that occult VUR is common despite neocystostomy techniques performed specifically to prevent this condition [24]. Whether or not transplant VUR increases the risk of UTI is unclear, but there is evidence among those with UTI that VUR increases the risk of both pyelonephritis and occult graft injury [24, 25]. In a recent study from Japan, nearly 30% of patients with neurogenic bladders prior to transplant had detectable reflux a year out from transplant, a finding that was associated with lower graft function [26]. A smaller pediatric study that did not select for a history of bladder dysfunction, found that 70% of tested children had reflux [24].

Other anatomic considerations in the evaluation of infection in a transplant recipient include peri-graft fluid collections, which represent potential sites of infection, and have been reported in between 36% and 49% of kidney transplant surgeries [27, 28]. The most common peri-nephric fluid collection is the lymphocele, arising from interruption of local lymphatic drainage. Less common are urinomas, which indicate interruption of the urinary tract, for example, from necrosis of the distal ureter. Hematomas and seromas are also common. Ultrasound and computerized tomographic studies (CT) are helpful identifying the source of fluid collection. However, aspiration for biochemical analysis (e.g., assay for creatinine concentration, complete blood count, gram stain, and culture) is often needed, though not always indicated, to make the diagnosis. Aspiration must be considered in the setting of unexplained fever, abdominal tenderness, and/or air in the collection.

For those who undergo simultaneous pancreas and kidney transplants (SPK) or pancreas after kidney transplants, it is important to consider the pancreas as a potential source of infection as well. The pancreas has both endocrine and exocrine function, and because of this requires not only a blood supply, but also drainage of secreted digestive enzymes. For the later, the pancreas may be anastomosed to the intestine or bladder, a decision that varies between patients, and often depends on the experience of the transplant center and surgeon. There is a significantly higher rate of UTI among those with bladder drained pancreases, with reports of more than 50% affected in the first year [29]. Intra-abdominal infections must be considered as well.

Immune Suppressants

The landscape of immune suppressants used in kidney transplantation has changed dramatically over several decades, with notable improvement in early graft survival at the expense of increased susceptibility to opportunistic infection [6]. For the "uncomplicated" transplant recipient, the intensity of the immune suppression regimen is typically maximal in the months immediately after the transplant, following one-time *induction* therapies and high dose *maintenance* immune suppression, and weans as the immune system reconstitutes itself and maintenance immune suppression is tapered. Important exceptions include those with allograft rejection or those receiving a second transplant (e.g., pancreas after kidney transplant or a second kidney transplant). These patients often receive additional boluses of steroids or lymphocyte depleting therapies (see next paragraph), or require intensification of their maintenance immune suppression. It is important to note however, that the infectious risk imposed by one's "cumulative exposure" to immune suppression is likely as significant as the intensity of the initial induction or maintenance regimens in defining ones risk for infection, and that this exposure can only be crudely estimated by routine surveillance of serum drugs concentrations and complete blood cell counts. At present, there is no well-validated assay that accurately assesses the overall inhibition or function of one's immune system (i.e., that weighs risk of rejection vs. risk of infection), though this is badly needed.

Induction therapy describes the use of bolus immune suppression at the time of the initial transplant event in order to prevent hyperacute or acute rejection. It historically has included intravenous steroids, and more recently has included a lymphocyte depleting antibody preparation such as anti-thymocyte globulin (Thymoglobulin), a polyclonal antibody preparation derived from rabbits directed against human thymocytes, or anti-CD52 (Alemtuzumab), a monoclonoal panlymphocytic antibody. An alternative to these lymphocyte depleting antibodies is the IL-2 receptor blocking antibody basiliximab [30]. In 1998 fewer than 40% of first-time kidney transplant recipients received any induction therapy, while in 2008 more than 80% did so. Nearly 29% of transplant patients received IL-2 RA, and 52.3% were on a T-cell depleting antibody [2]. Use of lymphocyte depleting induction therapies has been linked to a higher relative risk of post-transplant lymphoproliferative disorder (PTLD) ($RR = 1.78$, $p < 0.001$), a hematologic malignancy strongly associated with the Epstein-Barr virus (EBV) [31]. Further, a well-done meta-analysis in the Cochrane Library by Webster et al. describes a higher risk of CMV infection with anti-thymocyte globulin as compared to IL2-receptor antagonists, with no additional graft survival [32].

Maintenance immune-suppressive regimens have changed considerably the past 15 years, and must be reviewed in assessing a patient's risk for infection. Tacrolimus has largely replaced cyclosporine as the calcineurin inhibitor used post-operatively [2]. Mycophenolate mofetil has almost completely replaced azathioprine [2]. And, prednisone use is on the decline with less than 50% of first time kidney-only transplant recipients using it 1 year after transplant [2]. M-TOR inhibitor use following transplant (e.g., sirolimus and everolimus), which rose from approximately 1995 until around 2002, has been on the decline since.

Though it is appears that the net immune suppression of a particular regimen is at least as important as the specific agents used, some agents are associated with specific infections, and the side effects of each must be considered in the setting of suspected infection. For example, high dose corticosteroids have been associated with risk for developing pneumocystis carinii [33]. Sirolimus is associated with poor wound healing (7–20%) and lymphoceles (22–47%) [34] which may predispose to wound infections. Plasmapheresis, a therapy used to remove immunoglobulin directed against the allograft in order to facilitate incompatible transplants and for treatment of humoral rejection, may theoretically increase the risk of infection with encapsulated organisms.

It is also important to consider the side effects of common immune suppressants as well, as they may mimic infection in some cases. Mycophenolate mofetil for example, is associated with a high incidence of noninfectious diarrhea (12–30%) [35, 36], and sirolimus is associated with a noninfectious lymphocytic alveolitis (4–11%) that can look very much like pneumonia in the post-transplant course [37].

Preexisting Infection, Immunity, and Antimicrobial Prophylaxis

Knowledge of preexisting infections, immunity, and antimicrobial prophylaxis are helpful when assessing active infection in a kidney transplant recipient. In some cases previous infection poses a risk for reactivation following transplant, as in the case of infection with cytomegalovirus (CMV), varicella zoster virus, herpes simplex viruses, and EBV. Meanwhile established immunity through either past infection or vaccination is generally protective, mitigating susceptibility to future infection. Recent antimicrobial use directly influences the epidemiology of infectious pathogens, including antimicrobial resistance/sensitivity patterns. Each should be considered when devising an effective prevention strategy or assessing active infection.

Pre-existing infection and immunity can be found in the pre-transplant evaluation which includes a careful history, physical exam, extensive serologic testing and simple imaging, (Table 37.1) [38, 39]. Knowledge of this evaluation can help advise the risk of infection in the post-transplant period. For example, patients with evidence of circulating Hepatitis-C virus prior to transplant, but without advanced liver disease, appear to benefit from a transplant compared to remaining on dialysis [40–42], but are seemingly more likely to progress to cirrhosis in the setting of immune suppression [43] and therefore require special monitoring. Meanwhile, it has been suggested that the risks of kidney transplantation alone may be prohibitive in those with more advanced hepatitis-C liver disease [43]. Patients without evidence of previous exposure to the cytomegalovirus (CMV), a double-stranded DNA virus that takes up lifelong residence in an infected host, appear to be at high risk for primary CMV infection following transplant from a donor with past CMV exposure, due to the absence of established humoral or cellular immunity [44]. The absence of detectable immunity to the EBV in the recipient is a significant risk factor for post-transplant lymphoproliferative disorder (PTLD) in those with an EBV infected donor [45].

Vaccination is an important strategy to boost immunity and reduce the risk of infection following the transplant event. Several principles govern vaccination before and after the kidney transplantation, and are cited in the vaccination guidelines published by the American Society of Transplantation (AST) [46]. First, the initial immunologic response to vaccination appears to

Table 37.1 Common infection screening tests for kidney transplant donors and recipients

History and Physical Examination
Search for evidence of significant acute or chronic infections, and high-risk behaviors
Serologic Testing
Human immunodeficiency virus (HIV) antibody
Human T-cell lymphotropic virus (HTLV)-I/II antibody
Herpes Simplex Virus (HSV) IgG
Cytomegalovirus (CMV) IgG
Hepatitis C (Hep-C) antibody
Hepatitis B (Hep-B) surface antigen, core antibody (IgM and IgG, or total core), surface antibody (IgG)
Rapid plasma reading (RPR)
Toxoplasma antibody
Epstein-Barr Virus (EBV) viral capsid antigen (VCA) IgM and IgG
Varicella-zoster virus (VZV) antibody
Other Screening Tests
PPD or interferon gamma release assay for latent tuberculosis
Chest X-ray
Blood cultures, for potentially infected donors
Optional Screening Tests
West Nile Virus serology or nucleic acid testing (NAT)
Human herpesvirus-8 serology
Strongyloides, coccidioides serologic testing for recipients from endemic areas
Trypanosoma cruzi serologic testing for recipients and donors from endemic areas
Tetanus, diphtheria, measles, mumps, and pneumococcal titers optional to assess pre-transplant immunization
HIV, Hep-B, Hep-C NAT for recipients and donors at high risk with potential recent exposure[a]

This table summarizes the common pre-transplant infectious disease screening tests recommended by the American Society of Transplantation with slight modification [38, 39]. Additional testing should be considered in cases where additional pathogens are suspected

[a]High risk donors and recipients with potential recent exposure to HIV, Hep-B, or Hep-C should have nucleic acid testing performed to rule out acute infection prior to seroconversion

wane with advancing renal failure, and acutely following the transplant event [47–49]. Required vaccinations are therefore most effective if administered early in the course of progressive kidney disease and ideally given prior to transplant. Second, the response to vaccinations administered post-transplant appears to improve farther out from the event. AST vaccination guidelines indicate that most centers wait 3–6 months after transplant to administer additional vaccines, once the maintenance immune suppression regimen has been established, and recommends checking for serologic evidence of immunity as available and where well defined, a minimum of 4-weeks after vaccination [46]. Third, because of the theoretical risk that an attenuated virus may proliferate in an immune-suppressed individual, live attenuated vaccines (LAV) are contraindicated following transplant. It is recommended that live vaccines be avoided less than 4-weeks prior to transplant.

Table 37.2 provides a concise summary of AST's recommendation for vaccination in the adult kidney transplant recipient [46]. Although a detailed review of each vaccine is beyond the scope of this chapter, it is worth highlighting two recommendations commonly applied in the post-transplant setting. First, there is universal agreement among experts in the field that transplant recipients and close contacts receive annual vaccination against influenza virus [46, 50, 51]. As above, the live attenuated form of the influenza vaccine is contraindicated for transplant recipients, but may be used to immunize close contacts. Influenza vaccination has proven to be both efficacious and safe among transplant recipients with no associated increase in rejection rates nor rise in donor specific antibody levels [52, 53]. Second, with regards to the pneumococcal polysaccharide vaccine, in contrast to recommendations in the general population, where repeat administration has historically been recommended for immunocompetent persons over 65 years of age, in transplant recipients over 18 years it is recommended that a single revaccination be given if it has been 3–5 years since receipt of the first dose [46]. The AST guidelines also provide guidance for those anticipated to have close contact with transplant recipients as well. Specifically, healthcare workers, close contacts, and family members should be fully immunized, and may consider the use of live attenuated vaccines, with the exception of polio and small pox vaccines.

Multiple antibiotics are commonly used post-operatively to prevent infection, and exposure to

Table 37.2 Vaccinations for the adult kidney transplant candidate/recipient

Vaccine	Inactivated (I) or live attenuated (LA)	Recommended before transplant	Recommended after transplant
Hepatitis B[a]	I	Yes	Yes
Hepatitis A	I	Yes	Yes
Tetanus	I	Yes	Yes
Pertussis (Tdap)[b]	I	Yes	Yes
Inactivated polio	I	Yes	Yes
S. pneumoniae[c] (polysaccharide vaccine)	I	Yes	Yes
N. meningitides (MCV4)[d]	I	Yes	Yes
Human papilloma virus (HPV)[e]	I	Yes	Yes
Measles[f]	LA	Yes	No
Mumps[f]	LA	Yes	No
Rubella[f]	LA	Yes	No
Influenza	I LA	Yes No	Yes No
Varicella Varivax	LA	Yes	No
Varicella Zostavax[g]	LA	Yes	No
BCG[h]	LA	Yes	No

These vaccines are recommended for adult kidney transplant recipients, before and after transplant. A complete list of all vaccinations relevant to pediatric and adult transplant recipients is published by the American Society of Transplantation [46]. It is recommended all vaccinations be completed prior to transplant whenever possible, as those vaccines noted to be safe after transplantation may not be successful after the transplant in the setting of immune suppression. For patients who are incompletely vaccinated or unvaccinated prior to transplant, consultation with an infectious diseases specialist is recommended

[a]Hepatitis B surface antibody titers should be assessed before and after transplant to assess ongoing immunity

[b]If no tetanus booster in the past 10 years, Tdap should be administered. At least one dose of acellular pertussis should be given in adulthood

[c]This should be administered before transplantation and repeated once 3–5 years after initial vaccination

[d]Recommended for members of the military, travelers to high risk areas, properdin deficient terminal complement component deficient, those with functional or anatomic asplenia, and college freshman living on campus

[e]Recommended for all females aged 6–26 years

[f]Measles, mumps, and rubella should be given in childhood

[g]Vaccine is indicated for person >59 years

[h]Use of Bacillus Calmette-Guerin (BCG) in the United States are limited to instances in which exposure to tuberculosis is unavoidable and measures to prevent its spread have failed or are not possible

such antibiotics must be considered in determining the etiology and susceptibility of active infection. Perioperative prophylactic antibiotics are commonly used to prevent urinary tract and wound infections following the transplant event. This practice has been reported in nearly 90% of transplant centers [54]. The evidence for perioperative antibiotics specifically in kidney transplantation is somewhat limited, particularly in the modern era of transplant, though the literature for perioperative antibiotics in urologic surgery is much larger [55]. A single center report from a more remote era of immune suppression linked the use of perioperative broad-spectrum antibiotics to a significant reduction in wound-infection related sepsis [56]. This was followed by a limited randomized trial performed more than a decade later, which showed a small, but what the authors felt was significant reduction in wound infections in the first 14 days following surgery [57]. More recently single center, uncontrolled case series suggest that the incidence of wound infection is low (2–4%) without perioperative antibiotics, and that this practice is therefore perhaps unnecessary [54, 58, 59].

Two common prophylactic strategies include the use of trimethoprim-sulfamethoxazole (tmx-sulfa, or alternative if contraindicated due to allergy) for the prevention of UTI and pneumocystis pneumonia, and antivirals such as ganciclovir or valganciclovir for the prevention of cytomegalovirus (CMV) infection and CMV related disease. Use of the former is associated with a significantly reduced rate of urinary tract and pneumocystis pulmonary infections, although acquired UTI's are more often resistant to tmx-sulfa [60, 61]. Further, tmx-sulfa has activity against many urinary pathogens and some nocardia, toxoplasma, and listeria species. For patients with allergies to tmx-sulfa, dapsone, atovaquone, and inhaled pentamidine are potential alternatives for PCP prophylaxis, but they lack the same spectrum of antibacterial activity.

The choice of post-transplant CMV risk reduction strategy is based upon one's risk of de novo CMV infection or CMV reactivation following transplant, determined by the presence of anti-CMV IgG in the donor and recipient prior to transplant [44]. For those at moderate to high risk of infection, current guidelines suggest 3–6 months of antiviral coverage. One must consider the possibility of ganciclovir resistance in anyone with an extended exposure to antiviral medications and without prompt response to therapy [44].

Exposures to Potential Pathogens

It is important to consider the unique epidemiology of *exposures* to potential pathogens when working up active infection in a transplant recipient. These exposures may be considered logically as donor related, recipient related, and those encountered in community and health care environments.

Beginning with placement of the transplant organ, the recipient assumes the risk of *donor-derived infections*, as well as iatrogenic infections related to external contamination of the organ. The donor organ should be considered as a potential source for any infection occurring in the first several weeks to months after transplant. Potential living and deceased donors are screened scrupulously for infection prior to transplant, (Table 37.2) [38], though current screening methods are not foolproof. Potential pathogens include bacteria, fungi, mycobacterium, endemic parasites, and viruses. Typical screening tests include antibody testing for human immunodeficiency virus, herpes simplex, CMV, hepatitis C, Hepatitis B, rapid plasma reagin (RPR), EBV, and varicella zoster virus (VZV). Meanwhile, nucleic acid amplification testing is available for viruses such as HIV, Hepatitis C, and Hepatitis B if there is concern that a donor may be in the "window period," between acute infection and antibody seroconversion. In 2011, the Centers for Disease Control (CDC) published a case report of HIV transmission from a living donor who had no detectable anti-HIV antibodies by enzyme immunoassay testing performed 79 days prior to transplant, but later acquired the virus, prior to donation [62]. The precise screening strategy used for donors varies by organ procurement area, and in some cases screening tests performed prior to transplant may turn positive after the transplant event (e.g., donor blood cultures).

Although the donor may not have active infection at the time of donation, removal and transport of the donor organ presents the opportunity for contamination, and should be considered in a donor developing early postoperative infection. A single center examination of culture data collected from perfusate fluid, kidney swabs, and ureteric tissue of kidney transplants performed between 1990 and 2000 revealed 9.1% with evidence of contamination. Based upon clinical outcomes, the authors suggest lactose fermenting coliforms and fungi require preemptive treatment, while skin contaminants do not pose a risk to the graft [63].

Recipient derived exposures and subsequent infection may be deduced through knowledge of the pre-transplant serologies (see above) and a complete history, which should include a review of recent travel, animal contacts, substance abuse, and sexual contacts. Travel to endemic areas such as sub-Saharan Africa, India, China, Southeast Asia, and Micronesia can increase the risk of infection by mycobacterium tuberculosis. Domestic travel can increase the risk of infection by endemic fungi such as *Histoplasma capsulatum* and *Blastomyces dermatidis* (Mississipi, Ohio, and Saint Lawrence River valleys), and *Coccidioides immitis* (southwestern United States). Travel to developing countries can increase the risk of acquiring parasites including *Strongyloides stercoralis* and *Trypanosoma cruzi*. Animal contacts can raise the spectrum of zoonosis such as *Chlamydophila psittaci* and pneumoniae and *Cryptococcus neoformans* (birds), salmonella (reptiles, rodents, cats, chickens), and rabies. Depending on the route of entry, substance abuse can increase exposure to blood borne pathogens including HIV, hepatitis C, and hepatitis B. Marijuana can increase the risk of infection by *Aspergillus* species found in soil.

Finally, it is important to remember that transplant recipients have significant exposure to hospital-acquired pathogens, which often have a more complicated spectrum of antibiotic susceptibilities compared to community-acquired organisms. For example, recent decades have seen the emergence of Methicillin-resistant *Staphylococcus aureus* (MRSA) [64], Vancomycin-resistant *Enterococcus* species [65], and more recently multidrug-resistant (MDR) Gram-negative organisms including extended-spectrum beta-lactamase-producing *Escherichia coli* or *Klebsiella pneumoniae*, MDR *Pseudomonas aeruginosa* and *Acinetobacter baumannii* [66], and fluconazole resistant *Candida* [67]. The prevalence of such organisms varies between hospitals and health care settings, but must be considered, particularly in the perioperative period. *Clostridium difficile*, which is most often hospital acquired, and associated with antibiotic use, is most common in the first 3 months following transplant [68].

Case 1 Review

In the case outlined above, the patient has several unique susceptibilities to infection. These include several decades of diabetes, with secondary renal failure and bladder dysfunction requiring intermittent daily urinary catheterization, which in combination with the altered milieu of the urinary tract resulting from a bladder-drained pancreas, significantly increase the risk of UTI. His risk for infection is further compounded by significant exposures to immune suppression, including successive exposure to lymphocyte depleting induction therapies with consecutive kidney and pancreas transplants, and large cumulative exposure to steroids with recent empiric treatment for rejection and chronic steroid therapy. Available pre-transplant serologies suggest that the patient is at high risk for de novo CMV infection, given the absence of pre-transplant immunity and donation from a CMV infected donor. He had documented immunity to EBV pre-transplant, reducing the risk of primary infection.

Ultimately, CMV DNA was detected in circulation by polymerase chain reaction (PCR) at >100,000 copies/mL. In this case, the patient's hyponatremia and orthostasis resolved with aggressive IV fluid resuscitation. Urine and blood cultures revealed no growth. CT guided biopsy of the lung nodule (Fig. 37.2) demonstrated tissue invasive CMV initially, and later grew nocardia asteroids, present despite tmx-sulfa prophylaxis. Following 3 weeks of IV ganciclovir, the CMV viral load was undetectable, and the patient felt well. He was placed on high dose bactrim therapy

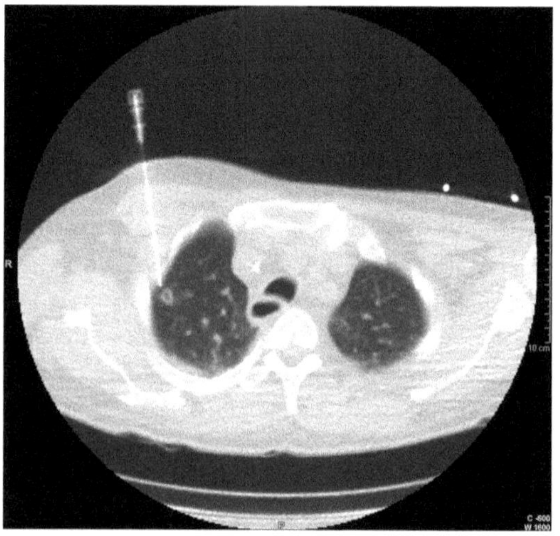

Fig. 37.2 *Lung nodule*. The patient in Case 1 had a lung nodule first identified on chest X-ray, later characterized in more detail by computerized-tomography (CT). CT guided biopsy of the lung nodule above demonstrated tissue invasive CMV initially, and later grew nocardia asteroids. Following 3 weeks of IV ganciclovir, the CMV viral load was undetectable, and the patient felt well. He was placed on high dose bactrim therapy for the nocardia, and had resolution of the pulmonary nodules at 1 year

for the nocardia, and had resolution of the pulmonary nodules at 1 year.

Important Pathogens and Clinical Syndromes

Case 2

A 67-year-old woman with a history of end-stage kidney failure attributed to hypertension presents to the transplant clinic 9-months following living donor kidney transplantation from her daughter with a serum creatinine of 1.8 mg/dL, up from a baseline of 0.9 mg/dL measured 8 weeks prior. She is a one-haplotype HLA match with her donor, received thymoglobulin and solumedrol for induction, and is maintained on 750 mg twice per day of mycophenolate mofetil, 5 mg per day of prednisone, and has tacrolimus troughs recorded at between 6 and 8 ng/mL. Her history is notable for 2 weeks of profound malaise, subjective low-grade fevers, and loose stools. Her physical exam is unremarkable. Her laboratory evaluation is notable for the absence of significant proteinuria or detectable anti-HLA antibodies, and transplant ultrasound is unremarkable. She has a white blood cell count of 2.0×10^9/L, detectable CMV and BK viremia by PCR with 4,900 copies/mL and 515,000 copies/mL respectively.

What is/are the most likely diagnoses, and what preventive and treatment options are available?

BK VIRUS

BK virus (BKV), named by the initials of the patient in whom it was first isolated, is a ubiquitous double-stranded circular DNA virus with a seroprevalence of approximately 80% in immunocompetent adults [69, 70]. Although the pathogenesis is not definitively understood, it is hypothesized that primary infection occurs via the respiratory tract [71] or oral route [72], followed by hematologic dissemination. The virus establishes latency in varies tissues, but most notably the epithelium of the urinary tract, and of the kidney in particular [73]. During active viral replication, epithelial cells are destroyed with subsequent end organ injury. Because BKV lies latent in urothelium, the virus may be present prior to transplant, or acquired after surgery, either from the donor organ or later in the community.

Despite the wide prevalence of BKV in the general population, clinical disease appears relatively unique to bone marrow and solid-organ transplant recipients, and is generally isolated to the urinary tract [73], though systemic involvement has been reported [74]. Hemorrhagic cystitis is well described among bone marrow transplant recipients [75], and ureteral stenosis and BK nephropathy (BKN) are widely reported among kidney transplant recipients [73]. BKN may also affect the native kidneys of other solid-organ transplant recipients, most commonly heart and lung recipients [76–78], but is generally considered a disease of the transplanted kidney.

The incidence of active infection is well described by a recent prospective clinical trial which had a strict BKV surveillance protocol. In this study, 35% of participants had detectable BKV viruria at 1 year, with a median onset of 40.5 days (range: 0–415 days) [79]. The incidence of viremia was 11.5%, with a median onset of 60 days (range: 18–276).

The incidence of clinically significant disease and outcomes vary between centers, even within single centers. This is illustrated by a single center review of 1,001 transplants between 1996 and 2003, in which BKN was diagnosed by biopsy alone in 2.3% of transplants done before 2001, with 62% graft failure. Meanwhile, using serum PCR and kidney biopsy as diagnostic tools, 7.9% of transplants done after 2001 were found to have BKN, with 36% graft failure [80]. The authors of this study attribute the higher rate of BKN and lower rate of graft loss in the later cohort to the introduction of a more aggressive screening protocol.

Regimented surveillance is important to prevent BKN, and current protocols are based upon the observation that detectable BKV moves reliably from urine, to blood, to kidney. In other words, viremia is not seen without concurrent viruria [79, 81]. BKN is generally not seen without concurrent BK viremia and viruria [72, 82]. Viruria is inferred by the presence of epithelial cells in the urine infected with BKV seen by light microscopy, so-called "decoy cells," or by the use of DNA PCR that gives a quantitative measure of viral DNA. PCR may be used to detect viral DNA in blood as well, which defines viremia. Meanwhile, electron-microscopic (EM) examination of urine can reveal tubular casts containing viral particles, so-called "Haufen," that is very specific for BKN [83], but may be limited in its clinical utility due to the need for EM.

In a seminal prospective observational study, the sensitivity of urinary decoy cells for BKN was 100%, while the specificity was 71%, and the positive and negative predictive values in this cohort was 29% and 100%, respectively. DNA PCR using blood had the same sensitivity as urinary decoy cells for BKN, but a specificity of 88%, and positive and negative predictive values of 88% and 100%. In a more recent paper, viral casts (i.e., Haufen) identified in the urine by EM was 100% sensitive and 99% specific for BKN, with 97% and 100% positive and negative predictive values. Despite the information provided by these test, kidney biopsy remained the gold standard for diagnosis of BKN, although it is subject to sampling error with a measurable false negative rate of between 10 and 30% [84, 85].

Histologically, BKN appears to move through progressive stages, although efforts to describe its evolution are confounded by the focal involvement in the graft, and by concurrent diagnosis such as acute cellular rejection and other viral nephropathies (e.g., CMV and adenovirus) that share similar light microscopic findings [84, 86, 87]. In the earliest stages of BKN, cytopathic and cytolytic changes are seen without significant inflammation or scarring. Typical findings include intranuclear basophilic viral inclusions and hyperchromasia, with immunohistochemical staining for viral antigens (e.g., SV40) revealing viral infected tubular cells. More advanced disease reveals interstitial inflammation with mononuclear and polymorphonuclear cells in areas of tubular injury, and active tubulitis, characterized by lymphocytes crossing the tubular basement membrane. The later finding can be difficult to distinguish from acute cellular rejection. As disease progresses, areas of inflammation are replaced by fibrosis. More advanced histopathology correlates with worse prognosis [84].

Early detection of viral replication and *preemptive* reduction of immune suppression appear to be successful strategies for limiting the harm of BKV, as there are currently no well validated antiviral therapies [85]. However, the risk of reducing immune suppression must be weighed against the risks of rejection on a case-by-case basis. Two recent prospective studies support the practice of preemptive reduction in immune suppression with early detection of BK viremia [88, 89]. The first, derived from a prospective clinic trial comparing tacrolimus vs. cyclosporine based IS regimens, screened for BKV using urine and plasma PCR weekly for the first 16-weeks post transplant, and then at months 5, 6, 9, and 12 [89]. Patients with BK viremia had their antimetabolite stopped (mycophenolate mofetil or azathioprine). If viremia failed to clear within 3–4 weeks, the calcineurin inhibitor was tapered to minimal acceptable levels. The authors report graft survival of 84%, acute rejection in 12%, and no BK nephropathy at 5-years.

In the second trial, patients were screened for BK with urine examination for decoy cells every 2 weeks until month 3, then at months 6 and 12, and yearly thereafter [88]. Those with decoy cells had plasma PCR for BKV performed. In those with sustained viremia, IS was reduced in a stepwise fashion until the viral load fell, beginning with an approximate 25% reduction in their CNI trough, followed by another 25% reduction in CNI trough, and ultimately MMF was reduced concurrently by 50%. These authors report an incidence of rejection of 8.6% following clearance of the virus, and conclude that this strategy was effective in preserving medium-term allograft function.

In cases where viremia persists despite acceptable levels of IS reduction, or in cases where there is profound BKN or concurrent BKN and rejection (which can be difficult to discern), adjuvant therapies may be considered. There is at least some evidence to support consideration of ciprofloxacin, leflunomide, intravenous immune-gamma globulin (IVIG), and/or cidofovir. Each has potential toxicities, and should be considered only on a case-by-case basis [85].

Based in part upon the cited evidence above, the AST has provided specific guidelines for the screening and management of BK infection, and the roll of adjuvant therapies, summarized in Table 37.3 [85]. In brief, based upon

Table 37.3 Screening and management of BK viremia and nephropathy

Screening test and frequency	Action
Urine (or serum) DNA PCR should be checked every 1–3 months for the first 2 years, then annually until year 5	If urine urine BKV loads >7 log geq/mL: Serum DNA testing should be performed
Serum (or urine) DNA PCR should be checked every 1–3 months for the first 2 years, then annually until year 5, and any time there is an unexplained rise in the serum creatinine or that a kidney biopsy is performed	If there is sustained plasma BKV DNA loads of >4 $\log_{10}$ geq/mL for >3 weeks: BK nephropathy is presumed Allograft biopsy should be considered for a definitive diagnosis
Kidney biopsy should be performed for any unexplained rise in serum creatinine or if there is sustained elevation in serum BKV DNA for >3 weeks. At least 2 cores should be obtained, preferably containing medullary tissue	If the kidney biopsy is negative for BK nephropathy: BK nephropathy is still presumed Immune suppression should be reduced[a] Serum creatinine should be checked weekly Serum BK DNA should be check every 2 weeks If the kidney biopsy is positive for BK nephropathy: BK nephropathy diagnosis is definitive Immune suppression should be reduced,[a] and in some cases, adjuvant treatment should be considered[b] If the kidney biopsy is positive for BK nephropathy and rejection is suggested[c]: Treatment should be considered on a case-by-case basis

The following screening and management strategies are reviewed in the American Society of Transplantation guidelines [85] and summarized in the text. It is recommended that recipients be screened using either urine or serum assays for BK virus every 1–3 months for the first 2 years post-transplant, and then annually for up to 5 years. If urine DNA testing reveals BKV loads >7 log geq/mL, serum BK DNA testing should be performed. If serum testing reveals sustained plasma BKV DNA loads of >4 $\log_{10}$ geq/mL for >3 weeks it is presumed the patient has BK nephropathy and a biopsy is recommended to confirm the diagnosis. Consideration should be given to reducing levels of immune suppression[a]. If BK nephropathy is confirmed, one may consider adjunctive therapy[b] in addition to reducing immune suppression. Serum creatinine and BK DNA should be followed closely, and if the BK viral load remains elevated, consideration should be given to adjunctive treatment[b]

[a]Two strategies have been described for reducing immune suppression. In strategy-1, dose reduction of the calcineurin inhibitor by 25–50% is done first, followed by reducing the antiproliferative drug by 50%; followed by discontinuing the latter if necessary. In strategy-2, the antiproliferative is reduced drug by 50% followed by reducing calcineurin inhibitors by 25–50% followed by discontinuing the antiproliferative drug if necessary. Prednisone is typically tapered to 10 mg or less daily dose. Immunosuppression is further adapted according to the course of serum creatinine concentration and the plasma viral loads. Responses may require several weeks

[b]Described Adjunctive therapies include ciprofloxacin, cidofovir, leflunomide, and IVIG. Given the absence of controlled data to support their use, and potential toxicities, these therapies should be reviewed in detail prior to prescribing

[c]Because tubulitis is common to both BK nephropathy and low grade acute cellular rejection, clinical judgement is required to determine if one, or both are present. Findings of arteritis, C4D positivity, fibrinoid necrosis, or glomerulitis are unique to rejection

the epidemiology of BK infection, it is recommended that recipients be screened using either quantitative urine or serum assays for BK virus every 1–3 months for the first 2 years post-transplant, and then annually for up to 5 years. If urine DNA testing reveals BKV loads >7 log geq/mL, because it has a relatively low positive predictive value for BK nephropathy, serum BK DNA testing should be performed. If serum testing reveals sustained plasma BKV DNA loads of >4 $\log_{10}$ geq/mL for >3 weeks it is presumed the patient has BK nephropathy, though a biopsy is recommended to confirm the diagnosis. In either case, consideration should be given to reducing levels of immune suppression as cited above, or outlined below. If BK nephropathy is confirmed or if high levels of BK virus persist, one may consider adjunctive therapy in addition to reducing immune suppression. Serum creatinine should be followed approximately weekly and BK DNA should be followed at least every other week. Because tubulitis is common to both BK nephropathy and low grade acute cellular rejection, clinical judgement is required to determine if one, or both are present. Findings of arteritis, C4D positivity, fibrinoid necrosis, or glomerulitis are unique to rejection

The AST guidelines described two strategies for reducing immune suppression. In strategy-1, dose reduction of the calcineurin inhibitor by 25–50% is done first, followed by reducing the antiproliferative drug by 50%; followed by discontinuing the latter if necessary. In strategy-2, the antiproliferative is reduced drug by 50% followed by reducing calcineurin inhibitors by 25–50% followed by discontinuing the antiproliferative drug if necessary. In either case, oral prednisone is typically tapered to 10 mg or less daily dose. Immunosuppression is further adapted according to the course of serum creatinine concentration and the plasma viral loads, but responses may require several weeks.

Cytomegalovirus

CMV has been called the most important pathogen in kidney transplantation [90], as infection following transplant is common and has been linked to worse graft and patient outcomes, as well as increased cost [91, 92]. First isolated in 1956 [93], CMV has a seroprevalence in the United States that varies by age, ranging from approximately 50% among 20 year olds, to near 90% for those over 70 years of age [94, 95]. In the transplant population, the seroprevalence has been noted to be around 60% among donors and recipients [91]. Donor and recipients' serologic status are typically referred to as D/R respectively, with a + or – following each letter connoting the presence (+) or absence (–) of circulating immunity (anti-CMV IgG).

As with other viruses in the Herpesvirus family (e.g., EBV, herpes simplex viruses, varicella-zoster virus), CMV is coded in linear double-stranded DNA. It establishes lifelong latency in the host following primary infection and therefore may reactivate in the setting of altered host immunity, for example with the initiation of immune suppressive medications required for solid-organ transplant [96]. CMV has been detected and/or may be transmitted through saliva, sexual contact, urine, breastfeeding, placental transfer, blood transfusion, and solid-organ transplant [96, 97]. As with BK, CMV may be present in the host prior to transplant, or acquired post-transplant, either through the donor kidney, or later in the community.

In kidney transplantation, CMV *infection* is differentiated from active *disease*, which is further considered in two distinct entities, as a *viral syndrome* or as *tissue invasive disease* [44]. *Infection* most commonly refers to the detection of virus in the blood by any of several molecular techniques, or isolation of the virus from cultured tissue or fluids. Two common methods of CMV detection include measurement of CMV pp65 antigen in host polymorpholeukocytes by *immunofluoresence*, and quantification of serum-, plasma-, and/or whole blood-viral DNA and/or RNA by *PCR*, which both can provide estimates of the detectable "viral load." Higher viral loads appear to correlate with disease, although disease may occur in the absence of a detectable viral load [44, 90]. Caution should be used in comparing results performed between two labs as significant variation may be seen between assays [44].

While infection is defined by detectable virus in the body alone, *disease* is defined by a combination of detectable virus and active signs and symptoms attributable to CMV infection [44]. The first category of disease, *CMV syndrome*, most often presents with fever, fatigue, and cytopenias, including leucopenia and thrombocytopenia. The second, *tissue invasive disease*, is defined by the presence of end organ infection and injury. This diagnosis is often dependent upon culture, histopathologic testing with immune-staining, or in situ DNA hybridization [90]. Exceptions to this are CMV retinitis that may be diagnosed by ophthalmologic exam, and CNS disease, which is extremely rare, but may be presumed in the appropriate clinical setting if CMV DNA is detectable in the cerebral spinal fluid (CSF) by PCR [98]. Additional manifestations of tissue invasive disease includes CMV colitis, hepatitis, pneumonitis, pancreatitis, myocarditis, cystitis, and nephritis, as CMV has a predilection to invade the transplant graft [44].

Of additional interest, CMV is felt to be immune-modulatory, predisposing to other infections including bacteremias, invasive fungal diseases, and EBV related disease [44], and is associated with a higher incidence of rejection [99, 100]. Because of its multiple clinical manifestations, CMV infection should be suspected in any transplant patient with undefined infection.

The risk of developing CMV disease is estimated prior to transplant, based upon the serologic status of the donor and the recipient (D/R, see first paragraph), which should be checked prior to transplant. Recipients with no evidence of past CMV exposure (R–) prior to transplant, receiving organs from previously infected recipients (D+) are considered "high-risk" for CMV disease following transplant. Presumably this is due to reactivation of acquired latent virus in the absence existing recipient immunity. In a seminal clinical trial from 1,999 examining valacyclovir prophylaxis for CMV, D-patients in the placebo group (i.e., no prophylaxis), receiving R+organs, had a 45% incidence of CMV infection (using culture detection methods) and disease at 6-months [99]. Using modern PCR detection, two recent studies described the incidence of viremia in this group at between 54 and 83% at 12-months [101, 102]. Nearly all episodes of infection in these trials occurred within the first 100 days.

As compared to high-risk recipients (D+/R–), recipients are considered "moderate-risk" disease if they have circulating immunity prior to transplant, regardless of the donors serologic status (D+/R+ or D–/R+). In the clinical trial from 1999 cited above, the incidence of disease at 6-months for this group was 6% [99]. Recipients without detectable immunity receiving organs from donors without evidence of previous exposure (D–/R–) are considered to be "low-risk" for subsequent infection, and have an incidence of disease cited as <5% [90]. Additional risk factors for CMV infection include receipt of induction immune suppression, particularly with lymphocyte depleting agents [32, 103], exposure to lymphocyte depleting therapies for rejection, and recipients' overall immune-suppressed status which correlates directly with increasing age, comorbidities, and total exposure to immune suppression [32, 44, 102, 104].

Two strategies are advocated to mitigate the harm associated with CMV infection—*preemptive treatment* or *universal prophylaxis* [44, 98, 104]. Preemptive treatment describes a regimen of close surveillance for viremia (e.g., checking serum PCR on a weekly basis), with prompt initiation of antiviral treatment following detection of circulating virus. Meanwhile, prophylaxis requires giving antiviral medication for a fixed period of time based upon recipients' risk of developing CMV related disease. There is no consensus in the field as to the preferred strategy, as both preemptive treatment and universal prophylaxis appear to have similar efficacy in reducing CMV disease in those at highest risk (i.e., D+/R– transplants) [105, 106], although there is some suggestion that universal prophylaxis alone reduces the risk of bacterial and fungal super-infection and death [106], and may prolong graft survival [107], a finding that varies between studies.

Specific protocols for both preemptive treatment and universal prophylaxis are outlined in recently published guidelines [44, 104, 108]. The AST guidelines are summarized in Table 37.4 [44]. A common approach for D+/R– transplants is to mandate either preemptive treatment or universal prophylaxis on a case-by-case basis. The former incurs the costs of serial viral load testing and requires intensive logistic support. It has the theoretical benefit of less exposure to antiviral medication, and therefore less risk of drug related side effects. The latter, which may employed with oral valganciclovir, IV ganciclovir, or oral valacyclovir is associated with higher drug related costs, but has potential benefits beyond prevention of CMV disease. Prophylactic antiviral use has been suggested for 3–6 months in the high risk population, with recent evidence suggesting added value extending this to 200 days. The recent IMPACT trial, a pharmaceutical industry sponsored, double-blind, randomized, controlled trial compared 100 days of valganciclovir 900 mg per day versus 200 day in D+/R– transplants. The rate of CMV viremia was

Table 37.4 Universal prophylaxis and preemptive treatment strategies post-transplant for CMV disease

CMV prevention strategy	Protocol
Universal Prophylaxis Stratified by Risk (Donor CMV-status/Recipient CMV-status)	
D+/R–, high risk	Valganciclovir (900 mg once daily), oral ganciclovir (1 g three times daily), or intravenous ganciclovir (5 mg/kg once daily), or valacyclovir (2 g four times daily) for 3–6 months
D– or D+/R+, intermediate risk	Valganciclovir, oral ganciclovir, intravenous ganciclovir or valacyclovir for 3 months
D–/R–, low risk	No prophylaxis is recommended
Preemptive treatment	CMV viral load testing or pp65 antigenemia assay is checked weekly for 12 weeks post-transplant. If the threshold for treatment is reached, preemptive therapy is initiated. Oral valganciclovir (900 mg two times a day) or intravenous ganciclovir (5 mg/kg two times a day) may be used. Therapy should be continued until viremia is undetectable

This is a summary of the American Society of Transplantation's guidelines for prevention of CMV disease [44]. At present, there is equipoise between Universal Prophylaxis and Preemptive Treatment strategies. In the former, the recipient's risk for CMV is determined based on their serologic status prior to transplant for CMV immunity, and that of the donor. Those at high or intermediate risk are given between 3 and 6 months of antiviral therapy. In the Preemptive Treatment strategy, recipients undergo weekly testing for CMV viremia, and begin therapy once it is detected above a defined threshold. Currently there is no standard for CMV detection, and therefore no recognized defined cutoff for initiating treatment. Treatment should continue until no viremia is detectable. Either strategy should be considered immediately after transplant and following treatment for acute rejection with lymphocyte depleting therapies (e.g., thymoglobulin)

51% at 12 months in the 100-day arm vs. 37% in those receiving 200-days of prophylaxis. The rate of CMV disease at 12 months was 36.8% in the 100-day group vs. 16.1% in the 200 day group, with the vast majority of disease defined as CMV syndrome at 97.6%. There was very little tissue invasive disease in either group at 12 months.

Treatment for CMV may be initiated at the onset of CMV viremia (e.g., with preemptive treatment strategy) or with symptomatic disease, either CMV syndrome or tissue invasive disease. Historically, intravenous ganciclovir has been cornerstone of treatment, and it remains the standard for severe or life-threatening disease. Ganciclovir works by inhibiting CMV DNA polymerase encoded by gene UL54, after it is phosporylated by a viral kinase encoded by the gene UL97. It is typically dosed at 5 mg/kg twice per day (adjusted based on renal function), for variable duration of 2–4 weeks, until the virus is undetectable [44]. More recently, oral valganciclovir, a highly bioavailable prodrug of ganciclovir has been used for treatment of mild to moderate disease. A randomized controlled trial published in 2007 showed that 3 weeks of oral valganciclovir (900 mg twice per day, adjusted for creatinine clearance) was non-inferior to IV ganciclovir for the treatment of mild to moderate CMV disease [109].

Mutations to the UL 97 and UL 54 genes predict resistance to standard therapies, and should be investigated in patients who develop disease following an extended period of prophylaxis, or if there is failure to respond promptly to standard treatment. Specific mutations to UL 97 may respond to high dose ganciclovir, while others require an alternative therapy, such as foscarnet. Consultation by an infectious disease specialist is suggested when any form of antiviral resistance is considered.

Case 2 Review

As above, BK and CMV viremia 9-months out from transplant is not uncommon. The former is more often associated with renal dysfunction, and the later with symptomatic disease. BK viremia in the setting of renal dysfunction is typically investigated by renal biopsy. CMV viremia in the

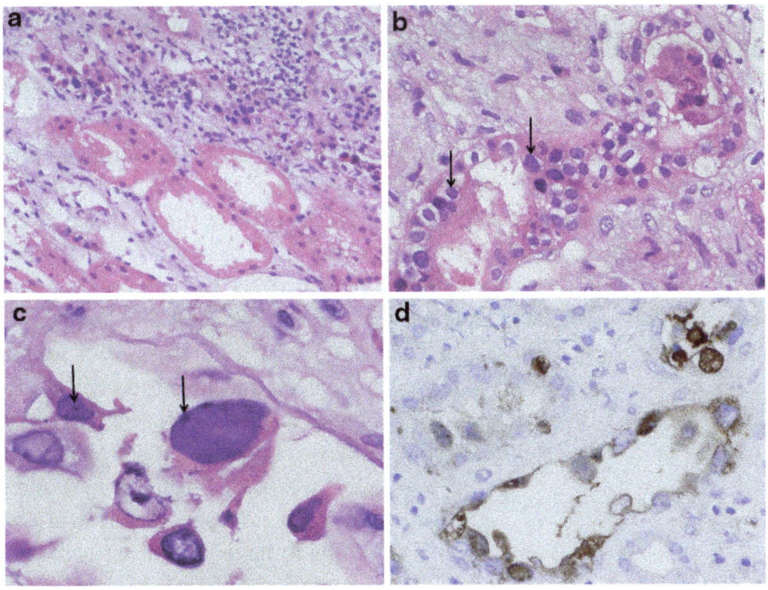

Fig. 37.3 (**a**) This is hematoxylin and eosin (H&E) stained renal cortex viewed by light microscopy at 200× magnification showing tubulointerstitial inflammation (*upper half of picture*). (**b**) Renal tubular epithelial cells are shown above on H&E stain at 400× magnification. The cells are notable for BK virus cytopathic effects, including intra-cellular inclusions (*black arrows*). (**c**) Renal tubular epithelial cells are viewed here in H&E stain at 1,000×. Large intranuclear viral inclusions are seen (*black arrows*). (**d**) At 400× magnification, renal tubular epithelial cells are seen with immunohistochemical staining for BK virus seen as brown discoloration of the cells cytoplasm

setting of fatigue, fever, and leucopenia are sufficient for a diagnosis of CMV syndrome. The history of loose stool raises the specter of invasive CMV colitis, though this element of the patient's history was not striking. For the diagnosis of CMV disease, the patient was treated with 3 weeks of renally dosed oral valganciclovir. Her CMV viral load became undetectable within 10 days, with prompt resolution of her symptoms. A renal biopsy was performed to investigate her renal dysfunction (Fig. 37.3). This revealed severe tubulitis and interstitial inflammation, along with moderate fibrosis. Intranuclear viral particles were visible by light microscopy and BK viral antigens were detected by immune histochemical staining. No CMV was detected. The diagnosis was advanced stage BK nephropathy. Because of the advanced histologic damage, the decision was made to stop the patient's mycophenolate mofetil, reduce her tacrolimus troughs to between 2 and 4 ng/dL, and initiate leflunomide 40 mg per day. She was kept on 5 mg of prednisone per day. The patient cleared her BK viremia over 1 year, and at 2–1/2 years post-transplant maintained a stable creatinine of between 1.6 and 1.8 mg/dL. Advanced BK nephropathy may be avoided in most cases with an intensive screening protocol, and preemptive reduction in the patient's IS with early viremia. Meanwhile, late onset CMV syndrome is not uncommon following cessation of CMV prophylaxis, and must always be considered in a transplant recipient with nonspecific symptoms of illness.

Case 3

A 25 year-old woman with a history of end-stage renal disease due to diabetes, now 1 year out from her deceased donor kidney transplant, comes to clinic complaining of a loss of appetite and night sweats over the preceding 4 months, and recent onset of numbness in her right arm and hand, blurred vision, and a mild headache. Her transplant course is notable for anti-thymocyte globulin induction at the time of transplant, with repeat use

4-months ago, following an episode of acute cellular rejection associated with medication non-adherence. She is maintained on prednisone 10 mg per day, mycophenolate mofetil 1 g twice per day, and has 12 h tacrolimus troughs between 5 and 7 ng/mL. On exam, she is thin, has lost 30 pounds over the past 3 months, and appears more subdued than usual. She has notable pronator drift, but otherwise no focal findings. Her laboratory evaluation reveals a creatinine is 1.0 mg/dL (at its baseline), new mild anemia, mildly elevated transaminases, and detectable EBV DNA in her plasma.

What is the relevance of EBV detected in her blood and what are the next steps in your evaluation?

Epstein-Barr Virus

EBV is a double-stranded DNA virus, a member of the gamma herpes virus family, whose infectivity is largely confined to humans. Viral transmission occurs via infected body fluids such as saliva, with primary infection most often involving the epithelium of the oropharynx, followed by later infection of B and T cell lymphocytes where the virus resides in a latent stage [110]. Because EBV takes up residence within lymphocytes, in the case of kidney transplantation, the virus also may be acquired through the donor organ or transfusion of non-leukocyte irradiated blood.

EBV infection is widely prevalent among kidney transplant recipients, as demonstrated by the presence of circulating anti-EBV antibodies prior to transplant. Among kidney transplant recipients enrolled in a large multinational cohort, the seroprevalence of EBV prior to transplant was upwards of 90% [111]. In this cohort, seroprevalence increased with age, with approximately 40% of those less than 10 years-old demonstrating seropositivity. Seropositivity was nearly 70% in those aged 10–19, 80% in those 30–39, and reached 90% in those over 30 [111].

EBV can cause a variety of clinical manifestations in the transplant recipient, from infectious mononucleosis to post-transplant lymphoproliferative disorders (PTLD). Mononucleosis is characterized at the onset by fatigue, headache, and low fevers, followed by the classic triad of enlarged tender symmetric cervical lymphadenopathy, pharyngitis with tonsillar exudate, and high fever [112, 113]. The diagnosis can be made on the basis of the clinical presentation with supportive laboratory evidence, which includes lymphocytosis, the presence of atypical lymphocytes on examination of the blood smear, and the development of heterophile antibodies, a group of IgM antibodies directed against various viral antigens which cross-react with antigens found on sheep and horse red cells, which are used in rapid testing [113]. In the general population, these antibodies may be absent in the first 1–2 weeks of infection. IgM and IgG antibodies directed more specifically against the viral capsid antigen have higher sensitivity early on and greater specificity for the diagnosis of EBV mononucleosis [114]. The prognosis of mononucleosis is good, but acute EBV infection in the transplant recipient can be a harbinger of more threatening disease later on, PTLD.

PTLD is a heterogeneous group of diseases that range from benign polyclonal lymphoproliferation in the setting of acute EBV infection to highly morbid diffuse lymphoma, but are linked by the shared finding of abnormal lymphocyte growth [115]. PTLD is most often derived from B-cells of the transplant recipient, and approximately 50–80% test positive for EBV [115]. However, PTLD can be of T-cell or NK-cell origin [116], can be derived from donor lymphocytes [117], and can occur independent of EBV [118], which explains in part the variable presentation and prognosis.

EBV-associated PTLD has been classified by the World health Organization (WHO) into four categories. The first three are most relevant to transplant [119]. *Early lesions* describes polyclonal lymphocytes dividing in response to EBV with minimal cellular atypia and intact architecture of involved tissue, and may be labeled as infectious mononucleosis or plasmacytic hyperplasia. *Polymorphic-PTLD* (*P-PTLD*) may be polyclonal or monoclonal, with increasing cytologic atypia, and involved tissue has some distortion of the architecture. *Monomorphic-PTLD* (*M-PTLD*) are overt malignant lymphomas of B- or T-cell lineage, with architectural and cytologic atypia. More than 85% of PTLD are from B-cells, 14% from T-cells, and 1% NK cells [119].

The incidence of PTLD following transplant is difficult to precisely define, due to the absence of a standardized definition, though a recent international cohort spanning 16 years, and including 145,104 kidney transplants, reported a 10 year incidence of non-Hodgkin lymphomas of 1.6%. Consistent with other studies, the highest rate of PTLD in this cohort was within the first year following the transplant event, though the median time of occurrence was nearly 5 years [120], highlighting that although the incidence of PTLD is highest early on, most cases of PTLD occur outside the first year. The incidence of lymphoma is highest in those less than 10 years of age and those over 60 [120].

The best-described risk factors for PTLD include patients who have a negative EBV serostatus prior having an EBV+donor, and the degree and type of immune suppression. The T-cell response of the immune system is important for containing EBV replication, even after integration of the virus into the host lymphocytes. In the EBV naïve transplant recipient without existing EBV directed T-cell population, primary EBV infection in the setting of immune suppression significantly increase the risk of PTLD. EBV seronegative patients have a 10- to 76-fold greater incidence of PTLD compared to seropositive recipients [121]. The lower seroprevalence of EBV in children may explain why PTLD rates are higher in this demographic.

Regarding the risk of immune suppression, the use of lymphocyte-depleting antibodies for either prevention of rejection (i.e., induction) or treatment of rejection is associated with a significant higher incidence of PTLD [31, 120]. Further, exposure to lymphocyte-depleting antibodies for treatment of rejection *after* initial exposure as induction, appears to have additive risk [120]. Some have suggested an increased risk for PTLD with the use of tacrolimus vs. cyclosporine [31, 120, 122], an inconsistent finding. Additionally, there is some evidence to suggest CMV presents a unique risk factor for developing PTLD [121].

Diagnosing PTLD requires clinical suspicion, as the findings may be subtle. This suspicion is often based upon the pre-existing risk factors listed above. Disease may be diffuse or localized, and as such, presenting symptoms may be nonspecific, including weight loss, night sweats, malaise, anorexia, or focal, including swollen lymph nodes, sore throat, abdominal pain, gastrointestinal bleeding, cough, headache, or neurologic symptoms [45]. In the case of donor derived PTLD, which is more often localized, graft infiltration by PTLD may present as renal dysfunction.

Indirect testing may further raise or lower suspicion for PTLD, though ultimately tissue examination is required to make the diagnosis and to determine appropriate treatment. CBC with differential may reveal anemia or lymphocytosis. Depending on end-organ involvement, abnormalities in liver function tests or renal function may be seen. EBV serologies are unreliable for making a diagnosis of PTLD, and the role of quantitative viral load determination as a screening test is undetermined, though in patients with overt signs and symptoms of PTLD, plasma viral load testing can have good positive and negative predictive values for EBV associated PTLD [123]. Importantly, EBV viral load testing is of little value for the detection of non-EBV associated PTLD and may miss donor derived PTLD or localized disease [45].

Chest, abdomen, and pelvic computerized tomography (CT scan) is most often used to look for bulky adenopathy or extranodal disease, and brain imaging with CT or magnetic resonance imaging (MRI) is an important part of staging, as CNS disease may substantially alter treatment and prognosis [45]. Positron emission tomography-computerized tomography (PET-CT) may be useful in diagnosis, or monitoring response to therapy. Pathology is the definitive gold standard for diagnosing PTLD and devising treatment with important distinctions often made on the basis of clonality, the presence of detectable EBV, and the cell type, although there is little consensus on how to treat PTLD.

Therapies for EBV associated PTLD have been nicely considered as T-cell therapies (e.g., restoration of host EBV T-cell immunity), B-cell directed therapies (e.g., those targeted at eliminating neoplastic B-cells), and antiviral agents (e.g., those directed at EBV control) (20576725, NDT 2010) [124]. Chief among the T-cell directed therapies is reduction of immune suppression, for the purpose of reviving the host cytotoxic T-cell response against EBV. This has been recommended as initial treatment for all forms of PTLD [125], but may have particular efficacy as a single intervention in *early lesions* and *polymorphic PTLD [*124], and is said to have a response rate of upwards of 50%, with evidence of clinical response seen in 2–4 weeks [45, 126]. B-cell directed therapies include Rituximab, an anti-CD20 antibody, which has shown to have efficacy in prospective trials, and is considered in many cases in CD20+ tumors if there is not a response to initial reduction of immune suppression [45, 127]. Additional cytotoxic chemotherapies, such as CHOP (cyclophosphamide, doxorubicin, vincristine, and prednisone) are used occasionally for more refractory disease, and surgery and radiation may be considered for localized disease, the later sometimes used for CNS disease and NK-cell lymphomas. Some centers consider adjunctive antiviral therapy such as ganciclovir and acyclovir [45], though these agents are more often advocated as prophylaxis agents in high-risk patients (EBV D+/R−) [128].

The prognosis for PTLD is variable given the heterogeneity of disease. Early lesions and early onset polymorphic EBV-associated PTLD often responds to reduction in immunosuppression, and has a favorable prognosis. Disease specific factors associated with worse prognosis include T- or NK-cell disease, EBV-negative PTLD, monoclonal disease, multisite or central nervous system involvement [45]. Several tools have been developed to better define the prognosis and response to treatment [129, 130].

Case 3 Review

The patients is highly immune-suppressed and her history is concerning for indolent infection or malignancy. Review of the patient's record revealed that she had no detectable immunity to EBV prior to transplant, while the donor had evidence of past infection (D+/R−). Her exam is most concerning for CNS disease and so brain imaging was pursued along with lumbar puncture. MRI of her brain revealed a mass lesion (see Fig. 37.4), and CT of her chest abdomen and pelvis revealed bulky mediastinal adenopathy. CSF

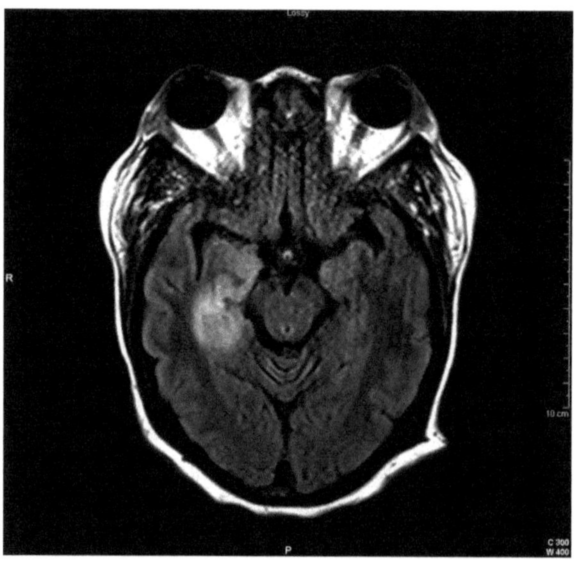

Fig. 37.4 The MRI above from Case 3 reveals abnormal enhancement concerning for infection versus malignancy. The tissue biopsy ultimately revealed EBV + B-cell lymphoma

revealed detectable EBV virus DNA, but no evidence of malignancy by cytology. The decision was made to perform a brain biopsy. This revealed monoclonal B-cell EBV-positive PTLD. Her tacrolimus and mycophenolate mofetil were promptly discontinued, and she received Rituximab therapy weekly for 4 weeks. The CNS lesion was reduced in size at 8 weeks, but the patient's course was complicated by the development of hospital acquire pneumonia, and she eventually died from sepsis syndrome.

Case 4

A 45-year-old man presents for consideration as a kidney transplant recipient. He has end-stage kidney disease due to diabetic nephropathy, and a history of Human Immunodeficiency Virus (HIV) infection going back to 2002, acquired through a job related needle stick. He wants to know if he is eligible for transplant given his HIV status.

How would you advise this gentleman?

Human Immunodeficiency Virus

Infection with the Human Immunodeficiency Virus (HIV) has been considered an absolute contraindication to transplant, until recently. This was in large part, due to the concern that the required immune suppression would accelerate progression to acquired immune deficiency syndrome (AIDS). With the advent of highly active antiretroviral therapy in the 1990s, the prognosis for HIV improved considerably [131], and in the last decade a good deal of work has been done performing kidney transplants in HIV infected individuals with kidney failure [132–134].

The largest such study is an NIH sponsored prospective nonrandomized trial, involving 150 HIV infected kidney transplant recipients. These transplants occurred between 2003 and 2009. Entry into the trial required a CD4+ T-cell count >200/mm^3 and undetectable plasma HIV RNA. Patient and graft survival were 88% and 74% at 3 years, though a higher rate of rejection was observed than expected. HIV infection remained well controlled with few HIV related complications. There is a profound drug interaction between many of the highly active antiretroviral medications (HAART), particularly between the protease inhibitors, and the calcineurin inhibitors (CNI), as the former inhibit enzymes of the cytochrome p-450 system, leading to much higher than predicted serum levels of CNI. As a result, nearly one third of enrolled patients in this trial were given their CNI at a frequency less than is typically recommended, in order to avoid supratherapeutic trough levels. It has been hypothesized that unintentional underdosing contributed to the higher than expected rate of rejection.

Kidney transplantation is now a reality in HIV+individuals, but must be undertaken on a multidisciplinary basis, with involvement of HIV infectious disease specialists, a knowledgeable pharmacist, and only after assuring excellent HIV control on a stable HAART regimen that has been reviewed and modified for anticipated drug interactions.

Case 4 Review

The man's HIV status alone is not a contraindication to kidney transplantation. His evaluation should include typical evaluation for occult cardiovascular disease, age appropriate malignancy screenings, and infectious serologies. With regards to his HIV status, most centers require the virus be undetectable and the potential recipient have CD-4 count >200/mm^3 for at least 6-months prior to transplant, on a stable antiviral regimen. Presuming this is the case, he is a potential candidate, and should be warned about the potential for drug interactions, the associated increased risk of rejection, and the typical outcomes listed above.

Case 5

A 58 year-old woman with history of Hepatitis-C infection acquired from remote blood transfusion presents to your transplant center for evaluation as a kidney transplant recipient. She has advanced chronic kidney disease attributed to hypertension and multiple available living donors. On exam she has no stigmata of liver disease and her labs reveal no detectable liver function test abnormalities.

What additional testing and treatments should be considered prior to transplant?

Hepatitis C

Hepatitis C (Hep-C) is an enveloped single-stranded RNA virus for which at least six genotypes have been identified throughout the world. Exposure leads to chronic infection in 85% of individuals. The prevalence of Hep-C in US hemodialysis units is around 7.8% [135] so that Hep-C infection has relevance both before and after kidney transplantation. Acute infection can unknowingly be transmitted through the donor organ, but current screening dramatically reduces this risk [136, 137]. For those in whom Hep-C is detected prior to surgery it must be determined if the risks of transplant outweigh the benefits and whether or not these risks can be mitigated to acceptable levels. Issues arising post-transplant include surveillance for progressive liver failure and Hep-C related kidney disease, and managing them if they arise.

Although no randomized prospective trials have examined survival in Hep-C infected patients receiving transplants versus remaining on dialysis, retrospective cohort studies suggest a measurable survival benefit with kidney transplantation for selected individuals [42, 138]. In making this assessment, it is important to recognize that Hep-C infection has been associated with accelerated liver disease following transplant [43], as well as worse graft outcomes and patient survival [139, 140]. Progression to cirrhosis appears to be more common in those with advanced liver disease prior to transplant, but is not inevitable, as a prospective study examining serial liver biopsies post-transplant documented stable disease and even disease regression in a small portion of their cohort [141]. The association of Hep-C infection with patient and graft outcomes is also inconsistent between studies, a fact attributed to differences in liver disease stage, and prevalence of comorbidities between study participants [142].

It is generally recommended that candidates for transplant with detectable circulating Hep-C virus undergo a liver biopsy prior to transplant in order to stage occult liver disease and assess the risk of progression following transplant [135]. A well-done summary of available data suggests that liver biopsy results may be used in the following way [142]. For those with mild to no fibrosis, Hep-C treatment may be considered if there are favorable predictors for response (e.g., viral genotype 2 or 3) or if there is Hep-C associated kidney disease. For those with moderate fibrosis, Hep-C treatment is recommended prior to transplant, moving forward with transplant if there is sustained viral response, or otherwise on a case by case basis. For those with cirrhosis, Hep-C treatment is recommended, followed by kidney transplantation alone or simultaneous liver and kidney transplants. In cases where there is no viral response, simultaneous liver kidney transplantation may be considered, or transplant may be contraindicated entirely. This algorithm is consistent with that recommended by the American Society of Transplantation [135].

The decision to treat Hep-C prior to transplant should be made on a case by case basis, taking into account many factors, including the stage of underlying liver disease, the likelihood of response to treatment, as well as the presence of comorbidities that can compromise treatment, such as end-stage kidney disease, cytopenias, and clinical depression. A full discussion of treatment options is beyond the scope of this paper, but well reviewed by others [142]. Treatment options for those without renal disease include interferon-alpha alone, or in combination with ribavirin, and for those with genotype 1 virus, a new class of protease inhibitors may be considered. For the pre-kidney transplant population, ribavirin is generally contraindicated and only considered for use in the context of a carefully monitored clinical trial, as the drug is renally cleared, and its metabolites are not removed by dialysis. A recent meta-analysis of 20 trials using interferon alpha alone in 459 dialysis patients reported a sustained viral response of 41% and treatment discontinuation rate of 26% [143].

Progressive liver failure or clinically significant Hep-C related renal disease, such as Hep-C associated vasculitis or cryoglobulin associated membranoproliferative glomerulonephritis (MPGN), are indications to consider Hep-C treatment following renal transplantation. Transplant recipients with detectable Hep-C must be followed closely for signs of end organ injury, including liver function test abnormalities, worsening renal function, or clinically significant proteinuria. The risk of interferon-based therapy in the setting of a functioning transplant includes rejection, with reported rates between 15 and 64% [143], but remains the standard of care.

Case 5 Review

Despite normal liver function tests, this candidate will require a liver biopsy prior to transplant to investigate occult liver disease, as laboratory testing alone is insensitive for significant disease. Additional testing should include viral genotyping to predict response to treatment, and consideration should be given to abdominal ultrasound if there is significant fibrosis in the biopsy, to investigate evidence of portal hypertension or ascites that would suggest more significant hepatic dysfunction. The patient would ideally be considered for Hep-C treatment prior to transplant, but this decision may be made on a case-by-case basis, most often in conjunction with a hepatologist. If the biopsy reveals cirrhosis, the decision to do a kidney transplant alone would be predicated on a successful response to therapy. In the setting of cirrhosis with decompensation (e.g., obvious synthetic dysfunction, ascites, significant portal hypertension), kidney transplantation would most often only be considered with a simultaneous liver transplant.

Case 6

A 55-year-old seen in the pre-transplant clinic completes his routine infectious serologic testing. He is found to have detectable Hepatitis-B surface antigen and core antibody, but no surface antibody or viral DNA is identified. His serum aminotransferases are just above the normal range.

What additional workup is required to assess the patient's candidacy and what additional care should be provided after the transplant event?

Hepatitis B

Hepatitis B is a partially double-stranded DNA virus that can cause fulminate or chronic liver disease. The most common clinical issues faced in kidney transplantation are the assessment and mitigation of progressive liver disease in those with chronic infection. Chronic Hep-B infection is associated with approximately 2.5 times the risk of death and 1.4 times the risk of allograft loss [144]. Fortunately, the burden of infection in the dialysis population has declined significantly over time as the result of intense infection control efforts, including routine vaccination in hemodialysis units. The prevalence of Hep-B infection among hemodialysis patients in the United States was around 3% in the late 1990s, ranging between 0 and 7% in developed countries worldwide [145].

Pre-transplant testing for circulating viral antigens and associated antibodies is standard to assess for remote Hep-B infection with resolution, active chronic infection, and/or successful vaccination. With initial infection, Hep-B surface antigen and viral DNA are detectable in circulation at high levels, and are often accompanied by elevations in serum liver enzymes. The host's early immune response is marked by the development of Hep-B core antibodies, followed by the development of Hep-B surface antibodies, which coincides with clearance of the Hep-B surface antigen from circulation. In those who ultimately clear the virus, testing reveals Hep-B core and surface antibodies, with no detectable surface antigen or viral DNA. In those with chronic infection, Hep-B surface antigen remains detectable with or without detectable viral DNA, often in the presence of Hep-B core antibody, but in the absence of surface antibody. Chronic hepatitis is marked by abnormal liver enzymes, and is differentiated from the chronic carrier in whom liver function tests are normal. Successful vaccination is marked by the presence of Hep-B surface antibodies, in the absence of core antibodies or surface antigen.

Chronic infection, defined by the presence of circulating Hep-B surface antigen more than 6-months after infection, is often first brought to the attention of the transplant team by routine pre-transplant serologies. It is not a contraindication to transplant, but requires more detailed assessment, including investigation with a liver biopsy, to differentiate those with occult cirrhosis, who may be considered ineligible for kidney transplant alone due to the risk of clinical decompensation post-transplant [135]. Among those with history of remote infection, evidence by detectable Hep-B surface and core antibodies, but without detectable surface antigen or viral DNA, the risk of viral reactivation is <5%, but has been reported [135].

Those without a history of Hep-B immunity should be vaccinated prior to transplant, ideally early in their course of renal failure to maximize their response to vaccination, as the seroconversion rate among patients on dialysis has been reported as between 50 and 60% [146]. In those completing the vaccination series without successful protective seroconversion, defined as a level of Hep-B surface antibody >10 mIU/mL, a booster series may be considered to try and establish protective immunity.

For those with chronic Hep-B infection (Hep-B surface antigen positive) who go on to transplant, it has been recommended that an antiviral agent be started prior to, or at the time of transplant, and continued indefinitely [135]. Limivudine is perhaps the best studied agent, but is associated with a high rate of resistance with long term exposure, and so other agents may be considered, including entecavir or tenofovir, among others. Those with remote resolved infection (Hep-B surface antigen negative, surface and core antibody positive) are at low risk for reactivation, and antiviral prophylaxis is optional but regular monitoring for Hep-B surface antigen, Hep B DNA, and ALT is recommended every 1–3 months with antivirals initiated if virus is detected by either assay [135].

Another important consideration in transplantation is the Hep-B status of the donor. For those receiving an organ from a Hep-B surface antigen positive donor, it is recommended that prophylactic Hep-B immunoglobulin (HBIG) and antiviral therapy be administered, regardless of host immunity, although it may be best to avoid transplant from an actively infected donor into a Hep-B naive recipient. It is suggested that if the recipient remains Hep-B surface antigen negative and Hep-B DNA negative, that consideration may be given to stopping HBIG after 6–12 months, though antiviral therapy should be given indefinitely [135]. For those with existing immunity receiving a Hep-B core positive, but surface antigen negative organ, the risk of infection is felt to be negligible and no prophylaxis is recommended. For those without immunity receiving a core positive, surface antigen negative organ, antiviral therapy or HBIG should be considered [135].

Case 6 Review

This patient has chronic Hep-B infection. His evaluation will require liver biopsy to assess for occult liver disease, which is suggested by his abnormal liver function tests. He is at risk for progressive liver disease following transplant, and so antiviral therapy and HBIG are recommended post-transplant. Additionally, it would be reasonable to follow the patient's liver function tests on a regular basis following the transplant event. Lumivudine has the most evidence to support its use in this situation, but with a high rate of resistance, around 20%, a more potent antiviral may be considered in those with a high viral load or advanced fibrosis [135]

Case 7

You are asked to consult on a transplant patient hospitalized with cough and altered mental status. He is 6 years out from liver transplant for alcoholic cirrhosis, and 6 months out from renal transplantation for end-stage kidney disease attributed to calcineurin inhibitor toxicity and multiple episode of acute kidney injury. His cough has been present for 6-weeks, and unresponsive to a 5-day course of azithromycin and a 10 day course of levofloxacin. On exam he is febrile to 38.2 °C, normotensive, somnolent, with a disconjugate gaze.

What pathogens should be considered and what are the next steps in his evaluation?

Central Nervous System Infection

The transplant physician must have a high clinical suspicion for CNS infection when evaluating patients with altered mental status, headache, or clinically apparent infection around the head and neck region. Viral pathogens to consider include CMV, herpes simplex (HSV), JC virus, and VZV. Common bacterial infections include pneumococcus, *Listeria monocytogenes*, nocardia, *Borrelia burgdorferi*, and risckettsial organisms. Metastatic fungi should be considered as well, and they include aspergillus, histoplasma, and importantly cryptococcus. Noninfectious causes of CNS symptoms should be considered as well, and include lymphoma or other malignancy or drugs, including calcineurin inhibitor toxicity.

With a broad differential, timely lumbar puncture and brain imaging are essential, along with peripheral blood cultures, and evaluation of any additional foci of infection, such as lung imaging. In the first year post transplant, when the patient is highly immune-suppressed and at risk for nosocomial and opportunistic infections, broad spectrum empiric treatment should be considered, and may include coverage for pneumococcus (e.g., ceftriaxone and vancomycin), HSV (e.g., acyclovir), cryptococcus (e.g., fluconazole or amphotericin), and listeria (e.g., ampicillin) while cultures are pending. Depending on the clinical circumstances, consideration should be given to reducing the patient's immune suppression, including cessation of their antimetabolite or calcineurin inhibitor.

In cases where CNS infection is suspected, timely consultation of an infectious disease specialist is recommended.

Respiratory Tract Infection

Given the diversity of organisms responsible for respiratory tract infection in the transplant population, a detailed discussion is beyond the scope of this chapter. However, several important principles are worth highlighting. First, as outlined in the opening section, it is important to consider the host's susceptibility to infection when generating the differential diagnosis, including recent use of immune suppressants and antibacterial prophylaxis. For example, high-dose steroids are a risk factor for pneumocystis pneumonia, but pneumocystis infection is rare in the setting of tmx-sulfa prophylaxis [147]. Second, given the breadth of potential pathogens and the possibility for multiple pathogens, it is important to consider early use of all available diagnostics in sick individuals and those with chronic progressive infection, including cross-sectional imaging, bronchosopy, and tissue biopsy, which may increase the sensitivity and specificity of the evaluation [148]. In *Case 1* presented earlier, lung biopsy provided a diagnosis of CMV pneumonitis and nocardia. Third, pay close attention to clinical clues that may suggest potential etiologies. For example, the acute onset of pulmonary infiltrate with fever is more consistent with bacterial infection, while the subacute development of multifocal infection suggests progression of more indolent diseases such as fungus or nocardia [149]. Cavitary lesions on imaging may suggest nocardia, aspergillus, staphylococcus, klebsiella, or pseudomonal infections [149].

Case 7 Review

This patient underwent detailed evaluation, guided by the focality of his symptoms, and prioritized by their urgency. Because of the broad differential diagnosis, and the possibility for multiple superimposed infectious processes, diagnoses were sought for each of the abnormal findings. Prompt noninvasive imaging including high-resolution CT imaging of his chest and magnetic-resonance imaging (MRI) of his brain were performed to

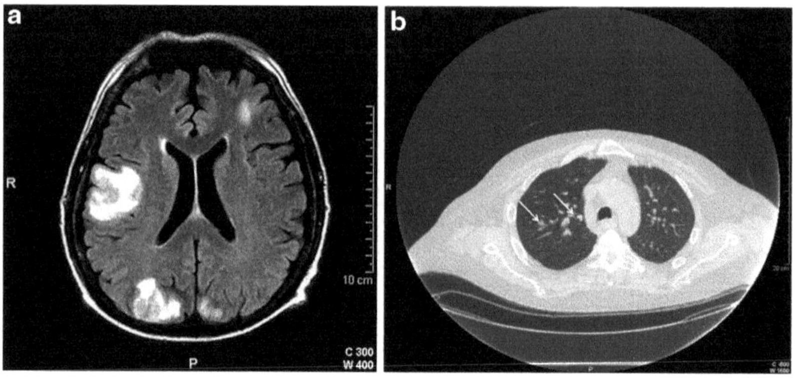

Fig. 37.5 (**a**) This brain MRI from Case 7 revealed several ring enhancing lesions, concerning for infection. The brain biopsy ultimately revealed nocardia. (**b**) This chest-CT from Case 7 reveals multiple cavitary lesions (*white arrows*). Biopsy revealed nocardia

assess his pulmonary symptoms and altered mental status. Chest imaging revealed multiple bilateral cavitating lesions, as did the brain MRI (Fig. 37.5). Broncoscopy, lumbar puncture, and ultimately brain biopsy were pursued.

This patient ultimately had a single diagnosis of disseminated nocardia identified on lung and brain pathology. He was started on therapy with high dose tmx-sulfa and concurrent meropenem directed by sensitivities. After 2 weeks, the patient was awake, alert, and interactive, with some improvement in his gaze.

Conclusion

It is important for the practicing nephrologist to have a sound understanding of common risk factors and causes of infection among transplant candidates and transplant recipients. In the pre-transplant population, this knowledge lends itself to identifying candidates who are eligible for transplant, including those with hepatitis B, hepatitis C, or HIV. Further, it may guide preparations for transplant, including administration of proper vaccinations. Following the transplant event, this information lends itself to reducing the risk of infection, as well as early diagnosis and treatment of active infection. In order to remain current with state-of-the-art prevention, diagnostic, and treatment strategies, and to the augment information provided in this chapter, the reader is encouraged to seek out the attached references, and to visit the Web sites of relevant professional organizations including the American Society of Transplantation (AST) and the Infectious Disease Society of America (IDSA).

References

1. Dharnidharka VR, Caillard S, Agodoa LY, Abbott KC. Infection frequency and profile in different age groups of kidney transplant recipients. Transplantation. 2006;81(12):1662–7.
2. U S Renal Data System, USRDS 2010 annual data report: atlas of chronic kidney disease and end-stage renal disease in the United States, National Institutes of Health, National Institute of Diabetes and Digestive and Kidney Diseases, Bethesda, MD, 2010.
3. Bender FH, Holley JL. Most nephrologists are primary care providers for chronic dialysis patients: results of a national survey. Am J Kidney Dis. 1996;28(1):67–71.
4. Israni AK, Snyder JJ, Skeans MA, Tuomari AV, Maclean JR, Kasiske BL. Who is caring for kidney transplant patients? Variation by region, transplant center, and patient characteristics. Am J Nephrol. 2009;30(5):430–9.
5. San Juan R, Aguado JM, Lumbreras C, et al. Incidence, clinical characteristics and risk factors of late infection in solid organ transplant recipients: data from the RESITRA study group. Am J Transplant. 2007;7(4):964–71.
6. Fishman JA. Infection in solid-organ transplant recipients. N Engl J Med. 2007;357(25):2601–14.
7. Parasuraman R, Samarapungavan D, Venkat KK. Updated principles and clinical caveats in the management of infection in renal transplant recipients. Transplant Rev (Orlando). 2010;24(2):43–51.
8. Fishman JA. Introduction: infection in solid organ transplant recipients. Am J Transplant. 2009;9 Suppl 4:S3–6.

9. Weinhandl ED, Snyder JJ, Israni AK, Kasiske BL. Effect of comorbidity adjustment on CMS criteria for kidney transplant center performance. Am J Transplant. 2009;9(3):506–16.
10. Menezes FG, Wey SB, Peres CA, Medina-Pestana JO, Camargo LF. Risk factors for surgical site infection in kidney transplant recipients. Infect Control Hosp Epidemiol. 2008;29(8):771–3.
11. Arozullah AM, Khuri SF, Henderson WG, Daley J. Development and validation of a multifactorial risk index for predicting postoperative pneumonia after major noncardiac surgery. Ann Intern Med. 2001;135(10):847–57.
12. Sallee M, Rafat C, Zahar JR, et al. Cyst infections in patients with autosomal dominant polycystic kidney disease. Clin J Am Soc Nephrol. 2009;4(7):1183–9.
13. Kabler RL, Cerny JC. Pre-transplant urologic investigation and treatment of end stage renal disease. J Urol. 1983;129(3):475–8.
14. Tsunoyama K, Ishida H, Omoto K, Shimizu T, Shirakawa H, Tanabe K. Bladder function of end-stage renal disease patients. Int J Urol. 2010;17(9):791–5.
15. Hurst FP, Neff RT, Falta EM, et al. Incidence, predictors, and associated outcomes of prostatism after kidney transplantation. Clin J Am Soc Nephrol. 2009;4(2):329–36.
16. Wasse H, Speckman RA, Frankenfield DL, Rocco MV, McClellan WM. Predictors of delayed transition from central venous catheter use to permanent vascular access among ESRD patients. Am J Kidney Dis. 2007;49(2):276–83.
17. Allon M. Dialysis catheter-related bacteremia: treatment and prophylaxis. Am J Kidney Dis. 2004;44(5):779–91.
18. U.S. Renal Data System, USRDS 2010 annual data report: atlas of end-stage renal disease in the United States, National Institutes of Health, National Institute of Diabetes and Digestive and Kidney Diseases, Bethesda, MD, 2009. http://www.usrds.org. Accessed 24 Mar 2011.
19. Marvin MR, Droogan C, Sawinski D, Cohen DJ, Hardy MA. Administration of rabbit antithymocyte globulin (thymoglobulin) in ambulatory renal-transplant patients. Transplantation. 2003;75(4):488–9.
20. Stamm WE. Catheter-associated urinary tract infections: epidemiology, pathogenesis, and prevention. Am J Med. 1991;91(3B):65S–71.
21. Rabkin DG, Stifelman MD, Birkhoff J, et al. Early catheter removal decreases incidence of urinary tract infections in renal transplant recipients. Transplant Proc. 1998;30(8):4314–6.
22. Wilson CH, Bhatti AA, Rix DA, Manas DM. Routine intraoperative ureteric stenting for kidney transplant recipients. Cochrane Database Syst Rev. 2005(4): CD004925.
23. Jolly EC, Adshead JM, Farrington K. The retained stent: forgotten but not gone. Kidney Int. 2010;77(3):260.
24. Coulthard MG, Keir MJ. Reflux nephropathy in kidney transplants, demonstrated by dimercaptosuccinic acid scanning. Transplantation. 2006;82(2):205–10.
25. Dunn SP, Vinocur CD, Hanevold C, Wagner CW, Weintraub WH. Pyelonephritis following pediatric renal transplant: increased incidence with vesicoureteral reflux. J Pediatr Surg. 1987;22(12):1095–9.
26. Inoue T, Satoh S, Saito M, et al. Correlations between pretransplant dialysis duration, bladder capacity, and prevalence of vesicoureteral reflux to the graft. Transplantation. 2011.
27. Khauli RB, Stoff JS, Lovewell T, Ghavamian R, Baker S. Post-transplant lymphoceles: a critical look into the risk factors, pathophysiology and management. J Urol. 1993;150(1):22–6.
28. Pollak R, Veremis SA, Maddux MS, Mozes MF. The natural history of and therapy for perirenal fluid collections following renal transplantation. J Urol. 1988;140(4): 716–20.
29. Sollinger HW, Odorico JS, Becker YT, D'Alessandro AM, Pirsch JD. One thousand simultaneous pancreas-kidney transplants at a single center with 22-year follow-up. Ann Surg. 2009;250(4):618–30.
30. Halloran PF. Immunosuppressive drugs for kidney transplantation. N Engl J Med. 2004;351(26):2715–29.
31. Bustami RT, Ojo AO, Wolfe RA, et al. Immunosuppression and the risk of post-transplant malignancy among cadaveric first kidney transplant recipients. Am J Transplant. 2004;4(1):87–93.
32. Webster AC, Ruster LP, McGee R, et al. Interleukin 2 receptor antagonists for kidney transplant recipients. Cochrane Database Syst Rev. 2010(1):CD003897.
33. Yale SH, Limper AH. Pneumocystis carinii pneumonia in patients without acquired immunodeficiency syndrome: associated illness and prior corticosteroid therapy. Mayo Clin Proc. 1996;71(1):5–13.
34. Tiong HY, Flechner SM, Zhou L, et al. A systematic approach to minimizing wound problems for de novo sirolimus-treated kidney transplant recipients. Transplantation. 2009;87(2):296–302.
35. A blinded, randomized clinical trial of mycophenolate mofetil for the prevention of acute rejection in cadaveric renal transplantation. The Tricontinental Mycophenolate Mofetil Renal Transplantation Study Group. Transplantation. 1996;61(7):1029–37.
36. Placebo-controlled study of mycophenolate mofetil combined with cyclosporin and corticosteroids for prevention of acute rejection. European Mycophenolate Mofetil Cooperative Study Group. Lancet. 1995;345(8961):1321–25.
37. Errasti P, Izquierdo D, Martin P, et al. Pneumonitis associated with mammalian target of rapamycin inhibitors in renal transplant recipients: a single-center experience. Transplant Proc. 2010;42(8):3053–4.
38. Fischer SA, Avery RK. Screening of donor and recipient prior to solid organ transplantation. Am J Transplant. 2009;9 Suppl 4:S7–18.
39. Kasiske BL, Cangro CB, Hariharan S, et al. The evaluation of renal transplantation candidates: clinical practice guidelines. Am J Transplant. 2001;1 Suppl 2:3–95.
40. Knoll GA, Tankersley MR, Lee JY, Julian BA, Curtis JJ. The impact of renal transplantation on survival in hepatitis C-positive end-stage renal disease patients. Am J Kidney Dis. 1997;29(4):608–14.

41. Roth D, Gaynor JJ, Reddy KR, et al. Effect of kidney transplantation on outcomes among patients with hepatitis C. J Am Soc Nephrol. 2011;22(6):1152–60.
42. Pereira BJ, Natov SN, Bouthot BA, et al. Effects of hepatitis C infection and renal transplantation on survival in end-stage renal disease. The New England Organ Bank Hepatitis C Study Group. Kidney Int. 1998;53(5):1374–81.
43. Zylberberg H, Nalpas B, Carnot F, et al. Severe evolution of chronic hepatitis C in renal transplantation: a case control study. Nephrol Dial Transplant. 2002;17(1):129–33.
44. Humar A, Snydman D. Cytomegalovirus in solid organ transplant recipients. Am J Transplant. 2009;9 Suppl 4:S78–86.
45. Allen U, Preiksaitis J. Epstein-barr virus and post-transplant lymphoproliferative disorder in solid organ transplant recipients. Am J Transplant. 2009;9 Suppl 4:S87–96.
46. Danzinger-Isakov L, Kumar D. Guidelines for vaccination of solid organ transplant candidates and recipients. Am J Transplant. 2009;9 Suppl 4:S258–62.
47. DaRoza G, Loewen A, Djurdjev O, et al. Stage of chronic kidney disease predicts seroconversion after hepatitis B immunization: earlier is better. Am J Kidney Dis. 2003;42(6):1184–92.
48. Birdwell KA, Ikizler MR, Sannella EC, et al. Decreased antibody response to influenza vaccination in kidney transplant recipients: a prospective cohort study. Am J Kidney Dis. 2009;54(1):112–21.
49. Gangappa S, Kokko KE, Carlson LM, et al. Immune responsiveness and protective immunity after transplantation. Transpl Int. 2008;21(4):293–303.
50. Weber DJ, Rutala WA. Immunization of immunocompromised persons. Immunol Allergy Clin North Am. 2003;23(4):605–34, v–vi.
51. General recommendations on immunization – recommendations of the Advisory Committee on Immunization Practices (ACIP). MMWR Recomm Rep. 2011;60(2): 1–64.
52. Scharpe J, Evenepoel P, Maes B, et al. Influenza vaccination is efficacious and safe in renal transplant recipients. Am J Transplant. 2008;8(2):332–7.
53. Candon S, Thervet E, Lebon P, et al. Humoral and cellular immune responses after influenza vaccination in kidney transplant recipients. Am J Transplant. 2009;9(10):2346–54.
54. Midtvedt K, Hartmann A, Midtvedt T, Brekke IB. Routine perioperative antibiotic prophylaxis in renal transplantation. Nephrol Dial Transplant. 1998;13(7):1637–41.
55. Bootsma AM, Laguna-Pes MP, Geerlings SE, Goossens A. Antibiotic prophylaxis in urologic procedures: a systematic review. Eur Urol. 2008;54(6):1270–86.
56. Tilney NL, Strom TB, Vineyard GC, Merrill JP. Factors contributing to the declining mortality rate in renal transplantation. N Engl J Med. 1978;299(24):1321–5.
57. Cohen J, Rees AJ, Williams G. A prospective randomized controlled trial of perioperative antibiotic prophylaxis in renal transplantation. J Hosp Infect. 1988;11(4):357–63.
58. Laftavi MR, Rostami R, Feng L, et al. The role of antibiotic prophylaxis in the new era of immunosuppression. Transplant Proc. 2011;43(2):533–5.
59. Stephan RN, Munschauer CE, Kumar MS. Surgical wound infection in renal transplantation: outcome data in 102 consecutive patients without perioperative systemic antibiotic coverage. Arch Surg. 1997;132(12):1315–18; discussion 1318–1319.
60. Fox BC, Sollinger HW, Belzer FO, Maki DG. A prospective, randomized, double-blind study of trimethoprim-sulfamethoxazole for prophylaxis of infection in renal transplantation: clinical efficacy, absorption of trimethoprim-sulfamethoxazole, effects on the microflora, and the cost-benefit of prophylaxis. Am J Med. 1990;89(3):255–74.
61. Green H, Paul M, Vidal L, Leibovici L. Prophylaxis for pneumocystis pneumonia (PCP) in non-HIV immunocompromised patients. Cochrane Database Syst Rev. 2007(3):CD005590.
62. HIV transmitted from a living organ donor – New York City, 2009. MMWR Morb Mortal Wkly Rep. 2011;60(10):297–301.
63. Sharma AK, Smith G, Smith D, et al. Clinical outcome of cadaveric renal allografts contaminated before transplantation. Transpl Int. 2005;18(7):824–7.
64. Garzoni C. Multiply resistant gram-positive bacteria methicillin-resistant, vancomycin-intermediate and vancomycin-resistant Staphylococcus aureus (MRSA, VISA, VRSA) in solid organ transplant recipients. Am J Transplant. 2009;9 Suppl 4:S41–9.
65. Munoz P. Multiply resistant gram-positive bacteria: vancomycin-resistant enterococcus in solid organ transplant recipients. Am J Transplant. 2009;9 Suppl 4:S50–6.
66. van Delden C, Blumberg EA. Multidrug resistant gram-negative bacteria in solid organ transplant recipients. Am J Transplant. 2009;9 Suppl 4:S27–34.
67. Pappas PG, Silveira FP. Candida in solid organ transplant recipients. Am J Transplant. 2009;9 Suppl 4:S173–9.
68. Dubberke ER, Riddle DJ. Clostridium difficile in solid organ transplant recipients. Am J Transplant. 2009;9 Suppl 4:S35–40.
69. Gardner SD, Field AM, Coleman DV, Hulme B. New human papovavirus (B.K.) isolated from urine after renal transplantation. Lancet. 1971;1(7712):1253–7.
70. Mengel M, Marwedel M, Radermacher J, et al. Incidence of polyomavirus-nephropathy in renal allografts: influence of modern immunosuppressive drugs. Nephrol Dial Transplant. 2003;18(6):1190–6.
71. Pahari A, Rees L. BK virus-associated renal problems – clinical implications. Pediatr Nephrol. 2003;18(8):743–8.
72. Nickeleit V, Klimkait T, Binet IF, et al. Testing for polyomavirus type BK DNA in plasma to identify renal-allograft recipients with viral nephropathy. N Engl J Med. 2000;342(18):1309–15.
73. Mylonakis E, Goes N, Rubin RH, Cosimi AB, Colvin RB, Fishman JA. BK virus in solid organ transplant

recipients: an emerging syndrome. Transplantation. 2001;72(10):1587–92.

74. Petrogiannis-Haliotis T, Sakoulas G, Kirby J, et al. BK-related polyomavirus vasculopathy in a renal-transplant recipient. N Engl J Med. 2001;345(17):1250–5.
75. Peinemann F, de Villiers EM, Dorries K, Adams O, Vogeli TA, Burdach S. Clinical course and treatment of haemorrhagic cystitis associated with BK type of human polyomavirus in nine paediatric recipients of allogeneic bone marrow transplants. Eur J Pediatr. 2000;159(3):182–8.
76. Schmid H, Burg M, Kretzler M, Banas B, Grone HJ, Kliem V. BK virus associated nephropathy in native kidneys of a heart allograft recipient. Am J Transplant. 2005;5(6):1562–8.
77. Munoz P, Fogeda M, Bouza E, Verde E, Palomo J, Banares R. Prevalence of BK virus replication among recipients of solid organ transplants. Clin Infect Dis. 2005;41(12):1720–5.
78. Egli A, Helmersen DS, Taub K, Hirsch HH, Johnson A. Renal failure five years after lung transplantation due to polyomavirus BK-associated nephropathy. Am J Transplant. 2010;10(10):2324–30.
79. Brennan DC, Agha I, Bohl DL, et al. Incidence of BK with tacrolimus versus cyclosporine and impact of preemptive immunosuppression reduction. Am J Transplant. 2005;5(3):582–94.
80. Vasudev B, Hariharan S, Hussain SA, Zhu YR, Bresnahan BA, Cohen EP. BK virus nephritis: risk factors, timing, and outcome in renal transplant recipients. Kidney Int. 2005;68(4):1834–9.
81. Babel N, Fendt J, Karaivanov S, et al. Sustained BK viruria as an early marker for the development of BKV-associated nephropathy: analysis of 4,128 urine and serum samples. Transplantation. 2009;88(1):89–95.
82. Hirsch HH, Knowles W, Dickenmann M, et al. Prospective study of polyomavirus type BK replication and nephropathy in renal-transplant recipients. N Engl J Med. 2002;347(7):488–96.
83. Singh HK, Andreoni KA, Madden V, et al. Presence of urinary Haufen accurately predicts polyomavirus nephropathy. J Am Soc Nephrol. 2009;20(2):416–27.
84. Drachenberg CB, Papadimitriou JC, Hirsch HH, et al. Histological patterns of polyomavirus nephropathy: correlation with graft outcome and viral load. Am J Transplant. 2004;4(12):2082–92.
85. Hirsch HH, Randhawa P. BK virus in solid organ transplant recipients. Am J Transplant. 2009;9 Suppl 4:S136–46.
86. Nickeleit V, Hirsch HH, Binet IF, et al. Polyomavirus infection of renal allograft recipients: from latent infection to manifest disease. J Am Soc Nephrol. 1999;10(5):1080–9.
87. Drachenberg RC, Drachenberg CB, Papadimitriou JC, et al. Morphological spectrum of polyoma virus disease in renal allografts: diagnostic accuracy of urine cytology. Am J Transplant. 2001;1(4):373–81.
88. Schaub S, Hirsch HH, Dickenmann M, et al. Reducing immunosuppression preserves allograft function in presumptive and definitive polyomavirus-associated nephropathy. Am J Transplant. 2010;10(12):2615–23.
89. Hardinger KL, Koch MJ, Bohl DJ, Storch GA, Brennan DC. BK-virus and the impact of pre-emptive immunosuppression reduction: 5-year results. Am J Transplant. 2010;10(2):407–15.
90. De Keyzer K, Van Laecke S, Peeters P, Vanholder R. Human cytomegalovirus and kidney transplantation: a clinician's update. Am J Kidney Dis. 2011;58(1): 118–26.
91. Schnitzler MA, Lowell JA, Hardinger KL, Boxerman SB, Bailey TC, Brennan DC. The association of cytomegalovirus sero-pairing with outcomes and costs following cadaveric renal transplantation prior to the introduction of oral ganciclovir CMV prophylaxis. Am J Transplant. 2003;3(4):445–51.
92. Sagedal S, Hartmann A, Nordal KP, et al. Impact of early cytomegalovirus infection and disease on long-term recipient and kidney graft survival. Kidney Int. 2004;66(1):329–37.
93. Brennan DC. Cytomegalovirus in renal transplantation. J Am Soc Nephrol. 2001;12(4):848–55.
94. Staras SA, Dollard SC, Radford KW, Flanders WD, Pass RF, Cannon MJ. Seroprevalence of cytomegalovirus infection in the United States, 1988–1994. Clin Infect Dis. 2006;43(9):1143–51.
95. Bate SL, Dollard SC, Cannon MJ. Cytomegalovirus seroprevalence in the United States: the national health and nutrition examination surveys, 1988–2004. Clin Infect Dis. 2010;50(11):1439–47.
96. Crough T, Khanna R. Immunobiology of human cytomegalovirus: from bench to bedside. Clin Microbiol Rev. 2009;22(1):76–98, Table of Contents.
97. Handsfield HH, Chandler SH, Caine VA, et al. Cytomegalovirus infection in sex partners: evidence for sexual transmission. J Infect Dis. 1985;151(2): 344–8.
98. Kotton CN, Kumar D, Caliendo AM, et al. International consensus guidelines on the management of cytomegalovirus in solid organ transplantation. Transplantation. 2010;89(7):779–95.
99. Lowance D, Neumayer HH, Legendre CM, et al. (1999) Valacyclovir for the prevention of cytomegalovirus disease after renal transplantation. International Valacyclovir Cytomegalovirus Prophylaxis Transplantation Study Group. N Engl J Med. 1999;340(19):1462–70.
100. Sagedal S, Nordal KP, Hartmann A, et al. The impact of cytomegalovirus infection and disease on rejection episodes in renal allograft recipients. Am J Transplant. 2002;2(9):850–6.
101. Reischig T, Jindra P, Hes O, Svecova M, Klaboch J, Treska V. Valacyclovir prophylaxis versus preemptive valganciclovir therapy to prevent cytomegalovirus disease after renal transplantation. Am J Transplant. 2008;8(1):69–77.
102. Khoury JA, Storch GA, Bohl DL, et al. Prophylactic versus preemptive oral valganciclovir for the management of cytomegalovirus infection in adult renal

transplant recipients. Am J Transplant. 2006;6(9):2134–43.

103. Tian JH, Wang X, Yang KH, Liu AP, Luo XF, Zhang J. Induction with and without antithymocyte globulin combined with cyclosporine/tacrolimus-based immunosuppression in renal transplantation: a meta-analysis of randomized controlled trials. Transplant Proc. 2009;41(9):3671–6.
104. Preiksaitis JK, Brennan DC, Fishman J, Allen U. Canadian society of transplantation consensus workshop on cytomegalovirus management in solid organ transplantation final report. Am J Transplant. 2005;5(2):218–27.
105. Small LN, Lau J, Snydman DR. Preventing post-organ transplantation cytomegalovirus disease with ganciclovir: a meta-analysis comparing prophylactic and preemptive therapies. Clin Infect Dis. 2006;43(7):869–80.
106. Kalil AC, Levitsky J, Lyden E, Stoner J, Freifeld AG. Meta-analysis: the efficacy of strategies to prevent organ disease by cytomegalovirus in solid organ transplant recipients. Ann Intern Med. 2005;143(12):870–80.
107. Kliem V, Fricke L, Wollbrink T, Burg M, Radermacher J, Rohde F. Improvement in long-term renal graft survival due to CMV prophylaxis with oral ganciclovir: results of a randomized clinical trial. Am J Transplant. 2008;8(5):975–83.
108. Andrews PA, Emery VC, Newstead C. Summary of the British Transplantation Society guidelines for the prevention and management of CMV disease after solid organ transplantation. Transplantation. 2011;92(11):1181–7.
109. Asberg A, Humar A, Rollag H, et al. Oral valganciclovir is noninferior to intravenous ganciclovir for the treatment of cytomegalovirus disease in solid organ transplant recipients. Am J Transplant. 2007;7(9):2106–13.
110. Andreone P, Gramenzi A, Lorenzini S, et al. Posttransplantation lymphoproliferative disorders. Arch Intern Med. 2003;163(17):1997–2004.
111. Opelz G, Daniel V, Naujokat C, Dohler B. Epidemiology of pretransplant EBV and CMV serostatus in relation to posttransplant non-Hodgkin lymphoma. Transplantation. 2009;88(8):962–7.
112. Kotton CN, Fishman JA. Viral infection in the renal transplant recipient. J Am Soc Nephrol. 2005;16(6):1758–74.
113. Luzuriaga K, Sullivan JL. Infectious mononucleosis. N Engl J Med. 2010;362(21):1993–2000.
114. Bruu AL, Hjetland R, Holter E, et al. Evaluation of 12 commercial tests for detection of Epstein-Barr virus-specific and heterophile antibodies. Clin Diagn Lab Immunol. 2000;7(3):451–6.
115. Nourse JP, Jones K, Gandhi MK. Epstein-Barr Virus-related post-transplant lymphoproliferative disorders: pathogenetic insights for targeted therapy. Am J Transplant. 2011;11(5):888–95.
116. Hsi ED, Picken MM, Alkan S. Post-transplantation lymphoproliferative disorder of the NK-cell type: a case report and review of the literature. Mod Pathol. 1998;11(5):479–84.
117. Petit B, Le Meur Y, Jaccard A, et al. Influence of host-recipient origin on clinical aspects of posttransplantation lymphoproliferative disorders in kidney transplantation. Transplantation. 2002;73(2):265–71.
118. Dockrell DH, Strickler JG, Paya CV. Epstein-Barr virus-induced T cell lymphoma in solid organ transplant recipients. Clin Infect Dis. 1998;26(1):180–2.
119. Mucha K, Foroncewicz B, Ziarkiewicz-Wroblewska B, Krawczyk M, Lerut J, Paczek L. Post-transplant lymphoproliferative disorder in view of the new WHO classification: a more rational approach to a protean disease? Nephrol Dial Transplant. 2010;25(7):2089–98.
120. Opelz G, Dohler B. Lymphomas after solid organ transplantation: a collaborative transplant study report. Am J Transplant. 2004;4(2):222–30.
121. Cockfield SM. Identifying the patient at risk for post-transplant lymphoproliferative disorder. Transpl Infect Dis. 2001;3(2):70–8.
122. Caillard S, Dharnidharka V, Agodoa L, Bohen E, Abbott K. Posttransplant lymphoproliferative disorders after renal transplantation in the United States in era of modern immunosuppression. Transplantation. 2005;80(9):1233–43.
123. Tsai DE, Douglas L, Andreadis C, et al. EBV PCR in the diagnosis and monitoring of posttransplant lymphoproliferative disorder: results of a two-arm prospective trial. Am J Transplant. 2008;8(5):1016–24.
124. Lim WH, Russ GR, Coates PT. Review of Epstein-Barr virus and post-transplant lymphoproliferative disorder post-solid organ transplantation. Nephrology (Carlton). 2006;11(4):355–66.
125. Paya CV, Fung JJ, Nalesnik MA, et al. Epstein-Barr virus-induced posttransplant lymphoproliferative disorders. ASTS/ASTP EBV-PTLD Task Force and The Mayo Clinic Organized International Consensus Development Meeting. Transplantation. 1999;68(10):1517–25.
126. Tsai DE, Hardy CL, Tomaszewski JE, et al. Reduction in immunosuppression as initial therapy for posttransplant lymphoproliferative disorder: analysis of prognostic variables and long-term follow-up of 42 adult patients. Transplantation. 2001;71(8):1076–88.
127. Choquet S, Leblond V, Herbrecht R, et al. Efficacy and safety of rituximab in B-cell post-transplantation lymphoproliferative disorders: results of a prospective multicenter phase 2 study. Blood. 2006;107(8):3053–7.
128. Darenkov IA, Marcarelli MA, Basadonna GP, et al. Reduced incidence of Epstein-Barr virus-associated posttransplant lymphoproliferative disorder using preemptive antiviral therapy. Transplantation. 1997;64(6):848–52.
129. Leblond V, Dhedin N, Mamzer Bruneel MF, et al. Identification of prognostic factors in 61 patients with posttransplantation lymphoproliferative disorders. J Clin Oncol. 2001;19(3):772–8.

130. Evens AM, David KA, Helenowski I, et al. Multicenter analysis of 80 solid organ transplantation recipients with post-transplantation lymphoproliferative disease: outcomes and prognostic factors in the modern era. J Clin Oncol. 2010;28(6):1038–46.
131. Palella Jr FJ, Delaney KM, Moorman AC, et al. Declining morbidity and mortality among patients with advanced human immunodeficiency virus infection. HIV Outpatient Study Investigators. N Engl J Med. 1998;338(13):853–60.
132. Roland ME, Barin B, Carlson L, et al. HIV-infected liver and kidney transplant recipients: 1- and 3-year outcomes. Am J Transplant. 2008;8(2):355–65.
133. Kumar MS, Sierka DR, Damask AM, et al. Safety and success of kidney transplantation and concomitant immunosuppression in HIV-positive patients. Kidney Int. 2005;67(4):1622–9.
134. Stock PG, Barin B, Murphy B, et al. Outcomes of kidney transplantation in HIV-infected recipients. N Engl J Med. 2010;363(21):2004–14.
135. Levitsky J, Doucette K. Viral hepatitis in solid organ transplant recipients. Am J Transplant. 2009;9 Suppl 4:S116–30.
136. Pereira BJ, Wright TL, Schmid CH, et al. Screening and confirmatory testing of cadaver organ donors for hepatitis C virus infection: a U.S. National Collaborative Study. Kidney Int. 1994;46(3):886–92.
137. Lonze BE, Dagher NN, Liu M, et al. Outcomes of renal transplants from Centers for Disease Control and Prevention high-risk donors with prospective recipient viral testing: a single-center experience. Arch Surg. 2011;146(11):1261–6.
138. Maluf DG, Fisher RA, King AL, et al. Hepatitis C virus infection and kidney transplantation: predictors of patient and graft survival. Transplantation. 2007;83(7):853–7.
139. Kokado Y, Takahara S, Ichimaru N, et al. Clinical outcome of HCV infection after renal transplantation. Transplant Proc. 2000;32(7):1940–3.
140. Mathurin P, Mouquet C, Poynard T, et al. Impact of hepatitis B and C virus on kidney transplantation outcome. Hepatology. 1999;29(1):257–63.
141. Kamar N, Rostaing L, Selves J, et al. Natural history of hepatitis C virus-related liver fibrosis after renal transplantation. Am J Transplant. 2005;5(7):1704–12.
142. Terrault NA, Adey DB. The kidney transplant recipient with hepatitis C infection: pre- and posttransplantation treatment. Clin J Am Soc Nephrol. 2007;2(3):563–75.
143. Gordon CE, Uhlig K, Lau J, Schmid CH, Levey AS, Wong JB. Interferon treatment in hemodialysis patients with chronic hepatitis C virus infection: a systematic review of the literature and meta-analysis of treatment efficacy and harms. Am J Kidney Dis. 2008;51(2):263–77.
144. Fabrizi F, Martin P, Dixit V, Kanwal F, Dulai G. HBsAg seropositive status and survival after renal transplantation: meta-analysis of observational studies. Am J Transplant. 2005;5(12):2913–21.
145. Burdick RA, Bragg-Gresham JL, Woods JD, et al. Patterns of hepatitis B prevalence and seroconversion in hemodialysis units from three continents: the DOPPS. Kidney Int. 2003;63(6):2222–9.
146. Propst T, Propst A, Lhotta K, Vogel W, Konig P. Reinforced intradermal hepatitis B vaccination in hemodialysis patients is superior in antibody response to intramuscular or subcutaneous vaccination. Am J Kidney Dis. 1998;32(6):1041–5.
147. Green H, Paul M, Vidal L, Leibovici L. Prophylaxis of Pneumocystis pneumonia in immunocompromised non-HIV-infected patients: systematic review and meta-analysis of randomized controlled trials. Mayo Clin Proc. 2007;82(9):1052–9.
148. Rano A, Agusti C, Jimenez P, et al. Pulmonary infiltrates in non-HIV immunocompromised patients: a diagnostic approach using non-invasive and bronchoscopic procedures. Thorax. 2001;56(5):379–87.
149. Morris PJ, Knechtle SJ. Kidney transplantation: principles and practice. 6th ed. Philadelphia, PA: Saunders/Elsevier; 2008.

Kidney Transplant Outcomes

38

Ankit Sakhuja, Neha Sehgal, Monica Vasudev and Brahm Vasudev

Case 1

A 25-year-old African-American man with past medical history of systemic lupus erythematosus (SLE) received a 0/6 HLA matched kidney transplant from a deceased donor. Four months post transplantation on routine screening his serum creatinine was elevated from a baseline value of 1.2 mg/dL–1.6 mg/dL. A kidney biopsy performed to elucidate the cause of transplant renal dysfunction revealed acute cellular rejection, BANFF 1a. He received three doses of IV solumedrol and 4 weeks later his serum creatinine was back to 1.2 mg/dL.

Case 2

A 65-year-old Caucasian woman with past medical history of Type 1 Diabetes Mellitus (T1DM) complicated by end stage renal disease (ESRD), status post 1/6 HLA match kidney transplant 6 years ago presented to the ER with chest pain and shortness of breath. She was diagnosed with an acute myocardial infarction. Her serum creatinine was stable at 1.4 mg/dL. She developed a fatal cardiac arrest in the ER.

Case 3

A 72-year-old African-American man with past medical history of ESRD secondary to hypertension status post 4/6 HLA match kidney transplant 8 years ago was seen in the clinic for follow-up. He was found have slowly progressive elevation of serum creatinine over the past 2 years from 1.8 mg/dL to a value of 4 mg/dL. He underwent a kidney biopsy which revealed calcineurin inhibitor (CNI) toxicity, severe interstitial fibrosis and tubular atrophy IFTA. Six months later he was restarted on dialysis.

Case 4

A 60-year-old Hispanic man with past medical history of ESRD secondary to diabetes and hypertension status post 3/6 HLA match kidney transplant 7 years ago was hospitalized with symptoms of hemoptysis and progressive weight loss. He had a history of 40 pack years of personal tobacco use. His serum creatinine was stable at 1.8 mg/mL. He was found to have

A. Sakhuja, M.D. • B. Vasudev, M.D. (✉)
Department of Internal Medicine, Medical College of Wisconsin,9200 W. Wisconsin Ave, Milwaukee, WI 53226, USA
e-mail: bvasudev@mcw.edu

N. Sehgal, M.D.
Division of Nephrology, Medical College of Wisconsin,9200 W. Wisconsin Ave, Milwaukee, WI 53226, USA

M. Vasudev, M.D.
Allergy and Clinical Immunology, Medical College of Wisconsin, 9200 W. Wisconsin Ave, Milwaukee, WI 53226, USA

E.V. Lerma and M. Rosner (eds.), *Clinical Decisions in Nephrology, Hypertension and Kidney Transplantation*, DOI 10.1007/978-1-4614-4454-1_38,

mediastinal lymphadenopathy and multiple lesions in his lung on his CT scan. The biopsy of the lesion showed small cell lung cancer. Given his poor prognosis he was discharged with home hospice.

Case 5

A 40-year-old Asian man had ESRD secondary to obstructive nephropathy status post 6/6 HLA matched living related kidney transplant 25 years ago from his brother, presented to the transplant clinic for routine follow-up. He was on prednisone and azathioprine for immunosuppression. His serum creatinine was stable at 1.3 mg/dL. His exam was stable. He was asked to come back for routine follow-up in 6 months.

Introduction

The transplantation of internal organs was not possible until Alexis Carrel invented the triangulation technique of vascular suture in the early 1900s. Despite such surgical advances, allotransplantation was uniformly unsuccessful. It was not until after the French immunologist Jean Dausset discovered the human leukocyte antigen (HLA) system in 1951 that physicians had a better understanding of the mechanisms responsible for allotransplantation failure. The proof of concept in humans came with the first successful kidney transplant that was performed between identical twins in 1954. It was around this time that the immunosuppressive properties of corticosteroids and azathioprine were discovered. Since then, there have been many advances in the field of kidney transplantation including improvement in surgical techniques and development of an armamentarium of immunosuppressive medications and immunological testing techniques [1].

Kidney transplantation was the first successful internal organ transplantation that was performed and today is the most common transplant performed worldwide. In the last three decades there have been substantial improvements in the short-term kidney graft survival and a steady improvement in the long-term kidney graft survival. Among the patients who are candidates for kidney transplantation, it is the best method of renal replacement therapy.

Short-Term and Long-Term Kidney Transplant Outcomes

In the early years, graft survival for HLA mismatched transplants was extremely poor. The major reason for graft failure in the first year after transplant was acute rejection, with others being primary non-function, recurrent renal disease, graft thrombosis, and death of the patient with a functioning graft. The availability of cyclosporine and muromonab-CD3 for prevention and treatment of acute rejections in 1980s greatly improved 1-year outcomes. Availability of newer maintenance immunosuppressive medications like mycophenolate mofetil (MMF) and tacrolimus in mid-1990s led to further reduction in episodes of acute rejection [2, 3]. In 1996, 51% of kidney transplant recipients were treated for acute rejection in the first year post transplantation, and in 2003 this number was down to 10–15% [4]. The reduction in acute rejection rates has been associated with significant improvements in 1-year graft as well as patient survival. According to the 2009 Organ Procurement and Transplantation Network (OPTN)/Scientific Registry of Transplant Recipients (SRTR) annual report the 1-year graft survival in US was 92% for standard criteria deceased donors and 96% for living donors. For the same time 1 year recipient survival was 96% for standard criteria deceased donor kidneys and 99% for living donors kidneys.

Death with a functioning kidney accounts for 40–45% cases of kidney transplant failure. The remaining 55–60% cases of transplant failure occur either early or late in the course of transplant. Common causes of early transplant failure include technical cause, acute rejection, recurrent disease, and BK virus nephropathy, while multifactorial interstitial fibrosis and tubular atrophy IFTA and calcineurin inhibitor toxicity are the common causes of late transplant failure.

Factors Affecting Kidney Transplant Outcomes

Primary Non-Function

The primary non-function of the kidney allograft can be related to technical issues related to surgery or due to thrombosis. With the improvement in the surgical techniques and the immunological and laboratory testing, this is now an uncommon cause of early transplant failure and accounts for less than 2% of the cases of transplant failure.

Delayed Graft Function

Delayed graft function (DGF) is defined as need for dialysis within the first week of transplantation. The risk factors for DGF include the warm and cold ischemia time (CIT), donor age, and donor comorbidities. Thus, extended criteria donor (ECD) kidneys and kidneys donated after cardiac death (DCD) have a higher risk of developing DGF. About 20% of deceased donor transplant recipients develop DGF and it has a negative impact on both short and long-term graft survival [5].

Acute Rejection

Acute rejection continues to be the major risk factor for chronic rejection, IFTA and kidney graft loss. With the availability of sensitive pre-transplant immunological testing like flow cytometry cross match, virtual cross match, use of pre-transplant plasmapheresis in cases of positive cross match, and use of potent induction and maintenance immunosuppressive agents, the incidence of both cellular and humoral rejection has decreased to 10–15% in the first year post transplant. This has lead to marked improvement in 1 year patient and graft survival. Clinically, acute rejection most often suspected due to elevated creatinine on routine post-transplant labs. The prognosis of cellular rejection is affected by factors like its histological grade, timing of diagnosis, promptness of treatment, degree of functional impairment, and response to treatment. Humoral rejections are generally more difficult to treat and tend to have a worse impact on transplant survival compared to cellular rejections. Subclinical rejection can be detected by performing protocol biopsies in early post-transplant period [6]. The past the frequency of subclinical rejection has been reported to be 1–17% at 3 months post transplant, but its incidence is lower with use of immunosuppressive agents like tacrolimus and MMF. Subclinical rejection at 6 months is an independent predictor of elevated creatinine at 2 years [7]. Subclinical and clinical rejections are thought to be the different stages of the same process and can lead to poor graft function and survival. Corticosteroid treatment of subclinical rejection is associated with decreased frequency of early and late acute rejection episodes, decrease in chronic tubulointerstitial score at 6 months, and preservation of graft function at 24 months in comparison to the control group [8]. Deceased donor transplants in whom subclinical rejection is diagnosed but not treated develop interstitial fibrosis and tubular atrophy. IFTA (previously called Chronic Allograft Nephropathy) is also strongly associated with number of acute rejection episodes in the first year post transplant.

Human Leukocyte Antigen

HLA antigens are inherited codominantly and matching is based on a total of six antigens; A, B, and DR inherited from each parent. Although six-antigen matched grafts are given priority by the UNOS registry, only 13% of deceased donor kidneys are well matched. Matching recipients and donors at the HLA A, B, and DR loci have been associated with improved long-term graft outcomes although other factors such as prolonged CIT, recurrence of underlying renal disease may negate short-term matching benefits. Currently, allograft survival has improved even with increasing antigen mismatches which is felt to be secondary to non-immunological factors (such as CIT, PRA, donor age) playing a more significant role in graft survival. Overall, however, it is shown that HLA matching exerts a favorable outcome on allograft survival likely due to decreased risk of IF/TA. Based on 2008 date from the Organ Procurement Transplant Network/Scientific Registry of Transplant Recipient (OPTN/SRTR) database, 5 year allograft survival between donor–recipient pairs with zero mismatches was higher in donor–recipient pairs with six mismatches (88% versus 70% in living donor kidneys, 75% versus 66% in deceased standard criteria donor kidneys, and 60% versus 55% in deceased ECD kidneys respectively).

Cold Ischemia Time

The time frame between organ procurement and organ transplantation when an organ is cooled with a cold perfusion solution is called the CIT. A longer CIT is associated with poorer long-term graft outcomes. The 2009 OPTN/SRTR report revealed that 22% of patients receiving deceased donor kidney transplants in 2006 had a CIT less than 11 h and 28% had a CIT of more than 21 h. The graft survival at 3 months, 1 year, and 5 year (transplanted in 2002) for those with CIT of 0–11 h, 22–31 h, and 42+ hours was 97%, 96%, and 94.1%; 93.4%, 92%, and 87.3%; and 73.1%, 71.1%, and 61%, respectively.

Medication Adherence

Adherence to immunosuppressive drug therapy plays a crucial role in favorable graft outcomes. Many studies which use electronic monitoring of medication intake have demonstrated that the rate of non-adherence ranges from 3 to 7%. Non-adherence is associated with acute and delayed rejection, increased financial burden, and decreased long-term survival of grafts. Factors which may play a role in non-adherence can be grouped as socioeconomic (cultural background, cost of medications), patient related (forgetfulness, depression), condition related (prior rejection, time since rejection, source of graft (e.g., deceased versus living related)), and health care related (relationship with providers, continuity of care). Identification of modifiable factors related to medication non-adherence may play a significant role in long-term graft survival.

BK Virus Nephritis

Since the 1990s there has been a progressive increase in the prevalence of BK virus (BKV) infection in kidney transplant patients. This relationship has been most strongly tied to induction therapy and tacrolimus/MMF combination regimen [9, 10]. In renal transplant patients roughly 30–50% recipients develop BK viruria within 3 months of transplant and 20% develop BK viremia within 12 months of transplant [9, 11]. The histological features of BK virus nephritis (BKVN) rather than the viral load correlate strongly with allograft outcome. Up to 5% of patients with viremia develop biopsy proven BKVN [9, 11] and irreversible allograft failure is seen in about 30% of these patients [12]. The treatment for BKVN in kidney transplant recipients is reduction of immunosuppression, which carries the risk of developing of acute rejection.

Recurrent Disease

The prevalence of recurrent disease increases with time post transplantation and is estimated to be 2.8% at 2 years, 9.8% at 5 years, and 18.5% at 8 years post transplantation. This is likely an underestimate since the diagnosis of recurrent disease is based on histology. It is important to understand that many patients with ESRD do not get native kidney biopsies. The diagnosis of recurrent disease is difficult because many patients have late presentation and the diagnosis requires electron microscopy and immunofluorescence. Clinicians are more likely to make a diagnosis of IFTA and CNI toxicity rather than recurrent disease in patients with progressive decline in renal function and proteinuria many years out from transplantation. Recurrent disease has an impact on transplant outcomes. Recurrent glomerulonephritis and is the third most common cause of late graft loss beyond the first year after transplantation after IFTA and Death with Functioning Graft [DWFG]. The risk of recurrence appears to be highest (almost 80%) for Membranoproliferative GN (MPGN type II) followed by MPGN type I, IgA nephropathy, Membranous GN, and Focal Segmental Glomerulosclerosis (FSGS) [13]. GN's like anti-glomerular basement disease recur rarely. Despite the high prevalence of recurrent disease, there is very little information regarding treating these patients. The choice of maintenance immunosuppressive drug does not have an impact on disease recurrence. Steroid free regimens are not associated with increased incidence of recurrent GN. Induction therapy with antithymocyte globulin has shown to reduce the risk of recurrent IgA nephropathy compared to no induction or use of anti CD-25 antibodies. Bilateral native nephrectomy is not helpful in reducing the incidence of recurrent disease and in fact may even increase the incidence of recurrent disease. The use of living versus deceased donors does not seem to have an impact on recurrence.

Death with Functioning Graft

Based on a study using the Scientific Registry of Transplant Recipients database, 42% of allograft loss was accounted for by death with functioning graft (DWFG) [14]. The most common cause of DWFG has been cardiovascular diseases which have been shown to cause up to 55% of DWFGs followed by infections and cancers. Development of post-transplant diabetes, hypertension, hyperlipidemia, anemia, proteinuria, and hypoalbuminemia has all been shown to be risk factors for cardiovascular disease and DWFG. This is very important as more elderly patients are now receiving kidney transplants. While there are no specific guidelines for prevention or screening of risk factors in these patients, aggressive management of risk factors is recommended at this time.

Calcineurin Inhibitor Toxicity

Introduction of CNIs with cyclosporine in 1980s and tacrolimus in 1990s led to significant improvement in the 1-year graft survival rates. CNIs are the backbone of present-day immunosuppression for kidney transplant recipients. Though CNIs have been associated with significantly improved 1 year allograft outcomes, they cause afferent arteriolar vasoconstriction. Chronic CNI use is associated with medial arteriolar hyalinosis, tubular atrophy, tubular microcalcifications, and striped interstitial fibrosis. CNIs have also been associated with post-transplant diabetes mellitus, hypertension, and hyperlipidemia. CNI avoidance studies have not surprisingly found increased incidence of biopsy proven acute rejection and graft dysfunction as manifested by progressive elevation in creatinine. CAESAR study [15] attempted to look at the effect of low dose cyclosporine, cyclosporine withdrawal or standard cyclosporine dose along with daclizumab, MMF, and corticosteroids. It did establish the safety and efficacy of low dose cyclosporine with daclizumab induction, MMF, and corticosteroids, but showed that cyclosporine withdrawal was associated with increased risk of rejection. The landmark Symphony trial by Ekberg et al. [16] showed the safety and efficacy of low dose CNI using the regimen of daclizumab induction, MMF, corticosteroids and low dose tacrolimus.

At this time, CNIs continue to be the most effective immunosuppressants currently available for prevention of acute rejection and their dose reduction likely reduces chronic nephrotoxicity.

Transplant Glomerulopathy—Interstitial Fibrosis and Tubular Atrophy—Chronic Allograft Nephropathy

Chronic allograft nephropathy (CAN) is the major cause of late loss of allograft [17]. CAN is defined as progressive allograft dysfunction occurring 3 months post transplantation [18]. It is histologically characterized by glomerulosclerosis, vasculopathy, tubular atrophy, and interstitial fibrosis, and its severity is graded by the Banff 97 classification [19, 20]. It appears to be a two-phase process [21] with early phase having an immune basis which manifests as subclinical rejection, tubulointerstitial disease and residua of previous episodes of acute rejection. The latter phase has a nonimmunologic basis like CNI toxicity, donor disease, glomerulosclerosis and tubulointerstitial disease associated with CAN. There is no specific therapy for CAN but both ACE inhibitors and ARBs have been shown to delay the deterioration of renal function attributed to CAN. Types of immunosuppressive regimens have also been shown to have effects on CAN outcomes. Regimens using tacrolimus instead of cyclosporine have been shown to confer some protection from CAN [22, 23].

Though the 1 year allograft outcomes have improved significantly, there has been only a modest improvement in long-term outcomes [24]. The major reason for graft failure on long-term follow-up is chronic allograft nephropathy (CAN), with others being death with functioning graft, recurrent disease, and CNI toxicity.

Post-Transplant Metabolic Syndrome

Kidney transplant recipients are at a higher risk for morbidity and mortality due to cardiovascular diseases. The incidence of cardiovascular disease is high in incident dialysis patients. The major risk factors for cardiovascular diseases in kidney transplant recipients are weight gain, hyperlipidemia, hypertension, and diabetes which characterize metabolic syndrome. Immunosuppressive medications contribute to the increased risk of components of metabolic syndrome. Forty-three percent of patients become obese within 1 year of transplantation with average weight gain of 10%. Increase in appetite due to resolution of uremia and removal of the dietary restriction is the main factor that contributes to weight gain. More than half of kidney transplant recipients are hypertensive. Calcineurin inhibitors especially cyclosporine are associated with hypertension probably because of vasoconstriction, increase in sympathetic nervous system activity, and increase in rennin angiotensin system activity. Steroids are also known to cause hypertension. Similarly over 60% of renal transplant recipients develop hyperlipidemia usually with elevated total cholesterol, elevated triglycerides, and high LDL levels. Post-transplant obesity, insulin resistance, corticosteroid therapy, and calcineurin inhibitor therapy all contribute to hyperlipidemia. Post-transplant diabetes mellitus is seen in 24% of patients at 36 months post transplant. Steroids, cyclosporine, and tacrolimus have been associated with development of post-transplant diabetes mellitus. Though the risk of glucose intolerance is higher with tacrolimus than with cyclosporine, but cyclosporine causes a higher risk of hyperlipidemia and hypertension, thus making management of metabolic syndrome and immunosuppression challenging. The development of post-transplant metabolic syndrome contributes to increased cardiovascular mortality and death with a functioning graft.

Post-Transplant Cancer

Kidney transplant recipients are at a high risk for developing cancers. Skin cancer is the most common cancer in kidney transplant recipients. Cancer is the third leading cause of death in renal transplant recipients. The incidence of cancer is increased two to fourfold in kidney transplant recipients but has been shown to be as high as 10 to 20-folds in younger recipients. According to a study using USRDS database, the risk of cancers was up to 20-fold for Kaposi's sarcoma, lymphomas, and skin cancer; up to 15-fold for kidney malignancies; up to three to fivefold for testicular, bladder, cutaneous melanoma, leukemia, liver, and gynecological tumors; and approximately twofold for colon, lung, prostate, breast, ovarian, and gastric cancers [25]. The increased risk of cancers in these patients is thought to result from the interplay of the conventional risk factors, disruption of antitumor surveillance and antiviral activity from immunosuppression, and direct DNA damage and reduced DNA repair due to immunosuppressive medications.

There are no guidelines or management protocols for management of post-transplant cancers in these patients; however, limited studies suggest that reduction in immunosuppression may be beneficial. The anti cancer properties of mTOR inhibitors like sirolimus are utilized in patients with Kaposi or non-melanoma skin cancer. The cancers tend to be aggressive in renal transplant patients and the prognosis of patients who develop solid tumors is uniformly poor.

Transplant Outcomes in the Elderly

With prevalence of ESRD on the rise we are encountering more and more elderly patients in need for renal replacement therapy. Kidney transplant is the treatment of choice even in the elderly patients and after kidney transplantation they are likely to have a much better life expectancy and quality of life than their counterparts who are on dialysis. Elderly recipients have lower rates of acute rejection than their younger counterparts. DWFG is the major reason for graft failure in the elderly and the death censored graft loss tends to get worse with increasing recipient age. Older donor kidneys transplanted into older recipients have a lower graft survival compared to younger donor kidneys transplanted into younger or older recipients.

The elderly transplant recipients have reduced cardiovascular mortality compared to elderly who remain on dialysis. Careful pre-transplant evaluation of cardiovascular diseases and aggressive post-transplant management of cardiovascular risk factors is important. Infections and malignancy are also more common in the elderly who receive a transplant and are important factors affecting transplant outcomes.

Donor Variables

The quality of the kidney used for transplantation has an impact on the long-term transplant outcome. According to the 2005 report of UNOS, kidneys from donors with age more than or equal to 65 years regardless of the type of donor (living or deceased) had poor long-term allograft survival in comparison to younger donors.

Older kidneys also have higher incidence of DGF. For unclear reasons, donor's race has an impact on survival in cases of deceased donor transplants. Survival of grafts from African Americans is poorer than that from Caucasians. Grafts from deceased woman donors fair slightly poorer compared to men, especially in *male* recipients. Kidneys from living donors have been associated with better allograft survival independent of donor age, race, HLA matching, CIT or delayed graft function [26]. Due to continuing shortage of living donors, deceased donor kidneys make up the major source of transplant pool. Due to mismatch in demand and supply of kidneys for transplant, there has been a growing interest in kidneys from Non-Heart-Beating Donors (NHBD)—Donation after Cardiac Death (DCD) kidneys and from deceased donors more than or equal to 60 years of age or with age 50–59 years but with two of following: hypertension, terminal serum creatinine >1.5 mg/dL or death from cerebrovascular disease—called as ECD kidneys. The DCD kidneys have been associated with delayed graft function; however, the allograft survival rates seem to be similar to heart-beating donors at 6 months, 1, 5, and 10 years with similar renal function especially after 3 months of transplant. ECD kidneys have been associated with poor outcomes compared to SCD kidneys [27, 28].

Recipient Variables

Increasing recipient age has been shown to be associated with worse graft survival especially when transplanted with old kidneys (>60 years of age) with the most common cause of graft loss being death with a functioning graft. However, elderly patients receiving transplant do better than elderly patients who stay on dialysis. African-American patients have an inferior graft survival compared to Caucasians; however, this gap is becoming narrower with currently available immunosuppressants. Male living kidney recipients tend to have better graft survival compared to female living kidney recipients possible due to higher sensitization to HLA or non-HLA antigens (related to pregnancy, transfusions). Patients who are highly sensitized (panel reactive antibody (PRA) >50%) have poorer graft survival compared to patients who are not sensitized likely due to increased risk of acute rejection or increased risk of infection/malignancy due to use of potent induction, plasmapheresis, and intensive immunosuppression to reduce the risk of rejection.

Time spent on dialysis prior to transplant has been shown to be an independent predictor of allograft outcome with worse outcomes with longer wait times for transplant on dialysis (especially >24 months) [29, 30]. Patients receiving preemptive transplant have also been shown to have a lower incidence of delayed graft function, which is an independent predictor of long-term allograft survival.

Development or worsening of metabolic syndrome post transplantation has been associated with increased cardiovascular risk and subsequent DWFG.

Recurrent disease in the transplanted kidney can lead to progressive decline in graft life. Kidney transplant recipients with hepatitis C antibody positivity have inferior transplant outcomes compared to recipients who are hepatitis C antibody negative mainly due to worsening liver disease. Despite this, carefully selected hepatitis C antibody positive patients who receive a transplant have a survival advantage over those who stay on dialysis. The availability of potent induction as well as maintenance immunosuppressive medications (mainly CNI's) has had a drastic impact on short-term kidney transplant survival. The most commonly prescribed immunosuppressive regimen in the United States is a combination of prednisone, MMF and a CNI. The CNI's form the backbone of our present immunosuppression but can cause both acute and chronic nephrotoxicity. Unfortunately CNI free regimens are associated with high rejection rates. Although the chronic nephrotoxicty from CNI's is debatable, it seems that dose reduction of these agents may have an impact on chronic nephrotoxcity. Initial results from trials using Belatacept seem very promising in terms of 1- and 3-year graft survival and improved metabolic profile but the long-term impact of this medication on graft survival and metabolic profile is yet to be determined.

References

1. Brennan DC. Long-term trends in allograft survival. Adv Chronic Kidney Dis. 2006;13(1):11–7.
2. Sollinger HW. Mycophenolate mofetil for the prevention of acute rejection in primary cadaveric renal allograft recipients. U.S. Renal Transplant Mycophenolate Mofetil Study Group. Transplantation. 1995;60(3):225–32.
3. Pirsch JD, Miller J, Deierhoi MH, Vincenti F, Filo RS. A comparison of tacrolimus (FK506) and cyclosporine for immunosuppression after cadaveric renal transplantation. FK506 Kidney Transplant Study Group. Transplantation. 1997;63(7):977–83.
4. Cohen DJ, St Martin L, Christensen LL, Bloom RD, Christensen RD, Sung RS. Kidney and pancreas transplantation in the United States, 1995–2004. Am J Transplant. 2006;6:1153–69.
5. Ojo AO, Wolfe RA, Held PJ, Port FK, Schmouder RL. Delayed graft function: risk factors and implications for renal allograft survival. Transplantation. 1997;63(7):968–74.
6. Rush D. Protocol transplant biopsies: an underutilized tool in kidney transplantation. Clin J Am Soc Nephrol. 2006;1(1):138–43.
7. Nickerson P, Jeffery J, Gough J, et al. Identification of clinical and histopathologic risk factors for diminished renal function 2 years posttransplant. J Am Soc Nephrol. 1998;9(3):482–7.
8. Rush D, Nickerson P, Gough J, et al. Beneficial effects of treatment of early subclinical rejection: a randomized study. J Am Soc Nephrol. 1998;9(11):2129–34.
9. Brennan DC, Agha I, Bohl DL, et al. Incidence of BK with tacrolimus versus cyclosporine and impact of preemptive immunosuppression reduction. Am J Transplant. 2005;5(3):582–94.
10. Rahamimov R, Lustig S, Tovar A, et al. BK polyoma virus nephropathy in kidney transplant recipient: the role of new immunosuppressive agents. Transplant Proc. 2003;35(2):604–5.
11. Bressollette-Bodin C, Coste-Burel M, Hourmant M, Sebille V, Andre-Garnier E, Imbert-Marcille BM. A prospective longitudinal study of BK virus infection in 104 renal transplant recipients. Am J Transplant. 2005;5(8):1926–33.
12. Hirsch HH, Brennan DC, Drachenberg CB, et al. Polyomavirus-associated nephropathy in renal transplantation: interdisciplinary analyses and recommendations. Transplantation. 2005;79(10):1277–86.
13. Fairhead T, Knoll G. Recurrent glomerular disease after kidney transplantation. Curr Opin Nephrol Hypertens. 2010;19(6):578–85.
14. Ojo AO, Hanson JA, Wolfe RA, Leichtman AB, Agodoa LY, Port FK. Long-term survival in renal transplant recipients with graft function. Kidney Int. 2000;57(1):307–13.
15. Ekberg H, Grinyo J, Nashan B, et al. Cyclosporine sparing with mycophenolate mofetil, daclizumab and corticosteroids in renal allograft recipients: the CAESAR Study. Am J Transplant. 2007;7(3):560–70.
16. Ekberg H, Tedesco-Silva H, Demirbas A, et al. Reduced exposure to calcineurin inhibitors in renal transplantation. N Engl J Med. 2007;357(25): 2562–75.
17. Peeters J, Roels L, Vanrenterghem Y. Chronic renal allograft failure: clinical overview. The Leuven

Collaborative Group for Transplantation. Kidney Int Suppl. 1995;52:S97–101.
18. Kaplan B. Overcoming barriers to long-term graft survival. Am J Kidney Dis. 2006;47(4 Suppl 2):S52–64.
19. Pascual M, Theruvath T, Kawai T, Tolkoff-Rubin N, Cosimi AB. Strategies to improve long-term outcomes after renal transplantation. N Engl J Med. 2002;346(8):580–90.
20. Racusen LC, Solez K, Colvin RB, et al. The Banff 97 working classification of renal allograft pathology. Kidney Int. 1999;55(2):713–23.
21. Schwarz A, Gwinner W, Hiss M, Radermacher J, Mengel M, Haller H. Safety and adequacy of renal transplant protocol biopsies. Am J Transplant. 2005;5(8):1992–6.
22. Kaplan B, Schold JD, Meier-Kriesche HU. Long-term graft survival with neoral and tacrolimus: a paired kidney analysis. J Am Soc Nephrol. 2003;14(11):2980–4.
23. Meier M, Nitschke M, Weidtmann B, et al. Slowing the progression of chronic allograft nephropathy by conversion from cyclosporine to tacrolimus: a randomized controlled trial. Transplantation. 2006;81(7):1035–40.
24. Meier-Kriesche HU, Schold JD, Kaplan B. Long-term renal allograft survival: have we made significant progress or is it time to rethink our analytic and therapeutic strategies? Am J Transplant. 2004;4(8):1289–95.
25. Kiberd BA, Rose C, Gill JS. Cancer mortality in kidney transplantation. Am J Transplant. 2009;9(8):1868–75.
26. Terasaki PI, Cecka JM, Gjertson DW, Takemoto S. High survival rates of kidney transplants from spousal and living unrelated donors. N Engl J Med. 1995;333(6):333–6.
27. Rosengard BR, Feng S, Alfrey EJ, et al. Report of the Crystal City meeting to maximize the use of organs recovered from the cadaver donor. Am J Transplant. 2002;2(8):701–11.
28. Pascual J, Zamora J, Pirsch JD. A systematic review of kidney transplantation from expanded criteria donors. Am J Kidney Dis. 2008;52(3):553–86.
29. Meier-Kriesche HU, Port FK, Ojo AO, et al. Effect of waiting time on renal transplant outcome. Kidney Int. 2000;58(3):1311–7.
30. Meier-Kriesche HU, Kaplan B. Waiting time on dialysis as the strongest modifiable risk factor for renal transplant outcomes: a paired donor kidney analysis. Transplantation. 2002;74(10):1377–81.

Part IX

Hypertension

Classification of Hypertension

39

William Burtnett and Eleanor D. Lederer

Case

A 37-year-old Caucasian man is seen in your office for routine physical examination. He is unaware of any medical problems but notes that he has gained approximately 25 pounds in the past year. He has a strong family history of hypertension, diabetes mellitus type II, and coronary artery disease. His physical exam shows an overweight man in no distress. His height is 71 in., weight 200 pounds, BMI 28. Waist circumference is 40 in. Blood pressure is 138/87, pulse 80/min, respiratory rate 12, and temperature 98.6 F orally. His general examination is unremarkable. He has no arteriolar changes on funduscopic examination; carotid or abdominal no bruits; cardiac exam shows no displacement of the point of maximal impulse and no gallop. Screening laboratory studies are completely normal including fasting blood sugar, electrolytes, kidney function, and urinalysis.

W. Burtnett, M.D.
Department of Nephrology, University of Louisville, Louisville, KY 40202, USA

E.D. Lederer, M.D., F.A.S.N. (✉)
Department of Medicine/Nephrology, University of Louisville, 615 S. Preston Street, Louisville, KY 40202, USA

Robley Rex VA Medical Center, 800 Zorn Avenue, Louisville, KY 40207, USA
e-mail: e.lederer@louisville.edu

Overview and Epidemiology

Hypertension is one of the most common, if not the most common, chronic disease in the world, estimated to affect 25% of the world's population. By the year 2025, it has been estimated that hypertension will affect 1.5 billion people. In the United States, hypertension has been identified in 30% of the population and the prevalence has been rising from 1988 to 2008 [1]. The rising prevalence has been attributed to a number of factors including the increase in obesity and dietary sodium ingestion. Epidemiologic studies show that the prevalence of hypertension increases with age, less than 10% in 18–39 age group and over 60% in the over 60 age group. Most recent studies suggest that the incidence in men and women is equivalent. Ethnicity, however, exerts a strong influence on hypertension prevalence with a 40% prevalence in African Americans as contrasted with a 25% prevalence in whites and Hispanics.

Hypertension is a major risk factor for cardiovascular disease, specifically left ventricular hypertrophy, heart failure, stroke, and kidney failure [2–19]. The identification of hypertension as a risk factor for these events has been established predominantly through epidemiologic studies showing an association between hypertension and cardiovascular outcomes and studies demonstrating that control of hypertension results in a reduction in the risk for these outcomes. The data are strongest for hypertension as a causative

E.V. Lerma and M. Rosner (eds.), *Clinical Decisions in Nephrology, Hypertension and Kidney Transplantation*, DOI 10.1007/978-1-4614-4454-1_39, © Springer Science+Business Media New York 2013

factor for stroke, left ventricular hypertrophy, and heart failure and weakest for hypertension as a cause of kidney failure. There is, however, clear evidence that control of hypertension ameliorates the progression of kidney failure.

Classification of Hypertension

Blood pressure is a continuous variable. In 1905 the Russian scientist Nikolai Korotkoff developed the methodology for measuring blood pressure as is performed now, paving the way for defining hypertension [20]. Although physicians had recognized that high blood pressure had deleterious effects on health for at least a century, the absence of effective means for lowering blood pressure discouraged rigorous classification or study into the causes and effects until the mid twentieth century. With the advent of thiazide diuretics and greater interest in epidemiology, an organized effort toward the recognition, classification, research, and treatment of hypertension culminated in the first Joint National Committee on Prevention, Detection, Evaluation, and Treatment of High Blood Pressure report in 1976 [21–23]. With this report came standardization of blood pressure definitions and the concept of the stepped care approach to treatment of hypertension. The subsequent seven reports have built upon this base, refining the definition of hypertension, the staging, and the treatment, drawing on the extensive work done over the last 35 years in this field [24]. Over time, the trend has been to lower the systolic and diastolic pressure definitions of hypertension, to promote aggressive treatment in all age groups, and, with the addition of the term "prehypertension," draw the line in the sand defining 120/80 as the upper acceptable limit of normal blood pressure. Of note, a lower limit of blood pressure has not been defined.

Hypertension has traditionally been classified either by either severity or pathophysiology. Occasionally, "age" of the patient has been suggested as a third classification. At its base this is an attempt to clarify pathophysiology, especially in isolated systolic hypertension. Younger individuals tend to have more arteriolar constriction compared to the predominant atherosclerotic disease of larger arteries found in older individuals.

Classification by Severity

Prior to the Joint National Commission classification system, severity of hypertension was poorly defined. Oversimplification into malignant and benign(!) hypertension has been replaced with a system of well-defined, if arbitrary strata (Table 39.1). If systolic and diastolic values fall into different categories, the higher category should be assigned. The use by JNC VII of the term prehypertension seems appropriate at this time, as the great majority of these patients will develop stage I hypertension [24]. Blood pressures in the prehypertensive range also place the patient at higher risk of cardiovascular events [25–27]. However, while pharmacologic therapy is clearly of benefit for stage I and higher, it is unclear if medications reduce risk in prehypertension [28, 29].

Classification by Pathophysiology

Elevated blood pressure can be secondary to cardiac or vascular issues (Table 39.2). Either the "pump" must produce more force or the "tubes" must provide greater resistance, otherwise pressure cannot rise. Obviously this represents an oversimplification as complex feedback mechanisms are in place to blunt the ultimate changes in pressure. "Pump" force relates directly to cardiac output. Multiple diseases increase cardiac output through increased heart rate or, more importantly, stroke volume. These

Table 39.1 JNC VII Classification of Hypertension

Category	Systolic (mmHg)	Diastolic (mmHg)
Normal	<120	<80
Prehypertension	120–139	80–89
Stage I Hypertension	140–159	90–99
Stage II Hypertension	≥160	≥100

Table 39.2 Mechanisms of Hypertension

Increased Cardiac Output	Increased Vascular Resistance
Increased Preload	Increased Sympathetic Activity
• Salt sensitive states	• Pheochromocytoma
• Minerallocorticoid excess	• Stress
• Chronic kidney disease	• Cocaine use
• Excessive salt intake	• CNS insults
Increased Pulse	Increased Angiotensin II Activity
• Thyrotoxicosis	• Reninoma
• Beri beri	• Chronic kidney disease
• Pheochromocytoma	• Renovascular disease
• Cocaine use	

include thyrotoxicosis, fever, and hyperkinetic heart syndrome. "Tube" resistance is determined as a ratio of tubular volume to tubular size. Many common pathways produce concurrent alterations to both tubular volume and size. The most common example is angiotensin II which increases arteriolar smooth muscle activity, but also stimulates aldosterone which results in volume expansion.

Many classification systems for hypertensions exist (Table 39.3). Perhaps the best known attempt to classify hypertension by pathophysiology was articulated by John Laragh, the physician scientist who first described the role of the renin angiotensin aldosterone system in control of sodium and potassium homeostasis and blood pressure [30–34]. This classification system was based on measurement of the plasma renin activity level as low, normal, and high which would then direct initial antihypertensive therapy. In general populations of hypertensives, approximately 27% of individuals had low renin activity, 16% had high renin activity, and 57% had "normal" renin activity [30]. Low renin individuals theoretically should respond to diuretics as they have salt sensitive/dependent hypertension. Conversely, individuals with high renin levels should respond to beta blockers which inhibit renin release. In clinical practice, low renin hypertension predominates in African Americans, older individuals, and women. This classification system failed to gain wide acceptance clinically for a number of reasons including variability in methodologies for measurement of plasma renin activity, lack of reproducibility in findings, and the general failure to demonstrate that stratification based on renin profiling was more predictive than clinical assessment of age and ethnicity in response to therapy [35]. However, high renin levels have been identified as a specific risk factor for cardiovascular complications. More recently, interest in using renin profiling for the evaluation, characterization, and therapy of hypertension has enjoyed a resurgence [36] and may yet become a common therapeutic tool. Currently, routine use of renin profiling is not recommended. However, the epidemiologic information obtained from these studies has persisted in clinical practice. Diuretics continue to be considered first line therapy for African Americans and the elderly.

Classification by Etiology

A common clinical device for classifying hypertension is to determine whether a patient has "essential" or primary hypertension or secondary hypertension. Greater than 90% of hypertensives will be unable to be classified beyond primary/essential hypertension.

The primary disorder leading to hypertension, however, may lie outside the cardiovascular system [37–44]. These secondary causes of hypertension are important to identify for a number of reasons. First, treatment of the underlying disorder can alter the natural history of secondary hypertension, even, at times, obviating the need for antihypertensive medications. Second, identification of a secondary cause of hypertension can uncover genetic causes of hypertension that were previously unrecognized. Third, defining the cause of hypertension may alert the clinician to other complications of the underlying disorder. Although blood pressure classically is felt to be related to cardiac output and peripheral vascular resistance, multiple physiologic processes including the renal, endocrine, and neurologic systems all contribute substantively to the

Table 39.3 Alternative Classification of Hypertension

Classification	Subtypes	Examples
Renin-based	High renin	Reninoma Renal artery stenosis
	Low renin	Liddle syndrome Salt-dependent hypertension
Pathophysiology-based (see Table 39.2)	Increased peripheral vascular resistance	Pheochromocytoma Hypercalcemia
	Increased cardiac output	Chronic kidney disease Thyrotoxicosis
Primary vs Secondary	Primary	Essential
	Secondary	Acute and chronic kidney disease Renovascular disease Minerallocorticoid mediated Hyperparathyroidism Hyper/hypothyroidism Spinal cord injury Obstructive sleep apnea
Ambulatory monitoring based	Masked hypertension White Coat hypertension Dipper vs nondipper	
Pregnancy-associated	Chronic hypertension Pre-eclampsia Pre-eclampsia superimposed on chronic hypertension Gestational hypertension	
Severity-based	Stable hypertension Hypertensive urgency Malignant hypertension Resistant hypertension	

level of vascular resistance and cardiac output. Thus, primary renal disease, hyper- or hypothyroidism, adrenal disorders, pituitary disorders, and primary neurologic injury may result in the development of hypertension. Pulmonary disease may lead to isolated pulmonary hypertension. In sleep apnea, neurologic stimulation may chronically elevate systemic pressures [45]. The most common impetus to investigate for secondary causes of hypertension is resistant hypertension, defined as blood pressure that is uncontrolled on optimal doses of four medications. One of these medications must be a diuretic and the patient must be adherent to the regimen. The most common causes of resistant hypertension include hyperaldosteronism, sleep apnea, substance use/abuse (including caffeine, tobacco, and alcohol), renal artery stenosis, and iatrogenic.

Additional Classes of Hypertension

Increased use of ambulatory blood pressure monitoring has shown that both white coat hypertension and masked hypertension are common [46–52]. White coat hypertensives will have repeatedly high blood pressures in medical care environments, but normal pressures on ambulatory monitoring. Initially thought to be benign, recent evidence has suggested that these patients are also at an increased risk of cardiovascular complications. White coat hypertension may affect over 10% of the population. Studies have demonstrated a higher anxiety index in individuals who have white coat hypertension, suggesting that the elevation in blood pressure in the physician office may be a "conditioned response." Masked hypertension is the converse phenomenon where the stimulation to elevated blood pressures is present in the patient's daily activities (emotional stress or extrinsic adrenergic stimulants such as alcohol, tobacco, or caffeine use). As the patient is away from these effects when visiting medical professionals, office blood pressures will be normal. Awareness of the prevalence of masked hypertension has been raised by the more widespread use of ambulatory blood pressure monitoring. Masked hypertension may affect as many as 20% of adults not otherwise identified as having hypertension. Triggers for higher out of the office blood pressures include smoking, physical exercise, caffeine, and stress. Additionally, some individuals may habitually skip taking their medications until just prior to an office visit, thus presenting to the office with a normal blood pressure while experiencing generally elevated blood pressures during their usual days. Like white coat hypertension, masked hypertension is also associated with increased cardiovascular risk [53–55]. For both white coat and masked hypertension, a home daytime blood pressure measurement of 135/85 is defined as hypertension, as opposed to 140/90 generally accepted for blood pressures measured in the office practice.

Ambulatory blood pressure monitoring has also disclosed variants in blood pressure circadian rhythms [56–62]. Normotensive individuals tend to experience the peak blood pressure in the early morning with a dip of 15.9 mmHg systolic and 13.5 mmHg diastolic at night according to one study of blood pressure variability in an international population. The nocturnal drop in blood pressure tends to be greater in the very young and the very old, greater in men than women. The drop in blood pressure corresponds to sleep/wake cycles as shift workers acquire sleep associated blood pressure drop within 24 h of changing shifts, suggesting the dip is dependent on sleep/arousal patterns, not endogenous circadian rhythms. Several studies have documented loss of the nocturnal decline in blood pressure in a subpopulation of hypertensive patients, resulting in the classification of hypertensive into so-called dippers and non-dippers. The association between non-dipping status and an increased risk of stroke first suggested that the absence of the nocturnal decline in blood pressure may be an independent risk factor for cardiovascular disease and turned attention to the study of this phenomenon. Whether the heightened risk is attributable to non-dipping versus the level of nocturnal blood pressure has not been definitively determined. Likewise the utility of focusing efforts on decreasing nocturnal blood pressure specifically has not been determined.

Isolated systolic hypertension is a relatively common finding in certain populations [63–66]. Patients with hyperthyroidism, beriberi, or aortic insufficiency frequently will have isolated systolic hypertension. This form of hypertension is the most common form of hypertension in those over 50 years of age, and certainly in the elderly. Isolated diastolic hypertension is more commonly seen in younger individuals. Differences in pathogenesis explain the altered presentations. Systolic hypertension is thought to be a result of progressive stiffening of the major arteries through vascular calcification and smooth muscle remodeling. In contrast, diastolic hypertension is attributed to vasoconstriction of small arterioles. Both conditions are indications for treatment, though treatment choices may differ.

Malignant hypertension and hypertensive emergency refer to evidence of acute organ damage clinically with extremely high blood pressures. This may be manifest most recognizably by acute kidney injury, encephalopathy, or visual disturbances. These disorders are discussed in a later chapter.

Pseudohypertension is a common finding in individuals with highly calcified arteries. In these patients, the brachial artery may be poorly compressible from wall calcifications rather than interior pressure. Artificially high sphygmomanometer readings are the ultimate result, even if invasive readings demonstrate normal pressures. Unfortunately, brachial artery palpation is not a reliable way to monitor for this.

Pregnancy and Hypertension

Hypertension during pregnancy warrants a classification of its own [67, 68]. During a normal pregnancy, blood pressure declines early in the first trimester then returns to normal levels at delivery. While the mechanisms responsible for these hemodynamic changes are not entirely understood, studies have demonstrated an increase in nitric oxide production, an increase in prostacyclin and prolactin levels, and peripheral vasodilation with resistance to the vasoconstrictive effects of angiotensin but concomitant responsiveness to the salt retaining properties of aldosterone. Hypertension during pregnancy is defined similarly to the non-pregnant individual as systolic greater than 140 and/or diastolic greater than 90 mmHg.

Hypertension during pregnancy can be classified into four major categories. Chronic hypertension is hypertension occurring either before pregnancy or diagnosed prior to the 20th week of pregnancy. Preeclampsia is defined as the development of hypertension, proteinuria, and edema generally after the 32nd week of pregnancy, though it can occur sooner than that in women with underlying hypertension. As opposed to chronic hypertension complicating pregnancy, preeclampsia resolves generally within 2 weeks of delivery. A third classification of hypertension of pregnancy is development of preeclampsia superimposed on chronic hypertension. The fourth category is gestational hypertension where hypertension develops in the absence of proteinuria after the 20th week and resolves after delivery. Hypertension occurring only during pregnancy was previously considered a circumscribed event without long-term consequences. More recent studies, however, suggest that the development of hypertension during pregnancy is a risk factor for subsequent development of fixed hypertension [69, 70].

Case Discussion

The patient presented likely has prehypertension; however, on the basis of one reading, you cannot make this diagnosis. A recently published report suggests that the diagnosis of hypertension is most reliable with at least five readings of hypertension [71]. This particular individual is at high risk for the development of hypertension due to his overweight status, his eating habits, and his family history. The physical examination shows no evidence of end organ damage, and thus, immediate pharmacologic therapy would not be warranted. In addition to advising him to adopt significant lifestyle changes including weight loss and dietary sodium restriction, you would inquire regarding substance use including alcohol, stimulants, and non-steroidal anti-inflammatory drugs. Another consideration would be having the patient undergo 24 h blood pressure monitoring. Should the measurements demonstrate greater than 25% of the readings over 120/80 or an absence of nocturnal dipping of the blood pressure by 15%, you would confirm the diagnosis of pre hypertension (or hypertension if the daytime pressures exceeded 140/90). You would advise this man of his high risk for progression to stage I hypertension and consequent cardiovascular complications. At this time, there would be no indication for initiating an investigation into secondary causes of hypertension.

References

1. Egan BM, Zhao Y, Axon RN. US trends in prevalence, awareness, treatment, and control of hypertension, 1988-2008. JAMA. 2010;303(20):2043–50.
2. The ACCORD Study Group. Effects of intensive blood pressure control in type II diabetes mellitus. N Engl J Med. 2010;362(17):1575–85.
3. Jamerson KA, Townsend RR. The attributable burden of hypertension: focus on CKD. Adv Chronic Kidney Dis. 2011;18(1):6–10.
4. Dawood T, Schlaich MP. Mediators of target organ damage in hypertension: focus on obesity associated factors and inflammation. Minerva Cardioangiol. 2009;57(6):687–704.
5. He FJ, Burnier M, MacGregor GA. Nutrition in cardiovascular disease: salt in hypertension and heart failure. Eur Heart J. 2011;32(24):3073–80.
6. Andrikou E, Tsioufis C, Dimitriadis K, Flessas D, Chatzistamatiou V, Grassos C, Papavasiliou M, Papadopoulos D, Stefanadis C. Parallel deterioration of albuminuria, arterial stiffness and left ventricular mass in essential hypertension: integrating target organ damage. Nephron Clin Pract. 2011;119(1): c27–34.

7. Cuspidi C, Vaccarella A, Negri F, Sala C. Resistant hypertension and left ventricular hypertrophy: an overview. J Am Soc Hypertens. 2010;4(6):319–24.
8. Georgiopoulou VV, Kalogeropoulos AP, Raggi P, Butler J. Prevention, diagnosis, and treatment of hypertensive heart disease. Cardiol Clin. 2010;28(4):675–91.
9. Chrysant SG, Chrysant GS. Effectiveness of lowering blood pressure to prevent stroke versus to prevent coronary events. Am J Cardiol. 2010;106(6):825–9.
10. Cuspidi C, Giudici V, Negri F, Sala C. Nocturnal non-dipping and left ventricular hypertrophy in hypertension: an updated review. Expert Rev Cardiovasc Ther. 2010;8(6):781–92.
11. Pimenta E, Oparil S. Prehypertension: epidemiology, consequences and treatment. Nat Rev Nephrol. 2010;6(1):21–30.
12. Fagard RH, Celis H, Thijs L, Wouters S. Regression of left ventricular mass by antihypertensive treatment: a meta-analysis of randomized comparative studies. Hypertension. 2009;54(5):1084–91.
13. Gaddam KK, Verma A, Thompson M, Rohit A, Ventura H. Hypertension and cardiac failure in its various forms. Med Clin North Am. 2009;93(3):665–80.
14. Verma A, Solomon SD. Diastolic dysfunction as a link between hypertension and heart failure. Med Clin North Am. 2009;93(3):647–64.
15. Kannel WB. Hypertension: reflections on risks and prognostication. Med Clin North Am. 2009;93(3):541–8.
16. Khosla N, Kalaitzidis R, Bakris GL. The kidney, hypertension, and remaining challenges. Med Clin North Am. 2009;93(3):697–715.
17. Wong ND, Thakral G, Franklin SS, L'Italien GJ, Jacobs MJ, Whyte JL, Lapuerta P. Preventing heart disease by controlling hypertension. Am Heart J. 2003;145(5): 888–95.
18. Shimbo D, Muntner P, Mann D, Barr RG, Tang W, Post W, Lima J, Burke G, Bluemke D, Shea S. Association of left ventricular hypertrophy with incident hypertension: the multi-ethnic study of atherosclerosis. Am J Epidemiol. 2011;173(8):898–905.
19. Saini M, Shuaib A. Blood pressure lowering and stroke. Expert Rev Neurother. 2010;10(2):225–41.
20. Booth J. A short history of blood pressure measurement. Proc R Soc Med. 1977;70:793–9.
21. Esunge PM. From blood pressure to hypertension: the history of research. J R Soc Med. 1991;84:621.
22. Hamdy RC. Hypertension: a turning point in the history of medicine… and mankind. South Med J. 2001;94(11): 1045–7.
23. Report of the Joint National Committee on Detection. Evaluation and treatment of high blood pressure: a Cooperative Study. JAMA. 1977;237:255–61.
24. Seventh Report of the Joint National Committee on Detection. Evaluation and treatment of high blood pressure. JAMA. 2003;289(19):2560–72.
25. Wei GS, Coady SA, Goff Jr DC, Brancati FL, Levy D, Selvin E, Vasan RS, Fox CS. Blood pressure and the risk of developing diabetes in african americans and whites: ARIC, CARDIA, and the Framingham Heart Study. Diabetes Care. 2011;34(4):873–9.
26. Egan BM, Lackland DT, Jones DW. Prehypertension: an opportunity for a new public health paradigm. Cardiol Clin. 2010;28(4):561–9.
27. Fuchs FD. Prehypertension: the rationale for early drug therapy. Cardiovasc Ther. 2010;28(6):339–43.
28. Fuchs FD, Fuchs SC, Moreira LB, Gus M, Nóbrega AC, Poli-de-Figueiredo CE, Mion D, Bortoloto L, Consolim-Colombo F, Nobre F, Coelho EB, Vilela-Martin JF, Moreno Jr H, Cesarino EJ, Franco R, Brandão AA, de Sousa MR, Ribeiro AL, Jardim PC, Neto AA, Scala LC, Mota M, Chaves H, Alves JG, Filho DC, Pereira e Silva R, Neto JA, Irigoyen MC, Castro I, Steffens AA, Schlatter R, de Mello RB, Mosele F, Ghizzoni F, Berwanger O. Prevention of hypertension in patients with prehypertension: protocol for the PREVER prevention trial. Trials. 2011;12:65.
29. Thompson AM, Hu T, Eshelbrenner CL, Reynolds K, He J, Bazzano LA. Antihypertensive treatment and secondary prevention of cardiovascular disease events among persons without hypertension: a meta-analysis. JAMA. 2011;305(9):913–22.
30. Brunner HR, Laragh JH, Baer L, Newton MA, Goodwin FT, Krakoff LR, Bard RH, Bühler FR. Essential hypertension: renin and aldosterone, heart attack and stroke. N Engl J Med. 1972;286(9):441–9.
31. Bühler FR, Laragh JH, Baer L, Vaughan Jr ED, Brunner HR. Propranolol inhibition of renin secretion: a specific approach to diagnosis and treatment of renin-dependent hypertensive diseases. N Engl J Med. 1972;287(24):1209–14.
32. Gavras H, Brunner HR, Laragh JH, Sealey JE, Gavras I, Vukovich RA. An angiotensin converting-enzyme inhibitor to identify and treat vascoconstrictor and volume factors in hypertensive patients. N Engl J Med. 1974;291(16):81821.
33. Dunn MJ, Tannen RL. Low renin hypertension. Kidney Int. 1974;5:317–25.
34. Laragh JH. Renin profiling for diagnosis, risk assessment, and treatment of hypertension. Kidney Int. 1993;44:1163–75.
35. Preston RA, Materson BJ, Reda DJ, Williams DW, Hamburger RJ, Cushman WC, Anderson RJ. Age-race subgroup compared with renin profile as predictors of blood pressure response to antihypertensive therapy. Department of Veterans Affairs Cooperative Study Group on Antihypertensive Agents. JAMA. 1998;280:1168–72.
36. Turner ST, Schwartz GL, Chapman AB, Beitelshees AL, Gums JG, Cooper-DeHoff RM, Boerwinkle E, Johnson JA, Bailey KR. Plasma renin activiy predicts blood pressure responses to beta blocker and thiazide diuretic as monotherapy and add-on therapy for hypertension. Am J Hypertens. 2010;23(9):1014–22.
37. Viera AJ, Neutze DM. Diagnosis of secondary hypertension: an age-based approach. Am Fam Physician. 2010;82(12):1471–8.
38. Stabouli S, Papakatskika S, Kotsis V. Hypothyroidism and hypertension. Expert Rev Cardiovasc Ther. 2010;8(11):1559–65.

39. Gupta D, Chaudhary K, Nistala R. Stenting renal artery stenosis: what is the fuss all about? Rev Recent Clin Trials. 2010;5:28–34.
40. Quack I, Vonend O, Rump LC. Familial hyperaldosteronism I-III. Horm Metab Res. 2010;42(6):424–8.
41. Textor SC, Lerman L. Renovascular hypertension and ischemic nephropathy. Am J Hypertens. 2010;23(11): 1159–69.
42. Anagnostis P, Karagiannis A, Tziomalos K, Athyros VG, Kita M, Mikhailidis DP. Endocrine hypertension: diagnosis and management of a complex clinical entity. Curr Vasc Pharmacol. 2010;8(5):646–60.
43. Udani S, Lazich I, Bakris GL. Nat Rev Nephrol. 2011;7(1):11–21.
44. Ritz E. Hypertension and kidney disease. Clin Nephrol. 2010;74 Suppl 1:S39–43.
45. Baqai K. Obstructive sleep apnea, stroke, and cardiovascular diseases. Neurologist. 2010;16(6):329–39.
46. Wexler R. Ambulatory blood pressure monitoring in primary care. South Med J. 2010;103(5):447–52.
47. Obrien E. Twenty-four-hour ambulatory blood pressure measurement in clinical practice and research: a critical review of a technique in need of implementation. J Intern Med. 2011;269:478–95.
48. Pickering TG, Shimbo D, Haas D. Ambulatory blood pressure monitoring. N Engl J Med. 2006;354:2368–74.
49. Owens P, Atkins N, O'Brien E. Diagnosis of white coat hypertension by ambulatory blood pressure monitoring. Hypertension. 1999;34:267–72.
50. O'Brien E. Unmasking hypertension. Hypertension. 2005;45:481–2.
51. Ogedegbe O, Pickering TG, Clemow L, Chaplin W, Spruill TM, Albanese GM, Eguchi K, Burg M, Gerin W. The misdiagnosis of hypertension. Arch Intern Med. 2008;168(22):2459–65.
52. Pickering TG, Davidson D, Gerin W, Schwartz JE. Masked hypertension. Hypertension. 2002;40:795–6.
53. Khattar RS, Senior R, Lahiri A. Cardiovascular outcome in white coat versus sustained hypertension: a 10 year follow up study. Circulation. 1998;98:1892–7.
54. Mancia G, Bombelli M, Facchetti R, Madotto F, Quarti-Trevano F, Friz HP, Grassi G, Sega R. Long term risk of sustained hypertension in white coat or masked hypertension. Hypertension. 2009;54: 226–32.
55. Ogedegbe O, Agyemang C, Ravenell JE. Masked hypertension: evidence of the need to treat. Curr Hypertens Rep. 2010;12(5):349–55.
56. Staessen JA, Bieniaszewski B, O'Brien E, Gosse P, Hayashi H, Imai Y, Kawasaki T, Otsuka K, Palatini P, Thijs L, Fagard R on behalf of the 'Ad Hoc' Working Group. Nocturnal blood pressure fall on ambulatory monitoring in a large international database. Hypertension. 1997;29:30–9.
57. Hansen TW, Li Y, Boggia J, Thijs L, Richart T, Staessen JA. Predictive role of the nighttime blood pressure. Hypertension. 2011;57:3–10.
58. De la Sierra A, Redon J, Banegas JR, Segura J, Parati G, Gorostidi M, de la Cruz JJ, Sobrino J, Llisterri JL, Alonso J, Vinyoles E, Pallares V, Sarria A, Aranda P, Ruilope RM. Prevalence and factors associated with circadian blood pressure patterns in hypertensive patients. Hypertension. 2009;53:466–72.
59. Routledge FS, McFetridge-Durdle JA, Dean CR. Night time blood pressure patterns and target organ damage: a review. Can J Cardiol. 2007;23(2):132–8.
60. Birkenhager AM, van den Meieracker AH. Causes and consequences of a non-dipping blood pressure pattern. Neth J Med. 2007;65:127–31.
61. Tsioufis C, Andrikou I, Thomopoulos C, Syrseloudis D, Stergiou G, Stefanidis C. Increased nighttime blood pressure or nondipping profile for prediction of cardiovascular outcomes. J Hum Hypertens. 2011;25: 281–93.
62. White WB. Importance of blood pressure control over a 24-hour period. J Manag Care Pharm. 2007;13(8 Suppl B):S34–S9.
63. Pinto E. Blood pressure and ageing. Postgrad Med J. 2007;83:109–14.
64. Dao HH, Essalihi R, Bouvet C, Moreau P. Evolution and modulation of age-related medial elastocalcinosis: impact on large artery stiffness and systolic hypertension. Cardiovasc Res. 2005;66:307–17.
65. O'Rourke MF, Nichols MW. Aortic diameter, aortic stiffness, and wave reflection increase with Age and isolated systolic hypertension. Hypertension. 2005;45:652–8.
66. Van Zwieten PA. Drug treatment of isolated systolic hypertension. Nephrol Dial Transplant. 2001;16: 1095–7.
67. Krane NK, Hamrahian M. Pregnancy: kidney diseases and hypertension. Am J Kidney Dis. 2007;49(2): 336–45.
68. Fabry IG, Richart T, Chengz X, Van Bortel LM, Staessen JA. Diagnosis and treatment of hypertensive disorders during pregnancy. Acta Clin Belg. 2010;65(4):229–36.
69. Williams D. Long term complications of pre-eclampsia. Semin Nephrol. 2011;31(1):111–22.
70. Staff AC, Dechend R, Pijnenborg R. Learning from the placenta: acute atherosis and vascular remodeling in preeclampsia-novel aspects for atherosclerosis and future cardiovascular health. Hypertension. 2010;56(6):1026–34.
71. Powers BJ, Olsen MK, Smith VA, Woolson RF, Bosworth HB, Oddone EZ. Measuring blood pressure for decision making and quality reporting: where and How many measures? Ann Intern Med. 2011;154: 781–8.

40 Pharmacologic Treatment of Hypertension

Nina Vasavada and Eleanor D. Lederer

Case 1

A 47-year-old African-American man presents to your outpatient clinic after learning that his blood pressure (BP) was 180/95 mmHg at a public health screening. He has been feeling well overall and does not take any medications regularly. He is anxious about his future risk of kidney disease, as his father recently has been initiated on hemodialysis for end stage kidney disease related to hypertension. Your patient is currently employed as a police officer and notes that on many work days he eats several fast food meals. His physical examination is pertinent for a seated BP of 176/89 mmHg, a pulse of 86 beats per minute, and a laterally displaced PMI on cardiac examination. Funduscopic exam reveals focal narrowing of retinal arterioles. He has no peripheral edema. The rest of the physical examination is unremarkable. He is wondering what medication he can take to help control his BP and is worried about side effects that might interfere with his work performance.

Case 2

A 52-year-old African-American man presents to your office for follow-up of hypertension. Ten days prior, he was prescribed Lisinopril 10 mg daily for an elevated blood pressure (BP) of 163/88 mmHg. On that visit, serum creatinine was 1.3 mg/dl; this value was consistent with laboratory values over the last 2 years. He has been compliant with the medication and has been feeling well since his last office visit. On physical examination, his BP is 148/78 mmHg and pulse is 74 beats per minute. He has no peripheral edema. The rest of the physical examination is unremarkable. Laboratory evaluation demonstrates a serum creatinine of 1.7 mg/dl. Serum potassium is 4.3 mg/dl. He would like to know if the new medication is helping control his BP, and concerned about potential side effects.

What Are Some Issues to Consider When Deciding What Antihypertensive Agent to Prescribe?

The stage of hypertension describes the degree of BP elevation. The selection of an agent to treat elevated BP begins with the designation of stage of hypertension and the patient's BP goal. Normal systolic BP is <120 mmHg and diastolic BP is <80 mmHg. Prehypertension describes systolic BP between 120 and 139 mmHg or diastolic BP 80–89 mmHg. Prehypertension is a designation

N. Vasavada, M.D. (✉)
Department of Medicine, University of Louisville, 615 South Preston Street, Louisville, KY 40202, USA
e-mail: n0vasa01@gwise.louisville.edu

E.D. Lederer, M.D., F.A.S.N.
Department of Medicine, University of Louisville, 615 South Preston Street, Louisville, KY 40202, USA

Robley Rex VA Medical Centre, 800 Zorn Avenue, Louisville, KY 40206, USA

E.V. Lerma and M. Rosner (eds.), *Clinical Decisions in Nephrology, Hypertension and Kidney Transplantation*, DOI 10.1007/978-1-4614-4454-1_40,

of patients at risk for developing hypertension; these individuals do not need pharmacologic therapy, but are candidates for lifestyle modifications. Stage 1 hypertension describes patients whose systolic BP is 140–159 mmHg or diastolic BP is 90–99 mmHg. Stage 2 hypertension describes patients whose systolic BP is ≥160 mmHg or diastolic BP is ≥100 mmHg [1].

Therapeutic goals for BP reduction differ for different patient populations. In the general population, goal BP is <140/90 mmHg. In patients with chronic kidney disease or diabetes mellitus, the BP goal is lowered to <130/80 mmHg [1]. Guidelines for pregnant patients with hypertension are more variable, but overall suggest that medications are indicated if systolic BP ≥150–160 mmHg and diastolic BP ≥95–100 mmHg [2, 3].

What Have We Learned from Recent Trials Regarding Initial Drug Selection for Hypertension?

Pharmacological reduction of elevated BP is appropriate when lifestyle modifications have failed to reduce BP to current treatment goals. Current treatment guidelines recommend thiazide diuretics as a first line therapeutic option, based on the results of several large randomized clinical trials (RCT) [1, 4].

Certain comorbid conditions may benefit from specific initial BP therapy. Current treatment guidelines note specific high-risk comorbidities that may benefit from specific BP reducing agents. These include heart failure [renin-angiotensin system (RAS) blockers, beta-blockers, diuretic]; post myocardial infarction (RAS blockers, beta-blockers), diabetes [thiazide diuretics, beta-blockers, RAS blockers, calcium channel blockers (CCB)], chronic kidney disease (RAS blockers), and recurrent stroke prevention [angiotensin converting enzyme (ACE) inhibitors, thiazide-type diuretics].

Long-acting thiazide diuretics are not inferior to CCBs and ACE inhibitors for BP reduction and cardiac outcomes. The Antihypertensive and Lipid-Lowering Treatment to Prevent Heart Attack Trial (ALLHAT) was a double-blinded RCT designed to evaluated the effect of chlorthalidone, lisinopril, or amlodipine on the incidence of fatal coronary heart disease and nonfatal myocardial infarction in over 33,357 participants aged 55 years or older with hypertension and other risk factors for coronary heart disease, including type 2 diabetes mellitus. After a mean follow-up of 4.9 years, non-inferiority was demonstrated between the three treatment groups. Analysis of secondary outcomes such as incidence of heart failure over 6 years was worse in the amlodipine group compared with the chlorthalidone group, and incidence of cardiovascular disease events over 6 years was higher in the lisinopril group when compared with the chlorthalidone group [4]. This large RCT has encouraged the current clinical recommendation of thiazide diuretics as first-line BP reducing agents [1].

Alpha-1 blockers are less effective than other agents in lowering incidence of cardiovascular disease in patients with hypertension. The ALLHAT study was initially designed with a fourth arm to evaluate the effect of doxazosin, an alpha-1 blocker, on the incidence of fatal coronary heart disease and nonfatal myocardial infarction. After a median follow-up of 3.3 years, the incidence of heart failure and major CVD events was significantly higher in the study cohort receiving doxazosin. These findings led to the early termination of the doxazosin study arm [5].

Long acting thiazide diuretics are not inferior to CCBs and ACE inhibitors for BP reduction and cardiac outcomes in patients with the metabolic syndrome. The subgroup of study participants in the ALLHAT trial with metabolic syndrome (at least 2 of the following: hyperglycemia, obesity, hyperlipidemia) revealed equivalent rates of cardiovascular disease across treatment groups. These results demonstrated that although classes of antihypertensive agents such as ACE inhibitors are thought to have a more favorable metabolic profile, thiazide diuretics are not inferior to other agents tested in preventing adverse clinical outcomes [6].

Short-acting thiazides such as hydrochlorothiazide may be less effective than other agents at BP reduction. A recent meta-analysis revealed that hydrochlorothiazide at a dose of 50 mg, but not 12.5–25 mg daily, reduced 24 h ambulatory BP comparably to other BP agents [7]. These findings may be attributed to discrepancies in pharmacokinetic profiles of hydrochlorothiazide versus longer-acting thiazide diuretics such as chlorthalidone [8].

CCB are not inferior to beta-blockers in hypertensive patients with coronary heart disease. The INVEST trial (International Verapamil SR-Trandolapril) was an open label RCT of 22,000 hypertensive patients with coronary artery disease aged 50 years or older randomized to receive either verapamil sustained release or atenolol for BP reduction. An ACE inhibitor (trandolapril) was also added if subjects had kidney disease, heart failure, or diabetes. Hydrochlorothiazide was added on to subjects who required additional lowering to BP goal. Over almost 3 years of follow-up, BP control was equivalent in both study cohorts. Treatment with a verapamil-sustained release–based or an atenolol-based strategy was equivalent for reducing adverse outcomes (death, nonfatal myocardial infarction, or nonfatal stroke) [9]. These findings were applicable to the subset of study participants with prior myocardial infarction as well [10].

RAS blockade in white elderly patients with essential hypertension may lower cardiovascular event rates. A RCT involving 6,083 mostly white hypertensive subjects ages 65–84 years old were randomly assigned to the ACE-inhibitor group or the diuretic group. After a median follow-up of 4 years, both study cohorts had similar reductions in BP, but the cohort receiving the ACE inhibitors had significantly lower rates of all cardiovascular events or death from any cause [11].

BP reduction in very elderly patients reduces the risk of stroke, heart failure, and death. The Hypertension in the Very Elderly Trial (HYVET) was a double-blinded, RCT evaluating hypertensive subjects ages 80 years of age or older to determine the effect of BP reduction on risk of fatal and nonfatal stroke. Subjects received either the thiazide-like diuretic indapamide with add-on ACE inhibitor perindopril as needed for BP reduction (target BP was 150/80 mmHg) or placebo. After a median follow-up of 1.8 years, the rates of stroke, heart failure, and death was significantly decreased in the treatment group, and the trial was thus terminated early [12].

What Have We Learned from Recent Trials Evaluating Combination Therapy for Hypertension?

Approximately two-thirds of patients require two or more drugs to achieve goal BP [1, 13, 14]. If the systolic BP is >20 mmHg or diastolic BP > 10 mmHg above BP goal, combination drug therapy is a prudent initial treatment plan [1].

Overall, adding a second BP agent is more effective that increasing the dose of a single agent. A meta-analysis on 11,000 participants from 42 trials evaluated the BP reduction produced by monotherapy versus two-drug combination therapy from the following classes: thiazide diuretics, CCBs, beta-blockers, and ACE inhibitors. The additional BP reduction from combining drugs from two different classes was approximately five times greater than doubling the dose of a single drug [15].

In hypertensive patients at high risk for cardiovascular events, combination therapy with RAS blockade/CCB protects against cardiovascular events better than combination therapy with RAS blockade/diuretic. The ACCOMPLISH (Avoiding Cardiovascular Events Through Combination Therapy in Patients Living With Systolic Hypertension) trial sought to compare the effect of combination BP reducing therapy in subjects with hypertension at high risk for cardiovascular events (history of coronary events, myocardial infarction, revascularization, or stroke; impaired renal function; peripheral arterial disease; left ventricular hypertrophy; or diabetes mellitus) on future cardiovascular events. Eleven thousand five hundred and six subjects were assigned to receive either the ACE inhibitor benazepril and the CCB amlodipine, or benazepril and the diuretic hydrochlorothiazide. After a mean follow-up of nearly 3 years, reduction in BP from baseline was similar between the two treatment groups. Risk of the primary outcome event (composite of a cardiovascular event and death from cardiovascular causes) was significantly less in the benazepril–amlodipine group as compared benazepril–hydrochlorothiazide group [16].

What Have We Learned About Adverse Effects of Therapeutic Agents for Hypertension?

Systemic BP reduction induced by RAS blockade modulates renal autoregulation, resulting in decreased glomerular filtration rate [17]. In the normal kidney, vasoreactivity of afferent and efferent arterioles in response to changes in systemic arterial pressure maintains intraglomerular pressure relatively constant, through the process of renal autoregulation. In the presence of chronic BP elevation, impaired renal autoregulation detrimentally increases intraglomerular pressure. RAS blockade vasodilates afferent and efferent arterioles, yielding reduced renal perfusion pressure and resultant reduced glomerular pressure. This benefit occurs at the expense of diminished glomerular filtration rate. Clinically, an increase in serum creatinine of ≤30% 1–2 weeks after initiating RAS blockade demonstrates successful hemodynamic-medicated reduction of intraglomerular pressure, and continuation of RAS blockade is associated with long-term kidney benefits. However, when serum creatinine rises greater than 30%, the patient should discontinue RAS blockade and be evaluated for additional causes of acute kidney injury [17].

Dual RAS Blockade leads to increased risk of adverse events including hypotension, renal impairment, and hyperkalemia, without significant benefit on cardiovascular outcomes. The ONgoing Telmisartan Alone and in Combination with Ramipril Global Endpoint Trial (ONTARGET) study was designed to determine if RAS blockade monotherapy or combination therapy might prevent vascular events in high-risk patients. This RCT evaluated 25,620 patients with coronary, peripheral, or cerebrovascular disease or diabetes with end-organ damage. Study participants were randomized to receive the ACE inhibitor ramipril, the angiotensin receptor blocker (ARB) telmisartan, or both as combination therapy. The primary outcome measure was a composite outcome of death from cardiovascular causes, myocardial infarction, stroke, or hospitalization for heart failure [18]. After a median follow-up of 4.7 years, the primary outcome occurred similarly in all three treatment groups, with no significant added benefit of combination therapy. However, risks of hypotension, syncope, renal impairment and hyperkalemia were both significantly increased in the combination therapy group, prompting the authors to conclude that the risks of combination therapy in this patient population do not outweigh any significant benefit over RAS blocker monotherapy [19].

Aldosterone receptor antagonism may reduce proteinuria, but carries safety concerns in patients with CKD. Cell culture and animal models of the kidney demonstrate the presence of mineralocorticoid receptors in vascular endothelial cells, vascular smooth muscle cells, podocytes, mesangial cells, and kidney fibroblasts. The expression of these receptors may be modulated by hypertension and proteinuria, as well as aldosterone levels. Increased aldosterone may occur during therapy with RAS blockade, termed aldosterone "escape," and is estimated to occur in up to 50% of patients within 12 months after the initiation of RAS blockade. Therefore, treatment with aldosterone receptor antagonists may yield a more complete inhibition of aldosterone effect. Resultant improvement in proteinuria may be independent of BP reduction [20]. After controlling for BP, dietary sodium and protein intake, a recent clinical trial involving patients with hypertension, diabetes, and CKD treated with ACE inhibitors demonstrated persistent significant reductions in proteinuria when given the aldosterone receptor antagonist spironolactone over nearly 1 year. Unfortunately these patients also demonstrated a greater incidence of hyperkalemia, although renal function was similar between treatment groups [21]. These safety issues have tempered the overall enthusiasm for combining RAS blockade and aldosterone receptor antagonism in patients with CKD.

Non-dihydropyridine CCBs reduce proteinuria when used in conjunction with RAS blockade. Antiproteinuric differences exist between subclasses of CCBs in spite of similar BP reduction potential [22]. Dihydropyridine CCBs and non-dihydropyridine (nonDHP) CCBs may exert different effects on glomerular protein permeability as well as renal autoregulation [22]. Dihydropyridine CCBs do not reduce proteinuria in patients with diabetic nephropathy [23] and hypertensive nephrosclerosis [24]. On the other hand, when combined with RAS blockade, nonDHP CCBs reduce proteinuria to a greater degree than either agent alone in patients with diabetic nephropathy [25]. This effect has been noted overall in the absence of diabetes as well [22].

Peripheral edema secondary to CCB treatment can be mitigated by combination therapy with RAS blockade. A recent meta-analysis of RCTs comparing calcium channel blocker monotherapy with calcium channel blocker and RAS blockade combination found significantly lower risk of peripheral edema with combination therapy than with calcium channel blocker monotherapy [26].

Characteristics of Individual BP Reducing Agents

Classes of BP reducing medications are presented in Table 40.1, along with specific examples, mechanisms of action, indications, and potential side effects [8].

Losartan, an ARB, uniquely reduces serum uric acid though increased urinary uric acid excretion. Uric acid is freely filtered at the glomerulus, and subsequently extensively reabsorbed and secreted by renal tubules. The rate of urinary uric acid excretion is directly correlated to plasma concentration. Clinical trials involving the ARB losartan have noted significant decreases in serum uric acid concentration in patients with essential hypertension as well as chronic kidney disease, primarily through augmented urinary excretion. This phenomenon appears to be unique to losartan, and is not observed with other ARBs [27].

BP reducing medications have variable effects on lipid metabolism. Several classes of BP reducing medications have effects on serum cholesterol. Thiazide diuretics have been noted to increase serum lipids by up to 10% [28]. Within the thiazide diuretic class, chlorthalidone may have more favorable effects on total cholesterol and low-density lipoprotein cholesterol than hydrochlorothiazide [29]. Beta-blockers have varying effects on lipids; nonselective and beta-1- blockers may induce up to 10% reduction in high-density lipoprotein (HDL) cholesterol and, especially with nonselective agents, up to 40% rise in triglycerides [28]. Interestingly, carvedilol, a combination nonselective beta-blocker and alpha-1 antagonist, has a more beneficial effect on total cholesterol and triglycerides when compared with metoprolol in patients with hypertension and diabetes [30]. This may be related to the finding that overall, alpha-blockers have a small but favorable effect on lowering total cholesterol and triglycerides while increasing HDL [28]. RAS blockers, CCBs, direct vasodilators, and centrally acting agents have minimal overall effects on serum lipids concentration [28].

Treatment of Hypertension in Special Populations

Black patients likely require multiple antihypertensive medications to achieve target BP.

Black patients exhibit excessive prevalence, earlier onset, and greater BP mediated target-organ injury relative to white patients with hypertension. Potential contributing factors include a higher prevalence of obesity, RAS activation, lack of a nocturnal fall in BP, and salt sensitivity. Recent guidelines published by the International Society on Hypertension in Blacks emphasize several recommendations for the management of hypertension in Blacks. These guidelines recommend a target BP of 135/85 mmHg. When BP is near goal levels, monotherapy with a diuretic or a CCB carries a greater likelihood of attaining goal BP when compared with a beta-blocker and RAS blocker. When the systolic BP is >15 mmHg and/or diastolic BP is >10 mmHg above goal levels, a two-drug combination therapy should be initiated. Most patients will likely require multiple BP reducing drugs to reach 135/85 mmHg [31].

Table 40.1 Classes of BP-reducing medications

Class	Drug	Mechanism	Indications	Side effects
Diuretics	Loop: bumetanide, furosemide Torsemide Ethacrynic acid	Inhibition of NKCC2, Na-K-2Cl symporter on the loop of Henle apical membrane	HT in edematous states	Hypotension, hyponatremia, hypokalemia, hypocalcemia, hypomagnesemia, hyperuricemia, ototoxicity (high doses), metabolic alkalosis
	Thiazide: Hydrochlorothiazide, Chlorthalidone, Indapamide, Metolazone	Inhibition of NC, Na-Cl cotransporter on the distal tubule apical membrane	First line agents for essential HT Hypercalciuria	Hypotension,hypokalemia, hyponatremia, hypochloremia, metabolic alkalosis, hypomagnesemia, hypercalcemia, hyperuricemia., metabolic alkalosis
	Potassium sparing: Spironolactone Eplerenone	Competitive antagonism of mineralocorticoid receptor	Primary aldosteronism Resistant HT Heart failure	Hyperkalemia Gynecomastia (spironolactone)
	Potassium-sparing: Triamterene Amiloride	Inhibition of ENaC, epithelial sodium channel on collecting tubule apical membrane	Amelioration of K losses with other diuretics	Hyperkalemia, kidney stones (triamterene)
Renin angiotensin blockers	Angiotensin converting enzyme inhibitors: Captopril, Enalapril, Lisinopril, Trandolapril, Benazepril, Fosinopril, Quinapril, Ramipril, Moexipril, Perindopril	Inhibition of conversion of angiotensin I to angiotensin II	HT, left ventricle systolic dysfunction, diabetic nephropathy, chronic kidney disease with proteinuria, acute myocardial infarction, scleroderma renal crisis	Cough, hyperkalemia, acute kidney injury, skin rash, angioedema, teratogenic potential
	Angiotensin receptor blockers: Candesartan, Irbesartan, Valsartan, Losartan, Olmesartan, Telmisartan, Eprosartan	Inhibition of the interaction between angiogensin II and its receptor	HT (all), left ventricle systolic dysfunction (valsartan), diabetic nephropathy (irbesartan and losartan); stroke prophylaxis (losartan)	Hyperkalemia, acute kidney injury, skin rash, angioedema, teratogenic effects
	Renin antagonists: Aliskaren	Direct inhibition of renin release	HT, especially in setting of hypokalemia	Hyperkalemia, acute kidney injury, skin rash, angioedema, teratogenic effects

Sympatholytic agents	Beta blockers: Propranolol, Nadolol, Timolol, Pindolol (nonselective) Metoprolol, Atenolol, Acebutolol, Esmolol, Bisoprolol, Nevibolol (selective beta-1)	Antagonism of beta adrenergic receptors: reduces myocardial contractility, heart rate, and cardiac output. reduces renin secretion	HT, angina, heart failure	Hypotension, bradycardia, decreased cardiac output, bronchospasm (nonselective beta blockers), sexual dysfunction, hypoglycemia unawareness
	Alpha- 1 blockers: Prazosin, Terazosin, Doxazosin	Selectively block alpha-1 adrenergic receptors yielding vasodilatation through reduced arteriolar resistance and increase venous capacitance	HT,benign prostatic hyperplasia (terazosin, doxazosin)	Hypotension (especially after first dose)
	Combined alpha-1 and alpha-2 blockers: Phentolamine, Phenoxybenzamine	Block alpha-1 and alpha-2 receptors leading to a decrease in peripheral vascular resistance and an increase in cardiac output (partially due to reflex sympathetic nerve stimulation)	Preoperative antihypertensive treatment for pheochromocytoma	Hypotension and tachycardia
	Combined alpha and beta blockers: Labetalol, carvedilol	Block alpha-1, beta-1, and beta-2 adrenergic receptors: Vasodilatation Reduced myocardial contractility, heart rate, cardiac output. Decreased renin secretion. Antioxidant and antiproliferative effects(carvedilol)	HT, heart failure (Carvedilol), left ventricular dysfunction post myocardial infarction (Carvedilol)	Hypotension, dizziness, fatigue
	Central alpha 2 agonists: Clonidine, Methyldopa, Guanabenz, Guanfacine	Activation of alpha-2 receptors in the cardiovascular control centers of the central nervous system (CNS), suppresses the outflow of sympathetic nervous system activity from the CNS reducing systemic vascular resistance	Hypertension, hypertension in pregnancy (methyldopa only)	Hypotension, dry mouth, sedation, sexual dysfunction, liver damage (methyldopa)
Calcium channel blockers	Dihydropyridine: Nifedipine, Amlodipine, Felodipine, Isradipine, Nicardipine, Nisoldipine, Nimodipine Nondihydropyridine: Diltiazem, Verapamil	Inhibit calcium entry into myocardial cells and vascular smooth muscle cells. Inhibits the contractile processes of cardiac and vascular smooth muscle. Nondihydropyridine agents directly decrease myocardial contractility and heart rate.	HT, angina, supraventricular tachycardias (verapamil, diltiazem), vasospasm associated with subarachnoid hemorrhage (nimodipine). Monotherapy for patients with isolated systolic hypertension	Hypotension, peripheral edema, gastroesophageal reflux, constipation, urinary retention, severe life threatening hypotension (immediate-release nifedipine), bradycardia (verapamil, diltiazem), cardiac conduction abnormalities (verapamil, diltiazem)

(continued)

Table 40.1 (continued)

Class	Drug	Mechanism	Indications	Side effects
Direct vasodilators	Hydralazine, Minoxidil, Sodium Nitroprusside, Diazoxide	Hydralazine and unknown molecular mechanisms. Minoxidil activates potassium channels in vascular smooth muscle. Sodium nitroprusside acts by releasing nitric oxide.	HT, hypertensive emergencies (intravenous sodium nitroprusside, intravenous diazoxide), hyperinsulinemic hypoglycemia (oral diazoxide)	Hypotension, fluid and sodium retention (hydralazone, minoxodil, diazoxide), drug-induced lupus syndrome (hydralazine), headache, nausea, flushing, hypotension, palpitations, tachycardia, dizziness, electrocardiographic T waves changes (minoxidil), hypertrichosis (minoxidil), toxic accumulation of cyanide leading to altered mental status and severe lactic acidosis (sodium nitroprusside) pericardial effusion (minoxidil)
Central acting agents	Reserpine, Guanethidine	Decrease the storage and release of norepinephrine and dopamine by central and peripheral adrenergic neurons	HT	Hypotension, altered mental status, psychotic depression (rare)

Pregnant patients with hypertension should be treated with medications if systolic BP ≥150–160 mmHg and diastolic BP ≥95–100 mmHg [2, 3]. Guidelines for the treatment of hypertension in pregnant patients differ than those for the general population. Hypertensive disorders in pregnancy may be related to one of four etiologies: preeclampsia-eclampsia, preexisting hypertension, preeclampsia superimposed upon preexisting hypertension, or gestational hypertension. In these disorders, aggressive BP reduction results in fetal growth restriction [32] and therefore goal BP is established to avoid secondary complications such as cerebral or cardiac decompensation [2]. Medications that may be used are (1) methyldopa, (2) labetolol, (3) sustained release nifedipine, and (4) hydralazine [2]. Hydrochlorothiazide has traditionally been avoided in pregnancy; however, a review of randomized trials showed similar pregnancy outcomes among women with hypertension who took thiazide diuretics and those who took no antihypertensive medication [3].

Thiazide diuretics are recommended for initial therapy in elderly patients with uncomplicated hypertension. A recent consensus statement on hypertension in the elderly published by the American College of Cardiology Foundation and the American Heart Association made several recommendations. Most elderly persons with hypertension will need at least two BP reducing medications. When BP is >20/10 mmHg above goal, consideration should be given to starting with a two-drug regimen. As in the general population, in the elderly population thiazide diuretics are effective first line agents for BP reduction. Individualization of therapy is recommended when comorbidities exist. If stable angina or prior myocardial infarction is present, beta-blockers should be the initial BP reducing therapy, followed by long-acting dihydropyridine CCBs. In the presence of reduced LV ejection fraction, RAS blockade with an ACE inhibitor should be included in the BP reducing regimen. In the absence of hyperkalemia or advanced kidney disease, elderly patients with hypertension and systolic heart failure should receive a diuretic, beta-blocker, ACE inhibitor, and an aldosterone receptor antagonist [33].

How Will Antihypertensive Agents Fit into This Patient's Overall Treatment Plan?

It is important to emphasize to this patient that the pharmacological treatment of hypertension should accompany lifestyle modification measures such as excess weight reduction, dietary measures such as sodium and fat restriction, increases in physical activity, and moderation of alcohol intake [1].

References

1. Chobanian AV, Bakris GL, Black HR, Cushman WC, Green LA, Izzo Jr JL, Jones DW, Materson BJ, Oparil S, Wright Jr JT, Roccella EJ. The seventh report of the Joint National Committee on prevention, detection, evaluation, and treatment of high blood pressure: the JNC 7 report. JAMA. 2003;289:2560–72.
2. Lindheimer MD, Taler SJ, Cunningham FG. Hypertension in pregnancy. J Am Soc Hypertens. 2010;4:68–78.
3. Seely EW, Ecker J. Clinical practice. Chronic hypertension in pregnancy. N Engl J Med. 2011;365:439–46.
4. ALLHAT Collaborative Research Group. Major outcomes in high-risk hypertensive patients randomized to angiotensin-converting enzyme inhibitor or calcium channel blocker vs diuretic: the antihypertensive and lipid-lowering treatment to prevent heart attack trial (ALLHAT). JAMA. 2002;288:2981–97.
5. ALLHAT Collaborative Research Group. Major cardiovascular events in hypertensive patients randomized to doxazosin vs chlorthalidone: the antihypertensive and lipid-lowering treatment to prevent heart attack trial (ALLHAT). JAMA. 2000;283:1967–75.
6. Wright Jr JT, Harris-Haywood S, Pressel S, Barzilay J, Baimbridge C, Bareis CJ, Basile JN, Black HR, Dart R, Gupta AK, Hamilton BP, Einhorn PT, Haywood LJ, Jafri SZ, Louis GT, Whelton PK, Scott CL, Simmons DL, Stanford C, Davis BR. Clinical outcomes by race in hypertensive patients with and without the metabolic syndrome: antihypertensive and lipid-lowering treatment to prevent heart attack trial (ALLHAT). Arch Intern Med. 2008;168:207–17.
7. Messerli FH, Makani H, Benjo A, Romero J, Alviar C, Bangalore S. Antihypertensive efficacy of hydrochlorothiazide as evaluated by ambulatory blood pressure monitoring: a meta-analysis of randomized trials. J Am Coll Cardiol. 2011;57:590–600.

8. Goodman LS, Gilman A, Brunton LL, Lazo JS, Parker KL. Goodman & Gilman's the pharmacological basis of therapeutics. 11th ed. New York: McGraw-Hill; 2006.
9. Pepine CJ, Handberg EM, Cooper-DeHoff RM, Marks RG, Kowey P, Messerli FH, Mancia G, Cangiano JL, Garcia-Barreto D, Keltai M, Erdine S, Bristol HA, Kolb HR, Bakris GL, Cohen JD, Parmley WW. A calcium antagonist vs a non-calcium antagonist hypertension treatment strategy for patients with coronary artery disease. The international verapamil-trandolapril study (INVEST): a randomized controlled trial. JAMA. 2003;290:2805–16.
10. Bangalore S, Messerli FH, Cohen JD, Bacher PH, Sleight P, Mancia G, Kowey P, Zhou Q, Champion A, Pepine CJ. Verapamil-sustained release-based treatment strategy is equivalent to atenolol-based treatment strategy at reducing cardiovascular events in patients with prior myocardial infarction: an INternational VErapamil SR-Trandolapril (INVEST) substudy. Am Heart J. 2008;156:241–7.
11. Wing LM, Reid CM, Ryan P, Beilin LJ, Brown MA, Jennings GL, Johnston CI, McNeil JJ, Macdonald GJ, Marley JE, Morgan TO, West MJ. A comparison of outcomes with angiotensin-converting–enzyme inhibitors and diuretics for hypertension in the elderly. N Engl J Med. 2003;348:583–92.
12. Beckett NS, Peters R, Fletcher AE, Staessen JA, Liu L, Dumitrascu D, Stoyanovsky V, Antikainen RL, Nikitin Y, Anderson C, Belhani A, Forette F, Rajkumar C, Thijs L, Banya W, Bulpitt CJ. Treatment of hypertension in patients 80 years of age or older. N Engl J Med. 2008;358:1887–98.
13. Cushman WC, Ford CE, Cutler JA, Margolis KL, Davis BR, Grimm RH, Black HR, Hamilton BP, Holland J, Nwachuku C, Papademetriou V, Probstfield J, Wright Jr JT, Alderman MH, Weiss RJ, Piller L, Bettencourt J, Walsh SM. Success and predictors of blood pressure control in diverse North American settings: the antihypertensive and lipid-lowering treatment to prevent heart attack trial (ALLHAT). J Clin Hypertens (Greenwich). 2002;4:393–404.
14. Hansson L, Zanchetti A, Carruthers SG, Dahlof B, Elmfeldt D, Julius S, Menard J, Rahn KH, Wedel H, Westerling S. Effects of intensive blood-pressure lowering and low-dose aspirin in patients with hypertension: principal results of the hypertension optimal treatment (HOT) randomised trial. HOT Study Group. Lancet. 1998;351:1755–62.
15. Wald DS, Law M, Morris JK, Bestwick JP, Wald NJ. Combination therapy versus monotherapy in reducing blood pressure: meta-analysis on 11,000 participants from 42 trials. Am J Med. 2009;122:290–300.
16. Jamerson K, Weber MA, Bakris GL, Dahlof B, Pitt B, Shi V, Hester A, Gupte J, Gatlin M, Velazquez EJ. Benazepril plus amlodipine or hydrochlorothiazide for hypertension in high-risk patients. N Engl J Med. 2008;359:2417–28.
17. Palmer BF. Renal dysfunction complicating the treatment of hypertension. N Engl J Med. 2002;347:1256–61.
18. Teo K, Yusuf S, Sleight P, Anderson C, Mookadam F, Ramos B, Hilbrich L, Pogue J, Schumacher H. Rationale, design, and baseline characteristics of 2 large, simple, randomized trials evaluating telmisartan, ramipril, and their combination in high-risk patients: the ongoing telmisartan alone and in combination with ramipril global endpoint trial/telmisartan randomized assessment study in ACE intolerant subjects with cardiovascular disease (ONTARGET/TRANSCEND) trials. Am Heart J. 2004;148:52–61.
19. Yusuf S, Teo KK, Pogue J, Dyal L, Copland I, Schumacher H, Dagenais G, Sleight P, Anderson C. Telmisartan, ramipril, or both in patients at high risk for vascular events. N Engl J Med. 2008;358:1547–59.
20. Bertocchio JP, Warnock DG, Jaisser F. Mineralocorticoid receptor activation and blockade: an emerging paradigm in chronic kidney disease. Kidney Int. 2011;79:1051–60.
21. Mehdi UF, Adams-Huet B, Raskin P, Vega GL, Toto RD. Addition of angiotensin receptor blockade or mineralocorticoid antagonism to maximal angiotensin-converting enzyme inhibition in diabetic nephropathy. J Am Soc Nephrol. 2009;20:2641–50.
22. Bakris GL, Weir MR, Secic M, Campbell B, Weis-McNulty A. Differential effects of calcium antagonist subclasses on markers of nephropathy progression. Kidney Int. 2004;65:1991–2002.
23. Lewis EJ, Hunsicker LG, Clarke WR, Berl T, Pohl MA, Lewis JB, Ritz E, Atkins RC, Rohde R, Raz I. Renoprotective effect of the angiotensin-receptor antagonist irbesartan in patients with nephropathy due to type 2 diabetes. N Engl J Med. 2001;345:851–60.
24. Agodoa LY, Appel L, Bakris GL, Beck G, Bourgoignie J, Briggs JP, Charleston J, Cheek D, Cleveland W, Douglas JG, Douglas M, Dowie D, Faulkner M, Gabriel A, Gassman J, Greene T, Hall Y, Hebert L, Hiremath L, Jamerson K, Johnson CJ, Kopple J, Kusek J, Lash J, Lea J, Lewis JB, Lipkowitz M, Massry S, Middleton J, Miller III ER, Norris K, O'Connor D, Ojo A, Phillips RA, Pogue V, Rahman M, Randall OS, Rostand S, Schulman G, Smith W, Thornley-Brown D, Tisher CC, Toto RD, Wright Jr JT, Xu S. Effect of ramipril vs amlodipine on renal outcomes in hypertensive nephrosclerosis: a randomized controlled trial. JAMA. 2001;285:2719–28.
25. Bakris GL, Weir MR, DeQuattro V, McMahon FG. Effects of an ACE inhibitor/calcium antagonist combination on proteinuria in diabetic nephropathy. Kidney Int. 1998;54:1283–9.
26. Makani H, Bangalore S, Romero J, Wever-Pinzon O, Messerli FH. Effect of renin-angiotensin system blockade on calcium channel blocker-associated peripheral edema. Am J Med. 2011;124:128–35.
27. Sica DA, Schoolwerth AC. Part 1. Uric acid and losartan. Curr Opin Nephrol Hypertens. 2002;11:475–82.
28. Kasiske BL, Ma JZ, Kalil RS, Louis TA. Effects of antihypertensive therapy on serum lipids. Ann Intern Med. 1995;122:133–41.
29. Dorsch MP, Gillespie BW, Erickson SR, Bleske BE, Weder AB. Chlorthalidone reduces cardiovascular events compared with hydrochlorothiazide: a retro-

spective cohort analysis. Hypertension. 2011;57:689–94.

30. Bakris GL, Fonseca V, Katholi RE, McGill JB, Messerli FH, Phillips RA, Raskin P, Wright Jr JT, Oakes R, Lukas MA, Anderson KM, Bell DS. Metabolic effects of carvedilol vs metoprolol in patients with type 2 diabetes mellitus and hypertension: a randomized controlled trial. JAMA. 2004;292:2227–36.
31. Flack JM, Sica DA, Bakris G, Brown AL, Ferdinand KC, Grimm Jr RH, Hall WD, Jones WE, Kountz DS, Lea JP, Nasser S, Nesbitt SD, Saunders E, Scisney-Matlock M, Jamerson KA. Management of high blood pressure in Blacks: an update of the International Society on Hypertension in Blacks consensus statement. Hypertension. 2010;56:780–800.
32. von DP, Ornstein MP, Bull SB, Logan AG, Koren G, Magee LA. Fall in mean arterial pressure and fetal growth restriction in pregnancy hypertension: a meta-analysis. Lancet. 2000;355:87–92.
33. Aronow WS. Black Cardiologists, and European Society of Hypertension. J Am Soc Hypertens. 2011;5:259–352.

Primary Hypertension

41

Eleanor D. Lederer

Case

A 47-year-old woman presents for establishment of primary care. She has not seen a physician in over 20 years and has been urged to seek medical attention for check up by her children. She is unaware of any medical problems and takes no medications. Her history is notable for four pregnancies, two of which were complicated by hypertension. Her family history is notable for diabetes mellitus, hypertension, and coronary artery disease. She has worked as a data entry technician for the past 25 years, generally eats packaged foods for all meals, and participates in no exercise program. Physical examination shows an overweight woman with BMI 26, BP 150/97, pulse 70/min, respiratory rate 18/min, and temperature 98.6 °F. Her general physical examination is unremarkable. Screening labwork, EKG, and chest radiograph are all unremarkable.

Questions:

1. Can you make the diagnosis of hypertension in this woman?
2. How would you confirm a diagnosis of essential hypertension?
3. What further testing would you do?
4. What nonpharmacologic measures would you recommend?
5. What pharmacologic agents would you recommend if hypertension is confirmed?

Definition and Epidemiology

Hypertension is the most common chronic non-communicable disease in the world, affecting as many as 25% of people world-wide. In the United States alone, it is estimated that nearly 70 million people have hypertension [1]. Many of those people do not know they have hypertension. Primary hypertension, also known as essential or benign hypertension, is defined as blood pressure greater than 140/90 with no identifiable secondary cause. Approximately 90% of hypertensives will fall into this category.

The prevalence of hypertension increases with age [1, 2]. There is almost a 100% chance of developing hypertension by the age of 90. Factors contributing to the increase in hypertension in the older population include increased stiffness and thickness of the arterioles and in some cases enhanced sodium retention. It has been suggested that arteriolar changes in the kidney may be critical in triggering hypertensive signaling mechanisms [3]. Many investigators attribute the rising prevalence of hypertension with age to a chronically high salt diet with secondary effects on sympathetic nervous system activity and vascular remodeling [4–7], reviewed in Chap. 42). In particular, an increase in the systolic blood pressure

E.D. Lederer, M.D., F.A.S.N. (✉)
Department of Medicine/Nephrology, University of Louisville, 615S. Preston Street, Louisville, KY 40202, USA

Robley Rex VA Medical Center, 800 Zorn Avenue, Louisville, KY 40207, USA
e-mail: e.lederer@louisville.edu

E.V. Lerma and M. Rosner (eds.), *Clinical Decisions in Nephrology, Hypertension and Kidney Transplantation*, DOI 10.1007/978-1-4614-4454-1_41,

out of proportion to the diastolic blood pressure has been noted and is strongly correlated with the development of cardiovascular complications [1, 2].

Hypertension is more common in African Americans than it is in individuals of Caucasian descent [1, 2, 8–10]. The reasons for this discrepancy are being actively investigated. Some of the suggested factors include a greater prevalence of obesity and variations in nephron endowment, sodium handling, and sympathetic reactivity. Other ethnic minorities such as Hispanics and Native Americans also tend to have a higher incidence of hypertension than Caucasians, again attributed in large part to the higher incidence of obesity, metabolic syndrome, and a "pro-hypertensive diet" [11]. A newer intriguing theory suggests that prenatal events may condition individuals to the development of hypertension through an influence on several aspects of metabolism that increase the propensity for obesity, insulin resistance, and chronic kidney disease [12, 13]. Specifically, low birth weight or prematurity, pregnancy-associated complications that are more common in minority populations, are associated with the subsequent development of hypertension and metabolic syndrome in some studies.

Individuals of lower socioeconomic status also have hypertension more often than those of higher socioeconomic status [14–16]. Although access to care is clearly a contributory factor to the lower rate of control of hypertension in these populations, the reasons for the genesis of hypertension in these individuals is not as clear. Lifelong ingestion of a diet relatively high in fat and salt and relatively low in fruits, vegetables, and fiber has been suggested as a major factor.

Hypertension is a component of the metabolic syndrome, a clinical condition that has been increasing in frequency over the past two to three decades parallel to the increase in obesity [17–21]. Various sources differ somewhat on the precise definition of metabolic syndrome but features common to all definitions include abdominal obesity, glucose intolerance (insulin resistance), high blood pressure, and atherogenic dyslipidemia. The frequency of the occurrence of most or all of these components in a single individual suggests the possibility of a common etiology; however, not all investigators feel that hypertension is an intrinsic component of the syndrome. Obesity very likely also explains the rapidly rising incidence of hypertension in the pediatric population [22]. The impact of these demographic changes in hypertension frequency on cardiovascular morbidity in this country is yet to be appreciated.

Table 41.1 Diagnosis of Hypertension

Conditions for Blood Pressure Measurement
Seated with back and arm supported
At rest for 15 minutes in quiet setting
Absence of smoking or eating for 30 minutes
Use of appropriate sized blood pressure cuff
Diagnostic Criteria
BP>140/90 on two separate occasions

Diagnosis

The definition of hypertension is standardized as is the methodology for measuring blood pressure [1, 23] (Table 41.1). Conventionally, hypertension is diagnosed by measurement in the office under standard conditions: the individual sitting with feet flat on the floor, arm at the height of the heart resting on a comfortable surface, at rest for 5 min, in a quiet space, with an appropriately sized cuff, i.e., the bladder being approximately 80% of the circumference of the arm. The individual should not have eaten or smoked a cigarette within the prior 15 min and should not speak during the actual measurement of the blood pressure. Generally, two blood pressures exceeding 140/90 in the office on separate occasions will suffice to make a diagnosis of hypertension. The definition applies to blood pressures obtained by mercury sphygmomanometer or electronic device. For individuals found to have high blood pressure, blood pressure should be measured in both arms and in the supine, sitting, and upright positions. Significant discrepancy between right and left arm blood pressures has been associated with greater cardiovascular sequelae [24, 25].

Recognition that blood pressure fluctuates during the day under a variety of circumstances and that isolated blood pressure measurements in the office may not reflect the typical blood pressure for an individual has led to a variety of alternative approaches to diagnosing blood pressure (Table 41.2) [26–33]. A recent study published in the Annals of Internal Medicine suggested that six measurements of blood pressure in the office more accurately defined hypertension than the standard two measurements [28]. Many studies suggest that the measurement of blood pressure out of the office may yield a more accurate picture of an individual's cardiovascular status, as ambulatory blood pressure tends to correlate more closely with cardiovascular morbidity [26, 27]. Intermittent home blood pressure monitoring is now quite feasible as accurate home blood pressure devices have been developed. Devices for the measurement of 24 h ambulatory blood pressure have also been studied. Hypertension is diagnosed as blood pressure greater than 135/85 using these measurement approaches. An interesting hybrid approach combining the extended features of ambulatory blood pressure measurement and the controlled environment of the in office measurement is the 30 min office blood pressure measurement. Using one of several devices now on the market, the practitioner can measure the patient's blood pressure in the office setting every 5 min for 30 min. Studies demonstrate a close correlation between 30 min office blood pressure measurement and ambulatory blood pressure measurement. The advantages of the 30 min method over the 24 h ambulatory method are numerous including the ability to obtain a number of blood pressure measurements within a reasonable time span, maintenance of the equipment within the office, the simplicity of analysis, and patient comfort. Disadvantages include the time and space required within the practitioner's office and by the patient. The in office measurement protocol also does not allow

Table 41.2 Methods for Blood Pressure Measurement

Method	Diagnostic Criteria	Advantages	Disadvantages
Intermittent Office Measurement: standard	>140/90 × 2	Timely, controlled environment	Does not measure usual BP Does not identify circadian variability Does not diagnose masked hypertension
Intermittent Office Measurement: proposed	>140/90 × 6	Timely, controlled environment	Same as above
Extended Office Blood Pressure Measurement	>140/90 averaged over 6 measurements at one time	Controlled environment	Requires extended time in office Requires specialized equipment
Intermittent Home Blood Pressure Measurement	>135/85	Better correlation with cardiovascular outcome Better reflection of ambient usual blood pressure May promote better medication compliance through constant and immediate feedback	Uncontrolled environment/equipment Dependence on patient compliance
24 hour Ambulatory Blood Pressure Monitor	>135/85	Better correlation with cardiovascular outcome Better reflection of ambient usual blood pressure Ability to diagnose white coat and masked hypertension Ability to assess circadian rhythm and determine "dipper" status	Requires specialized equipment Applicability for routine evaluation and follow up

the provider to determine whether a patient is a nocturnal "non-dipper" versus a "dipper" and may not allow the practitioner to identify white coat hypertension or masked hypertension. Both extended time approaches require specialized blood pressure equipment. Although these methods for blood pressure measurement may be ideal, whether they will supplant the standard intermittent office based blood pressure measurement remains to be seen. The practical applicability and the ability to predict cardiovascular sequelae will be the major determinants of which of these methods become the recommended one(s).

Initial evaluation of the patient with hypertension should be directed toward determining whether there is a secondary cause of hypertension, whether there are detectable sequelae of hypertension, and whether there are co-morbidities that may influence the choice of treatment for hypertension (Table 41.3) [1, 23, 34, 35]. Aspects of the initial work up include a complete history and physical examination to include medication and family history; funduscopic and cardiac examination, weight, anthropomorphic measurements, and calculation of BMI; measurement of electrolytes, kidney function, fasting glucose and lipid profile, and urinalysis. Electrocardiogram and chest radiograph are also frequently included. Prior history of high blood pressure, treated or not, suggests a history of chronic hypertension. Gestational hypertension or preeclampsia has also been associated with the development of hypertension later in life [36]. Features on evaluation that suggest chronicity to the hypertension, and therefore validity of labeling the individual as hypertensive, include the finding of arteriolar

Table 41.3 Initial Evaluation of the Hypertensive Patient

Type of Evaluation	Factors	Findings suggestive of sustained chronic hypertension	Findings suggestive of secondary hypertension
Medical history	Family history	HT in first degree relatives	HT in autosomal dominant pattern or no family history of HT
	Medication use	Past use of antiHT agents	Chronic use of illicit drugs, herbal supplements, NSAIDs
	Other medical illnesses	Diabetes mellitus, Obesity, Metabolic Syndrome, Heart Failure, Dyslipidemia	Diseases associated with CKD Symptoms suggestive of sleep apnea
	Lifestyle	Sedentary,	Illicit drug use, use of herbal supplements
Physical Examination	Blood Pressure	Sustained BP > 140/90	Widely variable BP, differences in BP between arms
	Funduscopic exam	Arteriolar narrowing	Severe arteriolar changes, papilledema
	Cardiac exam	Findings of LVH	Severe findings of LVH and heart failure
	Pulses	Peripheral bruits or diminished pulses	Abdominal bruit
	Anthropomorphic	Obesity, increased weight circumference	Morbid obesity, asthenia
Ancillary findings	Laboratory	Normal electrolytes Normal kidney function Normal urinalysis Normal calcium Dyslipidemia common Impaired glucose tolerance common	Hypernatremia Hypokalemia Metabolic alkalosis Elevated BUN and Cr Hypercalcemia
	EKG	Normal or left ventricular hypertrophy, arrhythmias	Left ventricular hypertrophy, arrhythmias
	CXR	Normal, mild cardiomegaly	Severe LVH, rib notching

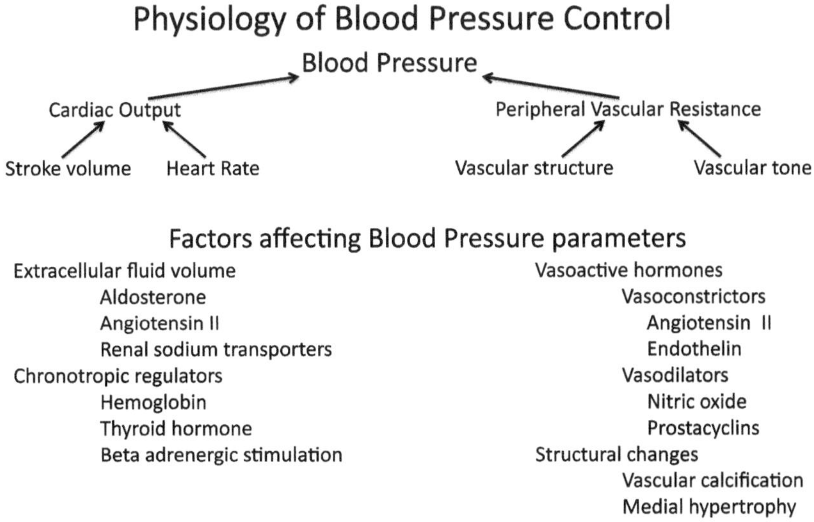

Fig. 41.1 Physiology of blood pressure control

narrowing on funduscopic exam, the identification of findings of left ventricular hypertrophy such as a displaced point of maximum impulse or an S4 gallop, and microalbuminuria. Findings that suggest a secondary cause of hypertension are also reviewed in Chap. 43 Secondary Hypertension.

Pathogenesis

Classic physiology has defined blood pressure as a function of cardiac output and peripheral vascular resistance (Fig. 41.1) [37]. In a normotensive individual, factors that increase one or the other are offset by a decrease in the other factor, countering a sustained elevation in blood pressure. One of the best examples is blood pressure regulation in pregnancy. During pregnancy, total body salt and water increase enormously with a subsequent increase in cardiac output. However, pregnant individuals are not hypertensive and in fact have lower than normal blood pressure because of a marked decrease in peripheral vascular resistance. When this decrease in peripheral vascular resistance does not occur, hypertensive syndromes of pregnancy occur. This suggests that the development of sustained hypertension must involve both modulators of blood pressure regulation, peripheral vascular resistance and cardiac output. An initiating factor can be identified for several forms of hypertension, particularly secondary hypertension. For example, primary hyperaldosteronism causes sodium retention, leading to an increase in extracellular fluid volume and cardiac output and clinically apparent hypertension. However, studies have demonstrated that the degree of hypertension actually correlates better with the level of vascular resistance. Thus, the clinical syndrome of hypertension is a result of pathology in both cardiac output and peripheral vascular resistance [38].

One interesting approach to understanding the pathogenesis of hypertension is to divide the risk factors for hypertension into genetic and environmental factors [37]. Genetic factors would be those factors defined by an individual's genetic and epigenetic makeup. Monogenic gene defects have demonstrated, for example, that defects in renal sodium transporters have profound effect on blood pressure [39–45]. Patients with Bartter and Gitelman syndrome who exhibit defective sodium transport are generally hypotensive while patients with Liddle syndrome who exhibit unchecked sodium transport are quite hypertensive. These rare diseases are autosomal recessive so the individuals have two copies of a defective gene for the respective sodium transporters.

However, even expression of a single mutant copy of one of these genes results in clinically significant differences in susceptibility to hypertension and cardiovascular disease. This observation suggests that subtle variations in the function of renal sodium transporters may contribute to the development of hypertension. Other genes implicated in the development of hypertension include α adducin which regulates the activity of the sodium pump; angiotensinogen, angiotensin converting enzyme, renin binding protein, components of the renin–angiotensin–aldosterone system; potassium channels which regulate aldosterone release; β adrenergic receptors, and the insulin receptor. Genome wide association studies which have identified many of these associations between gene polymorphisms and hypertension generally suggest that these genetic differences make only a very small contribution to an individual's blood pressure. However, in combination and in the context of other environmental factors, these genetic variations may play essential roles in the development of hypertension [46–48].

Several of the environmental or non-genetic factors that may contribute to the development of hypertension have been discussed [11–22], also reviewed in Chap. 42). Obesity, insulin resistance, metabolic syndrome, and a high salt diet have all been implicated. Additional dietary components that may play a role include excessive phosphate, saturated fat, uric acid, and high fructose corn syrup. Sedentary lifestyle and cigarette smoking are associated with the development of hypertension. Studies suggest that even environmental factors such as excessive noise may play a contributory role in the development of hypertension [49]. Although each of these genetic and non-genetic factors contribute very modestly to blood pressure control, the totality of factors at work over decades can certainly explain the progressive increase in prevalence of hypertension with age and may explain why the development of hypertension appears to be all but inevitable for individuals achieving very advanced old age.

Clinical Presentation, Symptoms and Signs, Natural History

Hypertension is called the "silent killer" for good reason. The vast majority of people with hypertension have no symptoms whatsoever. In fact, the absence of specific symptomatology likely accounts, at least in part, for the fact that some 30% of patients with hypertension are not aware that they have it. Some common complaints include headache and fatigue, but these symptoms are nonspecific and correlate poorly if at all with the presence or degree of hypertension. The few individuals who do present with symptoms generally fall into the category of hypertensive urgency or hypertensive emergency. These conditions are covered in depth in the chapter on hypertensive emergencies (Chap. 44). Briefly, some of the more common presentations of hypertensive emergencies include severe headache, blindness, altered mental status, chest pain, dyspnea, hematuria, or acute kidney injury. To emphasize, however, these patients represent the minority of individuals with hypertension. Most hypertensive individuals present asymptomatically in the context of other medical care, similarly to the case presented. In the early stages, particularly in patients with prehypertension, there may be no other manifestations of chronic hypertension such as left ventricular hypertrophy, arteriolar narrowing of retinal vessels, an S4 gallop, or microalbuminuria.

The natural history of hypertension is generally dominated by the persistent need for one or more medications [50–52]. Hypertension rarely remits spontaneously, likely reflecting the fact that the changes in the vasculature in key organs such as heart and kidneys are substantive structural sequelae of the accumulated effects of the genetic and non-genetic forces discussed in the prior section. With very remarkable lifestyle changes in diet, physical activity, and life circumstances (e.g., diminution in social/emotional stress), select individuals may be able to discontinue antihypertensive medications. Weight loss to achieve a BMI within the normal range; ingestion of a diet low in sodium, fat, phosphate, and uric acid and high in calcium, potassium, whole grains, fruits, and vegetables; participation in a daily exercise program that challenges the cardiovascular system; and elimination of stress have proven efficacy in ameliorating cardiovascular risk factors. Unfortunately, most studies suggest that only a minority of patients are able to achieve these goals over the long term. In effect, hypertension is a chronic lifelong disease.

Approximately 2% of patients with hypertension will develop the syndrome of resistant hypertension, defined as hypertension that is not controlled by optimal doses of four medications, one of which is a diuretic [53]. According to a recently published study of over 200,000 hypertensive patients, risk factors for the development of resistant hypertension included male gender, older age, and diabetes mellitus and tended to manifest within 1.5 years of diagnosis. Hypertensive urgencies and emergencies account for approximately 3% of all emergency room visits and affect approximately 1–2% of all hypertensives. A recent publication showed an increase in the number of hospital admissions for hypertensive emergencies but a decrease in mortality [54].

These figures suggest that the majority of hypertensives should be controllable; however, interestingly, only approximately 50% of hypertensives are controlled in accord with JNC VII guidelines [1]. This shortfall in achieving blood pressure goals has occurred in the setting of increased public awareness of hypertension. The reasons for the failure to achieve greater success are largely unknown but undoubtedly include patient related issues such as pill burden, economic issues, and inability to comply with nonpharmacologic prescriptions for lifestyle changes as well as provider related issues such as provider inertia, inability to deliver effective counseling, and failure to recognize appropriate goals.

Complications

Blood pressure is a continuous variable. Although it was recognized for centuries that blood pressure level correlated with cardiovascular risk, it was only in the mid to late twentieth century with the availability of devices for the measurement of blood pressure and pharmacologic agents for treatment that the definition of hypertension became standardized [55]. The risk for cardiovascular morbidity and mortality rises with all degrees of increase in blood pressure. The decision to define hypertension as blood pressure greater than 140/90 was somewhat arbitrary but based on epidemiologic studies showing increased cardiovascular risk.

Chronic hypertension is the major risk factor for cardiovascular morbidity and mortality. The sequelae of hypertension include coronary artery disease, congestive heart failure, kidney failure, stroke, and other peripheral vascular disease. As alluded to previously, many patients with hypertension also have other risk factors for cardiovascular disease including metabolic syndrome, frank diabetes mellitus, hyperlipidemia, and tobacco use. Nonetheless, hypertension alone remains as a significant risk factor for cardiovascular illness. According to the Framingham study, hypertension increases the risk of heart failure by over twofold in the groups with highest versus the lowest blood pressures [1, 56, 57]. Likewise the risk of coronary artery disease and stroke were significantly elevated in hypertensives versus normotensive individuals. In a large meta-analysis [2], Lewington et al. showed that the risk for mortality for cardiovascular disease increased in a graded linear fashion with increasing degrees of systolic (from 115 to 180 mmHg) and diastolic (from 70 to 110 mmHg) blood pressure in individuals from age 40 to 89 years. In this study, the correlation between usual blood pressure and stroke was most pronounced. There was no evidence of a cutoff at any blood pressure down to systolic 115. The effect was present in the youngest versus the oldest group and slightly though not significantly greater for men. A similar relationship was found for ischemic heart disease. The correlation between death from ischemic heart disease and blood pressure was linear with increasing blood pressures without evidence of a threshold or cutoff at systolic 115 mmHg. In contrast to the findings in stroke, the effect of blood pressure on mortality in women was higher but not significantly so than in men. Other large epidemiologic studies such as MRFIT and NHANES have shown similar findings.

While the impact of hypertension on the development of and mortality from stroke, ischemic heart disease, and heart failure are relatively well established, the effect of hypertension on the development and progression of chronic kidney disease has been debated [58–60]. A recent study in over 40,000 patients, however, did confirm an increase in the risk of the development of chronic kidney disease in individuals with a systolic blood pressure over 120 mmHg.

Treatment

Treatment of hypertension decreases the risk of the development and reduces the total mortality, cardiovascular mortality, heart failure and stroke. Beginning with the 1967 publication of the Veterans Cooperative Study documenting a salutary effect of blood pressure treatment on cardiovascular outcomes, a continuous series of reports has continued to confirm that control of hypertension results in a decrease in cardiovascular mortality [1, 55, 56, 63–65]. The decades following this initial report produced studies showing that lowering systolic blood pressure by 6–10 mmHg decreased stroke by up to 40%, coronary artery disease by 25%, heart failure by 55%, and death by 25%. These studies were followed by a variety of studies examining the relative efficacies of different agents. By and large, the consensus is that the primary objective above and beyond the choice of specific antihypertensive agents should be achievement of a sustained blood pressure less than 140/90 for most individuals with essential hypertension. Diuretics have consistently shown efficacy, however, alone and in combination therapies. A recent meta-analysis demonstrated that treatment of hypertension with diuretics prevented the development of heart failure more effectively than inhibitors of the renin–angiotensin system, calcium channel blockers, or beta blockers. Other studies have demonstrated the advantages of more intensive therapy goals and specific pharmacologic agents for very specific groups of individuals such as diabetics or patients with chronic kidney disease; however, for uncomplicated patients with essential hypertension, diuretics remain the first line of therapy.

The Joint National Commission Groups introduced and popularized the algorithmic stepped care approach to the treatment of hypertension [55]. Although the reports have varied somewhat over their history vis-à-vis classification of hypertension, several recommendations have not changed over the 30 years of their sequential reports. Lifestyle modifications remain the first recommendation, including dietary salt restriction and increased physical activity [66]. The fact that most hypertensives require two or more medications to control their hypertension highlights the failure of nonpharmacologic measures for the general population of hypertensives. Diuretics of the thiazide family are first line pharmacologic agents when lifestyle changes alone do not result in the desired goal blood pressure. The choice of a diuretic as the first step is based on fundamental physiologic studies showing the importance of sodium homeostasis in blood pressure control and on the many studies demonstrating the efficacy of this class of agents in achieving blood pressure goals and in achieving reduction in cardiovascular events. Most hypertensives will benefit from a diuretic, but the choice of a second agent may be dictated by additional comorbidities as discussed in the chapter reviewing treatment of hypertension (Chap. 40). For example, patients with proteinuric kidney disease may benefit from the addition of an angiotensin converting enzyme inhibitor or an angiotensin receptor blocker. Patients with coronary artery disease may benefit from a beta blocker which can address blood pressure and potential arrhythmias. Calcium channel blockers have demonstrated particular efficacy in the elderly.

The uncontested goal of therapy is achievement of a blood pressure less than 140/90 with the fewest side effects. This goal pertains to all age groups, though some suggest that in the very elderly over 80 years, the systolic goal may be relaxed to 150 mmHg. Although some investigators in the field have promoted lowering these goals, strong empiric evidence to support this suggestion are lacking in "uncomplicated" essential hypertension [67, 68].

Case Discussion

Although this woman's blood pressure is clearly elevated, a single measurement is not sufficient to diagnose chronic hypertension and would require at least one additional in office measurement in the hypertensive range. That being said, she has a number of risk factors for chronic hypertension including her prior history of gestational hypertension, age, overweight status, family history, and lifestyle. In addition to a second blood pressure measurement, the clinician would do well to measure waist circumference, measure blood pressure in both arms, lipid profile, and perhaps glycosylated hemoglobin if metabolic syndrome is a serious consideration. The absence of any other identified abnormalities does not exclude the possibility of secondary hypertension but in view of the unremarkable initial evaluation and her risk factors for essential hypertension, no further testing would be warranted. Even before a diagnosis of essential hypertension is made, this woman would benefit from counseling on lifestyle issues such as adoption of the DASH diet and initiation of a consistent exercise regimen to effect weight loss. At this point, no pharmacologic therapy is mandatory. If hypertension is confirmed and nonpharmacologic measures do not decrease blood pressure to less than 140/90, a thiazide diuretic such as hydrochlorothiazide or chlorthalidone would be a reasonable initial therapy.

References

1. Chobanian AV, Bakris GL, Black HR, Cushman WC, Green LA, Iaao JL, Jones DW, Materson BJ, Oparil S, Wright JT, Roccella EJ. Seventh Report of the Joint National Committee on Prevention, Detection, Evaluation, and Treatment of High Blood Pressure. Hypertension. 2003;42:1206–52.
2. Prospective Studies Collaboration. Age-specific relevance of usual blood pressure to vascular mortality: a meta-analysis of individual data for one million adults in 61 prospective studies. Lancet. 2002;360:1903–13.
3. Tracy RE. Renal vasculature in essential hypertension: a review of some contrarian evidence. Contrib Nephrol. 2011;269:327–36.
4. Yang Q, Liu T, Kuklina EV, Flanders D, Hong Yuling H, Gillespie C, Chang M-H, Gwinn M, Dowling N, Khoury MJ, Hu FB. Sodium and potassium intake and mortality among US adults. Arch Intern Med. 2011;171:1183–91.
5. Adrogue HJ, Madias NE. Shared primacy of sodium and potassium on cardiovascular risk. Am J Kidney Dis. 2009;54:598–601.
6. Adrogue HJ, Madias NE. Sodium and potassium in the pathogenesis of hypertension. N Engl J Med. 2007;356:1966–78.
7. Blaustein MP, Leenen FHH, Chen L, Golovina VA, Hamlyn MJ, Pallone TL, Van Huysse JW, Zhang J, Wier WG. How NaCl raises blood pressure: a new paradigm for the pathogenesis of salt-dependent hypertension. Am J Physiol Heart Circ Physiol. 2012;302:H1031–49.
8. Brondolo E, Love EE, Pencille M, Schoenthaler A, Ogedegbe G. Racism and hypertension: a review of the empirical evidence and implications for clinical practice. Am J Hypertens. 2011;24:518–29.
9. Rostand SG. Vitamin D, blood pressure, and African Americans: toward a unifying hypothesis. Clin J Am Soc Nephrol. 2010;5:1697–703.
10. Flack JM, Sica DA, Bakris G, Brown AL, Ferdinand KC, Grimm RH, Hall WD, Jones WE, Kountz DS, Lea JP, Nasser S, Nesbitt SD, Saunders E, Scisney-Matlock M, Jamerson KA. Management of high blood pressure in Blacks: an update of the International Society on Hypertension in Blacks consensus statement. Hypertension. 2010;56:780–800.
11. Ventura H, Pina IL, Lavie CJ. Hypertension and antihypertensive therapy in Hispanics and Mexican Americans living in the United States. Postgrad Med. 2011;123:46–57.
12. Bertram JF, Douglas-Denton RN, Diouf B, Hughson MD, Hoy WE. Human nephron number: implications for health and disease. Pediatr Nephrol. 2011;26:1529–33.
13. Kett MM, Denton KM. Renal programming: cause for concern? Am J Physiol Regul Integr Comp Physiol. 2011;300:R791–803.
14. Minor D, Wofford M, Wyatt SB. Does socioeconomic status affect blood pressure goal achievement? Curr Hypertens Rep. 2008;10(5):390–7.
15. Grotto I, Huerta M, Sharabi Y. Hypertension and socioeconomic status. Curr Opin Cardiol. 2008;23(4):335–9.
16. Bale B. Optimizing hypertension management in underserved rural populations. J Natl Med Assoc. 2010;102(1):10–7.
17. Grundy SM, Brewer HB, Cleeman JI, Smith SC, LEnfant C. Definition of metabolic syndrome: report of National Heart, Lung, and Blood Institute/AHA conference on scientific issues related to definition. Circulation. 2004;109:433–8.
18. Potenza MV, Mechanick JL. The metabolic syndrome: definition, global impact, and pathophysiology. Nutr Clin Pract. 2009;24:560–77.

19. Alberti KG, Eckel RH, Grundy SM, Zimmet PZ, Cleeman JI, Dobnato KA, Fruchart JC, James WP, Loria CM, Smith SC. Harmonizing the metabolic syndrome: a joint interim statement for the International Diabetes Federation Task Force on Epidemiology and Prevention; National Heart Lung and Blood Institute; American Heart Association; World Heart Federation; International Atherosclerosis Society; and International Association for the Study of Obesity. Circulation. 2009;120: 1640–5.
20. Zalesin KC, Franklin BA, Miller WM, Peterson ED, McCullough PA. Impact of obesity on cardiovascular disease. Med Clin North Am. 2011;95(5):919–37.
21. Kurukulasaliya LR, Stas S, Lastra G, Manrique C, Sowers JR. Hypertension in obesity. Med Clin North Amr. 2011;95(5):903–17.
22. Feber J, Ahmed M. Hypertension in children: new trends and challenges. Clin Sci. 2010;119:151–61.
23. The 1984 Report of the Joint National Committee on The Detection, Evaluation, and Treatment of High Blood Pressure. Arch Intern Med. 1984;144:1045–1057
24. Clark CE, Talor RS, Shore AC. Association of a difference in SBP between arms with vascular disease and mortality: a systematic review and meta-analysis. Lancet. 2012;11:61710–8.
25. McManus RJ, Mant J. Do differences in blood pressure between arms matter? Lancet. 2012;11:61926–30.
26. White WB. Relating cardiovascular risk to out-of-office blood pressure and the importance of controlling blood pressure 24 hours a day. Am J Med. 2008;121(8 Suppl):S2–7.
27. Parati G, Faini A, Valentini M. Blood pressure variability: its measurement and significance in hypertension. Curr Hypertens Rep. 2006;8(3):199–204.
28. Powers BJ, Olsen MK, Smith VA, Woolson RF, Bosworth HB, Oddone EZ. Measuring blood pressure decision making and quality reporting: where and how many measures? Ann Intern Med. 2011;154:781–8.
29. Bosworth HB, Powers BJ, Olsen MK, McCant FM, Rubber J, Smith V, Gentry PW, Rose C, Van Houtven C, Wang V, Goldstein MK, Oddone EZ. Home blood pressure management and improved blood pressure control. Arch Intern Med. 2011;171:1173–80.
30. Van der Wel MC, Buunk IE, van Weel C, Thien TABM, Bakx JC. A novel approach to office blood pressure measurement: thirty minute office blood pressure vs daytime ambulatory blood pressure. Ann Fam Med. 2011;9:128–35.
31. Scherpbier-de Haan N, van der Wel M, Schoenmakers G, Boudewijns S, Peer P, van Weel C, Thien T, Bakx C. Thirty-minute compared to standardised office blood pressure measurement in general practice. Br J Gen Pract. 2011;61(590):e590–7.
32. O'Brien E. Twenty-four-hour ambulatory blood pressure measurement in clinical practice and research: a critical review of a technique in need of implementation. J Intern Med. 2011;269:478–95.
33. Wexler R. Ambulatory blood pressure monitoring in primary care. South Med J. 2010;103(5):447–52.
34. Ashwell M, Gunn P, Gibson S. Waist to height ratio is a better screen tool than waist circumference and BMI in adult cardiometabolic risk factors. Obes Rev. 2012;13:275–86.
35. Cepeda-Valery B, Pressman GS, Fiqueredo VM, Romero-Corral A. Impact of obesity on total and cardiovascular mortality—fat or fiction? Nat Rev Cardiol. 2011;8(4):233–7.
36. Drost JT, Maas AH, van Eyck J, van der Schouw YT. Preeclampsia as a female-specific risk factor for chronic hypertension. Maturitas. 2010;67(4):321–6.
37. Carretero OA, Oparil S. Essential hypertension: part 1: definition and etiology. Circulation. 2000;101:329–35.
38. Tarazi RC, Ibrahim MM, Bravo EL. Hemodynamic characteristics of primary hyperaldosteronism. N Engl J Med. 1973;289:1330–5.
39. Martinez-Aguayo A, Fardella C. Genetics of hypertensive syndrome. Horm Res. 2009;71:253–9.
40. Vehaskari VM. Heritable forms of hypertension. Pediatr Nephrol. 2009;24:1929–37.
41. Lifton RP, Gharavi AG, Geller DS. Molecular mechanisms of human hypertension. Cell. 2001;104:545–56.
42. Ji W, Foo JN, O'Roak BJ, Zhao H, Larson MG, Simon DB, Newton-Cheh C, State MW, Levy D, Lifton RP. Rare independent mutations in renal salt handling genes contribute to blood pressure variation. Nat Genet. 2008;40(5):592–9.
43. Coffman TM. Under pressure: the search for the essential mechanisms of hypertension. Nat Med. 2011;17:1402–9.
44. Herrera M, Coffman TM. The kidney and hypertension: novel insights from transgenic models. Curr Opin Nephrol Hypertens. 2012;21:171–8.
45. Coffman TM, Crowley SD. Kidney in hypertension. Guyton redux. Hypertension. 2008;51:811–6.
46. Johnson RJ, Herrera-Acosta J, Schreiner GF, Rodriguez-Iturbe B. Subtle acquired renal injury as a mechanism of salt-sensitive hypertension. N Engl J Med. 2002;346: 913–23.
47. Rafiq S, Anand S, Roberts R. Genome-wide association studies of hypertension: have they been fruitful? J Cardiovasc Trans Res. 2010;3:189–96.
48. Kraja AT, Hunt SC, Rao DC, Davila-Roman VG, Arnett DK, Province MA. Genetics of hypertension and cardiovascular disease and their interconnected pathways: lessons from large studies. Curr Hypertens Rep. 2011;13:46–54.
49. Paunovic K, Stansfeld S, Clark C, Belojevic G. Epidemiological studies on noise and blood pressure in children: observations and suggestions. Environ Int. 2011;37:1030–41.
50. Carretero OA, Oparil S. Essential hypertension: part 2: treatment. Circulation. 2000;101:446–53.
51. Hackam DG, Khan NA, Hemmelgarn BR, et al. The 2010 Canadian Hypertension Education Program recommendations for the management of hyperten-

sion: part 2—therapy. Can J Cardiol. 2010;26(5): 249–58.
52. Egan BM, Zhao Y, Axon RN. US trends in prevalence, awareness, treatment, and control of hypertension, 1988–2008. JAMA. 2010;303:2043–50.
53. Daugherty SL, Powers JD, Magid DJ, Tavel HM, Masoudi FA, Margolis KL, O'Connor PJ, Selby JV, Ho PM. Incidence and prognosis of resistant hypertension in hypertensive patients. Circulation. 2012; online
54. Zampaglione B, Pascale C, Marchisio M, Cavallo-Perin P. Hypertensive urgencies and emergencies. Prevalence and clinical presentation. Hypertension. 1996;27:144–7.
55. Moser M. From JNC I to JNC 7—what have we learned? Prog Cardiovasc Dis. 2006;48:303–15.
56. Mancia G. Blood pressure reduction and cardiovascular outcomes: past, present, and future. Am J Cardiol. 2007;100(suppl):3J–9.
57. Sciarretta S, Palano F, Tocci G, Baldini R, Volpe M. Antihypertensive treatment and development of heart failure in hypertension. Arch Intern Med. 2011;171:384–94.
58. Hanratty R, Chonchol M, Havranek EP, Powers JD, Dickinson M, Ho PM, Magid DJ, Steiner JF. Relationship between blood pressure and incident chronic kidney disease in hypertensive patients. Clin J Am Soc Nephrol. 2011;6:2605–11.
59. Appel LJ, Wright JT, Greene T, Agodoa LY, Astor BC, Bakris GL, Cleveland WH, Charleston J, Contreras G, Faulkner ML, Gabbai FB, Gassman JJ, Hebert LA, Jamerson KA, Kopple JD, Kusek JW, Lipkowitz MS, Massry SG, Miller ER, Norris K, Phillips RA, Pogue VA, Randall OS, Rostand SG, Smogorzewski MJ, Toto RD, Wang X. Intensive blood pressure control in hypertensive chronic kidney disease. N Engl J Med. 2010;363: 918–29.
60. Murea M, Freedman BL. Essential hypertension and risk of nephropathy: a reappraisal. Curr Opin Nephrol Hypertens. 2010;19:235–41.
61. Veterans Administration Cooperative Study Group on Antihypertensive Agents. Effects of treatment on morbidity in hypertension: results in patients with diastolic blood pressures averaging 115 through 129 mmHg. JAMA. 1967;202:1028–34.
62. Hansson L, Lindholm LH, Niskanen L, Lanke J, Hedner T, Niklason A, Luomanmaki K, Dahlof B, de Faire U, Morlin C, et al. Effect of angiotensin-converting-enzyme inhibition compared with conventional therapy on cardiovascular morbidity and mortality in hypertension: the Captopril Prevention Project (CAPPP) randomised trial. Lancet. 1999;353:611–6.
63. Turnbull F, Blood Pressure Lowering Treatment Triallists'Collaboration. Effects of different blood-pressure-lowering regimens on major cardiovascular events: results of prospectively-designed overviews of randomised trials. Lancet. 2003;362:1527–35.
64. Hermida RC, Ayala DE, Fernandez JR, Portaluppi F, Fabbian F, Smolensky MH. Circadian rhythms in blood pressure regulation and optimization of hypertension treatment with ACE inhibitor and ARB medications. Am J Hypertens. 2011;24:383–91.
65. Minutolo R, Gabbai FB, Borrelli S, Scigliano R, Trucillo P, Baldanza D, Laurino S, Mascia S, Conte G, De Nicola L. Changing the timing of antihypertensive therapy to reduce nocturnal blood pressure in CKD: an 8-week uncontrolled trial. Am J Kidney Dis. 2007;50:908–17.
66. Hedayati SS, Elsayed EF, Reilly RF. Non-pharmacologic aspects of blood pressure management: what are the data? Kidney Int. 2011;79: 1061–70.
67. Agawal R. Blood pressure goal in chronic kidney disease: what is the evidence? Curr Opin Nephrol Hypertens. 2011;20:229–32.
68. Hermida RC, Ayala DE, Fernandez JR, Calvo C. Chronotherapy improves blood pressure control and reverts the nondipper pattern in patients with resistant hypertension. Hypertension. 2008;51:69–76.

Lifestyle Modifications in the Treatment of Hypertension

42

Vibha S. Nayak, Dawn J. Caster, and Eleanor D. Lederer

Case

A 42-year-old woman presents for routine health maintenance examination. She is unaware of any medical problems but states that she has checked her blood pressure several times at local health fairs and has been advised that she has "borderline" high blood pressure and should seek medical attention. She recalls blood pressures ranging from 135/80 to 142/90. She takes no medications. She thinks that her mother had hypertension. She drinks socially, generally one or two glasses of wine on the weekends. She does not follow a specific exercise routine but states that she moves all the time. Breakfast is usually a Pop Tart with two cups of coffee. Lunch is a meal from McDonald's with two more cups of coffee. She and her husband eat out frequently for dinner because of their hectic schedules. On physical exam she is an overweight woman with BP 138/87 (checked at rest with an appropriately sized cuff), pulse 90/min, respiratory rate 12/min, height 64 in., weight 150 pounds, and BMI 27. Her waist circumference is 35 in. The remainder of her examination is within normal limits. Her screening chemistries and urinalysis are normal.

V.S. Nayak, M.D. (✉) • D.J. Caster, M.D.
Department of Medicine, Nephrology, University of Louisville, 615 South Preston Street, Louisville, KY 40202, USA
e-mail: vsnaya01@louisville.edu

E.D. Lederer, M.D., F.A.S.N.
Department of Medicine, Nephrology, University of Louisville, 615 South Preston Street, Louisville, KY 40202, USA

Robley Rex VA Medical Centre, 800 Zorn Avenue, Louisville, KY 40206, USA

Introduction

In May 2003 the NHLBI's Joint National Committee VII on High Blood Pressure released its recommendations for the diagnosis and management of Hypertension [1]. Among its practice guidelines is listed the role of lifestyle modifications in preventing and treating hypertension. Data from the NHANES study show that approximately 50 million people across the USA have HTN necessitating some form of therapy [2]. The World Health Report in 2002 estimated that around the globe approximately one billion people will suffer from HTN and approximately seven million people will die from HTN and its related complications [3]. This report also states that suboptimal BPs (defined as a SBP > 115 mmHg) is the number one attributable risk factor for death throughout the world. It is also strongly correlated with increased cardiovascular and cerebrovascular disease. In addition the USRDS data shows a strong correlation between HTN and ESRD [4].

The JNC report highlights the importance of lifestyle modifications in the treatment of HTN. Lifestyle modifications are recommended for all stages of HTN [1]. The guidelines state "the adoption of healthy lifestyles by all persons is critical for the prevention of high blood pressure and is an

E.V. Lerma and M. Rosner (eds.), *Clinical Decisions in Nephrology, Hypertension and Kidney Transplantation*,
DOI 10.1007/978-1-4614-4454-1_42, © Springer Science+Business Media New York 2013

indispensable part of the management of patients with Hypertension".Most Americans are not at goal blood pressures and the importance of lifestyle modifications cannot be ignored. The pathophysiology of HTN is complex and its pathogenesis and onset is likely influenced significantly by the interplay of genetic, environmental and lifestyle factors.The management of HTN, like several other diseases, depends heavily on the ability of the patient to self manage his disease as well as promote and maintain a healthy lifestyle.

The lifestyle modifications that have been recommended by JNC VII are diet, specifically the DASH diet or the Dietary Approaches to Stop Hypertension, exercise, weight loss, cessation of smoking and limitation of alcohol.

Dietary Approaches to Control of Blood Pressure

Hypertension and Diet

The relationship between diet and hypertension has been examined for several decades. Multiple large epidemiologic studies have shown a relationship between increased sodium intake and elevated blood pressure. The converse relationship has been demonstrated for potassium intake [5–8]. Low calcium and magnesium intake have also been associated with increased blood pressure in population studies [9, 10]

One of the earliest observations of the connection between dietary sodium and hypertension was made by Lewis Dahl in 1960 [11, 12]. He observed large differences in sodium intake among five different populations. Furthermore, he found a positive linear relationship between sodium intake and the prevalence of hypertension. In his observations Alaskan Eskimos had the lowest intake at 68 mmol/day and Northern Japanese had the highest intake at 462 mmol/day. In the Japanese population he observed a relationship between the regional sodium intake and hemorrhagic stroke deaths. In Northern Japan where the sodium intake was the highest the rate was more than double that of the Southern region [13].

The Intersalt study [5] was a large (32 countries, 52 centers, 10,079 subjects) epidemiologic investigation of the relationship between dietary intake of electrolytes as measured by urinary content and blood pressure. The study found positive associations between 24 h urine sodium or urinary sodium/potassium ratios and systolic blood pressure. The four centers with very low sodium excretion (2–50 mmol/24 h) all had very low systolic and diastolic blood pressures (95–110/61–68 mmHg). Notably, in these populations a statistically significant increase in blood pressure with age was not seen. The authors found that the results in these four centers had a large impact on the statistical analysis of the entire data and that, in fact, when these four centers were removed from the analysis, much of the significance between 24 h urinary sodium and blood pressure was lost, while the relationship between age and increase in blood pressure remained. The authors also found a very strong association between body mass index and high alcohol intake and the development of hypertension. It is on the basis of this and other studies that more recent public health initiatives to limit sodium intake have been developed.

As populations have become more developed, the sodium intake has also risen. In contrast, the potassium intake has declined. Most of this transformation is secondary to increased consumption of processed foods and decreased intake of fresh fruits and vegetables. Contrary to popular belief, the largest source of dietary sodium in the USA is not from salt added at the table, but from manufactured foods (approximately 75% of intake). Moreover, cereals and baked goods make up the single largest contribution to sodium intake in adults who reside in the USA and U.K. [14]. As the sodium intake has increased, the potassium intake has decreased, resulting in a 100 fold decrease in the ratio of dietary potassium intake to dietary sodium intake.

In contrast to what has been observed in most developed populations, the Yanomamo Indians have maintained a high ratio of dietary potassium to dietary sodium. The Yanomamo, an indigenous population in the Amazon, consume a diet is extremely low in sodium and high in potassium. The mean blood pressure is also significantly lower at 96/61 mmHg [7].

These observations have led to several clinical trials looking at the efficacy of dietary modification on blood pressure control. Of note, the concept of treating hypertension by diet modification is a very old one. In the mid to late 1930s, Walter Kempner, an internist at Duke University, developed the Rice Diet, so named because unsalted white rice was a staple of this diet and included in most meals [15]. While the appearance of effective pharmacologic therapy and the severely restricted nature of the diet pushed this approach out of the limelight of academic inquiry, the rice diet has not disappeared and, in fact, has enjoyed something of a commercial resurgence in a more recently published updated book [16] and a robust online presence (http://www.ricedietprogram.com/). As a proof of concept experiment, Dr. Kempner's original studies in patients with severe forms of hypertension demonstrated conclusively that dietary manipulations could lower blood pressure. However, the patients on this diet experienced substantial weight loss, not just a decrease in sodium intake; thus, whether the blood pressure lowering effects were due to either or both interventions cannot be distinguished. The largest of the recent clinical trials to determine efficacy of diet in the treatment of hypertension were the Trials of Hypertension Prevention (TOHP I and II) and the Dietary Approaches to Stop Hypertension (DASH). Many additional studies have incorporated ideas from the original DASH diet with variations to enhance the antihypertensive effect. The DASH diet is a diet rich in lean meat, fish, legumes, fruits, vegetables, nuts, and seeds. In 2010, Fang et al. from the division for Heart Disease and Stroke prevention, National Center for Chronic Disease Prevention and Health Promotion, CDC [17], assessed the prevalence of dietary intake of the recommended servings of fruits and vegetables using the Behavioral Risk Factor Surveillance System among the US population with HTN in 2003 and 2007. They determined that among hypertensives, between 2003 and 2007, less than a quarter are eating five or more servings of fruits and vegetables a day.

TOHP I

TOHP 1 was a large multi-center, randomized trial in pre-hypertensive patients that looked at several lifestyle modifications including sodium restriction, weight loss, and dietary supplements. For the sodium restriction intervention, the experimental arm ($n = 327$) received nutrition and behavioral counseling with the goal of reducing dietary sodium intake to 1,400 mg/day. The control arm ($n = 417$) received no intervention. At 18 months the net decrease from baseline urinary Na in sodium was 44 mmol/day in the treatment arm. The net decrease in systolic blood pressure was small (1.7 mmHg), but statistically significant ($P < 0.01$). Furthermore, in a 15-year follow-up study, the treatment group experienced a 25% reduction in cardiovascular events [18].

TOHP II

The second TOHP trial tested the effects of weight loss and sodium restriction on the blood pressure of pre-hypertensive patients (SBP < 140, DBP 83–89) over a 3 year period. It was a multi-center randomized trial that had 2,182 participants. The study was a 2×2 factorial study that examined four groups: (1) sodium restriction with weight reduction, (2) sodium restriction alone, (3) weight reduction alone, and (4) standard therapy. All treatment groups experienced the most dramatic results at the end of 6 months. Unfortunately, the effects diminished as the study went on. At the end of 3 years those in the combination arm experienced a net decrease in sodium excretion of 33 mmol/day and only a modest decrease in systolic blood pressure (1.1 mmHg). Those in the sodium restriction alone group experienced a net decrease in sodium excretion of 40 mmol/day and had a modest reduction in systolic blood pressure (1.2 mmHg) [19]. At 48 months those in the intervention groups were significantly less likely to develop hypertension (SBP > 140 or use of antihypertensive medication) [19].

DASH

Rather than focus on dietary sodium, the DASH study looked at the benefit of a diet rich in vegetables, fruits, and low fat dairy products. A total of

459 participants were randomized to three groups after going through an initial 3 week control phase (low fruits/vegetables). The three groups included the following diets: (1) increased fruits/vegetables, (2) increased fruits/vegetables combined with low fat dairy products and reduced saturated and total fat (combination diet), and (3) control diet (low fruit/vegetable) Those in the combination group experienced the largest reductions in blood pressure from baseline. Among the patients with hypertension, the combination diet reduced systolic and diastolic blood pressure by 11.4 and 5.5 mmHg more than the control diet [20].

Several permutations of the original DASH diet have subsequently been examined. In the Optimal Macronutrient Intake Trial to Prevent Heart Disease (OmniHeart trial), reduced carbohydrate (carbohydrate replaced with protein or unsaturated fat) versions of the DASH diet reduced blood pressures further than the higher carbohydrate version of the DASH diet [21]. The Exercise and Nutrition Interventions for Cardiovascular Health (ENCORE) study looked at the effect of a reduced calorie version of DASH and had impressive results. The reduced calorie DASH showed a reduction in systolic blood pressure of 16.1 mmHg and diastolic blood pressure 9.9 mmHg [22]. Reduced sodium diet combined with DASH has also been studied in the DASH-Sodium trial. DASH combine with low sodium diet led to a systolic blood pressure drop of 11.5 mmHg in those with hypertension and 7.1 mmHg in those without hypertension. This is similar to the effect of a single drug regimen [23]. Finally, in the Diet, Exercise, and Weight Loss Intervention Trial (DEW-IT) the DASH diet was studied in combination with weight loss and reduced sodium. The BP reduction was 9.5/9.3 mmHg [24].

Increased Potassium Intake

The INTERSALT study demonstrated a strong positive association between sodium and blood pressure and a reverse association between potassium intake and blood pressure [5–7]. One potential mechanism for this observation is through increased expression of long WNK1, a serine threonine kinase critical for the differential regulation of sodium and potassium transport in the distal nephron. In a state of potassium depletion, long WNK1 is upregulated and stimulates ROMK to reduce potassium secretion. Long WNK 1 also stimulates sodium reabsorption through ENaC and NCC. This, in turn, leads to increased sodium retention and further hypertension [8].

While the observational data are promising, clinical trials report conflicting results about potential benefits of increased potassium intake on blood pressure. In TOHP I potassium supplementation caused a modest reduction in BP at 3 months that was not significant at 6 months [25]. In a meta-analysis of 33 randomized controlled trials, potassium supplementation was associated with a significant blood pressure reduction of 3.11 mmHg systolic and 1.97 mmHg diastolic. Treatment effects were strongest in patients with underlying hypertension as well as high sodium diet [26]. One of the potential limitations to universal potassium supplementation is that many patients with hypertension already have advanced kidney disease and thus are not candidates for potassium supplementation or high potassium diets.

Increased Magnesium and Calcium Intake

Although low calcium and magnesium intake have been associated with hypertension, a reproducible effect of divalent cation supplementation on blood pressure has been difficult to parse out in clinical trials. The TOHP I study failed to demonstrate a blood pressure lowering effect with the 1 g/day calcium supplementation [25]. Some small trials have shown promising results for magnesium supplementation, while others show no effect [27–29]. However, the doses of magnesium administered in the various trials were not uniform so it is difficult to compare. A meta-analysis of 20 magnesium studies showed dose dependent decrease in blood pressure with supplementation; however, adequately powered trials with sufficient magnesium supplementation are needed to confirm this relationship [30].

Dietary Fiber and Protein

Epidemiologic studies indicate that a diet rich in protein and fiber can lower BP. He et al. and his colleagues found a 10 g higher intake of dietary fiber was significantly associated with a lower level of systolic (−2.2 mmHg) and diastolic (−2.1 mmHg) blood pressure in their Chinese cohort [31, 32]. However, most studies are likely confounded by the fact that high fiber diets are generally vegetarian diets rich in plant based foods, unrefined grains, fruits, and vegetables that are also rich in potassium, magnesium, PUFA and low in saturated fatty acids and cholesterol.

Dietary protein has also been found to have an inverse relationship with BP in several observational studies. However, RCT's examining this have not provided a similar confirmation. Most of these studies lacked the statistical power, sample size, short duration of follow-up, etc.

More RCTs are needed to examine the effects of fiber and protein on BP.

Uric Acid and Hypertension

The concept that hyperuricemia may play a role in hypertension was noted by Dr. Frederick Akbar Mohamed as far back as 1879 [33]. There is evidence through clinical and laboratory studies regarding the impact of increased uric acid on hypertension in both Juvenile and adult populations [34]. The Olivetti Heart study [35] found and showed an independent positive association between serum uricacid levels and development of hypertension after correcting for age, BMI, CHOL, and TG. Several other studies by Selby et al.; also found a positive correlation between high uric acid levels and hypertension [36]. The pathophysiology of hyperuricemia in hypertension is thought to be related to the impaired handling and subsequent impaired excretion of UA via the renal tubules. In obesity, hyperuricemia occurs due to the overproduction of UA, as well as insulin resistance and hyperinsulinemia that causes increased reabsorption of uric acid. However, the precise mechanism of hyperuricemia causing hypertension has still not been clarified [37–39]. It is reasonable to control risk factors leading to hyperuricemia, including restricting red meat, alcohol and weight loss. Persistent hyperuricemia may be treated with Xanthine Oxidase inhibitors.

Weight Loss

The relationship between obesity and HTN is well established. Systolic blood pressure rises ~3 mmHg and diastolic blood pressure ~2.3 mmHg for each 10 kg increase in body weight [40]. Several large interventional trails have demonstrated a decrease in the incidence of hypertension with loss of body weight.

The TONE study [41] examined the effect of physical activity and weight loss in participants aged between 60–80 years of age and subsequent weight loss of 4.5 kg (10 lbs) or greater. Exercise counselors experienced in lifestyle change techniques were responsible for the implementation of active interventions including providing the participants with the core knowledge and behavioral skills necessary to achieve and maintain the desired body weight. The trial found that an average reduction in body weight of about 3.5 kg decreased the need for antihypertensives by about 30%, an effect that persisted 4 years after the end of the trial [42]. Similarly, the TOHP I [18] in a younger cohort of 2,182 patients with a high normal DBP (80–89 mmHg) between 35 and 54 year olds; studied the effects of weight loss on HTN over an 18 month period. The weight reduction program also encompassed a moderate increase in caloric expenditure by walking at a brisk pace for 45 min, 4–5 times per week. An average reduction in body weight by 3.9 kg resulted in a reduction in SBP and DBP by 2.9 mmHg and 2.3 mmHg respectively. A recent 7-year follow-up on the TOHP I trial by He et al.; reported a mean reduction in the incidence of hypertension by 77% [43]. The TOHP II [19] corroborated these results in a randomized clinical trial of almost 2,382 overweight hypertensive patients with a BMI of 110–165% of ideal body weight; a 4% reduction in body weight over 3 years resulted in a reduction in SBP and DBP of 1.3/0.9 mmHg respectively. The group with the largest weight loss (>4.4 kg) had the largest reductions in SPB and DBPs of 7.0 and 5.0 mmHg respectively.

Exercise

Data exists suggesting that exercise independent of weight loss is beneficial in lowering arterial BP. A meta-analysis of 54 RCTs by Whelton et al. [44]; ($N=2,419$) reported the beneficial effect of aerobic exercise on BP reduction. They reported a statistically significant reduction in BP of 3.8/2.6 mmHg in SBP and DBP respectively between the intervention and control groups, the groups differed only in aerobic exercise. Moreover, this mean BP reduction was achieved in all participants including those that did not lose weight, i.e., overweight patients as well as in normotensive patients. All frequencies, intensities, and types of aerobic exercise lowered blood pressure.

While this concept is widely accepted, the underlying pathogenetic mechanisms mediating the beneficial effects of exercise on HTN remain rather obscure. The beneficial effects of regular exercise may be due to a reduction in oxidative stress, decreased plasma norepinephrine levels, increased prostaglandin E, increased nitric oxide availability, and improvement in the overall metabolic profile [45]. There may also be beneficial effects on the prothrombotic state associated with hypertension at least with moderate intensity exercise [46].All forms of exercise seemed to be effective in reducing blood pressure.

The JNC 7guidelines recommend engaging in regular aerobic exercise such as brisk walking, at least 30 min a day on most days of the week [1].

Alcohol

Several epidemiological studies have established a close association between alcohol intake and HTN. The cut off seems to be roughly over three drinks per day [47]. Mechanisms underlying the pathophysiology of HTN associated with the ingestion of alcohol are ambiguous. Some suggested mechanisms include stimulation of the sympathetic nervous system and the renin–angiotensin–aldosterone system, increased cortisol levels, inhibition of nitric oxide, increased intracellular calcium especially in vascular smooth muscle, changes in electrolyte transport, a genetic predisposition, and a hyperdynamic circulation [48]. More than likely an interplay of several different factors is involved in the pathophysiology of alcohol mediated HTN.

Clinical studies examining the effects of alcohol on HTN are limited by size, short duration and variable findings. In the PATHS study (Prevention and Treatment of Hypertension Study), 641 veterans with an average intake of >3 drinks/day and a DBP between 80 and 99 mmHg were randomized to a cognitive behavioral alcohol reduction intervention group or a control group [49]. The intervention group at 6 months had a nonsignificant reduction in BP (1.2/0.7 mmHg) than the control group.

On the other hand, Abramson et al. [50] showed that higher levels of total weekly alcohol consumption and binge drinking were associated with higher ambulatory BP in normotensive individuals. For those consuming 0, 1–2, and 3 or more alcoholic drinks per week, mean 24-h systolic ambulatory BP values were 112.2, 115.2, and 116.6 mmHg, respectively ($P=0.05$), and mean 24-h diastolic ambulatory ABP values were 70.6, 71.9, and 74.2 mmHg, respectively ($P=0.02$). Beer and liquor consumption showed stronger positive associations with ABP than did wine consumption.

Recently Fuchs et al. [51] studied the association between alcohol consumption and the incidence of hypertension in 8,334 participants between 45 and 64 years of age over a 6-year follow-up. All participants were free of hypertension at start of the study. The risk of developing HTN was higher in all those who consumed greater than 210 g of alcohol per week. They concluded that consumption of large amounts of ethanol is an independent risk factor for hypertension

Xin et al. [52] in a meta-analysis of 15 RCTs ($N=2,234$) in which alcohol reduction was the only intervention reported a significant decrease in SBP and DBP of 3.31 and 2.04 mmHg respectively. Effects of intervention were higher in those with higher baseline BPs. Taken together, reduction in alcohol consumption can be a safe and effective nonpharmacologic way of controlling HTN.

The JNC VII [1] recommends that men limit their intake of alcohol to less than 1 oz per day which is roughly equivalent to 2 drinks/day and to 1 drink/day for women.

Smoking

The relationship between smoking and HTN still needs to be established [1]. Sympathetic overactivity is implicated in the increased cardiovascular risk of cigarette smokers. Cigarette smoking induces arterial stiffness, likely contributing to the onset of hypertension. This effect can persist up to a decade after the cessation of smoking [53–55].The adverse effects of smoking are due to the presence of several chemicals in tobacco including nicotine. Both systolic and diastolic pressures are increased in people who smoke after a single cigarette [56]. The mean elevation in SBPs is up to 6 mmHg [55].One study demonstrated an average elevation in systolic pressure of 20 mmHg after the first cigarette [57]. Smoking was also found to be an independent risk factor for renal function decline in patients with severe essential hypertension [58]. In one study cigarette smoking was modestly associated with an increased risk of developing hypertension, with an effect that was strongest among those who smoked at least 15 cigarettes per day [59].

For all the above reasons cessation of smoking should be recommended as an important adjunctive to lifestyle modifications in the treatment of HTN.

Caffeine

An effect of coffee on the development of hypertension has long been suspected. A recent meta analysis by Jee et al. [60] of 11 RCTs with 522 participants, a median follow-up period of 56 days and a median dose of coffee intake of 5 cups/day found an increase in SBPs and DBPs of 2.4 and 1.2 mmHg, respectively. The pooled effect of drinking one cup of coffee was 0.8 mmHg for systolic pressure (*P*, 0.001) and 0.5 mmHg for diastolic pressure (*P*, 0.01). Klag et al. for the Johns Hopkins Precursors Study [61] also found a small increase in both systolic and diastolic blood pressure in chronic coffee drinkers. In contrast, however, a review of several RCTs [62] concluded that caffeine did not cause a persistent increase in BP. Furthermore, the authors concluded that individuals who do not regularly ingest caffeine may experience an increase in BP when drinking coffee, but that tolerance develops in 2–3 days with BP returning to initial levels. Nurminen and his colleagues concluded that regular coffee consumption may be cause a hypertensive response in older hypertensive subjects, but could find no hypertensive effect in younger individuals [63].

The effects on the cardiovascular system appear to be related to the caffeine in the coffee rather than another ingredient in coffee [64]. The pathogenetic mechanisms proposed include sympathetic over activation, adenosine receptor blockade, activation of the renin–angiotensin system, increased nor epinephrine release etc [63, 65, 66].

Given these studies, it is reasonable to advise limited caffeine consumption in older hypertensive individuals as part of lifestyle modifications therapy.

Fish Oil

Fish oil supplementation may prevent HTN. The trials involving the effect of fish oil on hypertension are small, observational epidemiologic studies. The meta-analysis by Appel et al. [67] concluded that the supplementation of relatively high doses of omega 3 PUFA (>3 g/d) can lead to clinically relevant BP reductions in individuals with untreated hypertension. Weighted, pooled estimates of SBP and DBP change (mmHg) were −5.5 (−8.1 to −2.9) and −3.5 (−5.0 to −2.1) in the trials of untreated hypertensives. Another analysis of randomized trials more recently found BP reductions of 1.7 mmHg (95% CI: 0.3, 3.1) and 1.5 mmHg (95% CI: 0.6, 2.3), respectively, with the most pronounced effects in older hypertensive subjects as opposed to younger non-hypertensive subjects [68]. In summary, the effect of supplementation of diet with omega 3 PUFA to prevent or improve BP control needs to be further evaluated. No firm recommendations can be made at this time.

Case Revisited

Nonpharmacologic approaches have enormous potential as a means to reduce blood pressure and control hypertension, thereby preventing the occurrence of ASCVD. The current challenge to health care providers, government officials, and the general public is to develop and implement effective clinical and public health strategies that lead to desirable lifestyle modification. The case described at the beginning of this chapter embodies many of the lifestyle issues that have been discussed. She has prehypertension as defined by the JNC VII Report, and this would mark an excellent time to effect multiple lifestyle modifications to prevent advancement to frank hypertension. Specifically, you could recommend initiation of a more healthful diet such as the DASH diet to limit intake of sodium and processed food and increase intake of fruits, vegetables, and grains. Weight loss of 10 kg could have a substantive salubrious effect on her blood pressure as well. Initiation of a scheduled exercise program could aid in weight loss efforts and have blood pressure lowering effects independently of weight loss. Enrollment in a structured program for exercise and weight loss with scheduled follow-up is more likely to lead to successful achievement of these goals than isolated discussions in the physician office and should be encouraged. Discontinuation of coffee and alcohol would not be warranted at this time.

Conclusion

The investigations into lifestyle modifications for the treatment of hypertension raise more questions than answers. Clearly, there is a relationship between a modern diet and lifestyle and the development of hypertension, as individuals from undeveloped cultures definitely have lower blood pressures than those in developed countries. However, the precise components of the modern diet and lifestyle that contribute to the increased risk of hypertension and whether alteration of these components can really effect major change in blood pressure remains to be seen. The data are most convincing for the efficacy of weight loss. Clearly, however, diets that result in weight loss are more likely to be lower in sodium, lower in saturated fats, and higher in nutrients such as potassium, magnesium, and fiber. The roles of smoking, sedentary state, and alcohol in the development of hypertension seem to be prominent in some individuals but clearly not in all. Despite the ambiguity of the data, it is without doubt worthwhile encouraging lifestyle changes as these may be additive with pharmacologic therapy and may confer other cardiovascular and metabolic benefits. A summary of the current recommendations have been tabulated in Table 42.1.

Table 42.1 Lifestyle modifications to manage hypertension

Modification	Recommendation	Approximate BP reduction in SBP mmHg
Consume DASH diet	Consume a diet rich in fresh fruits, vegetables, low fat dairy products with reduced content of saturated fats and total fats	8–14
Reduce sodium intake	≤100 mmol/day (i.e., 2.4 g of sodium or 6 g of sodium chloride)	2–8
Increase physical activity	Regular aerobic physical activity like brisk walking for at least 30 min for most days of the week	4–9
Moderate alcohol intake	Limit to ≤2 drinks[a]/day for men, ≤1 drinks/day for women.	2–4
Reduce weight	Maintain normal body weight (BMI, 18–24.9 kg/m^2))	0.5–2/1 kg weight loss

[a]1 drink is equivalent to 12 oz of beer, 5 oz of wine, 1.5 oz of 80 proof liquor; all approximately equivalent to 14 g of ethanol

References

1. The Seventh Report of the Joint National Committee on Prevention, Detection, Evaluation, and Treatment of High Blood Pressure. JNC VII. Available at http://www.nhlbi.nih.gov/guidelines/hypertension/jnc7full.pdf.
2. National Health and Nutrition Examination Survey. www.cdc.gov/nchs/nhanes.htm
3. World Health Organization. World Health Report 2002: reducing risks, promoting healthy life. Geneva, Switzerland: World Health Organization; 2002.
4. USRDS. http://www.usrds.org.
5. Intersalt Cooperative Research Group. Intersalt: an international study of electrolyte excretion and blood pressure. Results for 24 hour urinary sodium and potassium excretion. BMJ. 1988;297(6644):319–28.
6. The INTERSALT Co-operative Research Group. Sodium, potassium, body mass, alcohol and blood pressure: the INTERSALT study. J Hypertens Suppl. 1988;6(4):S584–6.
7. Mancilha-Carvalho JJ, de Oliveira R, Esposito RJ. Blood pressure and electrolyte excretion in the Yanomamo Indians, an isolated population. J Hum Hypertens. 1989;3(5):309–14.
8. Huang CL, Kuo E. Mechanisms of disease: WNK-ing at the mechanism of salt-sensitive hypertension. Nat Clin Pract Nephrol. 2007;3(11):623–30.
9. Witteman JC, Willett WC, Stampfer MJ, Colditz GA, Sacks FM, Speizer FE, Rosner B, Hennekens CH. A prospective study of nutritional factors and hypertension among US women. Circulation. 2007;80(5):1320–7.
10. van Mierlo LA, Arends LR, Streppel MT, Zeegers MP, Kok FJ, Grobbee DE, Geleijnse JM. Blood pressure response to calcium supplementation: a meta-analysis of randomized controlled trials. J Hum Hypertens. 2006;20(8):571–80.
11. Dahl LK. Salt, fat and hypertension: the Japanese experience. Nutr Rev. 1960;18:97–9.
12. Dahl LK. Effects of chronic excess salt feeding. Elevation of plasma cholesterol in rats and dogs. J Exp Med. 1960;112:635–51.
13. Dahl LK. Possible role of salt intake in the development of essential hypertension. 1960. Int J Epidemiol. 2005;34(5):967–72. discussion 972–964, 975–968.
14. Brown IJ, Tzoulaki I, Candelas V, Elliott P. Salt intakes around the world: implications for public. Int J Epidemiol. 2009;38(3):791–813.
15. Kempner W. The treatment of heart and kidney disease and of hypertensive and arteriosclerotic vascular disease with the rice diet. Ann Intern Med. 1949;31(5):821–56.
16. Rosati KG, Rosati R. The rice diet solution. New York, NY: Simon & Schuster; 2005.
17. Fang J, Keenan NL, Ayala C, Dai S, Valderrama AL. Fruits and vegetables intake and physical activity among hypertensives adults in the United States: behavioral risk factor surveillance system, 2003 and 2007. Am J Hypertens. 2010;23:762–6.
18. Cook NR, Cutler JA, Obarzanek E, Buring JE, Rexrode KM, Kumanyika SK, Appel LJ, Whelton PK. Long term effects of dietary sodium reduction on cardiovascular disease outcomes: observational follow-up of the trials of hypertension prevention (TOHP). BMJ. 2007;334(7599):885–8.
19. Hypertension Prevention Collaborative Research Group. Effects of weight loss and sodium reduction intervention on blood pressure and hypertension incidence in overweight people with high-normal blood pressure. The Trials of Hypertension Prevention, phase II. The Trials of Hypertension Prevention Collaborative Research Group. Arch Intern Med. 1997;157(6):657–67.
20. Appel LJ, Moore TJ, Obarzanek E, Vollmer WM, Svetkey LP, Sacks FM, Bray GA, Vogt TM, Cutler JA, Windhauser MM, Lin PH, Karanja N. A clinical trial of the effects of dietary patterns on blood pressure. DASH Collaborative Research Group. N Engl J Med. 1997;336(16):1117–24.
21. Appel LJ, Sacks FM, Carey VJ, Obarzanek E, Swain JF, Miller 3rd ER, Conlin PR, Erlinger TP, Rosner BA, Laranjo NM, Charleston J, McCarron P, Bishop LM, OmniHeart Collaborative Research Group. Effects of protein, monounsaturated fat, and carbohydrate intake on blood pressure and serum lipids: results of the OmniHeart randomized trial. JAMA. 2005;294(19):2455–64.
22. Blumenthal JA, Babyak MA, Sherwood A, Craighead L, Lin PH, Johnson J, Watkins LL, Want JT, Kuhn C, Feinglos M, Hinderliter A. Effects of the DASH diet alone and in combination with exercise and weight loss on blood pressure and cardiovascular biomarkers in men and women with high blood pressure: the ENCORE study. Arch Intern Med. 2010;170(2):126–35.
23. Sacks FM, Svetkey LP, Vollmer WM, Apppel LJ, Bray GA, Harsha D, Obarzanek E, Conlin PR, Miller 3rd R, Simons-Morton DG, Karanja N, Lin PH, DASH-Sodium Collaborative Research Group. Effects on blood pressure of reduced dietary sodium and the Dietary Approaches to Stop Hypertension (DASH) diet. DASH-Sodium Collaborative Research Group. N Engl J Med. 2010;344(1):3–10.
24. Miller 3rd ER, Erlinger TP, Young DR, Jehn M, Charleston J, Rhodes D, Wasan SK, Appel LJ. Results of the diet, exercise, and weight loss intervention trial (DEW-IT). Hypertension. 2002;40(5):612–8.
25. TOHP Collaborative Research Group. The effects of nonpharmacologic interventions on blood pressure of persons with high normal levels. Results of the trials of hypertension prevention, phase I. JAMA 1992;267(9):1213–1220
26. Whelton PK, He J, Cutler JA, Brancati FL, Appel LJ, Follmann D, Klag MJ. Effects of oral potassium on blood pressure. Meta-analysis of randomized controlled clinical trials. JAMA. 1997;277(20):1624–32.
27. Cappuccio FP, Markandu ND, Tucker FA, MacGregor GA. Lack of effect of oral magnesium on high blood pressure: a double blind study. Br Med J (Clin Res Ed). 1985;291(6490):235–8.
28. Kawano Y, Matsuoka H, Takishita S, Omae T. Effects of magnesium supplementation in hypertensive patients:

assessment by office, home, and ambulatory blood pressures. Hypertension. 1998;32(2):260–5.
29. Motoyama T, Sano H, Fukuzaki H. Oral magnesium supplementation in patients with essential hypertension. Hypertension. 1989;13(3):227–32.
30. Jee SH, Miller 3rd ER, Guallar E, Singh VK, Appel LJ, Klag MJ. The effect of magnesium supplementation on blood pressure: a meta-analysis of randomized clinical trials. Am J Hypertens. 2002;15(8):691–6.
31. He J, Whelton PK. Effect of dietary fiber and protein intake on blood pressure: a review of epidemiological evidence. Clin Exp Hypertens. 1999;21:785–96.
32. He J, Klag MJ, Whelton PK, Chen JY, Qian MC, He GQ. Dietary macronutrients and pressure in Southwest China. J Hypertens. 1995;13:1267–74.
33. Mohamed FA. On chronic Bright's disease, and its essential symptoms. Lancet. 1879;1:399–401.
34. Kawano Y. Uric acid and blood pressure. Circ J. 2011;75(12):2755–6.
35. Jossa F, Farinaro E, Panico S, Krogh V, Celentano E, Galasso R, Mancini M, Trevisan M. Serum uric acid and hypertension: the Olivetti heart study. J Hum Hypertens. 1994;8(9):677–81.
36. Selby JV, Friedman GD, Quesenberry CP. Precursors of essential hypertension: pulmonary function, heart rate, uric acid, serum cholesterol, and other serum chemistries. Am J Epidemiol. 1990;131:1017–27.
37. Cappuccio FP, Strazzulo P, Ferinaro E, Trevisan M. Uric acid metabolism and tubular sodium handling. JAMA. 1993;270:354–9.
38. Ter Maaten JC, Voorburg A, Heine RJ, Ter Wee PM, Donker AJ, Gans RO. Renal handling of urate and sodium during acute physiological hyperinsulinemia in healthy subjects. Clin Sci. 1997;92:51–8.
39. Quinones Galvan A, Natali A, Baldo FS, Sanna G, Ciociaro D, Ferrannini E. Effects of insulin on uric acid excretion in humans. Am J Physiol. 1995;268:E1–5.
40. Stanton JA, Lowenthal DT. The evidence for life style modification in lowering blood pressure in the elderly. Am J Geriatr Cardiol. 2000;9(1):27–33.
41. Whelton PK, Appel LJ, Espeland MA, Applegate WB, Ettinger Jr WH, Kostis JB, Kumanyika S, Lacy CR, Johnson KC, Folmar S, Cutler JA. Sodium reduction and weight loss in the treatment of hypertension in older persons: a randomized controlled trial of nonpharmacologic interventions in the elderly (TONE). TONE Collaborative Research Group. JAMA. 1998;279(11):839–46.
42. Kostis JB, Wilson AC, Shindler DM, et al. Persistence of normotension after discontinuation of lifestyle intervention in the trial of TONE, trial of non pharmacologic interventions in the elderly. Am J Hypertens. 2002;15(8):732–4.
43. He J, Whelton PK, Appel LJ, et al. Long term effects of weight loss and dietary sodium reduction on incidence of hypertension. Hypertension. 2000;35:544–9.
44. Whelton SP, Chin A, Xin X, He J. Effect of aerobic exercise on blood pressure: a meta-analysis of randomized controlled trials. Ann Intern Med. 2002;136:493–503.
45. Roberts CK, Vaziri ND, Barnard RJ. Effect of diet and exercise intervention on blood pressure, insulin, oxidative stress, and nitric oxide availability. Circulation. 2002;106:2530–2.
46. Lee KW, Lip GYH. Effects of lifestyle on hemostasis, fibrinolysis, and platelet reactivity: a systematic review. Arch Intern Med. 2003;163:2368–92.
47. Klatsky AL, Friedman GD, Siegelaub AB, Gerard MJ. Alcohol consumption and blood pressure Kaiser-Permanente Multiphasic Health Examination Data. N Engl J Med. 1977;296(21):1194–200.
48. Tomson J, Lip GY. Alcohol and hypertension. An old relationship revisited. Alcohol Alcohol. 2006;41(1):3–4.
49. Cushman WC, Cutler JA, Hanna E, et al. Prevention and treatment of hypertension study (PATHS): effects of an alcohol treatment program on blood pressure. Arch Intern Med. 1998;158:1197–207.
50. Abramson JL, Lewis C, Murrah NV. Relationship of self-reported alcohol consumption to ambulatory blood pressure in a sample of healthy adults. Am J Hypertens. 2010;23:994–9.
51. Fuchs FD, Chambless LE, Whelton PK, et al. Alcohol consumption and the incidence of hypertension. The Atherosclerotic risk in Communities Study. Hypertension. 2001;37:1242–50.
52. Xin X, Frontini MG, Ogden EG, et al. Effects of alcohol reduction on blood pressure. A meta-analysis of randomized control trials. Hypertension. 2001;38:1112–7.
53. Najem B, Houssiere A, Pathak A, et al. Acute cardiovascular and sympathetic effects of nicotine replacement therapy. Hypertension. 2006;47:1162.
54. Jatoi NA, Jerrard-Dunne P, Feely J, Mahmud A. Impact of smoking and smoking cessation on arterial stiffness and aortic wave reflection in hypertension. Hypertension. 2007;49(5):981–5.
55. Narkiewicz K, Maraglino G, Biasion T, Rossi G, Sanzuol F, Palatini P. Interactive effect of cigarettes and coffee on daytime systolic blood pressure in patients with mild essential hypertension. HARVEST Study Group (Italy). Hypertension Ambulatory Recording VEnetia STudy. J Hypertens. 1995;13(9):965–70.
56. Frohlich ED, Gifford Jr RW, Horan M, et al. Non pharmacologic approaches to the control of high blood pressure. Report of the Subcommittee on non pharmacologic therapy of the Joint National Committee on Detection, evaluation, and treatment of high blood pressure, 1984. Hypertension. 1986;8:444–67.
57. Groppelli A, Giorgi DM, Omboni S, Parati G, Mancia GJ. Persistent blood pressure increase induced by heavy smoking. Hypertension. 1992;10(5):495–9.
58. Regalado M, Yang S, Wesson DE. Cigarette smoking is associated with augmented progression of renal insufficiency in severe essential hypertension. Am J Kidney Dis. 2000;35(4):687–94.
59. Bowman TS, Gaziano JM, Buring JE, Sesso HD. A prospective study of cigarette smoking and risk of incident hypertension in women. J Am Coll Cardiol. 2007;50(21):2085–92.

60. Jee SH, He J, Whelton PK, Suh I, Klag MJ. Controlled clinical trials. The effect of chronic coffee drinking on blood pressure: a meta-analysis of controlled clinical trials. Hypertension. 1999;33:647–52.
61. Klag MJ, Wang NY, Meoni LA, Brancati FL, Cooper LA, Liang KY, Young JH, Ford DE. Coffee intake and risk of hypertension: the Johns Hopkins precursors study. Arch Intern Med. 2002;162(6):657–62.
62. Myers MG. Effects of caffeine on blood pressure. Arch Intern Med. 1988;148:1189–93.
63. Nurminen ML, Niittynen L, Korpela R, et al. Coffee, caffeine and blood pressure: a critical review. Eur J Clin Nutr. 1999;53:831–9.
64. Smits P, Thien T, van't Laar A. The cardiovascular effects of regular and decaffeinated coffee. Br J Clin Pharmacol. 1985;19:852–4.
65. Rall TW. Evolution of mechanism of action of methylxanthines: from calcium mobilizers to antagonists of adenosine receptors. Pharmacologist. 1982;24:277–87.
66. Robertson D, Frohlich JC, Carr RK, et al. Effects of caffeine on plasma renin activity, catecholamines and blood pressure. N Engl J Med. 1978;298:181–6.
67. Appel LJ, Miller ER, Seidler AJ, et al. Does supplementation of diet with Fish oil reduce BP? A meta-analysis of controlled clinical trials. Arch Intern Med. 1993;153:1429–38.
68. Geleijnse JM, Giltay EJ, Grobbee dE, Donders AR, Kok FJ. Blood pressure response to fish oil supplementation: metaregression analysis of randomized trials. J Hypertens. 2002;20(8):1493–9.

Secondary Hypertension

43

Eleanor D. Lederer

Case

A 47-year-old man presents to the office for a blood pressure check. He has had hypertension for at least 7 years, impaired glucose tolerance, and obstructive sleep apnea. Current medications include lisinopril 40 mg daily, metoprolol 25 mg twice daily, amlodipine 10 mg daily, hydrochlorothiazide 12.5 mg daily, and metformin 500 mg twice daily. On examination, BP is 170/95 mmHg, pulse 80/min, respiratory rate 16/min, and temperature 98.7°F He is obese with BMI 35. Funduscopic examination shows mild arteriolar narrowing without hemorrhages, jugular veins are not distended, lungs are clear, cardiac examination discloses an S4 gallop, and he has 1+ leg edema. Laboratory evaluation shows hemoglobin 13.7 g/L, hematocrit 40%, white blood count 7.6, Na 137 meq/L, K 3.6 meq/L, Cl 100 meq/L, 30 meq/L, BUN 27 mg/dL, creatinine 1.4 mg/dL, glycosylated hemoglobin 6.9%, and urinalysis shows 100 mg% protein without cells.

1. Could this man have a secondary form of hypertension? If so, what are the potential causes of his hypertension?
2. What additional testing would be indicated to evaluate the patient's hypertension?
3. What changes to his antihypertensive regimen would be most likely to result in blood pressure control to goal?

E.D. Lederer, M.D., F.A.S.N. (✉)
Department of Medicine/Nephrology, University of Louisville, 615 S. Preston Street, Louisville, KY 40202, USA

Robley Rex VA Medical Center, 800 Zorn Avenue, Louisville, KY 40207, USA
e-mail: e.lederer@louisville.edu

Introduction

Hypertension is the most common chronic noncommunicable disease in the world. While the majority of cases by far are considered "primary" or "essential" hypertension, at least 10% of hypertensives will have an identifiable cause of hypertension and therefore secondary hypertension. Classically, secondary hypertension has referred to a group of predisposing disorders including acute and chronic kidney disease, renovascular disease, diseases of true and apparent mineralocorticoid excess, Cushing syndrome, pheochromocytoma, and coarctation of the aorta [1–3]. A number of other conditions may also result in secondary hypertension including a variety of genetic diseases, endocrine disorders, and conditions of sympathetic overactivity. Some medications or drugs of abuse can produce hypertension as well. For some of these causes of secondary hypertension, simple interventions such as correction of renal arterial disease or removal of an offending medication can be curative. Some of these causes are relatively simple to recognize, whereas others can be more difficult to diagnose even with extensive testing. In this chapter, the causes of

E.V. Lerma and M. Rosner (eds.), *Clinical Decisions in Nephrology, Hypertension and Kidney Transplantation*, DOI 10.1007/978-1-4614-4454-1_43, © Springer Science+Business Media New York 2013

secondary hypertension will be reviewed with an emphasis on common presentations, clinical clues to the presence of a form of secondary hypertension, rational approaches to evaluation, and specific therapies (see Table 43.1).

Chronic Kidney Disease

Intrinsic kidney disease is the most common cause of secondary hypertension [4–17]. Most forms of kidney disease can be associated with hypertension including glomerular, tubulointerstitial, and vascular diseases (see Table 43.1); however, not all kidney diseases are associated with hypertension. Glomerular diseases such as membranoproliferative glomerulonephritis or focal segmental glomerulosclerosis commonly are accompanied by hypertension while minimal change disease, another kidney disease characterized by heavy proteinuria, is only rarely complicated by the development of hypertension. The same is true for tubulointerstitial diseases. Over 90% of patients with autosomal dominant polycystic kidney disease [9] but patients with lithium associated kidney disease may not.

Patients with intrinsic kidney disease most often are asymptomatic but may present with leg edema, especially those with glomerular disease and nephrotic range proteinuria. Identification of a family history of kidney disease or the presence of a disease which can affect kidney function such as diabetes mellitus can alert the clinician to the possibility of secondary hypertension due to kidney disease. Initial evaluation should include electrolytes, BUN and Cr, urinalysis, and kidney ultrasound. If these are all within normal limits, then a renal cause of hypertension is highly unlikely.

The interaction between hypertension and kidney disease is complex as hypertension alone can produce intrinsic kidney disease and kidney disease can produce hypertension [5, 6]. Furthermore, uncontrolled hypertension can accelerate the decline in kidney function. The recommendation for the goal of hypertension control in the face of intrinsic kidney disease is less than 130/70, although the evidence for this goal is best documented for proteinuric kidney diseases as opposed to tubulointerstitial or vascular causes of kidney disease [5, 7–10]. The choice of antihypertensive agent also in part depends on the type of kidney disease. Most kidney diseases that result in the development of hypertension do so in part by promoting an increase in sodium retention, even in patients without overt edema. Therefore, diuretics are a first line treatment for this form of secondary hypertension [11–17]. For patients with heavy proteinuria, inhibitors of the renin-angiotensin-aldosterone axis are also considered highly effective agents [14–17]. Studies suggest that either ACE inhibitors or angiotensin receptor blockers are acceptable choices and some investigators in the field recommend a combination of the two agents. However, the data to support routine use of both agents is not convincing enough to recommend this approach routinely. Nonpharmacologic interventions such as restriction of sodium intake, limitation of alcohol ingestion, and weight control are also recommended.

Renovascular Disease

The two major forms of renovascular disease are fibromuscular dysplasia and atherosclerotic renal artery stenosis [18–26]. The mechanisms for the development of renal arterial disease for these entities are quite different as are the approach and therapy. Therefore, they will be discussed separately.

Fibromuscular Dysplasia

Fibromuscular dysplasia refers to a group of disorders characterized by abnormal vascular modeling, resulting in varying degrees of arterial stenosis [19]. The major sites affected include renal arteries, carotids, and the abdominal arteries with renal involvement being the most common. Fibromuscular dysplasia is classified into four different types determined by the portion of the artery affected: medial or perimedial fibroplasia, medial hyperplasia, intimal and adventitial dysplasia. Medial fibroplasia is most common, pathologically demonstrating fibrous cords within the media, sparing intima and adventitia. Frequently occurring as a series of bands in the distal renal artery, the patches between the fibrotic bands often dilate, resulting in

Table 43.1 Medical Causes of Secondary Hypertension

Classification	Examples	Clinical Clues
Intrinsic Kidney Disease	Glomerular disease, e.g., membranoproliferative GN, focal glomerulosclerosis, post-streptococcal GN	Abnormal urinalysis, e.g., proteinuria
		Elevated creatinine
	Tubulo-interstitial disease, e.g., polycystic kidney disease, acute interstitial nephritis	Abnormal kidney imaging, e.g., multiple cysts, horseshoe kidney
	Microvascular disease, e.g., thrombotic thrombocytopenic purpura, polyarteritis nodosa, scleroderma	
Renovascular Disease	Fibromuscular hyperplasia	Young age (<40)
	Atherosclerotic renovascular disease	Abdominal bruit
		Signs or symptoms of peripheral vascular disease such as TIA, CVA, claudication
Minerallocorticoid excess	Primary hyperaldosteronism	Unprovoked hypokalemia
		Serum Na > 140 meq/L
		Metabolic alkalosis
		Hypomagnesemia with urine magnesium wasting
	Cushing syndrome	Striae, typical cosmetic features
	Licorice ingestion	Absence of typical risk factors
	Congenital adrenal hyperplasia (11 or 17-hydroxylase deficiency)	Ambiguous genitalia, early puberty (male) or delayed puberty (female)
		Family history
	Apparent minerallocorticoid excess	Family history
	Glucocorticoid remediable hypertension (Familial Hyperaldosteronism Type I)	Family history
	Familial Hyperaldosteronism Type II	
Neuroendocrine and neurologic disorders	Pheochromocytoma	Very labile HT
	Paraganglionoma	Episodic flushing, sweating
	Neurofibromatosis	Family history, characteristic physical exam features
	Increased intracranial pressure	Acute neurologic event
	Quadriplegia	Paralysis/paresis of extremities
Endocrine causes	Adrenal diseases (see above)	
	Hyper/hypothyroidism	Heat/cold intolerance
		Diarrhea/constipation
		Weight loss/gain
	Hyperparathyroidism	Kidney stones
		Bone pain
	Acromegaly	
	Renin producing tumors	High renin and aldosterone
Genetic causes	Disorders of sodium homeostasis, e.g., Liddle syndrome, Gordon syndrome	Young age
		Severe hypertension
	Disorders of adrenal hormones (see above)	
	Genetic kidney diseases, e.g., Alport syndrome, polycystic kidney disease	
		Family history of kidney disease
Miscellaneous causes	Obesity	Physical examination
	Sleep apnea	Excessive snoring, daytime fatigue
		Discrepancy in BP measurement between arms
	Coarctation of aorta	

the classic string of beads appearance. The pathogenesis of fibromuscular dysplasia is unknown.

Fibromuscular dysplasia accounts for less than 10% of renal artery stenosis causing hypertension but may occur in up to 5% of the population. The most common presentation is the sudden onset of hypertension in a young woman. Features that raise the suspicion for fibromuscular dysplasia include onset at a young age in the absence of known risk factors for hypertension and difficult to control hypertension. Differential diagnosis includes Ehlers-Danlos syndrome and large vessel vasculitis. In contrast to vasculitis, however, the lesions of fibromuscular dysplasia are not inflammatory. The diagnosis of fibromuscular dysplasia is made by imaging techniques. The gold standard is renal arteriography demonstrating the classic string of beads appearance. Alternative modalities include digital subtraction angiography, magnetic resonance imaging, Doppler ultrasound, and captopril renal scan, but generally are not as widely used due to decreased sensitivity and significant center to center efficacy.

The treatment of choice for hypertension associated with fibromuscular dysplasia is angioplasty at the time of arteriography which is frequently curative. Alternatively, for complex lesions, surgery may be required. If blood pressure is easily controlled, a trial of antihypertensive therapy with close observation of renal function may be warranted as progression of disease occurs in only about 30–35% of patients. No specific antihypertensive agent is indicated though ACE inhibitors are generally avoided secondary to the hemodynamic effects in the affected kidney.

Atherosclerotic Renal Artery Stenosis

Atherosclerosis is the major cause of hypertension due to renal artery stenosis [20–26]. It generally occurs in the setting of extrarenal vascular disease such as coronary disease, aortofemoral disease, and carotid artery atherosclerosis. Studies performed in patients undergoing renal arteriogram at the time of coronary angiography have demonstrated renal artery stenosis in up to 34% of cases and 25% of the time in patients with lower extremity arterial disease. The presence of widespread large vessel atherosclerosis and small vessel disease makes the diagnosis and treatment of atherosclerotic renal artery significantly less straightforward than is true for fibromuscular dysplasia. Atherosclerotic lesions generally affect the proximal portion of the renal artery in contrast to the more distal localization seen in fibromuscular dysplasia.

The most common presentations include difficult to control hypertension, recurrent hypertensive crises, flash pulmonary edema, acute kidney injury with the use of ACE inhibitors or angiotensin receptor inhibitors, or progressive kidney failure in an individual over the age of 60 with known extrarenal vascular disease. The major indications for diagnosis and treatment of atherosclerotic renal artery stenosis are to improve blood pressure control and to prevent progressive kidney failure. However, whether intervention actually accomplishes either of these goals has been the subject of intense study and ongoing controversy. As for fibromuscular dysplasia, the modality of choice for diagnosis is renal arteriography; however, interpretation of the results is considerably more nuanced for atherosclerotic disease. Determination of whether a lesion is hemodynamically significant is particularly challenging as some clinicians consider lesions of greater than 50% stenosis to be worthy of intervention while others have argued that the degree of stenosis alone is not sufficiently sensitive to predict whether intervention to dilate the stenotic lesion will improve renal function or blood pressure control. The only imaging technique that incorporates functional information is the captopril renal scan. The physiological basis for the test is the recognition that glomerular filtration is maintained in the face of functionally significant renal artery stenosis by efferent arteriolar vasoconstriction, thus increasing glomerular capillary pressure. Vasodilation of the efferent arteriole by acute captopril administration will result in a significant decrease in renal perfusion pressure. Thus, if a patient has a significant renal artery stenosis, the perfusion to the affected kidney should decrease after captopril relative to the unaffected kidney. Unfortunately, the sensitivity of this test decreases in the setting of bilateral renal arterial disease, disease in a single functioning kidney, and decreased renal function, limiting its utility in a large number of patients with atherosclerosis. Another diagnostic tool to predict response to correction of renal artery stenosis is selective renal vein renin measurements. In theory, a kidney affected by significant renal artery stenosis should produce markedly increased amounts of renin in response to the decrease in blood flow, resulting in suppression of renin release from the contralateral kidney. Because of the invasive nature of the test and the specific technical expertise required to perform this test accurately, it is now seldom used as a screening tool to determine if intervention has a high likelihood of successfully decreasing blood pressure. Some investigators have suggested that measurement of the pressure gradient over the stenotic lesion especially under conditions of maximal hyperemia may be predictive of a salutary blood pressure response to intervention but this test is also not widely used.

The American Heart Association has developed guidelines for intervention in renal artery stenosis. Patients with uncontrolled hypertension, recurrent pulmonary edema or hypertensive crises, and patients with sudden progressive loss of kidney function have a greater than 70% chance of responding to angioplasty with stent placement and should be considered for this therapy. There is considerable controversy as to whether intervention carries any advantage over medical intervention alone in patients with asymptomatic renal artery stenosis discovered incidentally during cardiac angiography. These patients are judged on an individual basis taking into account ability to control blood pressure optimally, presence of unstable angina, or progressive kidney injury. Clearly, one major distinction between atherosclerotic renal arterial disease and fibromuscular dysplasia is the greater uncertainty of the response to the amelioration of the stenotic lesion in the former disorder compared to the latter and therefore the inability to recommend intervention as wholeheartedly for atherosclerotic disease.

Mineralocorticoid Associated Hypertension

The common theme in mineralocorticoid associated hypertension is the enhancement of sodium retention mediated by any of a variety of substances with mineralocorticoid activity accompanied by suppression of renin activity [27–40]. The scope of these illnesses include primary disease of the adrenal gland, secondary activation of aldosterone or other mineralocorticoid, genetic disorders of dysregulation of the steroid pathway, and even exogenous agents. While volume expansion due to sodium retention is the underlying mechanism for the development of hypertension in these states, additional effects of the excessive mineralocorticoids or the sodium retention itself cannot be excluded. Although initially thought to be rare, recent studies suggest that mineralocorticoid excess may be present in up to 50% of patients referred for resistant hypertension.

The clinical hallmarks of mineralocorticoid associated hypertension are unprovoked hypokalemia and frequently resistant hypertension, and most patients are identified in the context of resistant hypertension. However, as many as 38% of patients may not have frank hypokalemia so a high index of suspicion for this group of entities is required to identify patients likely to benefit from specific therapy.

Primary Hyperaldosteronism

The two most common varieties of primary hyperaldosteronism are adrenal adenoma and idiopathic adrenal hyperplasia. Previous studies had suggested that adrenal adenomas were more common, but more recent studies suggest that adrenal hyperplasia accounts for as many as 75% of cases. Although high aldosterone levels are common to both adrenal adenoma and adrenal hyperplasia, the pathogenesis of each disorder is different as is the treatment [27–31].

These entities present most frequently in middle age as difficult to control hypertension. Unprovoked hypokalemia or an exaggerated hypokalemic response to diuretics is seen in over 60% of patients. A low normal potassium level in an individual taking two or three inhibitors of the renin angiotensin aldosterone system may also alert the clinician to the possibility of primary hyperaldosteronism. A common clinical scenario is the incidental discovery of an adrenal adenoma in a patient with diagnosed hypertension. While suggestive of the possibility that the patient may have primary hyperaldosteronism, as much as 10% of the general population may have nonfunctioning adrenal adenomas. Studies of incidentally found adrenal adenomas suggest that 70% are nonfunctioning, so the congruity of hypertension with an incidentally identified adenoma is not diagnostic for primary hyperaldosteronism. Other clinical clues to the potential for mineralocorticoid mediated hypertension include serum Na greater than 140 meq/L, metabolic alkalosis, and magnesium wasting, although these findings are much less common. Notably, these patients are not edematous due to the development of mineralocorticoid escape, a phenomenon whereby the sodium retaining effects of aldosterone are blunted, allowing excretion of the daily sodium load. Therefore, when measured, the urine Na is not low.

The first step in diagnosing primary hyperaldosteronisms once it is suspected is measurement of the plasma aldosterone to renin ratio. This screening test is based on the assumption that with primary hyperaldosteronism, aldosterone secretion is high and unregulated while renin secretion is suppressed and therefore cannot be stimulated. As these hormones exhibit circadian variation, this measurement should be performed in the morning around 8 am and after medications known to alter the renin angiotensin aldosterone system are discontinued. This list is large and includes diuretics, beta blockers, ACE inhibitors, angiotensin receptor antagonists, direct renin antagonists, dihydropyridine receptor calcium channel blockers, and mineralocorticoid receptor antagonists. The nondihydropyridine calcium channel blockers have little effect on this system and therefore are the preferred choice of antihypertensive agent to use while the patient is being screened. In general, an aldosterone to renin ratio of 20–25 to 1 is considered a positive screen and warrants further investigation. A variety of methods for assessing whether or not an elevated aldosterone level is suppressible and/or a renin level is not stimulatable, i.e., unregulated aldosterone secretion is present, are available and reviewed well in Uwaifo and Sarlis [27]. One commonly used method is the saline suppression test where the patient is admitted to an outpatient infusion center, saline 500 ml/h for 4 h is infused, and serum aldosterone level is measured before infusion and at 2 and 4 h. Failure to suppress aldosterone to less than 9 ng/dL is considered diagnostic of primary hyperaldosteronism.

The next step is to determine what type of primary hyperaldosteronism is present. The gold standard for diagnosis of primary hyperaldosteronism due to functioning adrenal adenoma is adrenal vein sampling. The theory behind this test is that if the elevated serum aldosterone is secondary to a hyperfunctioning, nonsuppressible adenoma, then the vein draining the adenoma containing adrenal gland will have markedly elevated aldosterone levels relative to the contralateral side. Important controls for this test are to measure the aldosterone in the inferior vena cava and the cortisol level from both adrenal veins and the inferior vena cava. The aldosterone to cortisol level ratio on the affected side should be four or five times greater than the unaffected side to conclude with confidence that an adenoma is functioning. This test is technically demanding and may not be available at all medical centers. For patients younger than 40 years with an adrenal mass of greater than 1 cm, adrenal vein sampling is not required. However, for older patients or those with smaller lesions, adrenal vein sampling should be performed as imaging alone correctly identifies the source of aldosterone in only about 50% of cases.

The treatment of choice for the adrenal adenoma is surgical removal, optimally by laparoscopic methods. Although generally all patients are cured of hypokalemia only about 60% are cured of their hypertension. Factors predicting successful cure of hypertension after adrenalectomy include degree of hypertension, size of the lesion, and several demographic factors including age, gender, and BMI. The treatment of choice for adrenal hyperplasia is medical treatment with mineralocorticoid antagonists.

Cushing Syndrome

Excessive glucocorticoids can also lead to hypertension and hypertension is present in 80% of patients with glucocorticoid excess [37–39]. The glucocorticoid cortisol circulates at concentrations 1,000 times higher than aldosterone. Although the mineralocorticoid receptor can be activated by either mineralocorticoids or glucocorticoids, the mineralocorticoid receptor in classic mineralocorticoid responsive tissues such as the cortical collecting tubule escapes glucocorticoid stimulation by the activity of the enzyme 11ß-hydroxysteroid dehydrogenase type 2 which converts cortisol to cortisone. However, the presence of greater than normal concentrations of glucocorticoids results in mineralocorticoid stimulation. Several other mechanisms contribute to the development of hypertension including stimulation of renin release, inhibition of nitric oxide and other substances that lower blood pressure, and increased sensitivity to angiotensin II and sympathetic stimulation. These patients may present with subtle evidence of the metabolic syndrome including hypertension, glucose intolerance, and weight gain. Hypokalemia, hyperglycemia, and hypertriglyceridem ia are relatively common laboratory abnormalities. However, none of these findings are particularly specific and often the diagnosis is not entertained until the more obvious cosmetic features appear including striae; redistribution of fat to the face (moon facies), upper back (dorsal fat pad or buffalo hump), and abdomen; and muscle weakness due to loss of muscle mass. The diagnosis is made by measurement of an elevated 24 h urine cortisol followed by failure of suppression by dexamethasone. Cushing syndrome can be secondary to overproduction of ACTH from a pituitary lesion or primary overproduction of cortisol from the adrenal gland. The two disorders are distinguished by measurement of serum ACTH and by high dose dexamethasone suppression. A clearly low ACTH level (<5 pg/ml) indicates an adrenal source for the cortisol and the next diagnostic step would be abdominal CT to look for an adenoma. A clearly elevated ACTH level (>20 pg/ml) is consistent with a pituitary or ectopic (paraneoplastic) cause for hypercortisolism. If the level of ACTH is intermediate, then the high dose, 8 mg, dexamethasone suppression test is indicated. Suppression of ACTH by 50% suggests a pituitary origin as opposed to an ectopic cause of excessive ACTH. A decrease of 90% in urinary cortisol is virtually diagnostic of pituitary hypercortisolism. Alternatively, to distinguish between pituitary and ectopic ACTH, a CRH stimulation test can be done. If the elevated ACTH originates from the pituitary, CRH will increase ACTH level, but not with ectopic sources for ACTH. Treatment of Cushing syndrome depends upon the cause. Adrenalectomy is indicated for adrenal causes while surgical excision of the source of ACTH is indicated.

Disorders of Steroid Metabolism

Licorice Ingestion

Certain types of licorice, generally not the usual grocery store variety, contain a substance that inhibits the activity of 11ß-hydroxysteroid dehydrogenase type 2, the enzyme that converts cortisol to the inactive metabolite cortisone. Thus, individuals ingesting licorice, tea, or herbal remedies containing glycyrrhetinic acid, the active inhibitory substance, may develop hypertension with a clinical presentation resembling aldosteronism. Clues that suggest this cause all come from the history—a lack of usual risk factors for hypertension, the absence of a family history of hypertension, often a young age at onset, and a history of the ingestion of the aforementioned substances. Predictably, serum aldosterone levels are suppressed. The treatment of choice is discontinuation of these ingestions. Interestingly, forms of glycyrrhetinic acid are common cosmetic additives; however, a recent report by the Cosmetic Ingredient Review Expert Panel deemed cosmetics as a minimal risk for excess exposure to these agents [40].

Apparent Mine alocorticoid Excess

Inactivating mutations of 11ß-hydroxysteroid dehydrogenas e type 2 result in hypertension with features of hyperaldosteronism called apparent mineralocorticoid excess as the presentation is similar to hyperaldosteronism but serum aldosterone levels are low. This rare disease is transmitted in an autosomal recessive manner and generally presents either in the neonatal or early childhood period. However, a milder form that presents in adulthood has also been described. The diagnosis is confirmed by genetic analysis.

Congenital Adrenal Hyperplasia

Two forms of congenital adrenal hyperplasia, 11-β or 17-α hydroxylase deficiency, are associated with hypertension. These uncommon autosomal recessive disorders generally present early in life but may be clinically inapparent until adulthood. Classically, 11β hydroxylase deficiency presents in male subjects as early virilization and hypertension while female subjects may present with ambiguous genitalia or failure of the development of secondary sexual characteristics. The enzyme deficiency results in failure of conversion of 11-deoxycortisol to cortisol, resulting in marked hypersecretion of ACTH which in turn stimulates production of deoxycorticosterone, a potent mineralocorticoid steroid metabolite. The syndrome responds to dexamethasone suppression.

17α hydroxylase deficiency, also a rare disorder, presents with absence of sex steroid production and hypertension. The pathogenesis of the hypertension, similar to what is seen with 11β hydroxylase deficiency, is due to a defect in cortisol production resulting in excessive stimulation of ACTH and overproduction of deoxycorticosterone. This syndrome also responds to dexamethasone suppression.

Glucocorticoid Remediable Hypertension

This genetic disorder, also known as familial hyperaldosteronism type I, is an autosomal dominant disorder caused by a chromosomal translocation whereby an ACTH response element in a promoter drives the production of aldosterone through stimulation of the production of aldosterone synthase. The presentation is variable, with hypertension and/or features of mineralocorticoid excess occurring during childhood or adulthood. Interestingly, though the renin level is suppressed, aldosterone levels are not necessarily elevated. Afflicted individuals have a higher than usual incidence of cerebrovascular events associated with hypertension, including aneurysms and hemorrhage. The disorder is rare but should be considered in young individuals presenting with a strong family history of hypertension at an early age. These individuals respond well to glucocorticoid therapy.

Familial Hyperaldosteronism Type II

Although the gene responsible for this disorder has not been identified, investigators in the field now suggest that FH II may be the most common genetic cause of hypertension. Similar to sporadic hyperaldosteronism, patients with FH II generally present in adulthood with hypertension. The strong family history of hypertension suggesting autosomal dominant transmission will alert the clinician to the possibility of this disorder. In contrast to FH I, the hypertension associated with FH II does not respond to glucocorticoid therapy.

Neuroendocrine and Neurologic Causes of Hypertension

Neuroendocrine and neurologic causes of hypertension are generally mediated by excessive sympathetic activity [41–46]. The excessive sympathetic activity results in peripheral vasoconstriction and increased vascular tone. Sympathetic stimulation may also increase renal sodium reabsorption.

Pheochromocytoma

Pheochromocytoma is an unusual cause of hypertension, accounting for less than 1% of hypertensive individuals. These tumors arise from chromaffin cells of the adrenal medulla, producing large amounts of catecholamines, primarily norepinephrine. The classic presentation is sporadic severe hypertension accompanied by diaphoresis, tachycardia and palpitations, and headache. However, many individuals will present with resistant hypertension which may not appear to be sporadic. Clinical clues to the presence of a pheochromocytoma include hypertension triggered by anesthesia, childbirth, opiates, cocaine, radiocontrast media, or some medications such as tricyclic antidepressants; unexplained cardiomyopathy; unexplained arrhythmias; or weight loss. A family history of pheochromocytoma will alert the clinician to the possibility of one of the multiple endocrine neoplasia disorders, specifically MEN 2A (pheochromocytoma, medullary cardinoma of thyroid, hyperparathyroidism, and Hirschsprung disease) and MEN 2B (pheochromocytoma, medullary carcinoma of thyroid, Hirschsprung disease, mucosal neurofibromatosis, intestinal paraganglionomas, and a marfanoid body habitus). Pheochromocytoma is also a feature of neurofibromatosis, von Hippel Lindau syndrome, tuberous sclerosis, and Sturge–Weber syndrome. The distinguishing features of each of these hereditary disorders allow clinical diagnosis of the syndromes, most often without genetic testing. However, in some cases, genetic testing for the affected gene may be pursued. The diagnosis of pheochromocytoma in an individual should be followed up by examination for the features of any of the hereditary syndromes as well as acquisition of a complete family history followed by appropriate diagnostic studies if indicated. One interesting aspect of familial pheochromocytoma is that the predominant secreted catecholamine is epinephrine, not norepinephrine, as is seen in the sporadic forms.

90% of pheochromocytomas are found in the adrenal gland. When located outside of the adrenal gland, they are often called paraganglionomas. Common sites for paraganglionoma occurrence include the bladder wall (attacks triggered by micturition), mediastinum, carotid body, glomus jugulare body, and the organ of Zuckerkandl. 90% of pheochromocytomas are benign; therefore, removal of the tumor permanently cures the underlying disease.

The diagnosis of pheochromocytoma is made by the demonstration of excessive catecholamine production. Plasma metanephrine level is a sensitive tool but may have a 15% false positive rate. The diagnosis is strengthened by the demonstration of high 24 h urine catecholamines, vanillylmandelic acid, and metanephrine excretion. (Urine creatinine should also be measured to ensure adequacy of the collection). This measurement should be done preferably in the absence of medications known to have an impact on catecholamine metabolism including tricyclic antidepressants, amphetamine, alcohol, sotalol, and centrally acting antihypertensives such as levodopa, clonidine, and reserpine. An additional laboratory tool is plasma chromogranin A level which is not as sensitive as plasma metanephrine but more specific. A high 24 h urine catecholamine level should then prompt imaging by MRI to detect an adrenal mass. MRI is more specific and sensitive than CT. CT is very accurate for lesions greater than 1 cm but considerably less so for smaller lesions. CT angiography has been used successfully in this circumstance as most pheochromocytomas are very vascular. When pheochromocytoma has been confirmed chemically but no lesion found by CT or MRI, radionuclide imaging with iodine-131 (^{131}I)–labeled metaiodobenzylguanidine (MIBG) or indium-111 (^{111}In) pentetreotide can be used.

The treatment of choice for pheochromocytoma is surgical excision. Patients need to undergo alpha blockade with phenoxybenzamine for 7–10 days followed by the addition of beta blockade up to and including the day of surgery to avoid anesthesia-induced hypertensive crisis. Plasma metanephrine then is measured 2 weeks after surgery to ensure adequate tumor removal.

Increased Intracranial Pressure and Intracranial Vascular Events

The epidemiology, evaluation, and treatment of systemic hypertension in the clinical context of stroke are reviewed extensively in the chapter Hypertensive Emergencies. While hypertension is a major risk factor for the development of both ischemic and hemorrhagic stroke, hypertension can also complicate the presentation of stroke and other intracranial events or trauma, although more commonly, hypotension accompanies traumatic brain injury [47, 48]. The current recommendations are for maintaining extracellular fluid volume status and a mean arterial blood pressure of >90 mmHg.

Quadriplegia

Spinal cord injury is frequently complicated by severe dysregulation of the autonomic nervous system and specifically blood pressure control [42]. The tendency toward ypertensive regimen that is tolerable. A variety of conditions can provoke hypertension including urinary retention, pressure ulcerations, constipation, and muscle spasm. The cornerstone of treatment, therefore, is eradication of the inciting event, not pharmacologic therapy. Of the commonly used antihypertensives, clonidine and nifedipine have a track record of efficacy in this disorder.

Endocrine Causes of Hypertension

Multiple endocrine disorders can produce hypertension. Disorders of the adrenal gland or of steroid hormone homeostasis have been discussed extensively [27–46]. The disorders discussed in this section are uncommon though well-recognized endocrine causes of hypertension.

Thyroid Disorders

Both hyper and hypothyroidism are associated with the development of hypertension [50, 51]. Hyperthyroidism causes an increase in cardiac output, the major contributory factor in hypertension associated with this disorder [51]. T3 decreases systemic vascular resistance, resulting in reflex renin secretion and enhanced sodium retention. There is an increase in systolic pressure and a widening of the pulse pressure. Additionally, T3 stimulates erythropoietin release, which can also contribute to the development of hypertension. Thus, the finding of isolated systolic hypertension may suggest the need to exclude a diagnosis of hyperthyroidism in the appropriate setting. Other disorders that may mimic hyperthyroid associated hypertension include Paget Disease, beriberi, and aortic regurgitation.

Hypothyroidism, in contrast to hyperthyroidism, results in T3 deficiency and an increase in peripheral vascular resistance through vasoconstriction and enhanced vascular stiffness [50]. These changes may be mediated by enhanced α adrenergic receptor density and activity on vascular smooth muscle as β adrenergic activity declines. Hypothyroid patients are for the most part very salt sensitive, with most patients exhibiting a low renin, high extracellular fluid volume state.

The diagnosis of thyroid disease associated hypertension is based on the identification of a hyper or hypothyroid state through clinical and chemical studies. The treatment of choice is treatment of the underlying disorder, which in many cases may alleviate the hypertension altogether.

Hyperparathyroidism

Hypertension is seen in roughly 50% of patients with primary hyperparathyroidism, somewhat higher than an age matched population [52–54]. Nonetheless, because both disorders are relatively common, the argument has been made that the co-association is purely coincidental. Multiple studies, however, have demonstrated a documented decrease in blood pressure after treatment for hyperparathyroidism. The mechanism is presumably an increase in vascular resistance associated with hypercalcemic vasoconstriction. In one study, levels of plasma renin activity, aldosterone, and norepinephrine were higher in hyperparathyroid patients than in control individuals. For some individuals with hyperparathyroidism, low vitamin D levels may play a contributory role in stimulating renin release, thus increasing both angiotensin II and aldosterone levels. Recognition of hyperparathyroidism is based on the finding of high calcium levels in the face of nonsuppressed PTH levels, although some variants of hyperparathyroidism (normocalcemic hyperparathyroidism) may also exist. The first treatment is treatment of the underlying hyperparathyroidism by surgery or by the calcium sensing receptor agonist, cinacalcet.

Acromegaly

Acromegaly, the disorder produced by growth hormone excess, is associated with hypertension in about 35% of cases [55, 56]. Although the mechanism is unknown, several possibilities include sodium retention due to growth hormone, the development of metabolic syndrome associated with insulin resistance, or hyperinsulinemic effects such as stimulation of renin production. The diagnosis is made by the recognition of the classic features and chemical confirmation. The treatment of choice is removal of the pituitary adenoma that produces excess growth hormone but medical therapies such as somatostatin analogs have also been used.

Renin Producing Tumors

This rare cause of hypertension is a result of secondary aldosterone production due to excessive renin production from a tumor of the juxtaglomerular cells. As distinguished from the previously discussed mineralocorticoid mediated causes of hypertension, patients with reninomas have elevated, not suppressed, levels of renin. The diagnosis is made by the finding of a high renin and aldosterone level followed by determination of unilateral renin secretion by renal vein sampling.

Genetic Causes of Hypertension

Hypertension complicates multiple forms of genetic kidney disease such as polycystic kidney disease and Alport syndrome through the mechanisms discussed previously. Likewise, the genetic disorders of steroid hormone metabolism resulting in multiple forms of mineralocorticoid induced hypertension have been discussed.

Two monogenic causes of hypertension are characterized by enhanced distal renal tubule sodium reabsorption but because of the different sodium transporters involved, the electrolyte pictures are totally divergent [32–35, 57, 58]. Liddle syndrome is caused by an activating mutation of the epithelial sodium channel in the distal, connecting, and collecting tubule of the kidney, which enhances cell expression of the sodium channel leading to unregulated absorption of sodium and severe hypertension. The syndrome is transmitted in an autosomal dominant fashion and characterized by the early onset of difficult to control hypertension, hypokalemia, metabolic alkalosis, and suppressed plasma renin and aldosterone levels. The diagnosis is based on the appropriate family history and clinical presentation and can be verified by genetic analysis. The treatment of choice is a direct epithelial sodium channel blocker such as amiloride or triamterene. Frequently very high doses of these drugs are required.

The second disorder, Gordon syndrome, also known as pseudohypoaldosteronism type II, is an autosomal dominant disorder caused by mutations in kinases responsible for the regulation of the sodium chloride cotransporter expressed in the distal tubule. The mutations result in constitutively elevated expression and activity of the transporter and resultant increase in sodium transport at that site. The enhanced sodium reabsorption leads to decreased sodium delivery to the tubule sites expressing the epithelial sodium channel. Thus, renal potassium and hydrogen ion excretion are compromised resulting in a clinical picture of salt sensitive hypertension with hyperkalemia and a normal anion gap metabolic acidosis. The treatment of choice for this disorder is thiazide diuretics which block the function of the sodium chloride cotransporter, thus blocking the excessive distal tubule sodium transport. The enhanced sodium delivery to the more distal nephron sites thus permits adequate potassium and hydrogen ion secretion. Interestingly, the immunosuppressive agent tacrolimus appears to cause hypertension similarly by increasing the activity of the sodium chloride transporter, suggesting that the hypertension associated with the use of this drug may respond better to thiazide diuretics than to loop diuretics [59].

Miscellaneous Causes of Secondary Hypertension

Coarctation of the Aorta

Coarctation of the aorta is a condition characterized by the narrowing of the aorta, generally distal to the take-off of the left subclavian artery [60]. The condition is surprisingly common, accounting for 5–10% of congenital cardiac disorders. If not identified during infancy, the disorder can be silent, manifesting as hypertension and headaches. The cornerstone of diagnosis is the demonstration of a significant differential in blood pressure between left and right arm. One third of patients with Turner syndrome have coarctation; thus, the diagnosis of Turner syndrome should prompt screening for aortic coarctation. This disorder is associated with a number of other cardiovascular abnormalities including bicuspid aortic valve, berry aneurysms around the Circle of Willis, and ventricular septal defect. When the diagnosis is suspected, the diagnostic test of choice is the echocardiogram. Cardiac MRI and cardiac catheterization are secondary diagnostic choices. Additional findings that may suggest the presence of coarctation include rib notching on plain film and esophageal indentation (E sign) on barium swallow. Surgical repair is indicated for patients with hypertension associated with aortic coarctation.

Sleep Apnea

Sleep apnea is a very common cause of secondary and resistant hypertension [61–69]. Hypertension is seen in nearly three quarters of the patients with sleep apnea. A recent study placed sleep apnea as the second most common cause of secondary hypertension. The mechanisms for hypertension associated with sleep apnea are numerous and include enhanced sympathetic stimulation, increased sodium retention, and development of the metabolic syndrome. Oftentimes, patients with sleep apnea are obese with attendant metabolic syndrome, hyperinsulinemia, and adipose tissue related cytokine release. Sleep apnea should be suspected in individuals with the typical symptoms of snoring, reported apneic spells, chronic headache, and daytime fatigue and drowsiness. Treatment of the underlying disorder is the treatment of choice for sleep apnea associated hypertension. For obese patients, consideration of bariatric surgery should be entertained [68, 69]. Continuous positive airway pressure moves have also been documented to improve the hypertension associated with sleep apnea [67].

Medications

A number of medications and herbal supplements [70] can contribute to hypertension through several mechanisms including enhanced sodium retention, increased cardiac output, or increased peripheral vascular resistance. These are listed in Table 43.2. Some medications such as the non-steroidal anti-inflammatory drugs are commonly used by patients, frequently resulting in a picture of resistant hypertension, by antagonizing the effects of antihypertensive agents. The treatment of choice is discontinuation of the offending agent or agents.

Case Discussion

This 47-year-old man shows substantial evidence of underlying kidney disease as at least a contributory factor in his hypertension. He has an elevated serum creatinine of 1.4 mg/dL and proteinuria on urinalysis. Although he does not carry the diagnosis of type II diabetes mellitus and his funduscopic examination did not disclose diabetic proliferative retinopathy, he may have diabetic nephropathy. Other considerations for intrinsic proteinuric kidney disease in this age group would be focal glomerulosclerosis, either idiopathic or secondary to obesity, and membranous glomerulopathy. Additional potential causes of secondary hypertension in this individual include atherosclerotic renovascular disease as he has multiple risk factors for atherosclerotic disease and mineralocorticoid associated hypertension as his serum potassium is relatively low despite his use of an ACE inhibitor. His obesity, sleep apnea, and peripheral edema are factors rendering his hypertension difficult to control. In fact, he fulfills the criteria for resistant hypertension.

Identifying likely potential causes for his hypertension is critical to permit focused evaluation in a cost and time sensitive manner (see Table 43.3). The patient's initial evaluation suggests that important diagnostic studies to perform would be renal ultrasound to assess kidney

Table 43.2 Medications associated with hypertension

Classification	Examples	Mechanism of hypertension
Sympathomimetics	Pseudoephedrine, phenylephrine, Ritalin, adderall, amphetamines	Increased sympathetic tone
Cyclo-oxygenase inhibitors	COX-1 inhibitors: ibuprofen, naproxyn, COX-2 inhibitors: celecoxib, rofecoxib	Enhanced renal sodium reabsorption
Adrenal steroids	Glucocorticosteroids: dexamethasone, hydrocortisone Minerallocorticoids fludrocortisone	Enhanced renal sodium reabsorption
Illicit drugs	Cocaine, PCP	Increased sympathetic tone
Growth factor agonists/ antagonists	Erythropoietin Beclizumab, vandetaib, alemtuzumab, rituximab	Endothelial damage, enhanced sympathetic tone
Calcineurin inhibitors	Cyclosporine, tacrolimus	Enhanced renal sodium reabsorption
Beta receptor agonists	Albuterol	Increased sympathetic tone
Sex steroids	Estrogens	Enhanced renal sodium reabsorption
Migraine medications	Zolmitriptan, sumatriptan, ergotamine, isometheptine	Increased sympathetic tone
Tricyclic antidepressants	Desipramine, imipramine, doxepin	Enhanced renal sodium reabsorption
Alcohol	Multiple preparations	Increased sympathetic tone
Herbal supplements	Ma huang, ginkgo biloba	Increased sympathetic tone, renal damage

size. Depending on the local radiologic expertise, consideration could be given to duplex ultrasound of the renal arteries, magnetic resonance angiography, or digital subtraction angiography if any evidence of peripheral vascular disease or coronary artery disease is uncovered, for example, carotid bruits, claudication, or angina. 24 h urine for protein and creatinine clearance, serum aldosterone and renin measurements, and thyroid function tests would also be reasonable tests to perform. Although not as likely in this age group, familial forms of hypertension should be considered and a thorough family history should be obtained.

Further diagnostic studies and therapy would depend heavily on the results of these studies. Identification of atherosclerotic renal artery stenosis that is critical would warrant further evaluation for potential intervention, either by captopril renal scan or selective renal vein renin studies. Some investigators suggest that going directly to renal angiography for visualization and balloon angioplasty would be the most appropriate next step; however, this stance is controversial. Measurement of an elevated aldosterone to renin ratio (greater than 25 to 1) would suggest the presence of hyperaldosteronism either due to an adrenal adenoma or adrenal hyperplasia. The next step to assess the presence of hyperaldosteronism would be an aldosterone suppression test instructing the patient to ingest a high salt diet for several days prior to repeat renin and aldosterone measurement or an intravenous saline suppression test with measurement of serum renin and aldosterone prior to and 2 and 4 h after saline administration. These studies would necessitate that the patient discontinue the diuretic and ACE inhibitor for a period of time before the measurement. Some would argue that the beta blocker should also be discontinued due to its inhibitory effects on renin secretion. Identification of an adenoma with biochemical evidence of enhanced production of aldosterone from that adrenal gland would suggest adrenalectomy as the treatment of choice. Identification of idiopathic adrenal hyperplasia would suggest medical management with a mineralocorticoid receptor antagonist such as spironolactone or eplerenone.

Even if other metabolic or structural abnormalities to explain his hypertension are discovered, efforts should be directed toward treating the renal disease, obesity, and sleep apnea. Although no specific therapy for diabetic nephropathy exists, measures to retard progression of

Table 43.3 Approach to the Diagnosis of Secondary Hypertension

Step 1: Basic Initial Evaluation

Complete history and physical examination
Renal Profile, glucose, calcium, phosphorus
Urinalysis
Consider EKG, Chest radiograph

Step 2: Decision Analysis Based on Results of Initial Evaluation

Findings	Diagnostic Consideration	Next Step in Evaluation
Completely normal	Essential Hypertension	None. Start Treatment Re-evaluate if develops resistant hypertension
Abnormal urinalysis Elevated BUN, Cr Family history of kidney disease	Intrinsic kidney disease	24 hour urine for protein and creatinine clearance Kidney ultrasound Additional studies as indicated, e.g., ANA, C3
Vascular bruits, esp abdominal	Renal artery stenosis	Low to moderate index of suspicion: renal arterial Doppler, CT angiography
Sudden onset age < 40	Fibromuscular dysplasia	High index of suspicion: renal arteriography
Symptoms of vascular disease such as TIA, CVA, claudication, CAD Flash pulmonary edema	Atherosclerotic renal arterial disease	
Unexplained hypokalemia Serum Na > 140 meq/L Metabolic alkalosis	Minerallocorticoid excess	AM aldosterone and renin
Wide BP fluctuations Sporadic hypertension Tachycardia, diaphoresis Behavior-triggered HT plus symptoms, e.g., HT associated with micturition	Pheochromocytoma	Plasma metanephrines
Skin changes Heat/cold intolerance Weight loss or gain Tachycardia/bradycardia	Hyper or hypothyroidism	Thyroid function tests
Bone pain Calcium kidney stones Hypercalcemia	Hyperparathyroidism	Intact PTH level
Family history of HT	Familial kidney disease such as PCKD	Kidney ultrasound
Family history of intracranial bleed	Liddle syndrome	Consider genetic testing, urine for steroid metabolites
Family history of hypo/hyperkalemia	Gordon syndrome Genetic causes of abnormal steroid hormone metabolism	
Discrepancy in blood pressure between right and left arms Delayed or severely diminished pulses in left arm or legs	Coarctation of aorta	Aortic imaging by CT
Daytime drowsiness Obesity Mildly elevated fasting glucose	Obstructive sleep apnea Metabolic syndrome	Sleep study HbA1c Lipid panel
Illicit medication use Herbal supplement use	Drug-induced hypertension Drug induced kidney injury	Full review of all oral agents Discontinuation of potential offending agent if possible
Immunosuppressive use Extensive OTC medication use		

kidney disease such as control of blood pressure and hyperlipidemia should be instituted. Additionally, encouragement to lose weight would help with both blood pressure control and treatment of sleep apnea. Some studies have suggested that use of nocturnal CPAP may help with blood pressure control. From a pharmacologic standpoint, some investigators have suggested that even in the absence of frank mineralocorticoid excess, many patients with resistant hypertension respond to mineralocorticoid antagonists. Finally, consideration for bariatric surgery should be entertained.

References

1. Onusko E. Diagnosing secondary hypertension. Am Fam Physician. 2003;67:67–74.
2. Viera AJ, Neutze DM. Diagnosis of secondary hypertension: an age-based approach. Am Fam Physician. 2010;82(12):1471–8.
3. Sukor N. Secondary hypertension: a condition not to be missed. Postgrad Med J. 2011;87:706–13.
4. Jamerson KA, Townsend RR. The attributable burden of hypertension: focus on CKD. Adv Chronic Kidney Dis. 2011;18:6–10.
5. Yano Y, Fujimoto S, Sato Y, Konta T, Iseki K, Moriyama T, Yamagata K, Tsuruya K, Yoshida H, Asahi K, Kurahashi I, Ohashi Y, Watanabe T. Association between prehypertension and chronic kidney disease in the Japanese general population. Kidney Int. 2012;81:293–9.
6. Johnson RJ, Herrera-Acosta J, Schreiner GF, Rodriguez-Iturbe B. Subtle acquired renal injury as a mechanism of salt sensitive hypertension. N Engl J Med. 2002;346:913–23.
7. Upadhyay A, Eareley AM, Haynes SM, Uhlig K. Systematic review: blood pressure target in chronic kidney disease and proteinuria as an effect modifier. Ann Intern Med. 2011;154:541–8.
8. McCullough PA, Steigerwalt S, Tolia K, Chen SC, Li S, Norris KC, Whaley-Connell A. Cardiovascular disease in chronic kidney disease: data from the kidney early evaluation program. Curr Diab Rep. 2011;11(1):47–55.
9. Chapman AB, Stepniakowski K, Rahbari-Oskoui F. Hypertension in autosomal dominant polycystic kidney disease. Adv Chronic Kidney Dis. 2010;17(2):153–63.
10. Ernst ME, Jordan MA. Diuretic therapy: key aspects in hypertension and renal disease. J Nephrol. 2010;23(5):487–93.
11. Gallagher H, de Lusignan S, Harris K, Cates C. Quality improvement strategies for the management of hypertension in chronic kidney disease in primary care: a systematic review. Br J Gen Pract. 2010;60(575): e258–65.
12. Segura J, Ruilope LM. Hypertension in moderate to severe nondiabetic CKD patients. Adv Chronic Kidney Dis. 2011;18:23–7.
13. Van Buren PN, Toto R. Hypertension in diabetic nephropathy: epidemiology, mechanisms, and management. Adv Chronic Kidney Dis. 2011;18: 28–41.
14. Hackam DG, Khan NA, Hemmelgarn BR, et al. The 2010 Canadian Hypertension Education Program recommendations for the management of hypertension: part 2 – therapy. Can J Cardiol. 2010;26(5):249–58.
15. Kouri Y, Steigerwalt SP, Alsamara M, McCullough PA. What is the ideal blood pressure goal for patients with stage 3 or higher chronic kidney disease? Curr Cardiol Rep. 2011;13(6):492–501.
16. Sica DA. Pharmacologic issues in treating hypertension in CKD. Adv Chronic Kidney Dis. 2011;18:42–7.
17. Lerma EV. Hydrochlorothiazide vs calcium channel blockers: what is the best add-on to a renin-angiotensin blocker for treating hypertension in people with renal disease? Curr Hypertens Rep. 2011;13(5):386–95.
18. Mehta AN, Fenves A. Current opinions in renovascular hypertension. Eur Nephrol. 2010;4:45–8.
19. Slovut DP, Olin JW. Fibromuscular dysplasia. N Engl J Med. 2004;350:1862–71.
20. O'Neill WC, Bardelli M, Yevzlin AS. Imaging for renovascular disease. Semin Nephrol. 2011;31:272–82.
21. Colyer WR, Eltahawy E, Cooper CJ. Renal artery stenosis: optimizing diagnosis and treatment. Prog Cardiovasc Dis. 2011;54(1):29–35.
22. Lao D, Parasher PS, Cho KC, Yeghiazarians Y. Atherosclerotic renal artery stenosis – diagnosis and treatment. Mayo Clin Proc. 2011;86(7):649–57.
23. ACC/AHA. Practice guidelines for the management of patients with peripheral arterial disease (lower extremity, renal, mesenteric, and abdominal aortic). Circulation. 2005;2006(113):e463–654.
24. Shetty R, Biondi-Zoccai GG, Abbate A, Amin MS, Jovin IS. Percutaneous renal artery intervention versus medical therapy in with renal artery stenosis: a meta-analysis. EuroIntervention. 2011;7(7):844–51.
25. Meier P. Atherosclerotic renal artery stenosis: update on management strategies. Curr Opin Cardiol. 2011;26(6):463–71.
26. White CJ. Management of renal artery stenosis: the case for intervention, defending current guidelines, and screening (drive-by) renal angiography at the time of catheterization. Progr Cardiovasc Dis. 2009;52:229–37.
27. Uwaifo GI, Sarlis NJ. Primary hyperaldosteronism. Emedicine/Medscape; 2012.
28. Mulatero P, Tizzani D, Viola A, Bertello C, Monticone S, Mengozzi G, Schiavone D, Williams TA, Einaudi S, La Grotta A, Rabbia F, Veglio F. Prevalence and characteristics of familial hyperaldosteronism. The PATOGEN study (Primary Aldosteronism in TOrino-GENetic forms). Hypertension. 2011;58:797–803.
29. Westerdahl C, Bergenfelz A, Isaksson A, Nerbrand C, Valdemarsson S. Primary aldosteronism among newly diagnosed and untreated hypertensive patients in a

Swedish primary care area. Scand J Prim Health Care. 2011;29:57–62.
30. Tritos NA. Diagnosis of primary hyperaldosteronism in a patient with an incidentally found adrenal mass. Nat Clin Pract Endocrinol Metab. 2007;3:547–51.
31. Mulatero P, Bertello C, Rossato D, Mengozzi G, Milan A, Garrone C, Giraudo G, Passarino G, Garabello D, Verhovez A, Rabbia F, Veglio F. Roles of clinical criteria, computed tomography scan, and adrenal vein sampling in differential diagnosis of primary hyperaldosterone subtypes. J Clin Endocrinol Metab. 2008;93:1366–71.
32. Hassan-Smith Z, Stewart PM. Inherited forms of mineralocorticoid hypertension. Curr Opin Endocrinol Diabetes Obes. 2011;18(3):177–85.
33. Khosla N, Hogan D. Mineralocorticoid hypertension and hypokalemia. Semin Nephrol. 2006;26(6):434–40.
34. Martinez-Aguayo A, Fardella C. Genetics of hypertensive syndrome. Horm Res. 2009;71:253–9.
35. Vehaskari VM. Heritable forms of hypertension. Pediatr Nephrol. 2009;24:1929–37.
36. Matsson C, Young WF. Primary aldosteronism: diagnostic and treatment strategies. Nat Clin Pract Nephrol. 2006;2(4):198–208.
37. Hammer F, Stewart PM. Cortisol metabolism in hypertension. Best Pract Res Clin Endocrinol Metab. 2006;20:337–53.
38. Stewart PM. Cortisol as a mineralocorticoid in human disease. J Steroid Biochem Mol Biol. 1999;69:403–8.
39. Saruta T. Mechanism of glucocorticoid induced hypertension. Hypertens Res. 1996;19:1–8.
40. Cosmetic Ingredient Review Expert Panel. Final report on the safety assessment of glycyrrhetinic acid, potassium glycyrrhetinate, disodium succinoyl glycyrrhetinate, glyceryl glycyrrhetinate, glycyrrhetinyl stearate, stearyl glycyrrhetinate, glycyrrhizic acid, ammonium glycyrrhizate, dipotassium glycyrrhizate, disodium glycyrrhizate, trisodium glycyrrhizate, methyl glycyrrhizate, and potassium glycyrrhizinate. J Toxicol. 2007;26 Suppl 2:79–112.
41. Zhang Y, Nose V. Endocrine tumors as part of inherited tumor syndromes. Adv Anat Pathol. 2011;18(3):206–18.
42. Jiang S, Dahia PL. Minireview: the busy road to pheochromocytomas and paragangliomas has a new member, TMEM127. Endocrinology. 2011;152(6):2133–40.
43. McNicol AM. Update on tumours of the adrenal cortex, phaeochromocytomas, and extra-adrenal paraganglionomas. Histopathology. 2011;58(2):155–68.
44. Waguespack SG, Rich T, Grubbs E, Ying AK, Perrier ND, Ayala-Ramirez M, Jimenez C. A current review of the etiology, diagnosis, and treatment of pediatric pheochromocytoma and paraganglioma. J Clin Endocrinol Metab. 2010;95(5):2023–37.
45. Young Jr WF. Clinical practice. The incidentally discovered adrenal mass. N Engl J Med. 2007;356(6):601–10.
46. de Jong WH, Eisenhofer G, Post WJ, Muskiet FA, de Vries EG, Kema IP. Dietary influences on plasma and urinary metanephrines: implications for diagnosis of catecholamine-producing tumors. J Clin Endocrinol Metab. 2009;94(8):2841–9.
47. Owens WB. Blood pressure control in acute cerebrovascular disease. J Clin Hypertens. 2011;13: 205–11.
48. Marik PE, Varon J, Trask T. Management of head trauma. Chest. 2002;122:699–711.
49. Mathias CJ. Orthostatic hypotension and paroxysmal hypertension in humans with high spinal cord injury. Prog Brain Res. 2006;152:231–43.
50. Fletcher AK, Weetman AA. Hypertension and hypothyroidism. J Hum Hypertens. 1998;12:79–82.
51. Prisant LM, Gujral JS, Mulloy AL. Hyperthyroidism: a secondary cause of isolated systolic hypertension. J Clin Hypertens. 2006;8:596–9.
52. Tordjman KM, Yaron M, Izhakov E, Osher E, Shenkerman G, Marcus-Perlman Y, Stern N. Cardiovascular risk factors and arterial rigidity are similar in asymptomatic normocalcemic and hypercalcemic primary hyperparathyroidism. Eur J Endocrinol. 2010;162:925–33.
53. Schiffl H, Lang SM. Hypertension secondary to PHPT: cause or coincidence? Int J Endocrinol. 2011:1–6.
54. Broulik PD, Broulika A, Adamek S, Libansky P, Tvrdon J, Broulikova K, Kubiny J. Improvement of hypertension after parathyroidectomy of patients with primary hyperparathyroidism. Int J Endocrinol. 2011:1–6.
55. Colao A, Pivonello R, Marzullo P, Auriemma RS, De Martino MC, Ferone D, Lombardi G. Severe systemic complications of acromegaly. J Endocrinol Invest. 2005;28(5 Suppl):65–77.
56. Berg C, Petersenn S, Lahner H, Herrmann BL, Buchfelder M, Droste M, Stalla GK, Strasburger CJ, Roggenbuck U, Lehmann N, Moebus S, Jöckel KH, Möhlenkamp S, Erbel R, Saller B, Mann K, Investigative Group of the Heinz Nixdorf Recall Study and the German Pegvisomant Observational Study Board and Investigators. Cardiovascular risk factors in patients with uncontrolled and long-term acromegaly: comparison with matched data from the general population and the effect of disease control. J Clin Endocrinol Metab. 2010;95(8): 3648–56.
57. Stowasser M, Pimenta E, Gordon RD. Familial or genetic primary aldosteronism and Gordon syndrome. Endocrinol Metab Clin North Am. 2011;40(2):343–68.
58. Uchida S. Pathophysiological roles of WNK kinases in the kidney. Pflugers Arch. 2010;460:695–702.
59. Hoorn EJ, Walsh SB, McCormick JA, Fürstenberg A, Yang CL, Roeschel T, Paliege A, Howie AJ, Conley J, Bachmann S, Unwin RJ, Ellison DH. The calcineurin inhibitor tacrolimus activates the renal sodium chloride cotransporter to cause hypertension. Nat Med. 2011;17(10):1304–9.
60. Kenny D, Hijazi ZM. Coarctation of the aorta: from fetal life to adulthood. Cardiol J. 2011;18:487–95.
61. Potenza MV, Mechanick JL. The metabolic syndrome: definition, global impact, and pathophysiology. Nutr Clin Pract. 2009;24:560–77.
62. Alberti KG, Eckel RH, Grundy SM, Zimmet PZ, Cleeman JI, Dobnato KA, Fruchart JC, James WP,

Loria CM, Smith SC. Harmonizing the metabolic syndrome: a joint interim statement for the International Diabetes Federation Task Force on Epidemiology and Prevention; National Heart Lung and Blood Institute; American Heart Association; World Heart Federation; International Atherosclerosis Society; and International Association for the Study of Obesity. Circulation. 2009;120:1640–5.

63. Gopalakrishnan P, Tak T. Obstructive sleep apnea and cardiovascular disease. Cardiol Rev. 2011;19:279–90.
64. Mokhlesi H. Obesity hypoventilation syndrome: a state of the art review. Respir Care. 2010;55: 1347–62.
65. Flynn JT, Falkner BE. Obesity hypertension in adolescents: epidemiology, evaluation, and management. J Clin Hypertens. 2011;13:323–31.
66. Pedrosa RP, Drager LF, Gonzaga CC, Sousa MG, de Paula LKG, Amaro ACS, Amodeo C, Bortolotto LA, Krieger EM, Bradley TD, Lorenzi-Filho G. Obstructive sleep apnea: the most common secondary cause of hypertension associated with resistant hypertension. Hypertension. 2011;58:811–7.
67. Sharma SK, Agarwal S, Damodaran D, Sreenivas V, Kadhiravan T, Lakshmy R, Jagia P, Kumar A. CPAP for the metabolic syndrome in patients with obstructive sleep apnea. N Engl J Med. 2011;365:2277–86.
68. Kaul A, Sharma J. Impact of bariatric surgery on comorbidities. Surg Clin North Am. 2011;91:1295–312.
69. Dumon KR, Murayama KM. Bariatric surgery outcomes. Surg Clin North Am. 2011;91:1313–8.
70. Vivekanand J. Herbal medicines and chronic kidney disease. Nephrology. 2010;15:10–7.

Hypertensive Emergencies and Resistant Hypertension

44

Lina Mackelaite and Eleanor D. Lederer

Introduction

According to the American Heart Association (AHA), hypertensive emergency is defined as severely elevated blood pressure (>180/120 mmHg) with target organ damage [1], which includes left ventricular failure and pulmonary edema, acute myocardial infarction, ischemic stroke, intracranial hemorrhage, aortic dissection, acute kidney injury, encephalopathy, or eclampsia (Tables 44.1 and 44.2). Approximately 25% of patients that present to the emergency department with hypertensive emergency have no previous history of hypertension [1]. The American Heart Association recommends a reduction of mean arterial blood pressure by not more than 25% within the first hour and then, if clinically stable, to about 160/100 mmHg within next 2–6 h. Hypertensive emergencies are treated with intravenous blood pressure medications (Tables 44.3 and 44.4).

Malignant hypertension is a term that is often used synonymously with hypertensive emergency. Classically, however, malignant hypertension requires the presence of papilledema in addition to evidence of other end-organ damage [2]. Malignant hypertension is characterized by a distinctive pathology, fibrinoid necrosis of the small arterioles in any of several tissues including heart, kidney, or brain. The appearance of papilledema on funduscopic examination results from edema of the optic disk, not necessarily from an increase in intracranial pressure. Clinically, in addition to the presence of papilledema, patients with malignant hypertension exhibit hematuria and microangiopathic hemolytic anemia with thrombocytopenia and schistocytes in addition to other end-organ damage.

Hypertensive urgency is a severe (upper levels of stage II hypertension) elevation of blood pressure without target organ damage. Patients with hypertensive urgencies can have anxiety, headache, shortness of breath, or epistaxis. In case of hypertensive urgency (when there is no end-organ damage) blood pressure can be managed using oral agents [3].

Resistant hypertension refers to the condition where an individual continues to have blood pressure measurements in the hypertensive range despite taking at least three antihypertensive medications at optimal dosages, one of which will generally be a diuretic [4]. Hypertensive emergencies may occur in the setting of resistant hypertension; however, they are different entities.

Any of the above hypertensive conditions can occur as complications of either primary or secondary hypertension. Generally, as discussed in the chapter addressing secondary hypertension, the occurrence of any of these hypertensive events will raise the suspicion of a secondary form of hypertension.

L. Mackelaite, M.D. (✉)
Division of Nephrology, University of Louisville, 615 South Preston Street, Louisville, KY 40202, USA
e-mail: l0mack01@louisville.edu

E.D. Lederer, M.D.
Division of Nephrology, University of Louisville, 615 South Preston Street, Louisville, KY 40202, USA

Robley Rex VA Medical Centre, 800 Zorn Avenue, Louisville, KY 40206, USA

E.V. Lerma and M. Rosner (eds.), *Clinical Decisions in Nephrology, Hypertension and Kidney Transplantation*, DOI 10.1007/978-1-4614-4454-1_44, © Springer Science+Business Media New York 2013

Table 44.1 Definitions

Hypertensive emergency	Severely elevated blood pressure with target organ damage (acute myocardial infarction, aortic dissection, pulmonary edema, etc.)
Hypertensive urgency	Severe (upper levels of stage II hypertension) elevation of blood pressure without target organ damage
Malignant hypertension	Severely elevated blood pressure with papilledema
Resistant hypertension	Blood pressure that is not at goal despite use of 3 antihypertensive medications from different classes (ideally, one of them being diuretic)

Table 44.2 Symptoms, physical, and laboratory findings associated with specific end-organ damage in hypertensive emergency

End-organ damage	Symptoms	Laboratory/radiology findings
Stroke	Focal neurologic deficits, slurred speech, visual problems	MRI is preferred over CT unless there is a contraindication to it (like pacemaker)
SAH	Severe headache—especially the one that awakens patient at night, nausea, vomiting	CT scan without contrast will demonstrate clot in the subarachnoid space in 92% of the cases if performed within 24 h
Heart failure	Shortness of breath, orthopnea, paroxysmal nocturnal dyspnea, swelling	Chest X-ray showing pulmonary edema
Renal failure	Decreased urine output, frothy, "tea colored" urine, swelling	Elevated creatinine/BUN, hematuria, proteinuria
Acute coronary syndrome	Chest pain, diaphoresis, nausea	Elevated cardiac enzymes, EKG changes (ST-T depressions or elevations)
Aortic dissection	Severe abdominal pain, radiating to the back	CT angiogram showing "false lumen" in the aorta

Table 44.3 Preferred antihypertensive medications depending on end-organ damage

End-organ damage	Preferred medication	Avoid
Stroke	Labetalol, nicardipine	Nitroprusside—can increase intracranial pressure
Aortic dissection	Esmolol, labetalol. IF BP not controlled with beta-blocker alone—add nicardipine or nitroprusside	Nitroprusside or nicardipine without beta-blocker can cause reflex tachycardia
Pulmonary edema with systolic CMP	Nitroglycerin and loop diuretic, can add nitroprusside or nicardipine if BP still high	
Pulmonary edema with diastolic CMP	Esmolol, labetalol, verapamil. Low dose nitroglycerin and loop diuretic	High dose nitroglycerin or loop diuretic—can decrease preload
Acute coronary syndrome	Esmolol or labetalol with nitroglycerin	Nitroprusside—can cause "coronary steal syndrome"
Acute kidney failure	Nicardipine, fenoldopam	Nitroprusside—risk of cyanide toxicity
Preeclampsia, eclampsia	Labetalol, hydralazine, nicardipine	ACE inhibitors—renal malformation, nitroprusside—cyanide toxicity to the baby
Cocaine	Intravenous benzodiazepines, nitroglycerine, nitroprusside	β blockers secondary to unopposed α blockade

CMP cardiomyopathy, *ACE* angiotensin-converting enzyme

Case 1: Hypertensive Emergency with Cerebrovascular Involvement

As the senior resident on call, you are notified by the emergency room physician that a 57-year-old woman with long-standing resistant hypertension is being admitted for a hypertensive emergency. Her blood pressure is 200/140 mmHg and she is complaining of a severe headache. The remainder of the physical examination is unremarkable as is

Table 44.4 Parenteral antihypertensive medications used in hypertensive emergencies

Medication	Mechanism	Dose	Onset of action	Duration of action	Side effects
Labetalol	α1, α2, β2 antagonist	20 mg bolus, can repeat bolus every 10 min to a max dose of 300 mg or infusion at 05–2 mg/min	5–10 min	3–6 h	Bronchospasm, bradycardia, dizziness, nausea, vomiting, orthostatic hypotension
Esmolol	B1 antagonist	500 mcg/kg bolus followed by 50 mcg/kg/min infusion, titrated up to a max of 300 mcg/kg/min	Within 60 s	10–20 min	Bradycardia, hypotension, bronchospasm, nausea
Fenoldopam	DA-1 agonist	0.1–0.3 mg/kg/min infusion	<5 min	30–60 min	Tachycardia, dizziness, nausea, flushing, headache
Nicardipine	L-type calcium channel blocker (dihydropiridine)	5–15 mg/h infusion	1–5 min	15–30 min	Tachycardia, headache, nausea, flushing, edema, dizziness
Clevidipine	L-type calcium channel blocker (dihydropiridine)	1–21 mg/h infusion	2–4 min	5–15 min	Reflex tachycardia,nausea, headache, vomiting
Nitroglycerine	Vasodilator	5 mcg/min, titrated by 5 mcg/min every 5 min to max of 60 mcg/min	2–5 min	5–10 min	Headache, dizziness, tachyphylaxis
Nitroprusside	Vasodilator (arterial and venous)	0.5–10 mcg/kg/min	Immediate	2–3 min	Cyanide and thiocyanate intoxication, muscle twitching, vomiting, nausea, vomiting
Enalaprilat	ACE inhibitor	1.25 mg over 5 min, repeat every 4–6 h, maximum 5 mg every 6 h	Within 30 min	12–24 h	Variable response, hypotension, headache, dizziness
Phentolamine	α Adrenergic receptor blocker	5–15 mg IV bolus	1–2 min	10–30 min	Tachycardia, flushing, headaches

her initial laboratory screening studies. You ask yourself the following questions as you are heading down to the emergency room

1. What is the difference between a hypertensive emergency and simple severely elevated blood pressure?
2. Are the terms hypertensive emergency and malignant hypertension synonymous?
3. What is resistant hypertension and how is that different from a hypertensive emergency?
4. Are all hypertensive emergencies treated the same?

Case Discussion

The patient in question would fall under the category of hypertensive urgency, not emergency, as she does not exhibit specific end-organ damage. As the admitting resident, you would want to ensure that the patient had no evidence of cerebrovascular compromise, cardiac decompensation, or acute kidney injury. Your physical examination would be focused on mental status assessment, funduscopic examination, cardiopulmonary assessment, and evaluation of volume status. Laboratory values of interest would be the peripheral smear, renal function profile, urinalysis, and, if suggested by the history, toxin screen for cocaine ingestion. Initial therapy with oral agents would be appropriate if examination and laboratory evaluation were both normal.

Presentation and Findings

The patient who presents with symptoms and signs of cerebrovascular compromise and severe hypertension is defined as having a hypertensive emergency with cerebrovascular involvement [2, 3, 5]. Common symptoms would include headache, blurred vision or loss of vision, dizziness, confusion, or focal loss of motor or sensory function. Headache alone can be seen with a hypertensive urgency, so more tangible evidence of true cerebrovascular deficit would be required to define a hypertensive emergency. Some common signs would be altered mental status, seizure, papilledema, or unilateral loss of cranial nerve or sensorimotor function. These signs and symptoms may accompany cerebrovascular ischemia, hemorrhage, or even subarachnoid bleeding. Because the treatment of the underlying disorder and the approach to hypertension differ between these causes of cerebrovascular hypertensive emergencies, the clinician should first determine what type of cerebrovascular event has occurred. Most commonly, brain CT or MRI are employed to make this determination.

Treatment

According to current American Stroke Association (ASA) guidelines, hypertension should not be treated in patients with ischemic stroke unless systolic blood pressure (SBP) is more than 220 mmHg and diastolic blood pressure (DBP) is more than 120 mmHg. Lowering blood pressure may decrease perfusion in the penumbra (ischemic neuronal tissue surrounding necrotic area), thus worsening the neurologic deficit. Aggressive blood pressure management in ischemic stroke is associated with worse neurologic outcomes and increased mortality [6–8]. An exception is patients receiving thrombolytic therapy, in which case blood pressure should be lowered to at least 180/105 mmHg to decrease the risk of bleeding [9]. There is no data supporting use of any particular antihypertensive medication in patients with stroke. Possible choices include intravenous labetalol or nicardipine infusion.

In contrast to ischemic stroke, recent studies using PET and MRI scans in patients with intracranial hemorrhage (ICH) showed that there was no ischemic penumbra surrounding the hemorrhage [10]. Therefore, lowering of the blood pressure does not place remaining brain tissue at risk for further ischemia. In fact, the risk of death and dependency in patients with ICH correlates with the degree of hypertension on admission [11, 12]. AMAP greater than120 mmHg is associated with early hematoma expansion and increased mortality [11]. Based on these observations, ASA currently recommends maintaining MAP less than 130 mmHg in patients with ICH and history of hypertension and less than 100 mmHg in patients with no previous history of hypertension. MAP should not be decreased to less than 90 mmHg.

Blood pressure lowering is controversial in patients with subarachnoid hemorrhage. A MAP greater than 130 mmHg or less than 70 mmHg is associated with increased mortality and disability [13]. *AHA guidelines do not recommend routine blood pressure lowering in patients with subarachnoid hemorrhage.*

Case 2: Hypertensive Emergency with Aortic Dissection

A 57-year-old African-American man with a past medical history of poorly controlled hypertension, noncompliance with medications, and CKD stage 4 (baseline creatinine 2.4 mg/dL) presents to the emergency room (ER) with severe chest pain, radiating to the back. The initial set of cardiac enzymes was normal and EKG demonstrated no signs of myocardial infarction. His creatinine in the ER was 2.1 mg/dL. Emergent CT angiography demonstrated aortic dissection extending from the left subclavian artery to the level of the renal arteries,

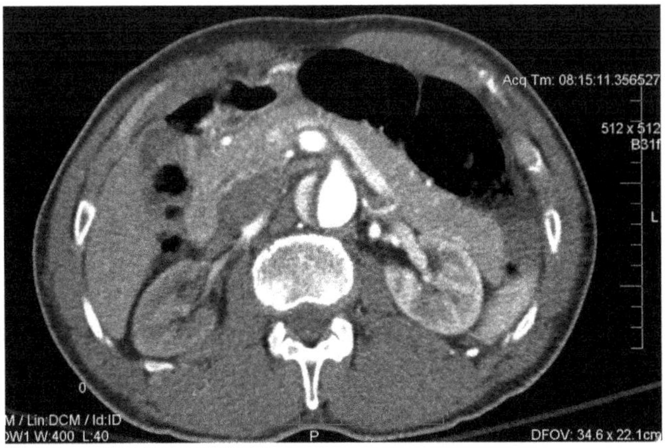

Fig. 44.1 Acute aortic dissection terminating just below the renal arteries

compromising blood flow to the left kidney (Fig. 44.1). After initial therapy with parenteral esmolol, his heart rate decreased to 50s but blood pressure remained elevated at 160/95.

Presentation and Findings

Tearing chest pain radiating to the back is the classic presentation for an aortic dissection, but up to 10–20% of patients may have no pain [14, 15]. Common nonpainful presentations include syncope and hypotension. Because of the very high mortality associated with unrecognized, and even recognized, aortic dissection, clinicians need to be aware of the common presentations and findings in order initiate early therapy. The common risk factors for aortic dissection include older age, history of hypertension, and underlying atherosclerosis. However, pregnancy, cocaine abuse, congenital bicuspid aortic valve, large vessel vasculitis, and connective tissue disorders such as Marfan syndrome are also associated with the development of aortic dissection. Common physical findings include aortic regurgitation in over 30%, and pulse deficit in 15%. A thorough examination of the peripheral pulses and measurement of the blood pressure in both upper extremities can disclose significantly asymmetric findings, suggesting to the clinician the potential diagnosis of aortic dissection. Type A aortic dissections (involving the ascending aorta) are frequently associated with hypotension while Type B aortic dissections almost always present with hypertension. The most commonly used modality for diagnosis is CT angiography but dissections can also be identified using transesophageal echocardiography or magnetic resonance angiography. Mediastinal enlargement on plain chest X-ray may be an important clue to the presence of a dissection.

Treatment

Type A dissections are treated surgically since mortality approaches 1–2% per hour after the onset of symptoms [16, 17]. Type B aortic dissections can be treated medically unless there is extravasation of blood or signs of end organ hypoperfusion [18]. The blood pressure goal in patients with aortic dissection is to lower blood pressure quickly to less than 120 mmHg and decrease heart rate to less than 60/min. These measures decrease left ventricular ejection force (dP/dt) and prevent propagation of dissection. β blockers are preferred antihypertensives: intravenous labetalol can be given as infusion at 0.5–2 mg/min or as a bolus of 20 mg IV which can be repeated every 10 min to a maximum total dose of 300 mg. Esmolol is a short-acting intravenous β blocker given as an initial 80 mg bolus over 30 s and then followed by 150 mcg/kg/min infusion and titrated up to 300 mcg/kg/min. If target systolic blood pressure is not achieved with β blockers alone, vasodilators like nitroprusside, fenoldopam, or nicardipine can be used [19].

Vasodilators should never be used alone since they can increase heart rate and left ventricular ejection force.

Case Discussion

In contrast to the first case discussed, this patient clearly fulfills the criteria for experiencing a hypertensive emergency, specifically hypertension complicated by an aortic dissection. Initial therapy would be with a beta blocker to decrease both pulse and blood pressure in order to decrease ventricular ejection force and shear stress. 500 mcg/kg bolus of esmolol followed by a constant infusion at the rate of 150 mcg/kg/min is an ideal choice in this situation. Although the patient's heart rate response reached the goal of therapy with the beta blocker alone, his blood pressure remained elevated beyond the target range. Addition of a vasodilator such as nicardipine 5 mg/h drip would then be indicated to decrease blood pressure to 120/70. Note that the primary objective is to decrease the force of ventricular ejection and shear stress on the aorta in order to decrease the likelihood of further dissection. Therefore, the administration of the beta blocker precedes the administration of a primary vasodilator.

Left Ventricular Failure and Pulmonary Edema

Presentation and Findings

Both patients with systolic and diastolic heart failure can present with severe hypertension and pulmonary edema [2, 3, 5]. Typically, the presenting symptom is dyspnea but may also be chest pain or discomfort. Physical examination should be directed toward the cardiac and pulmonary systems, looking for evidence of volume overload as manifested by rales, peripheral edema, or an S3 gallop and for evidence of cardiac strain as manifested by the presence of severe left ventricular enlargement, a gallop, or a hyperdynamic precordium. Chest X-ray may show evidence of pulmonary vascular congestion, pleural fluid, or cardiac enlargement.

Treatment

Treatment of hypertensive emergencies differs depending of the type of heart failure. Up to 40% of patients who present with symptoms of heart failure have preserved left ventricular systolic function but impaired diastolic relaxation [20–22]. Uncontrolled hypertension increases after load in these patients and can precipitate pulmonary edema [21]. On the other hand, patients with diastolic dysfunction are preload dependent, so diuretics and nitroglycerin have to be used with caution since they can potentially decrease stroke volume and cardiac output. β blocking agents can be effective in patients with diastolic heart failure and hypertensive emergency. By decreasing heart rate beta blockers allow for more complete left atrial emptying.

Patients with systolic heart failure, who present with severe hypertension and pulmonary edema, should be treated with intravenous diuretics and nitroglycerin or nitroprusside infusion. Nitroprusside is a potent vasodilator which increases cardiac index, decreases pulmonary vascular resistance and decreases pulmonary artery systolic pressure in patients with systolic heart failure. Even patients with heart failure and aortic stenosis (who are preload dependent) improve with nitroprusside treatment [20]. Nicardipine and fenoldopam are also effective [3].

Acute Coronary Syndrome

Presentation and Findings

Patients with severe hypertension complicating an acute coronary syndrome will generally present with chest pain; however, the presenting symptoms for an acute myocardial infarction are pleomorphic. Other common presenting symptoms include nausea, dyspnea, diaphoresis, arm pain, jaw pain, or even abdominal pain. The symptoms of the severe hypertension alone, i.e., headache, may predominate; thus, checking for evidence of cardiac ischemia is important in patients presenting with severe hypertension. Electrocardiogram and rapid cardiac enzyme screen should be performed in all patients presenting with severe hypertension.

Treatment

Patients presenting with myocardial infarction (MI) and systemic hypertension are at increased risk of death, left ventricular failure, and arrhythmias compared to normotensive patients with acute MI. Labetalol blocks both α and β adrenergic receptors and causes a decrease in systemic blood pressure, heart rate, and left ventricular end diastolic pressure (LVEDP), all of which decrease oxygen demand in myocardium [23]. Esmolol is another intravenous medication that can be used in patients with MI and hypertension. It is a cardioselective β-1 blocker with a very short plasma elimination half-life (9 min). It effectively lowers heart rate and blood pressure in patients with acute myocardial ischemia [24]. The advantage of esmolol is its short duration of action. If a patient develops hypotension with esmolol infusion, it reverses quickly after the drug is discontinued.

Nitroprusside should not be used in patients with MI since it increases mortality if administered early after myocardial infarction [25]. Nitroprusside can cause reduction of regional blood flow to coronary arteries known as coronary steal. Labetalol or esmolol infusion with nitroglycerin is preferred in acute coronary syndromes with severe hypertension.

Case 3: Acute Kidney Injury

A 25-year-old previously healthy Caucasian male was found to have a blood pressure of 230/120 and retinal hemorrhages at an ophthalmologist's office, where he sought care for blurred vision. On admission to the hospital his creatinine was 4.7 mg/dL. The patient had not received medical care for the prior 10 years and did not have a known history of kidney disease. Urine analysis showed 3+ protein, but no RBCs. Urine protein to creatinine ratio was 6.5 g/g. Renal ultrasound demonstrated slightly echogenic 10 cm kidneys bilaterally with no hydronephrosis. The patient was initially treated with intravenous nicardipine drip and subsequently switched to oral medications. His renal function did not improve and a renal biopsy was performed (Fig. 44.2).

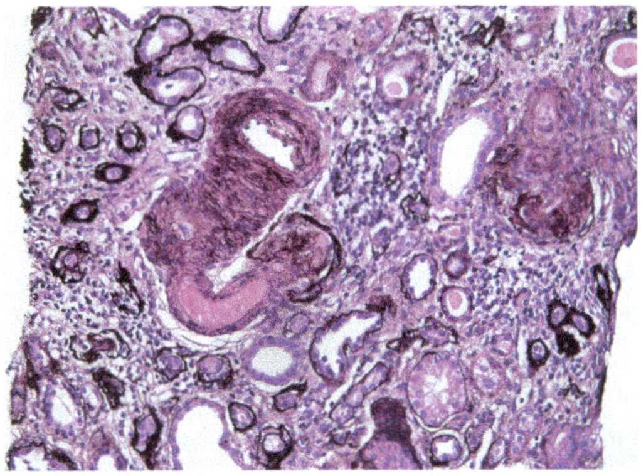

Fig. 44.2 Arterioles with medial thickening (onion-skinning), interlobular arteries with mucoid changes in the intima, and fibrinoid necrosis, consistent with malignant hypertension. Provided and interpreted by Dr Agnes B. Fogo, Vanderbilt University Medical Center, department of pathology

Presentation and Findings

Acute and chronic kidney diseases are common causes of hypertension. Conversely, severe hypertension can result in both acute kidney injury and chronic kidney disease. Because the symptoms and signs of kidney disease are frequently nonspecific, even patients with very advanced kidney disease may present without any specific complaints that would point toward a renal origin of hypertension. A family history of kidney disease; a history of illnesses associated with kidney involvement such as rheumatologic diseases like systemic lupus erythematosis, infectious diseases such as hepatitis C, or pulmonary hemorrhage; use of known nephrotoxins such as nonsteroidal anti-inflammatory drugs; a history of urinary tract obstruction; or sudden onset of peripheral edema can suggest the possibility of an underlying kidney disease as the cause of hypertension. Urinalysis, blood urea nitrogen, and serum creatinine measurement should be part of any assessment of a patient presenting with severe hypertension. The presence of heavy proteinuria and/or hematuria or the finding of small kidneys on renal ultrasound suggests kidney disease as a cause of severe hypertension. However, both proteinuria and hematuria can complicate hypertensive emergencies even in the absence of chronic kidney disease.

Treatment

Nicardipine and fenoldopam are the medications of choice in hypertensive emergencies with renal failure. Fenoldopam mesylate is a selective dopamine-1 (DA1) receptor agonist that acts as an arterial vasodilator and a diuretic. It has been approved by US Food and Drug Administration (FDA) for a short-term (up to 48 h) management of severe hypertension in inpatient setting. Fenoldopam is cleared primarily by the liver, and it can be safely used in patients with renal insufficiency. It increases renal blood flow and natriuresis in hypertensive patients [26]. When used at a dose of 0.04–0.8 mcg/kg/min it has no significant side effects, but at a dose higher than 0.8 mcg/kg/min it causes tachycardia, nausea, vomiting, and headache [27].

Nicardipine is usually started at a rate of 5 mg/h and can be increased to a maximum dose of 15 mg/h. It is as efficacious as intravenous nitroprusside in lowering blood pressure [28]. The disadvantage of nicardipine is a relatively long duration of action, so if patient develops side effects the latter may persist even after the infusion is discontinued. The main side effects seen with nicardipine infusion are tachycardia, headache, and flushing.

Nitroprusside should be avoided in renal failure due to increased risk of cyanide toxicity. Nitroprusside contains 44% cyanide. Cyanide is metabolized to thiocyanate in the liver and then excreted through the kidneys. Patients with hepatic or renal insufficiency can develop encephalopathy, seizures, and coma from accumulation of cyanide [29, 30].

Case Discussion

This patient presents something of a conundrum. The findings on ultrasound suggest that he has long-standing kidney disease with relatively small echogenic kidneys, so the hypertensive presentation may be simply a result of kidney failure. On the other hand, uncontrolled sudden worsening of his secondary hypertension may have produced acute kidney injury superimposed on chronic kidney disease. The findings on biopsy suggest the possibility of some reversibility of his kidney failure; however, the small size of his kidneys point toward significant chronic kidney damage that would not be reversible. The optimal approach would be to bring his blood pressure into the goal range for a proteinuric kidney disease, less than 135/75, and monitor kidney function. The heavy proteinuria suggests that an inhibitor of the renin–angiotensin–aldosterone system such as an angiotensin-converting enzyme inhibitor or an angiotensin receptor blocker may be considered. Because of the advanced nature of his kidney disease, however, such therapy would need to be initiated at low dose and his kidney function and serum potassium followed closely.

Preeclampsia and Eclampsia

Preeclampsia is defined as systolic BP $\geq$ 140 or diastolic BP $\geq$ 90 with proteinuria (>300 mg/24 h) after 20 weeks gestation. Eclampsia is diagnosed when in addition to hypertension and proteinuria pregnant woman develops seizures. The definite treatment for preeclampsia or eclampsia is delivery. Lowering blood pressure in preeclampsia decreases the risk of cerebrovascular accidents in the mother but can also decrease placental perfusion and cause lower birth weight [31, 32]. Antihypertensive medications should be initiated if systolic BP is $\geq$160 or diastolic BP is $\geq$110 to prevent stroke in pregnant women. The medication of choice in severe preeclampsia is intravenous labetalol. It is effective and safe in pregnant women [33]. Intravenous nicardipine or hydralazine can also be used.

Sympathetic Crises

Patients can develop severe hypertension with end-organ damage due to sympathetic overstimulation after suddenly stopping clonidine or β-blockers. Sympathetic crisis can also develop due to cocaine or amphetamine use.

After stopping clonidine abruptly patients develop hypertension that exceeds pretreatment blood pressure levels secondary to increased activity of sympathetic nervous system. Urinary norepinephrine and normetanephrine levels increase above baseline after clonidine discontinuation. Rebound hypertension can be more pronounced in a patient who is taking β blocker at the same time due to unopposed α blockade [34]. Treatment of hypertensive emergency caused by clonidine withdrawal is reinstitution of a drug. Combined β and α blocker like propranolol can also be used.

Withdrawal of a β blocker can cause severe hypertension and exacerbation of ischemic heart disease. Chronic β blocker use increases numbers of postsynaptic β receptors and creates hypersensitivity to catecholamines. β blocker should not be stopped abruptly, especially in a patient taking it for ischemic heart disease.

Cocaine use can cause hypertensive emergency with myocardial ischemia, aortic dissection, CVA, heart failure and renal insufficiency. Cocaine works by blocking reuptake of norepinephrine and dopamine in preganglionic sympathetic nerve endings and increasing release of epinephrine and norepinephrine in the adrenal glands. Hypertension and myocardial ischemia from cocaine use should be treated with intravenous benzodiazepines and nitroglycerin. Nitroprusside or calcium channel blockers are also effective and safe for the treatment of hypertension caused by cocaine [35]. The use of β blockers is controversial. Current AHA guidelines recommend avoiding β blocker use in the acute setting. The concern is unopposed α stimulated vasoconstriction and worsening hypertension and myocardial ischemia.

Case 4: Resistant Hypertension

A 68-years-old Caucasian female was referred to nephrology clinic by her primary care physician for the treatment of "resistant hypertension." She persistently had BP measurements between 160 s/90s to 180 s/100 s mmHg in her physician's office despite being on Amlodipine 5 mg daily, lisinopril 10 mg daily, and hydralazine 25 mg twice a day. After getting more detailed history and examining her, you find out that she prefers to eat in "fast food" restaurants, has BMI of 32, and takes Ibuprofen 600 mg orally almost every day for generalized body aches.

According to AHA definition, resistant hypertension is high blood pressure in spite of the use of three antihypertensive medications from different classes (one of them being diuretic) at optimal doses [36]. Uncontrolled hypertension due to suboptimal management or noncompliance is not considered resistant hypertension. Analysis of ALLHAT study revealed that the most important patient characteristics, associated with resistant *hypertension*, include older age, obesity, higher baseline blood pressure, left ventricular hypertrophy (LVH), and elevated baseline creatinine [37]. Before making diagnosis of resistant hypertension, one has to make sure that blood pressure is measured using correct size of a blood pressure cuff and that patient does not have "white coat" hypertension [38]. Also, patients should be screened for secondary causes of hypertension, including obstructive sleep apnea, primary aldosteronism, pheochromocytoma, Cushing's syndrome, renal artery stenosis, and CKD.

Treatment of resistant hypertension consists of lifestyle changes, discontinuation of any medications that can potentially increase blood pressure, and pharmacologic treatment.

Suggested approach to the treatment of a patient with suspected resistant hypertension:

- *Increase adherence to treatment* by asking patient to record his blood pressure measurements at home, simplify medication regimen, use timed medication reminders, and dietitian/nurse counseling [39].
- *Encourage lifestyle changes*, including weight loss, decreased sodium intake, and increased physical activity. Although not as dramatically as thought before, losing weight can decrease diastolic blood pressure by approximately 4.6 mmHg and systolic blood pressure by 6.0 mmHg [40].
- *Discontinue any medications that can potentially worsen hypertension*, including NSAIDs, Sympathomimetic agents (decongestants, dietary pills), stimulants (like methylphenidate), oral

contraceptives, some herbal supplements (like ephedra), cyclosporine, etc.

- *Pharmacological treatment*. Failure to control blood pressure is often due to lack of or suboptimal use of diuretic. Adding diuretic, increasing its dose or changing it to another class (patients with GFR less than 30 ml/min may not respond to thiazides) can improve blood pressure control. There are few randomized controlled studies comparing different medication combinations. Veterans Affairs Single Drug Therapy Cooperative Study demonstrated that adding thiazide diuretic (compared to other classes of antihypertensives) works better for blood pressure control in patients who previously were on one antihypertensive medication and still had diastolic blood pressures above 90 mmHg [41]. Other strategies that can be utilized in patients with resistant hypertension are switching from pure β-blocking agent to a combined α-β blocker or adding mineralocorticoid receptor antagonist [42].

Case Discussion

First of all, at this point we cannot say that patient really has resistant hypertension—her antihypertensive regimen does not include diuretic and all other medications that she is taking are not yet at optimal doses. You advise patient to discontinue her Ibuprofen, decrease sodium intake, and lose weight. Patient's calculated GFR is 68, so you add Chlorthalidone 25 mg orally daily during the same visit. Simplifying her medication regimen by discontinuing hydralazine and increasing the dose of Lisinopril to 20 mg daily is one strategy to improve compliance with her medical regimen. One week after being on the thiazide diuretic, blood pressure in your office is still 158/95. During the next couple of visits to your office you increase the dose of Amlodipine to 10 mg daily and Lisinopril to 40 mg daily. If she is still unable to achieve goal blood pressure on this regimen, you can say that patient really has resistant hypertension. An appropriate next step would be to add Spironolactone 25 mg po daily.

Conclusion

The majority of individuals with hypertension are not controlled; however, not every uncontrolled hypertensive patient is experiencing an acutely emergent condition. It is important for the clinician to recognize the differences between uncontrolled hypertension, hypertensive urgency, and hypertensive emergency (Table 44.1). The first two conditions can be managed most often in the outpatient setting with oral medications and close follow-up. In contrast, hypertensive emergencies mandate an aggressive approach. The first step in distinguishing these hypertensive conditions is recognizing the types of hypertensive emergencies, the patients at risk, and the evaluation required (Table 44.2). Patients presenting with uncontrolled hypertension should undergo a complete history, physical examination, specific laboratory, and radiologic evaluation. Based on these findings, the examining physician can make a determination of the urgency of the clinical condition and formulate a patient-specific management regimen (Tables 44.3 and 44.4).

References

1. Chobanian AV, Bakris GL, Black HR, Cushman WC. Seventh report of the Joint National Committee on prevention, detection, evaluation, and treatment of high blood pressure. Hypertension. 2003;42:1206–52.
2. Rodriguez MA, Kumar SK, De Caro M. Hypertensive crisis. Cardiol Rev. 2010;18(2):102–7.
3. Marik PE, Varon J. Hypertensive crises challenges and management. Chest. 2007;131:1949–62.
4. Calhoun DA, Jones D, Textor S, Goff DC, Murphy TP, Toto RD, White A, Cushman WC, White W, Sica D, Ferdinand K, Giles TD, Falkner B, Carey RM. Resistant hypertension: diagnosis, evaluation, and treatment. A scientific statement from the American Heart Association Professional Education Committee of the Council for High Blood Pressure Research. Hypertension. 2008;51:1403.
5. Hebert CJ, Vidt DG. Hypertensive crises. Prim Care Clin Office Pract. 2008;35:475–87.
6. William B, Owens MD. Blood pressure control in acute cerebrovascular disease. J Clin Hypertens. 2010: 1–7.
7. Ahmed N, Nasman P, Wahlgren NG. Effect of intravenous nimodipine on blood pressure and outcome after acute stroke. Stroke. 2000;31:1250–5.
8. Wahlgen NG, MacMahon DG, DeKayeser J. The Intravenous Nimodipine West European Trial

(INWEST) of nimodipine in the treatment of acute inschemic stroke. Cerebrovasc Dis. 1994;4:204–10.
9. Gilligan AK, Markus R, Read S, Srikanth V, Hirano T, Fitt G. Baseline blood pressure but not early computed tomography changes predicts major hemorrhage after streptokinase in acute ischemic stroke. Stroke. 2002;33:2236–42.
10. Herweh C, Juttler EJ, Schellinger PD, Klotz E, Jenetzky E. Evidence against a perihemorrhagic penumbra provided by perfusion computed tomography. Stroke. 2007;38:2941–7.
11. Fogelholm R, Avikainen S, Murros K. Prognostic value and determinants of first-day mean arterial pressure in spontaneous supratentorial intracerebral hemorrhage. Stroke. 1997;28:1396–400.
12. Becker KJ, Alexander B, Bybee HM, DI T, Abouelsaad T, Wendy A. Extravasation of radiographic contrast is an independent predictor of death in primary intracerebral hemorrhage. Stroke. 1999;30:2025–32.
13. Claassen J, Vu A, Kreiter KT, Kowalski RG, Du EY, Ostaokovich N. Effect of acute physiologic derangements on outcome after subaracnoid hemorrhage. Crit Care Med. 2004;32:832–8.
14. Karthikesalingam A, Holt PJE, Hinchliffe RJ, Thompson MM, Loftus IM. The diagnosis and management of aortic dissection. Vasc Endovascular Surg. 2010;44:165–9.
15. McMahon MA, Squirrell CA. Multidetector CT of aortic dissection: a pictorial review. Radiographics. 2010;30:445–60.
16. Tsai TT, Nienaber CA, Eagle KA. Acute aortic syndromes. Circulation. 2005;112:3802–13.
17. Hirst AE, Johns VJ, Kime SW. Dissecting aneurysm of the aorta: a review of 505 cases. Medicine. 1958;37:217–79.
18. Suzuki T, Mehta RH, Ince H, Nagai R, Sakomura Y, Weber F, Sumiyoshi T, Bossone E, Trimarchi S. Clinical profiles and outcomes of acute type b aortic dissection in the current era: lessons from the International Registry of Aortic Dissection (IRAD). Circulation. 2003;108:312–7.
19. Hoshino T, Ohmae M, Sakai A. Spontaneous resolution of a dissection of the descending aorta after medical treatment with a beta blocker and calcium antagonist. Br Heart J. 1987;58:82–4.
20. Bonow RO, Udelson JE. Left ventricular diastolic dysfunction as a cause of congestive heart failure. Ann Intern Med. 1992;117:502–10.
21. Khot UN, Novaro GM, Popovic ZB, Mills RM, Thomas JD, Tuzeu M, Manner D, Nissen SE, Francis GS. Nitroprusside in critically ill patients with left ventricular dysfunction and aortic stenosis. N Engl J Med. 2003;348:1756–63.
22. Gandhi SK, Powers JC, Nomeir AM, Fowle K, Kitzman DW, Rankin KM, Little WC. The pathogenesis of acute pulmonary edema associated with hypertension. N Engl Med. 2001;344:17–22.
23. Marx PG, Reid DS. Labetalol infusion in acute myocardial infarction with systemic hypertension. Br J Clin Pharmacol. 1979;8:223–38.
24. Kirshenbaum JM, Kioner RA, Antman EM, Braunwald E. Use of an ultrashort acting beta blocker in patients with acute myocardial ischemia. Circulation. 1985;72:873–80.
25. Cohn JN, Franciosa JA, Francis GS. Effect of short-term infusion of sodium nitroprusside on mortality rate in acute myocardial infarction complicated by left ventricular failure: results of a Veterans Administration cooperative study. N Engl J Med. 1982;306:1129–35.
26. Shusterman NH, Elliot WJ, White WB. Fenoldopam, but not nitroprusside, improves renal function in severely hypertensive patients with impaired renal function. Am J Med. 1993;95:161–8.
27. Murphy MB, Murray C, Shorten GD. Fenoldopan – a selective peripheral dopamine-receptor agonist for the treatment of severe hypertension. N Engl J Med. 2001;345:1548–57.
28. Neutel JM, Smith DH, Wallin D, Cook E, Ram CV, Fletcher E, Maher KE, Turlepaty P, Grandy S, Lee RS. A comparison of intravenous nicardipine and sodium nitroprusside in the immediate treatment of severe hypertension. Am J Hypertens. 1994;7:623–8.
29. Pasch T, Schulz V, Hoppenshauser G. Nitroprusside-induced formation of cyanide and its detoxification with thiosulphate during deliberate hypotension. J Cardiovasc Parmacol. 1983;5:77–85.
30. Hall VA, Guest JM. Sodium nitroprusside-induced cyanide intoxication and prevention with sodium thiosulphate prophylaxis. Am J Crit Care. 1992;2:19–27.
31. Martin JN, Thigpen BD, Moore RC, Rose CH, Cushman J, May W. Stroke and severe preeclampsia and eclampsia: a paradigm shift focusing on systolic blood pressure. Obstet Gynecol. 2005;105:246–54.
32. Dadelszen P, Magee LA. Fall in mean arterial pressure and fetal growth restriction in pregnancy hypertension: an updated metaregression analysis. J Obstet Gynaecol Can. 2002;24:941–5.
33. Duley L, Henderson-Smart DJ, Meher S. Drugs for treatment of very high blood pressure during pregnancy. Cochrane Database Sys Rev. 2006;3:CD001339.
34. Karachalios GN, Charalabopoulos A, Papalimneou V, Kiortsis D, Dimicco P, Kostoula OK, Charalabopoulos K. Withdrawal syndrome following cessation of antihypertensive drug therapy. Int J Clin Pract. 2005;59:562–70.
35. Maraj S, Figueredo VM, Morris L. Cocaine and the heart. Clin Cardiol. 2010;33:264–9.
36. Calhoun DA, Jones D, Textor S, Goff DC, Murphy TP, Toto RD, White A, Cushman C, White W, Sica D, Ferdinand K, Giles TD, Falkner B, Carey RM. Resistant hypertension: diagnosis, evaluation and treatment. A scientific statement from the American Heart Association professional education committee of the council for high blood pressure research. Hypertension. 2008;51:1403–19.
37. ALLHAT officers and coordinators for that ALLHAT Collaborative Research Group, The Antihypertensive and Lipid Lowering Treatment to Prevent Heart Attack Trial. Major outcomes in moderately hypercholesterolemic, hypertensive patients randomized to pravastatin

vs usual care: The Antihypertensive and Lipid-Lowering Treatment to Prevent Heart Attack Trial (ALLHAT-LLT). JAMA. 2002;288(23):2998–3007.

38. Dawe MG, Bartlett G, Juszczak E. Comparing the effects of white coat hypertension and sustained hypertension on mortality in UK primary care setting. Ann Fam Med. 2008;6(5):390–6.
39. Ogedegbe G, Schoenthaler A. A systematic review of the effects of home blood pressure monitoring on medication adherence. J Clin Hypertens. 2006;8:174–80.
40. Aucott L, Poobalan A, Smith WC, Avenell A, Jung R, Broom J. Effects of weight loss in overweight/obese individuals and long-term hypertension outcomes: a systematic review. Hypertension. 2005;45:1035–41.
41. Materson BJ, Reda DJ, Cushman WC, Henderson WG. Results of combination anti-hypertensive therapy after failure of each of the components. Department of Veterans Affairs Cooperative Study Group on Anti-hypertensive Agents. J Hum Hypertens. 1995;9(10):791–6.
42. Nishizaka MK, Zaman MA, Calhoun D. Efficacy of low-dose spironolactone in subjects with resistant hypertension. Am J Hypertens. 2003;16:925–30.

Part X

Kidney Disease Associated with Underlying Systemic Disease

45 Diabetic Kidney Disease

Raimund H. Pichler, Ian H. de Boer, Miguel F. Palma Diaz, and Maryam Afkarian

Case 1

A 35-year-old man with a 12 year history of type 1 diabetes presents with a new onset lower extremity edema and proteinuria. The patient had noted a 25 lb weight gain in a period of 8 weeks and had experienced headaches and blurry vision. He did carry a diagnosis of proliferative diabetic retinopathy in the past and also had had diabetic neuropathy on his feet. His only medication was insulin thought to be administered through an insulin pump. On exam his blood pressure was noted to be 154/100 mmHg. Physical exam was notable for pitting, bilateral lower extremity edema up to his thighs. A renal ultrasound revealed 13 cm measuring kidneys with slightly increased echogenicity. Laboratory testing showed a serum creatinine of 1.2 mg/dl, a serum albumin of 2.6 mg/dl, a total cholesterol of 592 mg/dl, a HbA1C of 18.3%, and 7 g of protein on a 24 h urine collection. The patient's urine sediment was notable for oval fat bodies and for 5–10 red blood cells per high power field, some of which had dysmorphic features. Does this patient have diabetic kidney disease (DKD)? What argues for DKD? Are there any red flags? Should this patient undergo a renal biopsy? How should this patient be managed? What is his prognosis?

Case 2

A 62-year-old gentleman presents to establish care at a diabetic care center. He has an 8-year history of type 2 diabetes mellitus and a 5-year history of hypertension and a history of hyperlipidemia. His medications include Glimepiride, Ramipril 5 mg, Aspirin, and Ranitidine. On exam his blood pressure is found to be 130/80 mmHg and except for some decreased sensitivity to a 1 g Monofilament on the soles of his feet has an unremarkable physical examination. An ophthalmologist does not note diabetic retinopathy. Laboratory testing reveals a serum creatinine of 2.7 mg/dl giving him an estimated GFR of 27 mL/min. Other laboratory testing is significant for a total cholesterol of 237 mg/dl, a hemoglobin of 10.7 mg/dl, a HbA1C of 6.8%, a parathyroid hormone of 236 pg/dl, a 25-hydroxyvitamin D concentration of 7 ng/mL, and a urinary albumin–creatinine ratio (ACR) of 4,800 mg/g. A urinalysis is

R.H. Pichler, M.D. (✉) • I.H. de Boer, M.D., M.S.
Division of Nephrology, Department of Medicine, University of Washington, 1159 NE Pacific Street, Box 356421, Seattle, WA 98195-6521, USA
e-mail: rpichler@u.washington.edu

M.F.P. Diaz, M.D.
Department of Pathology & Laboratory Medicine, David Geffen School of Medicine at UCLA, Los Angeles, CA 90095, USA

M. Afkarian, M.D., Ph.D.
Department of Medicine, Kidney Research Institute, Seattle, WA 98104, USA

E.V. Lerma and M. Rosner (eds.), *Clinical Decisions in Nephrology, Hypertension and Kidney Transplantation*,
DOI 10.1007/978-1-4614-4454-1_45, © Springer Science+Business Media New York 2013

unremarkable except for 2+protein. A renal ultrasound reveals 10 cm measuring kidneys with echogenic cortex. Does this patient have DKD? What additional workup should be done? How should the patient be treated and what is his prognosis?

Overview

Diabetes is the leading cause of chronic kidney disease (CKD) and end stage renal disease (ESRD) in developed countries and is rapidly becoming the leading cause of CKD in developing countries as a result of the global increase of type 2 diabetes mellitus [1]. The recent KDOQI clinical practice guidelines have defined DKD as the presumptive diagnosis of kidney disease caused by diabetes. The term *diabetic glomerulopathy* is reserved for biopsy proven kidney disease caused by diabetes [2].

Epidemiology

In 2003–2006, approximately 20 million people in the USA had diabetes mellitus, or 9.6% of all adults ages ≥ 20 years. This increase, from 7.4% of adults ages ≥ 20 years in 1988–1994, was driven by aging of the US population as well as the increasing prevalence of obesity, sedentary lifestyle, and unfavorable diet. 90–95% of diabetes cases are due to type 2 diabetes [3]. Over the course of their lifetime, approximately 40% of persons with diabetes develop DKD, as manifested by albuminuria and/or impaired glomerular filtration rate (GFR) [2, 4–7]. Most of these patients will not survive to develop ESRD (see Sect. "Prognosis and Complications" below). However, some survive and progress, and DKD now accounts for about 45,000 of new patients requiring renal replacement therapy in the USA every year. These patients account for approximately half of all incident ESRD cases in the USA [8]. Also in Canada, diabetes has risen to now comprise 51% of the incident dialysis population [9]. Medicare spending on the US ESRD program reached $26.8 billion in 2008.

Etiology/Pathophysiology

A number of different factors appear to be important for the development of DKD. Support for involvement of these pathways has come from animal models of DKD as well as evidence from clinical studies in humans. Chronic hyperglycemia is thought to be a central factor, contributing to development of DKD both directly (e.g., by stimulating overproduction of mesangial matrix proteins and promoting mesangial cell apoptosis) or indirectly (e.g., generation of advanced glycation end-products, AGE, by nonenzymatic glycation of proteins). AGE accumulation has been extensively linked with diabetic complications, for example by modification of glomerular basement membrane proteins [10]. Activation of renin–angiotensin–aldosterone axis is also implicated in pathogenesis of DKD [11] and is in fact supported by the beneficial effect of pathway inhibitors on progression of DKD. Dysregulated expression of cytokines and growth factors (e.g., TGF-β, VEGF, and EGF) [12], oxidative stress [13] and increased activation of Protein Kinase C and the polyol (or aldose reductase) pathway are among other pathophysiological mechanisms important in DKD.

Clinical Features

The two chief signs of DKD are increased urinary albumin excretion and reduced kidney function, as measured by estimated Glomerular Filtration Rate (eGFR) based on serum creatinine. Related clinical features include hypertension and other microvascular diabetes complications.

(a) *Urine albumin excretion*: Higher levels of urine albumin excretion are continuously correlated with worse kidney disease, but thresholds are commonly used to categorize severity of DKD (Table 45.1). Microalbuminuria, defined as an ACR of 30–300 mg/g, occurs in 20–30% of diabetics after ~5–15 years of disease [14–16]. Macroalbuminuria, defined as an ACR ≥300 mg/g, is usually seen after

Table 45.1 Classification of urine albumin excretion

	Albumin–creatinine ratio (ACR)	Albumin excretion rate (AER)
Normal	< 30 mg/g	< 30 mg/24 h
Microalbuminuria	30–299 mg/g	30/299 mg/24 h
Macroalbuminuria	≥300 mg/g	≥300 mg/24 h

~10 years of disease and gradually increases with time [15, 17].

(b) *Glomerular filtration rate (GFR)*: Impaired GFR is the second (and usually later) manifestation of DKD and represents a complementary measure of kidney damage. DKD is defined by a reduction in GFR and/or increase in urine albumin excretion in diabetic patients. While it was previously thought that DKD generally manifested with abnormal urine albumin excretion rate, it is now shown that in a subset of diabetics, it presents by a reduction in GFR in setting of normal urine albumin excretion [18–20].

(c) *Hypertension*: In type 1 diabetics, increase in urine albumin excretion is closely correlated with the onset of hypertension. The blood pressure begins to rise around the time microalbuminuria develops and continues to rise with worsening kidney function. In comparison, ~40% of type 2 diabetics are hypertensive at diagnosis of diabetes and in nearly half of these patients, hypertension predates microalbuminuria. Furthermore, among type 2 diabetics, hypertension is strongly associated with obesity.

(d) *Other microvascular complications (retinopathy, neuropathy)*: Most type 1 diabetics with DKD have diabetic retinopathy (DR) which usually precedes kidney disease (reverse is not the case, i.e., most DR patients do not have DKD). Association between DR and DKD is less certain in type 2 diabetes. There is a close association between DR and presence of Kimmelstiel–Wilson nodules on kidney biopsy. Type 2 diabetics with DR and proteinuria are most likely to have DKD, while ~30% of type 2 diabetics without DR may have kidney disease due to other etiology.

(e) *Pathology*: Pathologic anomalies may be observed long before onset of microalbuminuria and include mesangial expansion, glomerular basement membrane thickening, and glomerular sclerosis (compare the normal glomerulus depicted in Fig. 45.1 to the typical changes of diabetic glomerulopathy in Figs. 45.2 and 45.3). Renal Pathology Society has developed the following classification for glomerular lesions in type 1 and type 2 DKD [21]:

Class I—GBM thickening. No mesangial expansion, increased mesangial matrix or global glomerulosclerosis in >50% of glomeruli

Class II—Mild (IIa) or severe (IIb) mesangial expansion (see Fig. 45.2)

Class III—≥1 Kimmelstiel–Wilson lesion (nodular intercapillary glomerulosclerosis), but less than 50% glomerulosclerosis (see Fig. 45.3)

Class IV—advanced sclerosis. >50% glomerulosclerosis attributable to DKD.

Similar classification schemes have been developed for the interstitial and vascular components of DKD as well [21].

Diagnosis

Urine Albumin Excretion

Urine albumin excretion should be measured annually in all diabetic patients, starting at diagnosis for type 2 diabetes and 5 years after diabetes onset in type 1 diabetes. Urine albumin excretion should be measured using an ACR in a random urine sample. ACR indexes urine albumin to urine creatinine concentration, which corrects for changes in urine dilution. ACR is also preferable to albumin excretion rate as the latter requires a timed urine collection, which is cumbersome and error-prone. ACR can be transiently increased in the setting of fever, exercise, poor glycemic control, uncontrolled hypertension, decompensated congestive heart failure, and high dietary protein intake, and in the presence of urinary tract infections. Therefore, an abnormal urine albumin excretion should be confirmed by two to three repeat ACRs over the subsequent 3–6 months.

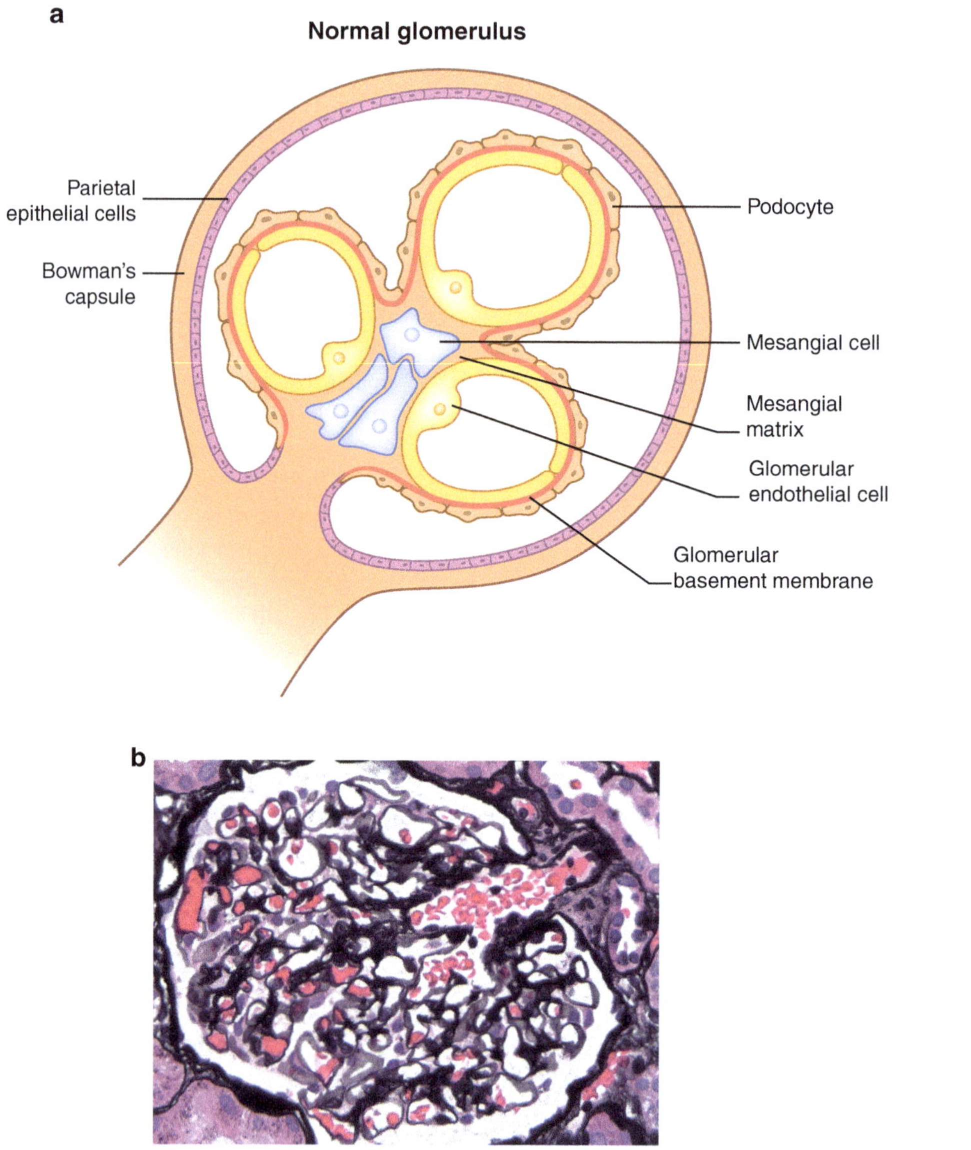

Fig. 45.1 Normal glomerulus. (**a**) Schematic view of a normal glomerulus depicting the cells of the glomerular tuft (mesangial cells, endothelial cells, and podocytes), capillary loops with basement membrane in red and Bowman's capsule lined by visceral epithelial cells. (**b**) Light photomicrograph of a normal glomerulus with the vascular pole, widely patent capillary loops demonstrating normal thickness of glomerular basement membrane and with normal mesangial cell size and matrix (JMS stain)

Urine dipstick is not an appropriate test because it only detects urine albumin excretion exceeding 300–500 mg/L and furthermore is sensitive to urine volume and dilution.

Limitations of Urine Albumin Excretion

- The ideal time for measuring ACR is not certain. As such and in light of clinical convenience,

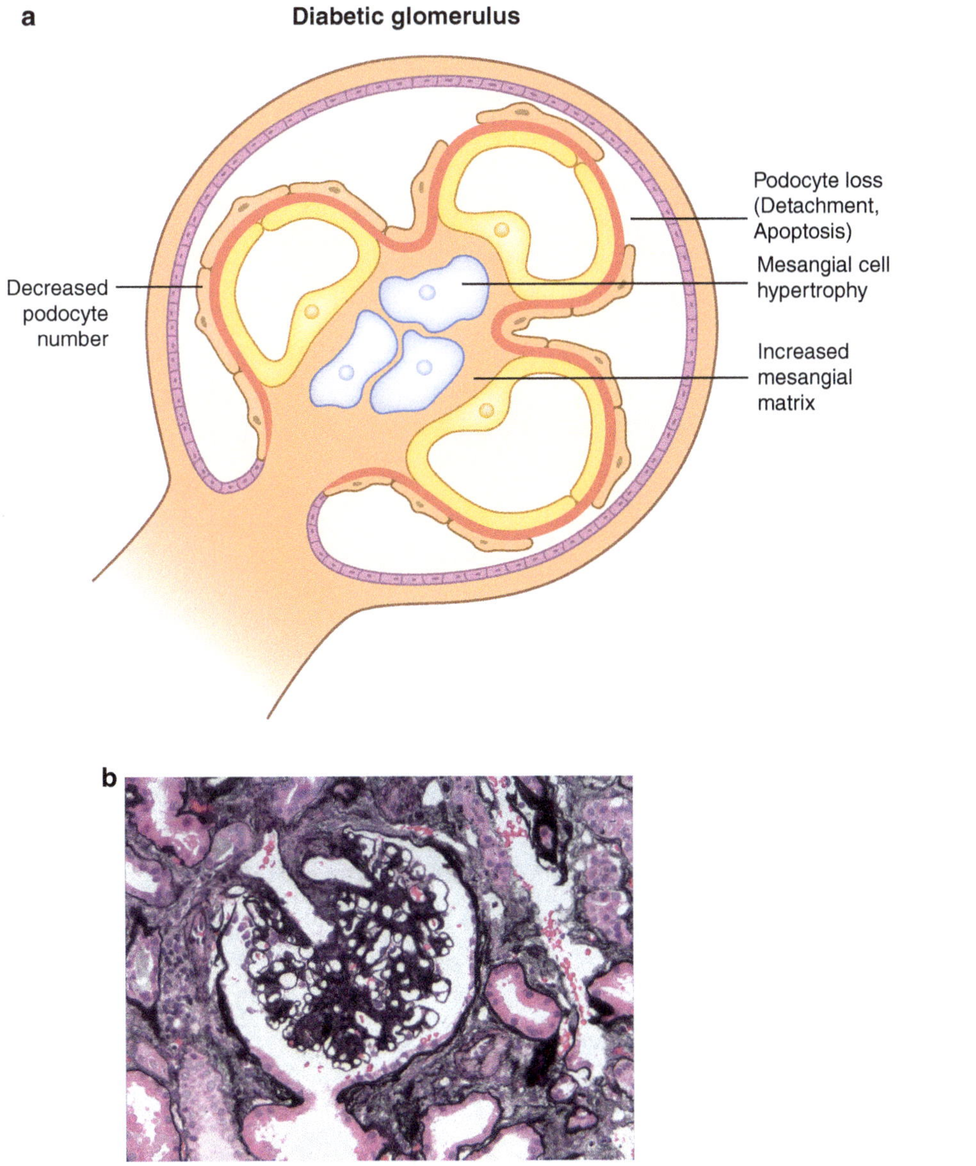

Fig. 45.2 Diabetic glomerulopathy. (**a**) Schematic view of a diabetic glomerulus depicting changes of diabetic glomerulopathy including thickening of the glomerular basement membrane, increase in mesangial matrix, and loss of podocytes. (**b**) Light photomicrograph of a glomerulus with diabetic glomerulopathy demonstrating an increase in mesangial matrix and thickened glomerular basement membranes (JMS stain)

ACR measurement is recommended in random voided urine samples.

- Accurate conversion of ACR to absolute daily albumin excretion depends on the assumption that 1 g of creatinine is excreted in the urine daily. Extreme departures from the 1 g daily creatinine excretion tends to over- or underestimate daily albumin excretion in individuals with much lower or higher daily creatinine excretion, respectively. For example, for a heavily muscled young man excreting 2–3 g creatinine per day, the urine ACR (in mg/g)

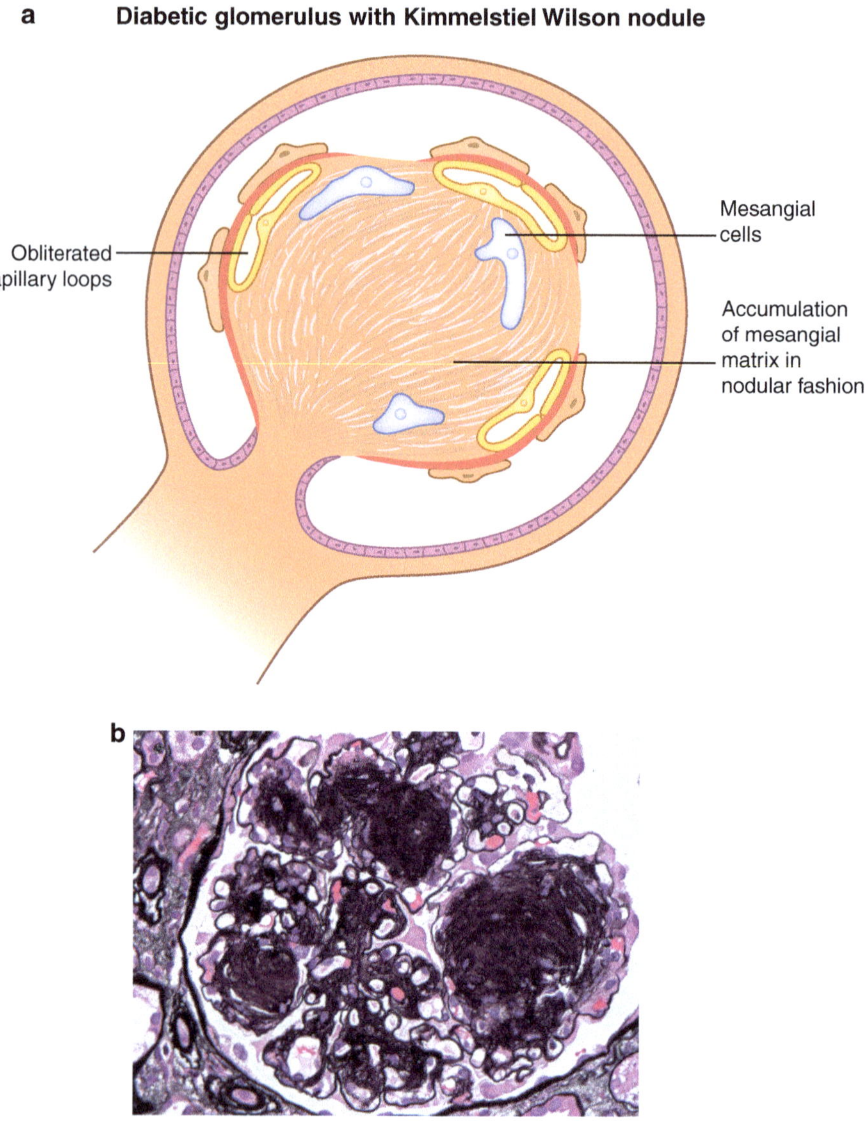

Fig. 45.3 Advanced diabetic glomerulopathy. (**a**) Schematic view of a glomerulus with advanced diabetic glomerulopathy with severe expansion of the mesangial matrix and obliteration of capillary loops. (**b**) Light photomicrograph of a diabetic glomerulus demonstrating the severe accumulation of mesangial matrix in a nodular fashion (Kimmelstiel–Wilson nodules) and obliteration of capillary loops. Note the mesangial layering in some of the nodules (JMS stain)

will be two to three times lower than the daily urine albumin excretion (in g/d).

- There are racial/ethnic- and gender-based differences in albumin and creatinine excretion. Daily creatinine excretion in higher in men compared to women and in African Americans and Mexicans compared to non-Hispanic whites. However, these differences are less important in clinical practice where relative change in individual patients over time affects management more than small differences in absolute albumin excretion at a given time.

Glomerular Filtration Rate

Serum creatinine should be measured yearly starting at diagnosis for type 2 diabetes and 5 years after diabetes onset for type 1 diabetes, with changes to medications known to affect or be affected by kidney disease, and with acute illness. Serum creatinine should be used to estimate GFR using a validated estimating equation (currently MDRD). Estimated GFR<60 mL/min/1.73 m^2 is abnormal and is used to grade severity of DKD [2].

(a) The MDRD-estimated GFR is imprecise and less useful in the "normal" range (≥60 mL/min/1.73 m2).

(b) Approaches using serum cystatin C have been suggested as a more precise alternative to estimating GFR in the "normal" range, but at this time the role of cystatin C in clinical care is poorly defined and cystatin C is not routinely available in clinical laboratories.

Urinalysis

Urinalysis is an informative, noninvasive, and inexpensive test and should be performed in all patients with kidney disease. Relevant information gleaned from urinalysis includes presence of hematuria (red urinary pellet, RBC in microscopy), urinary tract infections (WBC, bacteria, leukocyte esterase, etc.), crystals and an active urine sediment (cellular casts, dysmorphic red blood cells). The urinary sediment in patients with DKD tends to be bland, though microscopic hematuria can be present. This can potentially include dysmorphic red blood cells and reflects glomerular damage.

Kidney Imaging

Renal ultrasound is advisable if rise in serum creatinine is suspected to be due to urinary tract obstruction. It is also helpful for evaluation of baseline kidney size and disease chronicity. For example, kidneys are frequently enlarged early in the course of DKD, as manifest by normal or high GFR with or without albuminuria, probably reflecting hyperfiltration. Small echogenic kidneys with high resistive indices suggest chronic irreversible disease. Ultrasound with Doppler is used to evaluate renal vascular flow, for example if deterioration of renal function is suspected to be due to renal arterial stenosis (e.g., rapid rise in serum creatinine with RAAS blockade).

Retinopathy Evaluation

In type 1 diabetics, prevalence of other microvascular diabetic complications such as retinopathy and neuropathy correlates with the degree of albuminuria. For example, proliferative retinopathy was reported in 12%, 28%, and 58% of patients with normo-, micro-, and macroalbuminuria, respectively [22]. Presence of DR also corroborates the diabetic etiology of kidney disease. Therefore, concomitant retinopathy evaluation is prudent in both type 1 and type 2 diabetic patients.

Referral to Nephrologist

Per K/DOQI guidelines, patients with GFR below 30 mL/min should be referred to a nephrologist for education and planning for renal replacement therapy and close management of CKD complications [23]. In addition, patients should be referred to a nephrologist if their clinical course is not consistent with DKD or if they display signs of other causes of kidney disease.

Kidney Biopsy

Kidney biopsy is not commonly performed in diabetic patients with kidney disease unless their clinical course is not consistent with DKD (e.g., acute loss of kidney function or rise in proteinuria) or if they display signs of other causes of kidney disease (e.g., hematuria, an active urinary sediment). Some of the relative contraindications for kidney biopsy are small hyperechoic kidneys (<9 cm) which suggest chronic irreversible disease (and likely fibrosed and pathologically uninformative tissue), solitary native kidney, severe hypertension, and uncorrectable bleeding diatheses.

Differential Diagnosis

Other Kidney Diseases in Differential

(a) *Differential diagnoses of proteinuric kidney disease* in diabetic patients includes other proteinuric glomerular diseases, such as Focal Segmental Glomerulosclerosis, IgA nephropathy, Membranous glomerulonephritis Minimal change disease, Amyloid kidney disease, lupus nephritis, HIV nephropathy, HCV/HBV-associated kidney disease, etc.

(b) *Differential diagnosis for non-proteinuric kidney disease* falls along pre-renal, renal, and post-renal categories, as detailed in the section on diagnosis of acute kidney injury. However, a few conditions that are frequently responsible for acute increases in serum creatinine in diabetic patients include volume depletion (e.g., due to diuretics) particularly in the setting of RAAS blockade, urinary obstruction, and medications (e.g., Bactrim, over-the-counter NSAIDs).

Red Flags Suggesting Non-DKD Etiologies for Kidney Disease in Diabetic Patients

- Albuminuria <5 year after the onset of type 1 diabetes
- Nephrotic-range proteinuria (ACR>3 g/g or AER >3 g/24 h)
- Acute drop in GFR or rise in ACR
- Refractory hypertension
- Hematuria (or active urine sediment, e.g., dysmorphic RBCs and cellular casts)
- Absence of diabetic retinopathy in type 1 diabetics (DKD is seen in absence of diabetic retinopathy in as many as half of type 2 diabetic patients in small series)
- >30% GFR drop in 2–3 months after RAAS blockade
- Signs/symptoms of other systemic disease

Management

Glucose Control

The DCCT trial and the UKPDS study have shown that glucose control plays an important role in the development of DKD in both type 1 and type 2 diabetes. Therefore, tight glucose control is very important in the management of patients with kidney disease. The American Diabetes Association currently recommends a HbA1C target of <7%. While targeting HbA1c <6% reduced the risk of albuminuria development and progression, it may also increase the risk of mortality. Tight glucose control to this degree is not currently recommended.

Some authors have suggested that not only average glucose levels (reflected in HbA1C) but also glucose variability may be an important treatment target, but outcomes trials investigating this are currently lacking. A human biopsy study involving type 1 diabetics with classical changes of diabetic glomerulopathy who underwent pancreas transplantation has demonstrated resolution of the glomerular changes with successful pancreas transplantation (resulting in very tight glucose control with minimal variability) over a 10 year period [24].

With regards to the usefulness and accuracy of using HbA1C in patients with reduced GFR it has been shown that CKD, ESRD and treatment with Erythropoiesis stimulating agents (ESAs) are associated with decreased red blood cell survival or an increase in red blood cell production/turnover, thereby causing artificially low HbA1C levels in some of these patients. Other reports have shown an increase of HbA1C in CKD through possibly carbamylation of hemoglobin or acidosis. As a result HbA1C levels may not be as accurate in assessing glycemic control in patients with CKD or ESRD.

With advanced GFR loss, typically<20 mL/min/1.73 m^2 or ESRD, insulin catabolism is diminished and gluconeogenic capacity by the kidney is impaired. Therefore, glucose-lowering therapy often requires reduction to avoid hypoglycemia.

Blood Pressure Control and Blockade of the Renin–Angiotensin System

Blood pressure is another crucial part of the management of these patients. The JNCVII and ADA guidelines recommend a *blood pressure goal* for patients with diabetes of <130/80 mmHg. Angiotensin converting enzyme inhibitors (*ACE-I*) and Angiotensin Receptor Blockers (*ARBs*) are the *first choice* of antihypertensive treatment in any hypertensive diabetic patient. Several studies have demonstrated prevention of microalbuminuria [25], progression from micro- to macroalbuminuria [26] and also progression to ESRD [27, 28] with use of ACE-I or ARBs. Nevertheless, in normotensive, normoalbuminuric type 1 diabetics neither ACE-I or ARBs have been shown to provide renoprotection [29].

The *majority of* our *hypertensive diabetics require more than one agent* to get to a blood pressure goal of <130/80 mmHg. ACE-I and ARBs are most effective in terms of blood pressure reduction when combined with either a diuretic or a calcium channel blocker.

Diuretics and RAAS inhibitors are synergistic in terms of effect on BP, i.e., the combined effect of agents from these classes on BP is equal to or greater than the sum of individual effects of each medication. Patients with diabetes and normal or near-normal GFR usually respond to thiazide-type diuretics. In the diabetic subgroup of ALLHAT, chlorthalidone reduced the primary endpoint of fatal coronary heart disease and myocardial infarction to the same degree as lisinopril or amlodipine and was superior for prevention of heart failure [30].

Dihydropyridine calcium channel blockers (CCBs). Dihydropyridine CCBs (e.g., amlodipine, felodipine) as a sole agent have been shown to increase proteinuria in the IDNT study [26], but are thought to be safe if used in combination with an ACE-Inhibitor or ARB. In fact, the ACCOMPLISH study has demonstrated superiority with regards to progression of CKD of the combination of an ACE-Inhibitor with a dihydropyridine CCB as compared to the ACE-Inhibitor combined with hydrochlorothiazide [31].

Non-dihydropyridine CCBs (e.g., diltiazem, verapamil) reduce proteinuria in short-term studies but have not been demonstrated to prevent the development or progression of DKD or cardiovascular disease. In the BENEDICT study, Verapamil did not show a protective effect in terms of preventing the development of microalbuminuria [25]. Non-dihydropyridine CCBs tend to have less potent effects on BP than dihydropyridine CCBs.

Beta blockers have proven benefit for comorbidities that often accompany diabetes, including coronary artery disease, stroke, and congestive heart failure, and are often indicated for these conditions. In the absence of these conditions, the utility of beta blockers for BP control in diabetes is not clear. Beta blockers and RAAS inhibitors are not synergistic in terms of effect on BP, i.e., the combined effect of agents from these classes on BP is often less than the sum of individual effects of each medication. Beta blockers also have been shown to be problematic in diabetic patients as they can mask signs of hypoglycemia.

Some providers elect to combine two agents that block the renin–angiotensin system (*Dual RAAS Blockade*) in patients with >1 g of proteinuria on a fully dosed ACE-I or ARB to utilize the additive antiproteinuric effect in patients with severe proteinuria. While a number of short-term studies have demonstrated additional albuminuria/proteinuria reduction as a surrogate endpoint when combining multiple agents that block the Renin–Angiotensin system, none of such studies have shown an improvement of hard endpoints, such as doubling of serum creatinine or dialysis. In fact, a recent post-hoc analysis of the ON TARGET trial in patients with macroalbuminuria and an eGFR<60 mls/min/1.73 m^2 (about 80% of which were diabetics) showed an increased risk to develop renal failure or to require dialysis even in this patient population [32]. As a result, dual RAAS blockade should not be routinely applied for patients at low risk of progressive renal disease (urine albumin excretion<300 mg/day or normal eGFR). Clinical trials are currently evaluating whether dual RAAS blockade improves outcomes for patients at high risk of progressive renal disease (urine albumin excretion>300 mg/day and impaired eGFR) [33, 34]. Until results of these trials are available, dual RAAS blockade should be avoided or used with caution on an individual bases for such patients [35].

Lipid Control

Hyperlipidemia is common in diabetic patients with renal disease. Treatment with a statin reduces cardiovascular disease risk and may reduce albuminuria [36, 37] and risk of GFR loss in CKD. Therapy with a statin should be considered if the LDL cholesterol is>100 mg/dl with an LDL treatment goal of <100 mg/dl. An LDL treatment goal of <70 mg/dl is optional.

Dietary Considerations

For diabetics with CKD, a moderate protein restriction of 0.8 g/kg body weight per day has been shown to reduce the risk of progression of albuminuria/proteinuria and loss of GFR [2]. For other dietary interventions in patients with CKD, please see Chap. 27 on nutrition.

Lifestyle Changes

Smoking has been demonstrated to contribute to the rapidity of GFR loss in diabetic patients with kidney disease. Therefore, smoking cessation should be strongly considered for any diabetic patient. Regular exercise can lead to weight loss, reduction in creatinine, and albuminuria and should be encouraged. Normalization of the BMI (18.5–24.9) should be a treatment goal [2].

Utilization of Team Care

Care of the diabetic patient can be complex and challenging and may require the involvement of a whole team of healthcare providers. Team composition will vary according to patient needs, patient load, clinical setting, and professional skills. In general team care requires at least a "core" team, which involves a physician, nurse, and dietician, at least one of whom is a certified diabetes educator. Many other healthcare professionals can and need to be team members or collaborative consultants if needed. The team can minimize the patient's health risk by assessment, intervention and surveillance to prevent and identify problems early and start treatment.

Prognosis and Complications

In longitudinal cohorts of type 1 diabetes, long-term survival has been shown to be dependent on presence and proportional to severity of DKD [38, 39]. Type 1 diabetic subjects had several-fold higher mortality than age- and sex-matched general population. However, this excess mortality was confined to the individuals with DKD. The remarkable impact of DKD on survival may be in part due to the synergistic negative influences of diabetes and kidney disease on other major risk factors such as cardiovascular disease (CVD). Diabetes is one of the most important risk factors for cardiovascular disease (CVD), posing equivalent cardiovascular risk to history of a prior MI [40]. CKD also imparts an extremely high risk of cardiovascular disease. For those affected by both diabetes and CKD the outlook is far worse than for those affected by either condition alone. The relationship between CKD severity and cardiovascular risk is continuous. People with diabetes and microalbuminuria have twice the CVD risk of those with normoalbuminuria [41] and as albuminuria increases and GFR decreases, CVD risk increases progressively [42]. More people who reach CKD stage 3 will die, primarily of CVD, than progress to kidney failure, especially if they also have diabetes [2].

Preventive Measures/Prophylaxis

Tight glucose control administered early in the course of either type 1 or type 2 diabetes has been proven to prevent the development of

DKD, specifically of microalbuminuria and macroalbuminuria [43–45]. As a result, tight glycemic control is a cornerstone of clinical guidelines for the care of persons with diabetes [2, 4]. Risk factors for DKD other than hyperglycemia have been well described and include older age, male gender, long duration of diabetes, smoking, obesity, elevated blood pressure, and genetic predisposition [15, 46–51]. While RAAS inhibitors reduce the risks of progressive GFR loss and death among persons with established DKD, they do not prevent the histologic changes of diabetic glomerulopathy in type 1 diabetes [29]. In uncomplicated type 2 diabetes, RAAS inhibitors prevent or suppress albuminuria, but their long-term impact on prevention of clinical DKD outcomes remains unproven [25, 52]. Once DKD is diagnosed, clinical care should focus on preventing progression of kidney disease and, more importantly, on prevention of cardiovascular disease, as discussed above.

Case Discussion

The patient in *Case 1* had a number of features that pointed towards DKD (presence of retinopathy, poorly controlled diabetes, presence of neuropathy) but also had some red flags (seemingly rapid onset of severe nephrotic range proteinuria, hematuria with active appearing urine sediment). While we felt that DKD was most likely, we also felt it was prudent not to miss an additional, possibly superimposed glomerular disease process and the patient did undergo an ultrasound guided renal biopsy. The renal biopsy did indeed reveal classic diabetic glomerulopathy with multiple Kimmelstiel–Wilson nodules, thickened glomerular basement membranes, and mesangial matrix expansion (see Fig. 45.3). With regards to the management of this patient glucose control and blood pressure control were the two most pressing issues. It turned out that the patient's insulin pump had not been working properly and he was provided with a new one. The patient was also started on an ACE-Inhibitor and a loop diuretic. His ACE-Inhibitor was titrated to maximal dose and with furosemide his edema resolved. The patient did in addition require a dihydropyridine calcium channel blocker to get to a goal blood pressure of < 130/80 mmHg. A statin was started for his significant hyperlipidemia. With the above measures his proteinuria decreased to 750 mg/24 h in a 6 month period and his creatinine remained stable.

The patient in *Case 2* was a surgeon and was somewhat concerning for some potential red flags given the seemingly short duration of diabetes mellitus that also appeared to be relatively well controlled. Nevertheless, this patient had relocated from a different state and previous records were not available. Given also the presence of anemia and some neuropathy, serum and urine electrophoresis were performed and unrevealing. A recent biopsy series in patients with type 2 diabetes mellitus showed a relatively high incidence of nondiabetic renal disease (NDRD) of 38.5% [53]. Clinical characteristics suggestive of NDRD were short duration of diabetes and absence of retinopathy [53]. This patient also underwent ultrasound guided renal biopsy, which again showed Diabetic Glomerulopathy. Upon further questioning the patient did finally endorse "elevated blood sugars" dating back 18 years prior to presentation and prolonged periods without medical attention preceding his formal diagnosis of diabetes mellitus. The patient was managed by increasing his ACE-Inhibitor to maximal dose, treatment of his vitamin D deficiency and the addition of a statin, a protein restriction of 0.8 g/kg/day, and weight loss. With the above measures the patient's proteinuria improved to 500 mg/day within 6 months although his GFR decreased to about 22 mL/min in the same period.

Key Points

1. *Clinical features*. The two cardinal features of DKD are increased urinary albumin excretion and reduced kidney function. Other clinical features of DKD include hypertension, presence of other diabetic microvascular complications (e.g., retinopathy)
2. *Diagnosis*. Diagnosis of DKD relies on assessment of urine albumin excretion and kidney

function. Urine albumin excretion is best evaluated by measurement of the ratio of urine albumin to creatinine in a random urine sample (ACR). Renal function is assessed by calculation of estimated GFR from serum creatinine and a validated estimating equation (e.g., MDRD formula). Urine albumin excretion should be measured annually in all diabetic patients, starting at diagnosis for type 2 diabetics and 5 years after diabetes onset in type 1 diabetics. Serum creatinine should be measured yearly starting at diagnosis for type 2 diabetes and 5 years after diabetes onset for type 1 diabetes, with changes to medications known to affect or be affected by kidney disease, and with acute illness. DKD patients should be referred to a nephrologist if their clinical course is not consistent with DKD or when their GFR drops below 30 mL/min.

3. *Differential diagnosis*. Red flags for non-DKD causes for kidney disease should elicit a comprehensive search for other causes of kidney disease. Some of these red flags include early (sooner than 5 years after type 1 diabetes onset) albuminuria, nephrotic-range proteinuria (ACR > 3 g/g or AER > 3 g/24 h), acute drop in GFR or rise in ACR, hematuria (or active urine sediment, e.g., dysmorphic RBCs and cellular casts), absence of diabetic retinopathy in type 1 diabetics, a greater than 30% GFR drop in 2–3 months after RAAS blockade, or signs/symptoms of other systemic disease.

References

1. Zimmet P, Alberti KG, Shaw J. Global and societal implications of the diabetes epidemic. Nature. 2001;414(6865):782–7.
2. KDOQI. KDOQI clinical practice guidelines and clinical practice recommendations for diabetes and chronic kidney disease. Am J Kidney Dis. 2007;49(2 Suppl 2):S12–154.
3. Cowie CC, Rust KF, Byrd-Holt DD, Gregg EW, Ford ES, Geiss LS, et al. Prevalence of diabetes and high risk for diabetes using A1C criteria in the U.S. population in 1988–2006. Diabetes Care. 2010;33(3): 562–8.
4. Standards of medical care in diabetes–2010. Diabetes Care. 2010;33 Suppl 1: S11–61.
5. Garg AX, Kiberd BA, Clark WF, Haynes RB, Clase CM. Albuminuria and renal insufficiency prevalence guides population screening: results from the NHANES III. Kidney Int. 2002;61(6):2165–75.
6. Nathan DM, Zinman B, Cleary PA, Backlund JY, Genuth S, Miller R, et al. Modern-day clinical course of type 1 diabetes mellitus after 30 years' duration: the diabetes control and complications trial/epidemiology of diabetes interventions and complications and Pittsburgh epidemiology of diabetes complications experience (1983–2005). Arch Intern Med. 2009;169(14):1307–16.
7. de Boer IH, Rue TC, Cleary PA, Lachin JM, Molitch ME, Steffes MW, et al. Long-term renal outcomes of patients with type 1 diabetes mellitus and microalbuminuria: an analysis of the diabetes control and complications trial/epidemiology of diabetes interventions and complications cohort. Arch Intern Med. 2011;171(5):412–20.
8. Williams ME. Diabetic CKD/ESRD 2010: a progress report? Semin Dial. 2010;23(2):129–33.
9. Lok CE, Oliver MJ, Rothwell DM, Hux JE. The growing volume of diabetes-related dialysis: a population based study. Nephrol Dial Transplant. 2004;19(12): 3098–103.
10. Bohlender JM, Franke S, Stein G, Wolf G. Advanced glycation end products and the kidney. Am J Physiol Renal Physiol. 2005;289(4):F645–59.
11. Hollenberg NK. Diabetes, nephropathy, and the renin system. J Hypertens Suppl. 2006;24(1):S81–7.
12. Navarro-Gonzalez JF, Mora-Fernandez C. The role of inflammatory cytokines in diabetic nephropathy. J Am Soc Nephrol. 2008;19(3):433–42.
13. Brownlee M. Biochemistry and molecular cell biology of diabetic complications. Nature. 2001;414(6865): 813–20.
14. Orchard TJ, Dorman JS, Maser RE, Becker DJ, Drash AL, Ellis D, et al. Prevalence of complications in IDDM by sex and duration. Pittsburgh Epidemiology of Diabetes Complications Study II. Diabetes. 1990;39(9):1116–24.
15. Hovind P, Tarnow L, Rossing P, Jensen BR, Graae M, Torp I, et al. Predictors for the development of microalbuminuria and macroalbuminuria in patients with type 1 diabetes: inception cohort study. BMJ. 2004;328(7448):1105.
16. Warram JH, Gearin G, Laffel L, Krolewski AS. Effect of duration of type I diabetes on the prevalence of stages of diabetic nephropathy defined by urinary albumin/creatinine ratio. J Am Soc Nephrol. 1996;7(6):930–7.
17. Krolewski AS, Warram JH, Christlieb AR, Busick EJ, Kahn CR. The changing natural history of nephropathy in type I diabetes. Am J Med. 1985;78(5): 785–94.
18. Fioretto P, Mauer M, Brocco E, Velussi M, Frigato F, Muollo B, et al. Patterns of renal injury in NIDDM patients with microalbuminuria. Diabetologia. 1996;39(12):1569–76.

19. Lane PH, Steffes MW, Mauer SM. Glomerular structure in IDDM women with low glomerular filtration rate and normal urinary albumin excretion. Diabetes. 1992;41(5):581–6.
20. Perkins BA, Ficociello LH, Ostrander BE, Silva KH, Weinberg J, Warram JH, et al. Microalbuminuria and the risk for early progressive renal function decline in type 1 diabetes. J Am Soc Nephrol. 2007;18(4):1353–61.
21. Tervaert TW, Mooyaart AL, Amann K, Cohen AH, Cook HT, Drachenberg CB, et al. Pathologic classification of diabetic nephropathy. J Am Soc Nephrol. 2010;21(4):556–63.
22. Parving HH, Hommel E, Mathiesen E, Skott P, Edsberg B, Bahnsen M, et al. Prevalence of microalbuminuria, arterial hypertension, retinopathy and neuropathy in patients with insulin dependent diabetes. Br Med J (Clin Res Ed). 1988;296(6616):156–60.
23. K/DOQI clinical practice guidelines for chronic kidney disease: evaluation, classification, and stratification. Am J Kidney Dis. 2002;39(2 Suppl 1):S1–266.
24. Fioretto P, Steffes MW, Sutherland DE, Goetz FC, Mauer M. Reversal of lesions of diabetic nephropathy after pancreas transplantation. N Engl J Med. 1998;339(2):69–75.
25. Ruggenenti P, Fassi A, Ilieva AP, Bruno S, Iliev IP, Brusegan V, et al. Preventing microalbuminuria in type 2 diabetes. N Engl J Med. 2004;351(19):1941–51.
26. Parving HH, Lehnert H, Brochner-Mortensen J, Gomis R, Andersen S, Arner P. The effect of irbesartan on the development of diabetic nephropathy in patients with type 2 diabetes. N Engl J Med. 2001;345(12):870–8.
27. Lewis EJ, Hunsicker LG, Clarke WR, Berl T, Pohl MA, Lewis JB, et al. Renoprotective effect of the angiotensin-receptor antagonist irbesartan in patients with nephropathy due to type 2 diabetes. N Engl J Med. 2001;345(12):851–60.
28. Brenner BM, Cooper ME, de Zeeuw D, Keane WF, Mitch WE, Parving HH, et al. Effects of losartan on renal and cardiovascular outcomes in patients with type 2 diabetes and nephropathy. N Engl J Med. 2001;345(12):861–9.
29. Mauer M, Zinman B, Gardiner R, Suissa S, Sinaiko A, Strand T, et al. Renal and retinal effects of enalapril and losartan in type 1 diabetes. N Engl J Med. 2009;361(1):40–51.
30. Lasagna L. Diuretics vs alpha-blockers for treatment of hypertension: lessons from ALLHAT. Antihypertensive and Lipid-Lowering Treatment to Prevent Heart Attack Trial. JAMA. 2000;283(15):2013–4.
31. Bakris GL, Sarafidis PA, Weir MR, Dahlof B, Pitt B, Jamerson K, et al. Renal outcomes with different fixed-dose combination therapies in patients with hypertension at high risk for cardiovascular events (ACCOMPLISH): a prespecified secondary analysis of a randomised controlled trial. Lancet. 2010;375(9721):1173–81.
32. Tobe SW, Clase CM, Gao P, McQueen M, Grosshennig A, Wang X, et al. Cardiovascular and renal outcomes with telmisartan, ramipril, or both in people at high renal risk: results from the ONTARGET and TRANSCEND studies. Circulation. 2011;123(10):1098–107.
33. Fried LF, Duckworth W, Zhang JH, O'Connor T, Brophy M, Emanuele N, et al. Design of combination angiotensin receptor blocker and angiotensin-converting enzyme inhibitor for treatment of diabetic nephropathy (VA NEPHRON-D). Clin J Am Soc Nephrol. 2009;4(2):361–8.
34. Parving HH, Brenner BM, McMurray JJ, de Zeeuw D, Haffner SM, Solomon SD, et al. Aliskiren trial in type 2 diabetes using cardio-renal endpoints (ALTITUDE): rationale and study design. Nephrol Dial Transplant. 2009;24(5):1663–71.
35. Pichler RH, de Boer IH. Dual renin-angiotensin-aldosterone system blockade for diabetic kidney disease. Curr Diab Rep. 2010;10(4):297–305.
36. Nakamura T, Ushiyama C, Hirokawa K, Osada S, Inoue T, Shimada N, et al. Effect of cerivastatin on proteinuria and urinary podocytes in patients with chronic glomerulonephritis. Nephrol Dial Transplant. 2002;17(5):798–802.
37. Nakamura T, Ushiyama C, Hirokawa K, Osada S, Shimada N, Koide H. Effect of cerivastatin on urinary albumin excretion and plasma endothelin-1 concentrations in type 2 diabetes patients with microalbuminuria and dyslipidemia. Am J Nephrol. 2001;21(6):449–54.
38. Groop PH, Thomas MC, Moran JL, Waden J, Thorn LM, Makinen VP, et al. The presence and severity of chronic kidney disease predicts all-cause mortality in type 1 diabetes. Diabetes. 2009;58(7):1651–8.
39. Orchard TJ, Secrest AM, Miller RG, Costacou T. In the absence of renal disease, 20 year mortality risk in type 1 diabetes is comparable to that of the general population: a report from the Pittsburgh Epidemiology of Diabetes Complications Study. Diabetologia. 2010;53(11):2312–9.
40. Haffner SM, Lehto S, Ronnemaa T, Pyorala K, Laakso M. Mortality from coronary heart disease in subjects with type 2 diabetes and in nondiabetic subjects with and without prior myocardial infarction. N Engl J Med. 1998;339(4):229–34.
41. Dinneen SF, Gerstein HC. The association of microalbuminuria and mortality in non-insulin-dependent diabetes mellitus. A systematic overview of the literature. Arch Intern Med. 1997;157(13):1413–8.
42. Adler AI, Stevens RJ, Manley SE, Bilous RW, Cull CA, Holman RR. Development and progression of nephropathy in type 2 diabetes: the United Kingdom Prospective Diabetes Study (UKPDS 64). Kidney Int. 2003;63(1):225–32.
43. Effect of intensive therapy on the development and progression of diabetic nephropathy in the Diabetes Control and Complications Trial. The Diabetes

Control and Complications (DCCT) Research Group. Kidney Int. 1995;47(6):1703–20.
44. Sustained effect of intensive treatment of type 1 diabetes mellitus on development and progression of diabetic nephropathy: the Epidemiology of Diabetes Interventions and Complications (EDIC) study. JAMA. 2003;290(16):2159–67.
45. Intensive blood-glucose control with sulphonylureas or insulin compared with conventional treatment and risk of complications in patients with type 2 diabetes (UKPDS 33). UK Prospective Diabetes Study (UKPDS) Group. Lancet. 1998;352(9131):837–53.
46. Andersen AR, Christiansen JS, Andersen JK, Kreiner S, Deckert T. Diabetic nephropathy in Type 1 (insulin-dependent) diabetes: an epidemiological study. Diabetologia. 1983;25(6):496–501.
47. Seaquist ER, Goetz FC, Rich S, Barbosa J. Familial clustering of diabetic kidney disease. Evidence for genetic susceptibility to diabetic nephropathy. N Engl J Med. 1989;320(18):1161–5.
48. Coonrod BA, Ellis D, Becker DJ, Bunker CH, Kelsey SF, Lloyd CE, et al. Predictors of microalbuminuria in individuals with IDDM. Pittsburgh Epidemiology of Diabetes Complications Study. Diabetes Care. 1993;16(10):1376–83.
49. Chaturvedi N, Bandinelli S, Mangili R, Penno G, Rottiers RE, Fuller JH. Microalbuminuria in type 1 diabetes: rates, risk factors and glycemic threshold. Kidney Int. 2001;60(1):219–27.
50. Rossing P, Hougaard P, Parving HH. Progression of microalbuminuria in type 1 diabetes: ten-year prospective observational study. Kidney Int. 2005;68(4):1446–50.
51. de Boer IH, Sibley SD, Kestenbaum B, Sampson JN, Young B, Cleary PA, et al. Central obesity, incident microalbuminuria, and change in creatinine clearance in the epidemiology of diabetes interventions and complications study. J Am Soc Nephrol. 2007;18(1):235–43.
52. Haller H, Ito S, Izzo Jr JL, Januszewicz A, Katayama S, Menne J, et al. Olmesartan for the delay or prevention of microalbuminuria in type 2 diabetes. N Engl J Med. 2011;364(10):907–17.
53. Huang F, Yang Q, Chen L, Tang S, Liu W, Yu X. Renal pathological change in patients with type 2 diabetes is not always diabetic nephropathy: a report of 52 cases. Clin Nephrol. 2007;67(5):293–7.

Lupus Nephritis

46

Maaz A. Abbasi and Leah A. Haseley

Case 1

A 31-year-old African-American woman presents for evaluation of proteinuria. Several months earlier she was seen by her primary care physician for facial rash and pleuritic chest pain, and serologic evaluation revealed positive antinuclear antibodies (ANA) by immunofluorescence. In your office she complains of lower extremity swelling and foamy urine. The blood pressure is 155/90, and the exam is notable for the presence of oral ulcers and 3+ lower extremity edema. The urinalysis tests 3+ for protein and many dysmorphic red cells are seen on the microscopic examination of the sediment. Other testing reveals a serum creatinine of 1.3 mg/dl, serum albumin 2.9 g/dl, and her 24 h urine protein excretion is 4.5 g/day.

Does this patient meet the criteria for lupus? What additional testing should be done?
What would you be likely to see at renal biopsy?
What treatment choices would you consider?

M.A. Abbasi, M.D. (✉)
Nephrology Private Practice,2651 Bolton Boone Drive, DeSoto, TX 75115, USA
e-mail: maaz@uw.edu

L.A. Haseley, M.D.
Department of Medicine, University of Washington Medical Center, Harborview Hospital, Seattle, WA 98104, USA

Case 2

A 41-year-old Asian woman presents to an emergency room with a chief complaint of a 1 month of lower extremity edema. She also endorses an occasional headache, decreased exercise tolerance, arthralgias, and photosensitivity. Her physical examination is significant for a blood pressure of 178/112, JVP is elevated, bibasilar crackles are auscultated and dependent edema is 2+. No rash or synovitis is appreciated. Dipstick examination of her urine reveals 3+ protein and sediment shows numerous dysmorphic red blood cells. Additional laboratory testing includes a serum creatinine of 3.8 mg/dl, serum albumin is 2.6 g/dl, and hematologic testing revealed pancytopenia with a WBC count of 2.9 K/uL, hemoglobin of 7.8 g/dl, and a platelet count of 45 K/uL. Additional serologic testing included a complement 3 of 45 mg/dl and a complement 4 of 5 mg/dl, ANA 1:640 by IF, and anti-dsDNA is significantly elevated. A kidney biopsy shows 5% global sclerosis, and the remaining glomeruli show mesangial and endocapillary proliferation, extensive subendothelial deposition of immune complexes, fibrinoid necrosis. One cellular crescent is also seen. Cortical parenchyma exhibits a moderate patchy interstitial fibrosis and tubular atrophy. Immunofluorescence exam shows a "full house" pattern (positive staining for IgM, IgG, IgA, C3, and C1q).

In additional to IV pulse methylprednisone, what would you use for induction therapy?

E.V. Lerma and M. Rosner (eds.), *Clinical Decisions in Nephrology, Hypertension and Kidney Transplantation*, DOI 10.1007/978-1-4614-4454-1_46, © Springer Science+Business Media New York 2013

What agent would you use for maintenance therapy and for how long?

Overview

The kidney is the most common internal organ affected in systemic lupus erythematosus (SLE). The majority of patients with SLE will have an abnormal urinalysis at some point in the course of their disease, and clinical nephritis will affect up to 55% of patients depending on ethnicity [1]. Among lupus patients, renal disease is an independent predictor of mortality [2].

In SLE, multiple pathways of immune dysfunction lead to renal injury. Clinical manifestations vary greatly and can range from mild hematuria to rapidly progressive (crescentic) glomerulonephritis. While most kidney disease begins with immune complex deposition within the glomerulus, a minority of patients will have a renal manifestation of the antiphospholipid syndrome.

The majority of lupus patients are young, and treatment must aim to minimize long-term toxicity while maximizing outcome. In this chapter, we address key clinical points regarding lupus nephritis and highlight recent advances in treatment.

Epidemiology

In the United States, the prevalence of SLE is approximately 1:2,000 in the general population. Worldwide prevalence rates vary greatly, ranging 8–159/100,000 population [3, 4]. The disease affects women more often than men, at a ratio of roughly 10:1. Both incidence and prevalence rates are two to three times higher among people of African or Asian descent. The majority of patients present with symptoms between the ages of 16 and 55, with African-American women tending to present earlier.

The epidemiology of nephritis varies greatly by population and the diagnostic criteria for renal involvement. In a US cohort study, 69% of African Americans exhibited signs of nephritis, in contrast to 14% of Caucasians [5]. Globally, the incidence is highest among those of African or Asian dissent (50–55%) followed by those of Hispanic (43%) or Caucasian (17%) lineage [1]. Renal disease is often apparent within the first year of the diagnosis of SLE, but can occur as late as 8 years out [2]. Risk factors for early development of nephritis include male sex, age less than 33, and non-European lineage [6]. Blacks and Asians are particularly vulnerable to severe nephritis. Furthermore, poverty is an independent risk factor for progression of nephritis [7].

Etiology/Pathophysiology

The pathogenesis of lupus nephritis begins with the formation of antibodies directed at native nuclear antigens released from dead or dying cells (dsDNA, histones, and nucleosomes). The resulting immune complexes can deposit in the kidney during the normal filtration process, or form in situ within the mesangium or capillary loop. Thereafter, complement is activated, resulting in an inflammatory cascade that ultimately disrupts glomerular architecture, leading to proteinuria and renal impairment. Urinary evidence of inflammation includes hematuria, pyuria, and cellular casts.

While this common pathway of inflammation is well understood, the factors leading to autoantibody generation and impairments in immune complex processing are obscure and clearly multifactorial. The etiology of lupus nephritis involves a strong genetic predisposition enabled by immunologic, hormonal, and environmental factors.

Many genetic polymorphisms associate with SLE. The highest hazard ratio is seen among those with hereditary complement deficiencies (leading to impaired immune complex clearance) or mutations in TREX1 (required for the normal degradation of DNA) [8].

Table 46.1 outlines a sample of the many etiologic factors involved in SLE. Whereas classically oral contraceptives were felt to be contraindicated in lupus, a recent study supports their safety among patients with stable disease [9]

Table 46.1 Pathophysiology of SLE

Genetic	Environmental	Hormonal	Immunologic
Deficient C1q, C4A, C4B	UV light	Early menarche	Loss of self-tolerance
Mutated TREX1	Viruses (e.g., EBV)	Oral contraceptive pills	Impaired phagocytosis
HLA DR2, DR3	Mycobacterial infections	Nulliparity	Polyclonal B cell activation
Stat4, IRAK1 (interferon effects)	Trypanosomiasis	Breastfeeding (may decrease risk)	Abnormalities in Toll-like receptors
LYN, BLK (lymphocyte signaling)			Fetal microchimerism
FcgammaRIIA polymorphism			Dysfunctions in T and B cell signaling
TLR7, TLR9 (innate immunity)			

Clinical Features

Kidney disease is usually detected within the first year of a lupus diagnosis. Nephritis can be the presenting manifestation of SLE, or occur in the context of systemic symptoms such as rash, oral ulcers, Raynaud's, or serositis. Early diagnosis is often made on the basis of asymptomatic hematuria and/or proteinuria. Other patients present with classic features of *nephritic* (RBC casts, azotemia, hypertension, variable proteinuria), or *nephrotic* (protein excretion >3.5 g/24 h, edema, hypoalbuminemia, hyperlipidemia, lipiduria) syndromes. In any given patient, these symptoms and signs can overlap considerably.

Patients may complain of foamy urine, an indicator of proteinuria. Periorbital and lower extremity edema are common. In severe nephrosis, the abdominal wall and genitalia may become edematous, and the patient may develop ascites and pleural effusions. The presence of unilateral edema should raise consideration of venous thrombosis due to the nephrotic state, or underlying antiphospholipid antibodies (aPL).

While imprecise, the clinical presentation can often correlate with biopsy findings (Table 46.2). Nephritis limited to the mesangium is typically mild and is characterized by microhematuria and mild proteinuria. Membranous lupus tends to present with nephrotic syndrome and a bland urine sediment, and serologies can be negative including normal complement levels. In contrast, more aggressive proliferative lesions generally manifest in an active urine sediment, hypertension, and variable degrees of azotemia. In this setting, autoantibody levels are high and hypocomplementemia frequent.

It is important to note that SLE patients often present with mixtures of nephritic and nephrotic features. Moreover, chronic proteinuria can persist for years after treatment, despite histologic absence of disease activity.

Rarely, lupus patients with aPL can present with microangiopathic renal failure in the absence of immune complex disease. However, even in the presence of high aPL titer, a lupus patient is more likely to have an immune complex glomerulonephritis, albeit with a more poor prognosis [10]. Finally, tubular deposition of immune complexes can lead to renal tubular acidosis and hyperkalemia.

Diagnosis and Biomarkers

Nephrologists are often on the "front line" of diagnosing SLE. In this regard, it is helpful to review the current American College of Rheumatology (ACR) criteria for lupus, which are composed of both clinical and serologic findings. The presence of four of these findings establishes a diagnosis of SLE (Table 46.3).

Lupus patients elaborate a variety of autoantibodies, many of which associate with distinct organ systems (Table 46.4) [11]. Antibodies to dsDNA are the prototype, being both sensitive

Table 46.2 Clinical pathologic correlations in pts with SLE

Lupus class	Hematuria	Proteinuria	Azotemia	HTN	edema
Mesangial	+	+	–	–	–
Proliferative	++	++	++	++	++
Membranous lupus	+/–	++++	+	+	+++
Advanced sclerosing	+/–	++	+++	+/–	+/–

Table 46.3 American College of Rheumatology criteria for SLE

Clinical	Serologic
Malar	Positive ANA
Discoid Rash	Positive anti-dsDNA *or* positive anti-Sm antibody *or* positive antiphospholipid antibody (aPL)
Photosensitivity	
Oral ulcers	
Arthritis	
Hematologic (hemolytic anemia, leukopenia or lymphopenia on two or more occasions, thrombocytopenia)	
Serositis	
Renal disease (Protein Excretion > 0.5 g/day or cellular casts)	
Neurologic disorder	
SLE is diagnosed if any four criteria are positive	

Table 46.4 Autoantibody specificities in SLE

Antibody	Prevalence in SLE	Organ system
ANA	95–100%	All
Anti-dsDNA	40–80%	Nephritis
Anti-C1q	30–60%	Nephritis
Anti-Chromatin	50–90%	Nephritis
Anti-Ribosomal P	8–42%	CNS disease, nephritis
Anti-Sm	30%	Specific for SLE (more common in AA)
Anti-RNP	10–40%	Arthritis, Raynauds, MCTD
Anti-RO (SS-A)	24–60%	Photosensitivity, lung disease, neonatal lupus
Anti-LA (SS-B)	6–35%	Neonatal LE
Antiphospholipid	50%	Thrombosis, APS
Anti GP IIB-IIIA	10–62%	Thrombocytopenia
Anti-neuronal	33–75%	Neuropsychiatric lupus

(70–80%) and specific (95%) for SLE. Hypocomplementemia, due to consumption of complement proteins by immune complex deposition, is also a frequent finding which has been shown to track with activity of nephritis [12].

With regard to renal disease, recent investigations have focused on biomarkers that correlate with activity of lupus nephritis [13]. An ideal marker would track tightly with histologic and clinical activity, and have the capacity to predict a renal flare far earlier than conventional clinical markers (GFR, urinary protein, complement levels). Optimal biomarkers would have the capacity to identify subsets of patients likely to respond to particular treatment regimens. Both serum and urine biomarkers are under investigation, several of which are discussed below:

Anti-chromatin antibodies. While the pathophysiology of lupus nephritis is complex, recent literature has highlighted the important role played by nucleosomes released from dying cells [14]. These DNA–histone complexes can elicit an antibody response while in the circulation, or after lodging in the glomerulus. This antibody class is known as anti-chromatin antibodies.

Anti-chromatin antibodies have a sensitivity of 48–100% and a specificity of 90–99% for the detection of SLE [15]. With regard to renal disease, both cross-sectional and short longitudinal studies have shown a relationship between titers of these antibodies and clinical activity of nephritis. However, their ability to predict renal flares do not appear to be superior to anti-dsDNA antibodies [13].

Anti-C1q antibodies. Antibodies to the collagen-like-region of C1q, the first component of the classical complement pathway, have been found to associate with lupus nephritis in multiple case series [16]. After binding to C1q, pathogenic autoantibodies may amplify the immune response, or deplete complement components needed for proper immune complex clearance.

The prevalence of anti-C1q antibodies among SLE patients approximates 40% in most cross-sectional studies. Antibody titers correlate with renal disease activity with sensitivities ranging from 44 to 100% and specificities from 70 to 92% [13, 17]. In a prospective study, titers of anti-C1q antibodies were elevated in all of 15 patients that went on to develop renal disease. Moreover, high anti-C1q titers had a 100% negative predictive value for the development of proliferative nephritis [18].

In a recent longitudinal study, Petri et al. compared the ability of different biomarkers to distinguish between large changes in renal disease activity among individual patients [19]. Specifically, each patient's sera was tested at a time of high or low renal activity score, including the presence or absence of proteinuria. In this study, antibodies to C1q were the *only* marker that correlated significantly with activity of nephritis, as compared to anti-dsDNA, anti-chromatin antibodies, C3, C4, and levels of the adhesion molecules ICAM and VCAM.

Despite these promising data, anti-C1q titers have not outperformed more traditional nephritic markers in every study, and assays for these antibodies are not available in most commercial labs [20].

Urinary Biomarkers

Monocyte chemoattractant protein-1 (MCP-1) is a potent chemokine currently under study as a potential biomarker for acute kidney injury [21]. Among patients with SLE, urinary levels of MCP-1 have been shown to be specific for nephritis and to correlate with severity of proliferative disease [22]. Levels have been found to increase 2–4 months prior to a renal flare, and to fall slowly with clinical improvement [22]. In a separate small study, the combination of urinary MCP-1 level with serum creatinine was shown to correlate with interstitial injury in a sample of 64 SLE biopsies [23].

TNF-like weak inducer of apoptosis (TWEAK) is a multifunctional cytokine which plays a clear pathogenic role in rodent models of lupus nephritis [24]. Among lupus patients, urinary levels of TWEAK correlate with disease activity and are superior to anti-dsDNA for differentiating lupus pts with or without renal disease [25]. They have not yet been shown useful for prediction of flares.

Other promising urinary biomarkers under study include hepcidin, osteoprotegerin (OPG), and neutrophil gelatinase associated lipocalin (NGAL) [13]. It is likely that some combination of biomarkers will be needed to accurately predict nephritic flares and guide treatment decisions with or without the need for tissue.

Despite the evolution of more sophisticated biomarkers, the kidney biopsy remains the gold standard for diagnosing and classifying lupus nephritis. Findings at biopsy can establish an early diagnosis of SLE and inform prognosis. Guidelines for treatment of nephritis are derived from studies in which patients were stratified by pathologic findings. Thus, most nephrologists will not make treatment decisions without a biopsy.

Pathology

Light Microscopy. The current classification of lupus nephritis assigns a glomerular pattern to each biopsy, with specific attention to whether the lesion affects part (segmental) or all (global) of the glomerulus involved and whether more than 50% (diffuse) or less than 50% (focal) of the glomeruli are involved (Table 46.4) [26]. In addition, an assessment of the activity and chronicity of the lesion is often reported. Although the prognostic value of these features is not consistent, data supports the presence of chronic changes as being the greater risk factor for progression to ESRD. It is important to note that different morphologic patterns can exist within the same biopsy specimen. For example, class III and class V disease can be diagnosed on a single specimen.

Immunofluorescence staining is characteristically positive for IgG, IgM, and IGA containing immune complexes, reflecting the polyclonal nature of SLE. Glomeruli typically stain for both C3 and C1q, indicating local activation of the classical complement pathway. The presence of three immunoglobulins and two complement proteins is classically referred to as the "Full House" staining pattern seen in SLE.

Electron microscopy is likely to show numerous electron dense immune deposits in mesangial, subendothelial, and/or subepithelial sites. Even in membranous disease, immune deposits may be seen outside of the subepithelial space (which is unusual in idiopathic membranous nephropathy. Tubular reticular inclusions, thought to be a marker for local gamma-interferon production, can be seen within endothelial cells of patients with SLE, HIV, and rarely other viral infections.

Although patterns of glomerular injury tend to track with specific clinical findings (Table 46.2), the biopsy findings do not always correlate with the patient's symptoms and signs. Furthermore, it is not uncommon for serial biopsies to show evolution from one pattern to another. For example a patient with a histologic diagnosis of membranous lupus could develop hematuria, hypertension, and a rising creatinine. A second biopsy would be likely to show a new proliferative lesion.

Vascular lesions are not uncommon in lupus nephritis and can indicate the presence of aPL or a lupus anticoagulant. When severe, this can take the form of a thrombotic microangiopathic picture that conveys a worse prognosis [10].

Differential Diagnosis

The diagnostic criteria for SLE are clear-cut, although there is considerable overlap with other autoimmune diseases such as Rheumatoid Arthritis, Sjogren's, and mixed connective tissue disease. With regard to renal presentation, lupus nephritis can masquerade as many other glomerular diseases. In particular, diseases that commonly present with a mixture of nephritic and nephrotic features are listed in Table 46.5.

Table 46.5 ISN/RPS classification of lupus nephritis 2003

Class I	Minimal mesangial lupus nephritis
Class II	Mesangial proliferative lupus nephritis
Class III	Focal lupus nephritis
Class IV	Diffuse segmental (IV-S) or global (IV-G) lupus nephritis
Class V[a]	Membranous lupus nephritis
Class VI	Advanced sclerosing lupus nephritis

[a]Class V may occur in combination with class III or IV

Biopsy findings of lupus nephritis can share similarities with lesions seen in HIV disease, Hepatitis C and B infection, and other infections. Thrombotic vascular lesions in lupus are similar to those seen in malignant hypertension, hemolytic uremic syndrome/thrombotic thrombocytopenic purpura, or scleroderma renal crisis. Drug-induced lupus (hydralazine, procainamide) rarely affects the kidney [27].

Treatment

Treatment of lupus nephritis is best divided into an induction phase and a maintenance phase. The former usually deals severe life-threatening, often multi-organ, disease. The latter phase targets maintenance of remission and minimizing short and long-term toxicities of immunosuppressive treatments.

Non-immunomodulatory Treatment

The treatment for lupus nephritis is largely determined by the class of lupus nephritis. Only non-immunosuppressive treatments are usually required in Class I and II lupus nephritis; renal and patient survival is excellent (see Table 46.6). Patients with "pure" (no overlap with proliferative lupus) class V lupus without nephrotic range proteinuria and preserved renal functions also are managed without immunomodulatory agents.

The goal of treatment in severe lupus nephritis is resolution of immunological injury and

Table 46.6 Diseases that commonly present with a mixed nephritic and nephrotic picture

SLE
IgA nephropathy
Cryoglobulinemia
Membranoproliferative glomerulonephritis
Infection related GN

maintenance of remission. In the Lupus Nephritis Collaborative Study Group, complete remission was defined by a serum Cr ≤ 1.4 mg/dl and protein excretion ≤ 330 mg/day [28]. In other trials, the importance of attaining inactive urinary sediment was also emphasized [29]. Achieving clinical remission is closely linked with both renal and patient outcomes. Patients who achieved remission had a 95% patient survival and 94% renal survival at 10 years; those that did not achieve remission had a 10-year patient survival of 60% and a renal survival of 31% [28].

Monotherapy with Glucocorticoids

Glucocorticoid therapy is universally indicated for induction in severe lupus nephritis in combination with other agents. It is well established that monotherapy with steroid results in inferior renal outcomes [30].

In combination with other agents, 0.5–1.0 g of intravenous "pulsed" methylprednisolone is administered daily for 3 days followed usually by oral prednisone at a dose of 0.5–1.0 mg/kg/day for a minimum of 4 weeks. The prednisone dose is then tapered to the minimal dose required to control extra-renal disease (see Table 46.7) [30].

Pulsed Cyclophosphamide

The role of cyclophosphamide in severe lupus nephritis treatment is well established based on the results of several landmark trials from the NIH (see Table 46.7). One such trial enrolled 82 patients with proliferative lupus nephritis and preserved renal functions. Subjects were randomized to one of three regimens (all three arms received oral prednisone): pulsed IV cyclophosphamide for 6 months and then quarterly cyclophosphamide for 2 years; 1 year of monthly pulsed methylprednisolone or a combination of cyclophosphamide and methylprednisolone [31]. The initial dose of cyclophosphamide for patients with near normal renal functions was 0.75 g/m^2. Dose was titrated to achieve a nadir leukocyte count between 1,500 cells/mm^3 to 3,000 cells/mm^3 with a maximal dose of 1.0 mg/m^2 body surface area. Intravenous Mesna (2-mercaptoethanesulfonate) was used for bladder protection. After a median follow-up of 5 years, there was a higher rate (though not statistically significant) of remission with the combination therapy as compared to methylprednisolone treatment alone. The long-term effects of the different induction strategies were also reported by the same authors with an extended follow-up of 11 years [32]. For patients who completed the study protocol, significantly better renal outcomes (including less progression to ESRD) were noted with the cyclophosphamide and methylprednisolone combination treatment.

While cyclophosphamide was established as superior to monotherapy with steroids, significant toxicity was seen including premature ovarian failure (POF) and increased risk of avascular necrosis (see Table 46.8). More deaths were also seen in patients receiving cyclophosphamide. Subsequent studies evaluated protocols that decreased cyclophosphamide exposure. The Euro-Lupus trial evaluated the safety and efficacy of a low dose "Euro lupus" cyclophosphamide against a modified NIH protocol (higher dose) [33]. It bears emphasizing that the study population was pre-dominantly white with preserved renal functions. There was no difference in renal outcomes or treatment failure, a finding confirmed by long-term follow-up. Unfortunately an improved safety profile was not observed with the Euro lupus protocol.

Mycophenolate Mofetil

The best data for the use of mycophenolate mofetil (MMF) comes from the ALMS trial [29] where 370 patients were randomized to either

Table 46.7 Major clinical trials in lupus nephritis

Trial name	Pub year	Group 1	Group 2	Group 3	Pt no	Ethnicity	Mean Cr	Mean protein excretion	Duration of follow-up	Primary endpoint	Other outcomes
Controlled trial of pulse methylprednisolone versus two regimens of pulse cyclophosphamide in severe lupus nephritis [30]	1992	IV MP 1.0 g/m^2 q mth × 6 (MP alone)	Iv CP q mth × 6 (short course)	IV CP q mth × 6 then q 3 mths × 8 (long course)	65	Black 28	1.86 mg/dl	4.7 g/day	> 5 year	Doubling of Cr more frequent with MP only (12/25) than short course CP (7/20) or long course CP (3/20)	27% risk of POF with CP treatment. More relapses with short course CP than long course CP ($p=0.09$)
Methylprednisolone and cyclophosphamide, alone or in combination, in patients with lupus nephritis [31]	1996	IV MP 1.0 g/m^2 q mth × 12 (MP alone)	Iv CP q mth × 6 then q 3 mths × 8 (CP alone)	Combination of IV MP and CP (combination therapy)	82	57 white, 18 black	101	3.9 g/day	> 5 year	Significantly more renal remission with combination therapy (17/28) and IV CP alone (13/27) then MP alone (7/27)	55% risk of POF with CP. More relapse with MP alone. 3/55 deaths seen with CP treatment, none with MP alone
Combination therapy with pulse cyclophosphamide plus pulse methylprednisolone improves long-term renal outcome without adding toxicity in patients with lupus nephritis [32]	2001	IV MP 1.0 g/m^2 q mth × 12 (MP alone)	Iv CP q mth × 6 then q 3 mths × 8 (CP alone)	Combination of IV MP and CP (combination therapy)	82	57 white, 18 black	101	3.9	>10 year	Treatment failure (Doubling of creatinine, need for additional immunosuppression or death) more likely with MP alone then CP alone or combination therapy	Risk of doubling of serum Cr lowest with combination therapy (4/20) compared to MP alone (8/20) or CP alone (8/20). 10/55 patients receiving CP died, only 1/27 deaths with MP alone

Immunosuppressive therapy in lupus nephritis: the Euro-Lupus Nephritis Trial, a randomized trial of low-dose versus high-dose intravenous cyclophosphamide [33]	2002	0.5–1.0 g/m^2 IV CP qmth × 6 then q3mth × 2 then Aza to complete 30 months	Fixed dose 500 mg IV CP q 15 days × 6 then Aza to complete 30 months	n/a	90	76 White	1.15	3.04 g/day	Up to 60 months	No difference in risk of treatment failure (composite of doubling of Cr, lack of complete remission and steroid resistant flare-up)	Cumulative dose of CP 8.5 g (high dose) vs. 3 g (low dose). No difference observed in Cr, Proteinuria, leukopenia, or gonadal toxicity
Mycophenolate mofetil versus cyclophosphamide for induction treatment of lupus nephritis [29]	2009	MMF target dose 1.5 g twice a day	0.5–1.0 g/m^2 IV CP qmth × 6	n/a	370	147 White, 123 Asian, Black 46	1.1 mg/dl	4.1 g/g	24 weeks	No difference in primary end point (decrease in proteinuria and stabilization of Cr). Primary endpoint 2.4 times more likely in Blacks and Hispanics with MMF (60% vs. 39%)	No difference in Cr and Proteinuria and severe infections. Nine deaths with MMF, 5 with IV CP
Sequential therapies for proliferative lupus nephritis [38]	2004	Induction therapy with four to seven cycles of NIH protocol IV CP (remission achieved in 83% patients)			59	Black 27 Hispanic 29	1.6 mg/dl	5.0 g/g	5 year	Lowest event free survival (composite of death or renal failure) with CP. 4 deaths with CP, 1 with MMF	Amenorrhea and infections more with CP. 4/5 deaths observed with CP. Risk of relapse lowest with MMF. More prednisone needed with CP
		AZA 1–3 mg/kg/day upto 3 years	MMF (0.5–3 g/day) upto 3	q3 months IV CP upto 3 years							

(continued)

Table 46.7 (continued)

Trial name	Pub year	Group 1	Group 2	Group 3	Pt no	Ethnicity	Mean Cr	Mean protein excretion	Duration of follow-up	Primary endpoint	Other outcomes
Azathioprine versus mycophenolate mofetil for long term immunosuppression in lupus nephritis: results from the MAINTAIN nephritis trial [39]	2010	Induction therapy with 6 pulses of IV CP at 500 mg			105	83 white	1.01 mg/dl	3.4 g/day	48 months	Primary end-point of renal flare-up similar with MMF (19%) and AZA (25%). End of follow-up Cr, c3, albumin, protein excretion not different. Doubling of Serum Cr similar also (4/52 with AZA and 3/53 with MMF)	Serum Cr, C3, Albumin, protein excretion similar at end of follow-up. Doubling of Serum Cr also similar. More leukopenia and anemia with AZA. 8/53 patients stopped MMF to plan pregnancy
		AZA target dose 2 mg/kg/day for atleast 3 years	MMF target dose 2 g/day for atleast 3 year	n/a							

Table 46.8 Non-immunosuppressive treatment in lupus nephritis

ACE inhibitors may delay occurrence of kidney disease in patients with lupus
Indicated in all classes of lupus nephritis
Only treatment required in Class I/II lupus and pure membranous lupus with sub-nephrotic proteinuria and preserved renal functions
Anti-proteinuric treatment with ACE inhibitor
Systolic blood pressure goal between 110 and 129 mmHg [44]
Lipid lowering therapy
Influenza and pneumococcal vaccination
Smoking cessation [45]

MMF (target dose of 1.5 g twice a day) or 6 monthly infusions of cyclophosphamide using the NIH protocol. Follow-up was relatively short at 24 weeks. Primary outcome was a reduction in proteinuria. Hispanics, Asians and blacks were over-represented in the trial. With short term follow-up, the major renal outcomes were similar, though MMF was superior in achieving primary response in black and Hispanic populations. There was no significant decrease in major adverse events; more deaths were seen in patients treated with MMF and more patients discontinued MMF treatment. This study corroborated the observation from several smaller trials comparing induction with MMF versus cyclophosphamide. It should be noted that these trials have only reported on short term follow-up and that MMF has been studied primarily in patients with preserved renal functions. For example, the average serum creatinine in the ALMS trial was 1.1 mg/dl and almost 75% patients had a GFR ≥ 60 ml/min per 1.73 m^2;

Based on these findings, MMF is considered equivalent to cyclophosphamide for induction in proliferative lupus nephritis and probably superior in black or Hispanic patients. A lower dose of MMF is more appropriate for Asian patients given the higher incidence of death seen in Asian patients receiving 3.0 g per day of MMF.

Cyclophosphamide remains the agent with the most experience in management of patients with life-threatening renal and non-renal organ failure such as severe renal failure needing dialysis, diffuse alveolar hemorrhage, systemic vasculitis or patients with central nervous system disease.

Rituximab

There has been some recent interest in the use of the anti-CD 20 human/mouse chimeric monoclonal antibody Rituximab. Observational studies have suggested a role for rituximab in lupus nephritis resistant to MMF or cyclophosphamide. The largest of these case series describes 22 patients treated with 0.5–1.0 g of rituximab on day 1 and 15 of treatment [34]. Patients were refractory to either MMF or cyclophosphamide (but not both agents). At 3 month follow-up, proteinuria was significantly reduced and renal functions were nonsignificantly improved. Complete remission was seen in five patients and partial remission in another seven patients.

Data from randomized controlled trials has been disappointing. The LUNAR trial [35], presented in abstract form at 2009 scientific meeting of the ACR, evaluated the efficacy and safety of rituximab plus mycophenolate versus placebo plus mycophenolate in SLE patients with proliferative nephritis for primary induction. Preliminary results showed that rituximab plus mycophenolate was not superior to mycophenolate alone. Recent data from a small prospective trial using Rituximab and cyclophosphamide in combination for induction treatment showed encouraging short term results [36].

Larger studies are needed to define the role of rituximab in management of refractory and/or relapsing disease as well as the initial agent for induction in proliferative lupus nephritis.

Tacrolimus

There has been recent interest in the use of tacrolimus for induction immunosuppression in proliferative lupus nephritis in Asian populations. The largest trial [37] enrolled 81 Chinese patients with lupus nephritis of which 61 patients had Class III or IV pathology and another 11 had proliferative lupus nephritis in combination with Class V lupus.

The majority of patients had preserved renal functions and <1 g/day of protein excretion. Patients were randomly assigned to either tacrolimus (titrated to a trough level of 5–10) plus prednisone for 6 months or intravenous cyclophosphamide using the "NIH protocol" for 6 months. There was no statistical difference in the probability of achieving the primary end point which was complete remission (52.4% vs. 38.5%, $p=0.2$). Overall tacrolimus was well tolerated with statistically less leukopenia but without an associated decrease in infection risk.

Maintenance Immunosuppression

With current induction regimens, complete or partial remission is achieved in the majority of patients with proliferative lupus nephritis. The risk of relapse following reduction or withdrawal or initial immunosuppression remains high. In addition, "smoldering" disease in the kidney may result in chronic injury.

Glucocorticoids are usually continued for an extended duration, for both renal and extra-renal indications. Similar to induction immunosuppression, glucocorticoids are used with other immunosuppressive agents.

Mycophenolate Mofetil or Azathioprine

In the maintenance phase of treatment, the use of mycophenolate mofetil (MMF) or azathioprine, as compared to quarterly treatments with cyclophosphamide· increases event-free survival rate (composite end point of death or chronic renal failure) as well as decreases relapse rate [38]. This strategy is considered standard of care for maintenance regardless of the choice of induction agent.

In the MAINTAIN trial [39], 105 (primarily Caucasian patients) were randomized to MMF (2 g/day) or Azathioprine (2 mg/kg/day) after induction with Euro lupus protocol intravenous cyclophosphamide. At 3 year follow-up, there was no significant difference in renal relapse or adverse events except for leukopenia and anemia (more common with azathioprine).

In the ALMS trial, patients who achieved remission with MMF or IV cyclophosphamide were randomized to maintenance with azathioprine or MMF for 36 months. A composite renal outcome was significantly better with MMF then azathioprine (preliminary data only).

Based on this data, MMF 1 g twice a day is equivalent, and maybe superior, to azathioprine for maintenance therapy. This decision may be affected by patient factors, such as desire to achieve fertility in women. While both azathioprine and MMF are Category D drugs in pregnancy, MMF carries a boxed warning because of increased risk of teratogenicity. Azathioprine is generally considered safer in pregnancy and there is a large body of data from transplant literature regarding the safety of azathioprine in pregnancy [40]

Treatment of Class V Lupus

Immunosuppressive treatment is recommended in Class V lupus with patients with nephrotic range proteinuria despite RAAS blockade, patients with renal dysfunction or patients with concurrent proliferative lupus (treatments targeting proliferative lupus are used). Based on regimens successful for idiopathic membranous nephropathy, 42 patients with pure membranous lupus and a mean protein excretion of 5.4 g/day with preserved GFR were randomized to treatment with cyclosporine (5 mg/kg/day) with steroids versus pulsed cyclophosphamide administered every other month with steroids versus monotherapy with steroids alone [41]. At 1 year there was a significantly higher rate of remission with cyclosporine (83%) and cyclophosphamide (60%) compared to prednisone alone (27%). After extended follow-up for 10 years, the risk for relapse was higher with cyclosporine compared to cyclophosphamide. The ALMS, where pulsed cyclophosphamide was compared with MMF for induction, included 60 patients with pure membranous lupus. Outcomes were equivalent at the end of 24 weeks of follow-up [29].

Based on these findings, there is little evidence indicating superiority between cyclosporine, pulsed IV cyclophosphamide or MMF. An individualized decision, based on patient factors such as desi re to maintain fertility, is recommended.

Prognosis of Proliferative Lupus Nephritis

Both renal and patient survival has continued to improve over the last several decades. In the 1950s and 1960s, the 5-year patient survival of Class IV lupus nephritis was about 17% [42]; by the 1990s patient survival had significantly improved [42]. In an extended follow-up of 86 patients with severe lupus nephritis in the Lupus Nephritis Collaborative Study Group [43], patient survival was 80% at 5 years and 75% at 10 years; renal survival was 68% at 5 years and 59% at 10 years. Prognosis improves significantly for patients who achieve remission with induction therapy (RR 8.2) and for patients who presented with preserved renal functions (RR 2.0). Factors associated with increased likelihood of achieving remission include white race, Chronicity Index <4, preserved renal functions and lower proteinuria. Increased probability of remission has been seen in some studies with Class IV LN as compared to Class III lupus nephritis (RR 8.2). There is also significant morbidity and mortality associated with immunosuppressive therapy (see Table 46.9) and strategies to reduced complications from therapy are crucial in improving survival (see Table 46.10)

Case 1 Revisited

The patient meets criteria for SLE based on the findings of 4 ARA criteria: Malar rash, serositis, positive ANA, and proteinuria. It would be helpful to test for antibodies to double-stranded DNA which are more specific for lupus nephritis. The findings of low levels of C3 *and* C4 would confirm activation of the classical complement pathway and help rule out other diseases that present with a mixed nephritic and nephrotic picture, such as IgA nephropathy. Based on the heavy proteinuria, membranous lupus (WHO Class V) is a possibility, but the presence of hematuria, HTN, and azotemia suggests a proliferative GN (Class 3 or 4). It is also possible that she has a mixture of these patterns.

Table 46.9 Major side-effects of immunosuppressive drugs used in lupus nephritis

Drug	Major side-effects	Contraindications
Pulse cyclophosph-amide	Hemorrhagic cystitis, bladder and other malignancies, amenorrhea and ovarian failure, bone marrow suppression, infections Pulmonary fibrosis and cardiotoxicity usually only seen with oncology dosages	Pregnancy/ Lactation (teratogenic). Active neutropenia History of bladder cancer
Glucocorticoids	Infections, HTN, weight gain, insulin resistance, osteoporosis, avascular necrosis, Cushing syndrome, upper GI bleeding, neuropsychiat-ric side-effects. Possible teratogenic effects (cleft palate)	
Mycophenolate mofetil	Dose limiting GI side effects, bone marrow suppression, infections Decreased absorption with Magnesium and Aluminum containing antacids	Pregnancy (increased risk of first trimester pregnancy loss, congenital malformations)

Table 46.10 Decreasing risk of adverse events with cyclophosphamide used with steroids

PCP prophylaxis (Bactrim, dapsone for sulfa allergy)
GI prophylaxis with H2 blockers or PPI
Bone prophylaxis with Ca/Vitamin D
Consider bisphosphonate use in patients with preserved renal functions
Dose titration based on renal functions and nadir leukocyte counts
Consider Mesna use
Long-term surveillance for bladder injury

The patient is young and has preserved renal functions. MMF would be preferable to cyclophosphamide in order to limit long-term toxicity, in particular the risk for premature ovarian failure. Evidence suggests that MMF may be superior to cyclophosphamide in African-American women. In addition, the patient should receive steroids and aggressive management of her hypertension.

Case 2 Revisited

This 41-year-old Asian female presented with severe renal failure and pancytopenia. Serologies and renal biopsy were both consistent with active Class IV lupus nephritis. Compared to MMF, intravenous cyclophosphamide is better studied in patients with severe renal dysfunction and/or life-threatening extra-renal manifestations. The Euro-lupus protocol studied in primarily Caucasian patients with preserved renal functions and the results may not be generalizable to this Asian female. In addition, MMF has been associated with increased mortality in Asian populations. After induction with four to seven monthly pulses of intravenous cyclophosphamide, MMF and prednisone should be used for maintenance therapy for 3 years.

References

1. Ortega LM, Schulz DR, Lenz O, Pardo V, Contreras GN. Lupus nephritis: pathologic features, epidemiology, and a guide to therapeutic decisions. Lupus. 2010;19:557–74.
2. Cerversa R, Kamashta MA, Font J, Sebastini GD, Gil A, LaVilla P, et al. Morbidity and mortality in systemic lupus erythematosus during a 10-year period: a comparison of early and late manifestations in a cohort of 1,000 patients. Medicine (Baltimore). 2003;82:299–308.
3. Pons-Estel GJ, Alarcan GS, Scofield L, Reinib L, Cooper GS. Understanding the epidemiology and progression of systemic lupus erythematosus. Semin Arthritis Rheum. 2010;39:257–68.
4. Danchenko N, Satia JA, Anthony MS. Epidemiology of systemic lupus erythematosus: a comparison of worldwide disease burden. Lupus. 2006;15:308–18.
5. Bastian HM, Roseman JM, McGwin Jr G. Systemic lupus erythematosus in three ethnic groups. XII. Risk factors for lupus nephritis after treatment. Lupus. 2002;11(3):152–60.
6. Seligman VA, Lum RF, Olson JL, Li H, Criswell LA. Demographic differences in the development of lupus nephirits: a retrospective analysis. Am J Med. 2002; 112(9):726.
7. Barr RG, Seliger S, Appel GB, et al. Prognosis in proliferative lupus nephritis: the role of socioeconomic status and race/ethnicity. Nephrol Dial Transplant. 2003;18(10):2039–46.
8. Sestak AL, Fürnrohr BG, Harley JB, Merrill JT, Namjou B. The genetics of systemic lupus erythematosus and implications for targeted therapy. Ann Rhem Dis. 2011;70 Suppl: i37–43.
9. Petri M, Kim MY, Kalunian KC, et al. Combined oral contraceptives in women with systemic lupus erythematosus. N Engl J Med. 2005;353:2550–8.
10. Moroni G, Ventura D, Riva P, Panzeri P, Quaglini S, Banfi G, Simonini P, Bader R, Meroni PL, Ponticelli C. Antiphospholipid antibodies are associated with an increased risk for chronic renal insufficiency in patients with lupus nephritis. Am J Kidney Dis. 2004;43:28–36.
11. Sherer Y, Gorstein A, Fritzler M, Shoenfeld Y. Autoantibody explosion in systemic lupus erythematosus: more than 100 different antibodies found in SLE patients. Semin Arthritis Rheum. 2004;34: 501–37.
12. Julkunen H, Ekblom-Kullberg S, Miettinen A. Nonrenal and renal activity of systemic lupus erythematosus: a comparison of two anti-C1q assays and complement C3 and C4. Rheumatol Int. 2011.
13. Mok CC. Biomarkers for lupus nephritis: a critical appraisal. J Biomed Biotechnol. 2010;2010:638413.
14. Hedberg A, Mortensen ES, Rekvig OP. Chromatin as a target antigen in human and murine lupus nephritis. Arthritis Res Ther. 2011;13(2):214.
15. Gomez-Puerta JA, Burlingame RW, Cervera R. Anti-chromatin (anti-nucleosome) antibodies: diagnostic and clinical value. Autoimmun Rev. 2008;7(8): 606–11.
16. Kallenberg CG. Anti-C1q antibodies. Autoimmun Rev. 2008;7(8):612–15.
17. Sinico RA, Rimoldi L, Radice A, et al. Anti-C1q autoantibodies in lupus nephritis. Ann N Y Acad Sci. 2009;1173:47–51.

18. Meyer OC, Nicaise-Roland P, Cadoudal N, et al. Anti-C1q antibodies antedate patent active glomerulonephritis in patients with systemic lupus erythematosus. Arthritis Res Ther. 2009;11(3):R87.
19. Akhter E, Burlingame RW, Seaman AL, Magder L, Petri M. Anti-C1q antibodies have higher correlation with flares of lupus nephritis than other serum markers. Lupus. 2011;20(12):1267–74.
20. Heidenreich U, Mayer G, Herold M, Klotz W, Stemfl Al-Jazawi K, Lhotta K. Sensitivity and specificity of autoantibody tests in the differential diagnosis of lupus nephritis. Lupus. 2009;18:1276–80.
21. Munshi R, Johnson A, Siew ED, et al. MCP-1 gene activation marks acute kidney injury. J Am Soc Nephrol. 2001;22(1):165–75.
22. Rovin BH, Song H, Birmingham DJ. Urine chemokines as biomarkers of human systemic lupus erythematosus activity. J Am Soc Nephrol. 2005;16(2):457–73.
23. Zhang X, Nagaraja H, Nadasdy T, et al. A composite urine biomarker reflects interstitial inflammation in lupus nephritis kidney biopsies. Kidney Int. 2011. doi: 10.1038/ki.2011.354.
24. Sanz AB, Sanchez-Nino MD, Ortiz A. TWEAK, a multifunctional cytokine in kidney injury. Kidney Int. 2011;80(7):708–18.
25. Schwartz N, Rubinstein T, Burkly L, et al. Urinary TWEAK as a biomarker of lupus nephritis: a multicenter cohort study. Arthritis Res Ther. 2009;11(5):R143.
26. Weening JJ, D'agai VD, Schwartz MM, Seshan SV, Alpers GB, Balow JE, et al. The classification of glomerulonephritis in systemic lupus erythematosis revisited. J Am Soc Nephrol. 2004;15(2):241–50.
27. Vasoo S. Drug-induced lupus: an update. Lupus. 2006;15:757.
28. Levey AS, Lan SP, Corwin HL, et al. Progression and remission of renal disease in the Lupus Nephritis Collaborative Study. Results of treatment with prednisone and short-term oral cyclophosphamide. Ann Intern Med. 1992;116(2):114–23.
29. Appel GB, Contreras G, Dooley MA, et al. Mycophenolate mofetil versus cyclophosphamide for induction treatment of lupus nephritis. J Am Soc Nephrol. 2009;20(5):1103–12.
30. Boumpas DT, Austin III HA, Vaughn EM, et al. Controlled trial of pulse methylprednisolone versus two regimens of pulse cyclophosphamide in severe lupus nephritis. Lancet. 1992;340(8822):741–5.
31. Gourley MF, Austin III HA, Scott D, et al. Methylprednisolone and cyclophosphamide, alone or in combination, in patients with lupus nephritis. A randomized, controlled trial. Ann Intern Med. 1996;125(7): 549–57.
32. Illei GG, Austin HA, Crane M, et al. Combination therapy with pulse cyclophosphamide plus pulse methylprednisolone improves long-term renal outcome without adding toxicity in patients with lupus nephritis. Ann Intern Med. 2001;135(4):248–57.
33. Houssiau FA, Vasconcelos C, D'Cruz D, et al. Immunosuppressive therapy in lupus nephritis: the Euro-Lupus Nephritis Trial, a randomized trial of low-dose versus high-dose intravenous cyclophosphamide. Arthritis Rheum. 2002;46(8):2121–31.
34. Vigna-Perez M, Hernandez-Castro B, Paredes-Saharopulos O, et al. Clinical and immunological effects of Rituximab in patients with lupus nephritis refractory to conventional therapy: a pilot study. Arthritis Res Ther. 2006;8(3):R83.
35. Furie R, Looney RJ, Rovin B, et al. Efficacy and safety of rituximab in subjects with active proliferative lupus nephritis (LN): results from the randomized, double-blind Phase III Lunar study (Abstract). Presented at the 2009 scientific meeting of the ACR.
36. Melander C, Sallee M, Trolliet P, et al. Rituximab in severe lupus nephritis: early B-cell depletion affects long-term renal outcome. Clin J Am Soc Nephrol. 2009;4(3):579–87.
37. Chen W, Tang X, Liu Q, et al. Short-term outcomes of induction therapy with tacrolimus versus cyclophosphamide for active lupus nephritis: a multicenter randomized clinical trial. Am J Kidney Dis. 2011;57(2): 235–44.
38. Contreras G, Pardo V, LeClercq B, et al. Sequential therapies for proliferative lupus nephritis. N Engl J Med. 2004;350(10):971–80.
39. Houssiau FA, D'Cruz D, Sangle S, et al. Azathioprine versus mycophenolate mofetil for long-term immunosuppression in lupus nephritis: results from the MAINTAIN Nephritis Trial. Ann Rheum Dis. 2010;69(12):2083–9.
40. Bouattar T, Hakim H, Rhou H, Benamar L, Bayahia R, Ouzeddoun N. Pregnancy in renal transplant recipients. Transplant Proc. 2009;41(5):1586–8.
41. Austin III HA, Illei GG, Braun MJ, Balow JE. Randomized, controlled trial of prednisone, cyclophosphamide, and cyclosporine in lupus membranous nephropathy. J Am Soc Nephrol. 2009;20(4):901–11.
42. Feehally J, Floege J, Johnson RJ, editors. Comprehensive clinical nephrology. 3rd ed. In chapter 24 lupus nephritis, page 298. 2007. ISBN 0-323-04602-9.
43. Korbet SM, Lewis EJ, Schwartz MM, et al. Factors predictive of outcome in severe lupus nephritis. Am J Kidney Dis. 2000;35:904–14.
44. Jafar TH, Stark PC, Schmid CH, et al. Progression of chronic kidney disease: the role of blood pressure control, proteinuria, and angiotensin-converting enzyme inhibition: a patient-level meta-analysis. Ann Intern Med. 2003;139(4):244–52.
45. Ghaussy NO, Sibbitt Jr W, Bankhurst AD, Qualls CR. Cigarette smoking and disease activity in systemic lupus erythematosus. J Rheumatol. 2003;30(6):1215–21.

Viral Diseases and the Kidney

47

German T. Hernandez and Rudolph A. Rodriguez

Case

A 49-year-old white man with known human immunodeficiency virus (HIV) infection presented to his primary care physician due to a 1-month history of lower extremity swelling. He had a CD4+ lymphocyte count of 0.270×10^9/L (normal range 0.36–1.26 10^9/L) and a HIV-1 RNA viral load of 506,000 copies/mL. He was antiretroviral treatment naïve due to compliance issues. His physical examination was significant for a blood pressure of 170/90 mmHg and pitting edema of the legs extending to the sacrum. His initial testing revealed a serum creatinine of 1.8 mg/dL and a spot urine albumin of 4,800 mg per gram of creatinine. His urinalysis was significant for 3+ proteinuria, 20 red blood cells per high power field, and no red blood cell casts but many dysmorphic red blood cells. His cholesterol was 340 mg/dL and his albumin was 2 g/dL. In addition to his HIV infection, he was coinfected with Hepatitis C virus (HCV) and Hepatitis B Virus (HBV). Other notable serologic testing included complement three levels of 55 mg/dL (75–135 mg/dL), complement 4 levels of 10 mg/dL (12–72 mg/dL), HBsAg+, HBeAg+, HCV antibody positive, and HCV RNA undetectable.

Is this patient's presentation typical of HIV associated nephropathy?

Is a kidney biopsy necessary or could a clinical diagnosis be made with the available data?

What are the treatment options?

G.T. Hernandez, M.D.
Division of Nephrology & Hypertension, Department of Internal Medicine, Paul L. Foster School of Medicine, Texas Tech University Health Center at El Paso, El Paso, TX 79905, USA

R.A. Rodriguez, M.D. (✉)
Department of Nephrology, Puget Sound Veterans Affairs Medical Center, 1660S. Columbian Way, Seattle, WA 98108, USA
e-mail: Rudolph.rodriguez@va.gov

Overview of Viral Infections and Kidney Disease

Many active viral infections are associated with glomerular diseases. The classic associations include HIV infection and collapsing focal segmental glomerulosclerosis (HIV associated nephropathy or HIVAN), HCV and membranoproliferative glomerulonephritis, and HBV and membranous nephropathy. In additional to these classic presentations, viral infections may present with a variety of other renal disorders (Table 47.1) [1–8]. The mechanism of viral induced kidney injury is not well established but a variety of mechanisms have been described including cytopathic effects of the virus, circulating immune complexes, and in situ immune complex formation. A common theme is that active viral infection and replication exists when these glomerular lesions develop, and the clinical renal manifestations remit or stabilize when remission of the viral infection occurs either spontaneously or in response to antiviral therapy.

E.V. Lerma and M. Rosner (eds.), *Clinical Decisions in Nephrology, Hypertension and Kidney Transplantation*, DOI 10.1007/978-1-4614-4454-1_47, © Springer Science+Business Media New York 2013

Table 47.1 Viral infections and associated renal disorders

Viral infections	Renal disorders
Cytomegalovirus	Interstitial nephritis in kidney transplant patients Thrombotic microangiopathy in HIV-infected patients
Hantavirus	Interstitial nephritis Acute tubular necrosis [4]
Hepatitis B virus	Membranous nephropathy Membranoproliferative glomerulonephritis Polyarteritis nodosa with renal arteriolar vasculitis and glomerular ischemia Heroin nephropathy (in IV drug users)
Hepatitis C virus	Membranoproliferative glomerulonephritis with or without cryoglobulinemia Membranous nephropathy Serum Amyloid A nephropathy (from heroin skin popping) Heroin nephropathy (in IV drug users) Focal and segmental glomerulosclerosis Fibrillary glomerulonephritis Kidney transplant thrombotic microangiopathy with anticardiolipin antibodies
Human Immunodeficiency virus	Acute tubular necrosis (with use of aminoglycosides, amphotericin B, cidofovir, foscarnet, indinavir, pentamidine, ritonavir) Tubular crystal deposition (with use of acyclovir IV, atazanavir, ciprofloxacin, indinavir, sulfadiazine) Proximal tubular dysfunction (with use of abacavir, adefovir, cidofovir, didanosine, tenofovir) Interstitial nephritis due to drug allergy (with use of allopurinol, beta lactams, ciprofloxacin, nonsteroidal anti-inflammatory agents, phenytoin, proton pump inhibitors, rifampin, trimethoprim/sulfamethoxazole) Interstitial nephritis associated with the immune reconstitution inflammatory syndrome Interstitial nephritis due to reactivation of polyoma BK virus in AIDS HIV Associated Nephropathy (collapsing FSGS) Immune complex glomerulonephritis Membranoproliferative glomeruolnephritis +/− cryoglobulinemia (with Hepatitis C co-infection or with use of enfuviritide) Thrombotic microangiopathy Minimal change nephropathy (with use of non-steroidal anti-inflammatory agents) Membranous nephropathy (with Hepatitis B co-infection) IgA nephropathy Fibrillary/immunotactoid glomerulonephritis Serum Amyloid A nephropathy (from heroin skin popping)
Polyoma BK virus	Interstitial nephritis in kidney transplant patients

This chapter focuses on HIVAN along with a brief overview of the essentials of the renal manifestations of HCV and HBV infections in non-HIV-infected patients.

Epidemiology

HIV and Kidney Disease

HIVAN predominately affects African American individuals. In 1984 the original report of HIVAN described 11 African Americans with AIDS in New York City and subsequent kidney biopsy series have repeated this observation that HIVAN predominantly occurs in African Americans [9–11]. The United States Renal Data System, a national registry of patients requiring renal replacement therapy, reports that 90% of HIV-infected patients requiring renal replacement therapy are African Americans [12]. The prevalence of HIVAN is unknown. The diagnosis of HIVAN requires a kidney biopsy for confirmation, but kidney biopsies are not performed routinely in this patient population. In kidney biopsy case series among HIV-infected individuals, HIVAN is present in approximately 40–60% of the kidney biopsies performed [13, 14]. An autopsy study of HIV-infected persons in Texas found that the overall prevalence of HIVAN was 6.9%, while a screening protocol for HIVAN based on biopsies in HIV-infected patients with >1.5 g/day of proteinuria have found an overall prevalence of 3.5% [15, 16]. Recent epidemiologic studies have further characterized the marked racial differences in end stage renal disease (ESRD) incidence among HIV-infected individuals. A study from the Veterans Affairs health care system ascertained rates of ESRD among 2 million patients and compared rates between HIV-infected and uninfected groups. Among African Americans, rates of ESRD were equivalent between those with HIV infection versus diabetes. In contrast, among white individuals, HIV was not associated with an increased risk of ESRD when compared to patients without HIV or diabetes [17, 18].

Given the predilection for HIVAN among African Americans with HIV, a study from South Africa made some interesting observations. Kidney biopsies of HIV-infected individuals in South Africa suggest that HIVAN may be present even in the presence of mild kidney disease manifested with only microalbuminuria [19]. Blacks are the largest and fastest growing racial group with HIV in the United States and worldwide 63% of all persons with HIV-infection live in sub-Saharan Africa. These demographic trends in HIV infection have provided the basis for the growing concern that ESRD prevalence may increase dramatically in the future.

HBV and HCV Associated Kidney Disease

HBV is endemic in parts or Asia and Africa due to vertical transmission. The renal manifestations of HBV are mostly seen in these endemic areas and are less common in non-endemic areas such as the United States and Europe. The reported renal associations among HBV infected patients include membranous nephropathy, membranoproliferative glomerulonephritis, and polyarteritis nodosa (Table 47.1).

The National Health and Nutrition Examination Survey was used to estimate the prevalence of HCV infection in the United States and the prevalence of antibodies to HCV was 1.6% which translated to an estimated 4.1 million persons in the United States [20]. The prevalence of renal disease in persons with HCV infection is unknown but it is likely that renal glomerular lesions are present even in the absence of clinical manifestations such as proteinuria or chronic kidney disease [21, 22]. The common renal associations reported include membranoproliferative glomerulonephritis with or without mixed essential cryoglobulinemia and membranous nephropathy (Table 47.1).

Etiology and Pathophysiology

HIV and Kidney Disease

There is substantial evidence that HIVAN is caused by direct HIV infection in renal tissue. Polymerase chain reaction techniques have detected DNA from the HIV genome in all renal cell types except interstitial cells in HIV-infected patients with proteinuria, but the HIV DNA was also present in kidney tissue from HIV-infected patients without renal disease [23, 24].

The important role of HIV viral products in the pathogenesis of HIVAN have been demonstrated in studies using a transgenic mice model which contains a noninfective HIV construct encoding the envelope glycoproteins gp41 and gp120 but lacking the *gag* and *pol* genes. This mice model develops a renal syndrome closely resembling HIVAN [25, 26]. This transgenic mouse model was used to confirm that renal disease develops from intrinsic renal factors and not systemic factors related to HIV infection [27]. In one experiment, kidneys were cross-transplanted between normal and transgenic mice. HIVAN then developed in the transgenic kidneys transplanted into the non-transgenic mice, whereas the normal kidneys remained disease free when transplanted into the transgenic mice. This study implies that HIVAN in this model is caused by a direct effect of HIV gene expression rather than the systemic effects of HIV infection. In addition, this model demonstrated that the HIV transgene is expressed in renal glomerular and tubular epithelial cells, and this renal epithelial cell transgene expression was necessary for the development of the HIVAN phenotype [25, 26].

The mechanism for HIV infection of the kidney remains elusive because kidney tissue does not express CD4 and chemokine co-receptors required for HIV entry into cells. However, studies in humans have confirmed the presence of HIV in renal epithelial cells and the ability of HIV to generate full-length mRNA in the kidney [28]. A case report which described a patient with undetectable viral levels in the serum but expression of HIV in renal epithelial cells provided evidence that the kidney appears to be a reservoir for HIV [29]. Active replication of HIV may occur in renal epithelium despite well controlled HIV infection, possibly producing HIV strains in the kidney microenvironment that differ from HIV circulating in the blood [30].

HBV and HCV Associated Kidney Disease

Viral proteins and antigens have been detected in glomerular capillary walls in patients with Hepatitis B and separately in those with HCV related glomerular disease [31–33]. This indirect evidence supports the theory that these viral infections play a pathogenetic role in the development of these renal diseases, but the exact mechanism remains unknown.

Clinical Features

HIV and Kidney Disease

Patients with HIVAN typically present with significant proteinuria and rapidly progressive loss of kidney function in the setting of poorly controlled HIV infection [13, 34]. It is notable that most patients with HIVAN do not have significant edema or hypertension [35, 36]. Abdominal ultrasound usually reveals large, echogenic kidneys. Serologic testing such as ANA and ANCA is of limited utility because false-positive serologies are more common in HIV-infected versus uninfected patients [37].

HBV and HCV Associated Kidney Disease

HBV related membranous nephropathy usually presents with nephrotic syndrome in adults, and unlike pediatric cases which tend to undergo spontaneous remission, adult patients tend to have progressive renal disease [38].

Although the classic association of HCV related kidney disease is membranoproliferative glomerulonephritis, the clinical presentation is variable ranging from minimal clinical symptoms to acute glomerulonephritis [39]. In a quarter of patients with HCV related renal disease, the initial presentation will be nephrotic syndrome while another 25% of patients will present with acute nephritic syndrome with significant hematuria and hypertension. Mixed cryoglobulinemia may present with a number of non-renal manifestations including palpable purpura, arthralgias, peripheral neuropathy, lymphadenopathy, and hepatoslenomegaly [40]. Abnormal renal function will also be present in 50% of patients [41]. It is important to note that HCV also seems to be an important risk factor for ESRD regardless of the etiology of the renal disease [42].

Diagnosis

The common theme among viral infections and renal disease is that active viral replication is present concurrently with active glomerular disease. Therefore, if viral replication is undetectable then it is unlikely that an active glomerular process is due to viral disease despite the presence of antibodies to HIV, HBV, or HCV.

Table 47.2 Prevalence of positive serologic tests in HIV-infected patients

Serologic test	Prevalence of positive test
Antinuclear antibodies	0–23%
Antineutrophil cytoplasmic antibodies	12–33%
Anti-myeloperoxidase antibodies	0–25%
Anti-proteinase three antibodies	0–7%
Anti-glomerular basement membrane antibodies	17%
Antinuclear antibodies	0–23%
Cryoglobulins	33%
Hepatitis C virus negative	17%
Hepatitis C virus positive	42%
Lupus anticoagulant	20–71%
Rheumatoid factor	19–60%

Adapted from Hernandez GT, Critchfield JM, Rodriguez RA. Nat Clin Pract Nephrology 2006; 2: 708–12

HIV and Kidney Disease

The diagnosis of a glomerular renal lesion in an HIV-infected patient with proteinuria and hematuria can be challenging without a kidney biopsy. The interpretation of serologic tests in an HIV-infected patient with kidney disease is especially problematic because as compared to HIV-negative individuals, HIV-infected patients have a higher prevalence of other autoantibodies such as rheumatoid factor, antinuclear antibodies, anticardiolipin antibodies, lupus anticoagulant, and cryoglobulins despite the absence of disease (Table 47.2) [43–46]. These false positive tests can be misleading and could lead to inappropriate therapy without a confirmatory tissue diagnosis.

Renal tissue obtained by a kidney biopsy is used to diagnosis HIVAN which is associated with characteristic glomerular, tubulointerstitial, and ultrastructural lesions. These characteristic findings include collapsing focal segmental glomerular sclerosis, cystic tubular dilatation, interstitial edema, cellular infiltrates, and dilated tubules filled with pale-staining amorphous casts (Fig. 47.1). Electron microscopy often reveals tubuloreticular inclusions in endothelial cells [47, 48].

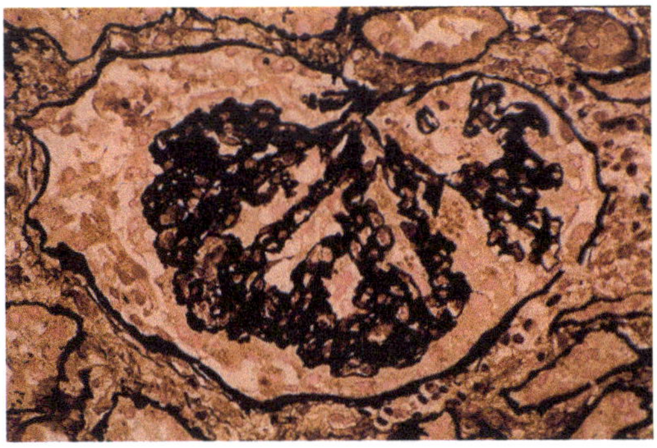

Fig. 47.1 HIV-associated nephropathy. A glomerulus displaying global collapse of glomerular basement membrane with hypertrophy and hyperplasia of the overlying podocytes. (Silver stain) Courtesy of Roberto Nicosia, MD

HBV and HCV Associated Kidney Disease

Patients with HBV related renal disease usually will have serologic tests revealing circulating HBsAg, HBeAg, and confirmatory HBV DNA all consistent with active viral replication. From a liver perspective, patients are likely to be asymptomatic except for mild to moderate elevations of serum liver enzymes if abnormal at all [38]. A kidney biopsy is necessary to differentiate between HBV related membranous nephropathy and membranoproliferative glomerulonephritis. Polyarteritis nodosa is associated with HBV, and this diagnosis can be made by tissue biopsy of an affected organ or radiologic imaging of affected vascular beds.

The classic teaching is that HCV related membranoproliferative glomerulonephritis occurs in patients with hematuria, low complements, RF, and cryoglobulinemia. However, cryoglobulins are detected in 50–70% of patients with membranoproliferative glomerulonephritis although the majority, but not all, will have low complements [49]. Some have argued that a kidney biopsy is not necessary in patients presenting with the typical findings of serologic evidence of active HCV (HCV RNA), low complements, hematuria, RF, and cryoglobulins, and that a clinical diagnosis of HCV related membranoproliferative glomerulonephritis can be made in these patients. However, a kidney biopsy and confirmation of the HCV-associated

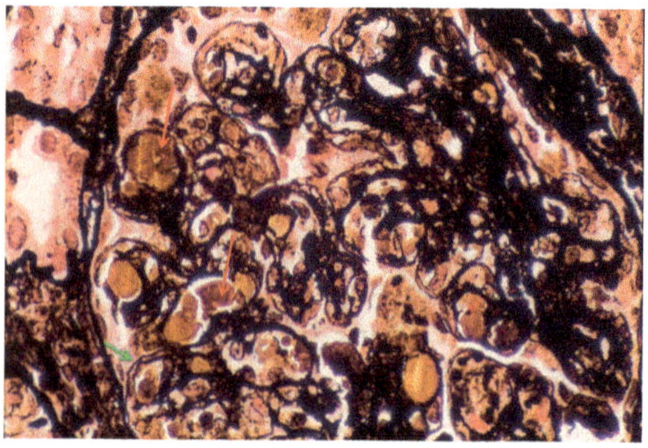

Fig. 47.2 Membranoproliferative glomerulonephritis. The glomerulus exhibits increased lobularity, cellularity, splitting of capillary basement membranes (*green arrow*), and "hyaline thrombi" (cryoglobulin deposits, *red arrows*). (Silver Stain) Courtesy of Roberto Nicosia, MD

renal disease may be useful in patients who would not otherwise be considered candidates for interferon treatment due to a lack of indications for treatment from a hepatic perspective. The typical pathology findings of membranoproliferative glomerulonephritis are shown in Fig. 47.2.

Differential Diagnosis

HIV and Kidney Disease

A variety of renal abnormalities have been described in HIV-infected patients (Table 47.1) [6]. These include HIVAN, HIV-related immune complex disease including lupus like glomerulonephritis, interstitial nephritis secondary to antiretroviral therapy or antibiotics, thrombotic microangiopathy, or diseases related to common comorbidities such as amyloidosis from heroin skin-popping, and hepatitis C related membranoproliferative glomerulonephritis.

HBV and HCV Associated Kidney Disease

Patients with active hepatitis B infection are also at risk for membranoproliferative glomerulonephritis and polyarteritis nodosa. One of the main risk factors for HCV infection is intravenous drug use and this population is also at risk for HIVAN, heroin nephropathy, amyloidosis due to skin-popping, and focal segmental glomerulosclerosis.

Management

HIV and Kidney Disease

Prior to the modern era of antiretroviral therapy, the overall incidence of ESRD due to HIV increased annually. However, since 1995, after protease inhibitors came into use, the incidence of ESRD secondary to HIV/AIDS declined and has since remained constant [12]. Observational data has now established HIV antiretroviral therapy as first line therapy for HIVAN. Other treatment options include angiotensin converting enzyme inhibitors (ACE-inhibitors), corticosteroids, and renal replacement therapy.

Antiretroviral Therapy

The Strategies for Management of Antiretroviral Therapy (SMART) study provided important insights into the value of antiretroviral therapy in treating HIV-related kidney disease. In this study, 5,472 HIV-infected patients who had $CD4^+$ counts of more than 350 per mm [3] were randomly assigned to continuous or episodic use of antiretroviral therapy and were followed for a mean of 16 months. Compared with continuous antiretroviral therapy, investigators found that planned treatment interruptions guided by $CD4^+$ counts significantly increased the risk of opportunistic disease and death from any cause. In addition, the investigators found an increased risk for fatal or nonfatal ESRD (hazard ratio 4.5; 95% confidence interval: 1.0–20.9) in the treatment interruption arm. Although this study was not statistically powered to detect a difference in renal outcomes, the high incidence of renal disease in the treatment interruption group suggests that antiretroviral therapy and sustained viral suppression are important factors in preventing and slowing progression of kidney disease [50, 51].

There are no controlled clinical trials on the effect of antiretroviral therapy on kidney disease progression due to the obvious ethical implications of nontreatment of HIV infection. Therefore, the evidence is obtained from several case series which have suggested a benefit of antiretroviral therapy in patients with HIVAN. A cohort of 53 patients with biopsy-proven HIVAN from the Johns Hopkins renal clinic were found to have better renal survival when treated with HAART compared to patients who did not receive HAART (adjusted hazard ratio 0.30; 95% confidence interval: 0.09–0.98) [52]. In a retrospective study of 19 patients with a clinical diagnosis of HIVAN, a significant association was found between protease inhibitor usage and a slower decline in renal function [53]. There have been some impressive case reports of patients responding with dramatic renal function recovery after initiation of antiretroviral therapy [29]. However, a dramatic recovery of renal function is not the rule and many patients may progress to ESRD despite antiretroviral therapy [54]. Based on observational data and the current understanding of the pathogenic role HIV infection, the Infectious Diseases Society of America guidelines recommend antiretroviral therapy as the first-line treatment of HIVAN [55]. Antiretroviral therapy is recommended in this setting irrespective of other indications for treatment of HIV such as level of $CD4^+$ count or HIV RNA level.

Angiotensin Converting Enzyme Inhibitors

Angiotensin II causes podocyte injury in HIVAN models and it increases the cellular synthesis of transforming growth factor-β, which has been implicated in the pathogenesis of HIVAN [56]. Due to the many beneficial effects of ACE-inhibitors in other proteinuric renal disease and possible specific benefits in HIVAN, ACE-inhibitors have been proposed as a logical therapy for HIVAN. In a study of 18 patients with HIVAN, 9 were treated with captopril, while 9 controls were identified by matching for age, race, gender, and level of serum creatinine concentration [57]. Renal survival was enhanced in the captopril treated group compared with controls (mean renal survival, 156±71 days versus 37±5 days, $P<0.002$). In a single center, prospective cohort study of 44 patients with HIVAN, 28 patients received fosinopril, 10 mg/day, and 16 were followed as controls [58]. The median renal survival of treated patients was 479.5 days, with only one patient developing ESRD while the untreated control patients had a median renal survival of 146.5 days ($p<0.0001$). Despite the limitations of these studies, they provide evidence that ACE-inhibitors should play a role in the treatment of HIVAN.

Steroids

Several observational studies support the use of steroids in treating HIVAN [59, 60]. An early study prospectively enrolled 20 patients with HIVAN to receive treatment with corticosteroids. Most patients had improvements in kidney function, and most had a reduction in 24 h urinary protein excretion with an average reduction from 9.1±1.8 g per day to 3.2±0.6 g per day ($p<0.005$) [61]. Another study of steroid therapy found similar results with no increased risk of infection in the steroid group [60]. Corticosteroids are considered second line therapy for patients with HIVAN with a possible role in treating patients with a recent rapid deterioration in kidney function, without current antiretroviral therapy, and with biopsy proven HIVAN. A short course of prednisone may be considered with a goal of allowing for stabilization of renal function until antiretroviral therapy is initiated.

HBV and HCV Associated Kidney Disease

Antiviral medications are also the mainstay of treatment for both HBV and HCV related renal disease, and the theme which has emerged from small trials, case reports, and case series is that proteinuria improves if antiviral medication is effective in reducing viral replication. Mono-therapy with corticosteroids provides little benefit when used alone. Antiviral agents such as interferon and lamivudine have been studied in a small number of subjects with active hepatitis B viral infection and these studies showed that the disappearance of HBV DNA is usually accompanied with remission of proteinuria [62, 63]. In 2008 the Kidney Disease: Improving Global Outcomes (KDIGO) clinical practice guidelines for HCV related chronic kidney disease were published [64]. These guidelines acknowledge that the treatment of HCV is evolving rapidly as new agents are developed and that these agents must be used with caution in patients with chronic kidney disease. For example, the clearance of pegylated interferon is reduced in patients on hemodialysis and limited information is available regarding the clearance of the drug with other late stages of chronic kidney disease [65]. Ribavirin is an agent used in combination with interferon and is critical in achieving the highest rates of sustained HCV remission. However, when ribavirin has been used in patients with an eGFR < 50 mL/min/1.73 m^2, severe cases of hemolytic anemia have been reported. The KDIGO guidelines reflect these limitations for the treatment of HCV related kidney disease. These guidelines suggest the following treatments: (1) for an eGFR > 50 mL/min/1.73 m^2, pegylated interferon and ribavirin, (2) for an eGFR of 15 to below 50 mL/min/1.73 m^2, monotherapy with peglylated interferon, and (3) for an eGFR less than 15 mL/min/1.73 m^2 monotherapy with non-pegylated interferon with dose adjustment.

Prognosis and Complications

HIV and Kidney Disease

In the 1980s newly diagnosed patients with ESRD and AIDS were dying an average of 1–3 months after starting hemodialysis, an observation made mostly in patients late in the course of their HIV disease with advanced opportunistic infections [2]. With the introduction of antiretroviral therapy, the survival of HIV patients with ESRD has steadily improved over the last decade. By 1999 the 1-year survival of HIV-infected dialysis patients was equivalent to the general dialysis population in the US and in Europe [66, 67]. In the most current United States Renal Data System report, the incidence of ESRD caused by AIDS has decreased since 1996–1998, while prevalent rates have more than doubled indicating the patients are living longer on dialysis [12]. Currently there is no reason to withhold renal replacement therapy from patients solely on the basis of HIV infection [17].

Hemodialysis, peritoneal dialysis, and transplantation are all potential options for renal replacement therapy for HIV-infected patients, and each modality has advantages and disadvantages. In general, preparation for renal replacement therapy should begin with a referral for kidney transplant evaluation for patients with well-controlled HIV infection and an eGFR < 25 mL/min/1.73 m^2 [68].

Hemodialysis

The most common renal replacement modality for HIV-infected patients is hemodialysis. Potential disadvantages of hemodialysis include risk of infections from temporary catheters and grafts, and risk to dialysis providers of blood and needlestick exposure. Early surgical referral for placement of a native arteriovenous fistula is advised due to the inferior outcomes for AV grafts among HIV-infected patients [69]. The outcomes for native arteriovenous fistulas in HIV-positive patients are comparable to that reported for HIV-negative patients [70].

Peritoneal Dialysis

Clinical patient outcomes among hemodialysis and peritoneal dialysis patients are equivalent among HIV-infected individuals, and therefore, patients should be offered a choice of either modality [71]. One advantage of peritoneal dialysis is the elimination of the risk of hemodialysis needlestick accidents among dialysis personnel. Among the potential disadvantages of peritoneal dialysis include albumin loss in the peritoneal dialysis fluid and the potential for severe peritonitis. The incidence and spectrum of peritonitis has been reported in several small series of HIV-infected patients. The largest series studied 39

HIV-infected patients on peritoneal dialysis and found a higher overall risk of peritonitis and more attributed to Pseudomonas species and fungi than in HIV-negative patients [72, 73]. However, the higher peritonitis rate in this study could have been due to HIV infection or other factors such as low socioeconomic status and drug use could have contributed. Overall, these studies suggest that the survival of patients is equivalent among peritoneal dialysis and hemodialysis HIV-infected patients [71].

HBV and HCV Associated Kidney Disease

HBV related membranous nephropathy is mostly observed in children and the prognosis is excellent due to the high incidence of spontaneous remission of active HBV. As previously mentioned, the prevalence of HCV in the US general population is relatively high [20]. However, the long-term prognosis and the incidence of extrahepatic manifestations such as membranoproliferative glomerulonephritis are not known due to the complexities of studying the natural history of an infection which evolves over decades. Nevertheless, HCV infection seems to worsen the prognosis of other renal diseases such as diabetic nephropathy [42, 74, 75].

Preventive Measures/Prophylaxis

HIV and Kidney Disease

Infection Control in Dialysis

In general, management of dialysis in the HIV-infected patient requires no special precautions besides careful adherence to universal body substance precautions. HIV-infected patients do not require special isolation precautions during hemodialysis, and dialyzer-reuse programs are permitted in HIV-infected patients. Precautions such as isolation of HIV-infected patients from other dialysis patients are unnecessary and could violate medical confidentiality. The size of the HIV particle is much larger than most dialyzer membrane pore sizes, and therefore, HIV particles are unlikely to cross the dialyzer membrane into the dialysate or ultrafiltrate. Despite a small decrease in plasma HIV RNA levels during hemodialysis, one study could not measure HIV RNA in the ultrafiltrate of 10 HIV-infected hemodialysis patients [76]. However, given the lack of definitive studies, dialysate should be treated as a potentially contaminated body fluid especially when counseling a health care worker after an exposure. HIV has been identified in peritoneal dialysate fluid, which should also be handled as a contaminated body fluid [77].

Kidney Transplantation

HIV infection should no longer be considered a contraindication to kidney transplantation. A relatively large prospective, nonrandomized trial of kidney transplantation in HIV-infected candidates demonstrated that HIV-infected kidney transplant recipients have patient and graft survival rates that are comparable to other high risk populations [68]. Patient survival rates at 1 year and 3 years were $94.6 \pm 2.0\%$ and $88.2 \pm 3.8\%$ (±SD), respectively, and the corresponding mean graft-survival rates were 90.4% and 73.7%. However, acute rejection episodes occurred at higher than expected rates, and long-term follow-up data are needed to determine the consequences of acute rejection. $CD4^+$ T cell counts and HIV RNA levels remained stable despite the complicated drug interactions between antiretroviral therapy and immunosuppressant medications, and this study reported few HIV-associated complications [68].

More information can be found about this National Institutes of Health sponsored ongoing study of kidney and liver transplantation at http://www.hivtransplant.com. The study is closed to new patients but many centers are now offering kidney transplants to HIV patients meeting the criteria. Inclusion criteria for the trial included $CD4^+$ T cell count ≥ 200 per mm^3 in adults and undetectable HIV RNA viral load. Patients requiring renal replacement therapy should be referred for kidney transplant. Patients not on dialysis but whose eGFR rate is <25 mL/min/1.73 m^2 should be referred for evaluation, although patients cannot start to accumulate time on the waiting list until their eGFR is <20 mL/min/1.73 m^2.

HBV and HCV Associated Kidney Disease

Similar to HIV, only universal body substance precautions are necessary among patients with HCV infections requiring hemodialysis. However, patients with active HBV infection are considered at a higher infectious risk. Care of these hemodialysis patients with active HBV infection require special precautions which include the following: (1) Isolation of HBsAg positive patients in a designated separate hemodialysis room along with dedicated machines, equipment, instruments, supplies, and medications, (2) dedicated staff (staff should not care for susceptible patients at the same time), and (3) dialyzers should not be reused on HBsAg positive patients [78].

The previously mentioned KDIGO clinical practice guidelines for HCV related chronic kidney disease recommend monotherapy with standard interferon for HCV-infected dialysis patients who are transplant candidates [64]. This recommendation is based on observations that interferon-treated dialysis patients have better clinical outcomes with subsequent kidney transplantation [79, 80].

Case Discussion

The patient's presentation is not typical of HIVAN and the atypical features include the patient's white race, significant hypertension and edema, and the presence of hematuria with dysmorphic red blood cells. Given the lack of specificity of serologic tests in HIV infection, the patient's atypical presentation, and his coinfection with HCV and HBV, a kidney biopsy was crucial in making the correct diagnosis. The patient underwent a kidney biopsy which revealed membranoproliferative glomerulonephritis. Although HCV is the classic association with membranoproliferative glomerulonephritis, this patient was also HBsAg positive and HBeAg positive with a negative HCV viral load. The decision was made to start HIV antiretroviral therapy with a regimen including lamuvidine which has activity against HBV. The patient responded well to his antiretroviral therapy with an undetectable HIV viral load after 3 months and conversion to negative HBAg and undetectable HBV DNA. His proteinuria improved to <500 mg per day and his creatinine remained stable in the 1.5 mg/dL range.

Key Points

1. HIV and Kidney Disease
   (a) HIVAN (Collapsing Focal Segmental Glomerulosclerosis) is predominately seen in African American patients with HIV infection.
   (b) In addition to HIVAN, a large number of other renal lesions have been reported in patients with HIV and Kidney Disease (Table 47.1).
   (c) Treatment of HIVAN consists of antiviral therapy and ACE-inhibitors or ARB's.
2. HCV and Kidney Disease
   (a) Membranoproliferative glomerulonephritis with or without the presence of circulating cryoglobulins is the characteristic lesion associated with chronic HCV infection.
   (b) The presence of HCV infection is a risk factor for progressive kidney disease irrespective of the cause of the kidney disease.
   (c) Remission of HCV with antiviral therapy is associated with a reduction in proteinuria.
3. HBV and Kidney Disease
   (a) HBV related membranous is mostly seen in children in HBV endemic areas.
   (b) As seen in other virus related kidney disease, spontaneous remission of HBV or in response to treatment is usually accompanied by a reduction in the degree of proteinuria.

References

1. Berns JS, Bloom RD. Viral nephropathies: core curriculum 2008. Am J Kidney Dis. 2008;52:370–81.
2. Ferluga D, Vizjak A. Hantavirus nephropathy. J Am Soc Nephrol. 2008;19:1653–8.
3. Maslo C, Peraldi MN, Desenclos JC, et al. Thrombotic microangiopathy and cytomegalovirus disease in patients infected with human immunodeficiency virus. Clin Infect Dis. 1997;24:350–5.
4. Peters CJ, Simpson GL, Levy H. Spectrum of hantavirus infection: hemorrhagic fever with renal syndrome

and hantavirus pulmonary syndrome. Annu Rev Med. 1999;50:531–45.

5. Hirsch HH. Polyomavirus BK nephropathy: a (re-) emerging complication in renal transplantation. Am J Transplant. 2002;2:25–30.
6. Roling J, Schmid H, Fischereder M, Draenert R, Goebel FD. HIV-associated renal diseases and highly active antiretroviral therapy-induced nephropathy. Clin Infect Dis. 2006;42:1488–95.
7. Waldman M, Marshall V, Whitby D, Kopp JB. Viruses and kidney disease: beyond HIV. Semin Nephrol. 2008;28:595–607.
8. Chacko EC, Surrun SK, Mubarack Sani TP, Pappachan JM. Chronic viral hepatitis and chronic kidney disease. Postgrad Med J. 2010;86:486–92.
9. Carbone L, D'Agati V, Cheng JT, Appel GB. Course and prognosis of human immunodeficiency virus-associated nephropathy. Am J Med. 1989;87:389–95.
10. Laurinavicius A, Hurwitz S, Rennke HG. Collapsing glomerulopathy in HIV and non-HIV patients: a clinicopathological and follow-up study. Kidney Int. 1999;56:2203–13.
11. Rao TK, Filippone EJ, Nicastri AD, et al. Associated focal and segmental glomerulosclerosis in the acquired immunodeficiency syndrome. N Engl J Med. 1984;310: 669–73.
12. US Renal Data System. Annual data report. 2011. National Institute of Diabetes and Digestive and Kidney Diseases. http://www.usrds.org.
13. Szczech LA, Gupta SK, Habash R, et al. The clinical epidemiology and course of the spectrum of renal diseases associated with HIV infection. Kidney Int. 2004;66:1145–52.
14. Haas M, Kaul S, Eustace JA. HIV-associated immune complex glomerulonephritis with "lupus-like" features: a clinicopathologic study of 14 cases. Kidney Int. 2005;67:1381–90.
15. Ahuja TS, Borucki M, Funtanilla M, Shahinian V, Hollander M, Rajaraman S. Is the prevalence of HIV-associated nephropathy decreasing? Am J Nephrol. 1999;19:655–9.
16. Shahinian V, Rajaraman S, Borucki M, Grady J, Hollander WM, Ahuja TS. Prevalence of HIV-associated nephropathy in autopsies of HIV-infected patients. Am J Kidney Dis. 2000;35:884–8.
17. Rodriguez RA, Mendelson M, O'Hare AM, Hsu LC, Schoenfeld P. Determinants of survival among HIV-infected chronic dialysis patients. J Am Soc Nephrol. 2003;14:1307–13.
18. Choi AI, Rodriguez RA, Bacchetti P, Bertenthal D, Volberding PA, O'Hare AM. Racial differences in end-stage renal disease rates in HIV infection versus diabetes. J Am Soc Nephrol. 2007;18: 2968–74.
19. Han TM, Naicker S, Ramdial PK, Assounga AG. A cross-sectional study of HIV-seropositive patients with varying degrees of proteinuria in South Africa. Kidney Int. 2006;69:2243–50.
20. Armstrong GL, Wasley A, Simard EP, McQuillan GM, Kuhnert WL, Alter MJ. The prevalence of hepatitis C virus infection in the United States, 1999 through 2002. Ann Intern Med. 2006;144:705–14.
21. McGuire BM, Julian BA, Bynon Jr JS, et al. Brief communication: glomerulonephritis in patients with hepatitis C cirrhosis undergoing liver transplantation. Ann Intern Med. 2006;144:735–41.
22. Arase Y, Ikeda K, Murashima N, et al. Glomerulonephritis in autopsy cases with hepatitis C virus infection. Intern Med. 1998;37:836–40.
23. di Barbiano BG, Genderini A, Vago L, Parravicini C, Bertoli S, Landriani N. Absence of HIV antigens in renal tissue from patients with HIV-associated nephropathy. Nephrol Dial Transplant. 1990;5:489–92.
24. Kimmel PL, Ferreira-Centeno A, Farkas-Szallasi T, Abraham AA, Garrett CT. Viral DNA in microdissected renal biopsy tissue from HIV infected patients with nephrotic syndrome. Kidney Int. 1993;43:1347–52.
25. Kopp JB, Klotman ME, Adler SH, et al. Progressive glomerulosclerosis and enhanced renal accumulation of basement membrane components in mice transgenic for human immunodeficiency virus type 1 genes. Proc Natl Acad Sci USA. 1992;89:1577–81.
26. Rosenstiel P, Gharavi A, D'Agati V, Klotman P. Transgenic and infectious animal models of HIV-associated nephropathy. J Am Soc Nephrol. 2009;20: 2296–304.
27. Bruggeman LA, Dikman S, Meng C, Quaggin SE, Coffman TM, Klotman PE. Nephropathy in human immunodeficiency virus-1 transgenic mice is due to renal transgene expression. J Clin Invest. 1997;100: 84–92.
28. Bruggeman LA, Ross MD, Tanji N, et al. Renal epithelium is a previously unrecognized site of HIV-1 infection 3. J Am Soc Nephrol. 2000;11:2079–87.
29. Winston JA, Bruggeman LA, Ross MD, et al. Nephropathy and establishment of a renal reservoir of HIV type 1 during primary infection. N Engl J Med. 2001;344:1979–84.
30. Marras D, Bruggeman LA, Gao F, et al. Replication and compartmentalization of HIV-1 in kidney epithelium of patients with HIV-associated nephropathy. Nat Med. 2002;8:522–6.
31. Ohba S, Kimura K, Mise N, et al. Differential localization of s and e antigens in hepatitis B virus-associated glomerulonephritis. Clin Nephrol. 1997;48: 44–7.
32. Cao Y, Zhang Y, Wang S, Zou W. Detection of the hepatitis C virus antigen in kidney tissue from infected patients with various glomerulonephritis. Nephrol Dial Transplant. 2009;24:2745–51.
33. Sansonno D, Gesualdo L, Manno C, Schena FP, Dammacco F. Hepatitis C virus-related proteins in kidney tissue from hepatitis C virus-infected patients with cryoglobulinemic membranoproliferative glomerulonephritis. Hepatology. 1997;25:1237–44.
34. Winston JA, Klotman ME, Klotman PE. HIV-associated nephropathy is a late, not early, manifestation of HIV-1 infection. Kidney Int. 1999;55:1036–40.
35. Perinbasekar S, Brod-Miller C, Mattana J. Absence of edema in HIV-infected patients with end-stage renal

disease. J Acquir Immune Defic Syndr Hum Retrovirol. 1996;13:368–73.
36. Guardia JA, Ortiz-Butcher C, Bourgoignie JJ. Oncotic pressure and edema formation in hypoalbuminemic HIV-infected patients with proteinuria. Am J Kidney Dis. 1997;30:822–8.
37. Hernandez GT, Critchfield JM, Rodriguez RA. Interpretation of serologic tests in an HIV-infected patient with kidney disease. Nat Clin Pract Nephrol. 2006;2:708–12.
38. Lai KN, Li PK, Lui SF, et al. Membranous nephropathy related to hepatitis B virus in adults. N Engl J Med. 1991;324:1457–63.
39. Galossi A, Guarisco R, Bellis L, Puoti C. Extrahepatic manifestations of chronic HCV infection. J Gastrointestin Liver Dis. 2007;16:65–73.
40. Iannuzzella F, Vaglio A, Garini G. Management of hepatitis C virus-related mixed cryoglobulinemia. Am J Med. 2010;123:400–8.
41. Daghestani L, Pomeroy C. Renal manifestations of hepatitis C infection. Am J Med. 1999;106:347–54.
42. Tsui JI, Vittinghoff E, Shlipak MG, et al. Association of hepatitis C seropositivity with increased risk for developing end-stage renal disease. Arch Intern Med. 2007;167:1271–6.
43. Bonnet F, Pineau JJ, Taupin JL, et al. Prevalence of cryoglobulinemia and serological markers of autoimmunity in human immunodeficiency virus infected individuals: a cross-sectional study of 97 patients. J Rheumatol. 2003;30:2005–10.
44. Klaassen RJ, Goldschmeding R, Dolman KM, et al. Anti-neutrophil cytoplasmic autoantibodies in patients with symptomatic HIV infection. Clin Exp Immunol. 1992;87:24–30.
45. Ng VL. B-lymphocytes and autoantibody profiles in HIV disease. Clin Rev Allergy Immunol. 1996;14:367–84.
46. Savige JA, Chang L, Horn S, Crowe SM. Anti-nuclear, anti-neutrophil cytoplasmic and anti-glomerular basement membrane antibodies in HIV-infected individuals. Autoimmunity. 1994;18:205–11.
47. Cohen AH, Nast CC. HIV-associated nephropathy. A unique combined glomerular, tubular, and interstitial lesion. Mod Pathol. 1988;1:87–97.
48. Chander P, Soni A, Suri A, Bhagwat R, Yoo J, Treser G. Renal ultrastructural markers in AIDS-associated nephropathy. Am J Pathol. 1987;126:513–26.
49. Meyers CM, Seeff LB, Stehman-Breen CO, Hoofnagle JH. Hepatitis C and renal disease: an update. Am J Kidney Dis. 2003;42:631–57.
50. El-Sadr WM, Grund B, Neuhaus J, et al. Risk for opportunistic disease and death after reinitiating continuous antiretroviral therapy in patients with HIV previously receiving episodic therapy: a randomized trial. Ann Intern Med. 2008;149:289–99.
51. El-Sadr WM, Lundgren JD, Neaton JD, et al. CD4+ count-guided interruption of antiretroviral treatment. N Engl J Med. 2006;355:2283–96.
52. Atta MG, Gallant JE, Rahman MH, et al. Antiretroviral therapy in the treatment of HIV-associated nephropathy. Nephrol Dial Transplant. 2006;21:2809–13.
53. Szczech LA, Edwards LJ, Sanders LL, et al. Protease inhibitors are associated with a slowed progression of HIV-related renal diseases. Clin Nephrol. 2002;57: 336–41.
54. Bige N, Lanternier F, Viard JP, et al. Presentation of HIV-associated nephropathy and outcome in HAART-treated patients. Nephrol Dial Transplant. 2011.
55. Gupta SK, Eustace JA, Winston JA, et al. Guidelines for the management of chronic kidney disease in HIV-infected patients: recommendations of the HIV Medicine Association of the Infectious Diseases Society of America. Clin Infect Dis. 2005;40:1559–85.
56. Ideura H, Hiromura K, Hiramatsu N, et al. Angiotensin II provokes podocyte injury in murine model of HIV-associated nephropathy. Am J Physiol Renal Physiol. 2007;293:F1214–21.
57. Kimmel PL, Mishkin GJ, Umana WO. Captopril and renal survival in patients with human immunodeficiency virus nephropathy. Am J Kidney Dis. 1996;28:202–8.
58. Wei A, Burns GC, Williams BA, Mohammed NB, Visintainer P, Sivak SL. Long-term renal survival in HIV-associated nephropathy with angiotensin-converting enzyme inhibition. Kidney Int. 2003; 64:1462–71.
59. Briggs WA, Tanawattanacharoen S, Choi MJ, Scheel Jr PJ, Nadasdy T, Racusen L. Clinicopathologic correlates of prednisone treatment of human immunodeficiency virus-associated nephropathy. Am J Kidney Dis. 1996;28:618–21.
60. Eustace JA, Nuermberger E, Choi M, Scheel Jr PJ, Moore R, Briggs WA. Cohort study of the treatment of severe HIV-associated nephropathy with corticosteroids. Kidney Int. 2000;58:1253–60.
61. Smith MC, Austen JL, Carey JT, et al. Prednisone improves renal function and proteinuria in human immunodeficiency virus-associated nephropathy. Am J Med. 1996;101:41–8.
62. Tang S, Lai FM, Lui YH, et al. Lamivudine in hepatitis B-associated membranous nephropathy. Kidney Int. 2005;68:1750–8.
63. Conjeevaram HS, Hoofnagle JH, Austin HA, Park Y, Fried MW, Di Bisceglie AM. Long-term outcome of hepatitis B virus-related glomerulonephritis after therapy with interferon alfa. Gastroenterology. 1995;109:540–6.
64. Covic A, Abramowicz D, Bruchfeld A, et al. Endorsement of the kidney disease improving global outcomes (KDIGO) hepatitis C guidelines: a European Renal Best Practice (ERBP) position statement. Nephrol Dial Transplant. 2009;24:719–27.
65. Rendina M, Schena A, Castellaneta NM, et al. The treatment of chronic hepatitis C with peginterferon alfa-2a (40 kDa) plus ribavirin in haemodialysed patients awaiting renal transplant. J Hepatol. 2007;46:768–74.
66. Ahuja TS, Grady J, Khan S. Changing trends in the survival of dialysis patients with human immunodeficiency virus in the United States. J Am Soc Nephrol. 2002;13:1889–93.
67. Tourret J, Tostivint I, du Montcel ST, et al. Outcome and prognosis factors in HIV-infected hemodialysis patients. Clin J Am Soc Nephrol. 2006;1:1241–7.

68. Stock PG, Barin B, Murphy B, et al. Outcomes of kidney transplantation in HIV-infected recipients. N Engl J Med. 2010;363:2004–14.
69. Curi MA, Pappas PJ, Silva Jr MB, et al. Hemodialysis access: influence of the human immunodeficiency virus on patency and infection rates. J Vasc Surg. 1999;29:608–16.
70. Obialo CI, Robinson T, Brathwaite M. Hemodialysis vascular access: variable thrombus-free survival in three subpopulations of black patients. Am J Kidney Dis. 1998;31:250–6.
71. Ahuja TS, Collinge N, Grady J, Khan S. Is dialysis modality a factor in survival of patients with ESRD and HIV-associated nephropathy? Am J Kidney Dis. 2003;41:1060–4.
72. Kimmel PL, Umana WO, Simmens SJ, Watson J, Bosch JP. Continuous ambulatory peritoneal dialysis and survival of HIV infected patients with end-stage renal disease. Kidney Int. 1993;44:373–8.
73. Tebben JA, Rigsby MO, Selwyn PA, Brennan N, Kliger A, Finkelstein FO. Outcome of HIV infected patients on continuous ambulatory peritoneal dialysis. Kidney Int. 1993;44:191–8.
74. Cacoub P, Renou C, Rosenthal E, et al. Extrahepatic manifestations associated with hepatitis C virus infection. A prospective multicenter study of 321 patients. The GERMIVIC. Groupe d'Etude et de Recherche en Medecine Interne et Maladies Infectieuses sur le Virus de l'Hepatite C. Medicine (Baltimore). 2000;79: 47–56.
75. Soma J, Saito T, Taguma Y, et al. High prevalence and adverse effect of hepatitis C virus infection in type II diabetic-related nephropathy. J Am Soc Nephrol. 2000;11:690–9.
76. Ahuja TS, Niaz N, Velasco A, Watts III B, Paar D. Effect of hemodialysis and antiretroviral therapy on plasma viral load in HIV-1 infected hemodialysis patients. Clin Nephrol. 1999;51:40–4.
77. Farzadegan H, Ford D, Malan M, Masters B, Scheel Jr PJ. HIV-1 survival kinetics in peritoneal dialysis effluent. Kidney Int. 1996;50:1659–62.
78. Recommendations for preventing transmission of infections among chronic hemodialysis patients. MMWR Recomm Rep. 2001; 50: 1–43.
79. Campistol JM, Esforzado N, Martinez J, et al. Efficacy and tolerance of interferon-alpha(2b) in the treatment of chronic hepatitis C virus infection in haemodialysis patients. Pre- and post-renal transplantation assessment. Nephrol Dial Transplant. 1999; 14:2704–9.
80. Gordon CE, Uhlig K, Lau J, Schmid CH, Levey AS, Wong JB. Interferon treatment in hemodialysis patients with chronic hepatitis C virus infection: a systematic review of the literature and meta-analysis of treatment efficacy and harms. Am J Kidney Dis. 2008;51:263–77.

48 Pregnancy-Associated Kidney Injury

A. Eric Anderson and Sophia M. Rothberger Lannon

Case 1

A 23-year-old G1P0000 without prior past medical history is 31 weeks pregnant with prenatal care presents with complaints of worsening leg and face swelling for the past 2 days now seeks care because of headache, diarrhea, nausea, and vomiting. On exam she is found to have a blood pressure of 120/86, edema, and brisk deep tendon reflexes. Laboratory testing revealed hemoglobin 11.3 g/dl, platelet count 141,000/μl white blood count 18,000/μl, creatinine 1.1 mg/dl, aspartate aminotransferases (AST) 65 U/l, lactate dehydrogenase (LDH) 400 U/l, total bilirubin 1.1 mg/dl, prothrombin time (PT) 14.7 s, ammonia of 90 mcg/dl, blood glucose 139 mg/dl, calcium 7.3 mg/dl, and uric acid of 6.0 mg/dl. The urinalysis demonstrated WBC's 3–5/hpf, RBC's 3–5/hpf—non-dysmorphic, renal tubular epithelial cells were seen and a urine protein to creatinine ratio of 2. One day after hospitalization the patient's blood pressure was 145/87 with a similar blood pressure 6 h later.

Case 2

A 38-year-old G4P2022 at 32 weeks gestational age who presents to clinic for her scheduled prenatal visit, and her blood pressure is found to be 147/92. Urine dip was negative for protein. She returned the following day with a 24 h urine collection which was negative for proteinuria again and her blood pressure was 156/94. She denied headache, vision changes, abdominal pain, or peripheral edema. Laboratory testing revealed hemoglobin 10 g/dl, platelet count 79,000, white blood count 13,270, creatinine 1.9 mg/dl, AST 92 U/l, and alanine aminotransferases (ALT) 120 U/l, and LDH of 672 U/l. A peripheral smear was significant for moderate shistocytes. The patient was admitted and given antenatal corticosteroids for fetal lung development in anticipation of preterm delivery. On hospital day 3, the patient developed severe right upper quadrant (RUQ) pain. Laboratory values were repeated and revealed hemoglobin 10.5 g/dl platelet count 85,000, white blood count 11,360, creatinine 1.8 mg/dl, AST 94, and ALT 98.

Introduction

Kidney injury in pregnancy is not a rare phenomenon. However, kidney injury reaching the level to warrant nephrology involvement is. The cases of patients with preexisting kidney disease prior to pregnancy differs in the differential diagnosis

A.E. Anderson, M.D. (✉)
Outpatient, General Nephrology Clinic, Department of Medicine, University of Washington Medical Center, 1959 NE Pacific St., Seattle, WA 98195, USA
e-mail: iamerica@u.washington.edu

S.M.R. Lannon, M.D., M.P.H.
Department of Obstetrics & Gynecology, University of Washington, Seattle, WA 98195, USA

E.V. Lerma and M. Rosner (eds.), *Clinical Decisions in Nephrology, Hypertension and Kidney Transplantation*, DOI 10.1007/978-1-4614-4454-1_48,

from new onset kidney disease that develops because of pregnancy. The focus of this chapter is to review the evaluation of new onset kidney injury as a result of pregnancy. This chapter does not attempt to review the newly diagnosed patient with kidney disease that may be discovered during pregnancy, that in and of itself is not thought related to pregnancy. When kidney involvement occurs, from proteinuria alone to elevation of creatinine, pathologic systemic changes related to the fetal-placenta interaction provokes the obstetric provider to heighten their level of concern for the maturing fetus and the welfare of the mother. While the diagnosis of preeclampsia is easily the first consideration given how common it is, a broaden differential is employed. Before doing so, a discussion of kidney physiology during pregnancy is prudent as well as a review of the diagnostic tools used in kidney function assessment during pregnancy.

Kidney-Related Physiology During Pregnancy

Glomerular filtration rate (GFR) increases during pregnancy beginning in the first trimester after 6 weeks, the GFR increases [1]. This is before there is an increased placental blood supply or a decreased serum albumin and hence a lower glomerular oncotic capillary pressure that can explain this consequence. GFR continues to increase throughout pregnancy and a lower serum creatinine is evidence of this. A rise in serum creatinine will raise the suspicion of potentially dire systemic concerns. There are other physiologic perturbations that have accompanying laboratory changes seen during normal pregnancy that are shown in Table 48.1. This is not intended to be all-inclusive but present labs more germane to this review.

Anatomic changes in ureteral contraction and stasis from the gravid uterus will cause an anatomic anomaly that is normal in pregnancy with the ultrasound of the kidneys revealing hydronephrosis.

The plasma volume, cardiac output (CO), and GFR increase by 30–50% during pregnancy [1]. Additionally, the mean arterial pressure (MAP) decreases during pregnancy. This is related to the physics of an increased diversion of plasma volume through the uterus an organ that is in parallel with the other organs, so systemic vascular resistance (SVR) decreases. These hemodynamic changes of lower MAP, higher CO, and lower SVR occur beginning at 6 weeks [1]. Other reasons for decreased SVR and blood pressure are attributed to hormones such as relaxin.

Table 48.1 Laboratory changes in normal pregnancy

	First trimester	Third trimester
Albumin	↓	↓
Fibrinogen	↑	↑
PT	Normal [2]	Normal [2]
AST/ALT	Normal or slight ↓	Normal or slight ↓
Total bilirubin	Normal or slight ↓	Normal or slight ↓
Creatinine	↓	↓
Sodium	↓	↓
Uric acid	↓	Normal or slight ↓
GFR	↑	↑

Adapted from Creasy RK, Resnik R et al. Maternal-fetal medicine: principles and practice. 6th ed. Philadelphia, PA: Saunders/Elsevier; 2009

Kidney Function Testing

Practically assessing GFR during pregnancy has all the flaws as in the non-obstetric realm but has the added nuisances of increased GFR and urinary stasis. The best test was discerned by comparing inulin versus 24 h creatinine clearance as well as using the modification of diet in renal disease (MDRD) formula in healthy pregnant women and women with preeclampsia or chronic kidney disease (CKD) [3]. In healthy pregnant women the 24 h creatinine clearance was better than the MDRD by 40 cc/min. In women with preeclampsia or prior CKD the MDRD underestimated the GFR in both by 25 cc/min. Because the GFRs were >60 the MDRD formula loses its' integrity in this population. Following serum creatinines is certainly useful, but the absence of changes in creatinine may not be indicative of true GFR changes and so 24 h urine collections may be instructive.

Estimating proteinuria during pregnancy also has its limitations as in the non-obstetric world. If one assumes the urine protein to creatinine ratio (PCR) is expected to hold in pregnancy, it is useful for quantification for diagnosis of preeclampsia and monitor preexisting kidney disease. Urine dipsticks routinely have high rates of false positives and negatives compared to 24 h urines and do not take into consideration the specific gravity in the guidelines when assessing proteinuria such as in preeclampsia. Most nephrologists do not speak in terms of urine protein dipsticks. However, urinary stasis complicates the utility of the urine PCR. There is sufficient data in the literature that demonstrates that the spot urine PCR has been shown to correlate well with 24 h urine collections [4, 5]. Certainly, if the cutoff value is questionable, a 24 h urine collection for creatinine and protein should be done.

Acute Kidney Disease Resulting from Pregnancy

The evaluation schema for this differential diagnosis is similar to the nonpregnant patient but with diagnoses that are only related to the pregnant condition (Table 48.2). Most kidney injury associated with increased creatinine is related to hypovolemia or hemorrhage. Most kidney injury with proteinuria is related to preeclampsia. With both of these presentations, nephrology involvement is rare. The obstetric provider will manage these scenarios without the need for specialized consultation. Additionally, the nephrologist may not be as aware of the other obstetric pathologic diseases that involve the kidney.

Table 48.2 Pregnancy-associated kidney injury

Prerenal
Anatomic—none
Physiologic
Hyperemesis gravidarium
Obstetrical hemorrhage
Abruptio placentae
Postpartum
Liver Failure
AFLP
Intrahepatic cholestasis
Viral hepatitis
Cardiomyopathy
Milk alkali syndrome
Post-renal
Gravid uterus and ureteral obstruction
Postpartum surgical clips of ureters
Nephrolithiasis
Intrinsic
Glomerular
Nephrotic
Preeclampsia/HEELP
Nephritic
PIGN
Tubular—Acute tubular necrosis
Ischemic
Cortical necrosis
Protracted volume depletion
Sepsis/SIRS
Septic abortion
Puerperal
Chorioamionitis
Endometritis
Pyelonephritis
Toxins
Endogenous
Rhabdomyolysis
Cocaine
Methamphetamine
Baking soda
CPT deficiency
Uric Acid
Sickle cell disease/trait
Exogenous
Tocolytics
NSAIDS
Interstitial nephritis
Vascular
TTP/HUS

Abbreviations: *AFLP* acute fatty liver of pregnancy, *HELLP* hemolysis elevated liver enzymes low platelets, *PIGN* post-infectious glomerular nephritis, *SIRS* systemic inflammatory response syndrome, *CPT* carnitine palmitoyl transferase, *TTP/HUS* thrombotic thrombocytopenia purpura/hemolytic uremic syndrome

Prerenal

Hyperemesis Gravidarium

Prerenal causes of kidney disease during pregnancy are mainly of the physiologic type as opposed to anatomical causes, i.e. renal artery stenosis. Prerenal kidney disease is defined as reversible hypoperfusion where the kidney injury recovers after the underlying problem is reversed within 24–48 h. Examples of this would be volume resuscitation in the setting of hyperemesis gravidarium (HG). HG is severe nausea and vomiting beginning ≤12 weeks of gestation, ketonuria, and >5% loss of pre-pregnancy body weight without a known cause. It tends to improve in the later part of pregnancy but may persist up until delivery. The etiology of this is not well elucidated. Patients develop severe volume depletion potentially leading to kidney injury. An increase in transaminases is seen in up to 50% of cases. They are usually elevated from 2 to 10 times the upper limit of normal.

Obstetrical Hemorrhage

Obstetrical hemorrhage occurs when there is a blood loss of greater than 500 ml with vaginal delivery or 1,000 ml with cesarean delivery. Any number of pregnancy diagnoses can cause an obstetrical hemorrhage, most commonly uterine pathology such as uterine atony, inappropriate placental separation, and placental retention. Obstetrical hemorrhage can occur during pregnancy, immediately postpartum or delayed postpartum. Severe cases can cause hemorrhagic shock, thus leading to renal hypoperfusion and oligouria. Identifying and correcting the source of bleeding is the mainstay of treatment, as is aggressive replacement of blood products. These strategies will also correct renal function unless the bleeding is protracted and then the patient may have superimposed acute tubular necrosis (ATN).

Acute Fatty Liver of Pregnancy

Acute fatty liver of pregnancy (AFLP) is a rare but potentially fatal complication of the third trimester occurring from 1 in 10,000 to 20,000 pregnancies [6]. The median gestation is 36 weeks reportedly occurring between 22 and 40 weeks. The classic presentation of this rare disease is hypoglycemia, transaminitis, elevated coagulation studies, hypofibrinogenemia, kidney injury, and fatty infiltration of the liver. However, the exclusion of these signs does not rule out the diagnosis. The largest series of AFLP studied to date came from a population of over 1.1 million deliveries in the United Kingdom Obstetric Surveillance System Study between 2005 and 2006 [6]. Providers diagnosed only 61 women with AFLP, 90% of which were retrospectively confirmed by the authors using the previously described Swansea criteria [7] (see Table 48.3). Of the 57 women meeting the criteria for the diagnosis of AFLP, 1 woman died; and of the 67 infants, there were 7 deaths, yielding a perinatal mortality rate of 104 per 1,000 births.

Table 48.3 Criteria for diagnosis of AFLP [6, 7]

Six or more of the following features in the absence of another explanation
Vomiting
Abdominal pain
Polydipsia/polyuria
Encephalopathy
Elevated bilirubin (>0.8 mg/dl)
Hypoglycemia (72 mg/dl)
Elevated urate (5.7 mg/dl)
Leucocytosis (11,000/μl)
Ascites or bright liver on ultrasound scan
Elevated transaminases (AST or ALT > 42 U/l)
Elevated ammonia (>80)
Renal impairment (>1.7 mg/dl)
Coagulopathy (PT > 14 s or aPTT > 34 s)
Microvesicular steatosis on biopsy

Liver ultrasound is not typically very helpful when performed, and in the aforementioned study showed evidence of disease by ascites or echogenicity in only 27% of women. Liver biopsies are seldom performed, as the maternal condition is typically too unstable. However, autopsies have shown swollen pale hepatocytes with central nuclei and positive fat staining.

The pathogenesis of AFLP has been better elucidated. There is a subset of AFLP that has been linked to long-chain 3-hydorxyacyl-coenzyme A dehydrogenase (LCHAD) deficiency, a transport protein for long-chain fatty acids [8]. This is an autosomal recessively inherited condition that results in the inability of the fetus to transport free fatty acids (FFA) into the liver mitochondria, thereby preventing its metabolism. Fetuses homozygous for LCHAD deficiency return high levels of FFA to maternal circulation, yielding excess levels of FFA. High levels of FFA in the already mildly comprised maternal heterozygous liver puts a strain on maternal hepatic activity, resulting in AFLP. Infants with LCHAD deficiency are commonly born to mothers diagnosed with AFLP [8].

Consequences of fat deposition in the maternal liver include inadequate fibrinogen synthesis and impeded bilirubin conjugation. Coagulation factor synthesis may decrease as fat deposits in the liver. Because the fetus is unable to oxidize the long-chain fatty acids, the fetal glucose demand increases and the mother may become hypoglycemic. Hypoglycemia is not required for the diagnosis of AFLP and excluding it in the setting of euglycemia may delay the diagnosis. Our case #1 presented with complaints of nausea and vomiting and meets six of the diagnostic criteria for AFLP: elevated AST, bilirubin, PT, WBC, ammonia, and uric acid level. Management of such patients requires hospitalization, close monitoring, and urgent delivery. However, because the signs and symptoms are nonspecific, other etiologies must be entertained.

The resulting elevated creatinine and renal injury is not well understood, because kidney biopsies are rarely performed in the setting of coagulopathy and impending delivery (similar to reason liver biopsies are not performed). However, severe liver dysfunction frequently results in renal hypoperfusion and thus ATN.

Intrahepatic Cholestasis of Pregnancy

Intrahepatic cholestasis of pregnancy (ICP) is a disease of unknown etiology that occurs in the second and third trimester with pruritus alone or accompanied by icterus. Symptoms of liver dysfunction are uncommon. Serum bilirubin may be elevated but usually less than 5 mg/dl and alkaline phosphatase may be increased. Serum aminotransferases are also elevated and may reach values tenfold normal [9]. Severe cholestasis may lead to steatorrhea and loss of fat soluble vitamins with vitamin K deficiency and prolonged PT. Decreased creatinine clearance with increased serum creatinines along with decreased urine output and decreased NH_4^+ urinary excretion invoke kidney involvement as well [10]. The maternal outlook is excellent but fetal prematurity is of concern and demise occurs rarely. It is unlikely our patient in case #1 had this without the symptom of pruritus, elevation of bilirubin, and with such an elevated creatinine, which is atypical for ICP. The diagnosis, if entertained, would require an 8-h fast with elevated bile acids.

Viral Hepatitis

Acute viral hepatitis with fulminant hepatic failure associated with high viral loads of Hepatitis E in developing countries is associated with poor pregnancy outcomes including intrauterine demise and maternal death particularly in the third trimester [11]. Kidney involvement was not discussed by this aforementioned paper, but likely occurs. The pathogenesis of kidney failure is likely due to systemic and intrarenal hemodynamic changes leading to hepatorenal syndrome (HRS), but ATN could also occur.

Herpes simplex virus (HSV) is a rare but commonly fatal condition with mortality in untreated individuals >80% [12]. It is most common in the third trimester of pregnancy. HSV causing hepatitis occurred in 132 patients noted in the literature from 1969 to 2006 [12]. Twenty three percent of the patients were pregnant. The majority of these patients, 98%, had fever, 97% developed coagulopathy, 80% encephalopathy, and acute kidney injury in 65%. Herpetic rash was detected in only 44% of patients, of which 61% were mucocutaneous and 39% were disseminated. Liver transaminases in HSV hepatitis generally increase 100 to 1,000-fold above normal [12]. It is most common in the third trimester of pregnancy [13]. When suspected, polymerase chain reaction (PCR) testing is done and prophylactic treatment is begun with parenteral acyclovir while awaiting the results. Kidney biopsies are prohibitive in these setting with fulminant liver failure so the kidney pathogenesis is speculative. The kidney pathology is presumptive in these cases being either prerenal or ATN.

Cardiomyopathy

Peripartum cardiomyopathy is defined as a condition that occurs in the last gestational month and first 5 months after delivery in the absence of another identifiable cause of heart failure and absence of recognizable heart disease prior to the last month of pregnancy. Also, left ventricular systolic dysfunction demonstrated by classic echocardiographic criteria, such as depressed shortening fraction or ejection fraction below 45% is present [14, 15]. Undiagnosed heart failure can lead to prerenal disease in pregnancy, as it does in the nonpregnant state.

Milk Alkali Syndrome

Pregnant women have an increased susceptibility to developing milk/calcium alkali syndrome if there is hyperemesis causing volume depletion and enhanced kidney absorption of calcium in that setting [16]. The need for fetal calcium is satiated by maternal increases in intestinal calcium absorption by twofold, probably through an increase twofold of 1,25-dihydroxyvitamin and vitamin D independent mediated affects along with prolactin and placental lactogen [17]. This renders the mother susceptible to hypercalcemia. With increased use of calcium and vitamin D supplements to treat osteoporosis and when used to treat gastroesophageal reflux (GERD) exacerbated by pregnancy, milk alkali syndrome occurs [18]. GERD is a common problem in pregnancy occurring in 30–56% of all pregnancies and therefore with indiscriminate use of calcium products lead to the syndrome [19]. The kidney injury from hypercalcemia has several mechanisms. It causes afferent arteriolar vasoconstriction and decreases renal blood flow and GFR. Increased calcium binds to calcium-sensitive receptors in the medullary thick ascending limb and inhibits Na-K-2Cl cotransporter and blocks sodium reabsorption leading to volume depletion. Increased calcium in the tubulointerstitium can affect kidney function as well. The treatment is avoidance of calcium and vitamin D, control of emesis and volume resuscitation. Our patient was normocalcemic.

Post-Renal

Gravid Uterus and Ureteral Obstruction

As previously mentioned, hydronephrosis and hydroureter are not uncommon findings in pregnancy. Several factors are thought to contribute to these physiologic changes that most commonly do not lead to renal injury. Progesterone reduces ureteral tone and contractility. Enlarged blood vessels in the pelvis may cause ureteral compression, especially at the pelvic brim. The enlarging uterus displaces the ureters laterally, and on rare occasions can directly compress the ureters. The resulting urinary obstruction is marked by severe abdominal pain and inability to void. Resolution with maternal position changes aids in making the diagnosis. In these severe cases ureteral stents can relieve the ureteral compression, but in case of stent failure, delivery may be required.

Ureters can also be injured during delivery, most commonly during a challenging cesarean delivery. Lacerations of the uterine incision that extend into the lateral lower uterine segments, cervix or vagina are at highest risk for lacerating the ureters. Repair of uterine extensions that are in close proximity to the ureter could inadvertently obstruct them. Women with ureteral injury or obstruction will present with abdominal pain and possibly hematuria. The diagnosis does not require an elevated creatinine or signs of renal failure, as ureteral injury is commonly unilateral. CT scan showing urinary obstruction or urinoma is diagnostic, and this requires surgical correction.

Nephrolithiasis

Nephrolithiasis in pregnancy poses risks to the mother and fetus. Renal colic from ureteral obstruction in pregnancy may induce hypertension, premature labor, preeclampsia and may be associated with urinary-tract infections [20–22]. The incidence is similar to the nonpregnant childbearing women despite hypercalciuria with normal serum calcium levels, hyperuricosuria with normal to low serum uric acid levels and increased urinary citrate, magnesium and glycoproteins which exert a protective effect against stone formation and aggregation [20]. Most symptomatic stone episodes occur during the second or third trimesters when ureteral dilation and compression by the gravid uterus is more likely [20]. The symptoms are similar to the nonpregnant patient with abdominal or flank pain, nausea, vomiting, and hematuria with 42% of these patients having pyuria on urinalysis [23]. The most appropriate first-line test is renal ultrasound and management is conservative if possible, with analgesia and intravenous volume. A majority of the patients, 84%, passed the stones spontaneously during pregnancy [23]. Obstruction of the ureter above or below the level of the pelvic brim with tapering of the ureter to a normal caliber is suggestive of pathologic obstruction [20]. The risk of acute kidney injury is low, given the unilateral presentation.

Intrinsic Kidney Injury

Glomerular: Nephrotic

Preeclampsia and Hemolysis Elevated Liver Enzymes Low Platelets Syndrome

Preeclampsia is a systemic syndrome that occurs in 3–14% of pregnancies worldwide and 5–8% of pregnancies in the USA. It manifests after 20 weeks gestation with new onset hypertension and proteinuria. It is a leading cause of maternal and neonatal morbidity and mortality. Placental anti-angiogenic factors are upregulated and disrupt maternal endothelium damaging target organs; glomerular endotheliosis, cerebral edema, liver injury, and the vasculature of other organs are thereby impacted. Preeclampsia is a spectrum of disease with eclampsia and hemolysis elevated liver enzymes low platelets (HELLP) syndrome on the severe end of it. In pregnancy, preeclampsia is the third leading cause of death after bleeding and infection and accounts for 20% of maternal deaths [24]. Women affected by preeclampsia have a 20% risk of developing cardiac disease years later as well as microalbuminuria [25]. Cardiovascular and cerebrovascular disease double in women with preeclampsia and may be a risk factor for CKD.

Because the pathophysiology of the disease is not well known, diagnosis depends on the presence of clinical signs of disease. Strict criteria for the diagnosis presented in Table 48.4 have been established for clinical consistency. However, it should be noted that the pathophysiological changes of preeclampsia may be present in the absence of hypertension and proteinuria, as in the HELLP syndrome. Note that evidence of systemic vascular involvement without hypertension or proteinuria does not exclude preeclampsia as a diagnosis.

Table 48.4 Preeclampsia

1. New onset of hypertension and proteinuria after 20 weeks gestation • Systolic blood pressure (SBP) ≥ 140 mmHg or diastolic blood pressure (DBP) ≥ 90 mmHg, on two occasions at least 6 h apart
• Proteinuria of 3 g or greater in a 24-h urine specimen
• Preeclampsia before 20 weeks, consider molar pregnancy
2. Severe preeclampsia in addition must have one of the following • Symptoms of central nervous system dysfunction = Blurred vision, scotomata, altered mental status, severe headache
• Symptoms of liver capsule distention = Right upper quadrant or epigastric pain
• Nausea, vomiting
• Hepatocellular injury = Serum transaminase levels ≥ 2× normal
• SBP ≥ 160 mmHg or DBP ≥ 110 mmHg on two occasions at least 6 h apart
• Thrombocytopenia < 100,000 platelets/μl
• Proteinuria ≥ 5g in 24 h
• Oliguria = <500 mL in 24 h
• Severe fetal growth restriction
• Pulmonary edema or cyanosis
• Cerebrovascular accident

Reprinted with permission from ACOG practice bulletin No. 33: diagnosis and management of preeclampsia and eclampsia, Obstet Gynecol 2002;99:159–167

HELLP syndrome is a diagnosis based on clinical findings rather than pathophysiology. The incidence is 1–2 per 1,000 live births and acute renal failure occurs in 4% of these women [26]. The progression of disease and its termination with delivery suggest its relation to preeclampsia. There are degrees to the extent of the laboratory abnormalities seen with HELLP. Extremes of thrombocytopenia, elevated AST, and LDH levels are distinguished by some authorities as complete HELLP with all of the following AST > 70 IU/l, platelets < 100,000, and

LDH>600. Partial HELLP may manifest with milder or incomplete laboratory abnormalities such as AST>40, platelets<150,000, and hemolysis present or absent [7, 26].

The physiologic invasion of placental vascularization into the uterine spiral arteries requires VEGF and TGF-β1 to maintain endothelial health in several tissues, including the kidney and the placenta. During normal pregnancy, vascular homeostasis is maintained by physiologic levels of VEGF and TGF-β1 signaling in the vasculature. In preeclampsia, excess placental secretion of sFLT1 and sENG, two endogenous circulating anti-angiogenic proteins, inhibits VEGF and TGF-β1 signaling. This results in endothelial cell dysfunction, leading to hypertension, proteinuria, and other systemic manifestations.

The most frequent and pronounced renal changes from preeclampsia occur in the glomerulus. The kidney injury is glomerular capillary endothelial cell swelling (endotheliosis) and vacuolization and loss of capillary space with subendothelial deposits of fibrin [27]. Capillary lumen occlusion is thought to render the glomeruli nonfunctional, thus leading to a lower GFR seen in preeclampsia. With increased glomerular damage, there is an increase in the permeability of the glomeruli, likely the cause of proteinuria in preeclampsia. These glomerular changes regress postpartum. Not all patients with preeclampsia have proteinuria that reaches the level of nephrotic syndrome; it depends on the severity. The pathogenesis of preeclampsia is likely multifactorial and is beyond the scope of this review.

The renin–angiotensin system is suspected to play a role in preeclampsia, although research in this area is limited. Plasma renin activity, plasma renin concentration, and angiotensin levels are all decreased in preeclampsia compared to normal pregnancy [28, 29]. Women with preeclampsia are suspected to be more sensitive to angiotensin. Urinary sodium excretion is reduced in preeclampsia and returns to normal postpartum. Although the mechanism of renal changes in preeclampsia are not clear, they could all be explained by decreased renal perfusion.

Preeclampsia should certainly be on the differential diagnosis for case #1. Although her initial blood pressure was below the cut-off for preeclampsia at 120/86, it subsequently increased to 145/87 and remained elevated 6-h later. Her blood pressure in combination with her proteinuria was adequate for the diagnosis of preeclampsia. Hyperreflexia and elevated uric acid are also consistent with the diagnosis of preeclampsia, but these measurements are nonspecific. Measuring SFLT-1 and sENG may have been insightful, but at this time are not standardly performed.

Glomerular: Nephritis

Post-Infectious Glomerular Nephritis

Pregnant women with exposure to children aged 5–7 years are at risk for parvovirus B19 infection during pregnancy [30]. A case report of a patient in the tenth week of pregnancy developed parvovirus B19 IgM positive and 2 weeks later developed hypertension, nephrotic range proteinuria and evidence of pure red cell aplasia. The kidney biopsy revealed diffuse proliferative glomerulonephritis with immunofluorescent and electron microscopic changes consistent with post-infectious glomerulonephritis. The kidney function and blood pressure recovered by the 16th week gestation and the delivery was at term with a healthy infant [31].

Several case reports of pregnant patients developing (PIGN) appear in the literature. The classic findings of antecedent infection with resolution and then development of gross hematuria and the urinalysis confirming proteinuria and red blood cell casts along with serology with low C3. In one case, the biopsy demonstrated proliferative and exudative glomerular lesions along with immunofluroescence demonstrating coarse staining of C3 along the capillary loops and mesangium [32]. There was IgG staining as well. The electron microscopy demonstrated subepithelial electron dense deposits and humps, all the findings consistent with PIGN. The patient required dialysis but recovered without residual kidney injury with a creatinine peak of 4.9–0.9 mg/dl 1 week after discharge. As in previously reported cases with biopsy-proven post-infectious glomerular nephritis (PIGN), the disease had remitted [24, 33–36].

Hematuria

In a prospective case–control study pregnant women following in an antenatal care clinic in Australia enrolled to have routine urinalysis performed and were referred to nephrology clinic for investigation if dipstick microscopic hematuria was detected more than once before 32 weeks gestation [37]. Of 902 women (20%) had dipstick hematuria on at least two occasions in pregnancy. Sixty-six of 126 women (53%) who had hematuria before 32 weeks followed up with nephrology where the hematuria was confirmed in 40 women. Microscopic hematuria persisted in half (15 women) of those who followed up after 3 months postpartum. They concluded from their results that dipstick hematuria is common during pregnancy but rarely signifies a disorder such as preeclampsia, hypertension, or small for gestational age infants. Kidney biopsies and follow up was not reported. Antecedent hematuria prior to pregnancy was not assessed or commented on.

ATN: Ischemia

Cortical necrosis is a devastating insult to the kidneys with the cardinal signs and symptoms of abrupt onset anuria, flank pain, and gross hematuria. It is severe kidney ischemia from hypoperfusion or disseminated intravascular coagulopathy that is seen with abruption of the placenta, prolonged intrauterine fetal death, or amniotic fluid embolism. It is diagnosed by ultrasound or noncontrast CT scan demonstrating hypoechoic areas in the cortex or renal calcifications, which is a late finding. This disease is not usually reversible and treating the underlying problems may prevent extensive damage. Cocaine has been reported to cause abruption of the placenta and cortical necrosis leading to end stage renal disease (ESRD) [38].

ATN: Sepsis

Peurperal sepsis is a leading cause of maternal death worldwide, accounting for over 80,000 deaths per year [39], although uncommon in the USA, it remains a top cause of maternal death. Women are especially at risk for infection during the peripartum period, as labor and delivery exposes the typically sterile uterine environment to the multitude of bacteria harbored in the vagina. Undiagnosed or undertreated chorioamnionitis and postpartum endometritis can both lead to fulminant sepsis, threatening a woman's future fertility and life. Peurperal sepsis is most often a polymicrobial in nature, but coliform bacteria such as *Escherichia coli* and *Enteroccocus* are known pathogens as are *Staphylococcus* and *Streptococcus*.

Similarly, pregnancy is a risk factor for pyelonephritis. Asymptomatic bacteriuria occurs in approximately 5% of pregnant women; similar to nonpregnant women [40], but more commonly leads to pyelonephritis (40% of untreated bacteriuria develop acute urinary tract infection (UTI) or pyelonephritis) [41]. This is likely a result of the increased urinary stasis and ureteral dilation which allows ascent of lower urinary tract bacteria [42]. Approximately 2% of women with pyelonephritis develop acute renal failure which may or may not be reversible [43]. If biopsied, microabscesses may be found. Treatment is with empiric i.v. antibiotics until culture results are available, and until the patient is 24–48 h afebrile. Recurrence during pregnancy is not uncommon, thus prophylactic/suppressive antibiotics after diagnosis are standard of care. Of note, unlike other forms of sepsis and infection, volume resuscitation should be performed with caution, as women with pyelonephritis are at quite susceptible to ARDS. Prevention of infectious complications may be mitigated by universal screening for UTIs at the first prenatal visit and treated accordingly.

ATN: Toxins

Endogenous Toxins: Rhabdomyolysis

Rhabdomyolysis is muscle injury from ischemia or metabolic perturbations that leads to release of myoglobin that is a tubular toxin. Pregnant patients are at risk for rhabdomyolysis similar to the general population. Coma induced by alcohol and opioid overdose leads to immobilization and compartment syndrome that may lead to muscle injury. Cocaine causes rhabdomyolysis as well [38]. Cocaine-induced hyperthermia with excess muscle energy demands may lead to this. Methamphetamine use may occur in pregnancy, as it is known that 3% of pregnant women in the USA had used illicit substances in the preceding month and methamphetamine is associated with rhabdomyolysis [44, 45].

A case of baking soda ingestion in a woman at 31 weeks gestation developed severe hypokalemic metabolic alkalosis and rhabdomyolysis with elevation in serum transaminases and hypertension and 1 g of proteinuria on a 24 h urine collection [46]. She presented as though she had preeclampsia until further history was obtained that she was ingesting large amounts of baking soda.

Patients with carnitine palmitoyl transferase (CPT) type 2 deficiency are at risk of rhabdomyolysis. The disorder of mitochondrial fatty acid oxidation during pregnancy creates a situation where energy stores are inadequate, such as may occur during labor and women are at risk of rhabdomyolysis [47]. It is an autosomal recessive disorder. Normal functioning of the CPT system is required to ensure long-chain fatty acyl CoA is transported to the mitochondrial matrix where it is needed for B-oxidation. Deficiencies of both CPT1 and two leave patients unable to create energy from fatty acid oxidation and after immediate glucose and glycogen stores are exhausted, hypoglycemia may occur leading to rhabdomyolysis and if severe, acute kidney injury. Patients present with dark urine, from myoglobinuria, increased serum creatinine phophokinase, hypertension, low platelets, and elevated liver enzymes. Attentive glucose and volume management may help avoid this along with avoidance of strenuous exercise and labor.

Endogenous Toxins: Sickle Cell Disease/Trait

People with sickle cell disease (SCD) are living longer with advances in medical technology. Improved pregnancy outcomes no longer warrant avoidance or termination of pregnancy [48]. The kidney is at risk for tubulointerstitial injury in patients with SCD and sickle cell trait (SCT). Volume depletion that may occur for a variety of reasons during pregnancy may increase the risk for further tubular injury in these patients. SCD increases the risk of pyelonephritis, and the incidence of pyelonephritis in pregnant women with SCD is 5–7% in pregnancy [48, 49]. Patients with SCT are also at increased risk for urinary tract infections or pyelonephirits [50]. Another potential cause of kidney injury in this population is the use of nonsteroidal anti-inflammatory drugs (NSAIDS) for pain crisis which may lead to ATN, minimal change disease or interstitial nephritis.

Endogenous Toxins: Uric Acid

Acute uric acid nephropathy in pregnancy was reported in a 38-year-old primigravid woman who was admitted for vomiting and oliguria during the 30th week of gestation with a creatinine of 6.7 mg/dl and serum uric acid of 19 mg/dl [51]. After volume resuscitation, the creatinine was 0.8 mg/dl and the serum uric acid dropped to 3.1 mg/dl. A similar episode occurred 3 weeks later. The etiology of the hyperuricemia was unclear.

Exogenous Toxins

Rhabdomyolysis seemingly provoked by exogenous toxins has been reported during pregnancies. Ritodrine, a potent $beta_2$ stimulant that produces direct relaxation of the uterine smooth muscle and decreases the force and frequency of uterine contractions is used as a tocolytic. There are a few case reports in the literature and one by the referenced authors who noted a CK value of 25,000 IU/l (normal range 40–190) without another explanation [52, 53]. The urinary myoglobin was elevated but the creatinine was normal. The mechanism for the cause of rhabdomyolysis is speculative, but hypokalemia may arise from potassium shifting intracellularly and thus causing rhabdomyolysis.

Another tocolytic and B_2-adrenoceptor agonist, terbutaline, has been reported to cause rhabdomyolysis [54]. This case occurred after receiving terbutaline i.v. and magnesium sulfate during her 25th week of pregnancy to manage premature labor. Her labor was controlled and she was started on oral terbutaline and then because of muscle weakness was noted to have an elevated creatinine kinase up 14,330 U/dl and a creatinine of 1.1 mg/dl. An EMG was consistent with inflammatory myopathy and a muscle biopsy was consistent with acute polymyositis (PM). The patient was treated with prednisone and tocolytics withheld. She had new onset PM after the use of tocolytics.

Indomethacin use as a tocolytic in three cases may have been responsible for reversible acute kidney injury [55]. Other medical circumstances in these patients may have predisposed them to renal vasoconstriction and the vasodilatory protaglandin inhibition of indomethacin in these patients may have exacerbated the acute kidney injury. Cautious use of this medication when patients have potential compromise of hemodynamic perfusion of the kidneys should be considered.

Interstitial Nephritis

A case report of magnesium dypirone (metamizol), a nonsteroidal anti-inflammatory agent used as an analgesic and antipyritic, caused oligohydramnios and acute renal failure [56]. The patient took a high dose of this medication and her creatinine was 3.7 mg/dl. The patient developed a rash and had proteinuria with 0.8 g/24 h and the urinalysis demonstrated leucocytouria and three red blood cells. After discontinuation of the medication the rash resolved and creatinine returned to normal. Magnesium dypirone is a prostaglandin synthetase inhibitor that may cause ischemia or interstitial acute interstitial nephritis.

Vascular

As a way of categorizing vascular involvement as a cause of intrinsic acute kidney injury, one may distinguish this entity from both large and small vessels. The large renal arteries, when occluded, may be defined as prerenal kidney failure. When the small capillaries in the glomerular are primarily involved, this is nephritis or nephrosis. When the interlobular arteries are involved, we speak of intrinsic vascular involvement. Thrombotic microangiopathy (TMA) is an intrinsic cause of renal vascular disease. It is composed of the syndromes thrombotic thrombocytopenic purpura and hemolytic uremic syndrome (TTP-HUS), both of which are seen in pregnancy. The pathology does overlap, with thrombi in the glomeruli, and injury to the interlobular arteries is seen as intimal thickening and onion skinning. The pathogenesis relates to Von Willebrand Factor (VWF) maintenance by ADAMTS-13 enzyme molecules [57]. The VWF multimeric structures are secreted from stimulated endothelial cells. When the activity of ADAMTS-13 is absent or reduced, VWF cleavage does not occur and platelets adhere and aggregate onto the uncleaved VWF molecules forming microvascular platelet thrombi. Severe congenital deficiency of ADAMTS-13 caused by gene mutations or inhibition of the enzyme caused by acquired autoantibodies, inflammatory cytokines, estrogen or bacterial toxins, results in TTP [57]. HUS is described in association with infections by the Shiga toxin-producing hemorrhagic strains of *E. coli* [58]. HUS presents with a greater degree of kidney injury, potentially requiring renal replacement therapy. TTP-HUS is extremely rare during pregnancy and postpartum. They afflict <1 case in 100,000 pregnancies [59]. One review of the literature from 1955 to 2006, only noted 166 cases of TTP, distinguished from HUS by creatinines <3 mg/dl, and 55% of the cases occurred in the second trimester, whereas 33% occurred after 28 weeks [60]. The classic diagnosis of TTP/HUS includes the pentad of thrombocytopenia, Coombs negative hemolytic anemia, kidney injury, neurologic abnormalities, and fever but not all of these findings are present. The ADAMTS-13 activity is absent to markedly reduced in 33–100% of patients with TTP but in HUS that is not the case [59]. TTP-HUS has similarities with HELLP that may confuse the diagnosis and therefore the management. TTP/HUS should be favored as a diagnosis if the patient has a past history of TTP/HUS, ADAMTS-13 activity <5%, severe hemolytic anemia, markedly reduce platelets, a bloody diarrheal prodrome, congenital TTP-HUS, or presentation in the first trimester. Plasma exchange with fresh frozen plasma should be considered if a HELLP-like syndrome persists beyond 3 days postpartum and/or sooner if there is life-threatening microangiopathy. Our case #1 had diarrhea, but the platelets were only modestly reduced and the LDH was only modestly increased and there were no shistocytes on the smear, making TTP-HUS less likely. In case #2, the moderate shistocytes and more elevated creatinine raises the specter of TTP-HUS more so and thus plasma exchange should be considered as the patient is followed.

Case 1 Revisited

This patient is at the gestational age consistent with preeclampsia and has significant proteinuria. The creatinine of 1.1 mg/dl appears normal for a nonpregnant patient but is noticeable elevated for pregnancy. The initial blood pressure does not meet the defined criteria for this disease but that is not always necessary and certainly blood pressures may fluctuate. The patient does have other constitutional signs consistent with a systemic process, and the subsequent blood pressures became consistent with preeclampsia. Other considerations for her presentation are AFLP as the patient meets six or more of the Swansea criteria, those being vomiting, elevated bilirubin, uric acid, ammonia, AST, PT, and leukocytosis. If the patient has HELLP, it is likely considered partial as the AST is not >70 U/l, the platelet count is not <100,000, the LDH is not >600 U/l and there was no hemolysis seen on the peripheral smear. TTP is unlikely without hemolysis but this and HUS should be followed after delivery. Our patient was felt to have preeclampsia and she was delivered after being given antenatal corticosteroids for fetal lung development in anticipation of preterm delivery. The patient's creatinine, liver function tests, and urinalysis normalized.

Case 2 Revisited

This case illustrates the difficulty in clinically distinguishing HELLP syndrome from TTP-HUS. This patient has elevated blood pressures without proteinuria, thus she does not meet criteria for preeclampsia. Proteinuria is *not* necessary for the diagnosis of HELLP syndrome, and in such circumstances the diagnosis is known as "atypical HELLP." She has several features of HELLP syndrome including severe right upper quadrant pain, evidence of hemolysis, mildly elevated liver enzymes, and low platelets. But the clinical picture is confused by renal insufficiency which is a sign of possible TTP-HUS. Whereas the clinical picture for HELLP and TTP-HUS is very similar, treatment strategies are quite different. Delivery for this patient is indicated, as preeclampsia or some variant (such as HELLP), cannot be completely excluded. Given the elevated liver function tests (LFTs) and RUQ pain, HUS is an unlikely diagnosis, but should be considered, especially if the patient does not improve clinically within 48 h after delivery. Postpartum, the patient's AST and ALT continued to rise peaking in the 300 s and her platelets fell to a nadir of 32,000 on postpartum day 1 with a stable creatinine. In this case, a multidisciplinary team with seasoned expert consultants can be helpful in determining if plasma exchange is necessary. She made a full recovery by her 1-week postpartum visit, confirming the diagnosis of HELLP syndrome.

Conclusion

New onset kidney injury during pregnancy that is not coincidentally discovered because of preexisting kidney disease first noticed on medical evaluation of the newly pregnant patient has a broad differential that is well known to the experienced healthcare professional. The commonly anticipated complications of pregnancy warrant more than a cavalier assessment of the patient and the fetus to avoid the kidney organ injury that is usually reversible upon supportive management of the mother or modifiable with expectant delivery avoiding the dire consequences of preeclampsia, HELLP, AFLP, and sepsis. The nephrologist is not as familiar with the management of these entities as the obstetric provider but the rare presentation of TTP/HUS falls in the preview of their specialty and a collaborative approach with the primary maternal caregiver will enhance everyone's experience and potentially improve patient care in these rare predicaments.

Key Points

Pregnancy associated kidney injury is not uncommon during pregnancy, nephrology involvement is

Reversible kidney injury is probably the rule with delivery of the fetus

Catastrophic consequences involving life-threatening kidney failure may arise if simple laboratory assessment is neglected and common untoward symptoms are dismissed without considering the differential outlined herein

References

1. Chapman AB, Abraham WT, Zamudio S, Coffin C, Merouani A, Young D, Johnson A, Osorio F, Goldberg C, Moore L, Dahms T, Schrier RW. Temporal relationships between hormonal and hemodynamic changes in early human pregnancy. Kidney Int. 1998;54:2056–63.
2. Szecsi PB, Jorgensen M, Klajnbard A, Andersen MR, Colov NP, Stender S. Haemostatic reference intervals in pregnancy. Thromb Haemost. 2010;103:683–873.
3. Smith MC, Moran P, Ward MK, Davison JM. Assessment of glomerular filtration rate during pregnancy using the MDRD formula. Br J Obstet Gynaecol. 2008;115:109–12.
4. Price CP, Newll RG, Boyd JC. Use of protein: creatinine ratio measurements on random urine samples for prediction of significant proteinuria: a systematic review. Clin Chem. 2005;51(9):1577–86.
5. Ganesan C, Maynard SE. Acute kidney injury in pregnancy: the thrombotic microangiopathies. J Nephrol. 2011;24(5):554–63.
6. Knight M, Nelson-Piercy C, Kurinczuk JJ. A prospective national study of acute fatty liver of pregnancy in the UK. Gut. 2008;57:951–6.
7. Ch'ng CL, Morgan M, Hainsworth I, Kingham JGC. Prospective study of liver dysfunction in pregnancy in Southwest Wales. Gut. 2002;51:876–80.
8. Bellig LL. Maternal acute fatty liver of pregnancy and the associated risk for long-chain 3-hydroxyacyl-coenzyme A dehydrogenase (LCHAD) deficiency in infants. Adv Neonatal Care. 2004;4(1):26–32.
9. Davies MH, Elias E. Intrahepatic cholestasis of pregnancy: pathogenesis and management. Trop Gastroeneterol. 1993;14(3):79–86.
10. Smolarczyk R, Wojcicka-Jagodzinska J, Piekaarski P, Romejko E, Czjkowski K. The biochemical functions of the renal tubules and glomeruli in the course of Intrahepatic cholestasis of pregnancy. Eur J Obstet Gynecol Reprod Biol. 2000;89:35–9.
11. Bose PB, Das BC, Kumar A, Gondal R, Kumar D, Kar P. High viral load and deregulation of the progesterone receptor signaling pathway: association with hepatitis E-related poor pregnancy outcome. J Hepatol. 2011;54(6):1107–13.
12. Norvell JP, Blei AT, Jovanovic BD, Levitsky J. Herpes simplex virus hepatitis: an analysis of the published literature and institutional cases. Liver Transpl. 2007;13:1428–34.
13. Thurman RH, Konig K, Watkins A, Weerasiri T, Permezel M. Fulminant herpes simplex virus hepatic failure in pregnancy in pregnancy requiring liver transplantation. Aust N Z J Obstet Gynaecol. 2010;50:491–8.
14. Pearson GD, Veille JC, Rahimtoola S, Hsia J, Oakley CM, Hosenpud JD, Ansari A, Baughman KL. Peripartum cardiomyopathy: National Heart, Lung, and Blood Institute and Office of Rare Disease (National Institutes of Health) workshop recommendations and review. JAMA. 2000;283(9):1183–8.
15. Demakis JG, Rahimtoola SH, Sutton GC, et al. Natural course of peripartum cardiomyopathy. Circulation. 1971;44:1053–61.
16. Patel AM, Goldfarb S. Got calcium? Welcome to the calcium-alkali syndrome. J Am Soc Nephrol. 2010;21:1440–3.
17. Kovacs CS, Kronenberg HM. Maternal-fetal calcium and bone metabolism during pregnancy, puerperium and lactation. Endocr Rev. 1997;18:832–72.
18. Kolnick L, Harris BD, Choma DP, Choma NN. Hypercalcemia in pregnancy: a case of milk-alkali syndrome. J Gen Intern Med. 2011;26(8):939–42.
19. Fill Malfertheiner S, Malfertheiner MV, Monkemuller K, Rohl FW, Malfertheiner P, Costa DS. Gastroesophageal reflux disease and management in advanced pregnancy: a prospective survery. Digestion. 2009;79(2):115–20.
20. Thomas AA, Thomas AZ, Campbell SC, Palmer JS. Urologic emergencies in pregnancy. Pediatr Urol. 2010;76:453–60.
21. Swanson SK, Hellman RL, Eversman WG. Urinary tract stones in pregnancy. Surg Clin North Am. 1995;75(1):123–42.
22. Srirangam SJ, Hickerton B, Cleynenbreugel BV. Management of urinary calculi in pregnancy: a review. J Endourol. 2008;22:867–75.
23. Stothers L, Lee LM. Renal colic in pregnancy. J Urol. 1992;148(5):1383–7.
24. Chang J, Elam-Evans LD, et al. Pregnancy-related mortality surveillance—United States, 1991–1999. MMWR Surveill Summ. 2003;52(2):1–8.
25. Bellamy L, Casas JP, Hingorani AD, Williams DJ. Pre-eclampsia and risk of cardiovascular disease and cancer in later life: systematic review and meta-analysis. BMJ. 2007;335(7627):974.
26. Audibert F, Friedman S, Frangieh AY, Sibai BM. Clinical utility of strict diagnostic criteria for the HELLP syndrome. Am J Obstet Gynecol. 1996;175:460–4.
27. Spargo BH, McCartney CP, Winemiller R. Glomerular capillary endotheliosis in toxemia of pregnancy. AMA Arch Pathol. 1959;68:593.
28. Hanssens M, Keirse MJ, Spitz B, et al. Angiotensin II levels in hypertensive and normotensive pregnancies. Br J Obstet Gynecol. 1991;98:155.
29. Brown MA, Zammit VC, Mitar DA, et al. Renin-aldosterone relationships in pregnancy-induced hypertension. Am J Hypertens. 1992;5:366.
30. Valeur-Jensen AK, Pedersen CB, Westergaar T, Jensen IP, Lebech M, Andersen PK, Aaby P, Pedersen BN,

Melbye M. Risk factors for parvovirus B19 infection in pregnancy. JAMA. 1999;281(12):1099–105.
31. Podymow T, Muhtadie L. Pregnancy-associated parovirus B19 infection causing postinfectious glomerulonephritis. Hypertens Pregnancy. 2010;29(4): 429–33.
32. Fervenza F, Green A, Lafayett RA. Acute renal failure due to postinfectious glomerulonephritis during pregnancy. Am J Kidney Dis. 1997;29(2):273–6.
33. Singson E, Fisher KF, Lindheimer MD. Acute poststreptococcal glomerulonephritis in pregnancy: case report with an 18 year follow-up. Am J Obstet Gynecol. 1980;137:857–8.
34. Kincaid-Smith P, Fairley KF, Bullen M. Kidney disease and pregnancy. Med J Aust. 1967;2:1155–9.
35. Nadler N, Salinas-Madrigal L, Charles AG, Pollak VE. Acute glomerulonephritis during late pregnancy: report of a case. Obstet Gynecol. 1969;34:277–83.
36. Fukuda O, Ito M, Nakayama M, Matsui K, Fujisaki S, Okamura H. Acute glomerulonephritis during the third trimester of pregnancy. Int J Gynecol Obstet. 1988;26:141–4.
37. Brown MA, Holt JL, Mangos GJ, Murray N, Curtis J, Homer C. Microscopic hematuria in pregnancy: relevance to pregnancy outcome. Am J Kidney Dis. 2005;45(4):667–73.
38. Lampley EC, Williams S, Myers SA. Cocaine-associated rhabdomyolysis causing renal failure in pregnancy. Obstet Gynecol. 1996;87(5):804–6.
39. Maternal mortality in 2005: estimates developed by WHO, UNICEF, UNFPA and the World Bank. Geneva, World Health Organization, 2007, at (http://www.who.int/reproductive-health/publications/maternal_mortality_2005/index.html).
40. Whalley P. Bacteriuria of pregnancy. Am J Obstet Gynecol. 1967;97:723–38.
41. Smaill F, Vazquez JC. Antibiotics for asymptomatic bacteriuria in pregnancy. Cochrane Database Syst Rev. 2007;(2):CD000490.
42. Dafnis E, Sabatini S. The effect of pregnancy on renal function: physiology and pathophysiology. Am J Med Sci. 1992;303:184–205.
43. Hill JB, Sheffield JS, McIntire DD, Wendel Jr GD. Acute pyelonephritis in pregnancy. Obstet Gynecol. 2005;105:18–23.
44. Winslow BT, Voorhees KI, Pehl KA. Methamphetamine abuse. Am Fam Physician. 2007;76:1169–74.
45. Pregnancy and substance use. NSDUH Report January 2 2004, at http://www.oas.samhsa.gov/2k3/pregnancy/pregnancy.htm.
46. Groteut CA, Dandolu V, Katari S, Whiteman VE, Geifman-Holtzman O, Teitelman M. Baking soda pica: a case of hypokalemic metabolic alkalosis and rhabdomyolysis in pregnancy. Obstet Gynecol. 2006; 107(2 Pt2):484–6.
47. Slater PM, Grivell R, Cyna AM. Labour management of a woman with carnitine palmitoyl transferase type 2 deficiency. Anaesth Intensive Care. 2009;37:305–8.
48. Sun PM, Wilbrun W, Raynor BD, Jamieson D. Sickle cell disease in pregnancy: twenty years of experience at Grady Memorial Hospital, Atlanta, Georgia. Am J Obstet Gynecol. 2001;184(6):1127–30.
49. Villers MS, Jamison MG, De Castro LM, James AH. Morbidity associated with sickle cell disease in pregnancy. Am J Obstet Gynecol. 2008;199:125. e1–125.e5.
50. Hassell K. Pregnancy and sickle cell disease. Hematol Oncol Clin North Am. 2005;19:903–16.
51. Alexopoulos E, Tampakoudis P, Bili H, Mantalenakis S. Acute uric acid nephropathy in pregnancy. Obstet Gynecol. 1992;80:488–9.
52. Verriello L, D'Amico D, Pauletto G, Gigli GL, Bergonzi P. Rhabomyolysis caused by tocolytic therapy with Ritodrine hydrochloride. Neuromuscul Disord. 2009;19:718–20.
53. Matsuda Y, Nagayoshi Y, Kirihara N. Rhabdomyolysis during prolonged intravenous tocolytic therapy. J Perinat Med. 2002;30(6):476–9.
54. Ditzian-Kadanoff R, Reinhard JD, Thomas C, Segal AS. Polymyositis with myoglobinuria in pregnancy: a report and review of the literature. J Rheumatol. 1988;15:513–4.
55. Steiger RM, Boyd EL, Powers DR, Nageotte MP, Towers CV. Acute maternal renal insufficiency in premature labor treated with indomethacin. Am J Perinatol. 1993;10(5):381–3.
56. Sanchez de la Nieta MD, Rivera F, de la Torre M, Alcazar R, Caparros G, Paz Alcaide M, Vozmediano C, Sanchez A. Acute renal failure and oligohydramnios induced by magnesium dypirone (metamizol) in a pregnant woman. Nephrol Dial Transplant. 2003;8(8): 1679–80.
57. Moake J. Thrombotic thrombocytopenia purpura and other thrombotic microangiopathies. Best Pract Res Clin Haematol. 2009;22:567–76.
58. Stella CL, Dacus J, Guzman E, Dhillon P, Coppage K, How H, Sibai B. The diagnositic dilemma of thrombotic thrombocytopenic prupura/hemolytic uremic syndrome in obstetric triage and emergency department: lessons from 4 tertiary hospitals. Am J Obstet Gynecol. 2009;200:381. e1–e6.
59. Sibai B. Imitators of severe pre-eclampsia. Semin Perinatol. 2009;33:196–205.
60. Martin JN, Bailey AP, Rehberg JF, Owens MT, Keiser SD, May W. Thrombotic thrombocytopenic purpura in 166 pregnancies: 1955–2006. Am J Obstet Gynecol. 2008;199(2):98–104.

49 Genetic Diseases of the Kidney

Scott D. Bieber and J. Ashley Jefferson

Case

A 48-year-old woman comes to the clinic to establish medical care and for routine physical examination. Her past medical history is notable for elevated blood pressure. She is currently not taking any medications. Her family history is unremarkable; her mother lived into her 80s with no apparent medical problems. Her father passed away at a young age in a motor vehicle accident. She has three brothers and one sister who are apparently healthy. Review of systems is notable for increasing abdominal fullness over the past few years, early satiety and leg cramps. Physical exam reveals a blood pressure of 152/92, heart rate 81, respiratory rate 14, temperature of 36.4°C. Abdominal exam is remarkable for bilateral palpable kidneys. Laboratory studies reveal a serum creatinine of 2.5 mg/dL and blood urea nitrogen 37 mg/dL. Urinalysis reveals 1+ blood and trace protein. Urine microscopy is noted to be bland. Abdominal CT scan without contrast reveals bilaterally enlarged kidneys with numerous cysts and several small calculi (Fig. 49.1). The liver is also noted to have several cysts.

What is the most likely diagnosis? What is the prognosis? Is this a familial disease and do family members need to be screened? Does this disease affect other organ systems? What can be done to prevent progression of the disease?

S.D. Bieber, D.O. (✉)
Division of Nephrology, University of Washington, Kidney Research Institute, 325 9th Ave. Box 359606, Seattle, WA 98104, USA
e-mail: scbieber@u.washington.edu

J.A. Jefferson, M.D., F.R.C.P.
Division of Nephrology, University of Washington, Seattle, WA 98195, USA

Autosomal Dominant Polycystic Kidney Disease

Overview

Autosomal dominant polycystic kidney disease (ADPKD) is the most common inherited kidney disease and the fourth commonest cause of end stage renal disease (ESRD), behind diabetes hypertension and glomerulonephritis. The estimated prevalence of ADPKD is between 1:400 and 1:1,000 live births with 5,000–6,000 new cases each year in the USA [1]. It affects males and females equally, and there is no racial predilection [2].

Clinical Features

Patients with ADPKD often present as a result of screening following the diagnosis in a family member, or as a result of incidental findings on scans performed for other reasons. Typical clinical features may be divided into renal and extra-renal manifestations (Table 49.1).

E.V. Lerma and M. Rosner (eds.), *Clinical Decisions in Nephrology, Hypertension and Kidney Transplantation*, DOI 10.1007/978-1-4614-4454-1_49, © Springer Science+Business Media New York 2013

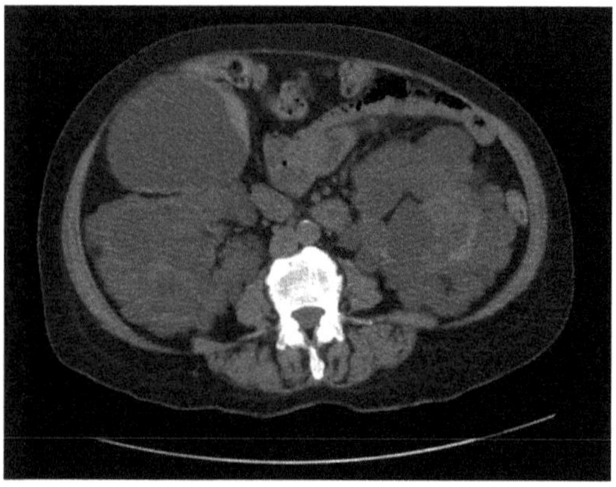

Fig. 49.1 Non-contrast abdominal CT scan of a patient with ADPKD shows enlarged kidneys with numerous bilateral cysts

Table 49.1 Clinical manifestations of ADPKD

Renal	Non-renal
Hypertension	Left ventricular hypertrophy
Hematuria (cyst bleeding/rupture)	Mitral valve prolapse
Nephrolithiasis	Intracranial aneurysms
Cyst infection	Hernias (inguinal, umbilical, hiatal)
Renal colic/chronic pain	Diverticulosis (particularly in ESRD)
Urinary concentrating defect	Liver cysts
	Pancreatic cysts
	Other cysts (spleen, arachnoid membrane, seminal vesicles, ovarian)
	Dilation of aortic root
	Dissection of thoracic aorta

Renal Manifestations

Progressive Renal Dysfunction. Renal function is typically normal for many years, but as the cysts enlarge they compress the adjacent normal renal tissue and renal injury develops. By the time the serum creatinine starts to rise, greater than 50% of the renal parenchyma is probably destroyed [3]. The average rate of renal decline is 4–5 mL/min/year, although kidneys that are markedly enlarged on ultrasound may have a faster rate of progression [2]. Other risk factors for progression include male sex, hypertension before age 35, gross hematuria before age 30 in men and more than three pregnancies [1]. The course of the chronic kidney disease is somewhat dependent on the underlying genetic mutation (see genetics section below). Individuals that carry a mutation in polycystin 1 (*PKD1*) tend to develop cysts in their 20s, and typically reach ESRD by time they are in their 50s. By comparison, those with polycystin 2 (*PKD2*) mutations typically do not reach ESRD until they get into their 70s and may survive the duration of their lives without noticeable kidney problems [3].

Local renal complications. Renal colic or loin pain is a common complaint in patients with ADPKD. Acute severe episodes of pain should be evaluated for evidence of cyst rupture, cyst bleeding, cyst infection, or kidney stones. Occasionally bleeding into the urinary tract can cause renal colic as clots are passed. Usually acute pain from ADPKD is self-limited and will improve within days. Patients with ADPKD can also develop chronic pain which can be difficult to manage.

Gross hematuria due to cyst rupture may be the presenting complaint in ADPKD. Cyst rupture can be spontaneous or associated with a traumatic event of injury such as in contact sports or a motor vehicle accident [3].

Nephrolithiasis is twice as common in ADPKD patients compared to the normal population [3]. Approximately 20% of patients with ADPKD have problems with stones [1]. The stone composition is usually uric acid or calcium oxalate. Structural deformities resulting in areas of stasis of tubular flow created by enlarging cysts are believed to contribute to stone formation.

Hypertension is a common feature of ADPKD and can start in childhood. It occurs in 60% of patients despite normal renal function [2]. Hypertension in ADPKD is often secondary to upregulation of the renin–angiotensin–aldosterone system (RAAS) due to cysts compressing and stretching blood vessels causing renal ischemia. In certain patients there may also be ectopic renin production from the cysts themselves [1].

Decreased renal concentrating ability with polyuria may be an early sign of cystic renal disease [2]. The concentrating defect in ADPKD is unique when compared to diabetes insipidus because it occurs despite over-expression of vasopressin V2 receptors and aquaporin 2 in the cortical collecting duct [4]. Proteinuria is not typically a prominent feature of ADPKD with microalbuminuria described in 35% of patients, dipstick positive proteinuria in less than 18% of patients. The total amount of proteinuria in patients in ADPKD usually measures less than 1 g/24 h.

Extra-Renal Manifestations

Liver cysts are the most common extra-renal manifestation of ADPKD and are seen in 80% of patients. Massive cystic enlargement of the liver may occur and is more common in women due to estrogen stimulation of cyst growth [3]. Unlike renal cysts, liver cysts usually do not result in hepatic failure and hepatic synthetic function is typically maintained despite large cyst burden. Of note, there is a different cystic disease which involves the liver alone, not causing renal cysts, which is termed autosomal dominant polycystic liver disease. Pancreatic cysts occur in 10% of patients, but are usually not clinically significant. Cysts are also rarely found in the spleen, arachnoid membrane, and the seminal vesicles [1].

Berry aneurysms of the cerebral vasculature are the most concerning extra-renal manifestation because of the risk of subarachnoid hemorrhage. These aneurysms occur in approximately 8% of ADPKD patients, compared with a prevalence of 1–2% in the general population, but this increases to 16–20% prevalence in patients with a family history of intracranial aneurysm or subarachnoid hemorrhage. Patients with berry aneurysms may present with headache, cranial neuropathies (diplopia), or other neurologic symptoms. Although berry aneurysms are associated with ADPKD, it is worth noting that hypertensive hemorrhage or ischemic infarcts are more common etiologies of stroke in patients with ADPKD [5]. Screening for berry aneurysms (preferably with magnetic resonance angiography, MRA) is recommended for patients with ADPKD who have a family history of aneurysm, stroke, or sudden death and those with severe or new onset headaches or neurologic signs. Routine screening for aneurysms in the absence of family history or symptoms is not recommended [3], though some clinicians would advocate for screening in high risk occupations for example, airline pilots. Aneurysms discovered on imaging that are larger than 10 mm may require surgical intervention [2].

Other extra-renal manifestations include mitral valve prolapse (about 30% of patients) and abdominal hernias (about 45% of patients) [1]. Hernias can be in the umbilical, hiatal, or inguinal location. Diverticular disease of the colon has been associated with ADPKD, especially in patients with ESRD. Massive cyst growth can lead to abdominal distension and rarely to compression of the inferior vena cava or iliac veins leading to thrombus formation and pulmonary embolism. ADPKD patients are at increased risk for pulmonary embolism post kidney transplantation [1]. Similar to other populations with renal disease, cardiovascular disease is the commonest cause of death in patients with ADPKD [2].

Genetics

The majority (85%) of cases of ADPKD are due to mutations in a large gene on chromosome 16 called *PKD1* (46 exons), which encodes a protein called polycystin-1 (~4,000 amino acids). Approximately 10–15% of cases are due to mutation in *PKD2* on chromosome 4, a smaller gene (15 exons) encoding polycystin-2, although a few families have been described that are not linked to either *PKD1* or *PKD2*. There are more than 300 *PKD1* mutations and 70 *PKD2* mutations described and most mutations are unique to a single family [1]. *PKD1* mutations are associated with a more severe phenotype with increased numbers of cysts and earlier renal failure than *PKD2* [3]. The genotype–phenotype relationship for *PKD1* is not strong, although mutations in the 5′ region of the gene may have a milder disease course [1]. A family history cannot be established in around 25% of patients, and a spontaneous mutation is estimated to occur in about 5–7% of cases.

Polycystin 1 (PC1) is found on the basolateral membrane of epithelial cells and is involved in cell–cell interactions at adherens junctions and in cell binding to the underlying basement membrane. It is also expressed in hepatic ductules and pancreatic ducts. Polycystin 2 (PC2) is a member of the TRP family of ion channels and plays a role in calcium signaling and cell proliferation. It is mostly an intracellular protein, but notably is expressed with PC1 in the primary cilium where it likely forms a common signaling pathway (see below).

ADPKD is an example of a "two-hit" mechanism of genetic disease. Every cell in the body inherits a mutation in one allele of the gene in the germ line, but a second somatic mutation occurs in tubular cells leading to loss of function of the normal allele. This hypothesis is supported by the observation that cysts affect only a fraction of the renal tubules and the disease manifests later in life. Environmental factors may affect the timing and frequency of these second hits and may partly account for the variability in disease progression.

Pathophysiology

The renal cysts in ADPKD form at multiple sites along the nephron (proximal tubule, loop of Henle, distal tubule, and collecting duct), but arise in less than 10% of the nephrons. By comparison, in autosomal recessive polycystic kidney disease the cysts arise from collecting ducts only [4]. As the cysts enlarge, they compress the normal parenchyma resulting in renal dysfunction. The cysts are initially in continuity with the renal tubule and are filled by the glomerular filtrate, but as they enlarge, they become disconnected from the tubule, and enlarge through fluid secretion from the tubular cells lining the cyst. Tubular epithelial cells normally absorb fluid, but in ADPKD they alter their polarity and secrete fluid into the cysts. Translocation of Na-K-ATPase pumps and chloride channels (CFTR) from the basolateral to luminal membranes may facilitate this. The CFTR channel is activated by elevated levels of cyclic AMP (cAMP). The epithelial cells lining the walls of the cyst also proliferate allowing the cyst to expand. This may be promoted through upregulation of the Ras signaling pathway and by growth factors such as epidermal growth factor and insulin-like growth factor (Fig. 49.2).

Dysfunction of primary cilium. The primary cilium is a hair-like structure found on renal tubular epithelial cells that projects into the lumen of the tubule and is involved in sensing tubular flow of filtrate. Both polycystin 1 and polycystin 2 are expressed in the primary cilium and may form a complex which acts as a mechanosensor that reacts to shear stress by increasing intracellular calcium. Impaired signaling by this PC1/PC2 complex may promote fluid secretion and

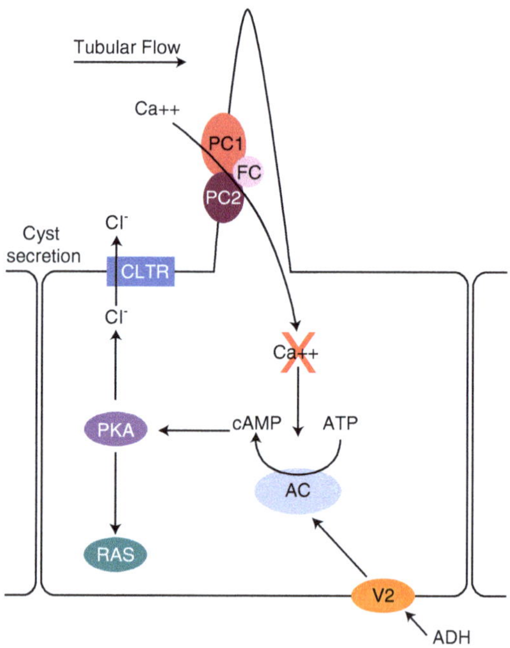

Fig. 49.2 Disease mechanisms involving the primary cilium in ADPKD. Tubular flow displaces the primary cilium causing calcium to enter the cell via polycystin 2 (PC2). Note that PC2 is complexed with polycystin 1 (PC1) and fibrocystin (FC). In ADPKD, defects in the PC1/PC2/FC complex inhibit calcium entry, which upregulates adenylate cyclase leading to increased intracellular cAMP levels. Subsequent activation of protein kinase A (PKA) stimulates cell proliferation through activation of Ras. PKA signaling also promotes the expression of chloride channels (CTFR) which increases tubular secretion of chloride, with resultant sodium and water secretion. Also note that vasopressin (ADH) binding to vasopressin 2 (V2) receptors increases cAMP

Table 49.2 Sonographic criteria for the diagnosis of ADPKD [1, 7]

Age	Criteria	PPV	NPV
Revised unified diagnostic criteria			
15–29	≥3 cysts unilateral or bilateral	100	85.5
30–39	≥3 cysts unilateral or bilateral	100	96.4
40–59	≥2 cysts in each kidney	100	94.8
≥60	≥4 cysts in each kidney	100	100
Revised criteria for exclusion of diagnosis			
15–29	≥1 cyst	96.6	90.8
30–39	≥1 cyst	94.0	98.3
40–59	≥2 cysts	96.7	100
≥60	≥4 cysts in each kidney	100	100
Revised Ravine criteria including family history			
	Positive family history	Negative family history	
<30	2 cysts unilateral or bilateral	5 cysts bilaterally	
30–60	4 cysts bilaterally	5 cysts bilaterally	
>60	8 cysts bilaterally	8 cysts bilaterally	

PPV positive predictative value, *NPV* negative predictative value

tubular cell proliferation. Notably, several other inherited cystic diseases of the kidney (e.g., autosomal recessive polycystic disease, nephronophthesis) are due to mutations in genes encoding proteins that localize to the primary cilium.

Diagnosis

The diagnosis of ADPKD is usually made by imaging (ultrasound or CT scanning) which reveals bilateral renal cysts which enlarge the kidney. Simple cysts may also be bilateral, occur spontaneously, and become more common with age. Diagnostic criteria for ADPKD have been developed which take into account the number of cysts and the age of the individual (revised Ravine criteria, Table 49.2). In addition, there are other causes of renal cystic disease which need to be differentiated from ADPKD (Table 49.3) [6].

Renal ultrasound can determine kidney size and detect cysts down to 1 cm in diameter. Cysts in the liver can also be identified on routine abdominal ultrasonography (US). Computed tomography (CT) or magnetic resonance imaging (MRI) are more sensitive (can detect cysts down to 3 mm in diameter), but US is cheaper, noninvasive and does not involve radiation exposure or administration of contrast agents. A normal renal US without cysts has a greater negative predictive value with increasing age (Table 49.2).

Genetic testing may be performed for diagnosis in uncertain cases or for screening of at risk relatives. Although this can be done by DNA linkage analysis within large families, mutation analysis by direct sequencing is more commonly performed. It should be recognized that mutation analysis is technically difficult due to the large size and complexity of the *PKD1* gene (46 exons), and due to regions of genomic duplication on chromosome 16, where multiple copies of PKD-like genes are found. Direct sequencing can detect mutations in 85–90% of patients with ADPKD; however, as most mutations are unique to individual families, it can be difficult to be certain that the sequence variations are truly pathogenic. Therefore, genetic testing, may be associated with significant rates of false-negative and false-positive results, depending on the techniques used.

Screening for ADPKD may be offered to persons 18 years or older with a positive family history for diagnostic or family planning purposes. However, as there are currently no proven treatments to slow the progression of the disease, great thought needs to be given to genetic screening, as this may have an adverse effect on the patient's ability to secure insurance, despite new laws designed to protect patients from discrimination [7]. Screening of asymptomatic children is usually not recommended. It is important to note that screening recommendations are likely to change in the near future as researchers develop new ways to treat ADPKD.

Management

Measures to Slow Progression of Kidney Disease

Unfortunately no specific therapies to date have been proven to slow progression of ADPKD, but a number of general measures are recommended based on studies in animal models. Arginine vasopressin (AVP) activates cAMP which can stimulate cyst growth and secretion, and many

Table 49.3 Renal cystic conditions other than ADPKD [6, 19]

Condition	Associated features
Simple renal cysts	Associated with normal aging, number of cysts increases with age. Prevalence of one or more cysts: <30 years: 0.2% 30–49 years: 2% 50–70 years: 11.5% >70 years: 22%
Acquired renal cystic disease (ACKD)	Cysts that are seen in patients with CKD (7% of patients) and ESRD (20% of patients). Despite cysts, kidney size is usually normal or small due to underlying CKD and loss of renal mass. The progression of ACKD may exist along a spectrum where cystic lesions evolve from simple to complex and on to form cancer. The prevalence of RCC in dialysis patients is noted to be 1–2%, about 40 times higher than the general population.
Autosomal recessive polycystic kidney disease	Usually presents in utero or shortly after birth. Oligohydramnios, enlarged echogenic kidneys, hypertension, and hyponatremia can develop. Associated with hepatic fibrosis; complications related to liver failure are usually the predominant clinical problems. Frequently progresses to ESRD, usually by adolescence.
Medullary sponge kidney	Dilated medullary and papillary collecting ducts form multiple cysts usually measuring 1–8 mm giving the kidney a spongy appearance. May be asymptomatic but can present with hyperuricemia, gout, hypercalciuria, stones, hematuria, or urinary tract infection. IVP shows retention of contrast in ectatic ducts. Long-term prognosis is good and progression to ESRD is rare. Presents in adulthood. Developmental defect, occurs frequently in persons with other developmental defects (Marfans, Ehlers-Danlos, etc.). Usually not familial and no clear genetic link identified.
Tuberous sclerosis complex	Results from inactivation mutations in either gene TSC1 or TSC2 (adjacent to PKD1). TSC1/TSC2 function as tumor suppressor genes. Patients can have skin lesions (facial angiofibromas, hypomelanotic macules, Shagreen patches, periungal fibromas). Can be associated with mental retardation, autism, seizures. Tumors can form in the brain, retina, kidneys, and heart. Renal angiomyolipomas (AMLs) are present in 80% of patients and can convert to renal cell carcinomas. Risk for spontaneous retroperitoneal bleeding from AMLs. Renal cysts also frequently present but less common than AMLs. Autosomal dominant inheritance but 2/3 of cases due to sporadic mutations.
Von Hippel-Lindau syndrome	Results from mutation in VHL gene (tumor suppressor gene). Associated with tumors in multiple areas, retinal and CNS hemangioblastomas, renal cell carcinomas (can be multiple RCCs), pheochromocytoma, papillary cystadenomas of the epididymis, multiple pancreatic cysts. Renal cysts usually bilateral but abnormal to have multiple cysts or to have cysts severe enough to affect renal function. Autosomal dominant inheritance. Familial 80%, sporadic 20%.
Orofaciodigital syndrome	Oral (hyperplastic frenula, cleft tongue, cleft lip or palate, malposed teeth), Facial (broad nasal root, hypoplasia of nasal alae, and malar bones), and digital anomalies. X-linked dominant inheritance, lethal in males.
Isolated glomerulocystic disease (GCKD)	Cystic dilation involving Bowman's space and initial portion of the proximal tubule. Cysts < 1 cm in size, limited to the cortex. Can occur as a familial condition (usually autosomal dominant) or in association with ADPKD.
COL4A1 nephropathy (HANAC syndrome)	Systemic disease recently characterized due to mutation in genes that code for $\alpha 1$ subtype of type IV collagen. Described as a hereditary angiopathy with nephropathy. Patients prone to aneurysms, muscle cramps. Renal manifestations: hematuria or large bilateral renal cysts, impaired GFR. Ultrastructural evaluation of renal tissue reveals basement membrane abnormalities "basket-weaving" of Bowman's capsule and tubules (similar to the abnormalities seen in GBM of Alports syndrome). Can have elevated CPK levels, retinal vessel tortuosity, Reynaud's phenomenon, cardiac arrhythmias.

clinicians recommend an increased water intake (3 L/day) to decrease the osmotic stimulus for AVP secretion. Caffeine and other medications (e.g., theophylline, beta-agonists) that increase cAMP levels should also be avoided. Avoidance of estrogens is recommended as estrogen can stimulate cyst growth, particularly, liver cyst growth [3]. The Consortium for Radiographic Imaging Studies of Polycystic Kidney Disease (CRISP) is an ongoing observational study that should help establish measures of disease progression in early ADPKD.

Future potential therapies in ADPKD are mostly directed against the deregulated secretory function or augmented proliferative capacity of tubular cells. Cyclic AMP is known to stimulate fluid secretion and is upregulated in ADPKD, possibly by the vasopressin V2 receptor. Tolvaptan, a V2 receptor antagonist, markedly decreases renal cyst formation in animal models and is currently being studied in a phase 3 clinical trial [8]. Other antisecretory therapies may include long-acting somatostatins, CFTR inhibitors, and potassium channel (KCa3.1) inhibitors. Several anti-proliferative therapies have shown promise in experimental models and are progressing to clinical trials. Sirolimus and everolimus were strong candidates as blockade of the mammalian target of rapamycin (mTOR) pathway theoretically inhibits cell growth and cyst proliferation. In a retrospective study of kidney transplant patients, those treated with sirolimus had a reduction in the size of their native kidneys. However, recent clinical studies of mTOR inhibitors in ADPKD have not demonstrated clinical efficacy in late disease [9]. At this time, there is no specific medical therapy that can be recommended to slow cyst growth.

Management of Hypertension

Most clinicians recommend treatment of hypertension to a level less than 130/80 in adults with ADPKD, though the supportive evidence is flimsy. Hypertension is often mediated by activation of the RAAS; therefore, angiotensin-converting enzyme inhibitors (ACEI) or angiotensin receptor blockers (ARB) are considered the preferred agents. Patients are frequently plasma volume expanded and may need diuretics and sodium restriction. Unfortunately, although good blood pressure control has been associated with reversal of left ventricular hypertrophy [1, 10], there is little evidence that RAAS blockade or blood pressure control actually slows down the progression of ADPKD. The ongoing HALT-PKD study should help to clarify the role of ACEI/ARBs and blood pressure control in ADPKD.

Management of Other Renal Complications: Hematuria/Pain/Cyst Infection/Stones

Hematuria secondary to ruptured or bleeding renal cysts is a frequent complication of ADPKD. Cysts can rupture and cause retroperitoneal bleeding and flank pain. In general, management is supportive with rest, analgesics, hydration, and avoidance of contact sports. Pain may occur as a result of the rupture of the cysts themselves or due to renal colic caused by clots in the collecting system. Urinary flow should be maintained at about 2–3 L daily to help prevent clotting and obstruction. Renal stones in patients with ADPKD are managed in a similar fashion to stones in other conditions (see Chapter XX). Urinary tract infections in ADPKD patients can be more serious as they have the potential to involve the cyst and form abscesses. Antibiotic therapy in cases of cyst infection should be selected carefully to ensure that the drug is able to penetrate the cyst and reach the site of infection. Examples of antibiotics with good cyst penetration include trimethoprim–sulfamethoxazole,floroquinalones, and vancomycin. Longer courses of antibiotics (up to 4 weeks) may be required for clearance of cyst infections and occasionally intervention to drain pockets of infection is necessary. Chronic pain is also a complication of ADPKD and can be difficult to treat. Narcotic medications should be avoided in the management of chronic pain. Patients may need referral to a pain specialist and consideration for alternative therapies. Renal denervation, local injection of anesthetics, laparoscopic and surgical cyst unroofing have been used with limited success [3].

Dialysis/Transplant

Both peritoneal dialysis and hemodialysis can be considered in ADPKD patients who progress to ESRD. The frequent rate of hernias in ADPKD patients may complicate peritoneal dialysis. If patients are prone to cyst rupture and bleeding, heparin given during hemodialysis can worsen bleeding episodes. Following renal transplantation, patients with ADPKD have better outcomes with regards to allograft survival compared to other patients with ESRD. They also have lower rates of infectious complications but are complicated more frequently by hypertension and thromboembolic events [11].

Pregnancy

Pregnancy in patients with ADPKD is generally uncomplicated, as the renal function usually remains good at child bearing ages. The risk of hypertensive complications during pregnancy and the risk of preeclampsia are higher when chronic HTN and renal insufficiency are already present. ADPKD patients may also be at increased risk of ectopic pregnancies [2].

Hereditary Nephritis

The term hereditary nephritis encompasses a range of disorders mainly due to structural abnormalities in the glomerular basement membrane (GBM) that often present with familial hematuria and varying degrees of renal dysfunction (Table 49.4). Most are due to abnormalities in type IV collagen, which is the major component of the GBM and have therefore been termed "type IV collagenopathies."

Table 49.4 Hereditary disorders of the glomerular basement membrane [15, 20, 21]

Condition	Associated features
Hereditary nephritis (Alport's)	Presents with hematuria, proteinuria, and occasionally hearing and visual defects. Mutations on the α3, α4, or α5 subunit of type IV collagen. α5 mutations most common, X-linked. Mutations in α3 or α4 autosomal recessive.
Thin basement membrane disease	Microscopic hematuria. Mostly asymptomatic. Autosomal dominant in 2/3, de novo mutation in 1/3. Genetic defect in type IV collagen, the α3 or α4 subunits. LM is normal, EM reveals uniformly thin GBM (thickness of less than 200–250 nm).nm
Nail patella syndrome	Mutation in LMX1B gene which is involved in gene transcription of type IV collagen. Tetrad of absent or hypoplastic toe or fingernails, absent or hypoplastic patellae, elbow dysplasia, iliac horns, and triangular lunulae. Hematuria can be present. LM usually is unremarkable, EM glomerular basement membrane with irregular thickening, deposits in the lamina densa and/or patchy lucent "moth-eaten" areas. Minority (5–10%) progress to nephrotic range proteinuria and ESRD.
MYHIIA syndromes	Defects in non-muscle myosin heavy chain 9 genes (MYH9) which encode non-muscle myosin heavy chain IIA (MYHIIA). Autosomal dominant disorders. Platelet disorder characterized by macrothrombocytopenia with leukocyte inclusions. Can have sensorineural deafness, cataracts, nephritis. Also known as Fetchner syndrome, Epstein syndrome, and Alport's syndrome with marcothrombocytopenia.

Glomerular Basement Membrane

The normal GBM is a 300–400 nm thick gel-like structure which lies between the glomerular endothelial cells and the podocytes in the capillary loop within the glomerulus. It is part of the glomerular filtration barrier, allowing high flux hydraulic permeability, whilst retarding the passage of cells and larger molecular weight proteins such as albumin. It consists predominantly of type IV collagen, laminin 521 (α5β2γ1), nidogen and heparan sulfate proteoglycans.

Type IV collagen is the main collagen in basement membranes throughout the body and is composed of six different alpha chains (α1–α6) that assemble into trimers, the building blocks of the three type IV collagen networks, α1–α1–α2(IV), α3–α4–α5(IV), and α5–α5–α6(IV). These different type IV collagen networks have different expression patterns in adults (Table 49.5). The GBM is initially composed primarily of the α1–α1–α2(IV) network derived from endothelial cells, but during glomerular development, it is replaced by more robust α3–α4–α5(IV) network, produced by podocytes, which is more resistant to stress and proteolysis due to multiple cross-linking (see Fig. 49.3).

Table 49.5 Type IV collagen networks [15]

Network	Location
α1–α1–α2	Expressed throughout the body. Also seen in the glomerular basement membrane early on in development and later replaced by α3–α4–α5(IV) during embryogenesis. Found in Bowman's capsule and tubular membranes along with α5–α5–α6(IV).
α3–α4–α5	Glomerular basement membrane, lung, eye, lens, ear.
α5–α5–α6	Bowman's capsule, tubular basement membranes, esophagus, skin, smooth muscle cell basement membranes.

Alport Syndrome

Alport syndrome (AS) is an inherited disorder of type IV collagen leading to GBM abnormalities, hematuria and renal dysfunction. AS is often associated with deafness. The prevalence of AS is about 1:10,000 and it accounts for 1–2% of patients with ESRD [2].

Clinical features. AS is most commonly inherited in an X-linked pattern (85%) due to mutations in the COL4A5 gene encoding the α5 chain

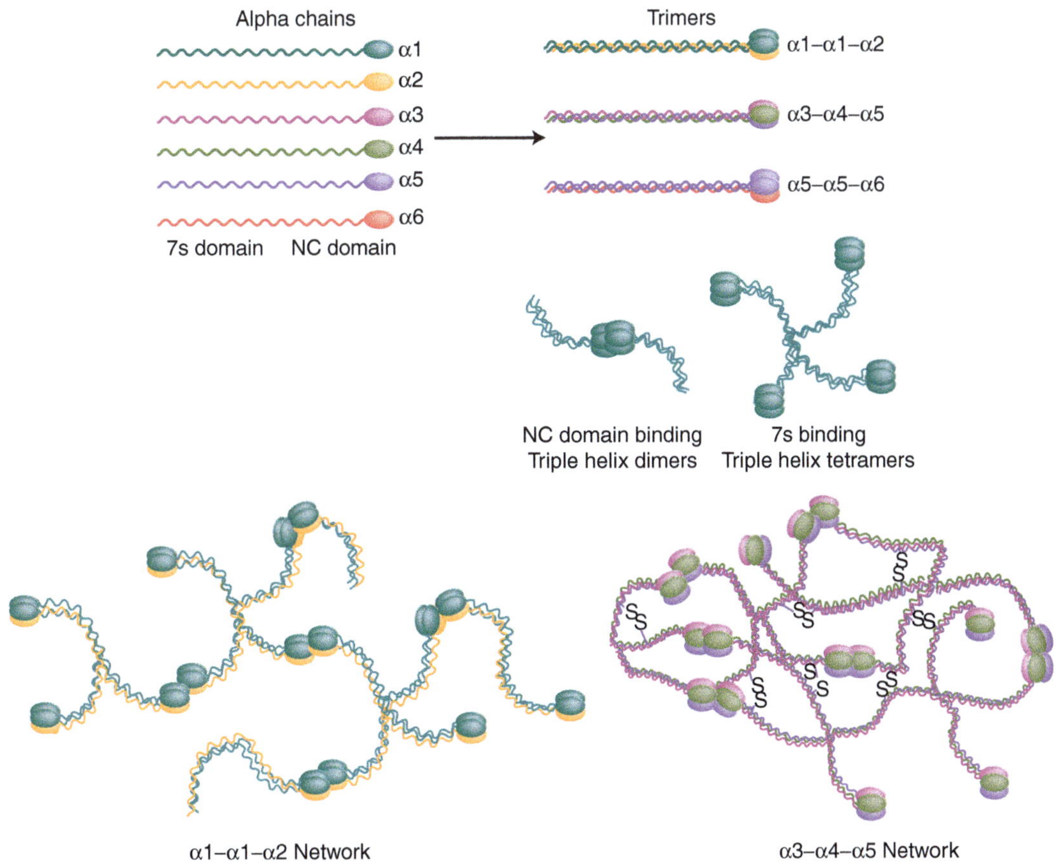

Fig. 49.3 Collagen networks. Single helix alpha chains come together to form triple helix trimers in type four collagen. There are three different trimers, α1–α1–α2, α3–α4–α5, and α5–α5–α6. Networks of collagen are formed in basement membranes. The trimers are bound by their noncollagenous domains (NC) as triple helix dimers and by their 7s domains as triple helix tetramers. In the golmerular basement membrane, the α1–α1–α2 network is found early in development and later replaced by the α3–α4–α5. Compared to the α1–α1–α2 network, the α3–α4–α5 network is more robust due to multiple disulfide bridge cross-linking

of type IV collagen. Macro or microscopic hematuria is present in nearly all patients with AS, and proteinuria is usually modest, although nephrotic range proteinuria can occur. Males are typically more severely affected and often present with hematuria in early childhood, develop renal impairment in their teens, and progress to ESRD in their 20s–40s. Affected females are hemizygous and carry a normal copy of the COL4A5 gene. A majority of females have persistent microscopic hematuria and do not progress to ESRD, but due to skewing of lyonization, the random inactivation of the X chromosome, some may have a more severe clinical course similar to males. As the α3–α4–α5(IV) network is also found in the basement membranes of the ear and eye, affected patients classically suffer from a high tone sensorineural deafness, and develop characteristic signs on eye examination including anterior lenticonus and dot and fleck retinopathy, although blindness is uncommon. The severity of disease is partly related to the mutation that is inherited.

An autosomal recessive form of AS occurs due to mutations in COL4A3 or COL4A4 encoding the α3 and α4 chains of type IV collagen. The phenotype is very similar to the X-linked disease, as abnormalities in any of the α3, α4, or α5 chains affect the formation of the α3–α4–α5 trimers and failure to replace the original α1–α1–α2(IV) network. Males and females are equally affected in the autosomal recessive disease. There is also a rare autosomal dominant form of AS due to mutations in COL4A3 or COL4A4.

Renal Pathology. The characteristic features of AS are noted on renal biopsy. Although light microscopy may show nonspecific glomerular disease with negative immunofluorescence, electron microscopy reveals irregular thickening and splitting of the GBM. The absence of α3, α4, and α5 can be detected by special immunostaining. Due to the α5–α5–α6(IV) network expression in the skin, the X-linked form of AS in male patients can be diagnosed by skin biopsy.

Treatment. Unfortunately, there is no specific treatment which will correct the underlying pathophysiology. Current treatment options focus on control of blood pressure and reduction of glomerular pressure and proteinuria through the use of ACEI or ARB. Kidney transplantation should be considered for those who progress to ESRD. After kidney transplantation, 20–30% of patients with AS develop alloantibodies to epitopes on the α3 chain of type IV collagen due to the de novo presentation of this protein in the graft. In a small percentage (~5%), these antibodies lead to anti-GBM disease in the allograft which is associated with a high rate of graft loss [2, 12, 13].

Thin Basement Membrane Nephropathy

Thin basement membrane nephropathy (TBMN) is a very common renal disorder believed to affect about 1% of the population. It leads to persistent microhematuria, which is often familial, but rarely progresses to renal dysfunction, and has previously been called benign familial hematuria.

Clinical Features

Patients with TBMN usually present following the detection of hematuria on routine urinalysis. The cells are often dysmorphic on urine sediment exam, but red cell casts are uncommon. Patients are asymptomatic and typically do not develop renal dysfunction. Proteinuria is usually minimal or absent, but approximately 5% may develop more significant proteinuria associated with the development of focal segmental glomerulosclerosis [14].

Genetics

TBMN is an inherited disorder with autosomal dominant transmission and 2/3 of patients have a family member with hematuria. Up to 1/3 of the mutations in TBMD are de novo. In the majority of cases, the genetic defect is a heterozygous mutation in COL4A3 or COL4A4 encoding the α3 and α4 chains of type IV collagen, although families not linked to the type IV collagen loci have been described. In TBMN, compared to AS, the alteration in type IV collagen is less severe. Gene mutations usually involve a single amino acid substitution and do not involve more crucial segments of the gene such as the promoter region.

Renal Pathology

On renal biopsy, light microscopy is often normal. Electron microscopy reveals a homogenous uniformly thinned GBM. It is important to keep in mind that normal GBM thickness varies among institutions and technique. In general, GBM thickness of less than 200–250 ηm is considered consistent with TBMN. Notably, in early stages of AS, the GBM may appear thin before the development of the more characteristic thickening and splitting. Therefore, in patients with a diagnosis of TBMN who progress to more severe kidney disease, an alternate diagnosis of AS should be entertained [15].

Treatment

The prognosis for TBMN is excellent and usually no specific therapy is required. In such cases, tight control of blood pressure and consideration for treatment with ACEI or ARB agents is recommended.

Fabry Disease

Fabry disease is an X-linked disorder caused by a deficiency of the lysosomal enzyme α-galactosidase A (α-gal A), an important enzyme in the metabolism of glycosphingolipids. Deficiency of α-gal A leads to a buildup or increased storage of glycosphingolipids in lysosomes eventually leading to cellular malfunction, inflammation, and subsequent fibrosis.

Clinical Features

Symptoms usually start in early childhood. Burning neuropathic pain in extremities is a common presenting symptom. Patients can also develop pronounced vascular disease (cardiomyopathy, stroke at an early age), decreased sweating (hypohidrosis), corneal opacities (whirls), hearing loss, gastrointestinal upset, and angiokeratomas [16]. Renal impairment tends to develop later in life (in the 30s–50s) with roughly 50% of males and 20% of females developing ESRD [17]. Proteinuria is usually the first sign of renal impairment. Diagnosis can be confirmed by sequencing of the defective gene or by measuring plasma α-gal A activity.

Renal Pathology

Deposition of glycosphingolipids occurs in podocytes, mesangium, capillary walls, and tubular cells. Electron microscopy reveals lysosomes full of lamellar structures also known as Zebra bodies or Myelin bodies.

Treatment

Includes control of blood pressure and ACE inhibition to reduce proteinuria. Enzyme replacement therapy via infusions of recombinant α-gal A is available and has been shown to be safe and effective in improving disease severity [18].

Other hereditary diseases of the kidney are reviewed in Table 49.6.

Case Discussion

The patient described in the case report has autosomal dominant polycystic kidney disease (ADPKD). The diagnosis is confirmed by the presence of multiple bilateral kidney cysts (>3 bilaterally) and cysts in the liver. Though our patient does not have a family history of polycystic kidney disease, it is possible that her father carried a gene mutation for PKD which did not manifest as he passed away at a young age. It is also possible that our patient had a de novo mutation, as is the case in 5–7% of patients with ADPKD. The natural history of a person who has a mutation in the PKD1 gene results in reaching ESRD in her 50s, as opposed to the milder PKD2 gene defects in which patients usually do not reach ESRD until they are in their 70s. Due to the lack of effective interventions to treat ADPKD, most clinicians would not routinely screen family members unless it is for family planning purposes. The patient is at risk for developing all of the complications for ADPKD described in Table 49.1. There is no family history of sudden death, stroke, CNS aneurysms, or patient symptoms to suggest an aneurysm so routine imaging to screen for brain aneurysms is not indicated.

Table 49.6 Other hereditary kidney diseases [22, 23]

Condition	Associated features
Nephronophthisis	Due to defects in genes that are associated with the primary cilium on renal tubular epithelial cells. Cysts are usually located in the corticomedullary junction and appear in later stages of the disease. Predominantly tubulointerstital process with tubular damage and thickening or disintegration of tubular basement membranes. Diagnosis can be made by detecting a gene mutation in NPHP1 which is seen in 20–40% of cases or by screening for mutations in other NPHP genes. Renal manifestations of polyuria, polydipsia, secondary enuresis, and anemia. Extra-renal: retinitis pigmentosa, mental retardation, cerebellar ataxia, bone abnormalities, or liver fibrosis. Symptoms present in the first few decades of life. Usually the serum creatinine level is elevated by age 9 and ESRD develops by the teen years. Autosomal recessive disorder.
Medullary cystic kidney disease	Triad of tubular basement membrane irregularities, tubular atrophy, interstitial inflammation, and fibrosis. Age of onset in the 30s–40s. Not associated with extra-renal manifestations. Associated with defects loci at *MCKD1* and *MCKD2*. *MCKD2* more severe phenotype with ESRD in 30s, *MCKD1* less severe with ESRD in the 60s. Also associated with mutations in *UMOD*, gene that encodes uromodulin or Tamm-Horsefall protein. May be linked to familial juvenile hyperuricemic nephropathy. Autosomal dominant, may have variable penetrance.

Unfortunately, there is no specific treatment for ADPKD outside of routine CKD management. If the patient progresses to ESRD, hemodialysis, peritoneal dialysis, or renal transplant are all acceptable forms of renal replacement therapy. Peritoneal dialysis can be complicated by a higher rate of abdominal hernias. Hemodialysis can be complicated by increased severity of cyst bleeding due to anticoagulation with heparin. In general, patients with ADPKD have better transplant outcomes when compared with patients with other types of renal disease.

Key Points

1. Simple cysts are common with aging, and may be bilateral, but are of little clinical importance. Patients with chronic kidney disease may have a higher degree of acquired cyst burden.
2. Autosomal polycystic kidney disease (ADPKD) is the most common cause of ESRD in the USA (behind diabetes hypertension and glomerulonephritis).
3. ADPKD patients with a family history of CNS aneurysm, stroke, or sudden death have a 16–20% chance of having CNS aneurysms and should be screened by MRA to detect the presence of aneurysms.
4. Cystic disease in ADPKD is not associated with a higher risk of renal cell carcinoma. This compares with acquired renal cystic disease, such as that seen in patients with ESRD, where there is an increased risk for malignant transformation to renal cell carcinoma.
5. Thin basement membrane nephropathy is a common cause of asymptomatic hematuria. It is believed to be present in 1% of the population.
6. Patients with Alport syndrome present with hematuria, variable proteinuria and renal dysfunction, often associated with hearing loss.
7. Alport syndrome is a disease of type IV collagen which affects basement membranes. The most common X-linked form is due to a defect in the $\alpha 5$ subunit of type IV collagen. Autosomal forms are usually due to mutations in the $\alpha 3$ or $\alpha 4$ subunit of type IV collagen.

References

1. Braun WE. Autosomal dominant polycystic kidney disease: emerging concepts of pathogenesis and new treatments. Cleve Clin J Med. 2009;76(2): 97–104.
2. Rizk D, Chapman AB. Cystic and inherited kidney diseases. Am J Kidney Dis. 2003;42(6):1305–17.
3. Grantham JJ. Clinical practice. Autosomal dominant polycystic kidney disease. N Engl J Med. 2008;359(14): 1477–85.

4. Torres VE, Harris PC. Mechanisms of disease: autosomal dominant and recessive polycystic kidney diseases. Nat Clin Pract Nephrol. 2006;2(1):40–55. quiz 55.
5. Chow CL, Ong AC. Autosomal dominant polycystic kidney disease. Clin Med. 2009;9(3):278–83.
6. Feehally J, Floege J, Johnson RJ. Comprehensive clinical nephrology. 3rd ed. Philadelphia, PA: Mosby/ Elsevier; 2007.
7. Torres VE, Harris PC. Autosomal dominant polycystic kidney disease: the last 3 years. Kidney Int. 2009; 76(2):149–68.
8. Torres VE. Vasopressin antagonists in polycystic kidney disease. Semin Nephrol. 2008;28(3):306–17.
9. Walz G, Budde K, Mannaa M, et al. Everolimus in patients with autosomal dominant polycystic kidney disease. N Engl J Med. 2010;363(9):830–40.
10. Patel V, Chowdhury R, Igarashi P. Advances in the pathogenesis and treatment of polycystic kidney disease. Curr Opin Nephrol Hypertens. 2009;18(2): 99–106.
11. Jacquet A, Pallet N, Kessler M, et al. Outcomes of renal transplantation in patients with autosomal dominant polycystic kidney disease: a nationwide longitudinal study. Transpl Int. 2011;24(6):582–7.
12. Heidet L, Gubler MC. The renal lesions of Alport syndrome. J Am Soc Nephrol. 2009;20(6):1210–5.
13. Gross O, Kashtan CE. Treatment of Alport syndrome: beyond animal models. Kidney Int. 2009;76(6): 599–603.
14. Tryggvason K, Patrakka J. Thin basement membrane nephropathy. J Am Soc Nephrol. 2006;17(3):813–22.
15. Gubler MC. Inherited diseases of the glomerular basement membrane. Nat Clin Pract Nephrol. 2008; 4(1):24–37.
16. Zarate YA, Hopkin RJ. Fabry's disease. Lancet. 2008;372(9647):1427–35.
17. Ramaswami U, Najafian B, Schieppati A, Mauer M, Bichet DG. Assessment of renal pathology and dysfunction in children with Fabry disease. Clin J Am Soc Nephrol. 2010;5(2):365–70.
18. Schiffmann R, Kopp JB, Austin 3rd HA, et al. Enzyme replacement therapy in Fabry disease: a randomized controlled trial. JAMA. 2001;285(21):2743–9.
19. Plaisier E, Gribouval O, Alamowitch S, et al. COL4A1 mutations and hereditary angiopathy, nephropathy, aneurysms, and muscle cramps. N Engl J Med. 2007;357(26):2687–95.
20. Heath KE, Campos-Barros A, Toren A, et al. Nonmuscle myosin heavy chain IIA mutations define a spectrum of autosomal dominant macrothrombocytopenias: May-Hegglin anomaly and Fechtner, Sebastian, Epstein, and Alport-like syndromes. Am J Hum Genet. 2001;69(5):1033–45.
21. Lemley KV. Kidney disease in nail-patella syndrome. Pediatr Nephrol. 2009;24(12):2345–54.
22. Salomon R, Saunier S, Niaudet P. Nephronophthisis. Pediatr Nephrol. 2009;24(12):2333–44.
23. Hildebrandt F, Zhou W. Nephronophthisis-associated ciliopathies. J Am Soc Nephrol. 2007;18(6): 1855–71.

Further Reading

Grantham JJ. Clinical practice. Autosomal dominant polycystic kidney disease. N Engl J Med. 2008; 359(14):1477–85.

Rizk D, Chapman AB. Cystic and inherited kidney diseases. Am J Kidney Dis. 2003;42(6):1305–17.

Gubler MC. Inherited diseases of the glomerular basement membrane. Nat Clin Pract Nephrol. 2008;4(1): 24–37.

Multiple Myeloma and the Kidney

50

Fionnuala C. Cormack and Robert E. Richard

Case 1

RG, a 60-year-old African-American man, presents to your clinic with a 6-week history of fatigue and right hip pain, which he attributes to a fall a few months ago. He has not seen a physician in years because he has felt well. However, he did visit the ER a week ago for his hip pain and labs showed a creatinine of 1.9 mg/dL. He has been taking 800–1,200 mg of ibuprofen daily for the last 2 weeks. His physical examination is notable for pain over the right hip. Laboratory studies show a creatinine of 4.6 mg/dL, calcium of 11 mg/dL, and hemoglobin of 7.2 g/dL. Plain films of the right hip show osteolytic lesions. Urine dipstick is negative for protein.

What is the most likely diagnosis?
What is the most likely reason for RG's kidney injury?
What further studies would you obtain?
How would you manage this patient in the acute setting?

F.C. Cormack, M.D. (✉)
Division of Nephrology, Department of Medicine, University of Washington, 325 Ninth Avenue, Seattle, WA 98104, USA
e-mail: dubh@u.washington.edu

R.E. Richard, M.D.
Department of Hematology, VA – Puget Sound Health Care System, University of Washington School of Medicine, 1660 S. Columbian Way, Seattle, WA 98180,USA
e-mail: rrichard@u.washington.edu

Case 2

Mr. AF, a 42-year-old Caucasian man, presents with generalized fatigue. He does not take any over-the-counter or prescribed medications. Physical examination is unremarkable. Laboratory studies show a normal serum glucose, non-anion gap acidosis and hypophosphatemia. Urinalysis is positive for protein and glucose.

What is the most likely diagnosis?
What is the most likely pathophysiology underlying this presentation?

Introduction

A connection between bone marrow tumors and proteinuria was made in 1845 [1]. Dr. William Macintyre noted his patient, Alexander McBean, to have edema and an opaque urine sample with high specific gravity. Dr. Macintyre sent his patient's urine to Dr. Henry Bence Jones who concluded that the urine contained protein, an oxide of "albumen" [2]. At autopsy, the ribs were soft and brittle and drawings of the bone marrow cells examined retrospectively were consistent with plasma cells [1]. The cause of death was documented as "atrophy from albuminuria" [3].

The term "multiple myeloma" was first used in 1873 by J. von Rustizky in Kiev to describe soft, reddish tumors containing round vesicle-like cells on the autopsy of a 47-year-old man [1]. Professor Otto Kahler tied the story

E.V. Lerma and M. Rosner (eds.), *Clinical Decisions in Nephrology, Hypertension and Kidney Transplantation*, DOI 10.1007/978-1-4614-4454-1_50, © Springer Science+Business Media New York 2013

Table 50.1 The International Myeloma Working Group's diagnostic criteria for multiple myeloma

Multiple myeloma (all three criteria must be met)
Presence of serum or urinary monoclonal protein (no specific level of monoclonal protein is used as a cutoff value)
Presence of clonal plasma cells in the bone marrow or a plasmacytoma
Presence of end organ damage (1 or more)[a]
[C] elevated calcium, >10.5 mg/dL
[R] renal insufficiency, Cr > 2 mg/dL
[A] anemia, hemoglobin < 10 g/dL
[B] lytic bone lesions

[a]CRAB

together in 1889 when he evaluated a patient with grey-reddish masses or "multiple myeloma" in the ribs and urinary protein as described by Bence Jones [1]. In the 1950s, Korngold and Lipari further characterized these urinary proteins, leading to their present distinction as κ and λ after these investigators [4].

Multiple myeloma (MM) is a neoplastic clonal expansion of plasma cells producing a monoclonal protein (M protein) or paraprotein. Under normal circumstances, plasma cells produce immunoglobulins composed of two heavy chains and two κ or λ light chains; they are classified by the heavy chain component as either immunoglobulin (Ig) A, D, E, G, or M [5]. The M protein detected on serum or urine electrophoresis or immunofixation can be either intact immunoglobulin or light chain. In multiple myeloma, the excess secretion of monoclonal proteins causes renal and nonrenal disease. The International Myeloma Working Group's diagnostic criteria for multiple myeloma is outlined in Table 50.1 [5]. In this chapter, our focus is on renal damage in the setting of multiple myeloma since kidney injury is the most common and often earliest end organ manifestation of this systemic disease [6]. In fact, multiple myeloma is often diagnosed from the workup of unexplained renal disease [7].

Epidemiology

Multiple myeloma is a malignant plasma cell disorder that accounts for approximately 10% of all hematologic cancers [8]. It is twice as common in African Americans compared to Caucasians and slightly more common in men than in women. The median age of onset is 66 years; 2% of patients present under age 40 [9]. Renal involvement is present in 20–50% of cases at diagnosis and in over 50% during the course of myeloma [10]. The Durie–Salmon clinical staging system has been supplanted by the International Staging System (ISS) that uses only two lab measurements to determine prognosis: albumin and beta-2 microglobulin (B2M). Median survival of patients with stage I (B2M < 3.5 mg/L and serum albumin ≥ 3.5 g/dL) is 62 months, stage II (neither stage I nor stage III) 44 months, and stage III (B2M ≥ 5.5 mg/L) 29 months [11]. While creatinine does not factor into the ISS, studies show the presence of renal disease increases morbidity and mortality. The higher the creatinine on presentation, the lower the median survival [12]. With respect to kidney disease, according to the 2004 US Renal Data Systems (USRDS) report, the incidence of end-stage renal disease (ESRD) secondary to myeloma in 2004 was 1.1% [13]. Despite representing only 1% of all malignancies, MM contributes to over half of malignancy-related ESRD.

Pathophysiology

There are a number of patterns of renal disease in multiple myeloma. Clinical-pathologic presentations differ based on the type of protein involved—intact immunoglobulin, monoclonal light chains, heavy chains, truncated portions of these proteins—and its target in the renal parenchyma: tubules, interstitium, or glomerulus. Vascular lesions are rare, as is parenchymal infiltration by plasma cells.

Most renal injury in multiple myeloma is due to monoclonal light chains, as opposed to intact immunoglobulins or heavy chains [6, 14]. Light chains are metabolized primarily by the kidneys, therefore it is important to review renal handling of light chains. Because of their small size and cationic net charge, κ and λ light chains (LCs) are freely filtered at the glomerulus and actively endocytosed by the proximal tubule epithelial cells (PTECs) by binding receptors megalin and cubilin [15]. 90% of circulating LCs are reabsorbed and catabolized to their amino acid components which are returned to the circulation. In health, the average filtered load of light chains is 100–600 mg/24 h but ultimately <5 mg/24 h are excreted, reflecting the renal tubules' ability to handle a large filtered load [16]. As is the case in MM, the concentration of serum free light chains (FLCs) must increase manifold to overwhelm the PTECs' reabsorptive capabilities. In addition to excessive numbers of FLCs, structural variability among light chains influences nephrotoxicity [16]. Both κ and λ light chains can be nephrotoxic. Studies suggest that the variable region of the light chain determines its pathogenic nature and the specific type of renal damage caused. Mouse models reinforce that the type of renal disease one develops depends specifically on the monoclonal light chain. When light chains isolated from patients with MM were injected into mice, the mice developed the same renal lesions as the myeloma patients [17].

Table 50.2 Types of renal disease in multiple myeloma

Acute kidney injury
Cast nephropathy ("myeloma kidney")
Prerenal azotemia or acute tubular necrosis (ATN)
Hypercalcemia
NSAIDS
Volume depletion
Loop diuretics
Hyperuricemia
Contrast nephrotoxicity
Chronic kidney injury
Tubular or tubulointerstitial disorders
Fanconi's syndrome
Cast nephropathy
Glomerulopathies
AL-amyloidosis
Light chain deposition disease (LCDD)
Heavy chain deposition disease (HCDD)
Mixed chain deposition disease (MCDD)

Histopathology

The main categories of renal lesions are shown in Table 50.2. In a review of 118 patients with multiple myeloma, renal biopsy showed cast nephropathy in 41%, AL-amyloidosis in 30%, light chain deposition disease in 22%, and chronic tubulointerstitial nephritis in 10% [18].

Tubulointerstitial Disorders

Cast Nephropathy

The most common renal presentation is light chain cast nephropathy, also referred to as "myeloma kidney." It is a chronic tubulointerstitial nephropathy characterized by tubular atrophy and interstitial fibrosis [16]. The characteristic pathologic finding is large, waxy, fractured casts surrounded by giant cells in the lumen of distal and collecting tubules. Casts are composed of monoclonal light chains and Tamm–Horsfall protein (THP). When the concentration of clonal FLCs exceeds the reabsorptive capacity of PTECs, free light chains coprecipitate with THP produced in the thick ascending loop of henle causing distal intratubular obstruction [19, 20]. The binding between THP and light chains is augmented by conditions that commonly arise in patients with multiple myeloma: hypercalcemia/calciuria and/or use of loop diuretics, NSAIDs, or IV contrast material. The interstitium is characterized by edema, fibrosis, and often plasma cell infiltration [20]. The occurrence of distal obstructive casts does not explain the degree of tubulointerstitial inflammation, scarring, and fibrosis that occurs. There is a growing body of literature that exposure of PTECs to excess light chains causes apoptosis of these cells as well as cytokine release, recruitment of inflammatory cells and subsequent interstitial fibrosis [16].

Fanconi Syndrome

Fanconi syndrome is a classic renal presentation of multiple myeloma. It is a proximal tubular disorder attributed to the toxic effects of light chains on PTECs. In vitro studies show that the variable domain of the light chains producing this lesion resists degradation by proteases. Variable domain fragments accumulate and subsequent intracellular crystal formation inhibits transport of glucose, amino acids, and phosphate. Renal biopsies show crystalline or fibrillary-like inclusions of light chains in the PTECs as well as cellular desquamation, cytoplasmic vacuolization, and focal loss of microvilli [16]. The crystals usually consist of light chains that do not bind THP, which is why cast nephropathy and Fanconi syndrome rarely coexist.

Glomerularopathies

Within the glomeruli, pathologic light and heavy chains cause two distinct patterns of injury. Both can either deposit in the glomerular mesangium or form amyloid, a protein folding disorder in which fibrils are derived from light or heavy chains. Heavy chain deposition disease (HCCD) and AH-amyloidosis (amyloid associated with heavy chains) are exceeding rare. Only IgG and IgM AH-amyloidosis have been reported in the literature. Therefore, our discussion will primarily focus on light chain deposition disease (LCCD) and AL-amyloidosis (amyloid associated with light chains) [21].

There is much investigation into the mechanism by which nephrotoxic light chains induce LCDD versus AL-amyloidosis. While the understanding of the mesangial cell-light chain interaction remains under investigation, LCs have been shown to bind to a receptor on the mesangial cell. The divergent phenotypic presentations may be related to distinct cellular trafficking of the pathogenic light chain after binding to a mesangial cell receptor. AL-amyloid LCs are internalized to a lysosomal compartment where amyloid formation occurs, whereas LCDD LCs do not appear to be internalized [22]. Another critical difference in the pathogenesis of glomerular AL-amyloidosis versus LCDD seems to be a phenotypic transformation of the mesangial cell into a macrophage phenotype in AL-amyloidosis versus a myofibroblastic phenotype in LCDD [23].

LCDD

LCDD occurs in about 25% of patients with myeloma presenting with renal disease [10]. A striking feature of LCDD on light microscopy (LM) is the dramatic accumulation of extracellular matrix (ECM) that is responsible for glomerular and tubular basement membrane thickening, nodular glomerulosclerosis, and interstitial fibrosis [22]. The classic glomerular pattern in LCDD is nodular glomerulosclerosis in the mesangium, similar to the mesangial pathology seen in renal disease due to diabetes mellitus. The mesangial nodules are composed of normal constituents (collagen type IV, laminin, fibronectin, and tenascin) and light chains [22].

Light chains, predominantly κLCs, deposit along the glomerular basement membranes (GBM) and tubular basement membranes (TBM) [21]. The most characteristic ultrastructural feature is granular electron-dense deposits delineating the outer aspect of the TBM. In glomeruli, a nonfibrillar electron-dense material is seen in the mesangial nodules and along the GBM. Immunofluorescence (IF) shows LC fixation along tubular BM, a criterion for the diagnosis of LCDD. The tubular deposits stain strongly and predominate along the loops of Henle and distal tubules. In contrast, light chain deposition in the glomerulus is heterogeneous. In patients with nodular glomerulosclerosis, LCs are seen along the peripheral GBM and to a lesser extent in the nodules themselves. The staining in glomeruli typically is weaker relative to the TBM [22].

AL-Amyloidosis

The amyloidoses are a group of protein folding disorders sharing unique staining and a similar fibrillar ultrastructure [24]. By convention, the amyloid type is designated A (amyloid) followed by an abbreviation for the name of the amyloid fibril precursor protein. There are more than 20 types of precursor proteins. AL-amyloidosis or light chain amyloidosis is the most prevalent type of systemic amyloidosis [14]. In AL-amyloidosis, the mesangium is replaced by amyloid fibrils composed of light chains. As the disease progresses, amyloid deposits can extend to the interstitium and vasculature. Electron microscopic findings show randomly distributed non-branching fibrils 8–12 nm in diameter. LM is notable for a salmon-pink appearance on Congo Red staining and applegreen birefringence when viewed with polarized light microscopy. While LCDD is associated with κ light chain restriction, AL-amyloidosis is more associated with the λ isotype [25, 26].

AL-amyloidosis is a disease characterized by a decrease in ECM; extraneous material replaces the normal mesangial matrix. On binding amyloidogenic light chains, the normal smooth muscle phenotype of the mesangial cells changes into a macrophage phenotype. The LCs are internalized and delivered to lysosomal compartments where amyloid fibrils are formed. Metalloproteinases are activated, destroying the normal matrix, which is eventually replaced by amyloid fibrils [26].

It is critical to distinguish AL-amyloidosis from other glomerular diseases such as fibrillary glomerulonephritis (FGN) and immunotactoid glomerulopathy (ITG) in which pathogenic immunoglobulins form immune deposits in the mesangium or glomerular basement membrane. FGN and ITG are uncommon causes of glomerular disease; the main distinguishing feature between amyloidosis and these other immunoglobulin deposition diseases is the absence of reactivity with Congo Red in these other disorders [27–30]. Light microscopic findings are nondiagnostic and heterogeneous; diagnosis is based on ultrastructural findings. On electron microscopy (EM), FGN is characterized by glomerular accumulations of small, nonbranching, randomly arranged fibrils that are ultrastructurally indistinguishable from amyloid fibrils. Involvement of the TBM is uncommon. Immunofluorescence is usually positive for IgG, C3, and both kappa and lambda light chains [30]. ITG is characterized by glomerular deposits of immunoglobulins organized as large microtubules on electron microscopy [30]. Many patients have either a circulating paraprotein or monoclonal immunoglobulin deposition in the glomeruli by immunofluorescence microscopy with a restricted light chain, either kappa or lamda. In both disorders, the fibril or microtubule deposition is almost always limited to the kidney. The distinguishing histological and clinical features of these disorders are outlined in Table 50.3.

Clinical Features

The monoclonal gammopathies are a group of disorders associated with a neoplastic proliferation of plasma cells. The International Myeloma Working Group established a classification system for differentiating symptomatic multiple myeloma from other monoclonal gammopathies and clarified the difference among myeloma, smoldering myeloma, and monoclonal gammopathy of unknown significance (MGUS). The main distinction among multiple myeloma and other monoclonal gammopathies is the presence of end organ damage manifested by increased *c*alcium, *r*enal insufficiency, *a*nemia or *b*one lesions (*CRAB*) attributable to the plasma cell disorder (Table 50.1) [5]. MGUS and smoldering myeloma are differentiated by the amount of M protein and the percentage of plasma cells in the bone marrow. MGUS is defined by the presence of a serum monoclonal (M) protein <3 g/dL, bone marrow plasma cells $<10\%$, and absence CRAB findings. In smoldering myeloma, serum M protein is ≥ 3 g/dL or bone marrow plasma cells are $\geq 10\%$, and there are no CRAB findings. The distinction is important since treatment is only universally accepted for patients with multiple myeloma. There are ongoing studies to determine whether patients benefit from early treatment of smoldering myeloma.

Among the monoclonal gammopathies, another disease entity to consider in the differential diagnoses of multiple myeloma is Waldenström's macroglobulinemia (WM). It is characterized by a malignant proliferation of bone marrow cells with lymphocyte and plasma cell characteristics (lymphoplastmacytoid lymphoma or LPL) that produce circulating monoclonal IgM [31]. WM is a rare disease affecting patients in their mid-60s with symptoms related to direct tumor infiltration of hematopoietic tissues—anemia, lymphadenopathy, hepatosplenomegaly—and/or the effects of circulating IgM—hyperviscosity, peripheral neuropathy [31]. Renal involvement is exceedingly rare, but cases of IgM-related systemic amyloidosis with kidney involvement have been reported [32]. One

Table 50.3 Clinical and histological features of Ig-related kidney diseases

	Myeloma kidney "Cast nephropathy"	LCDD	AL-Amyloid	FGN[a]	ITG[b]	WM[c]
Mean age (years) at presentation	mid-60s	mid-60s	mid-60s	mid-50s	mid-50s	mid-60s
Proteinuria	Usu < 1 g/day	Occa < 1 g/day Usu > 3.5 g/day	>3.5 g/day	>3.5 g/day	>3.5 g/day	>3.5 g/day
Urine sediment	Bland	Bland/dysmorphic RBCs	Bland/dysmorphic RBCs	Bland/dysmorphic RBCs	Bland/dysmorphic RBCs	Bland/dysmorphic RBCs
LM	PAS stain of waxy, fractured tubular casts, chronic interstitial nephritis/fibrosis	Tubular basement membrane thickening, mesangialnodular glomerulosclerosis, instersti-tial fibrosis	Congo red-positive, amorphous, hyaline material in the mesangium and capillary loops	Nonspecific, variable, mesangial expansion	Nonspecific, variable, mesangial expansion	Renal involvement exceedingly rare AL-amyloidosis has been reported
IF	Intratubular κ or λ LCs	κ > λ LCs along GBM, tubular BM, in glomerular nodules	λ > κ in mesangium capillary walls	IgG, C3, λ, κ in Mesangium, capillary walls	Variable Usu IgG, C3 in mesangium, capillary walls	
EM Appearance	Casts have nonspecific appearance, may contain crystalline structures	Electron-dense deposits along tubular BM, nonfibrillar electron-dense material in mesangial nodules and GBM	Fibrils	Fibrils	Microtubules	
Fibril/microtubule size (nm)			8–12	18–20	>30	
Fibril arrangement			Random	Random	Parallel	
Location			Mesangium, capillary walls	Mesangium capillary walls	Mesangium, capillary walls	
Reaction with histochemical dyes Congo Red and Thioflavin T on LM	No	No	Yes	No	No	

[a] Fibrillary glomerulonephritis
[b] Immunotactoid glomerulopathy
[c] Waldenström's macroglobulinemia

series described 50 patients with an IgM monoclonal protein and systemic amyloidosis. Amyloid deposits consisted of a monoclonal immunoglobulin light chain, indicating that the amyloidosis was of the primary (AL) type [33].

Renal manifestations in myeloma vary depending on the disease process. While cast nephropathy can cause chronic tubulointerstitial nephritis, up to 50% of patients present acutely with oliguric renal failure without significant proteinuria [7]. These acute cases are often precipitated by volume depletion, infection, hypercalcemia, or nephrotoxic agents such as IV contrast, NSAIDs, or loop diuretics [34]. Patients often have a bland urine sediment with a urine dipstick negative for protein. It is important to keep in mind that the urine dipstick tests for albumin but not light chains. Historically, immunoglobulins were detected by adding sulfosalicylic acid (SSA) to the urine. Acidification causes immunoglobulins to precipitate, increasing the turbidity of the sample.

In cases of glomerular injury such as AL-amyloidosis and LCDD, kidney function may be normal, but patients often have nephrotic syndrome with >3.5 g of proteinuria (albuminuria), edema, and hypoalbuminemia. Hematuria is occasionally present. The presence of a monoclonal light chain in the urine of a patient with nephrotic-range proteinuria is indicative of AL-amyloidosis or LCDD. That said, a subset of patients with LCDD can present with proteinuria of <1 g/day which is more consistent with a tubulointerstitial process. AL-amyloidosis and LCDD are usually the presenting diseases that lead to the diagnosis of myeloma at an early stage; in most cases, renal function declines rapidly [21, 22].

Patients with AL-amyloidosis typically present with fatigue and weight loss. On ultrasound, kidneys may be enlarged. The clinical presentation in primary (AL) amyloidosis depends on the organs affected and may include nephrotic syndrome, restrictive cardiomyopathy, peripheral neuropathy, hepatomegaly, macroglossia, or purpura. Cardiac involvement may manifest as cardiac arrhythmias or congestive heart failure. Macroglossia is considered to be pathognomonic for AL, occurring in 20% of patients. The diagnosis requires histologic evidence of amyloid. A renal biopsy is diagnostic in >95% of patients with clinical evidence of renal disease [25].

Fanconi syndrome is a dysfunction of the proximal tubule leading to urinary excretion of amino acids, glucose, phosphate, and bicarbonate. Patients are often asymptomatic. Multiple myeloma should be high on the differential diagnosis of any adult presenting with proximal renal tubular acidosis.

Finally, hypercalcemia is both a common manifestation of multiple myeloma and a common cause of acute kidney injury in MM. Serum calcium levels between 12 and 15 mg/dL cause renal vasoconstriction and a natriuresis-induced volume contraction, thus lowering glomerular filtration rate and raising creatinine [35]. Patients with an acute rise in calcium levels may present with volume depletion, nausea, anorexia, constipation, and/or confusion.

Work-up

The definition of renal failure varies in the literature. Most studies use a creatinine of 2 mg/dl [36]. Per guidelines from the International Myeloma Working Group, both serum and urine should be evaluated for the presence of a monoclonal protein [37]. About 97% of patients with multiple myeloma have an M protein produced and secreted by the malignant plasma cells which can be detected by serum protein electrophoresis (SPEP) and/or urine protein electrophoresis (UPEP) from a 24-h urine collection. The M protein usually presents as a single narrow peak in the gamma, beta, or alpha-2 region on densitometer tracing or as a dense, discrete band on agarose gel. Serum immunofixation is the gold standard for identifying the specific monoclonal protein and distinguishing its heavy and light chain type. Immunofixation will detect a serum M-protein as low as 0.2 g/L and a urine M-protein of 0.04 g/L [37].

A serum free light chain (FLC) assay is recommended in all patients with suspected multiple myeloma, but especially in patients with renal insufficiency and a high clinical suspicion for multiple myeloma but low or nondetectable M protein on serum and urine immunofixation. Up to 20% of patients with myeloma do not demonstrate heavy chain expression in the M protein and are therefore considered to have light chain myeloma [38]. In health, the production of both kappa and lambda light chains is constant and the κ/λ ratio remains in a fixed range. Patients with renal impairment often have elevated κ FLC and λ FLC due to decreased renal clearance, however the κ/λ FLC ratio (rFLC) remains normal. Katzmann et al. defined the normal range for κ FLC as 3.3–19.4 mg/L and λ FLC as 5.7–26.3 mg/L and a normal diagnostic range for κ/λ FLC as 0.26–1.65 [39]. Patients with a κ/λ ratio > 1.65 are presumed to be producing clonal κ light chains and with < 0.26, excess λ light chains. An abnormal serum FLC has a high sensitivity and specificity for multiple myeloma [40].

Ultimately, the definitive workup for renal injury is a kidney biopsy, especially since immunofixation does not identify a monoclonal Ig component in 10–20% of patients. In most cases of cast nephropathy and nephrotoxic-induced injury (volume depletion, hypercalcemia, NSAIDS, IV contrast), diagnosis is based on the clinical presentation. In cases of suspected glomerular injury, biopsy is often pursued and leads to the diagnosis of multiple myeloma [7].

Treatment and Outcomes

According to the International Staging System, the median survival for patients diagnosed with MM ranges from 29 to 62 months. Renal insufficiency in the setting of multiple myeloma portends increased morbidity and mortality. It is one of the most common causes of death, second only to infection. Even with aggressive chemotherapy, the average time to initiation of dialysis in myeloma kidney is 3 months, 15 months with AL-amyloidosis, and 18 months with LCDD [34]. In several series, the median survival of patients with MM and renal failure is less than 2 years [12].

Acute cast nephropathy is associated with the poorest outcomes in all myeloma-related kidney disease and warrants aggressive intervention. The main goal of therapy is to reduce light-chain production. Initial treatment is volume resuscitation and minimizing factors leading to decreased GFR and cast precipitation: avoiding radiocontrast agents, NSAIDs, diuretics. Therapy should also be directed toward controlling the tumor burden. Given the role of inflammatory cytokines in the pathogenesis of myeloma kidney and the likelihood of hypercalcemia, steroids are a reasonable approach to target the renal aspect of the disease. These measures along with chemotherapy lead to renal recovery in 50% of cases and improve patient survival to that of patients without renal insufficiency [7].

Given that serum concentrations of monoclonal FLCs are typically several thousand times higher than normal in myeloma, a modality that rapidly removes light chains would theoretically limit or abrogate renal injury. Data for removal by plasma exchange has not borne this out. There are two small prospective studies showing benefit and one large prospective study showing no significant change in renal function or need for dialysis. While the larger study's findings were limited by lack of renal biopsies and free light chain measurements, on balance, plasma exchange is thought to be of no additional benefit in the management of acute kidney injury (AKI) in multiple myeloma [41–43]. A newer modality of treating AKI with extended hemodialysis using a high cut-off dialyzer (HCO-HD) is being explored but clinical utility has not been established [44].

Initial therapy of patients with symptomatic myeloma varies depending on whether patients are eligible for autologous stem cell transplantation (ASCT). Eligibility varies across countries and institutions. Generally, the principal characteristics determining eligibility are age, performance status, and/or the presence of comorbid conditions. The randomized trials showing benefit of ASCT over chemotherapy have mainly studied patients with serum creatinine <2.0 mg/dL. Induction therapies vary based on patient characteristics and institutional protocols but include agents such as bortezomib, lenalidomide, or thalidomide +/− dexamethasone given over

Table 50.4 Current treatment strategies in multiple myeloma

Myeloma [50–52]	Transplant candidate	Bortezemib and/or lenalidomide with dexamethasone followed by high-dose alkylating agents and autologous stem cell transplant
	Not a transplant candidate	Thalidomide or lenalidomide or bortezemib with melphalan and prednisone as initial treatment. Switch to other agent when the patient relapses
Amyloid (AL) [53]	Transplant candidate	Clinical trial preferably or high-dose melphalan with autologous stem cell transplant
	Not a transplant candidate	Clinical trial or melphalan/prednisone or dexamethasone. Consider bortezemib/lenalidomide depending on end organ damage and toxicity profile
Light chain deposition disease [28]		Data is limited Myeloma therapy is generally employed

2–4 months followed by autologous stem cell harvest [45, 46]. This approach has been associated with improved progression-free survival in several studies. With ASCT, response rates are as high as 85% and overall median survival increased by 12 months, compared with standard chemotherapy. In patients who attain remission, median overall survival ranges from 40–89 months compared to 26 months in nonresponders. Response to therapy and survival seem to be independent of renal function (creatinine >2 mg/dl) and ESRD, however ASCT-related mortality is higher in patients with kidney disease [47]. In a study of 59 dialysis-dependent patients with multiple myeloma, 24% recovered renal function following successful ASCT with high-dose melphalan as the induction agent [48]. Of note, in LCDD and AL-amyloidosis, clearance of LC deposits has been demonstrated after intensive chemotherapy with ASCT [22]. For patients deemed poor transplant candidates, treatment depends on a number of factors but common protocols include melphalan, prednisone and thalidomide (MPT) or bortezomib, melphalan, and prednisone (VMP) [49, 50]. Table 50.4 outlines current treatment strategies.

Case 1 Revisited

What is the most likely diagnosis? What is the most likely reason for patient's kidney injury? How would you manage this patient in the acute setting? What further studies would you obtain?

RG presents with a few critical features of end organ damage: C-hyper*C*alcemia, R-*r*enal insufficiency, A-*a*nemia and B-*b*one pain, suggesting osteolytic lesions. The presence of "CRAB" puts multiple myeloma high on the differential. Regarding patient's kidney injury, he has a subacute rise in creatinine in the setting of heavy NSAID use and a negative urine dipstick. Cast nephropathy is the most likely diagnosis. Initial treatment should be hospital admission with aggressive volume resuscitation. Ins and outs must be monitored closely as well as serum creatinine and calcium levels. Patient's high calcium should also respond to volume repletion, however caution should be taken in using loop diuretics as they can precipitate cast formation between light chains and THP. Steroids could be considered for managing RG's hypercalcemia. Once these initial therapies have been instituted, an SPEP and UPEP with immunofixation as well as serum FLCs should be ordered and hematology consult obtained to pursue a bone marrow biopsy.

Case 2 Revisited

What is the most likely diagnosis? What is the most likely pathophysiology underlying this presentation?

Mr. AF has generalized proximal tubular dysfunction or Fanconi syndrome. Multiple myeloma should be the primary consideration in any adult presenting with Fanconi syndrome.

High concentrations of κ or λ light chains are toxic to proximal tubular epithelial cells. In this setting, fragments of the light chains crystallize in the proximal cells, inhibiting reabsorption of bicarbonate, phosphate, glucose, amino acids, and other electrolytes. Patients with this generalized dysfunction of the proximal tubular cells typically present with polyuria, a non-anion gap renal tubular acidosis and hypophosphatemia. A spot urine sample will show glucosuria. This patient should be managed with volume repletion and electrolyte replacement and work-up for multiple myeloma should be initiated.

Key Points

- The most common cause of acute kidney injury in multiple myeloma is cast nephropathy
- Cast nephropathy should be suspected in older patients with a constellation of fatigue, acute kidney injury with creatinine >2.0 mg/dL, bland urine sediment, and a urine dipstick negative for proteinuria
- Initial work-up should include an SPEP, UPEP on a 24 h urine collection, measurement of serum FLCs, and a serum calcium level
- Initial treatment should be aggressive volume resuscitation and consideration of steroids in the setting of hypercalcemia
- Renal biopsy should be considered in patients with a bland urine sediment and nephrotic-range (>3.5 g) proteinuria
- Prompt hematology consultation should be obtained to guide further workup and management

References

1. Kyle RA. Multiple myeloma: an odyssey of discovery. Br J Haematol. 2000;111:1035–44.
2. Kyle RA, Rajkumar SV. Multiple myeloma. Blood. 2008;111:2962–72.
3. Clamp JR. Some aspects of the first recorded case of multiple myeloma. Lancet. 1967;290:1354–6.
4. Korngold L, Lipari R. Multiple-myeloma III. The antigenic relationship of BenceJones proteins to normal gammaglobulin and multiple-myeloma serum proteins. Cancer. 1956;9:262–72.
5. International Myeloma Working Group. Criteria for the classification of monoclonal gammopathies, multiple myeloma and related disorders: a report of the International Myeloma Working Group. Br J Haematol. 2003;121(5):749–57.
6. Herrara G. Renal lesions associated with plasma cell dyscrasias, practical approach to diagnosis, new concepts and challenges. Arch Pathol Lab Med. 2009; 133:240–67.
7. Korbet SM, Schwartz MM. Multiple myeloma. J Am Soc Nephrol. 2006;17:2533–45.
8. Kyle RA, Rajkumar SV. Multiple myeloma. N Engl J Med. 2004;351:1860–73.
9. Kyle RA, Gertz MA, Witzig TE, et al. Review of 1027 patients with newly diagnosed multiple myeloma. Mayo Clin Proc. 2003;78:21–33.
10. Lin J, Markowitz GS, Valeri AM, et al. Renal monoclonal immunoglobulin deposition disease: the disease spectrum. J Am Soc Nephrol. 2001;12:1482–92.
11. Greipp PR, San Miguel J, Durie BG, et al. International staging system for multiple myeloma. J Clin Oncol. 2005;23(15):3412.
12. Kyle RA, Therneau TM, Rajkumar SV. Incidence of multiple myeloma in Olmsted County, Minnesota: trend over 6 decades. Cancer. 2004;101:2667–74.
13. US Renal Data System: USRDS 2005 annual data report: atlas of end-stage renal disease in the United States. Bethesda, MD: National Institutes of Health, National Institute Diabetes and Digestive and Kidney Diseases; 2005.
14. Dimopoulos MA, Terpos E, Chanan-Khan A. Renal impairment in patients with multiple myeloma: a consensus statement on behalf of the international myeloma working group. J Clin Oncol. 2010;29: 4976–84.
15. Christensen EI, Brin H. Megalin and cubilin: synergistic endocytic receptors in renal proximal tubule. Am J Physiol Renal Physiol. 2001;280:F562–73.
16. Batuman V. Proximal tubular injury in myeloma. In: Herrera GA, editor. The kidney in plasma cell dyscrasias, Contribution to nephrology, vol. 153. Basel: Karger; 2007. p. 87–104.
17. Solomon A, Weiss DT, Kattine AA. Nephrotoxic potential of Bence Jones proteins. N Engl J Med. 1991;324:1845–51.
18. Monteseny JJ, Kleinknecht D, Meyrier A, et al. Long-term outcome according to renal histological lesions in 118 patients with monoclonal gammopathies. Nephrol Dial Transplant. 1998;13:1438–45.
19. Basnayake K, Ying WZ, Wang PX, et al. Immunoglobulin light chains activate tubular epithelial cells through redox signaling. J Am Soc Nephrol. 2010;21:1165–73.
20. Merlini G, Pozzi C. Mechanisms of renal damage in plasma cell dyscrasias: an overview. In: Herrera GA, editor. The kidney in plasma cell dyscrasias, Contribution to nephrology, vol. 153. Basel: Karger; 2007. p. 66–86.
21. Keeling J, Herrera GA. The mesangium as a target for glomerulopathic light and heavy chains: pathogenic

considerations in light and heavy chain-mediated glomerular damage. In: Herrera GA, editor. The kidney in plasma cell dyscrasias, Contribution to nephrology, vol. 153. Basel: Karger; 2007. p. 116–34.
22. Ronco P, Plaisier E, Mougenot B. Immunoglobulin light (heavy)-chain deposition disease: from molecular medicine to pathophysiology-driven therapy. Clin J Am Soc Nephrol. 2006;1:1342–50.
23. Keeling J, Teng J, Herrera GA. AL-amyloidosis and light chain deposition disease light chains induce divergent phenotypic transformations of human mesangial cells. Lab Invest. 2004;84:1322–38.
24. Westermark P, Benson MD, Buxbaum JN. Amyloid: toward terminology clarification. Amyloid. 2005;12: 1–4.
25. Falk RH, Skinner M. The systemic amyloidoses: an overview. Adv Intern Med. 2000;45:107–37.
26. Herrera GA. Renal manifestations of plasma cell dyscrasias: an appraisal from the patient's bedside to the research laboratory. Ann Diagn Pathol. 2000;4:174–200.
27. Dember LM. Light chains, casts, sheets and fibrils: monoclonal immunoglobulin diseases and immunotac toid/fibrillaryglomerulopathy. Clin J Am Soc Nephrol. 2006;1:1320–1.
28. Ganeval D, Noël LH, Preud'homme JL, et al. Light-chain deposition disease: its relation with AL-type amyloidosis. Kidney Int. 1984;26(1):1.
29. Korbet SM, Schwartz MM, Lewis EJ. Immunotactoidglomerulopathy (fibrillary glomerulonephritis). Clin J Am Soc Nephrol. 2006;1:1351–6.
30. Alpers CE, Kowalewska J. Fibrillary glomerulonephritis and immunotactoid glomerulopathy. J Am Soc Nephrol. 2008;19:34–7.
31. Dimopoulos MA, Panayiotidis P, Moulopoulos LA. Waldenström's macroglobulinemia: clinical features, complications, and management. J Clin Oncol. 2000;18:214–26.
32. Gerz MA, Kyle RA, Noel P. Primary systemic amyloidosis: a rare complication of immunoglobulin M monoclonal gammopathies and waldenström's macroglobulinemia. J Clin Oncol. 1993;11:914.
33. Veltman GA, van Veen S, Kluin-Nelemans JC. Renal disease in waldenström's macroglobulinaemia. Nephrol Dial Transplant. 1997;12:1256.
34. Penfield JG. Multiple myeloma in end-stage renal disease. Semin Dial. 2006;19:329–34.
35. Levi M, Ellis MA, Berl T. Control of renal hemodynamics and glomerular filtration rate in chronic hypercalcemia. Role of prostaglandins, renin-angiotensin system and calcium. J Clin Invest. 1983;71(6):1624.
36. Dimopoulos MA, Kastritis E, Rosinol L, et al. Pathogenesis and treatment of renal failure in multiple myeloma. Leukemia. 2008;22:1485–93.
37. Dimopoulos M, Kyle R, Fermand JP. Guidelines for standard investigative workup: report of the international myeloma workshop consensus panel 3. Blood. Prepublished online February 2, 2011:1–17.
38. Rajkumar VS, Kyle AK. Multiple myeloma: diagnosis and treatment. Mayo Clin Proc. 2005;80:1371–82.
39. Katzmann JA, Clark RJ, Abraham RS. Serum reference intervals and diagnostic ranges for free kappa and free lambda immunoglobulin light chains: relative sensitivity for detection of monoclonal light chains. Clin Chem. 2002;48:1437–44.
40. Pratt G. The evolving use of serum free light chain assays in haematology. Br J Haematol. 2008;141: 413–22.
41. Johnson WJ, Kyle RA, Pineda AA. Treatment of renal failure associated with multiple myeloma. Arch Intern Med. 1990;150:863–9.
42. Zuchelli P, Pasquali S, Cagnoli L, Ferrari G. Controlled plasma exchange trial in acute renal failure due to multiple myeloma. Kidney Int. 1998;33:1175–80.
43. Clark WF, Steart AK, Rock GA. Plasma exchange when myeloma presents as acute renal failure: a randomized, controlled trial. Ann Intern Med. 2005;132:777–84.
44. Hutchinson CA, Bradwell AR, Cook M. Treatment of acute renal failure secondary to multiple myeloma with chemotherapy and extended high cut-off hemodialysis. Clin J Am Soc Nephrol. 2009;4:745–54.
45. Gay F, Hayman SR, Lacy MQ, et al. Lenalidomide plus dexamethasone versus thalidomide plus dexamethasone as initial therapy for multiple myeloma: a comparative analysis of 411 patients. Blood. 2010;115:1343.
46. Jagannath S, Durie BG, Wolf J, et al. Bortezomib therapy alone and in combination with dexamethasone for previously untreated multiple myeloma. Br J Haematol. 2005;129:776.
47. Knudsen LM, Nielsen B, Gimsing P. Autologous stem cell transplantation in multiple myeloma: outcome in patients with renal failure. Eur J Haematol. 2005;75:22–33.
48. Lee CK, Zangari M, Barlogie B. Dialysis-dependent renal failure in patients with myeloma can be reversed by high-dose myeloablative therapy and autotransplant. Bone Marrow Transplant. 2004;33:823–8.
49. Palumbo A, Bertola A, Musto P, et al. Oral melphalan, prednisone, and thalidomide for newly diagnosed patients with myeloma. Cancer. 2005;104:1428.
50. San Miguel JF, Schlag R, Khuageva NK, et al. Bortezomib plus melphalan and prednisone for initial treatment of multiple myeloma. N Engl J Med. 2008;359:906.
51. Mehta J, Cavo M, Singhal M. How I treat elderly patients with myeloma. Blood. 2010;116:2215–23.
52. Stewart AK, Richardson PG, San-Miguel JF. How I treat multiple myeloma in younger patients. Blood. 2009;114:5436–43.
53. Comenzo RL. How I treat amyloidosis. Blood. 2009;114:3147–57.

Part XI

Nephrolithiasis

Nephrolithiasis

51

Kerry C. Cho, Grace J. No, Lowell J. Lo, and Andrew Lin

Case 1

A 24-year-old Hispanic woman with no medical history presents to the emergency department for the acute onset of left flank pain that radiated to the left lower quadrant. She had two episodes of non-bloody vomiting. She denied any prior episode of flank pain or nephrolithiasis, hematuria, pyuria, and dysuria. Her menstrual periods have been normal; her last menses was 7 days ago. She is in a monogamous relationship using barrier contraception. She denied sexually transmitted diseases, urinary tract infections, and any family history of kidney stones. Physical exam was notable for a non-tender left flank. Routine blood tests were unremarkable, including routine chemistries, creatinine, liver function tests, amylase, and lipase. Urinalysis revealed amber urine, specific gravity 1.020, pH 6.5, leukocyte esterase negative, nitrite negative, trace protein, five to ten white cells, and > 50 red cells per high powered field. Urine pregnancy test was negative. Stone protocol abdominal CT scan revealed a non-obstructing, 4 mm renal calculus in the distal left ureter. She received IV ketorolac and normal saline hydration with relief of her flank pain. As an outpatient, she spontaneously passed the stone. Chemical analysis revealed a calcium oxalate stone. Her primary care doctor told her to increase her urine output to at least 2 L per day and to reduce dietary sodium intake to 2,300 mg daily. Protein restriction to 0.8–1 g/kg body weight per day was also recommended.

K.C. Cho, M.D. (✉) • G.J. No, M.D. • L.J. Lo, M.D. • A. Lin, M.D.
Division of Nephrology, Department of Medicine, University of California San Francisco, 521 Parnassus Avenue, Box 0532, San Francisco, CA 94143, USA
e-mail: Kerry.cho@ucsf.edu

Introduction

Nephrolithiasis is a common, often recurrent, and occasionally morbid condition. The overall stone prevalence in the USA has doubled since the 1960s and 1970s with substantial increases through the 1990s. The prevalence of kidney stones increases with age such that 11% of men and 5.6% of women in the USA will have had a symptomatic kidney stone by age 70. According to a large study in 2000, the incidence of kidney stones was 1,116 per 100,000 reported in 18- to 64-year-old employees. The first episode of renal colic related to nephrolithiasis is most likely to occur between the ages of 20 and 30 years for women and 30–60 years for men. Urological intervention is required in approximately 20% of episodes of nephrolithiasis. Recurrence rates are as high as 50% within 5 years and 80% within 20 years.

Many health care providers will encounter nephrolithiasis in their clinical practice, including primary care physicians, nephrologists, urologists, interventional radiologists, and emergency department physicians. This review addresses the

E.V. Lerma and M. Rosner (eds.), *Clinical Decisions in Nephrology, Hypertension and Kidney Transplantation*, DOI 10.1007/978-1-4614-4454-1_51, © Springer Science+Business Media New York 2013

Table 51.1 Major stone types and frequency in adults

- Calcium oxalate (40–60%)
- Calcium phosphate (10–20%)
- Uric acid (10–15%)
- Magnesium ammonium phosphate (struvite, 10–15%)
- Cystine (<1%)
- Other: indinavir, triamterene, xanthine (<1%)

acute management of renal colic as well as the chronic management of nephrolithiasis with strategies for secondary prevention.

Types of Stones

There are five major types of kidney stones (in order of decreasing frequency): calcium oxalate, calcium phosphate, uric acid, magnesium ammonium phosphate (struvite), and cystine (see Table 51.1). An individual stone can have a mixed composition, for example, a nidus of one type and the remainder of another. Calcium stones (either oxalate or phosphate) are by far the most common, comprising up to 90% of stones in men and 70% in women. Stones from initial episodes of renal colic are often not collected for analysis; there is limited information about the frequency of stone types in this population. A small minority of stones (<1%) is composed of medications such as indinavir, acyclovir, and triamterene (see section on Medication-induced nephrolithiasis and Table 51.6).

Pathophysiology

Nephrolithiasis is a biophysical process of crystal nucleation from a supersaturated solution. Supersaturation is expressed as a ratio of a patient's ion activity product to the known solubility product for a particular stone composition. A supersaturation ratio > 1 promotes stone formation because the concentration product exceeds the solubility product, while a ratio < 1 favors stone dissolution. Various factors promote or inhibit the nucleation process. Under normal circumstances, urine may be supersaturated with the components of the most common kidney stones including calcium oxalate, calcium phosphate, and uric acid. Factors that promote stone formation include low urine volume and flow, urinary stasis, urine pH (depending on the type of stone), and the presence of a nidus to initiate crystal nucleation. Factors that inhibit stone formation include high urine volume and flow.

The complex pathogenesis of calcium stones is worth understanding since these stones will be the most frequently encountered in clinical practice. Calcium stones are thought to start in the medullary interstitium as calcium phosphate stones that erode through the renal papilla. Calcium oxalate is then deposited around the calcium phosphate nidus. Urinary citrate inhibits calcium stones formation by chelating calcium, decreasing the free calcium available for crystal formation with oxalate and phosphate. Urinary glycoproteins such as Tamm-Horsfall protein, bikunin, and nephrocalcin also inhibit calcium oxalate stone formation.

Several medical conditions predispose to calcium stones by affecting the balance of calcium, phosphate, oxalate, and citrate. Primary hyperparathyroidism and idiopathic hypercalciuria increase urinary calcium and the risk of calcium oxalate and calcium phosphate stones. Crohn's disease and other diseases of malabsorption increase fecal fat which binds luminal calcium, increasing the delivery of oxalate to the colon since calcium would ordinarily bind oxalate and prevents its absorption. An intact colon is needed to absorb the extra oxalate, producing enteric hyperoxaluria and predisposing to calcium oxalate stones. Dietary oxalate may increase urinary oxalate, especially in the presence of ascorbic acid which is a precursor of oxalate. Distal (or type 2) renal tubular acidosis (RTA) results increased citrate absorption (as a potential source of bicarbonate) and decreased urinary citrate to bind calcium. Metabolic acidosis from diarrhea and gastrointestinal bicarbonate losses will have a similar effect.

The pathogenesis of other stones depends on stone type. Uric acid stones form in persistently acidic urine (pH < 5.5). Dietary purine intake and endogenous uric acid production from purine turnover will increase urinary uric acid. Cystine stones form in patients with cystinuria, an autosomal recessive condition. Struvite stones form as a result of urinary tract infections with urea-splitting bacteria, such as *Proteus*, *Klebsiella* that produce the enzyme urease. The increased urine pH increases the risk of struvite stones.

Risk Factors

Risk factors for nephrolithiasis are genetic, medical, dietary, and environmental. Prevalence and incidence rates are highest for whites, followed by Hispanics, blacks, and Asians. There is a male to female predominance of 2–4:1. Approximately 50% of stone patients have first-degree relatives with stones. Stones in both members of a twin pair occur twice as frequently in monozygotic twins than dizygotic twins.

Stones are associated with weight gain, obesity, diabetes, gout, and the metabolic syndrome, all of which are increasing in industrialized countries. Diabetes increases the risk for calcium and uric acid stones. Urinary tract anomalies can result in stasis, slow urine flow, and stones in general, and more specifically urinary tract infections and struvite stones. Bowel pathology from inflammatory bowel disease and short gut syndrome may cause enteric hyperoxaluria and calcium oxalate stones. Ileostomy, bariatric surgery, sarcoidosis, gout, RTA, primary hyperparathyroidism, idiopathic hypercalciuria, myeloma, immobilization, untreated hyperthyroidism, and urinary stasis can all increase the risk for calcium stones, either calcium oxalate or calcium phosphate (see Table 51.2). Anatomic abnormalities such as ureteropelvic junction obstruction, horseshoe kidney, and polycystic kidney can cause urinary stasis, promoting stone formation.

Dietary factors associated with decreased risk include increased dietary calcium (but not supplemental calcium), fluid, and potassium. The exact mechanism why dietary, but supplemental, calcium is protective is not entirely clear. High risk dietary factors include animal protein, sodium, sucrose, and fructose.

Medications such as calcium supplements, alkali (bicarbonate or citrate), high-dose vitamin C, and vitamin D increase the risk of stones. Acetazolamide and topiramate increase urine pH and decrease urinary citrate excretion, increasing the risk for calcium phosphate stones.

Increased dietary sodium, oxalate, and animal protein may alter urine composition in favor of stone formation. Dietary calcium can precipitate intestinal oxalate, preventing its absorption and decreasing urinary oxalate excretion; low dietary calcium may increase the risk of calcium stones. Low urine volume increases the urine concentration of calcium salts and oxalate. Patients in hot climates and others with increased insensible losses from sweating may have decreased urine volumes and increased stone risk.

Clinical Presentation

Nephrolithiasis typically presents with renal colic, a paroxysmal pain that begins as the stone enters the ureter. The onset of pain is typically sudden, and the location of the pain will vary depending on the location of the stone within the ureter. Proximal ureteral stones may cause flank pain or upper abdominal pain, while more distal stones may cause groin, pelvic, testicular, or labial pain. Stones lodged at the ureterovesical junction may cause suprapubic pain, urinary urgency, and frequency. Patients may experience sudden and complete pain relief with passage of the stone into the bladder or out the urethra. Struvite stones can be intrarenal and remain relatively asymptomatic until obstruction occurs or the underlying urinary tract infection produces symptoms.

Nausea and vomiting are often present, but fever is not unless there is a superimposed urinary tract infection or pyelonephritis. Patients with stones often have microscopic or gross hematuria, but this finding is not universal. In one study, 9% of patients with nephrolithiasis did not have hematuria detectable by urine dipstick and microscopy. Other less common presentations include painless hematuria or persistent urinary tract infections.

Table 51.2 Summary of stone types, risk factors, and therapies

Stone type	Associated conditions	Metabolic abnormalities	Treatment
Calcium oxalate	1. Idiopathic hypercalciuria 2. Medullary sponge kidney 3. Granulomatous diseases 4. Malignancy-induced hypercalciuria 5. Malabsorption 6. Primary or enteric hyperoxaluria	For #1–4 Most common 24-h urinary finding will be hypercalciuria and hypocitraturia For #3 and 4 Serum calcium may be elevated or at high end of normal range For #5 and 6 Most common 24-h urinary finding will be (a) Hypocalciuria, (b) Hyperoxaluria, (c) Hypocitraturia, (d) Urine pH < 5.5	1. Treat underlying granulomatous disease or malignancy 2. Increase fluid intake to at least 2 L/day 3. Treat hypercalciuria: (a) Restrict dietary sodium intake < 2 g/day (b) Do NOT restrict dietary calcium intake (c) HCTZ 25–50 mg PO daily 4. Treat hypocitraturia: (a) Prescribe citrate salt (potassium, calcium, or sodium citrate) 10 mEq PO TID, increase dose until urinary citrate normalized. (b) Increase lemon or lime juice intake 5. Treat hyperoxaluria: (a) Restrict oxalate (b) Liberalize calcium intake (c) Moderate fruit and vegetable intake (d) Avoid vitamin C supplementation (e) Restrict oxalate intake to < 200 mg/day 6. Low urinary pH: Alkalinize urine with potassium citrate or calcium citrate
Calcium phosphate	1. Hyperparathyroidism 2. Distal renal tubular acidosis 3. Pregnancy	For #1 Most common findings are hypercalcemia and elevated PTH. Most common 24-h urinary finding is hypercalciuria. For #2 Most common findings are elevated urine pH and hypocitraturia	1. Treat underlying hyperparathyroidism or cause of distal rental tubular acidosis 2. Increase fluid intake to at least 2 L/day 3. Treat hypercalciuria: (a) <2 g/day dietary sodium intake (b) Do NOT restrict calcium intake (c) HCTZ 25–50 mg PO daily 4. Decrease phosphate intake 5. Urinary acidification with cranberry juice (at least 16 oz/day) or betaine hydrochloride 650 mg PO TID with meals
Uric acid	1. Metabolic syndrome 2. Gout 3. Myeloproliferative disorders 4. Lesch-Nyhan syndrome	Most common 24-h urinary finding will be hyperuricosuria and low urinary pH	1. Decrease dietary protein and caloric intake 2. Reduce alcohol intake 3. Alkalinize urine with potassium or calcium citrate 4. Allopurinol 300 mg PO daily; increase dose as tolerated to normalize serum uric acid level. Patients with chronic kidney disease will need dose reduction
Struvite	1. Urinary tract infection with urea-splitting organisms 2. Anatomical defects	Elevated urinary pH	1. Surgical intervention to correct any anatomical defects 2. Urinary acidification with cranberry juice (at least 16 oz/day) or betaine hydrochloride 650 mg PO TID with meals 3. Acetohydroxamine (urease inhibitor) 15 mg/kg in divided doses 3–4 times/day
Cystine	1. Cystine gene transporter defect	Elevated urinary cystine level	1. Decrease dietary intake of methionine (e.g., dairy products, eggs, meats, seafood, nuts, seeds, legumes, spinach, broccoli, asparagus) 2. Cystine binding agents 3. Tiopronin (divided into three daily doses), Children 15 mg/kg, Adults 800–1,000 mg/day 4. Penicillamine: 20–40 mg/kg/day

Differential Diagnosis

Renal colic from nephrolithiasis can mimic many abdominal and pelvic processes. The differential diagnosis includes

- Pyelonephritis
- Renal infarct
- Renal papillary necrosis with a sloughed papilla causing obstruction
- Renal cell carcinoma (e.g., renal colic from blood clots in the ureter)
- Ureteral obstruction from non-stone pathology, e.g., a sloughed papilla or thrombus
- Ureteral stricture
- Pelvic inflammatory disease, ovarian torsion, ectopic pregnancy
- Prostatitis, prostate cancer, testicular torsion
- Cholecystitis, e.g., a right sided stone at the ureteropelvic junction
- Appendicitis, e.g., a right ureteral stone crossing the pelvic brim
- Cystitis, e.g., a stone at the ureterovesical junction
- Peritonitis
- Intestinal obstruction
- Duodenal ulcer
- Abdominal aortic aneurysm
- Musculoskeletal pain
- Herpes zoster

Diagnostic Evaluation

The physical examination is nonspecific, but may exclude other pathology. The patient is typically in pain and uncomfortable. There may be ipsilateral costovertebral angle tenderness. With superimposed infection as such as pyelonephritis, there may be signs of sepsis including fever, tachycardia, and hypotension. Pelvic examination may be necessary in female patients to rule out obstetrical or gynecological pathology, while rectal examination may reveal prostate pathology in men.

The role of diagnostic testing is to confirm the diagnosis of nephrolithiasis, rule out indications for urgent intervention, and reveal any potential underlying causes. A basic diagnostic evaluation consists of

- Urinalysis with microscopy (and urine culture if evidence of infection)
- Serum electrolytes, BUN, creatinine, and calcium
- Complete blood count in cases of suspected infection
- Abdominal imaging (most commonly spiral abdominal CT without contrast) (Table 51.3)
- Stone analysis (if a specimen can be obtained)
- Tests to rule out alternate diagnoses: amylase/lipase (pancreatitis), urine pregnancy test (pregnancy complications), liver function tests (biliary disease)

The extent of additional diagnostic evaluation for patients presenting with their first stone is controversial. Since about 50% of patients may not have a second stone for 10 years or more, some experts favor a relatively limited diagnostic evaluation in a patient with an initial uncomplicated stone. Other experts recommend a thorough diagnostic evaluation even with the first stone given the high lifetime risk of recurrence. The NIH consensus guidelines for the prevention and treatment of kidney stones from 1988 recommended basic laboratory testing for first-time stone formers, while the European Association of Urology recommendations from 2008 also recommended limited evaluation for presenting with an initial, uncomplicated episode of renal colic. A discussion between patient and provider may be useful to determine which path to take. For example, if the patient is unwilling to make dietary modifications, a full metabolic workup may not be useful.

Complicated cases such as recurrent nephrolithiasis, solitary kidney, transplant kidney, heavy stone burden (e.g., staghorn calculus), chronic kidney disease, obstruction, and superimposed infection warrant a more thorough evaluation (Table 51.4). Patients who present with their first episode of renal colic, but have multiple stones should be considered to have recurrent disease. A more thorough diagnostic approach is discussed in Case 2.

Nephrocalcinosis refers to the deposition of calcium oxalate and calcium phosphate in the renal

Table 51.3 Imaging modalities for nephrolithiasis

Imaging modality	Comments	Advantages	Disadvantages
Abdominal X-ray	Useful for calcium stones, often detects cystine and struvite stones with some calcium component, never detects uric acid stones, detects stones > 5 mm diameter	Inexpensive, fast, low radiation exposure	May miss radiolucent/non-calcium stones, poor anatomical definition, may detect phleboliths and other calcium-based objects not in the urinary system
Intravenous pyelography	Detects stones of all compositions Gold standard for diagnosis of medullary sponge kidney which predisposes to stone formation	Inexpensive, low radiation exposure, may be considered during pregnancy	Contrast exposure and possible contrast nephropathy, time consuming to perform, has been replaced by abdominal CT in many hospitals
Abdominal CT	Detects stones of all compositions	Fast, anatomical definition, highest sensitivity, detects radiolucent, and radiopaque stones on plain films, may provide alternative diagnoses	Radiation exposure, unsafe for pregnant patients, expense
Ultrasound	Useful for stones in renal pelvis and proximal ureter	Low radiation exposure, may be used for longitudinal follow-up, can detect hydronephrosis, may suggest alternative diagnoses, may be considered during pregnancy	Will not detect distal ureteral stones

Table 51.4 Complete diagnostic evaluation of complicated or recurrent nephrolithiasis

1. Routine serum chemistries and uric acid: Rule out hypercalcemia, renal tubular acidosis, chronic kidney disease, and hyperuricemia. 25-hydroxyvitamin D and 1,25-dihydroxyvitamin D levels are indicated in hypercalcemic patients with normal or suppressed serum PTH
2. Serum PTH: primary hyperparathyroidism
3. Urinalysis: urine pH, evidence of urinary tract infection
4. Urine culture: urinary tract infection, especially with urea-splitting organisms
5. Urine microscopy: urine crystals may suggest stone type
6. 24 h Urine collection for total volume, pH, calcium, oxalate, phosphate, citrate, uric acid, sodium, magnesium, potassium, sulfate, ammonium, creatinine, urea nitrogen
7. Stone analysis for chemical composition
8. Spiral CT: rule structural abnormalities, branched stones consistent with struvite and cystine stones
9. Urinary cystine:
   (a) Pediatric patients
   (b) Patient with first or recurrent kidney stone with a family history of stone disease
   (c) Unknown composition of stone

parenchyma, while oxalosis refers specifically to calcium oxalate deposition. Nephrocalcinosis may be acute or chronic and associated with normal or reduced kidney function. Often noted incidentally on radiological imaging, including plain films, CT, or ultrasound, nephrocalcinosis may be diagnosed during the evaluation of nephrolithiasis. Although associated with some of the nephrolithiasis risk factors, nephrocalcinosis may occur without nephrolithiasis, and vice versa.

Risk factors for nephrocalcinosis include hypercalciuria with hypercalcemia (primary hyperparathyroidism, vitamin D therapy, sarcoidosis), hypercalciuria without hypercalcemia (distal/type I RTA, medullary sponge kidney, loop diuretics, neonatal nephrocalcinosis, congenital tubulopathies, and chronic hypokalemia), hyperphosphaturia (e.g., tumor lysis syndrome, oral sodium phosphate bowel preparations), and hyperoxaluria (i.e., primary, secondary, and enteric).

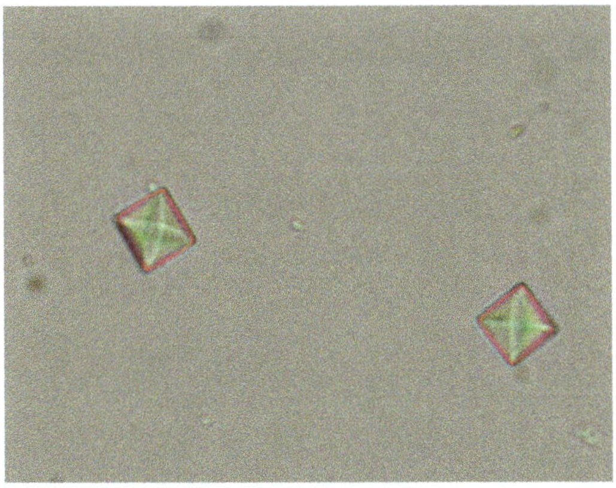

Fig. 51.1 Calcium oxalate dihydrate crystals in urine sediment (×40 original magnification; unstained), provided courtesy of Dr. Tracy Stokol from the Clinical Pathology Laboratory at Cornell University

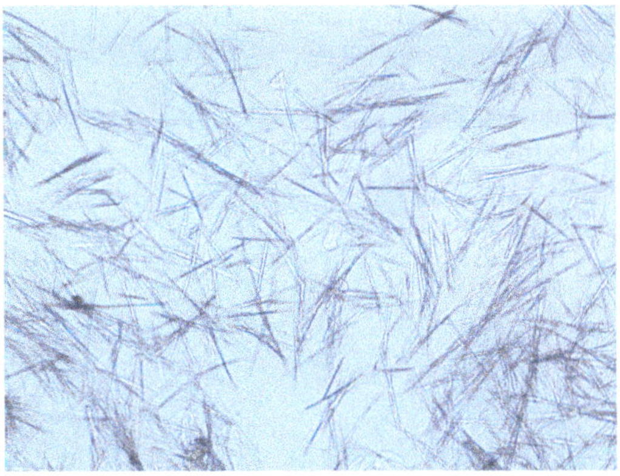

Fig. 51.2 Calcium phosphate crystals in urine sediment (×40 original magnification; unstained), provided courtesy of Dr. Tracy Stokol from the Clinical Pathology Laboratory at Cornell University

Treatment of nephrocalcinosis involves treating the underlying cause, but maintenance of adequate urine output (>2 L/day) may benefit all patients with nephrocalcinosis. Hypercalciuric patients may benefit from oral potassium citrate to increase solubility of calcium oxalate and dietary restriction of animal protein (<0.7 g/kg/day) and sodium (<2.3 g/day) along with liberalized potassium intake. Calcium deposition is typically irreversible, even if the underlying cause is corrected.

Urinalysis and Sediment Examination

Urine that is positive for hemoglobin on dipstick analysis and erythrocytes on microscopic examination supports the diagnosis of kidney stones. However, the lack of hematuria does not definitively rule out nephrolithiasis. Leukocytes in the urine suggest a urinary tract infection. If pyuria is present, a urine culture should also be obtained. Nephrolithiasis with associated pyelonephritis is an indication for urgent surgical evaluation and possible intervention.

Microscopic evaluation of urine for crystals may reveal the composition of the stone, although the absence of crystals does not rule out nephrolithiasis. Examination may yield crystals of calcium oxalate, calcium phosphate, uric acid, cystine, magnesium ammonium phosphate (struvite), or drug crystals. See Figs. 51.1, 51.2, 51.3, 51.4, and 51.5, which demonstrate microscopic finding seen with calcium oxalate, calcium phosphate, struvite, uric acid, and cystine crystals.

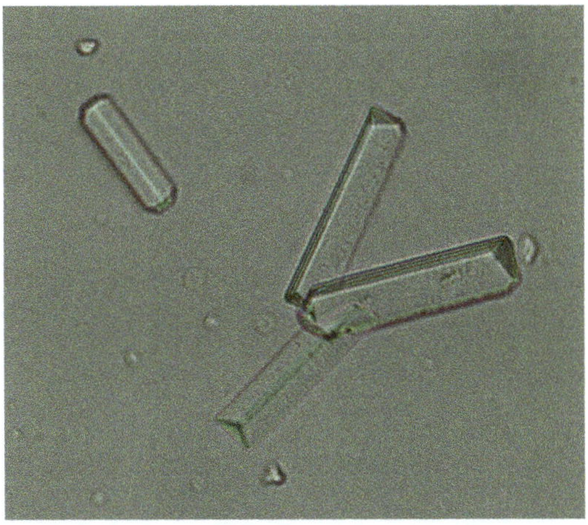

Fig. 51.3 Triple phosphate crystals (struvite crystals) in urine sediment (×40 original magnification; unstained), provided courtesy of Dr. Tracy Stokol from the Clinical Pathology Laboratory at Cornell University

Urinary pH may also be helpful in determining the cause of nephrolithiasis. Alkaline urine (pH>7.5) or pyuria can be caused by urinary tract infections with urea-splitting organisms; the alkaline urine promotes struvite stones. Acidic urine (pH<5.5) is associated with uric acid stones. An inappropriately high urine pH in the setting of metabolic acidosis may suggest RTA, which is a potential cause of kidney stones.

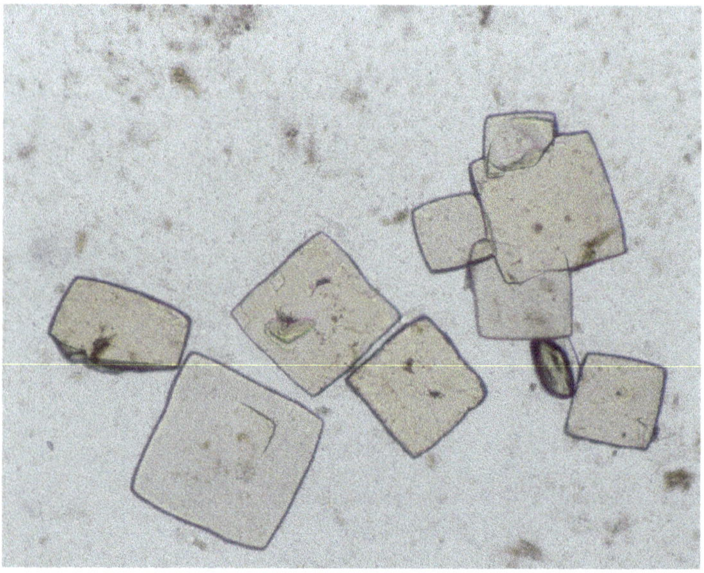

Fig. 51.4 Uric acid crystals in urine sediment (×40 original magnification; unstained), provided courtesy of Dr. Tracy Stokol from the Clinical Pathology Laboratory at Cornell University

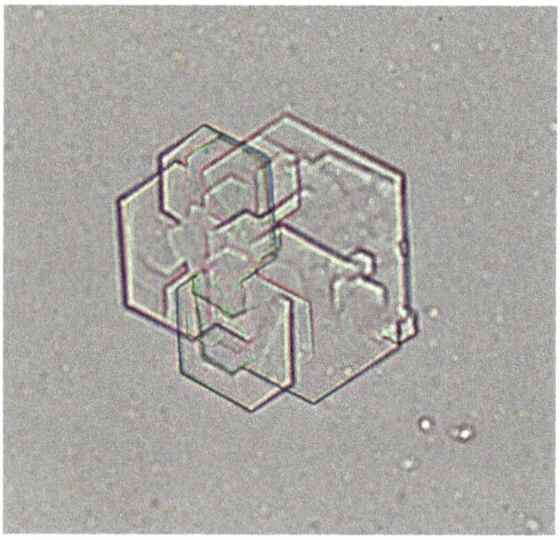

Fig. 51.5 Cystine crystals in urine sediment (×40 original magnification; unstained), provided courtesy of Dr. Tracy Stokol from the Clinical Pathology Laboratory at Cornell University

Electrolytes, Bun, and Creatinine

An acutely elevated creatinine in the setting of nephrolithiasis could be a sign of urinary obstruction and warrants urgent urological consultation. A low serum bicarbonate could suggest RTA, which can cause nephrolithiasis. Distal RTA is the type most commonly associated with nephrolithiasis. Other lab disorders such as hypokalemia and an inappropriately high urinary pH would also be suggestive of distal RTA. Nausea and vomiting may produce a metabolic alkalosis from volume contraction. Acute kidney injury with an elevated BUN and serum creatinine can accompany nephrolithiasis with obstruction.

Serum Calcium

Hypercalcemia may precipitate stone formation. If the serum calcium is elevated, a parathyroid hormone (PTH) level and serum phosphorus should be obtained to detect disorders such as primary hyperparathyroidism. The serum calcium is often only modestly elevated or at the high end of the normal range in primary hyperparathyroidism; the threshold for checking a serum PTH should be relatively low. Other etiologies of hypercalcemia include malignancy, vitamin D intoxication, and granulomatous diseases (e.g., sarcoidosis and tuberculosis).

Imaging Modalities (Table 51.3)

Diagnostic imaging is critical in the care of patients with nephrolithiasis. These modalities are summarized in Table 51.3. Representative images of various modalities are shown in Figs. 51.6, 51.7, 51.8, 51.9, and 51.10.

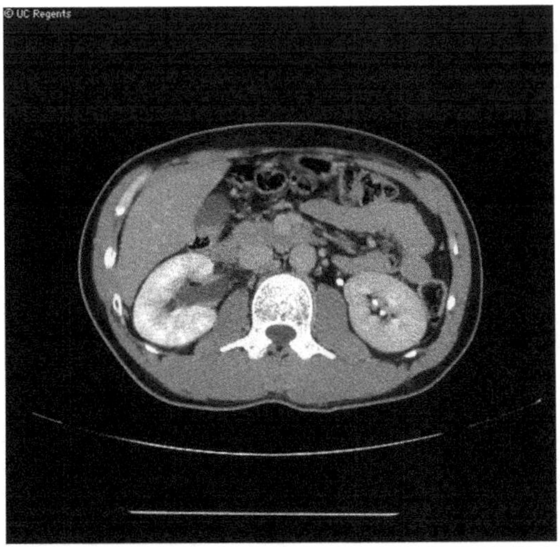

Fig. 51.6 CT abdomen with L-sided kidney stones, provided courtesy of Dr. Benjamin Yeh from Department of Radiology at UCSF

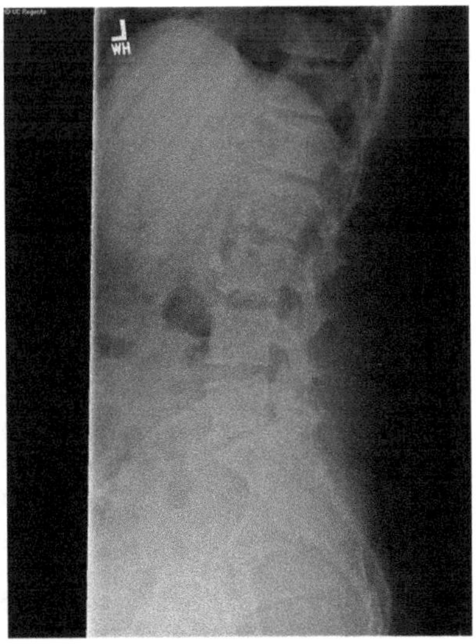

Fig. 51.8 KUB Lateral view with kidney stone, provided courtesy of Dr. Benjamin Yeh from Department of Radiology at UCSF

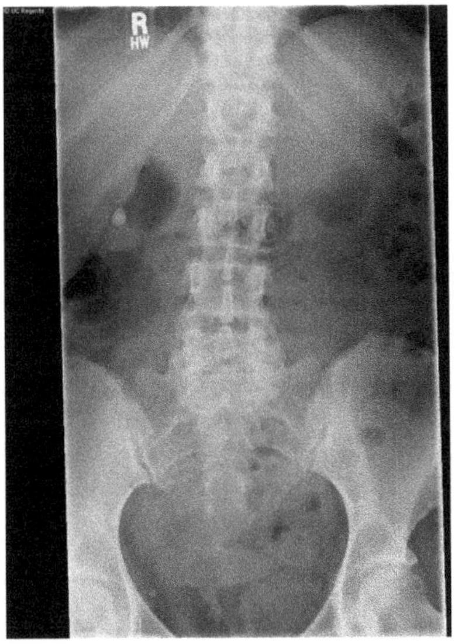

Fig. 51.7 KUB AP view with R-sided kidney stone, provided courtesy of Dr. Benjamin Yeh from Department of Radiology at UCSF

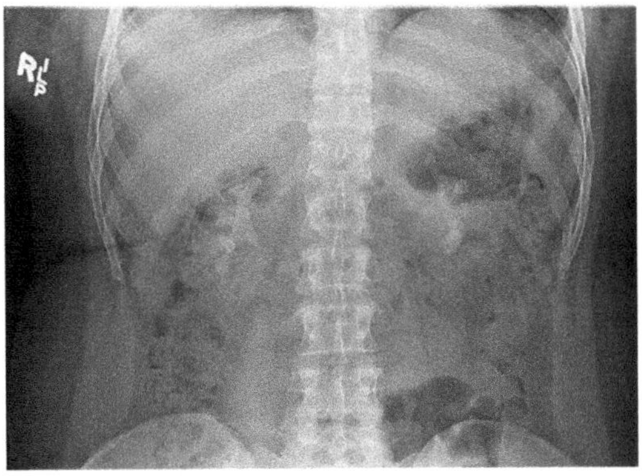

Fig. 51.9 KUB AP view with bilateral staghorn calculi, provided courtesy of Dr. Benjamin Yeh from Department of Radiology at UCSF

Abdominal Imaging

Spiral computed tomography (CT) of the abdomen without intravenous contrast is the imaging modality of choice for confirming nephrolithiasis. CT can detect stones as small as 1 mm in diameter. The sensitivity and specificity of noncontrast spiral CT are 98% and 100%, respectively, for the diagnosis of stones. CT can detect radiolucent stones such as uric acid and indinavir stones. CT provides information regarding location, size, number of stones, and any structural abnormalities predisposing to stone formation. CT also has the advantage of imaging structures outside the urinary system, which can be useful if stone disease has been ruled out. Low-dose CT may be available to minimize radiation exposure and may be nearly as effective as standard spiral CT, especially in non-obese patients.

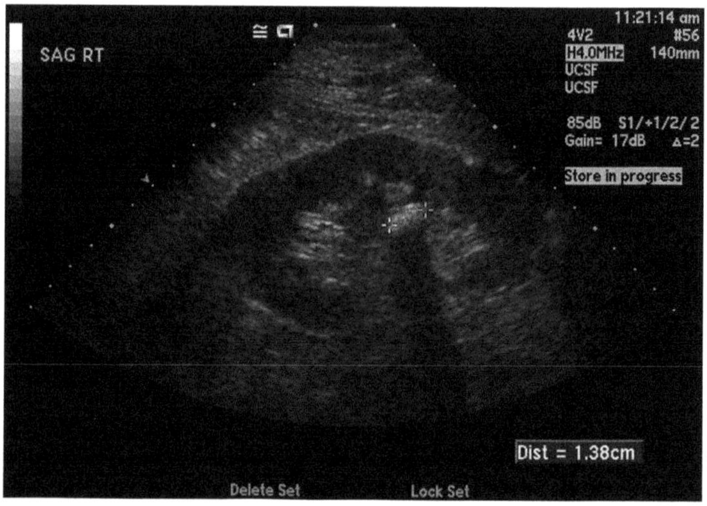

Fig. 51.10 Renal ultrasound with kidney stone in renal pelvis, provided courtesy of Dr. Benjamin Yeh from Department of Radiology at UCSF

Intravenous pyelography (IVP) should be rarely used in the evaluation of nephrolithiasis since it requires contrast administration and may miss small stones. IVP also takes more time to perform than CT. Some medical centers do not routinely perform IVP in the era of CT. IVP remains the gold standard for the diagnosis for medullary sponge kidney, a condition which may cause calcium oxalate and calcium phosphate stones and nephrocalcinosis. Spiral CT and CT urography can be used in lieu of IVP for the diagnosis of medullary sponge kidney.

Ultrasound is inferior to CT for visualization of stones, with a sensitivity of 24% and a sensitivity of 90% compared to spiral CT as the gold standard (Fowler et al. 2002). Ultrasound can only image the kidney and proximal ureter and may miss distal stones. Although a suboptimal imaging modality for nephrolithiasis, ultrasound does not use radiation and should be used in cases where radiation is contraindicated, such as pregnant patients. Intravenous pyelogram is generally not recommended for diagnosis of kidney stones, as spiral CT gives more structural information without exposure to intravenous contrast and the risk of contrast nephropathy.

Abdominal X-ray of the kidneys, ureters, and bladder (KUB) is inadequate since it may miss radiolucent stones and stones less than 5 mm in diameter. Calcium stones are radiopaque, while cystine and struvite stones are often, but not consistently, radiopaque. Uric acid stones are radiolucent unless they contain a calcium component. KUB also does not provide information about obstruction and hydronephrosis and yields limited information about surrounding anatomy. Magnetic resonance image is a poor modality for imaging stones.

CT should be avoided in children and pregnant women due to concerns of radiation exposure. Ultrasonography is the imaging study of choice in these patients. Limited or "3-shot" IVP utilizes a scout film, a 30-s film, and a 20-min film; this modality could be considered if the diagnosis remains uncertain after ultrasonography. Requiring relatively low radiation exposure compared to CT, 3-shot IVP does require IV contrast, which is not known to be teratogenic, but may cause thyroid abnormalities in the fetus. In cases where the mother receives IV contrast, the neonate should be tested for thyroid function after delivery (Thomas et al. 2010).

Stone Analysis

The patient should be given a urine strainer with the instructions to strain all urine until the stone has passed. A 4×4 gauze pad placed over a cup can be used to collect stone specimens if a urine strainer is not available. Collected fragments or stones can be sent for chemical analysis. A detailed discussion of management based on stone composition is included below.

Acute Medical Management

In general, stones larger than 10 mm typically do not pass spontaneously, while stones less than 5 mm will. Intermediate stones between 5 and 10 mm have variable outcomes. Distal ureter stones are more likely to pass than proximal stones. Patients with ureteral stones less than 10 mm in diameter in the absence of fever, infection, kidney injury, or other complications are candidates for conservative management with analgesia and hydration.

Nonsteroidal anti-inflammatory drugs (NSAIDs) and opiates are the two most commonly used classes of analgesics used for renal colic. NSAIDs have been shown to be at least as effective as opiates in controlling pain. Intravenous ketorolac is commonly used in the emergency department setting for effective analgesia with less sedation than opiates. The choice between NSAIDs and opiates largely depends on the side effect profile of the medication and the patient's comorbidities.

Hydration can correct hypovolemia associated with nausea and vomiting from nephrolithiasis. Forced intravenous hydration does not reduce pain medication requirements or facilitate stone passage compared to regular IV hydration. Increased oral fluid intake is recommended to increase urine flow and hasten stone passage. Patients are usually instructed to drink at least 2–3 L of fluid per day to maintain a urine output of at least 2.5 L per day. Increased urine output will decrease the solute supersaturation, leading to stone formation and growth; a more detailed discussion of dietary modifications is included below.

Expulsive Medical Therapy

Alpha$_1$-adrenergic blockers and calcium channel blockers have been used to facilitate passage of ureteral stones. These medications may relax the ureter and increase hydrostatic pressure proximal to the stone, resulting in stone passage. Both medications have been studied with and without concomitant corticosteroids. A 2006 meta-analysis showed that both tamsulosin and nifedipine were effective for stone expulsion. Both medications are generally well tolerated and may be considered for patients with smaller stones < 5 mm and/or stones located in the distal ureter. Expulsive medical therapy with tamsulosin or nifedipine has been shown to reduce time to stone passage, pain episodes, pain scores, and analgesic requirements. Tamsulosin may be preferred, since most trials show either a trend or a statistically significant benefit over nifedipine, although there are few head-to-head trials of these medications. Tamsulosin may cause less hypotension and lightheadedness than nifedipine. The usual doses are tamsulosin 0.4 mg daily and extended-release nifedipine 30 mg daily. Corticosteroids may have an additive benefit to both tamsulosin and nifedipine, but they may be contraindicated in particular patients given their side effect profile.

Outpatient Versus Inpatient Management

Routine uncomplicated cases of nephrolithiasis with small (<5 mm) and especially distal stones can be managed successfully in the outpatient setting. Patients can be diagnosed quickly in the emergency department on the basis of history and physical, urinalysis, basic laboratory testing, and spiral CT. Other pathology and complications can be ruled out, and the patient can receive adequate analgesia and hydration. The patient can be discharged from the emergency department with oral analgesics, expulsive medical therapy (tamsulosin or nifedipine), a urine strainer, and careful instructions to return for persistent symptoms, worsening pain, or fever. Appropriate follow-up with the primary care provider should be arranged.

Complicated cases including larger stones (> 5 mm), proximal stones, superimposed infection, pyelonephritis, obstruction (either unilateral with a solitary kidney or bilateral), acute kidney injury, and significant comorbidities may require hospitalization. Patients with larger stones requiring IV analgesics may require hospitalization for pain control. Consultation by urology or interventional radiology for stone removal or definitive drainage should be considered. Nephrology consultation may be necessary for risk factor identification, risk reduction for recurrent nephrolithiasis, and any concomitant acute and/or chronic kidney disease.

Indications for Surgical Intervention

The likelihood of spontaneous ureteral stone passage decreases as the size of the stone increases. One study found that the frequency of spontaneous passage was 78% for 1–4 mm stones, 60% for 5–7 mm stones, 39% for 8–10 mm stones, and 0 for stones > 10 mm. The same study found that proximal ureteral stones were less likely to pass spontaneously than distal ureteral stones.

Therefore, any of the following conditions should prompt urgent urological consultation: stones over 10 mm, proximal ureteral stones, pyelonephritis, urosepsis, urinary obstruction, acute kidney injury, and uncontrollable pain. Outpatient, nonurgent consultation should be considered if stone passage has not occurred after 4 weeks.

Case 2

A 32-year-old woman with Sjogren's syndrome presented to her primary care physician with new onset right flank pain radiating to the groin. She had a similar episode 5 months earlier which resolved after passing a small stone. She denied any hematuria, dysuria, or pyuria. She has not been sexually active for the past 2 years and has no history of sexually transmitted diseases. Her menstrual periods have been normal. Her mother has systemic lupus erythematosus. There is no family history of kidney disease or stones. Physical exam was notable for a lower right flank and right lower quadrant pain. Routine blood work revealed a serum bicarbonate level of 15 mEq/L. Urinalysis revealed amber urine, specific gravity 1.030, pH 7, leukocyte esterase negative, nitrite negative, trace protein, five to ten white cells, and >50 red cells per high powered field. Stone protocol abdominal CT scan demonstrated multiple small punctate kidney stones in the right kidney and a 5 mm stone at the distal ureter.

Diagnostic Evaluation for Recurrent Nephrolithiasis (Table 51.4)

Conservative management of a patient with an initial, uncomplicated episode with a calcium stone would include a limited evaluation: history and physical, urinalysis, urine microscopy, routine blood tests, and spiral CT. Routine chemistries can screen for hypercalcemia, chronic kidney disease, and distal RTA. Other possible tests in the basic evaluation include urine culture, PTH, and stone analysis. However, with recurrent disease, pediatric disease, or complicated disease, a more thorough evaluation is necessary to rule out systemic diseases associated with nephrolithiasis and to guide preventive therapy. Patients with medical conditions that predispose to nephrolithiasis deserve additional evaluation and may require ongoing therapy. Preventive therapy is important because recurrent stone disease is associated with chronic kidney disease and hypertension. Recurrent disease has potential complications and morbidity including pain, acute kidney injury, urosepsis, emergency department visits, and hospitalizations.

Additional testing for complicated or recurrent stone disease includes serum PTH for hyperparathyroidism and 24 h urine collection for metabolic analysis. Pediatric patients in particular should be screened for cystinuria and hyperoxaluria.

A 24 h urine collection for metabolic analysis is used to identify risk factors for stone formation and provide clues to the stone type if a stone specimen is not available. 24 h urine collections should be used in recurrent disease, pediatric cases, and complicated disease (e.g., large stones or stones requiring urological intervention). Physicians use the test results to provide specific dietary and pharmacological recommendations to reduce recurrent stone risk.

The 24 h urine is analyzed for total volume, pH, calcium, oxalate, phosphate, citrate, uric acid, sodium, magnesium, potassium, sulfate, ammonium, creatinine, and urea nitrogen. The collection should be done at least 6 weeks after the stone has passed. Some experts recommend two or three urine collections because of variability in the test results from dietary intake; utilizing multiple collections increases the sensitivity of detecting metabolic abnormalities to 92%. The creatinine index (mg of creatinine excreted per kg body weight per day) is used to determine the adequacy of the 24 h urine collection. An adult man should excrete 20–25 mg/kg/day of creatinine, while the creatinine index for an adult woman is 15–20 mg/kg/day. An undercollected urine sample will have a low creatinine index, while an overcollection will have a high creatinine index.

There is little evidence supporting the strict cutoffs for high risk or abnormal test results in 24 h urine samples. For example, total amounts of substances (rather than their concentrations) are reported as abnormal or high risk. As discussed earlier, urine volume and solute concentrations are important factors in the pathogenesis of stones. Cutoffs defined by amount per body weight (such as defining hypercalciuria as > 4 mg/kg/day) also do not make pathophysiological sense for stone formation.

Dietary Modification

Dietary modification is the cornerstone for secondary prevention of nephrolithiasis. Specific dietary recommendations depend on the patient's risk factors, type of stone, and results of a 24 h urine collection. For patients presenting with their first stone, recommendations for dietary modification should be made with the patient's input. Because many patients will not have another stone for years or may never have another stone, some may feel that the inconvenience of long-term dietary restrictions is not worth the potential benefit.

Increased fluid intake is useful in secondary prevention for all types of stones. Decreasing the urinary concentration of solutes should reduce supersaturation and stone formation and/or growth. Patients should drink 2–3 L of water per day, titrating oral fluid intake to keep urine output greater than 2.5 L per day. One consideration when prescribing increased fluid intake is that patients may develop increased urinary frequency which could be disruptive, particularly with nocturia. Some stone specialists recommend that patients drink water immediately prior to sleeping or even in the middle of the night to decrease the nocturnal urine concentration and supersaturation conditions. Under normal circumstances, patients produce the most concentrated urine of the day while sleeping since fluid intake is limited.

One controlled trial randomized 199 patients to high oral fluid intake with mean daily urine volume of 2 L or no intervention. Within 5 years, 12% of patients in the high-fluid intake group had a second stone event, compared to 27% of patients in the control group. Hence even in patients with only one stone event, increased fluid intake is recommended.

If the stone composition is not known, physicians often assume that the stones are calcium-based as they are by far the most common. Details regarding dietary modification for specific stone types can be found below.

Medications

If dietary therapy does not adequately modify a patient's risk profile (i.e., normalization of 24 h urine results), then medication may be indicated. The three most commonly used are thiazides, alkali, and allopurinol. Thiazides such as chlorthalidone and hydrochlorothiazide reduce urine calcium excretion. Alkali therapy increase urinary citrate excretion in hypocitraturic patients who form calcium stones. Furthermore, calcium oxalate supersaturation is independent of urinary pH, however calcium phosphate supersaturation increases with rise in urinary pH. Urine alkalinization may also be helpful for uric acid stones by increasing the solubility of uric acid, but there should be adequate urine flow around the stone. Allopurinol inhibits the enzyme xanthine oxidase, preventing the formation of uric acid and decreasing urine uric acid excretion. High urine uric acid levels are not associated with increased risk of stone formation in epidemiological studies, so the benefit of allopurinol in a randomized trial of patients with recurrent calcium oxalate stones and isolated hyperuricosuria is poorly understood. Specific recommendations for medication therapy are included below with each stone type.

Specific Recommendations Based on Stone Composition

Calcium Oxalate and Calcium Phosphate Stones

There are two types of calcium stones: calcium oxalate and calcium phosphate. Calcium stones tend to form in low urine volume states, especially in people on high salt diets or vitamin D or calcium supplements. The resultant hypercalciuria increases the supersaturation of calcium oxalate and calcium phosphate. Conditions associated with urinary stasis, such as ureteropelvic junction obstruction, horseshoe kidney, and polycystic kidney disease, increase the risk of calcium stone precipitation.

Calcium oxalate stones make up the majority, about 80% of calcium stones. They tend to form over regions of interstitial calcium phosphate deposits called Randall's plaques. Calcium phosphate stones are associated with crystal deposits in the inner medullary collecting ducts that contain apatite, a calcium carbonate-phosphate compound. Unlike calcium oxalate stones, calcium phosphate stones tend to form in alkaline urine (pH > 6.3) as is seen with distal RTA, either genetic or acquired. Primary hyperparathyroidism increases urinary calcium and phosphate excretion, predisposing to calcium phosphate stones. Interestingly, most patients with calcium phosphate stones do not have metabolic acidosis and the cause of the persistently alkaline urine is unclear. Overall, calcium phosphate stones are more common in women and have lower stone-free rates after percutaneous nephrolithotomy.

A low calcium diet has not been shown to prevent recurrent calcium stones. In fact, reducing dietary calcium may increase the risk of recurrent stones, although the exact mechanism is unclear. Calcium binds oxalate in the gastrointestinal tract; decreasing calcium intake increases oxalate absorption and leads to hyperoxaluria, which may increase calcium oxalate stones. A low sodium diet limits urinary calcium excretion, while protein restriction increases urinary citrate excretion and decreases calcium excretion. Additional dietary recommendations include avoiding high amounts of purines and protein, especially animal protein from meat, poultry, and seafood.

Goal oxalate intake should be < 100 mg daily and avoid taking more than 100 mg of ascorbic acid as well. Foods that are rich in oxalate that should be eaten in moderation include spinach, rhubarb, wheat bran, beets, miso, chocolate, and nuts. Dietary oxalate intake should be < 100 mg daily and avoid taking more than 100 mg of ascorbic acid as well. Oxalate-rich foods should be eaten in moderation, including spinach, rhubarb, wheat bran, beets, miso, chocolate, and nuts.

Some inhibitors of calcium oxalate crystallization can be used as well, including citrate or phosphate. Potassium citrate or orthophosphate (20–60 mg/kg/day divided in three to four doses) can also be used to decrease calcium absorption and calciuria.

The management of the many risk factors for calcium stones will now be discussed individually.

Hypercalciuria

There are many causes of hypercalciuria, including primary hyperparathyroidism, granulomatous diseases, vitamin D excess, corticosteroid treatment, distal RTA, hyperthyroidism, and malignancy (e.g., multiple myeloma). Idiopathic hypercalciuria is the most common. Patients with hypercalciuria tend to develop calcium oxalate and calcium phosphate stones, the latter more notably in patients with alkaline urine.

Idiopathic hypercalciuria can be further classified into three different types: absorptive, resorptive, and renal leak. Absorptive hypercalciuria is thought to be due to increased gastrointestinal absorption of ingested calcium. These patients will tend to have slightly decreased PTH, slightly elevated 1,25-dihydroxyvitamin D levels, elevated serum calcium, and slightly low serum phosphorus. The pathophysiology is thought to be either overproduction of vitamin D or increased sensitivity to vitamin D action. However, not all patients with absorptive hypercalciuria have increased gut absorption of calcium mediated by vitamin D. This finding is not fully understood, but suggests that there are other mechanisms for intestinal hyperabsorption of calcium. These patients tend to be poorly responsive to any dietary modifications in calcium.

Resorptive hypercalciuria occurs with increased bone resorption and turnover (typically from hyperparathyroidism), leading to increased urinary calcium excretion. Renal leak hypercalciuria is due to a primary defect in renal tubular transport causing inappropriate urinary calcium losses and secondary gastrointestinal calcium reabsorption and calcium mobilization from the bone. These patients have mild hypocalcemia and secondary hyperparathyroidism.

Interestingly, in most of the studies examining thiazide diuretics in calcium nephrolithiasis, patients did not have hypercalciuria. A study of patients with normal urinary calcium excretion showed that there was an increase in relative risk for kidney stone formation as urinary calcium excretion increased within the normal range.

Many patients who are initiated on thiazide diuretics for hypercalciuria are not on therapeutic doses of thiazides. Patients may require hydrochlorothiazide 50 mg daily to achieve significant decreases in calcium excretion; the prescribing physician should document decreased urinary calcium excretion with 24 h urine collections. Patients on thiazides should be monitored for hypokalemia since hypokalemia can decrease urinary citrate excretion and increase the risk for calcium stones. Hypokalemic patients should be supplemented with potassium citrate or start potassium sparing diuretics such as amiloride or spironolactone. Triamterene should be avoided because it is poorly soluble and can worsen stone disease.

Distal RTA

Patients that have distal RTA will usually present with nephrolithiasis due to excessive urinary calcium excretion, decreased urinary citrate excretion and persistently alkaline urine (2). They have a chronic metabolic acidosis which results in loss of bone calcium leading to hypercalciuria. In addition, the acidosis also contributes to hypocitraturia, which is an independent risk factor that increases risk for stone recurrence. Finally, the chronic alkaline urine promotes calcium phosphate precipitation.

Patients with hypercalciuria should limit dietary calcium to less than 2 g/day. Thiazide diuretics can decrease urinary calcium excretion by more than 50%, thereby decreasing supersaturation of calcium phosphate and calcium oxalate in the urine. The benefit of thiazides is most notable after more than 1 year of therapy. The mechanism of decreased urinary calcium excretion with thiazides is thought to be increased absorption of calcium in the proximal tubule due to volume contraction. Thiazide diuretics transiently decrease urinary magnesium excretion which may reduce stone formation. However, the effect on magnesium excretion lasts only for days to weeks. Diets high in sodium or carbohydrates increase urinary calcium excretion. Therefore low sodium and low carbohydrate diets are recommended.

These recommendations have changed more recently after a recent study looking at Italian men with hypercalciuria. These men were randomly assigned to diets low in calcium and oxalate and were compared to a control which involved a normal calcium diet. After 5 years, there was a 50% reduction in stone formation in the normal calcium group (1,200 mg daily of calcium) in comparison to those on a low calcium, low oxalate diet. Also of note, the calcium should be obtained from dietary sources rather than supplements. Moreover, calcium restriction in patients with hypercalciuria can result in decreasing bone mineral density and increased rate of fractures in this patient group and should be avoided.

Hypocitraturia

Citrate slows the growth of calcium crystals by chelating urinary calcium, preventing supersaturation and stone formation. Hypocitraturia can be idiopathic or associated with medical conditions, including distal RTA, hypokalemia, glycogen storage disease type I, and a high protein/low carbohydrate diet. Carbonic anhydrase inhibitors (acetazolamide, topiramate) alter urinary pH and decrease urinary citrate excretion in the urine.

Urinary citrate excretion is determined by tubular reabsorption of citrate that is increased in acidemia. Intracellular acidosis enhances proximal tubular transport of citrate by the brush border membrane. The opposite is seen in that urinary citrate excretion will increase in alkaline environments. However, despite extensive study attempting to understand the causes of hypocitraturia, the majority of patients with hypocitraturia have unknown cause.

In patients with hypocitraturia, increase urinary citrate by using potassium citrate or potassium bicarbonate. Try to avoid sodium-based medications to avoid the calciuric effect of sodium. Looking at two randomized control trials, comparing sodium-based and potassium-based citrate/bicarbonate, there was a substantial reduction in stone recurrence among the population on potassium-based medications and there was no clinically significant reduction in stone formation in the sodium-based medication group. However, it is important to avoid aggressive alkalinization of the urine. In patients with urine pH > 6.5 or in patients with calcium supersaturation levels that are high ≥ 1. Alkaline therapy lowers supersaturation of calcium phosphate by chelating calcium in the urine, inhibiting the growth of calcium-containing crystals.

Potassium citrate should be 10–20 mEq two to three times daily. Of note, orange juice and lemonade can also increase urinary citrate excretion. Even in patients that have normal urine citrate levels, if they have recurrent stones, consider starting citrate or bicarbonate therapy. Looking at one placebo-controlled trial, 63.6% of patients receiving placebo vs. 12.9% of patients receiving a combination of potassium and magnesium citrate developed recurrent stones at 3 years. The drug was effective regardless of whether or not urine citrate was low.

Unfortunately there are no trials that specifically look at the combination of alkaline therapy with thiazide-type diuretics compared to either agent alone, but they can be used safely in combination when indicated, especially in patients with hypercalciuria and hypocitraturia. All patients initiated on therapy should have a repeat 24 urine study in 4–6 weeks after initiating interventions to assess the efficacy of treatment and also to make sure patients do not become hypokalemic, which can actually worsen patients hypocitraturia.

Hyperoxaluria

Hyperoxaluria is frequently seen in patients who develop recurrent calcium stones. The differential diagnosis includes high dietary oxalate, malabsorptive states, and hyperoxalosis (primary or enteric).

Patients who eat a high protein diet, oxalate-rich diet (found in nuts, soybean, spinach), or large amounts of ascorbic acid can also have hyperoxaluria because of increased oxalate production. Patients who are on a low calcium diet can also have increased oxalate absorption and hyperoxaluria as a result. Preventive measures focus on a low fat and low oxalate diet, increasing calcium intake with meals to bind oxalate and prevent absorption from the gut, increased fluid intake, and avoiding a high protein and/or ascorbic acid-rich diet. There have been no randomized controlled studies of low oxalate diets in the prevention of stone recurrence in hyperoxaluric patients.

Patients with malabsorptive states can have increased enteric absorption of oxalate and present with hyperoxaluria, increased urine uric acid secretion and hyperuricosuria, and calcium oxalate stones. Normally, 90% of dietary oxalate binds dietary calcium in the small intestine and passes into the stool as calcium oxalate. 10% of dietary oxalate is absorbed in the colon and excreted in the urine. Patients that have enteric malabsorption have increased gut absorption of oxalate due to the excess enteric fat binding dietary calcium and allowing free oxalate to be absorbed. Chronic diarrhea, small bowel resection, ileostomy, roux-en-Y bypass surgery, and inflammatory bowel disease have been associated with enteric hyperoxaluria. A study looking at 1,436 roux-en-Y gastric bypass surgery patients noted that 60 patients developed calcium stones. 31 patients underwent urinary metabolic analysis and were found to have hyperoxaluria and hypocitraturia.

Primary hyperoxaluria, a recessive hereditary disorder of oxalate metabolism, should be suspected in patients who have early onset formation of calcium oxalate stones, nephrocalcinosis, and chronic kidney disease in childhood. Pyridoxine can be used as a possible treatment as it lowers oxalate production and excretion in some patients. Definitive treatment is liver transplantation which transfers a functional liver-specific alanine:glyoxylate aminotransferase enzyme.

Prolonged thiazide use (> 1 year) decreases urinary oxalate excretion. Some experts speculate that long-term thiazide use decreases intestinal calcium absorption, increasing oxalate binding with calcium in the gut. In another study looking at patients with recurrent calcium stones, at 3 years, 50–60% of patients on placebo compared to 15–30% of patients receiving thiazides had stone recurrence. Studies with less than 2 years of follow-up did not show any benefit. Indapamide and chlorthalidone are both effective and long-acting diuretics only requiring once-daily dosing while HCTZ requires twice-daily dosing.

Hyperuricosuria

Hyperuricosuria can be associated with calcium oxalate stones and uric acid stones. Patients that develop calcium oxalate stones have elevated urinary uric acid levels, which promote stone formation by reducing the solubility of calcium oxalate and increasing supersaturation of calcium oxalate in the urine. Patients with hyperuricosuria and idiopathic calcium oxalate nephrolithiasis should be started on allopurinol (100 mg daily which can be titrated to a maximum dose of 300 mg daily) to decrease stone recurrence. Though not explicitly studied in this patient population, a low protein/low purine diet may be beneficial in patients with recurrent idiopathic calcium oxalate nephrolithiasis and hyperuricosuria.

Uric Acid Stones

Comprising 10–15% of kidney stones, uric acid stones form in the setting of hyperuricosuria and decreased solubility at low urine pH. Uric acid nephrolithiasis is associated with obesity, metabolic syndrome, gout, chronic diarrhea, high protein diets, myeloproliferative disorders and hereditary inborn metabolism disorders such as Lesch-Nyhan syndrome. Patients with chronic diarrhea have lower urine pH because of the loss of alkali via stool and increased urinary H+ secretion.

Uric acid stones are radiolucent on plain films, but can be visualized on CT. Prevention and treatment involves alkalinization of the urine to pH 6–6.5 to increase uric acid solubility and adequate hydration to reduce supersaturation. Alkalinization consists of oral potassium citrate 10–20 mEq two to three times daily. Patients, especially diabetics, should be carefully monitored for hyperkalemia. A low animal protein diet is recommended to reduce acid production and the amount of alkali needed to increase the urine pH. Dietary sodium should be restricted to reduce urinary uric acid excretion.

High dietary intake of purines can result in hyperuricosuria, but these patients tend to have a more alkaline urine pH which protects against uric acid stones by increasing uric acid solubility. These patients typically have higher urine uric acid levels than patients with gout and uric acid stones. Patients that develop uric acid stones tend to have low urinary pH and a defect in renal ammonium secretion.

Allopurinol should be used in hyperuricosuria or when urine alkalinization is difficult or not well tolerated. Recurrent uric acid stones despite adequate urine alkalinization should be treated with allopurinol regardless of whether hyperuricosuria is present because most patients have low urine pH as their major risk factor and may not always have hyperuricosuria.

Before initiating therapy for recurrent stones, the urinary pH and citrate levels for these patients needs to be evaluated and if urinary citrate levels do not rise but urinary pH tends to rise, the degree of supersaturation worsens and patients can then develop calcium phosphate stones and alkaline therapy is unlikely to be beneficial in this patient group. However it is still recommended that these patients should adhere to increasing fluid intake to increase urinary output and should adhere to a low-salt and low-protein diet with normal calcium intake.

Patients with metabolic syndrome tend to have relative insulin resistance. Interestingly, insulin stimulates ammoniagenesis. A study of nondiabetic patients with recurrent uric acid stones found insulin resistance and the tendency to excrete acidic urine correlated with the degree of insulin resistance. Hence, uric acid stones may be another manifestation of the metabolic syndrome.

It is important to remember that hyperuricosuria can be associated with calcium oxalate stones and uric acid stones. Hyperuricosuria reduces the solubility of calcium oxalate, and thereby increasing supersaturation of calcium oxalate in the urine.

Patients with the inborn metabolism disorder Lesch-Nyhan syndrome have a deficiency in hypoxanthine–guanine phosphoribosyltransferase which leads to overproduction of uric acid. Treatment involves decreasing uric acid secretion in the urine by giving allopurinol at a dose of 4–10 mg/kg/day without exceeding a total daily dose of 300 mg.

Struvite Stones

Magnesium ammonium phosphate (struvite) stones make up 10–15% of stones. More common in women and patients with chronic urinary obstruction, struvite stones are usually associated with urinary tract infections with urease-producing organisms such as *Proteus*, *Klebsiella*, *Providencia*, *Pseudomonas*, enterococci, *Haemophilus*, and *Ureaplasma urealyticum*. The initial event in the pathogenesis of struvite stones may in fact be a calcium oxalate nidus infected with a urea-splitting organism. Urease hydrolyzes urea to ammonia and CO_2, resulting in a urine pH>7. Ammonia combines with water to form ammonium, resulting in an increased amount of ammonium in alkaline urine. Struvite precipitates with calcium carbonate to form large stones and staghorn calculi that can fill the renal pelvis. Struvite stones can progress rapidly over weeks to months. Untreated, struvite stones can cause acute and chronic kidney disease and end-stage renal disease.

The coffin-lid appearance of magnesium ammonium phosphate crystals on urine microscopy confirms the diagnosis. Staghorn calculi can be visualized on KUB or CT, although cystine stones are another potential cause of branched stones, especially in children and young adults.

Treatment involves antibiotics and concomitant stone removal to eradicate the infection and to remove the nidus. Medical therapy alone is rarely successful. According to the American Urological Association Nephrolithiasis Clinical Guidelines Panel, struvite stones should be removed via percutaneous nephrolithotomy and then patients should remain on suppressive low-dose antibiotics with sulfamethoxazole/trimethoprim or nitrofurantoin for 4–6 months. Open nephrolithotomy is rarely indicated in the modern era. Selected patients may require shock-wave lithotripsy, combination therapy with percutaneous nephrolithotomy and lithotripsy, or nephrostomy tube placement. A multidisciplinary approach with nephrology, a urology, and interventional radiology may be indicated.

Following successful stone removal, monitoring with periodic CT for recurrent disease is indicated, especially if an underlying urological condition predisposing to recurrent urinary tract infections has not been resolved. Patients should also be monitored for calcium stones as the initial step in the pathogenesis of recurrent struvite stones. Any risk factors for calcium stones should be addressed.

If stone removal is not possible, then medical therapy includes antibiotics and a urease inhibitor. Selected on the basis of urine culture sensitivity results, antibiotics may not eradicate the infection and sterilize the stone, but may slow stone progression. Acetohydroxamic acid, a urease inhibitor, has been used to slow or prevent stone growth. However, many patients have intolerable side effects, with up to 60% experiencing headache, nausea, vomiting, tremor, and rash. Acetohydroxamic acid is contraindicated in patients with moderate to severe chronic kidney disease. Patients on medical therapy should be closely followed with quarterly abdominal plain films to monitor stone growth.

Cystine Stones

Cystine stones are rare, comprising < 1% of stones, but are more common in pediatric patients. Patients have an autosomal recessive disorder that causes impaired reabsorption of dibasic amino acids including cystine, ornithine, arginine, and lysine in the small intestine and renal proximal tubule, resulting in increased urinary excretion. Only cystine is insoluble in the urine, producing radiopaque stones that present at an earlier age than calcium stones. The median age at onset is 12 years, although some will present in infancy. Large staghorn calculi of cystine can form. Patients may have decreased kidney function and diffuse interstitial fibrosis and plugging of collecting ducts with cystine crystals on kidney biopsy.

Cystine stones should be considered in children and young adults, patients with a family history of nephrolithiasis, and patients with stones of unknown composition. The diagnosis is made by family history of stone disease, hexagonal cystine crystals on urine microscopy, stone analysis, and a positive cyanide-nitroprusside screening test for urine cystine (which indicates a concentration > 75 mg/L; normal is less than 30 mg/L). Cystine stones are less radiopaque than calcium stones on plain films. Less common than struvite stones as the cause of staghorn calculi, cystine stones should be considered in a pediatric patient with a large branched stone.

Prevention focuses on hydration (urine volume of at least 3–3.5 L/day) and urine alkalinization to pH >7.0 to enhance solubility. Potassium citrate or potassium bicarbonate at 3–4 mEq/kg daily may be necessary for adequate alkalinization, but alkaline urine will also decrease the solubility of calcium phosphate and possibly increase calcium stones. Sodium salts of citrate and bicarbonate should not be used for alkalinization because sodium can increase renal cystine excretion.

Low protein and low salt diets decrease urinary cystine excretion. Protein is a source of methionine, the precursor to cystine. Protein intake can be restricted to 0.8–1 g/kg/day, while sodium should be limited to 100 mEq/day, but long-term outcomes with dietary modification are poorly studied.

If a patient has recurrent cystine stones despite conservative management, a cysteine-binding medication may be necessary. Cystine is a dimer of cysteine molecules linked by disulfide bond. Cysteine-binding drugs have sulfhydryl groups that form mixed disulfides with cysteine that are more soluble than cystine. Two regimens include D-penicillamine 1–2 g daily in three to four divided doses and tiopronin at 400–1,200 mg daily in three to four divided doses. Both medications have side effects including abdominal pain, dygeusia, leukopenia, fever, proteinuria, and rarely nephritic syndrome. Tiopronin tends to be better tolerated with fewer adverse reactions than D-penicillamine. Captopril is another cysteine-binding drug, but its use is limited by hypotension and its long-term efficacy is unproven. Thus, captopril should be used in patients unable to tolerate tiopronin or D-penicillamine.

D-Penicillamine and uncommonly tiopronin can cause vitamin B6 (pyridoxine) deficiency. Patients on D-penicillamine should take vitamin B6 50 mg daily. Monitoring for both drugs should include regular testing of liver function tests and complete blood counts. Patients on D-penicillamine should have annual abdominal plain films for the development of calcium stones, while annual abdominal ultrasounds are recommended for tiopronin.

Efficacy and safety of therapy can be monitored by serial 24 h urine collections for total volume, pH (to assess adequate alkalinization), cystine, calcium, oxalate, phosphate, and sodium. Urine microscopy should be used regularly to document the absence of cystine crystals.

Nephrolithiasis Related to Medications (Tables 51.5 and 51.6)

Drug-induced renal calculi comprise 1–2% of all stones. Medications can cause stone formation via two mechanisms. First, drugs can induce metabolic abnormalities that promote stone formation (e.g., loop diuretics, carbonic anhydrase inhibitors, laxatives). Second, poorly soluble medications with high urinary excretion can crystallize in urine, directly forming stones or a nidus for subsequent stone formation. Examples include ciprofloxacin, sulfa drugs, triamterene, indinavir, ephedrine, and magnesium trisilicate. Most drug calculi are radiolucent.

Risk factors for developing drug-induced nephrolithiasis include personal or family history of kidney stones, preexisting stone, urinary stasis (e.g., from benign prostatic hypertrophy or a urinary tract abnormality), underlying hypercalciuria/hypocitraturia, abnormal urine pH (high or low), urinary tract infections, low urine output, and warm climates. Some drug-specific risk factors include high daily dosing of medication, long-term treatment with the offending medication, high urinary excretion and/or low solubility of the drug and/or its metabolites, short half-life of the drug, and the size and morphology of drug crystals.

Medication-Induced Nephrolithiasis (Table 51.5)

Loop diuretics such as bumetanide and furosemide inhibit sodium and calcium reabsorption in the loop of Henle, causing a hypercalciuric state and increasing risk of calcium oxalate stone formation. Carbonic anhydrase inhibitors (acetazolamide) block reabsorption of $NaHCO_3$. Prolonged use can lead to hyperchloremic metabolic acidosis, an alkaline urine pH, hypocitraturia, and an increased risk for calcium phosphate stones. Topiramate, an antiepilepsy medication, inhibits isoenzymes of carbonic anhydrase (CA-II, CA-IV). According to one study, 1.5% of patients on topiramate developed urinary calculi. Inhibition of CA-II and CA-IV by topiramate results in a metabolic acidosis, hypocitraturia, and alkaline urine. Zonisamide, a sulfonamide agent, is an antiepileptic that blocks T-type calcium channels and GABA potentiation. This medication also has weak carbonic-anhydrase activity and causes hypercalciuria and alkaline

Table 51.5 Medication-induced nephrolithiasis

Medication	Mechanism of stone formation	Type of stone	X-ray findings	Treatment
Loop diuretics (e.g., furosemide, bumetanide)	Inhibition of Na and Ca reabsorption in loop of Henle → hypercalciuria	Calcium oxalate	Radiopaque	
Acetazolamide	Inhibition of $NaHCO_3$ reabsorption in proximal tubule → increased urine pH and decreased urine citrate	Calcium phosphate	Radiopaque	
Topiramate	CA-II and CA-IV inhibition by topiramate → metabolic acidosis with hypocitraturia and alkaline urine	Calcium phosphate	Radiopaque	High fluid intake, limit Na intake and increase citrate in diet
Zonisamide	Blocks T-type calcium channels and also acts as a weak CAI → hypercalciuria, alkaline urine	Calcium phosphate	Radiopaque	
Laxative abuse	Patients with chronic diarrhea have low urine volume and acidic urine. Supersaturation of ammonia and uric acid	Ammonium acid urate	Radiolucent	Cessation of laxatives and increase fluid intake
Calcium/vitamin D supplements	Hypercalciuria	Calcium oxalate	Radiopaque	
Antibacterials	Increased oxaluria → calcium oxalate supersaturation	Calcium oxalate	Radiopaque	

Table 51.6 Medication-induced nephrolithiasis

Medication	Mechanism of stone formation	Type of stone	X-ray findings	Risk factors	Treatment
Magnesium trisilicate	Excessive silica in the urine → silica stone formation	Silica	Poorly Radiopaque	Urine pH > 6.6, proteinuria	Discontinue medication
Ciprofloxacin	Ciprofloxacin forms crystals in alkaline urine (pH > 7.3)	Ciprofloxacin	Radiolucent	Alkaline pH, low urine output, high drug dose	Discontinue medication
Sulfa medications	Sulfonamides tend to have high urinary excretion and low solubility, crystallizing in acidic urine	Sulfa	Radiolucent	Low urine pH, low urine output, long term treatment at high doses	Increase urinary pH and increase hydration
Triamterene	Triamterene stones and mixed stones can be seen. Triamterene may act as a nidus for subsequent calculus growth. The pathophysiology is poorly understood	Triamterene	Poorly radiopaque	Urine pH < 6, dose > 150 mg/day, of uric acid lithiasis, h	Discontinue medication
Protease inhibitors (Indinavir, Nelfinavir)	Decreased solubility of indinavir in alkaline urine and increased plasma level of indinavir (high doses or dehydration)	Indinavir	Radiolucent	Decreased fluid intake < 1.5 L/day, alkaline urine pH > 5.5, coinfected HIV/HCV patients	Discontinue medication and hydration/analgesic tx for initial stone therapy
Ephedrine		Ephedrine	Radiolucent		
Allopurinol		Oxypurinol or mixed oxypurinol and allopurinol		Doses > 600 mg/day, acidic urine	Alklainize urine, adjust allopurinol dose
Ceftriaxone		Calcium ceftriaxone		Acidic pH, low urine output, high drug dose	Discontinue medication
Norfloxacin		Magnesium norfloxacin salt		Acidic pH, low urine output, high drug dose > 1,200 mg/day	Discontinue medication
Nitrofurantoin		Nitrofurantoin		Acidic pH, low urine output, high drug dose	Discontinue medication
Phenazopyiridine		Hydroxyphenazopyridine sulfate & other metabolites		Acidic pH, low urine output, high drug dose	Discontinue medication
Amoxicillin/ampicillin		Amoxicillin trihydrate, Ampicillin trihydrate		Acidic pH, low urine output, high drug dose	Discontinue medication
Aluminum hydroxide		Aluminum magnesium potassium urate			Discontinue medication
Guaifenesin		Calcium salt of Beta-2-methoxyphenoxy lactic acid			Discontinue medication

urine, resulting in a 4% incidence of renal calcium phosphate calculi.

Chronic laxative abusers are at risk for ammonium acid urate stones. The chronic diarrhea causes a hyperchloremic metabolic acidosis, leading to increased ammonia excretion from the proximal tubule. Uric acid solubility is dependent on urine pH, and chronic diarrhea patients have low urine volumes and acidic urine pH, factors which promote the formation of ammonium acid urate stones. Increased ammonium excretion can also be seen with dehydration, starvation, and high consumption of acid-forming foods.

Medication Nephrolithiasis (Table 51.6)

Triamterene, a potassium-sparing diuretic commonly used to treat hypertension, was one of the first medications known to cause nephrolithiasis. It inhibits the reabsorption of Na in exchange for potassium and hydrogen ions in the distal tubule. The mechanism for increased stone formation is poorly understood. One hypothesis is that triamterene precipitates and provides a scaffold for subsequent calculus growth as 21% of stones are pure triamterene and the rest are mixed stones.

Magnesium trisilicate, an over the counter medication for gastroesophageal reflux disease, can induce silica stone formation. Dietary silica is easily excreted in the urine, and excessive amount of magnesium trisilicate can lead to renal calculi. The fluoroquinolone ciprofloxacin is nearly insoluble in neutral or alkaline urine. When urine pH exceeds 7.3, ciprofloxacin crystalluria may be seen with oral doses of 1,000 mg. Sulfa medications include sulfadiazine and sulfamethoxazole–trimethoprim. Sulfonamide solubility decreases in low urinary pH and can crystallize and form calculi. By increasing urinary pH and hydration, sulfonamide-induced calculi can be avoided.

Protease inhibitors such as indinavir and nelfinavir are used to treat HIV infection. The incidence of indinavir nephrolithiasis is 7–12%. Some risk factors for indinavir stone formation include decreased fluid intake < 1.5 L/day, urine pH >5.5, and concomitant infection with hepatitis C. Co-infection with hepatitis C is thought to increase indinvair crystalluria due to decreased hepatic indinavir catabolism and increased renal excretion of the medication.

Allopurinol is used to treat hyperuricemia, gout, and uric acid nephrolithiasis. It can also cause nephrolithiasis, especially with doses > 600 mg/day. Allopurinol is rapidly metabolized by xanthine oxidase to the active metabolite oxypurinol, which has a prolonged half-life and inhibits xanthine oxidase. Patients taking allopurinol can develop oxypurinol or mixed oxypurinol–allopurinol stones. Ephedrine, either alone or in combination with guaifenesin, has also been known to cause nephrolithiasis. These calculi tend to be radiolucent on X-ray.

Rare and Unusual Stones

Certain medications may precipitate in the urine, causing nephrolithiasis. The HIV medication indinavir and the potassium sparing diuretic triamterene are two such medications. Patients with gout can sometimes develop xanthine stones due to the use of drugs such as allopurinol. The treatment would be focusing on switching to alternative agents for treatment of underlying diseases.

Ammonium acid urate stones are mostly seen in developing countries in children and present as bladder stones. Usually these stones are associated with diarrheal illnesses (laxative abuse, bowel resection, infection) and with hypokalemia. They are radiolucent as well. Treatment involves increased fluid intake, controlling diarrhea, and correcting hypokalemia.

Uric acid stones are the most common purine stones. Other purine stones are very rare, and there are two that are most common among them. Xanthine stones are radiolucent and tend to form in patients who have severe hyperuricemia and are taking allopurinol at the same time. They can also be seen in rare inherited forms of xanthinuria as well. 2,8-Dihydroxyadenine stones are also radiolucent and are due to a deficiency of adenine phosphoribosyltransferase. These patients can be treated with allopurinol.

Conclusion

Nephrolithiasis is a prevalent, frequently recurrent, and occasionally morbid condition associated with increased risk of bone disease, chronic kidney disease, and hypertension. Many physicians including family practitioners, internists, nephrologists, urologists, emergency room physicians, and interventional radiologists will see stone patients in their routine practice. Many underlying disorders have been associated with stone formation; recognizing these disorders is important in stone prophylaxis.

Bibliography

Borghi L, Meschi T, Amato F, et al. Urinary volume, water and recurrences in idiopathic calcium nephrolithiasis: a 5-year randomized prospective study. J Urol. 1996;155:839–43.

Brener ZZ, Winchester JF, Salman H, et al. Nephrolithiasis: evaluation and management. South Med J. 2011;104: 133–9.

Coll DM, Varanelli MJ, Smith RC. Relationship of spontaneous passage of ureteral calculi to stone size and location as revealed by unenhanced helical CT. AJR Am J Roentgenol. 2002;178:101–3.

Daudon M, Jungers P. Drug-induced renal calculi: epidemiology, prevention and management. Drugs. 2004; 64(3):245–75.

Dellabella M, Milanese G, Muzzonigro G. Randomized trial of the efficacy of tamsulosin, nifedipine and phloroglucinol in medical expulsive therapy for distal ureteral calculi. J Urol. 2005;174:167–72.

Fielding JR, Steele G, Fox LA, et al. Spiral computerized tomography in the evaluation of acute flank pain: a replacement for excretory urography. J Urol. 1997; 157:2071–3.

Fink HA, Akornor JW, Pranav SG, et al. Diet, fluid, or supplements for secondary prevention of nephrolithiasis: a systematic review and meta-analysis of randomized trials. Eur Urol. 2009;56(1):72–80.

Fowler KA, Locken JA, Dushesne JH, et al. US for detecting renal calculi with nonenhanced CT as a reference standard. Radiology. 2002;222:109–13.

Goldfarb DS. In the clinic: nephrolithiasis. Ann Intern Med. 2009;151:ITC2.

Griwan MS, Singh SK, Himanshu P, et al. The efficacy of tamsulosin in lower ureteral calculi. Urol Ann. 2010;2:63–6.

Hall PM. Nephrolithiasis: treatment, causes, and prevention. Cleve Clin J Med. 2011;78(5):332–42.

Holdgate A, Pollock T. Systematic review of the relative efficacy of non-steroidal anti-inflammatory drugs and opioids in the treatment of acute renal colic. Br J Med. 2004;328:1401.

Hollingsworth JM, Rogers MA, Kaufman SR, et al. Medical therapy to facilitate urinary stone passage: a meta-analysis. Lancet. 2006;368:1171–9.

Labrecque M, Dostaler LP, Rouselle R, et al. Efficacy of nonsteroidal anti-inflammatory drugs in the treatment of acute renal colic. Arch Intern Med. 1994;154:1381–7.

Li J, Kennedy D, Levine M, et al. Absent hematuria and expensive computerized tomography: case characteristics of emergency urolithiasis. J Urol. 2001;165:782–4.

Miller OF, Kane CJ. Time to stone passage for observed ureteral calculi: a guide for patient education. J Urol. 1999;162:688–91.

Romero V, Akpinar H, Assimos DG. Kidney stones: a global picture of prevalence, incidence, and associated risk factors. Rev Urol. 2010;12(2–3):e86–96.

Saiga CS, Joyce G, Timilsina AR, Urologic Diseases in America Project. Direct and indirect costs of nephrolithiasis in an employed population: opportunity for disease management? Kidney Int. 2005;68(4):1808–14.

Sarica K, Inal Y, Erturhan S, Yagci F. The effect of calcium channel blockers on stone regrowth and recurrence after shock wave lithotripsy. Urol Res. 2006;34:184–9.

Smith RC, Verga M, McCarthy S, et al. Diagnosis of acute flank pain: value of unenhanced helical CT. AJR Am J Roentgenol. 1996;166:97–101.

Thomas AA, Thomas AZ, Campbell SC, et al. Urologic emergencies in pregnancy. Urology. 2010;76:453–60.

Uribarri J, Oh MS, Carroll HJ. The first kidney stone. Ann Intern Med. 1989;111:1006–9.

Vincendeau SV, Bellissant E, Houlgatte A, et al. Tamsulosin hydrochloride vs placebo for management of distal ureteral stones. Arch Intern Med. 2010;170:2021–7.

Worcester EM, Coe FL. Calcium kidney stones. N Engl J Med. 2010;363:954–63.

Index

E.V. Lerma and M. Rosner (eds.), *Clinical Decisions in Nephrology, Hypertension and Kidney Transplantation*, DOI 10.1007/978-1-4614-4454-1, © Springer Science+Business Media New York 2013

N

P

T

CPSIA information can be obtained
at www.ICGtesting.com
Printed in the USA
LVHW062313191121
703578LV00002B/1

9 781461 444534